LIPPINCOTT'S REVIEW FOR
NCLEX-RN

Sixth Edition

Diane M. Billings, RN, EdD, FAAN

Professor of Nursing and Associate Dean of Teaching,
Learning and Information Resources
Indiana University
School of Nursing
Indianapolis, Indiana

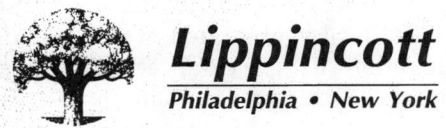

Lippincott
Philadelphia • New York

Acquisitions Editor: Susan M. Glover, RN, MSN
Assistant Editor: Bridget Blatteau
Project Editor: Gretchen Metzger
Production Manager: Helen Ewan
Production Coordinator: Kathryn Rule
Design Coordinator: Nicholas Rook

Edition 6

9 8 7 6 5 4 3 2 1

Library of Congress Cataloging-in-Publication Data

Billings, Diane McGovern.
    Lippincott's review for NCLEX-RN.—6th ed. / Diane M. Billings.
        p.   cm.
    Includes bibliographical references.
    ISBN 0-397-55452-4 (alk. paper)
    1. Nursing—Examinations, questions, etc.   I. Title.
    [DNLM: 1. Nursing—examination questions.   WY 18.2 B598L   1998]
RT55.M29   1998
610.73'076—dc21
DNLM/DLC
for Library of Congress   97-3490
                                                                  CIP

Care has been taken to confirm the accuracy of the information
presented and to describe generally accepted practices. However, the
authors, editors, and publisher are not responsible for errors or
omissions or for any consequences from application of the
information in this book and make no warranty, express or implied,
with respect to the contents of the publication.

The authors, editors, and publisher have exerted every effort to
ensure that drug selection and dosage set forth in this text are in
accordance with current recommendations and practice at the time of
publication. However, in view of ongoing research, changes in
government regulations, and the constant flow of information relating
to drug therapy and drug reactions, the reader is urged to check the
package insert for each drug for any change in indications and dosage
and for added warnings and precautions. This is particularly
important when the recommended agent is a new or infrequently
employed drug.

Some drugs and medical devices presented in this publication have
Food and Drug Administration (FDA) clearance for limited use in
restricted research settings. It is the responsibility of the health care
provider to ascertain the FDA status of each drug or device planned
for use in their clinical practice.

Contributors

Susan Bennett, RN, DNS

Associate Professor of Nursing
Indiana University School of Nursing
Indianapolis, Indiana

Carol Bostrom, RN, MSN, CS

Clinical Assistant Professor
Indiana University School of Nursing
Indianapolis, Indiana

Karen Cobb, RN, EdD

Assistant Professor of Nursing
Indiana University School of Nursing
Indianapolis, Indiana

Judith Halstead, RN, DNS

Assistant Professor of Nursing
University of Southern Indiana School of Nursing
  and Health Professions
Evansville, Indiana

Patricia Henry, RN, MSN

Lecturer
Indiana University School of Nursing
South Bend, Indiana

Virginia Richardson, RN, DNS, CPNP

Associate Professor of Nursing
Indiana University School of Nursing
Indianapolis, Indiana

Preface

Preparing thoroughly for examinations is necessary for obtaining satisfactory test scores. This book is written to assist nursing students in preparing for one of the most important examinations they will take—the licensing examination. Although this book is written primarily for students preparing to take the licensure examination, nurses who are preparing for challenge examinations, inactive nurses preparing to return to practice, practicing nurses transferring to a different clinical area, and nursing faculty will also find this book helpful.

The major features of this book are:

- A clear explanation of the licensure examination.
- A description of the current NCLEX-RN test plan of the National Council of State Boards of Nursing, Inc.
- Case studies with commonly encountered client situations.
- More than 3,000 test questions, with test items written for all clinical areas of nursing (nursing care of clients with psychiatric disorders and mental health problems, the childbearing family and their neonate, children and adults with medical and surgical health problems.)
- Review tests grouped by clinical area to facilitate study in specific content areas.
- Four comprehensive tests designed to resemble the format of the NCLEX-RN examination.
- Test items emphasizing current nursing practice in the areas of home care, health promotion, and community health.
- Test items written using the Agency for Health Care Policy and Research (AHCPR) guidelines.
- Test items written using current North American Nursing Diagnosis Association (NANDA) and Diagnostic and Statistical Manual of Mental Disorder (DSM-IV) stan-

dards as well as the latest protocols for drug and nutrition therapies.

- Test items based on current childhood immunization guidelines.
- Correct answers and rationale are given for all items in this book. The rationales explain why the correct answer is correct, as well as why the distractors are incorrect.
- A tear-out study plan and checklist to guide systematic preparation for the licensing examination.
- Sections on developing study skills, taking multiple choice examinations, and managing test anxiety.
- Answer grids at the end of each test can be used to identify areas for further study based on four content areas, step of the nursing process, and area of client need.
- A computer disk to practice taking computer adaptive tests.
- References at the end of each clinical section.
- Address and telephone number of the National Council of State Boards of Nursing, Inc., and for each state board of nursing.

I would like to acknowledge the item writers for this edition—Susan Bennett, Carol Bostrom, Karen Cobb, Judith Halstead, Patricia Henry, and Virginia Richardson—nationally recognized content experts and valued colleagues. Thanks also to Bill Collins for designing the answer grids and Louise Bowman for secretarial assistance. Donna Hilton and Susan Glover provided the editorial expertise that guided the development of this edition. Finally, thanks to my parents, John and June McGovern who taught me to review before all of life's "examinations."

Diane M. Billings, EdD, RN, FAAN

Contents

Contents

Introduction

ORGANIZATION AND USE OF THIS BOOK

This book has been developed to help you prepare for the National Council of State Boards of Nursing Licensing Examination for Registered Nurses (NCLEX-RN). The book is divided into two major sections. The first section contains practice exams that represent the four main clinical areas of nursing: psychiatric nursing, obstetric nursing, pediatric nursing, and medical-surgical nursing. Each test presents a variety of situations commonly encountered in nursing practice. The second section contains four comprehensive exams written to simulate the NCLEX-RN by placing test items in random order. A computer disk is also included to help you practice taking computerized adaptive tests.

You can begin your review by using the practice exams to identify areas of strength and areas needing further study. Each exam contains specific case study situations and miscellaneous questions written in the style of the NCLEX-RN. Answers with rationales, coded according to the NCLEX-RN test plan for the step of the nursing process, cognitive level, and client needs, are included at the end of each exam under the heading Correct Answers and Rationale.

To evaluate your results after completing each exam, divide the number of your correct responses by the total number of questions in the test and multiply by 100. For example, if you answered 72 of 90 items correctly, you would divide 72 by 90 and multiply by 100, for a result of 80%. If you answered more than 75% of the items in an area correctly, you are most likely prepared to answer questions in that area on the NCLEX-RN. But if you answered fewer than 75% of the questions correctly, you need to determine why. Did you answer incorrectly because of lack of content knowledge or because you did not read carefully? Use this information to guide your study.

Use the answer grid at the end of each exam to calculate the percentage of items you answered correctly for each area of the test plan (nursing process, cognitive level, and client needs). For example, calculate the percentage of correctly answered questions about the nursing diagnosis step of the nursing process; if you missed more than 75% of these questions, you should review information about formulating nursing diagnoses.

After reviewing the specific content areas in the practice exams, take the comprehensive exams. These exams more realistically reflect the NCLEX-RN, which is a comprehensive exam; that is, each test presents a variety of situations commonly encountered in nursing practice and across all clinical disciplines. Underlying knowledge, skills, and abilities related to the basic physiopsychosocial sciences, fundamentals of nursing, pharmacology and other therapeutic measures, communicable diseases, legal and ethical considerations, and nutrition are included in items as needed to plan nursing care for a specific client. The items in the comprehensive exams were also written to test competent nursing practice based on this knowledge and these skills and abilities.

After completing each exam, review the answers and rationales to evaluate your results. Use the diagnostic grids to determine the percentage of correct answers in each content area and NCLEX-RN test plan component.

Finally, if you have access to an IBM-compatible personal computer, use the computer disk accompanying this review book to simulate taking computerized adaptive tests. Note how the questions are presented on the computer screen, and practice answering questions without using a pencil.

ABOUT THE LICENSING EXAMINATION

The NCLEX-RN is administered to graduates of nursing schools to test the knowledge, abilities, and skills necessary for entry-level, safe and effective nursing practice. The examination is developed by the National Council of State Boards of Nursing, Inc., an organization with representation from all state boards of nursing. The same examination is used in all 50 states, the District of Columbia, and United States possessions. Students who have graduated from baccalaureate, diploma, and associate degree programs in nursing must pass this examination to meet licensing requirements in the United States.

THE TEST PLAN

The National Council of State Boards of Nursing, Inc. prepares the test plan used to develop the licensing examination.[1] The test plan, or framework of the examination, is based on the results of a job analysis, conducted every

3 years, of the entry-level performance of newly licensed registered nurses.[2] The questions are written by nurse clinicians and nurse educators nominated by the Council of State Boards of Nursing to serve as item writers and reflect nursing practice in all parts of the country.

The questions for the test are formulated on health care situations that registered nurses commonly encounter, addressing two components: 1) phases of the nursing process and 2) client needs. Representative items test knowledge of these components as they relate to specific health care situations. The questions developed for the test plan were written to test application and analysis of nursing knowledge at these levels of the cognitive domain. The following sections explain how the nursing process, client needs, and cognitive levels are used to formulate test questions.

The Nursing Process

The five phases of the nursing process are: 1) assessment; 2) analysis; 3) planning; 4) implementation; and 5) evaluation.

Assessment. Assessment involves establishing a data base. The nurse gathers objective and subjective information about the client, then verifies the data and communicates information gained from the assessment.

Analysis. Analysis involves identifying actual or potential health care needs or problems based on assessment data. The nurse interprets the data, collects additional data as indicated, and identifies and communicates the client's nursing diagnoses. The nurse also determines the congruency between the client's needs and the ability of the health care team members to meet those needs.

Planning. Planning involves setting goals for meeting the client's needs and designing strategies to attain those goals. The nurse determines the goals of care, develops and modifies the plan, collaborates with other health team members for delivery of the client's care, and formulates expected outcomes of nursing interventions.

Implementation. Implementation involves initiating and completing actions necessary to accomplish the defined goals. The nurse organizes and manages the client's care; performs or assists the client in performing activities of daily living; counsels and teaches the client, significant others, and health care team members; and provides care to attain the established client goals. The nurse also provides care to optimize the achievement of the client's health care goals; supervises, coordinates, and evaluates delivery of the client's care as provided by nursing staff; and records and exchanges information.

Evaluation. Evaluation determines goal achievement. The nurse compares actual with expected outcomes of therapy, evaluates compliance with prescribed or proscribed therapy, and records and describes the client's response to therapy or care. The nurse also modifies the plan, as indicated, and reorders priorities.

The five phases of the nursing process are equally important. Therefore, each is represented by an equal number of items on the NCLEX-RN.[1]

Client Needs

The health needs of clients are grouped under four broad categories: 1) safe, effective care environment; 2) physiologic integrity; 3) psychosocial integrity; and 4) health promotion and maintenance.[1]

Safe, effective care environment. The nurse meets the client's needs for a safe and effective environment by providing and directing nursing care that promotes attainment of client needs. These needs include coordinated care, quality assurance, goal-oriented care, environmental safety, preparation for treatments and procedures, and safe and effective treatments and procedures (Box 1).

Physiologic integrity. The nurse meets the physiologic integrity needs of clients with potentially life-threatening or recurring physiologic conditions, and clients at risk for the development of complications or untoward effects of treatments or management of modalities. The nurse meets the physiologic integrity needs of these clients by providing and directing nursing care that promotes achievement of needs such as physiologic adaptation, reduction of risk potential, mobility, comfort, and provision of basic care (Box 2).

Psychosocial integrity. The nurse meets the client's needs for psychosocial integrity in stress and crisis-related situations throughout the life cycle. The nurse does this by providing and directing nursing care that promotes achievement of the client's needs for psychosocial adaptation and coping (Box 3).

Health promotion and maintenance. The nurse meets the client's needs for health promotion and maintenance throughout the life cycle by providing and directing nursing care that promotes achievement, by the client and significant others, of such needs as continued growth and development, self-care, integrity of support systems, and prevention and early treatment of disease (Box 4).

Each category of client need is represented on the NCLEX-RN as follows[1]:

1. Safe, effective care environment   15% to 21%
2. Physiologic integrity   46% to 54%
3. Psychosocial integrity   8% to 16%
4. Health promotion and maintenance   17% to 23%

Cognitive Level of Questions

The cognitive level of questions refers to the type of mental activity required to answer the question as defined in a taxonomy of the cognitive domain.[3] Test questions can be written to test at all levels of the cognitive domain.

The lowest level of the taxonomy is the *knowledge* level, the ability to recall facts about principles, concepts, theories, terms, or procedures. Questions at this level ask you

BOX 1. SAFE, EFFECTIVE CARE ENVIRONMENT

Knowledge, Skills, and Abilities:

- Advance directives
- Basic principles of management
- Client rights
- Confidentiality
- Continuity of care
- Environmental and personal safety
- Expected outcomes of various treatment modalities
- General and specific protective measures
- Informed consent
- Interpersonal communications
- Knowledge and use of special equipment
- Principles of teaching and learning
- Principles of quality improvement
- Principles of group dynamics
- Spread and control of infectious agents
- Staff education

BOX 2. PHYSIOLOGIC INTEGRITY

Knowledge, Skills, and Abilities:

- Activities of daily living
- Body mechanics
- Comfort interventions
- Drug administration
- Effects of immobility
- Expected and unexpected response to therapies
- Intrusive procedures
- Managing emergencies
- Normal body structure and function
- Nutritional therapies
- Pathophysiology
- Pharmacologic actions
- Skin and wound care
- Use of special equipment

BOX 3. PSYCHOSOCIAL INTEGRITY

Knowledge, Skills, and Abilities:

- Accountability
- Behavior norms
- Chemical dependency
- Communication skills
- Community resources
- Cultural, religious, and spiritual influences on health
- Family systems
- Mental health concepts
- Principles of teaching and learning
- Principles of quality improvement
- Psychodynamics of behavior
- Psychopathology
- Treatment modalities

BOX 4. HEALTH PROMOTION AND MAINTENANCE

Knowledge, Skills, and Abilities:

- Adaptation to altered health states
- Birthing and parenting
- Communication skills
- Community resources
- Concepts of wellness
- Death and dying
- Disease prevention
- Family systems
- Family planning
- Growth and development, including aging
- Health care screening
- Lifestyle choices
- Principles of immunity
- Principles of teaching and learning
- Reproduction and human sexuality

BOX 5. PERSONAL STUDY PLAN (TEAR OUT)

ASSESS STUDY NEEDS

1. Review your success in nursing school.
   - ❑ I did best in these courses: _____.
   - ❑ I needed to study harder in these courses: _____.
   - ❑ I took these courses near the beginning of the curriculum: _____.
   - ❑ I scored best on these practice exams in this book: _____.
   - ❑ I am not satisfied with my scores on these practice exams in this book: _____.
   - ❑ I need further study in these content areas: _____.
   - ❑ I need further study in these areas of the nursing process: _____.
   - ❑ I need further study in these areas of client needs: _____.
   _____.

2. Review your test-taking skills.
   - ❑ I can identify the components of a test question.
   - ❑ I read questions carefully before answering.
   - ❑ I can make reasonable guesses if I am not certain of the correct answer.

3. Review your test anxiety management skills.
   - ❑ I can do relaxation and deep breathing exercises.
   - ❑ I can visualize success.
   - ❑ I can give myself positive feedback.
   - ❑ I can concentrate for extended periods of time.

4. Review your computer skills.
   - ❑ I am able to use a computer to read and answer test questions.
   - ❑ I have used the practice disk accompanying this book.

DEVELOP A STUDY PLAN

- ❑ I will study in this location: _____.
- ❑ I will study at these times and dates: _____.
- ❑ I have assembled all of the materials I need to study: _____.
- ❑ I will study with a study group: _____.

EVALUATE PROGRESS

- ❑ I have completed the practice tests in this book: _____.
- ❑ I have completed the comprehensive tests in this book: _____.
- ❑ I need to improve my scores in these areas: _____.
- ❑ I am prepared to take the NCLEX-RN examination: _____.

STRATEGIES FOR TAKING TESTS

- ❑ Read the question carefully.
- ❑ Anticipate the correct answer.
- ❑ Read for key words.
- ❑ Base answers on nursing knowledge.
- ❑ Identify the components of the test item.

STRATEGIES FOR MANAGING TEST ANXIETY

- ❑ Mental rehearsal
- ❑ Relaxation
- ❑ Deep breathing
- ❑ Positive self-talk
- ❑ Distraction
- ❑ Concentration

to define, identify, or select. *Comprehension* requires understanding data; questions ask you to interpret, explain, distinguish, or predict. *Application* involves using information in new situations. At this level, you are expected to solve problems, modify plans, manipulate data, and demonstrate appropriate use of information. *Analysis* requires recognizing relationships between parts. Questions at this level ask you to analyze, evaluate, select, differentiate, or interpret data from a variety of sources. The highest level of the cognitive domain is *synthesis*. Here you must put data together in new and meaningful ways.

The test items in the NCLEX-RN are written to test *application* and *analysis* of nursing knowledge. All items in this book have been coded according to the taxonomy of the cognitive domain. As you answer the questions and review your scores, you can determine whether you are able to answer questions at the levels of the cognitive domain tested on the NCLEX-RN.

For further information about the NCLEX-RN, write to the National Council of State Boards of Nursing, Inc. For information about the dates, requirements, and specifics of writing the examination in your state, contact your state board of nursing. The addresses and telephone numbers of the National Council of State Boards of Nursing, Inc. and each state board of nursing are provided in the Appendix.

TAKING THE EXAMINATION

Computer Adaptive Testing

Since April 1994, the NCLEX-RN has been administered using computer adaptive testing (CAT) procedures. CAT involves using a computer to randomly generate questions from an item pool to administer individually tailored examinations. CAT has several advantages. For example, an exam can be given in less time because there are potentially fewer questions for each candidate. CAT exams can also be administered frequently, allowing a graduate of a nursing program to take the exam close to graduation, receive the results quickly, and enter the work force as a registered nurse in less time than is possible with paper and pencil exams. Study results also show that because CAT is self-paced, there is less stress on the candidate.

CAT uses the memory and speed of the computer to administer a test for each candidate. The test is generated from a large pool of questions (a test item bank) based on the NCLEX-RN test plan. The examination begins as the computer randomly selects a question of medium difficulty for each candidate. The next question is based on the response to the previous question. If the question is answered correctly, an item of similar or greater difficulty is generated; if it is answered incorrectly, a less-difficult item is selected. Thus, the test is adapted for each candidate. Once competence has been determined, the exam is completed at a passing level. CAT for the NCLEX-RN has been field-tested and is psychometrically sound.

The exams for all candidates are derived from the same large pool of test items. They contain comparable questions for each component of the test plan. Although the questions are not exactly the same, they test the same knowledge, skills, and abilities from the test plan.

All candidates must meet the requirements of the test plan and achieve the same passing score. Each candidate, therefore, has the same opportunity to demonstrate competence. Although one candidate may answer fewer questions, all candidates have the opportunity to answer a sufficient number of questions to demonstrate competence.

Although each exam is individualized, the minimum number of questions is 75. The maximum number of questions is 265. Do not worry if others near you finish early or receive more questions. Focus on doing your best and working at a comfortable speed.

Because each exam is adapted for each candidate, the time taken to complete the exam can vary. The time also varies depending on how long it takes to finish each question. Enough time is allotted for each candidate to demonstrate competence. Most candidates complete the exam within the maximum 5 hours allotted.

Examination Locations

The Council of State Boards of Nursing contracts with vendors in each state to serve as exam sites. Your school of nursing can inform you of the location nearest you. You can also contact your state board of nursing for information. (See the Appendix for the address.)

The testing service that administers the NCLEX-RN CAT (Educational Testing Service) has formed a partnership with Sylvan/Kee Systems.[4] The NCLEX-RN is administered at more than 1,200 Sylvan/Kee learning centers nationwide and at various universities and colleges that meet testing site guidelines. Each center has about 10 computer stations equipped with adequate lighting and scratch paper for candidates' use. The computers have surge-protection devices to prevent data loss. Secured storage areas outside of the testing room are provided for storage of personal articles. Each testing center maintains comprehensive security, using audio and video camera monitoring.

The exam site is designed so that candidates can take breaks. There is a mandatory 10-minute break after 2 hours and an optional break 1.5 hours after that.

Scheduling the Examination

The first step is to apply to the state board of nursing in the state in which you plan to take the examination. Within about 30 days, you will receive a ticket of admission from the Educational Testing Service Data Center with information about available testing centers and procedures for making an appointment. Testing centers are open Monday through Saturday, about 15 hours each day.

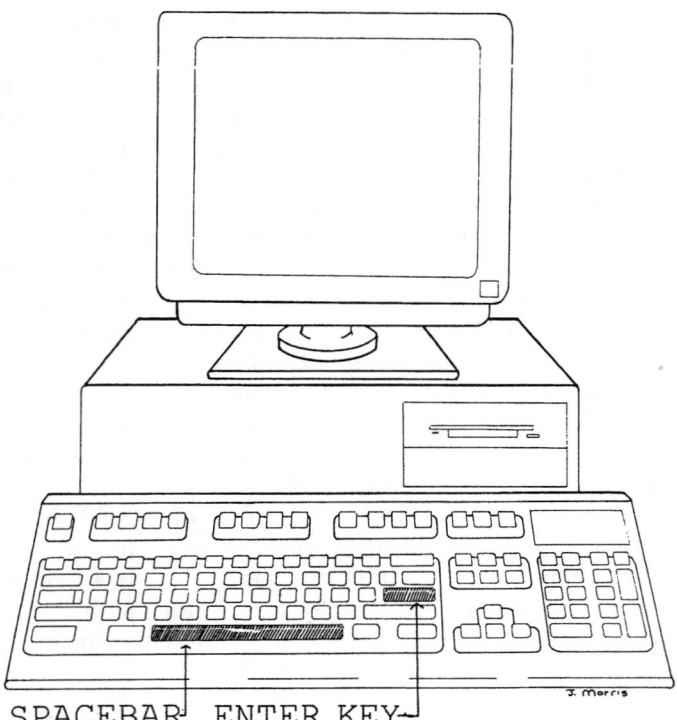

SPACEBAR ENTER KEY

Fig. 1. Computer screen (monitor) and keyboard.

Computer Use and Screen Design

Test questions are presented on the computer screen (monitor); you select your answer and use the keyboard to enter the response (Fig. 1). The keyboard is simplified to use only two color-coded keys: the space bar and the enter key. Press the space bar to highlight the answer, then press the enter key once to select your answer and a second time to enter your answer into the computer. If you have access to an IBM-compatible personal computer, you can use the practice disk included with this review book to practice selecting and entering answers.

At every testing site, written directions are provided at each computer exam station. There are also practice questions on the computer that you can use to be sure you understand how to use the computer before you begin the exam.

Field studies conducted by the Council of State Boards of Nursing find that previous computer experience or lack of it has no effect on exam performance. Candidates are able to acquire the necessary computer skills at the testing center.

PREPARING FOR THE EXAM

Studying for the NCLEX-RN requires careful planning and preparation. You can make the best use of your time and energy by developing a systematic approach to study that includes assessing your strengths and weaknesses, developing a study plan, and evaluating progress on a regular

DIFFERENCES BETWEEN PAPER AND PENCIL AND COMPUTER ADMINISTERED EXAMS

Exam Feature	Paper and Pencil Exams	Computer Administered Exams
Question layout	Linear	Blocked, with stem of the question or the case study on the left, options on the right
Question design	Case study with several related questions following the case study	All information related to the question is presented in the stem
Ability to read questions randomly	Yes	No, one question presented at a time
Ability to review or change answer to previous question	Yes	No
Ability to skip question if not sure of answer	Yes	No, must answer each question before receiving the next one
Ability to underline or circle key words; make margin notes	Yes	No
Scratch paper available	Yes	Yes
Proctor	Rotates among tables	Can observe all candidates simultaneously and video monitored
Ergonomics	Sit at desk	Sit at computer
Breaks	Yes	Yes

basis. Use the Personal Study Plan in Box 5 to help develop your own study plan.

Assessing Study Needs

The first step in developing a study plan is to determine which content areas you know well and which areas you need to review further. Follow these steps to assess your knowledge, skills, and abilities:

1. Review your success in nursing school. Review your record of achievement in courses in the nursing curriculum. Subjects in which you received high grades, that you found easy to learn, or in which you have had additional clinical practice or work experience are likely areas of strength. On the other hand, subjects you found difficult to learn or did not achieve high grades in should be areas for concentrated review. Also consider content areas that you have not studied for a while. Recent course work will be most familiar and, therefore, may require the least amount of study.

You can also use the practice exams in this book to identify areas needing further study. Begin with the subjects you find most difficult or in which you have the least confidence. Use the grids at the end of each test to determine areas for further study.

2. Assess your test-taking skills. Using effective test-taking skills contributes to exam success. What have you done in the past to make you confident about taking a test? How do you feel when you are in the exam situation? What has worked in the past to help you be successful? Review these strategies to build on past successes and work on problem areas. Consider additional strategies suggested in the following section, Test-Taking Strategies. You can practice these skills by simulating the testing situation using the practice tests and comprehensive exams in this review book.

3. Assess your skills for taking computer-administered exams. Although previous computer experience is not necessary to take the NCLEX-RN, you may wish to familiarize yourself with the differences between taking a paper and pencil exam and taking exams administered by the computer. Use the display, "Differences Between Paper and Pencil and Computer-Administered Exams" to review these differences. If you have not used a computer before, find a learning resource center at your college, university, library, or hospital where you can become familiar with basic computer keyboard skills. Use the disk accompanying this review book to simulate the experience of answering questions using a computer. Practice reading questions from the computer screen. If you are accustomed to underlining key words or making notes in the margins of paper and pencil tests, adapt these strategies to reading and answering the questions on the computer screen.

Developing a Study Plan

Once you have identified areas of strength and areas needing further study, develop a specific plan and begin to study regularly. Students who study a small amount of content over a longer period of time tend to have higher success rates than students who wait until the last few weeks before the exam and then "cram." Consider these suggestions:

1. Identify a place for study. The area should be quiet and have room for your books and papers. This area might be in your home, at your nursing school, or in a library. Be sure your friends and family understand the importance of not interrupting you when you are studying.

2. Establish regular study times. Make appointments with yourself to ensure a commitment to study. Frequent, short study periods (1–2 hours) are preferable to sporadic, extended study periods. Plan to finish your studying 1 week before the NCLEX-RN; last-minute cramming tends to increase anxiety.

3. Obtain all necessary resources. As you begin to study, it is helpful to have easy access to textbooks, notes, and study guides. Suggested readings are included at the end of each unit in this book.

4. Make the best use of your time. Make review cards that you can carry with you to study during free moments throughout the day. If possible, you may want to tape record review notes and listen to the tapes on the way to work.

5. Develop effective study skills. Study skills enable you to acquire, organize, remember, and use the information you need to take the NCLEX-RN. These skills include outlining, summarizing, reviewing, and practicing test-taking. Some students prefer to study alone, while others benefit from study groups; know which approach works best for you, and develop your study plan accordingly. You can use this book to learn, refine, and practice your study skills. Study skill suggestions include the following:

- Use study skills with which you are familiar and that have worked well for you in the past. Recall effective study behaviors that you used in nursing school, such as reviewing highlighted text, outlines, or content maps. What are your learning style preferences? Do you study best in a quiet room, or do you prefer music in the background? Are you most alert in the morning or evening? Do you like to eat while you study? Does it help you to concentrate and learn if you make notes as you study? Learn what works best for you, and use it to optimize your study plan.

- Study to learn, not to memorize. The NCLEX-RN tests application of knowledge. When reviewing content, continually ask yourself, "How is this information used in client care?"

- Anticipate questions. As you study, formulate questions around the content. Practice giving a rationale for your answer to these questions. If you work in a study group, have each member contribute questions.

- Study common, not unique, nursing care situations. The NCLEX-RN tests minimum competence for nursing practice; therefore, focus on common health problems and client needs.

- Simulate test-taking. The comprehensive tests in Section Two of this book are designed to simulate the random order in which questions appear in the NCLEX-RN. Use these tests to focus on areas of common concern in nursing care rather than on the traditional content delineations of adult, pediatric, psychiatric, and childbearing clients. Make additional copies of answer sheets, and retake the exams on which you had low scores.

- Give yourself positive feedback. Use positive self-talk strategies to build your confidence. Reward yourself as you study. Engage in a favorite activity after a successful study session.

Evaluating Your Progress

Periodically determine if you are on schedule with your study plan. Note if your scores on the practice and comprehensive tests improve. Do not spend time on content you have mastered, on areas in which you obtained high scores on the practice exam, or on areas with which you feel confident. Set priorities for study on areas needing additional review.

TEST-TAKING STRATEGIES

Knowing how to take a test is as important as knowing the content being tested. Strategies for taking tests can be learned and used to improve test scores.[5] Here are some suggestions for building a repertoire of effective test-taking strategies:

1. Understand the components of the test item. Typically, test items consist of a situation or background information, a question, and four possible answers[6] (Fig. 2).

The *background (situation)* is a client-based scenario that gives information about the client needed to answer the question. The questions that follow are based on the information given in the situation. As you answer the question, relate the answer to the background information. Pay particular attention to information about the client's age, family status, health status, ethnicity, or point in the care plan (eg, early admission versus preparation for discharge).

The *stem (question)* poses the problem to solve. The stem may be written as a direct question, such as "What should the nurse do first?" or as an incomplete sentence, such as "The nurse should . . ."

The *answers (options)* are possible responses to the stem. Each stem has one correct option and three incorrect options. The options may be written as complete sentences or may complete the sentence stated as a question.

2. Understand which step of the nursing process is being tested. Refer to page xii for an explanation of nursing process questions, and review your study grids. For example, as you read the question, determine whether the question is asking you to set priorities (planning) or judge outcomes (evaluation).

3. Understand client needs. As you read the question, consider the question in the context of client needs.

4. Read the question carefully. This is one of the most important aspects of effective test taking. Do not rush. Ask yourself, "What is this question asking?" and "What is the expected response?" If necessary, rephrase the question in your own words. Do not read meaning into a question that is not intended, and do not make a question more difficult than it is. If you do not understand the question, try to figure it out. If, for example, the question is asking about the fluid balance needs of a client with pheochromocytoma and you do not remember what pheochromocytoma is, then try to answer the question based on your knowledge of principles of fluid balance.

5. Look for key words that provide clues to the correct answer. For instance, words such as *except, not,* or *but* can change the meaning of a question; words such as *first, next,* and *most* ask you to establish a priority or use an order or sequence of steps.

6. Be certain you understand the meaning of all words in the question. If you see a word you do not know, try to figure out its meaning from a familiar base of the word or from the context of the question.

7. Attempt to answer the question before you see the answers, then look for the answer that is similar to the one you generated.

8. Base answers on nursing knowledge. Remember that the NCLEX-RN is used to test for safe practice and that you have learned the information needed to answer the question.

9. If you do not know the answer, make a reasonable guess. Hunches and intuition are often correct. If you do not know the answer, do not waste time and energy; give yourself permission to not know every question, and move

Background ⇓	⇓ Stem
SITUATION: The parents of children attending an elementary school and a high school invite the school nurse to attend some of their Parent-Teacher Association meetings to discuss common health problems related to their youngsters.	**QUESTION 1:** One parent asks about head lice (pediculosis capitis). The nurse discusses the symptoms with the parents. Which of the following symptoms is *most* common when a child has been infected with head lice? 1. Itching of the scalp. 2. Scaling of the scalp. 3. Serous weeping on the scalp surface. 4. Pinpoint hemorrhagic spots on the scalp surface.

⇑ Answers

Fig. 2. Sample test item, computer adaptive testing format: background (situation), stem (question), and answers (options).

on to the next one. In CAT, you must answer each question before the next item is administered, and since the level of difficulty will be adjusted as you answer each question, it is likely that you will know the answer to one of the next questions.

STRATEGIES FOR MANAGING TEST ANXIETY

All test takers experience some anxiety. A certain amount of anxiety is motivating, but be prepared to control unwanted anxiety. Develop the following anxiety management strategies, practice them while you are taking the comprehensive examinations in this book, and use them during the exam as needed.

- **Mental rehearsal.** Mental rehearsal involves reviewing the events and environment during the examination. Anticipate how you will feel, what the setting will be like, how you will take the exam, what the computer screen will look like, and how you will talk to yourself during the exam. Visualize your success. Rehearse what you will do if you have test anxiety.

- **Relaxation exercises.** Relaxation exercises involve tensing and relaxing various muscle groups to relieve the physical effects of anxiety. Practice systematically contracting and relaxing muscle groups from your toes to your neck to release energy for concentration. You can do these exercises during the exam to promote relaxation.

- **Deep breathing.** Taking deep breaths by inhaling slowly while counting to 5 and then exhaling slowly while counting to 10 increases oxygen flow to the lungs and brain. Deep breathing also decreases tension and helps manage anxiety by focusing your thoughts on the breathing and away from worries.

- **Positive self-talk.** Talking to yourself in a positive way serves to correct negative thoughts (eg, "I can't pass this test" and "I don't know the answers to any of these questions") and reinforces a positive self-concept. Replace negative thoughts with positive ones, telling yourself, "I can do this" and "I studied well and am prepared."

- **Distraction.** Thinking about something else can clear your mind of negative or unwanted thoughts. Think of something fun, something you enjoy. Plan now what you will think about to distract yourself during the exam.

- **Concentration.** During the exam, be prepared to concentrate. Have tunnel vision. Do not worry if others finish the test before you. Remember that everyone has their own speed for taking tests and that each test is individualized. Do not rush; you will have plenty of time. Focus; do not let noises from the keyboard next

to you divert your attention. Do not become overwhelmed by the testing environment. Use positive self-talk as you begin the exam.

FINAL WORDS

When you are fully prepared, you are ready to make your appointment to take the licensing exam. As you get ready to go to the exam site, consider these suggestions:

1. Make sure you know the date, time, and place the exam will be given; how to get to the exam site; know how long it takes to drive there; and where you can park. It may be helpful to visit the exam site and see the room where the exam will be given. Visualize yourself in the room, taking the test. Arrive on time for the exam.

2. Make sure you are physically prepared. Get enough rest before the examination; fatigue can impair concentration. If you are working, it may be advisable not to work the day before the exam; if you are working on a shift that is different from the time of the exam, adjust your work schedule several days ahead of time. Avoid planning time-consuming activities (eg, weddings, vacation trips) immediately before the exam. Do not use any drugs you usually do not use (including caffeine and nicotine), and do not use alcohol for 2 days before the exam. Eat regular meals before the exam. Remember that high-carbohydrate foods provide energy, but excessive sugar and caffeine can cause hyperactivity. Dress comfortably, in layers that can be added or removed according to your comfort level.

3. When you arrive at the site you will be asked to present your authorization to test. You will also need to provide two forms of identification, one of which must be a photo identification (eg, driver's license or passport). At the time of arrival you will be photographed and thumb-printed. You will then be oriented to the facilities and the use of the computer.

Best wishes! Your systematic review and preparation has given you a good foundation for a positive experience.

REFERENCES

1. National Council of State Boards of Nursing. (1995). *Test plan for the National Council Licensure Examination for Registered Nurses*. Chicago: Author.
2. National Council of State Boards of Nursing. (1994). Changes incorporated in the NCLEX-RN test plan. *Issues, 15*(4), 1.
3. Bloom, B.S. (1956). *Taxonomy of educational objectives. Handbook I: Cognitive domain*. New York: David McKay.
4. National Council of State Boards of Nursing. (1992). Walk-through of the computerized testing experience: What students will experience when taking NCLEX/CAT. *Issues, 13*(4), 1.
5. Sides, M.B., & Korcheck, N. (1996). *Nurses' guide to successful test-taking*. Philadelphia: Lippincott-Raven.
6. Gronlund, N.E. (1993). *How to make achievement tests and assessments*. Boston: Allyn & Bacon.

Section ONE

Practice Tests

Part I

The Nursing Care of Clients With Psychiatric Disorders and Mental Health Problems

Mood Disorders and Crisis Situations

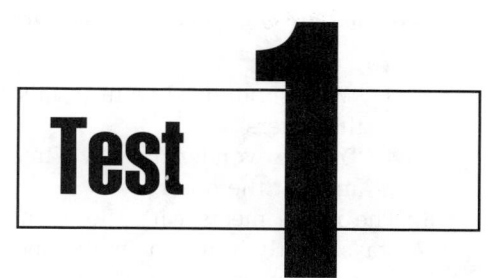

Test 1

- **The Client With Major Depression**
- **The Client With Bipolar Disorder, Manic Phase**
- **The Client With Major Depression and Suicidal Ideation**
- **The Client Who Attempts Suicide**
- **The Client in Crisis**
- **Correct Answers and Rationale**

Select the one best answer, and indicate your choice by filling in the circle in front of the option.

The Client With Major Depression

A 62-year-old client comes to the neighborhood health center for his annual physical examination.

1. While interacting with the nurse, the client states that he feels tired all of the time, has trouble sleeping, and has a problem with thinking. The best nursing action is to
   - ○ 1. inform the client about the normal aging process.
   - ○ 2. further assess the client's mental status and health history.
   - ○ 3. refer the client to a senior citizens' support group.
   - ○ 4. advise the client to discontinue daytime napping.
2. During the nurse's conversation with the client, the client states, "I have no reason to be sad. I have a great job and a wonderful wife and family." Which of the following comments would be best for the nurse to make at this time?
   - ○ 1. "Why do you think you're depressed?"
   - ○ 2. "Think about how fortunate you are."
   - ○ 3. "You have many positive qualities."
   - ○ 4. "Depression can be caused by a chemical imbalance in the brain."
3. The client is taking sertraline (Zoloft), 50 mg q AM. The nurse includes which of the following in the teaching plan about Zoloft?
   - ○ 1. Zoloft may cause erectile and ejaculatory dysfunction in some men.
   - ○ 2. It may be 3 to 4 weeks after starting Zoloft before the client feels better.

   - ○ 3. Zoloft causes lightheadedness or dizziness when rising.
   - ○ 4. Zoloft increases the appetite and causes weight gain.
4. The nurse meets with the client and his wife to discuss depression and the client's medication. Which of the following comments by the wife would indicate a correct understanding of her husband's illness and medication?
   - ○ 1. "His depression is almost cured."
   - ○ 2. "He's intelligent and won't need to depend on a pill much longer."
   - ○ 3. "It's important for him to take his medication so that the depression will not return or get worse."
   - ○ 4. "It's important to watch for physical dependency on Zoloft."

The client was admitted to the psychiatric unit yesterday. The nurse observes that his head is bowed in a dejected manner, his facial expression is sad, and he isolates himself in his room.

5. After a few minutes of conversation, the client wearily asks the nurse, "Why pick me to talk to when there are so many other people here?" Which reply by the nurse would be best?
   - ○ 1. "I'm assigned to care for you today, if you'll let me."
   - ○ 2. "You have a lot of potential, and I'd like to help you."

○ 3. "Why shouldn't I want to talk to you, as well as the others?"

○ 4. "You're wondering why I'm interested in you, and not the others?"

6. The nurse meets with the client daily. The client stays mostly in his room and speaks only when addressed, answering briefly and abruptly while keeping his eyes on the floor. In this stage of their relationship, the nurse focuses on the client's ability to

○ 1. make decisions.

○ 2. relate to other clients.

○ 3. function independently.

○ 4. express himself verbally.

7. Which of the following client behaviors would best indicate to the nurse that the relationship with the client is in the working phase?

○ 1. The client attempts to familiarize himself with the nurse.

○ 2. The client makes an effort to describe his problems in detail.

○ 3. The client tries to summarize his progress in the relationship.

○ 4. The client starts to challenge the boundaries or outer limits of the relationship.

8. The client is concerned that the information he gives to the nurse remains confidential. Which of the following comments would be best for the nurse to make in this situation?

○ 1. "If the information you share with me is important in relation to your care, I'll need to share it with the staff."

○ 2. "We can keep the information just between the two of us if you prefer."

○ 3. "I'll share the information with staff members only with your approval."

○ 4. "You can decide whether your physician needs this information for your care."

A client is admitted to the psychiatric unit with complaints of sleep disturbance, fatigue, feelings of uselessness, and inability to concentrate. The client was let go from her place of employment last month owing to her inability to keep up with the demands of her position.

9. On the day after an interview during which the client talked at length and tearfully about feeling useless and old, she failed to keep an appointment with the nurse. Which action would be best for the nurse to take?

○ 1. Assume that the client had a good reason for not coming and let her make the next move.

○ 2. Confront the client with her behavior and ask her to explain the reason for her absence.

○ 3. Seek out the client at the end of the scheduled interview time and tell her she was missed today.

○ 4. Arrange for another session with the client later the same day and say nothing about her absence.

10. The client speaks in a seemingly sincere manner about her former employer who replaced her with a younger person. "He was a wonderful boss. He was the most understanding boss I've ever had. It was a privilege to work for him." Which of the following defense mechanisms is the client most likely using?

○ 1. Sublimation.

○ 2. Suppression.

○ 3. Repression.

○ 4. Reaction formation.

11. The client begins to attend group sessions daily. She explains to the group how she lost her job. Which of the following statements by a group member would be most therapeutic for the client?

○ 1. "Tell us about what you did on your job."

○ 2. "It must have been very upsetting for you."

○ 3. "With your skills, finding another job should be easy."

○ 4. "The company must have had some reason for letting you go."

12. During an interaction with the nurse, the client states, "I have nothing to be depressed about. My husband has supported me throughout each of my many hospitalizations. He'll probably leave me this time. I'm an awful person and wife. I'm no good. I can't do anything right." Based on this information, the nurse should consider which of the following as an appropriate nursing diagnosis?

○ 1. Ineffective Individual Coping related to depression, as evidenced by withdrawal.

○ 2. Self Esteem Disturbance related to numerous hospitalizations, as evidenced by negative self-statements.

○ 3. Dysfunctional Grieving related to imagined loss of husband, as evidenced by negativity.

○ 4. Potential for Self-Directed Violence related to numerous failures, as evidenced by worthlessness.

13. The client has tearfully described her negative feelings about herself to the nurse during their last three interactions. Which of the following goals would be most appropriate for the nurse to include in the care plan at this time? The client will

○ 1. increase her self-esteem.

○ 2. write her negative feelings in a daily journal.

○ 3. verbalize her work-related accomplishments.

○ 4. verbalize three things she likes about herself.

The client with depression has been hospitalized for 3 days

on the psychiatric unit. This is the second hospitalization during the past year.

14. The physician orders a different drug, tranylcypromine sulfate (Parnate), when the client does not respond positively to a tricyclic antidepressant. Which of the following reactions should the client be cautioned about if her diet includes foods containing tyramine?
○ 1. Heart block.
○ 2. Grand mal seizure.
○ 3. Respiratory arrest.
○ 4. Hypertensive crisis.

15. While the client is taking tranylcypromine sulfate (Parnate), the nurse would teach her to avoid which food in particular because of its high tyramine content?
○ 1. Nuts.
○ 2. Aged cheeses.
○ 3. Grain cereals.
○ 4. Reconstituted milk.

16. The client obtains permission for a 24-hour pass to go home. Which of the following suggestions to the family in preparing for the visit indicates the best understanding of the client's needs?
○ 1. Plan to encourage the client to seek employment outside the home.
○ 2. Limit friends' visits so that the client can rest during the day.
○ 3. Schedule a day of interesting activities for the client outside the home.
○ 4. Plan to involve the client in usual at-home pursuits of the immediate family.

17. After a 2-month hospitalization, the client is preparing for discharge. Which of the following subjects would be most helpful to discuss when preparing to terminate the nurse–client relationship?
○ 1. The gains that the client has made during therapy.
○ 2. The plans that the client should make to find a job.
○ 3. The knowledge that the client's daughter is divorcing her husband.
○ 4. The conflicts the client has had with another staff member.

18. Which client reaction in terminating the relationship with the nurse should be considered the most healthy?
○ 1. A lack of response.
○ 2. A display of anger.
○ 3. An attempt at humor.
○ 4. An expression of grief.

A client is admitted involuntarily by court order to a psychiatric hospital for 90 days. Documents sent with her cite, among other things, that she will not eat because she feels her stomach is missing and her bowels have turned to jelly, and that she views this as "just punishment for my past wickedness and for the evil I've brought on my family."

19. To be evaluated as being legally committable, which of the following criteria did the client most likely have to meet?
○ 1. Presence of psychosis.
○ 2. Tried to harm herself or others.
○ 3. Unable to afford private treatment.
○ 4. Made threatening remarks to friends or relatives.

20. Which of the following rights did the client lose by being admitted involuntarily to a psychiatric hospital? The right to
○ 1. send and receive mail.
○ 2. vote in a national election.
○ 3. make a will or legally binding contract.
○ 4. sign out of the hospital against medical advice.

21. Through which of the following legal methods could the client seek release from the psychiatric hospital if she believed she was being improperly detained?
○ 1. Malpractice suit.
○ 2. Guardianship hearing.
○ 3. Writ of habeas corpus.
○ 4. Lien of property petition.

22. When the client expresses feelings of unworthiness, how would the nurse best respond?
○ 1. "Your family loves you even if you feel unworthy."
○ 2. "Your feelings of being unworthy are just your imagination."
○ 3. "It would be best to try to forget the idea that you are unworthy."
○ 4. "As you begin to feel better, your feelings of unworthiness will begin to disappear."

23. The client has not been eating. After serving the client her tray, which of the following actions by the nurse would be most likely to encourage her to eat?
○ 1. Leave the client's room without comment.
○ 2. Sit beside the client and place the fork in her hand.
○ 3. Tell the client that she will not recover unless she eats.
○ 4. Comment on how good the food looks.

24. The nurse notes that the client becomes restless and incoherent at night. Besides administering a prescribed medication, which of the following actions by the nurse would be most helpful for the client at this time?
○ 1. Encourage the client to talk about her family.

○ 2. Read to the client with the lights turned down low.

○ 3. Help the client take a cool shower before retiring.

○ 4. Sit quietly with the client until the medication takes effect.

25. The client demands to be left alone to die. She states, "If you try to cheat the avenger, you will suffer." Which of the following possible replies by the nurse would be best?

○ 1. "I won't let anything harm you."

○ 2. "It sounds like you're trying to frighten me."

○ 3. "I'm not trying to cheat anyone. What do you mean by that?"

○ 4. "I'll leave you alone for 15 minutes. Then I'll be back to see how you're doing."

A client is being admitted to the psychiatric unit. She responds to some of the nurse's questions with one-word answers. Her eyes are downcast, and her movements are very slow.

26. Later that morning, the nurse approaches the client and asks how she feels about being in the hospital. The client does not respond verbally and continues to gaze at the floor. Which of the following actions should the nurse take first?

○ 1. Spend time sitting in silence with the client.

○ 2. Leave the client alone and tell her that you will be back later to talk.

○ 3. Introduce another client to her and ask him to join you.

○ 4. Ask another staff member to include the client in an informal group discussion.

27. Which short-term goal should the nurse include in the client's care plan? The client will

○ 1. approach the nurse to engage in a one-to-one interaction by the end of the week.

○ 2. verbally interact with the nurse for 5 minutes in 1 week.

○ 3. problem solve with the nurse in 1 week.

○ 4. participate in milieu activities by the end of the week.

28. The nurse observes that the client has bathed, is wearing a clean blouse and slacks, and has combed her hair. Which statement by the nurse would be most helpful for the client?

○ 1. "You look good today."

○ 2. "I'm glad you're feeling better today."

○ 3. "I'm glad you combed your hair today."

○ 4. "I like your blouse and slacks."

A client with recurrent, endogenous depression has been hospitalized on the psychiatric unit for 3 days. He exhibits psychomotor retardation, anhedonia, and indecision.

29. Which goal of nursing care should have highest priority if the client demonstrates suicidal tendencies?

○ 1. Provide for contact between the client and his wife.

○ 2. Use measures to protect the client from harming himself.

○ 3. Reassure the client of his worthiness in a gentle manner.

○ 4. Maintain a calm environment in which the client can express his feelings and thoughts.

30. The nursing assistant approaches the nurse and states, "The client doesn't know what caused him to be so depressed. He must not want to tell me because he doesn't trust me yet." In responding to this staff member, which of the following statements by the nurse would most accurately describe the client's illness?

○ 1. "Endogenous depression is biochemical in nature and isn't caused by an outside stressor or problem. Therefore, the client cannot tell you why he's depressed because he really doesn't know."

○ 2. "Endogenous depression can be caused by various stressors. Perhaps the client isn't willing to tell you at this time."

○ 3. "Endogenous depression comes from within the person. It's a reaction to a loss. You need to give the client more time to identify the cause or loss."

○ 4. "Endogenous depression usually derives from past childhood conflicts. It really isn't important for the client to remember what happened years ago."

31. The client's condition improves, but he still remains alone in his room most of the time. Which of the following statements by the nurse would most likely help the client become involved with a unit activity?

○ 1. "Would you like to go to the movie with me today?"

○ 2. "I'll be back at 4 o'clock to take you to the movie."

○ 3. "I hope you go to the movie this afternoon. It will cheer you up."

○ 4. "You might want to go to the movie in the dayroom this afternoon."

32. The physician orders imipramine (Tofranil) for the client. The nurse explains the purpose of the medication to the client. The client asks the nurse, "If I start taking the pills, I'll have to take them the rest

of my life, won't I?" Which would be the nurse's most accurate and therapeutic reply?
- ○ 1. "Your condition determines the need for continued medication."
- ○ 2. "The medication prescribed is safe and routine."
- ○ 3. "After your symptoms decrease, the need for medication will be reevaluated."
- ○ 4. "Are you concerned about taking the medication?"

33. Which of the following health status assessments must be completed before the client starts taking imipramine (Tofranil)?
- ○ 1. Electrocardiogram (ECG).
- ○ 2. Urine sample for protein.
- ○ 3. Thyroid scan.
- ○ 4. Creatinine clearance test.

34. One nurse strongly believes that all psychiatric medication is a form of chemical mind control. When the client's wife asks about the efficacy of antidepressant medications, which of the following courses of action would be best for this nurse to take?
- ○ 1. Give an honest opinion of the treatment.
- ○ 2. Refer the client's wife to another knowledgeable person for information about the treatment.
- ○ 3. Explain that there are not enough current statistics about the efficacy of the treatment.
- ○ 4. Provide a package insert for the wife to read.

35. The nurse develops a medication teaching plan for the client. Which of the following plan components would be least important?
- ○ 1. A description of possible side effects.
- ○ 2. An opportunity for the client to express her fears and concerns about the therapy.
- ○ 3. A description of current research into antidepressant therapy.
- ○ 4. An explanation of why the first dose of medication is less than a full dose.

36. The client has been taking imipramine (Tofranil) at bedtime for 5 days. The nurse correctly judges that the medication is beginning to produce therapeutic effects when the client
- ○ 1. asks for a snack of cookies.
- ○ 2. sleeps 12 to 14 hours a night.
- ○ 3. states that she can feel her stomach getting better.
- ○ 4. asks to take the medication in the morning.

37. The client states that imipramine (Tofranil) is helping her feel less depressed but that she is still experiencing dry mouth. Which statement by the client would indicate the need for further teaching?
- ○ 1. "I've been chewing sugarless gum."
- ○ 2. "I'm sucking on ice chips."
- ○ 3. "I'm drinking a lot of water."
- ○ 4. "I'm sipping water often."

A client with depression has been taking fluoxetine (Prozac), 20 mg qd at 9 AM for 7 days.

38. Which of the following would be most important to report to the evening nursing shift?
- ○ 1. The client received Tylenol at 2 PM for a headache. He spent most of the day in his room.
- ○ 2. The client is still depressed. He refused to participate in group today.
- ○ 3. The client was weighed this morning; he has lost 4 pounds since admission last week.
- ○ 4. The client seemed much less depressed today and participated in a card game for the first time since his admission.

39. The nurse visits the client in a group home 1 week after discharge. He is prescribed fluoxetine (Prozac), 40 mg qd at 9 AM. The client states he is having problems concentrating, feels nervous, and has had diarrhea. The nurse appraises the client's symptoms to be
- ○ 1. important, probably suggesting a decrease in dosage or change to another medication.
- ○ 2. of no consequence because the client's symptoms are side effects of the Prozac.
- ○ 3. indicative of an exacerbation of the client's depression.
- ○ 4. unimportant and a method to elicit the nurse's empathy and attention.

The Client With Bipolar Disorder, Manic Phase

A client is admitted to the psychiatric unit accompanied by her husband. She brings six suitcases and three shopping bags. She orders the nurse to carry her bags. Her husband states she has been purchasing items that they cannot afford and has not slept for 4 nights.

40. Which additional information would be a priority for the nurse to seek from the client's husband?
- ○ 1. The client's fluid and food intake.
- ○ 2. Their current financial status.
- ○ 3. The client's usual sleeping pattern.
- ○ 4. Whether the client becomes agitated easily.

41. The husband apologizes to the nurse for his wife's demanding behavior. Which of the following possible replies by the nurse would be best?
- ○ 1. "I'm sure she's doing the best she can."
- ○ 2. "It's all right. We have been treated worse."
- ○ 3. "It must be hard for you to see her like this."
- ○ 4. "I understand. What happened to set her off like this?"

42. The client puts out her hand and says to the nurse, "Watch out! Here I come." She then puts her hand down and sits in a chair. After determining that the client is not about to harm anyone, the nurse should intervene by
○ 1. giving the client a book of her choice to read.
○ 2. placing the client in isolation to work out her aggression in private.
○ 3. taking the client to a punching bag for exercise to release excess energy.
○ 4. having the client continue to sit while holding her hands to help her gain control of herself.

43. The client is scheduled to go to the radiology department. Before taking the client for her x-ray examination, which of the following actions should the nurse take?
○ 1. Explain the x-ray procedure in simple terms.
○ 2. Provide a detailed explanation of the x-ray procedure.
○ 3. Say nothing before taking her to the x-ray department.
○ 4. Bring another staff member along in case she resists going to the x-ray department.

44. The nurse notes that the client is too busy investigating the unit and overseeing the activities of other clients to eat dinner. To help the client obtain sufficient nourishment, which of the following plans would be best?
○ 1. Serve foods that she can carry with her.
○ 2. Allow her to send out for her favorite foods.
○ 3. Serve food in small, attractively arranged portions.
○ 4. Allow her to enter the unit kitchen for extra food as necessary.

45. Later the same evening, the client appears at the nurses' station with brightly rouged cheeks, ornaments in her hair, and three pairs of false eyelashes, wearing a sheer nightgown, high heels, and bracelets up to her elbows. Which of the following actions should the nurse take in relation to the client's attire?
○ 1. Redirect the client to her room and help her put on proper apparel.
○ 2. Allow the client to wear what she likes and get her involved in a unit activity.
○ 3. Remind the client that she agreed to wear slacks and a shirt when out of her room.
○ 4. Ask the client to put on hospital pajamas until she can dress appropriately on her own.

A client with bipolar disorder, manic phase has just sat down to watch television in the lounge.

46. As the nurse approaches the lounge area, the client states, "The sun is shining. Where is my son? I love Lucy. Let's play ball." The client is displaying
○ 1. concreteness.
○ 2. flight of ideas.
○ 3. depersonalization.
○ 4. use of neologisms.

47. The client's speech pattern is related primarily to
○ 1. underlying hostilities.
○ 2. loose ego boundaries.
○ 3. feelings of anxiety.
○ 4. distortions in self-concept.

48. Which of the following responses by the nurse would be the most therapeutic for the client?
○ 1. "Let's talk about what you did today instead."
○ 2. "How does the sun shining relate to your son?"
○ 3. "You're talking nonsense. Try to stay on one subject?"
○ 4. "I can't follow you. It would help me if you'd speak a little slower."

49. The client is intrusive and disruptive to other clients. He constantly walks about the unit interrupting others. Which plan should the nurse institute first in this situation?
○ 1. Escort the client to his room and explain that he cannot come out until he gets permission.
○ 2. Set limits on the client's behavior. Explain what is expected and what the consequences will be if limits are violated.
○ 3. Ask another staff member to take the client to watch television for the next hour.
○ 4. Bargain with the client. Explain which privileges he can attain if he can control his behavior.

50. Which activity would be most therapeutic for channeling the client's hyperactive behavior? Allowing the client to
○ 1. lead some group activities.
○ 2. clean his room and the dayroom.
○ 3. read to patients who are depressed.
○ 4. exercise and move about as much as possible.

51. Which of the following feeling states is reflected by the client's behavior during a manic episode?
○ 1. Guilt.
○ 2. Anger.
○ 3. Mistrust.
○ 4. Hostility.

52. The client sometimes makes inappropriate requests. For example, he calls an office supply store to order many items and charges them to his account. Which of the following nursing interventions would be best in this situation?
○ 1. Tell the client that his request will be filled.
○ 2. Explain to the client that his request is denied.
○ 3. Suggest to the client that part of his request can be met.

○ 4. Call the store to cancel the request without telling the client.

53. The nurse evaluates the client's condition daily. During the client's period of euphoria, the nurse should be especially alert for which conditions?
○ 1. Gastritis and vertigo.
○ 2. Exhaustion and infection.
○ 3. Convulsions and dermatitis.
○ 4. Bradycardia and palpitations.

54. The client has been taking lithium carbonate (Lithane) for hyperactivity, as prescribed by his physician. While the client is taking this drug, the nurse should ensure that he has an adequate intake of
○ 1. sodium.
○ 2. iron.
○ 3. iodine.
○ 4. calcium.

55. Which of the following clinical manifestations would alert the nurse to lithium toxicity?
○ 1. Increasingly agitated behavior.
○ 2. Markedly increased food intake.
○ 3. Sudden increase in blood pressure.
○ 4. Anorexia with nausea and vomiting.

56. After 10 days of lithium therapy, the client's lithium level is 1.0 mEq/L. The nurse knows that this value indicates which of the following?
○ 1. A laboratory error.
○ 2. An anticipated therapeutic blood level of the drug.
○ 3. An atypical client response to the drug.
○ 4. A toxic level.

57. The client expresses the belief that he was born out of wedlock to a famous woman. When dealing with this delusion of grandeur, the nurse should first try to
○ 1. get the client to discuss another topic.
○ 2. involve the client in a simple group project.
○ 3. convince the client that he is wrong in his belief.
○ 4. satisfy the client's implied need to feel important.

A client is irritable and hostile. He becomes agitated and verbally lashes out when his personal needs are not immediately met by the staff.

58. When the client's request for a pass is refused by the physician, he utters a stream of profanities. Which of the following statements best describes the client's behavior? The client's anger is usually
○ 1. not intended personally.
○ 2. a reliable sign of serious pathology.
○ 3. an intended attack on the physician's skills.
○ 4. a sign that his condition is improving.

59. A goal of the client's treatment plan is to reduce his activity and aggression. Which of the following comments by the nurse when the client's anger escalates would best help him move toward his treatment goal?
○ 1. "You must go to your room or into seclusion now."
○ 2. "You're disturbing other clients. If you don't stop, you'll need to go into seclusion."
○ 3. "You have a choice of going to your room voluntarily or being escorted to your room."
○ 4. "Your behavior is disrupting the unit. Let's find a quiet place and talk about what is happening."

60. After 2 weeks of hospitalization, the client has improved with medication and therapy. Which statement made by the client indicates therapeutic gain and readiness for discharge?
○ 1. "I'm cured now and won't need my medicine when I go home."
○ 2. "I know that I'm getting sick when I get very angry."
○ 3. "My medicine really helps me. I'll be ready to go back to work in a few weeks."
○ 4. "I like feeling high from my illness. It helps me feel great and gives me a lot of energy."

61. The client's wife asks the nurse what she can do to help her husband at home. Which of the following actions by family members on behalf of the client would probably be least helpful?
○ 1. Try to keep the client free from worry and anxiety.
○ 2. Relieve the client of some home responsibilities he had.
○ 3. Develop effective communication techniques with the client at home.
○ 4. Learn to recognize when the client is showing signs of drug toxicity.

62. The client's illness is most likely related to which of the following factors?
○ 1. Having been molested as a preschool-age child.
○ 2. A family history of mood disorders.
○ 3. High levels of potassium in the brain.
○ 4. Excessive alcohol intake.

The client with bipolar disorder meets with the nurse at the community mental health center for follow-up care.

63. The client has been taking valproic acid (Depakene), 500 mg tid for 1 month. The serum blood level is 60 μg/mL. The client states that her stomach feels upset after she takes the medication. Which of the following statements by the nurse would be most helpful?

○ 1. "We'll adjust the dose of your medication."
○ 2. "Chew the tablet before swallowing it."
○ 3. "Take the valproic acid with meals or food."
○ 4. "We'll have you take your medication all at one time."

64. The client states her husband told her she must be a weak person because she cannot control her behavior and has to rely on pills to control her. Which of the following statements by the nurse would be most appropriate?

○ 1. "Bipolar disorder is a biochemical disorder that necessitates medication like Depakene to help control the symptoms and keep your mood stable."
○ 2. "Bipolar disorder is more prevalent in certain personality types."
○ 3. "Relying on pills temporarily is necessary to help your control your illness."
○ 4. "Your husband may be correct because stronger people are better able to control their symptoms."

65. The nurse would judge client education regarding valproic acid (Depakene) as effective if the client states

○ 1. "I can stop the Depakene because the serum level is normal."
○ 2. "I can take the Depakene only when I feel I need it."
○ 3. "Depakene is safe to use when I get pregnant."
○ 4. "I might need to take the Depakene for a long time."

The Client With Major Depression and Suicidal Ideation

A nurse who makes weekly visits to area boarding homes observes a client who was discharged from a psychiatric hospital. The client is irritable and walks about her room slowly and morosely. After 10 minutes, the nurse prepares to leave, but the client plucks at the nurse's sleeve and quickly asks for help in rearranging her belongings. She also anxiously makes inconsequential remarks to keep the nurse with her.

66. Which of the following statements provides the most likely explanation for the client's behavior? The client

○ 1. is lonely and looking for a way to pass the time.
○ 2. is self-centered and possessive of the nurse's time.

○ 3. needs attention paid to some as yet unknown concern.
○ 4. desires assistance to improve her room's appearance.

67. The nurse is careful not to act rushed or impatient with the client and gradually learns that the client is very down and feels worthless and unloved. In view of the fact that the client had previously made a suicidal gesture, which of the following interventions by the nurse would be a priority at this time?

○ 1. Ask the client frankly if she has thoughts of or plans for committing suicide.
○ 2. Avoid bringing up the subject of suicide to prevent giving the client ideas of self-harm.
○ 3. Outline some alternative measures to suicide for the client to use during periods of sadness.
○ 4. Mention others the nurse has known who have felt like the client and attempted suicide, to draw her out.

68. The nurse would be most concerned about the client's depression when the client states that she

○ 1. feels more tired than usual.
○ 2. has difficulty falling asleep and wakes up early in the morning.
○ 3. no longer watches her favorite television programs.
○ 4. is gaining weight.

69. The client's friend asks the nurse, "What is the best way to act around her when she's so blue?" When considering therapeutic ways to behave with the client, the nurse should recommend that the friend avoid behaving in a way that is

○ 1. firm.
○ 2. serious.
○ 3. cheerful.
○ 4. spontaneous.

During his admission to an inpatient psychiatric unit, a client tells the nurse that he has been experiencing headaches that have worsened in the past 2 weeks. He also has difficulty falling asleep and has nightmares when he does sleep. He states, "Nothing matters anymore. Life is nothing, and there's nothing left for me. My wife divorced me 3 months ago. No one will want me or love me anymore. I'm not good for anyone."

70. When documenting the admission data, which of the following statements should the nurse include in the client's chart?

○ 1. The client has been depressed since his wife divorced him 3 months ago. He stated, "No one will want or love me anymore." He also complained of headaches and nightmares.

○ 2. The client is suffering from feelings of depression. He complains of headaches and nightmares and exhibits suicidal ideation. He feels unloved and unwanted since his divorce 3 months ago.

○ 3. The client willingly related his recent stressors. Suicidal ideation was also present. His headaches and nightmares have increased during the past 2 weeks.

○ 4. The client verbalized feelings of worthlessness and lack of hope for the future. He exhibited suicidal ideation, stating, "Nothing matters anymore. Life is nothing. No one will want me or love me anymore."

The client was divorced 3 months ago. He has difficulty falling asleep and experiences nightmares and headaches, which have increased in the past 2 weeks.

71. From the information provided about this client, which nursing diagnosis would be least accurate?
○ 1. Disturbance in Self Esteem related to divorce, as evidenced by negative statements about self.
○ 2. Potential for Self Directed Violence related to lack of hope for the future, as evidenced by suicidal ideation.
○ 3. Sleep Pattern Disturbance related to depressed mood, as evidenced by difficulty falling asleep.
○ 4. Social Isolation related to feelings of worthlessness, as evidenced by withdrawal.

72. Regarding the nursing diagnosis of Potential for Self Directed Violence, which action should the nurse take first?
○ 1. Instruct the client to seek out staff when he has thoughts of harming himself.
○ 2. Have the client agree to a no-harm contract.
○ 3. Remove all potentially harmful objects from the client's environment.
○ 4. Assign the client to a double room occupied by another client.

73. The client admits to having thoughts of suicide. He is lethargic, withdrawn, and irritable. In conversations with the nurse, he stresses his faults. When he starts to point out the things he cannot do, which of the following responses by the nurse would provide the best intervention?
○ 1. "You can do anything you put your mind to."
○ 2. "Try to think more positively about yourself."
○ 3. "Let's talk about your plans for the weekend."
○ 4. "You were able to write a letter to your friend today."

The client visits a community mental health center for follow-up care after being discharged 1 week ago from an inpatient unit. The client was hospitalized with Major Depression With Suicidal Ideation for 1 week. He is taking venlafaxine (Effexor), 75 mg tid, and is planning to return to work.

74. The nurse asks the client if he is experiencing thoughts of self-harm. The client responds, "I hardly think about it anymore and wouldn't do anything to hurt myself." The nurse judges
○ 1. the client to be decompensating and in need of rehospitalization.
○ 2. the client to need an adjustment or increase in his dose of antidepressant.
○ 3. the depression to be improving and the suicidal ideation to be lessening.
○ 4. the presence of suicidal ideation to warrant a telephone call to the client's physician.

75. The client states, "I'm still feeling nauseous after I take Effexor. Maybe I need something else." Which of the following actions by the nurse would be most accurate? Advise the client to
○ 1. take the medication at mealtime.
○ 2. take Effexor only in the morning.
○ 3. cut the dose in half.
○ 4. take Effexor before bedtime.

76. The client states, "I'm looking forward to going back to work, but I wonder if I'll be able to keep up with the demands of my job." Which of the following statements by the nurse would be most helpful?
○ 1. "You'll do well. You have an excellent work record."
○ 2. "I wouldn't worry about it. The main thing to remember is that you can work."
○ 3. "You might need extra breaks at first until you feel better."
○ 4. "You sound concerned. I want to hear more about how you are feeling."

A 68-year-old client is nearing discharge from the inpatient psychiatric unit to live alone in her apartment. She has improved with medication and treatment and no longer has suicidal ideation. All her family members live out of state.

77. As the nurse helps the client plan an activity program on her return home, which plan of action would likely be most helpful for the client?
○ 1. Finding a volunteer to visit regularly at her apartment.

2. Arranging for Meals-on-Wheels.
3. Arranging transportation to a senior citizens' social group that meets near her apartment.
4. Asking a friend of the client to spend more time with her.

78. In general, it is difficult for a nurse to maintain effective relationships with depressed clients experiencing suicidal ideation because their
 1. pessimism arouses frustration and anger in others.
 2. poor personal grooming invites disgust and ridicule from others.
 3. independence prevents them from asking for assistance.
 4. laziness keeps them from putting forth the necessary effort to get well.

79. The nurse judges correctly that a client is experiencing an adverse effect from amitriptyline hydrochloride (Elavil) when the client demonstrates
 1. an elevated blood glucose level.
 2. insomnia.
 3. hypertension.
 4. urinary retention.

80. Which of the following variables should the nurse judge as least likely to indicate high risk when assessing a client's potential for suicide?
 1. Age.
 2. Angry behavior.
 3. Home environment.
 4. Previous suicidal gesture.

81. A client's goal is: Client will state two alternative actions to take when feeling suicidal in the future. Which of the following client outcomes would indicate the least progress toward meeting this goal?
 1. The client states that she will volunteer time at a senior day care center.
 2. The client has written down the telephone number of the suicide help-line and states that she will use it if necessary.
 3. The client has arranged to join a woman's support group at her church.
 4. The client is keeping a daily journal of her feelings and problems.

82. Which of the following statements is the best wording of a no-harm, no-suicide contract?
 1. "I will not think about killing myself."
 2. "I will not accidentally or on purpose kill myself during the next 24 hours."
 3. "I will not kill myself until after talking to my doctor."
 4. "I will not kill myself unless my wife dies."

83. The nurse correctly judges that the danger of a suicide attempt is greatest when the client's behavior indicates that he
 1. has resumed his former lifestyle.

2. has an increased energy level.
3. is at a point of deepest despair.
4. agrees to visit with an estranged brother.

The Client Who Attempts Suicide

An adolescent girl is brought to the hospital emergency room in a state of unconsciousness after having swallowed "a bottle of red pills" 45 minutes earlier. The pills are identified as secobarbital (Seconal). A suicide note is found that asks for forgiveness and states, "I can't live without my boyfriend. He has left me because I'm no good."

84. Which of the following measures should the nurse be prepared to carry out when this client is admitted?
 1. Forcing fluids.
 2. Giving a diuretic.
 3. Inducing vomiting.
 4. Lavaging the stomach.

85. Which of the following interventions should be of primary concern to the nurse after the client's physical condition is no longer critical?
 1. Providing the client with a safe environment.
 2. Ensuring that the client's diet is high in fiber.
 3. Providing the client with quiet periods for reflection.
 4. Ensuring that the client's fluid intake is generous.

86. After the client regains consciousness, she says to the nurse, "I can't even kill myself. I can't even do that right." Which of the following responses by the nurse would be most therapeutic at this time?
 1. "These feelings will pass."
 2. "Tell me more about how you are feeling."
 3. "Why would you feel that way?"
 4. "You have a great deal to live for."

87. When evaluating the effectiveness of the client's treatment, the nurse can judge that progress is being made when the client's behavior shows an improvement in her
 1. appetite.
 2. self-concept.
 3. activity level.
 4. gender identity conflict.

88. The client goes to her room and slams the door immediately after the first family therapy session. Later, she tells the nurse, "I'm so mad. The therapist didn't let me tell my side of the story. He just agreed with everything my parents said." Which of the following nursing actions would be most therapeutic in this situation?

14

○ 1. Consider terminating the therapy because it upsets the client.

○ 2. Redirect the client to the therapist to tell him how she feels.

○ 3. Allow the client to continue to ventilate her feelings to the nurse.

○ 4. Suggest to the therapist that he allow the client to tell her side of the story.

A client is brought to the inpatient psychiatric unit from the emergency room with a self-inflicted gunshot wound in his arm. He is escorted to the unit by emergency room staff, with his arm bandaged and in a sling.

89. A staff member states to the nurse, "He only hurt his arm, so he probably only wanted to manipulate someone or did it for attention." Which of the following responses by the nurse to the staff member would be most appropriate?

○ 1. "All suicide attempts or acts of self-harm are very serious and indicate a cry for help."

○ 2. "He really must not have wanted to kill himself, but he certainly injured his arm."

○ 3. "He didn't use a lethal method to kill himself, so he must not have been serious about taking his life."

○ 4. "It was probably a way to escape a serious problem. The hospital is a safe and secure environment."

90. What client data would be most important for the nurse to consider in deciding to institute suicide precautions because of high-risk behavior? The client

○ 1. states that he still has thoughts of harming himself but feels he can control them.

○ 2. states that he is worried about his child's reaction.

○ 3. expresses guilt and shame about trying to harm himself.

○ 4. has recently attempted suicide with a lethal method.

91. Later in the day, the client's wife visits and brings a bag of some of her husband's personal items. Which of the following actions by the nurse would be most appropriate?

○ 1. Direct another caregiver to inspect the bag and its belongings in the examining room.

○ 2. Ask the wife if the bag contains any dangerous items.

○ 3. Tell the wife that her husband's items will be locked.

○ 4. Inspect the bag and its contents in the presence of the client and his wife.

92. Which of the following items would the nurse keep in the locked area for client's belongings?

○ 1. bar of soap

○ 2. belt

○ 3. shoes

○ 4. trousers

The Client in Crisis

The nurse is employed at a crisis shelter that has several clients each day in a state of severe disorganization. An anxious teenage girl is brought to the interviewing room, sobbing and saying that she thinks she is pregnant but does not know what to do.

93. Which of the following nursing interventions would be the most appropriate at this time?

○ 1. Ask the client what she had thought of doing.

○ 2. Give the client some ideas about what to do next.

○ 3. Summarize what the nurse heard and ask the client to confirm the nurse's perceptions.

○ 4. Question the client in more detail about her feelings and about what her parents' reactions are likely to be.

94. The client says that she and her boyfriend have engaged in "mostly heavy petting and necking." Which of the following responses by the nurse to the client's comment would be best?

○ 1. "You mean you have had sexual intercourse?"

○ 2. "Describe what you mean by heavy petting and necking."

○ 3. "I think we need to talk about what's involved in sexual intercourse."

○ 4. "All you have been doing with your boyfriend is heavy petting and necking?"

95. The client says that she would "rather die than be pregnant." Which of the following responses by the nurse would be most helpful?

○ 1. "Try not to worry until after the pregnancy test."

○ 2. "Pregnancy is normal."

○ 3. "Why are you so upset?"

○ 4. "You're very upset now; it will be easier for you to talk about this if you can relax."

96. The results of the client's pregnancy test is negative. The nurse teaches her about sexual intercourse and contraception. "No more fooling around for me!" she states. Which of the following replies by the nurse would be best?

○ 1. "Just in case, why don't you try the pills for a while?"

○ 2. "The last person who said that ended up having a baby."

○ 3. "It's up to you, but if you change your mind, come back and we'll try to help you."

○ 4. "Aren't you being a little bit overconfident about it, as attractive as you must be to the fellows?"

The nurse is responsible for counseling clients who call a crisis shelter hot line. One night, the nurse talks to two 11-year-old boys on the telephone who think a friend sniffs glue. They say his breath sometimes smells like glue and he acts drunk. They ask if they should tell their parents about the friend.

97. When formulating a reply, the nurse should be guided by the knowledge that

○ 1. the boys probably fear punishment.

○ 2. sniffing glue is illegal.

○ 3. the boys' observations could be wrong.

○ 4. glue-sniffing is a minor form of substance abuse.

98. The nurse urges the boys to seek help for their friend and warns them that delaying treatment could result in the boy's death. A person who inhales noxious substances is most likely to die from

○ 1. brain lesions.

○ 2. malnutrition.

○ 3. cardiac failure.

○ 4. kidney damage.

The nurse is caring for a client who came to the crisis shelter frightened and behaving aggressively. From the client's friends, the nurse learns that he has been smoking cocaine for the last 3 hours. The client is having a severe reaction to the cocaine and seems to have lost touch with reality. He is very suspicious of his friends who came with him and does not want to talk to the nurse. Suddenly, he yells out, "I'll kill you before I'll let you take me."

99. The nurse should base intervention on knowledge that the client's primary need is

○ 1. physical contact with his friends.

○ 2. isolation from other clients.

○ 3. reassurance from the staff.

○ 4. protection from his own behavior.

100. Which of the following comments by the nurse would be most useful to help the client reestablish his self-control and orientation?

○ 1. "You have no need to be concerned. You're going to be all right."

○ 2. "You have taken a drug you shouldn't have, and it is making you sick."

○ 3. "You're reacting to the cocaine and will soon be past the main drug reaction. You're safe here."

○ 4. "You have a temporary psychosis from taking a psychedelic. Let's watch some television while we wait for it to pass."

101. For this client, using a tranquilizing drug, such as chlorpromazine hydrochloride (Thorazine), to shorten the drug reaction should be avoided because

○ 1. the major tranquilizers can cause a reuptake of the drug in the brain.

○ 2. flashbacks increase in severity when mediating drugs are used to treat the initial reaction.

○ 3. the client's emotions might stem from a source entirely different from the cocaine effects.

○ 4. other incompatible drugs may have been combined with the cocaine that, together with the tranquilizer, might be fatal.

A client has come to the crisis shelter because she wants to ask someone a question. In a matter-of-fact manner, she asks, "How would you feel if your girlfriend had been raped?" The nurse suspects that the client may have been sexually assaulted.

102. What would be the nurse's best reply to the client's question?

○ 1. "Before I answer, tell me what's really on your mind, okay?"

○ 2. "I haven't thought about it. How would you expect me to feel?"

○ 3. "I'd probably be upset and angry. Do you have a special reason for asking?"

○ 4. "It would bother me. But don't you think there's too much violence these days?"

103. The client reports that since being raped, she has constantly sought out brightly lit places and the company of friendly people. She also plans to move to another part of the city. When analyzing the client's behavior, the nurse correctly identifies the most likely goal for her maneuvers as

○ 1. self-defense.

○ 2. self-assertion.

○ 3. self-deception.

○ 4. self-gratification.

The nurse is responsible for teaching volunteers for a crisis hot line.

104. During one of the sessions, a volunteer asks, "What if I'm not sure why someone is calling?" Which of the following statements by the nurse would be most helpful?
- ○ 1. "Ask the caller to tell you why he or she is calling you today."
- ○ 2. "Tell the caller to make an appointment at the walk-in crisis clinic."
- ○ 3. "Instruct the caller to go to the nearest emergency room."
- ○ 4. "Tell the caller to let you speak to anyone else in the house."

105. The nurse judges that further education about crisis and intervention is needed when a volunteer states,
- ○ 1. "Callers to a crisis line use this service when they're overwhelmed and exhausted."
- ○ 2. "People use crisis hot lines when they're in the most pain and nothing is working for them."
- ○ 3. "Most people in crisis will be calling the line daily for a year."
- ○ 4. "One benefit of crisis intervention is that a person will know how to handle stressful situations better in the future."

The family members of the victims of a three-car accident have arrived at the emergency room.

106. A wife of one of the victims in the accident is sitting away from the others and crying. Which of the following actions by the nurse would be first?
- ○ 1. Leave the wife alone to cry.
- ○ 2. Sit next to the wife and offer her some tissues.
- ○ 3. Call the physician for a sedative.
- ○ 4. Ask the wife if she would like to speak to the social worker.

107. The victim's wife is admitted to the hospital after attempting to overdose on her antidepressant 3 months after his death. She states, "I can't live without him. It's no use. I just want to die." Which of the following nursing diagnoses is a priority in the plan of care for this client?
- ○ 1. Dysfunctional grieving.
- ○ 2. Powerlessness.
- ○ 3. Hopelessness.
- ○ 4. Potential for self-harm.

CORRECT ANSWERS AND RATIONALE

The letters in parentheses following the rationale identify the step of the nursing process (A, D, P, I, E); cognitive level (K, C, T, N); and client need (S, G, L, H). See the Answer Grid for the key.

The Client With Major Depression

1. 2. The client is exhibiting signs of possible depression. The nurse should explore his medical history and conduct a mental status examination to further assess and explore this possibility. He is not exhibiting signs and symptoms of the normal aging process. Referral to a senior citizens' support group may be appropriate later, depending on the client's needs and interests. Daytime napping should be discouraged if it interrupts nighttime sleeping. At this time, the nurse does not have enough information about the client's daily schedule to warrant napping being a problem. It is more important to first determine the source of his symptoms so that the client can be treated appropriately. (I, T, L)

2. 4. The biologic theory of depression indicates a neurotransmitter imbalance involving serotonin, norepinephrine, and possibly dopamine. Endogenous depression (depression coming from within the person) is biochemical in nature. Asking the client why he is depressed is nontherapeutic because there is no external cause or reason for the client's depression, and it will only increase the client's feelings of guilt for not being able to answer the nurse. Telling the client that he is fortunate and has positive qualities is not helpful and will not decrease his sadness or feelings of depression because it is biologically based. (I, T, L)

3. 1. To promote medication compliance and treatment of depression, it is important for the male client to know that Zoloft may cause loss of libido, erectile dysfunction, and ejaculatory dysfunction. A decrease in dosage can decrease these symptoms. Zoloft typically takes 1 to 2 weeks to work before benefits are noted. Tricyclic antidepressants take 3 to 4 weeks before the patient receives maximum benefit, cause postural hypotension, and may cause weight gain. (P, C, G)

4. 3. Medication compliance is essential to prevent a return or worsening of the symptoms of endogenous depression. Maintaining biochemical balance can occur with medication. Depression is not cured and is not dependent on the client's intelligence to will the illness away. Zoloft is not physically addicting. (E, N, L)

5. 4. The nurse is using a therapeutic technique of restatement when reiterating the client's comment in the form of a question. This technique best helps the client continue the conversation with an expression of his feelings. Telling the client that the nurse is assigned to care for him and why is impersonal and implies that the client is being uncooperative. Telling the client that the nurse is there because the client has potential for improvement implies that other clients perhaps do not have this potential. Asking the client a question with the word *why* challenges him and demands an explanation. None of these approaches is as effective as using the technique of restatement. (I, N, L)

6. 4. When working with a client who speaks little, answers briefly, and looks at the floor, the nurse should focus on the simplest type of behavior (ie, behavior requiring the least effort for the client). The relationship described in this item is the orientation phase. When self-expression and verbalization are more appropriate goals, then decision making, relating to others, and functioning independently may be pursued. (P, N, L)

7. 2. This nurse–client relationship is most probably in the working phase. The client's effort to describe his problems to the nurse illustrates that the client has gone beyond testing and acquainting himself with a new relationship and is now working on his problems. The relationship is in an orientation phase when the client attempts to familiarize himself with the nurse and challenges boundaries of the relationship. The relationship is in a termination phase when the client summarizes and evaluates his progress. (A, T, L)

8. 1. The nurse should make sure that the client understands that the nurse's need to discuss information given by the client when, in the nurse's judgment, the information is necessary in relation to his therapy. This is a judgment the client is unable to make with safety. Promising a client to keep information confidential places the nurse in a difficult position. If the client tells the nurse something that the nurse considers vital information for others on the health team, the nurse would need to break a promise to the client to share the information. (I, N, S)

9. 3. The responsibility for maintaining a relationship with a client rests with the nurse. If a client misses a scheduled interview, the nurse is assuming responsibility for the relationship by seeking her out

at the end of the scheduled interview time and telling her she was missed. To confront the client with her absence and ask her to explain it is nontherapeutic and threatening. To arrange another session with the client and to say nothing about the missed appointment does not keep to the terms of the nurse–client contract and offers little help to the client. The nurse makes an assumption without knowing the facts by thinking that the patient has good reason for not keeping her appointment. The nurse is not assuming responsibility by waiting for the client to make the next move in this situation. (P, N, L)

10. 4. Reaction formation is a defense mechanism that occurs when a person expresses an attitude or feeling opposite from his unconscious feelings or attitudes. The client compliments her employer when, unconsciously, she most likely does not like him because he fired her. Sublimation involves directing unacceptable impulses into constructive channels. Suppression is a conscious effort to overcome unacceptable thoughts or desires. Repression is a defense mechanism that occurs when a person excludes or bars painful experiences and thoughts from his or her state of consciousness. (A, T, L)

11. 2. It is most therapeutic when clients in group sessions help each other explore feelings further and when they demonstrate understanding of each other. In this situation, asking the client to describe her work and indicating that the company must have had a reason for firing her avoid discussing the client's feelings. Suggesting to the client that she will have no trouble finding another job offers false hope without full knowledge of the situation. (E, N, L)

12. 2. Negative self-statements are directly related to how the client views and feels about herself. The comments reflect a feeling of low self-esteem because of the psychopathology of the illness necessitating or related to her many hospitalizations. The negative view of self is a prominent theme underlying her verbalizations. Information concerning whether the client is withdrawn or is going to hurt herself is absent. The client only imagines that her husband will leave her because of her view of herself. (D, T, L)

13. 4. Describing and verbalizing feelings are necessary and normal because the client has usually repressed or blocked feelings, which is partly responsible for the client's pain. Expressing feelings are a prerequisite before the nurse can intervene in how the client thinks or behaves. Stating a goal like increasing self-esteem is too global and nonspecific. Writing feelings in a journal will not benefit the client since she has verbalized them to the nurse. Verbalizing work-

related accomplishments is too specific and focuses on only one client aspect. Focusing on what the client likes about herself is too broad for what the client thinks is important to her. Asking the client to identify only three qualities does not overwhelm the client. (P, N, L)

14. 4. Tranylcypromine sulfate (Parnate) is a monoamine oxidase (MAO) inhibitor. A client taking this drug in combination with foods or beverages rich in tyramine is likely to have a hypertensive crisis. The medication should be discontinued and the physician notified if the client exhibits symptoms related to an impending hypertensive crisis, such as headaches, diaphoresis, palpitations, pallor, nausea and vomiting, and chest pain. (D, K, L)

15. 2. Aged and strong cheeses are tyramine-rich foods and, when ingested in combination with MAO inhibitors, can cause a severe hypertensive crisis. Other foods and beverages rich in tyramine include aged meat and other nonfresh meat, liver, dried fish, any fermented high-protein food (eg, yeast extracts and concentrates), Italian broad beans (pods), green bean pods, wine, beer, and ale. In many instances, the following caffeine-containing foods and beverages are also restricted: coffee, tea, cocoa, chocolate, and caffeine-containing soft drinks. (I, T, L)

16. 4. Planning to involve the client in usual at-home pursuits of the immediate family is best when the client is to go home for a pass. There are no indications that this client requires extra rest or unusual activities. It is too early, and possibly inappropriate, for the client to start looking for employment. (P, N, L)

17. 1. Terminating a nurse–client relationship is a weaning process. Subjects such as plans for finding employment, divorce plans of a family member, and conflicts during hospitalization do not aid this weaning. Discussing the gains that the client has made during hospitalization does. The content focuses on gains made in treatment, feelings about termination, and saying goodbye. Introducing new material at termination may impede therapeutic termination. (P, T, L)

18. 4. Grief is a direct and appropriate response to termination of a positive relationship and indicates acceptance of termination. Anger is healthy when openly expressed but is a less healthy reaction than grief. A lack of response may be interpreted as indifference, but it represents a profound emotional reaction that the patient is unable to express. Humor may be a defense against feelings of loss. (E, C, L)

19. 2. A client is legally committable when she tries to harm herself or others. (D, T, S)

20. 4. A person who has been involuntarily committed to a hospital for the mentally ill loses the right to leave the hospital of his own accord. He does not necessarily lose rights to vote, make a will or contract, or send and receive mail. (D, T, S)

21. 3. A writ of habeas corpus is defined as an order requiring that a prisoner (in this case, the client) be brought before a judge or into court to decide whether he is being held lawfully. Its purpose is to obtain liberation of a person held without just cause. (D, T, S)

22. 4. When the client feels unworthiness, she reflects low self-esteem. Presenting another set of facts in a manner that is accepting of the client but avoids a power struggle is necessary. Telling the client that her feelings are imaginary, that her family still loves her, and that she should try to forget ideas of unworthiness disregard her feelings and may be perceived as rejection. (I, T, L)

23. 2. Sitting beside the client and placing the fork in her hand are likely to stimulate the depressed client to eat. Sitting with the client also conveys a message of having time for her and of caring. Leaving the client alone, telling her that she must eat to recover, and trying to encourage her by saying the food looks good are techniques that are less likely to interest the client in eating. (I, T, L)

24. 4. Doing something with or to this client is unlikely to help restlessness and incoherence. It is best to sit quietly with the client until the medication takes effect. A warm bath might be helpful, but not a cool shower. (I, T, L)

25. 4. When this client wants to be left alone to die, it is best to leave the client for a few minutes, then return to see how the client is getting along. This response acknowledges the client's request and also lets the client know that the nurse will be back shortly. It responds to reality. Telling the client that the nurse will not allow anything to hurt the client, that the nurse is not trying to cheat the client, and that the client may be trying to frighten the nurse all are responding to delusional material. (I, T, L)

26. 1. Sitting in silence with the client shows that the nurse accepts the client and cares about her. It also will help the client to get to know the nurse, initiate a feeling of comfort with the nurse, and lead to development of trust. The nurse would not persist in asking the client questions or attempt to engage her in conversation because these measures would only overwhelm the client at this time. Leaving the client alone does not promote comfort or trust with the nurse. Telling the client that the nurse will be back to talk later will only burden the client with the nurse's expectation to talk, which the client may not be likely to meet. Including the client in group discussion will increase her discomfort and anxiety and will not be therapeutic at this time. (I, T, L)

27. 2. The goal of nurse–client interaction for 5 minutes is a realistic one to work toward based on the severity of the client's illness. This implies that the client will have gained some measure of trust in the nurse. Expecting the client to take the initiative to approach the nurse to interact in 1 week is probably unrealistic. Participating in milieu activities and problem solving are unrealistic goals at this time. The client must first start talking with the nurse before she can tolerate groups or participate in group activities. The client would feel too anxious and overwhelmed if urged too soon to participate in groups. (P, T, L)

28. 3. Relating to the client that she combed her hair points out a visible accomplishment to the client and reinforces positive self-care behavior. Telling the client that she looks good today implies that the client did not look good yesterday. Expressing gladness that the client is feeling better today may be an erroneous interpretation. The client may feel just as depressed as before. If the nurse compliments the client's blouse and slacks, the client may infer that the nurse did not like the client's clothing before this time. (I, T, L)

29. 2. Whenever a client is suicidal, steps must be taken to prevent the client from harming herself. Other goals of care are less important than being sure the client does not carry out the threat of suicide. All threats of suicide should be taken seriously, and proper precautions should be taken to protect the client from self-harm. (P, T, L)

30. 1. The cause of endogenous depression is believed to be biochemical and not a reaction to a loss. It is caused by an imbalance or decreased availability of norepinephrine, serotonin, and possibly dopamine, so the client cannot identify a specific outside cause or a loss. Reactive depression is a reaction to a loss or a stressor. It is wrong to consider that lack of trust or slow thinking are reasons why the client will not identify the cause of his depression. Problems and stressors in the client's life are usually present, however, and he can discuss them with the staff when he is willing or able. (I, N, L)

31. 2. A depressed client is often ambivalent; that is, he both wants to and does not want to carry out an activity. This client should not be given choices that allow him to say no. His disinterest may not really indicate a wish to be left alone. Making an appointment to take a client to a unit activity is more helpful than allowing the client to say he does not wish to go or leaving it up to the client to decide on his own. (I, T, L)

32. 3. This response provides the most complete information about both the current and future treatment plans and answers the question asked by the client. (I, T, L)

33. 1. Because tricyclic antidepressants, such as imipramine (Tofranil), cause tachycardias and ECG changes, an ECG should be done before the client takes the medication. Other side effects include urinary retention, constipation, and drowsiness. Imipramine is administered cautiously to clients receiving thyroid medication. (A, C, L)

34. 2. When strongly opposed to a type of therapy, the nurse should refer people who ask about the therapy to another knowledgeable person for information. If the nurse gives the client and family an honest opinion, it may cause the client and family to lose confidence in prescribed therapy. It would be dishonest to tell the client and family that the nurse does not know enough about the treatment to be of help. Just providing a copy of the package insert is impersonal and likely to be of little help. (P, T, L)

35. 3. A medication teaching plan includes information relevant to the client's care. A description of current research about antidepressant therapy is not essential unless the client is participating in a research protocol. (P, T, L)

36. 1. Improved appetite and improved sleep patterns indicate that the medication is having a therapeutic effect. Oversleeping could indicate oversedation. (E, T, L)

37. 3. Dry mouth is a common side effect of tricyclic antidepressants. Drinking copious amounts of water does not eliminate this side effect and can be physiologically detrimental, possibly leading to electrolyte imbalance. (E, N, G)

38. 4. The client's lessening depression could indicate that the client has decided to commit suicide. Headache and loss of appetite are side effects of the medication and are not life-threatening. A full therapeutic effect could take up to 4 weeks, so a continuance of the depressive state would not be a cause for concern at this time. (E, N, L)

39. 1. Anxiety and diarrhea are side effects of Prozac and may be relieved by a decrease in dosage, or it may be necessary to change to another SSRI (selective serotonin reuptake inhibitor) or to a different class of antidepressants. The discomfort experienced by the client could lead to medication noncompliance and dehydration. The client's symptoms alone do not indicate a worsening of depression. Concluding that the client's symptoms are a means to seek attention is a grave error of judgment. Other behaviors or evidence would need to be present for the nurse to reach that conclusion. (E, N, G)

The Client With Bipolar Disorder, Manic Phase

40. 1. Assessing nutritional status is a priority in this situation. A client with bipolar disorder, manic phase commonly does not have time to eat or drink because of their state of constant activity and easy distractability. Altered nutritional status and constant physical activity can lead to malnutrition, weight loss, and physical exhaustion. These states can lead to death if appropriate intervention is not instituted. Financial status is neither important nor something that the nurse can modify. Clients with bipolar disorder, manic phase typically go on spending sprees, have disturbed sleep patterns, and exhibit hostility when their personal desires are limited. (A, N, L)

41. 3. When the client's husband apologizes for her behavior, it is best to focus on the husband's feelings and to be supportive of him. To say that the client is doing the best she can and that the nurse is used to being treated worse by clients ignores the husband's feelings. To ask what caused the client's behavior suggests criticism of the client and asks the husband for a judgment that he may not be able to make accurately. (I, T, L)

42. 3. If a client with overactive behavior acts aggressively, the nurse must first take measures to protect herself and others from harm. However, when the aggression subsides, efforts should be made to provide activity that is most likely to decrease tension and energy, such as using a punching bag. Reading a book, holding the client's hands, or placing her in isolation to work out aggression in private will not meet her needs to reduce energy and tension. However, when selecting an activity for a hyperactive client, care should be taken so that the activity does not overstimulate an already overactive client. (I, T, L)

43. 1. It is best to explain the x-ray procedure to the client in simple terms. Saying nothing or giving overly detailed explanations is inappropriate; the client needs some explanation, but details are unnecessary. There is no indication that additional help is needed for this client. (I, T, L)

44. 1. Because the client is very active, it would be best to give her food she can carry with her and eat as she moves. Allowing the client in the unit kitchen is impractical, and she most likely would be too busy to eat anyway. Allowing the client to send out for her favorite foods and serving food in small, attractively arranged portions do not meet the problem of ensuring that the active client has proper nourishment. (I, T, L)

45. 1. Explanations are unlikely to be of value for this client. It is best to assist the client into proper attire in a matter-of-fact way. At this point, the nurse needs to assist the client in setting limits on her behavior. (I, T, L)

46. 2. The client is demonstrating flight of ideas. Concreteness involves interpreting another person's words literally. Depersonalization refers to feelings of strangeness concerning the environment or the self. A neologism is a word coined by a client. (A, C, L)

47. 3. The anxiety the client feels gives rise to the distorted thinking displayed in such speech patterns as flight of ideas. Loose ego boundaries, underlying hostilities, and distortions in self-concept have little, if any, relation to the thought disorder described here. (D, T, L)

48. 4. The nurse takes responsibility for not being able to understand the client by asking the client to speak more slowly so that the nurse can follow the client's train of thought. This is least likely to arouse anxiety in the client. Although helping the client make adequate connections between events is desirable, the manner in which it is done (when the nurse asks how the sun shining relates to her son) offers a threat by requiring that the client analyze thoughts and describe why they occur. Changing the subject by suggesting that the client talk about what she did yesterday is not helpful and does not focus on the client's needs. Reprimanding the client by indicating that she is talking nonsensically also is not helpful for the client in this situation. (I, T, L)

49. 2. Setting limits on behavior and explaining consequences if the limits are violated informs the client about which behaviors are unacceptable and sets limits on manipulative behavior. The client becomes aware of what is expected and what will happen if he is not responsible for his own behavior. Taking the client to his room and telling him that he can come out when permitted does not teach him what behavior is acceptable, give him the opportunity to accept responsibility for himself, or clearly define the consequences of the inability to control himself. Asking a staff member to take the client to watch television is not appropriate because, in addition to the above, the client most likely cannot sit for an hour, and the television may be too stimulating. The nurse should never bargain, argue, or reason with this type of client. Rather, the nurse states what the limits are, what is expected, and what will occur if limits are not observed. (P, N, L)

50. 2. Channeling activities through constructive tasks, such as cleaning, allows the client to express aggressive behavior. During periods of client hyperactivity, it is generally advisable not to involve the client in activities with other clients because the technique tends to be nontherapeutic. Allowing the hyperactive client to exercise and move about as much as possible is likely to lead to exhaustion. (P, N, L)

51. 4. During a manic phase, the client is unlikely to show evidence of feelings of guilt, anger, or mistrust. Hostility is a more characteristic feeling. (D, C, L)

52. 2. Here, the nurse has a responsibility to deny the client's request because it is inappropriate and financially irresponsible. Limit-setting is also an important part of working with clients, especially those in a hyperactive phase of their illness. (I, T, L)

53. 2. The client should be observed for physical exhaustion, which predisposes to infections when a hyperactive client experiences euphoria and becomes overactive. (D, N, G)

54. 1. Sodium is necessary for renal excretion of lithium carbonate (Lithane). A low sodium intake results in retention of lithium and eventual lithium toxicity. (I, T, G)

55. 4. Clinical manifestations of lithium toxicity include anorexia, nausea and vomiting, diarrhea, coarse hand tremors, twitching, lethargy, decreased urine output, decreased blood pressure, and impaired consciousness. (D, T, G)

56. 2. The therapeutic blood level range for lithium is between 0.6 and 1.4 mEq/L for adults. A level of 1.0 mEq/L can be anticipated after 10 days of treatment. (D, T, G)

57. 4. When a client has delusions of grandeur, it is not helpful to change the topic of discussion, involve him in a group project, or try to convince him that his thoughts are erroneous. It is far better to try to satisfy his implied need to feel important because this recognizes the cause of the behavior and helps make him feel important. (I, N, L)

58. 1. Staff members sometimes are the recipients of a client's angry behavior because they are safe targets and are available for attack. The display of anger is rarely intended to be personal. Nor is such behavior necessarily a sign of serious pathology, an attack on a physician's skills, or a sign that the client's condition is improving. (E, N, L)

59. 3. Whenever possible, the client should first be given choices when action must be taken because of behavior. In this situation, this is best accomplished by telling the client that he has a choice of going to his room voluntarily or being escorted to his room. The client's room should be used first; if this does not help, then seclusion may be indicated. Because the client's anger is increasing, the situation is beyond discussion. (I, T, L)

60. 3. The client's statements reflecting cure and not needing medication are unrealistic and inaccurate. The presence of anger does not indicate illness. The feeling of anger is normal. Enjoyment of the state that mania produces implies that the client may not take his medication. It also implies that he does not understand the personal, family, medical, and social problems that the manic phase entails. (E, N, L)

61. 1. For the client going home, it is best to suggest that he be relieved of some home responsibilities, that better communication be developed, and that family members learn to recognize signs of toxicity while the client is on drug therapy. It is unrealistic and impractical to attempt to eliminate worry and anxiety from a client's environment. (I, N, L)

62. 2. A family history of mood disorders is commonly present. Histories of child molestation, high potassium levels in the brain, and drinking alcohol have not been found to be of etiologic significance for this illness. (D, T, L)

63. 3. Valproic acid can be taken with food or at mealtime to minimize gastrointestinal upset. The client's dosage of medication is appropriate, and the serum level is therapeutic between 50 and 100 μg/mL. The tablets should not be chewed because of the possibility of mouth and throat irritation. Valproic acid is given in two to four doses daily because of its short half-life (6–16 hours, peaking in less than 4 hours). (I, N, G)

64. 1. Bipolar disorder is biochemical in nature and can be treated effectively with lithium, tegretol, or valproic acid. The client cannot voluntarily control her symptoms of the illness, and the disorder does not affect one type of personality over another. The client is not to be blamed or held responsible for her illness. Telling the client to rely on pills temporarily is inaccurate and not helpful because the nurse cannot predict the length of time the client will need medication. (I, T, L)

65. 4. Because bipolar disorder is a biochemical disorder, the client needs to know that she may need medication for a length of time. Stopping the Depakene may cause a return of symptoms, and taking the Depakene on an as-needed basis may be harmful because of toxicity or may be inadequate to manage symptoms and to balance brain neurotransmitters. It is not safe to take when pregnant because of risk to the fetus. The client should inform the nurse and physician if she thinks she might be pregnant. (E, N, G)

The Client With Major Depression and Suicidal Ideation

66. 3. This client most likely needs attention paid to some unknown concern. Her behavior should be considered meaningful but not as yet fully understood. The client is also showing signs of agitated depression. Judging that the client is lonely and looking for a way to pass time, that she is self-centered and possessive of the nurse's time, or that she desires assistance to improve her room's appearance are conclusions or value judgments based on insufficient data in this situation. (D, N, L)

67. 1. Investigating the presence of suicidal thoughts and plans by overtly asking the client if she is thinking of or planning to commit suicide is a priority nursing action in this situation. Direct questioning about thoughts or plans related to self-harm does not give a person the idea to harm herself. Self-harm is an individual decision. To avoid the subject when a client appears suicidal is unwise; the safest procedure is to investigate. It would be premature in this situation to outline alternative measures to suicide or to describe other clients who have attempted suicide. (I, N, L)

68. 2. Sleep disturbances are markers of the biologic changes associated with depression and indicate increased severity. Feelings of fatigue, decreased interest in usual activities, and changes in appetite are common symptoms of depressed mood. (E, T, L)

69. 3. Cheerfulness and gaiety have a tendency to make a depressed person feel more guilty and unworthy. It is helpful to be firm and businesslike or serious with a depressed client and to behave naturally and spontaneously. (I, T, L)

70. 4. The nurse documents specific behavioral, emotional, and somatic clues, including objective and subjective data, as succinctly as possible to relate accurate and complete information about the client. This documentation is important not only when the client is admitted but also throughout the hospitalization. Charting information in vague terms leaves room for varied interpretations. (E, N, L)

71. 4. All four client problems and nursing diagnoses could apply to a client with depression and suicidal ideation. Social isolation is a typical problem of depressed clients; however, information is lacking regarding whether the client is withdrawn, and further assessment would be needed to consider it as a problem. (D, T, L)

72. 3. Client safety is the nursing priority. The nurse would remove potentially harmful objects from the environment to minimize the occurrence of self-harm. Instructing the client to seek out staff when he has thoughts of harming himself gives the staff an opportunity to intervene and provide relief in discussing his feelings. Having the client agree to a no-harm contract is important because the client is participating in being responsible for his own behavior. The nurse assigns the client to a double room so he is not alone. (I, T, L)

73. 4. Pointing out the client's progress by describing what he can now do is therapeutic. Telling the client that he can do anything he puts his mind to, encouraging him to think more positively about himself, and talking about weekend plans may prove more frustrating than helpful for a client who is already finding fault with himself. Also, suggesting that the client and nurse make plans for the client's weekend changes the subject that the client introduced in the conversation. (I, T, L)

74. 3. Evidence that suicidal ideation, although present, is decreasing; the client's statements about being in control of his behavior; and the client's plans to return to work indicate an improvement in depression. There is no evidence to support an increase or adjustment in the dose of Effexor or a call to the physician. Typically, the cognitive components of depression are the last symptoms eliminated. For the client to be experiencing some suicidal ideation in the second week of psychopharmacologic treatment is not unusual. (E, N, G)

75. 1. Nausea is a common side effect of Effexor; it should be taken at mealtime to minimize gastrointestinal discomfort. It is given in divided doses, and the amount should not be taken in one dose because of the drug's 3- to 7-hour half-life in adults. (I, N, G)

76. 4. Helping the client to express his feelings is an important client goal. Talking about feelings to an accepting, empathetic nurse fosters trust in the caregiver and allows client issues and concerns to surface. Telling the client that he'll do well, shouldn't worry about it, or that he may need extra breaks dismisses the client and minimizes his feelings and concerns. The client may interpret the nurse's statements as a message that the nurse does not want to hear or listen to him. (I, T, L)

77. 3. Arrangements for a volunteer visitor, a friend's visit, and Meals-on-Wheels all increase the client's activity but do not get her out of the house or increase her social resources as transportation to the senior group does. (P, T, H)

78. 1. Depressed clients are difficult to relate to because of their hopelessness and general apathy. The concomitant feelings of hopelessness and lack of success experienced by the nurse may lead her to withdraw or to feel angry with the client. Poor personal grooming is typical of clients with depression and suicidal ideation but can be managed by the nurse. Depressed clients are typically dependent on others. They are not motivated by laziness and are usually conscientious and dependable. (D, C, L)

79. 4. Depressed clients have sleep disturbances, and hence the property of sedation in a drug is valuable. Urinary retention is a serious problem in the elderly that should be reported promptly. Insomnia, elevated blood glucose level, and hypertension are not associated with amitriptyline hydrochloride (Elavil) therapy. (E, N, L)

80. 2. Anger is a low risk factor for suicide, certainly less significant than such factors as age, home envi-

ronment, and previous suicidal gestures. Anger turned outward is usually more positive than anger turned inward. (D, T, L)

81. 4. Recording feelings and problems daily would not be an adaptive action helpful to the client who feels suicidal. In fact, it probably would increase the client's focusing on negative thoughts and occurrences. Volunteering at a senior day care center will enhance the client's self-esteem, provide a measure of socialization outside of the home, and add structure to her day. Joining a woman's support group will provide the client with a support system. Expressing a willingness to call the suicide help line if necessary will provide the client with support and appropriate intervention. Concrete plans when thinking about suicide provide adaptive coping methods. (E, N, L)

82. 2. Agreeing to not kill oneself until after talking to a physician or unless one's spouse dies implies that self-harm is still possible. Not thinking about killing oneself does not eliminate the possible impulsive behavior or action of self-harm. Agreeing to not kill oneself purposely or accidentally for 24 hours implies agreement to be partly responsible for one's own behavior and safety. In this situation, the nurse would renew the contract each day, if necessary, after assessing the client. (E, T, L)

83. 2. Suicide attempts are more likely when the client has more energy to act on thoughts and impulses. A client may not have the energy to commit suicide during times of greatest depression. The client's energy level, rather than status, is related to the danger involved. (E, N, L)

The Client Who Attempts Suicide

84. 4. Stomach contents should be removed to prevent further absorption of the secobarbital. Lavage is preferred to induced vomiting in an unconscious client to prevent aspiration of stomach contents. Forcing fluids and giving a diuretic are inappropriate measures in this situation. (P, N, G)

85. 1. The primary nursing responsibility for a suicidal client is to provide a safe environment and to protect the patient from harming himself or herself. (P, T, G)

86. 2. When the client criticizes herself for not being able to commit suicide successfully, it is most therapeutic when the nurse makes a comment that encourages the client to elaborate and ventilate her feelings. To tell the client that her feelings will pass or that she has a great deal to live for discounts her feelings. A comment that includes the word *why* asks the client to defend her feelings and tends to be nontherapeutic. (I, T, L)

87. 2. An improved self-concept indicates that the client's therapy is effective. A poor self-concept is a common sign of depression and almost always occurs in the suicidal client. Appetite and activity level are not necessarily decreased in depression. Gender identity conflict is common in adolescence but is not a sign of depression. (E, T, L)

88. 2. Because self-responsibility is part of the focus of family therapy, direct communication between the people involved in the situation is encouraged. Learning to express oneself clearly and to give direct feedback is part of healthy communication. Here, terminating therapy because it upsets the client and suggesting to the therapist that the client be allowed to speak do not allow the client to deal directly with the person she is angry with and discourage the client from taking responsibility for her own feelings. It is satisfactory to allow a client to ventilate to a nurse, but in this situation, it would be best for the client to open communication with her therapist. (I, T, L)

89. 1. The nurse must always consider all suicide attempts as very serious. Even though the attempt may result in minimal injury, it is still a cry for help and an extremely dysfunctional method of coping. To think of a suicide attempt as a form of manipulation or means to gain attention is irresponsible and leads to unsafe nursing practice. It also minimizes the client's pain and disregards his intent. Even if a client is ambivalent about suicide, accidental suicide results in loss of life. Using a gun is a high-risk and lethal method of suicide. Other high-risk methods include jumping, hanging, carbon monoxide poisoning, and staging a car crash. (I, N, L)

90. 4. Suicide precautions are instituted for a client who has made a recent suicide attempt using a lethal method. The client is at high risk for suicide, and his life must be protected and safety maintained. Feelings of being in control of suicidal thoughts, expressing guilt and shame about the suicide attempt, and worrying about a child's reaction indicate a lower risk for suicide. Recent suicide attempt using a lethal method always indicates the need for suicide precautions. (E, N, L)

91. 4. The nurse would inspect the bag and its contents in the presence of the client and his wife to demonstrate respect to the client and family. It is an overt method that can be used to teach the client and his wife about what is allowed in the room and on the unit and why. Instructing another staff member to go through the contents of the bag is a covert method and invades the client's privacy unnecessarily. Because the nurse is responsible for the safety of all clients and staff on the unit, asking the wife about the contents of the bag is insufficient to en-sure safety. Locking all of the client's belongings diminishes his sense of identity and is not desirable. (I, T, S)

92. 2. The belt would be kept in a locked area because it can be used for harm directed at self or others. The nurse would not allow the client who has recently attempted suicide or who is actively suicidal to have or keep in his presence any article that knowingly could be harmful. (I, T, S)

The Client in Crisis

93. 3. For the client who believes she is pregnant and comes to a crisis center for help, it would be best for the nurse first to summarize the client's comments and ask the client to confirm her perceptions. The first step in the nursing process is assessment, which includes obtaining accurate information about the client. Other interventions can then follow. (I, T, L)

94. 2. When the client describes what she has been doing in sexual encounters with her boyfriend, the nurse's best and initial response is to gather data that will help her determine meanings of terms the clients uses. Other comments at this time are less effective because they assume an understanding of what the client has said. (I, T, L)

95. 4. Because people in the midst of emotional crises find it difficult to focus their thinking, the goal of the nursing intervention is to return the client to noncrisis functioning and to reduce anxiety. Pointing out the level of distress that the client is actually experiencing is the first step in attaining this goal. (I, T, L)

96. 3. When the client says she needs no more help because she is going to stop "fooling around," the nurse should make a comment that lets the client know the door is open for her to return. The nurse leaves the decision to the client, but does not threaten or push her own point of view. Nor does the nurse put the client down or ridicule her. (I, T, L)

97. 1. Telephoning the crisis shelter indicates that the boys are alarmed but are reluctant to talk with their parents. The nurse should focus on helping the boys talk with their parents. Because of their ages and the problem, the boys may fear that their parents will assume that they have been sniffing glue. (D, N, L)

98. 3. People who inhale noxious substances, such as glues, risk cardiac failure because of overexertion when under the influence of the substance. Respiratory failure is another cause of death from inhalant use. Liver and kidney damage may occur with prolonged use but are not the most common causes of death. (D, T, L)

99. 4. The client may be experiencing delusions secondary to cocaine intoxication, which diminish reality testing and make the client fearful. Because the client is a potential danger to himself and to others, he should be protected from his own behavior. (P, N, L)

100. 3. To help the client reestablish self-control and orientation, it would be best for the nurse to make a truthful statement about what is happening and to explain what to expect. Telling the client that he has no need for concern offers false assurance. It is not helpful to moralize by berating the client for what he did. A statement with technical terms that the client may not understand is futile. Television is generally contraindicated for a client suffering ill effects after using cocaine. (I, T, L)

101. 4. Major tranquilizers should not be given to shorten the drug reaction because of the danger (possibly fatal) of drug incompatibility. Street drugs are often combined with other substances. (D, N, L)

102. 3. When the client asks how the nurse would feel if her girlfriend had been raped, and the nurse believes that the question is most probably personal, the nurse should give a straightforward response while focusing on the client. It is better not to respond to the client's question with a probing question. A nurse who asks for the client's opinion on how the nurse should feel is asking the client to analyze the nurse's feelings rather than her own. The client's problem is ignored if the nurse changes the subject of the conversation. (I, T, L)

103. 1. A client who has been raped and who seeks out brightly lit places and the company of friends and plans to move to another part of the city is exhibiting self-defense to help avoid being raped again. (D, N, L)

104. 1. The crisis worker uses active focusing techniques to determine the crisis-precipitating event or the immediate problem. "Why are you calling today?" or "What is the immediate problem?" will assist the caller to focus on the specific need or event. Telling the client to make an appointment is irresponsible because the problem might be life-threatening. Telling the caller to go to the nearest emergency room is precipitous and may be unnecessary. Asking to speak to someone else in the home may be futile because the caller might be alone; this action also ignores the caller. (I, N, L)

105. 3. The concern that someone may call the crisis hot line everyday for a year indicates that further understanding about crisis and crisis intervention is needed. A crisis situation is time-limited and should be resolved in 4 to 6 weeks if handled effectively. If a person calls the line daily for a year, that person has not been properly dealt with or is probably in a highly disorganized state requiring an alternate intervention. The nurse would need to further review and clarify the material presented. (E, N, H)

106. 2. Conveying warmth, empathy, and support to the wife to encourage the release of feelings is a priority nursing action at this time. Leaving her alone to cry without offering help is inappropriate behavior by the nurse. Calling the doctor for something to sedate the wife and asking her if she would like to speak to the social worker are actions that may be necessary and appropriate later. (I, N, L)

107. 4. Potential for self-harm is the priority nursing diagnosis for a client who has attempted or verbalizes the intent to harm himself or herself. The client is depressed and feeling hopeless, powerless, and lonely. (D, N, L)

THE NURSING CARE OF CLIENTS WITH PSYCHIATRIC DISORDERS AND MENTAL HEALTH PROBLEMS

TEST 1: Mood Disorders and Crisis Situations

Directions: Use this answer grid to determine areas of strength or need for further study.

NURSING PROCESS	COGNITIVE LEVEL	CLIENT NEEDS
A = Assessment	K = Knowledge	S = Safe, effective care environment
D = Analysis, nursing diagnosis	C = Comprehension	G = Physiologic integrity
P = Planning	T = Application	L = Psychosocial integrity
I = Implementation	N = Analysis	H = Health promotion and maintenance
E = Evaluation		

Question #	Answer #	Nursing Process					Cognitive Level				Client Needs			
		A	D	P	I	E	K	C	T	N	S	G	L	H
1	2				I				T				L	
2	4				I				T				L	
3	1			P				C				G		
4	3					E				N			L	
5	4				I					N			L	
6	4			P						N			L	
7	2	A							T				L	
8	1				I					N	S			
9	3			P						N			L	
10	4	A							T				L	
11	2					E				N			L	
12	2		D						T				L	
13	4			P						N			L	
14	4		D				K						L	
15	2				I				T				L	
16	4			P						N			L	
17	1			P					T				L	
18	4					E		C					L	
19	2		D						T		S			
20	4		D						T		S			
21	3		D						T		S			
22	4				I				T				L	
23	2				I				T				L	
24	4				I				T				L	

ANSWER GRID: 1

NURSING PROCESS

A = Assessment
D = Analysis, nursing diagnosis
P = Planning
I = Implementation
E = Evaluation

COGNITIVE LEVEL

K = Knowledge
C = Comprehension
T = Application
N = Analysis

CLIENT NEEDS

S = Safe, effective care environment
G = Physiologic integrity
L = Psychosocial integrity
H = Health promotion and maintenance

Question #	Answer #	Nursing Process					Cognitive Level				Client Needs			
		A	D	P	I	E	K	C	T	N	S	G	L	H
25	4				I				T				L	
26	1				I				T				L	
27	2			P					T				L	
28	3				I				T				L	
29	2			P					T				L	
30	1				I					N			L	
31	2				I				T				L	
32	3				I				T				L	
33	1	A						C					L	
34	2			P					T				L	
35	3			P					T				L	
36	1					E			T				L	
37	3					E				N		G		
38	4					E				N			L	
39	1					E				N		G		
40	1	A								N			L	
41	3				I				T				L	
42	3				I				T				L	
43	1				I				T				L	
44	1				I				T				L	
45	1				I				T				L	
46	2	A						C					L	
47	3		D						T				L	
48	4				I				T				L	
49	2			P						N			L	
50	2			P						N			L	
51	4		D					C					L	
52	2				I				T				L	
53	2		D							N		G		
54	1				I				T			G		

NURSING PROCESS

A = Assessment
D = Analysis, nursing diagnosis
P = Planning
I = Implementation
E = Evaluation

COGNITIVE LEVEL

K = Knowledge
C = Comprehension
T = Application
N = Analysis

CLIENT NEEDS

S = Safe, effective care environment
G = Physiologic integrity
L = Psychosocial integrity
H = Health promotion and maintenance

Question #	Answer #	A	D	P	I	E	K	C	T	N	S	G	L	H
55	4		D						T			G		
56	2		D						T			G		
57	4				I					N			L	
58	1					E				N			L	
59	3				I				T				L	
60	3					E				N			L	
61	1				I					N			L	
62	2		D						T				L	
63	3				I					N		G		
64	1				I				T				L	
65	4					E				N		G		
66	3		D							N			L	
67	1				I					N			L	
68	2					E			T				L	
69	3				I				T				L	
70	4					E				N			L	
71	4		D						T				L	
72	3				I				T				L	
73	4				I				T				L	
74	3					E				N		G		
75	1				I					N		G		
76	4				I				T				L	
77	3			P					T					H
78	1		D					C					L	
79	4					E				N			L	
80	2		D						T				L	
81	4					E				N			L	
82	2					E			T				L	
83	2					E				N				L
84	4			P						N		G		

ANSWER GRID: 3

NURSING PROCESS

A = Assessment
D = Analysis, nursing diagnosis
P = Planning
I = Implementation
E = Evaluation

COGNITIVE LEVEL

K = Knowledge
C = Comprehension
T = Application
N = Analysis

CLIENT NEEDS

S = Safe, effective care environment
G = Physiologic integrity
L = Psychosocial integrity
H = Health promotion and maintenance

Question #	Answer #	Nursing Process					Cognitive Level				Client Needs			
		A	D	P	I	E	K	C	T	N	S	G	L	H
85	1			P					T			G		
86	2				I				T				L	
87	2					E			T				L	
88	2				I				T				L	
89	1				I					N			L	
90	4					E				N			L	
91	4				I				T		S			
92	2				I				T		S			
93	3				I				T				L	
94	2				I				T				L	
95	4				I				T				L	
96	3				I				T				L	
97	1		D							N			L	
98	3		D						T				L	
99	4			P						N			L	
100	3				I				T				L	
101	4		D							N			L	
102	3				I				T				L	
103	1		D							N			L	
104	1				I					N			L	
105	3					E				N				H
106	2				I					N			L	
107	4		D							N			L	
Number Correct														
Number Possible	107	5	20	16	46	20	1	6	59	41	6	13	86	2
Percentage Correct														

Score Calculation: To determine your **Percentage Correct,** divide the **Number Correct** by the **Number Possible.**

ANSWER GRID: 4

Schizophrenia and Other Psychoses, Cognitive Disorders, and Using a Therapeutic Milieu

- **The Client With Paranoid Schizophrenia**
- **The Client With Other Types of Schizophrenia and Psychotic Disorders**
- **The Client With Chronic Mental Illness**
- **The Client With a Cognitive Disorder**
- **Using a Therapeutic Milieu**
- **Correct Answers and Rationale**

Select the one best answer, and indicate your choice by filling in the circle in front of the option.

The Client With Paranoid Schizophrenia

A client scans the adult inpatient unit on his arrival at the hospital. He is neatly dressed and clutches a leather briefcase tightly in his arms.

1. The client refuses to let the nurse touch his briefcase or check it for valuables or contraband. Which of the following actions by the nurse would be best?
   - ○ 1. Obtaining help to take the briefcase away from the client.
   - ○ 2. Asking the client to open the briefcase while he describes its contents.
   - ○ 3. Inspecting the briefcase when the client is temporarily out of the room.
   - ○ 4. Telling the client that he must follow hospital policy if he wishes to stay.
2. As the nurse stands near the window in the client's room, the client shouts, "Come away from the window! They'll see you!" Which of the following responses by the nurse would be best?
   - ○ 1. "Who are 'they?'"
   - ○ 2. "No one will see me."

   - ○ 3. "You have no reason to be afraid."
   - ○ 4. "What will happen if they do see me?"
3. The nurse should recognize that moving away from the window quickly as the client requested is contraindicated because it would
   - ○ 1. reveal a lack of poise in the nurse.
   - ○ 2. make the client feel the nurse is only humoring him.
   - ○ 3. indicate nonverbal agreement with the client's false ideas.
   - ○ 4. let the client think he will have his way when he wishes.
4. The client thinks he is being followed by foreign agents who are after secret papers in his briefcase. What thought disorder does this indicate?
   - ○ 1. Idea of reference.
   - ○ 2. Idea of influence.
   - ○ 3. Delusion of grandeur.
   - ○ 4. Delusion of persecution.
5. The client's thoughts of being followed by foreign agents who are after secret papers indicates which nursing diagnosis?
   - ○ 1. Sensory-Perceptual Alteration: Visual related to increased anxiety, as evidenced by inappropriate responses.

31

- ○ 2. Alteration in Thought Processes related to increased anxiety, as evidenced by delusional thinking.
- ○ 3. Impaired Verbal Communication related to disordered thinking, as evidenced by loose associations.
- ○ 4. Social Isolation related to mistrust, as evidenced by withdrawal.

The client was admitted to the psychiatric unit yesterday evening.

6. In the morning, the client approaches the nurse and states, "The doctor and all of you nurses are conspiring against me. I've been warned and I know it's true. You know what I mean." Which of the following responses by the nurse would be most therapeutic?
- ○ 1. "That simply isn't true. Just stay calm."
- ○ 2. "I'll see if I can find your doctor for you."
- ○ 3. "I don't know what you mean, but you're secure here."
- ○ 4. "You must feel very frightened. You're safe here."

7. The client is suspicious of the staff members and other clients. To help establish a therapeutic relationship with the client, which of the following plans would be best?
- ○ 1. Initiate conversations with the client whenever he becomes agitated.
- ○ 2. Set aside specific times each day for conversations with the client.
- ○ 3. Allow the client to initiate conversations when he feels ready for them.
- ○ 4. Plan conversations with the client at frequent but unspecified times during the day.

8. During a conversation with the nurse, the client suddenly jumps up, begins pacing, and wrings his hands. The nurse should first
- ○ 1. take the client for a walk to help reduce his restlessness.
- ○ 2. change the subject of conversation.
- ○ 3. share the nurse's observations with the client and comment that he appears anxious.
- ○ 4. suggest that the nurse leave, and point out to him that he does not appear to want to talk now.

9. The nurse observes the client to be looking around the room with eyes darting to a chair in the corner. The client grimaces and then states, "bastard," under his breath. Which of the following nursing actions is most appropriate?
- ○ 1. Ignore the client since he appears to be hallucinating.

- ○ 2. Approach the client to interrupt the hallucinations.
- ○ 3. Suggest the client spend some time in his room.
- ○ 4. Remind the client that vulgar language is not appropriate in the hospital.

10. Which of the following observations about the client would warrant the most prompt reporting and the use of safety precautions? The client
- ○ 1. cries when he talks about his divorce.
- ○ 2. starts a petition to end the curfew hour.
- ○ 3. declines to attend a daily group therapy session.
- ○ 4. names another client as his adversary

11. The client is to receive haloperidol (Haldol). To prevent the client from possibly "cheeking" the medication, the drug should be given
- ○ 1. in liquid form.
- ○ 2. in capsule form.
- ○ 3. in suppository form.
- ○ 4. as an intramuscular injection.

12. After 3 days of taking haloperidol, the client shows an inability to sit still, is restless and fidgety, and paces around the unit. Of the following extrapyramidal adverse reactions, the client is showing signs of
- ○ 1. dystonia.
- ○ 2. akathisia.
- ○ 3. parkinsonism.
- ○ 4. tardive dyskinesia.

13. Which of the following medications can the nurse anticipate administering to treat the client's extrapyramidal side effects?
- ○ 1. Chlordiazepoxide (Librium).
- ○ 2. Benztropine mesylate (Cogentin).
- ○ 3. Imipramine hydrochloride (Tofranil).
- ○ 4. Thioridazine hydrochloride (Mellaril).

The 20-year-old client with paranoid schizophrenia is in the fourth day of hospitalization.

14. The client's parents visit, and state to the nurse, "What did we do wrong? What caused this awful thing to happen?" Which of the following explanations by the nurse is most accurate and therapeutic?
- ○ 1. "We really don't know. There are many theories about schizophrenia. Your daughter's physician has worked with this illness for many years."
- ○ 2. "Let's talk about your family background. Often, schizophrenia is genetic."
- ○ 3. "You didn't cause schizophrenia by doing something wrong. Schizophrenia is a biologic brain disease and can be caused by biochemical and structural changes in the brain."
- ○ 4. "Try not to worry. Paranoid schizophrenia has a good prognosis, and your daughter is receiving excellent treatment here."

15. The client's parents attend a family psychoeducation group in the hospital. Which of the following statements by the mother indicates that she is understanding her daughter's illness and management?
- ○ 1. "I know that I'll have to do everything for my daughter when she comes home."
- ○ 2. "Tasks as simple as getting out of bed and showering in the morning may be difficult for her."
- ○ 3. "I know that visits from her friends at home should be discouraged for a while."
- ○ 4. "Relapse will not occur if she takes her medicine."

16. The nurse conducts a home visit 1 week after the client's discharge from the hospital. The client's mother tearfully states, "I can hardly sleep because I'm so worried about my daughter. I'm afraid to leave her alone in the house. What if something should happen while I'm gone?" The nurse incorporates which of the following problems into the care plan?
- ○ 1. Caregiver role strain.
- ○ 2. Anxiety.
- ○ 3. Fear.
- ○ 4. Sleep pattern disturbance.

The nurse is conducting a mental status exam with a newly admitted client who has a diagnosis of Axis I Paranoid Schizophrenia.

17. During the interview, the client states, "I'm being followed; it's not safe. They're putting poison in my food." The nurse charts the client's statements in which area of the mental status exam?
- ○ 1. Thought content.
- ○ 2. Quality of speech.
- ○ 3. Insight.
- ○ 4. Judgment.

18. The client spends much of the morning in his room but seeks out the nurse for brief interactions throughout the morning. Which of the following expected outcomes would the nurse assist the client with achieving in the afternoon? The client will
- ○ 1. participate in the community meeting.
- ○ 2. volunteer to organize an evening of games with his peers.
- ○ 3. help put a puzzle together with the nurse.
- ○ 4. engage three of his peers in a card game.

19. The client's wife visits in the evening and states to the nurse, "Why isn't he eating? He's still talking about his food being poisoned." Which of the following appraisals by the nurse would be most accurate?

- ○ 1. The wife's inquiry is reasonable.
- ○ 2. Education about her husband's illness is needed.
- ○ 3. Her expectations of her husband are realistic.
- ○ 4. An increase in the client's medication is indicated.

The Client With Other Types of Schizophrenia and Psychotic Disorders

A client brought to the hospital by her husband is wearing a wrinkled dress with stains on the front. Her hair is disheveled, and she has an unpleasant body odor. She looks confused, exhibits a flat affect, and moves slowly and hesitantly.

20. The initial goal of the nurse who admits the client should be focused on
- ○ 1. making the client feel safe and accepted.
- ○ 2. helping the client get acquainted with others.
- ○ 3. giving the client information about the program.
- ○ 4. providing the client with clean and comfortable clothes.

21. When asked about herself during the admission interview, the client stares blankly at the nurse and mutters unintelligibly. The nurse would best chart this behavior as
- ○ 1. "not able to answer questions at this time."
- ○ 2. "uncooperative during admission procedure."
- ○ 3. "responded to questions with a blank look and incomprehensible mumble."
- ○ 4. "stared when asked questions and was disoriented and incoherent."

22. The client begins to express herself verbally on occasion. Which of the following nursing actions should be credited with helping a mute client express herself verbally?
- ○ 1. Asking questions that draw the client out.
- ○ 2. Using hand signals to entice the client to communicate.
- ○ 3. Making open-ended statements followed with silence.
- ○ 4. Expressing perceptions about what the client is experiencing.

23. The client often does the opposite of what she is requested to do. For example, if asked to stand up, she sits down; if asked to dress, she undresses. In view of the client's negativism, which of the following actions would be best for the nurse to take to get the client to the dining room for meals?
- ○ 1. Ask her to eat in her room away from the other clients.
- ○ 2. Wait for her to get hungry enough to come to the dining room by herself.

   ○ 3. Tell her it is time for lunch and lead her firmly by the arm to the dining room.

   ○ 4. Promise her a reward if she eats in the dining room and get help to take her there if she refuses.

24. When upset, the client curls into a fetal position in bed. The nurse judges the client to be exhibiting
   ○ 1. fixation.
   ○ 2. regression.
   ○ 3. substitution.
   ○ 4. symbolization.

25. Which short-term goal would be most therapeutic for the client with a nursing diagnosis of Self Care Deficit related to apathy, as evidenced by unwillingness to shower and dress self? By the end of 1 week, the client will
   ○ 1. verbalize the need to shower and dress self .
   ○ 2. recognize the need to shower and dress self.
   ○ 3. explain reasons why she should shower and dress self.
   ○ 4. shower and dress self.

The client is brought to the hospital from a group home where she became agitated and threw a chair at another client. She has refused medication for 8 weeks and refuses to care for her hygiene. The client exhibits a flat affect and has become increasingly withdrawn and asocial.

26. The physician orders risperidone (Risperdal) 1 mg PO bid for the client on admission to the hospital. The nurse judges this dose to be
   ○ 1. too high for the client.
   ○ 2. too low for the client.
   ○ 3. typical when initiating therapy.
   ○ 4. inadequate to be of therapeutic benefit.

27. The nurse predicts that pharmacologic treatment with risperidone will improve the client's negative symptoms of schizophrenia as well as the positive symptoms. Which of the client's negative symptoms would be affected?
   ○ 1. Apathy, affect, social isolation.
   ○ 2. Agitation, delusions, hallucinations.
   ○ 3. Hostility, ideas of reference, tangential speech.
   ○ 4. Aggression, bizarre behavior, illusions.

28. The client suddenly behaves in an impulsive, hyperactive, unpredictable manner. Which of the following approaches would be best for the nurse to use first if the client becomes violent?
   ○ 1. Provide a physical outlet for the client's energies.
   ○ 2. Let the client know that her behavior is not acceptable.
   ○ 3. Get help to handle the situation safely.
   ○ 4. Use heavy sedation to keep the client calm.

A client comes to the outpatient mental health clinic 2 days after being discharged from the hospital. The client was given a 1-week supply of clozapine (Clozaril).

29. The nurse reviews information about clozapine with the client. Which client statement indicates an accurate understanding of the nurse's teaching about this medication?
   ○ 1. "I need to call my doctor in 2 weeks for a checkup."
   ○ 2. "I need to keep my appointment here at the hospital this week for a blood test."
   ○ 3. "I can drink alcohol, can't I?"
   ○ 4. "I can take over-the-counter sleeping medication if I have trouble sleeping, can't I?"

30. The client tells the nurse that he has too much saliva and frequently needs to spit. The nurse appraises the client's statement as
   ○ 1. a delusion, requiring further assessment.
   ○ 2. an unusual reaction to clozapine.
   ○ 3. a side effect of clozapine.
   ○ 4. an unresolved symptom of schizophrenia.

The client, with a diagnosis of Axis I Schizophrenia, Undifferentiated Type, is acutely psychotic and exhibits religious delusions, hallucinations, loose associations, and concrete thinking.

31. The nurse offers the client her medication. The client states, "I don't need that. God will help me." Which of the following statements by the nurse would be best at this time?
   ○ 1. "God helps those who help themselves."
   ○ 2. "God wants you to take your medicine."
   ○ 3. "God is important in your life, but the medicine will help you too."
   ○ 4. "This medicine will help clear your thinking and decrease the voices."

32. The nurse hands the client the medication cup and tells the client to take her medicine. The client takes the cup and holds it in her hand. The nurse would
   ○ 1. tell the client to put the medicine in her mouth and swallow it with some water.
   ○ 2. instruct the client to sit in the dayroom and wait for the nurse to assist her.
   ○ 3. ask another staff member to stay with the client.
   ○ 4. say nothing and wait for the client to take the medication.

The client is admitted to the unit with a diagnosis of Axis I Delusional Disorder, Persecutory Type.

33. The nurse appraises the client's thought content to include nonbizarre delusions. Which of the following statements by the client validate the nurse's judgment?
- ○ 1. "The geezbots from outerspace are following me."
- ○ 2. "My neighbor is trying to steal my land. He is going to move his fence to impinge on my property."
- ○ 3. "My wife is being unfaithful and I have proof. She's seeing other men."
- ○ 4. "No one knows but I'm the President's most secret top adviser."

34. The nurse includes the diagnosis Defensive Coping Secondary to Suspiciousness as evidenced by the paranoid statement, "everyone's talking about me," in the client's care plan. Which of the following statements would be an expected outcome specific to the nursing diagnosis? The client will
- ○ 1. demonstrate an absence of hostile behavior.
- ○ 2. express own needs using assertive communication.
- ○ 3. use adaptive coping strategies.
- ○ 4. accurately interpret the behaviors of staff and clients in the milieu.

35. Which of the following actions would increase the client's anxiety and suspiciousness?
- ○ 1. Informing the client of schedule changes.
- ○ 2. Whispering with others where the client can observe.
- ○ 3. Gently informing the client that the nurse does not share the client's interpretation of an event.
- ○ 4. Inviting the client to join in leisure activities.

The nurse is meeting at the mental health clinic with a client who has Schizoaffective Disorder, Depressive Type.

36. Which of the following client behaviors would the nurse expect the client to have exhibited during the course of his illness?
- ○ 1. Hallucinations and delusions only.
- ○ 2. Active or residual symptoms of schizophrenia and major depression.
- ○ 3. Anhedonia, sleep disturbances, and mania.
- ○ 4. A brief psychosis.

37. The client tells the nurse that he doesn't go out much because he doesn't have anywhere to go and that he doesn't know anyone in the apartment where he's staying. Which of the following actions would the nurse recommend to the client at this time?
- ○ 1. Call his family to visit more often.

- ○ 2. Make an appointment for the client to see the nurse daily for 2 weeks.
- ○ 3. Consider rehospitalization for the client.
- ○ 4. Arrange to have the client attend day treatment at the clinic.

The Client With Chronic Mental Illness

38. The nurse working with the chronically mentally ill recognizes which of the following to be least helpful for this client population?
- ○ 1. Community-based treatment programs.
- ○ 2. Psychosocial rehabilitation.
- ○ 3. Employment opportunities.
- ○ 4. Better custodial care in long-term hospitals.

39. The nurse is offered a position as a psychiatric nurse in a psychosocial rehabilitation program. The nurse knows that the role would least likely include which of the following interventions?
- ○ 1. Teaching independent living skills.
- ○ 2. Assisting clients with living arrangements.
- ○ 3. Assisting clients in insight-oriented therapy.
- ○ 4. Linking clients with community resources.

A client in the program has worked as a hotel maid for the past 3 years. She tells the nurse she is thinking of quitting her job because "voices on television are talking about me."

40. What would be the nurse's initial action?
- ○ 1. Obtain information about the client's medication compliance.
- ○ 2. Remind the client that hearing voices is a symptom of her illness with which she can cope.
- ○ 3. Check with the client's employer about her work performance.
- ○ 4. Arrange for the client to be admitted to a psychiatric hospital for a short stay.

41. The client tells the nurse she stopped taking chlorpromazine hydrochloride (Thorazine) 2 weeks ago because she is better and wants "to make it on my own without this damned medicine." Which of the following would be the nurse's most therapeutic response?
- ○ 1. "You've told me about other times like this when you stopped taking your medication and got sick again. Please don't do it again this time."
- ○ 2. "You're a smart girl. You know what will happen if you don't take your medication. Why do you want to be so bad to yourself?"
- ○ 3. "I know you get tired of taking the medication,

especially when you're doing well. Is there any special reason you decided to stop right now?"

○ 4. "Maybe you're ready for a short holiday from the Thorazine. I'll talk it over with the physician. But you need to keep taking it until I talk with the doctor."

A nurse working at an outpatient mental health center primarily with the chronically mentally ill receives a telephone call from the mother of a client who lives at home. The client's mother reports that the client refuses to go to the sheltered workshop where she has worked for the last year, and that she has been taking her medication.

42. What should the nurse do first?
○ 1. Call the director of the sheltered workshop for information about the client.
○ 2. Reserve an inpatient bed in the hospital.
○ 3. Ask to speak to the client.
○ 4. Make an appointment to see the client.

43. The director of the sheltered workshop tells the nurse that the client had done well until last week when a new person started at the workshop. This new person worked faster than the client and took her place as leader of the group. Based on this information, which of the following would be the most appropriate nursing intervention?
○ 1. Make a home visit and tell the client that if she does not return to the workshop, she will lose her place there.
○ 2. Ask the director to assign the client to another work group when she returns to the workshop.
○ 3. Make an appointment to meet the client at the mental health center and ask her about the situation.
○ 4. Arrange placement for the client in a skill training program.

44. The nurse invites the client's parents to attend the psychoeducational program for families of the chronically mentally ill. The program would be least likely to help the family
○ 1. feel less guilty about the client's illness.
○ 2. develop a support network with other families.
○ 3. manage their finances.
○ 4. recognize the client's strengths more accurately.

A client who has not left the bus station for 3 days is brought to the mental health center by a police officer because she had been bothering other people. She denies this, will not give her name, and holds tightly to her purse.

She refuses to talk to anyone except to say, "You have no right to keep me here. I have money, and I can take care of myself." The police can hold her for disturbing the peace but think she needs psychiatric evaluation.

45. Which of the following factors would be most relevant to a decision about this client's disposition?
○ 1. She seems able to care for herself.
○ 2. She has no known family.
○ 3. She is not known to the mental health center.
○ 4. She has $500 in cash and says she will go to a hotel.

46. The decision is made to admit the client involuntarily on an emergency basis. The nurse on the inpatient unit explains the involuntary hospitalization process to the client, who listens quietly. Which of the following statements made by the nurse would be inaccurate?
○ 1. "You're in the hospital because the psychiatrist who saw you earlier thinks that you are unable to care for yourself right now."
○ 2. "You're free to talk to a lawyer if you'd like to do so."
○ 3. "You cannot leave the hospital until the doctor or a judge thinks you can take care of yourself."
○ 4. "You cannot have any visitors while you're here involuntarily."

47. The nurse informs the staff members that the physician is discharging the client because involuntary commitment is not indicated. Another nurse states, "How can her physician be so cruel? She should stay in the hospital instead of the bus station." Which of the following responses would be best for the nurse to make to her peer?
○ 1. "I agree with you. She does have symptoms of mental illness."
○ 2. "Even though the client may have a mental illness, she is not gravely disabled or dangerous to herself or others."
○ 3. "The client wants to leave, so the physician is not going to put her through the commitment process."
○ 4. "The client has a home to go to and family to support her. She doesn't need to be here."

48. As the nurse helps the client prepare for discharge, the client says, "You know, I've been in lots of hospitals and I know when I'm sick enough to be there. I'm not that sick now. You don't need to worry about me." Which of the following would be the most therapeutic response by the nurse?
○ 1. "We're concerned about you. How can we help you now?"
○ 2. "We could have helped you more if you had told us more."

○ 3. "You told us you were a visitor here. Is there any information you need before you leave the hospital?"

○ 4. "How do you know when you need to be in the hospital?"

49. The nurse has been asked to develop a medication education program for clients in the rehabilitation program. When developing the course outline, which of the following topics would be least helpful?

○ 1. A categorization of a wide variety of psychotropic drugs.

○ 2. Interventions for common side effects of psychotropic drugs.

○ 3. The role of medication in treating chronic illness.

○ 4. The effects of combining common street drugs with psychotropic medication.

50. The nurse at the mental health center has been asked to develop an in-service program for the staff about young adult, chronically mentally ill clients. Which of the following characteristics would the nurse most likely find common to this group of clients?

○ 1. They have minimal experience with lengthy periods of hospitalization.

○ 2. They accept the client role easily.

○ 3. They have a low incidence of substance abuse.

○ 4. They have lower expectations of achieving social goals of employment and relationships than do older chronically mentally ill clients.

The Client With a Cognitive Disorder

Mrs. Jones, a 72-year-old client, is brought by ambulance to the hospital's psychiatric unit from a nursing home where she has been a client for 3 months. Transfer data indicate that she has become increasingly confused, disoriented, and a management problem.

51. In which of the following ways should the hospital admission routine be modified for the client? The client should be

○ 1. left alone to promote recovery of her faculties and composure.

○ 2. medicated to ensure her calm cooperation during the admission procedure.

○ 3. allowed sufficient extra time in which to gain an understanding of what is happening to her.

○ 4. given a tour of the unit to acquaint her with the new environment in which she will live.

52. The client is to undergo a series of diagnostic tests to determine whether her dementia is treatable. Which of the following forms of dementia is nonreversible?

○ 1. Cerebral abscess.

○ 2. Multiple sclerosis.

○ 3. Syphilitic meningitis.

○ 4. Electrolyte imbalance.

53. The client's mental condition is found to be due to cerebral arteriosclerosis. Because no known cure exists for this disorder, which of the following attitudes should the nursing staff use to influence the client (and each other) to adopt?

○ 1. A hopeful attitude.

○ 2. A resigned attitude.

○ 3. A concerned attitude.

○ 4. A nonchalant attitude.

54. In addition to disturbances in her mental awareness and in her orientation to reality, the client is also likely to show loss of ability in

○ 1. speech.

○ 2. judgment.

○ 3. endurance.

○ 4. balance.

55. The client states to the nurse, "I know you. You're Margaret, the girl who lives down the street from me." Which of the following responses by the nurse would be most therapeutic?

○ 1. "Mrs. Jones, I'm Rachel, a nurse here at the hospital"

○ 2. "Now Mrs. Jones, you know who I am."

○ 3. "Mrs. Jones, I told you that my name is Rachel and that I didn't live down the street from you."

○ 4. "I think you forgot that I'm Rachel, Mrs. Jones."

56. The client exhibits memory loss, confusion, and wandering behavior. Of the following comments by the nurse, which would provide the best reality orientation for the client when she first awakens in the morning?

○ 1. "Do you remember who I am or what day it is today?"

○ 2. "Hello, did you sleep well? Which dress would you like to wear today, the yellow or the green one?"

○ 3. "Here I am again, your favorite nurse. Today is Tuesday, so there will be pancakes for breakfast this morning."

○ 4. "Good morning. This is your second day in Memorial Hospital and I'm your nurse for today. My name is Rachel."

57. Because of the client's age and cognitive impairment, which of the following courses of action should most certainly be included in the plan of care?

○ 1. Have two people accompany the client when she is up and about.

○ 2. Make sure all objects that the client could trip over are removed from her path.

○ 3. Put the client's favorite belongings in a safe place so that she will not lose them.

○ 4. Give the client her medications in liquid form to make certain that she swallows them.

58. The client roams about the hospital unit at night, disturbing the sleep of other clients. When asked why she walks about, she complains of being lost and unable to sleep. A large sign is posted on the door of her room to help her locate it. Which of the following programs would be best for dealing with the client's insomnia?

○ 1. A daily afternoon nap to prevent overtiredness at night.

○ 2. Administration of a hypnotic drug at bedtime.

○ 3. Enough active exercise daily so she will be comfortably tired at night.

○ 4. A cup of hot tea with lemon before bed to promote a feeling of well-being.

59. The client's daughter says that her mother wore the same dirty, worn-out undergarments for weeks at home. Of the following techniques, which would be best for the nurse to follow with the client during hospitalization to prevent further regression in her personal hygiene habits?

○ 1. Accept her need to go without bathing if she so desires.

○ 2. Make her assume responsibility for her own physical care.

○ 3. Encourage her to do as much self-care as she can.

○ 4. Do most of her physical care while letting her think she did it herself.

60. A nurse on the unit often avoids the client's company, preferring to associate with clients of her own age group or younger. Which of the following factors is most likely responsible for this nurse's extreme discomfort with older clients and her unconscious avoidance of them?

○ 1. Fears and conflicts about aging.

○ 2. Dislike of physical contact with older people.

○ 3. A desire to be surrounded by beauty and youth.

○ 4. Recent experiences with her mother's elderly friends.

61. One day when she is more alert than usual, the client asks the nurse to help her make out her will. Which of the following possible responses by the nurse would be best in this situation?

○ 1. "I'm not a lawyer, but I'll do what I can for you."

○ 2. "You have a long way to go before you'll need to do that. Let's wait on it a while, shall we?"

○ 3. "I don't believe in getting involved in legal matters, but maybe I can find another nurse who'll help you."

○ 4. "You need to consult an attorney because I'm not trained in such matters. Is there a family lawyer I can call for you?"

62. The client is allowed to reminisce about her past life. What effect can reminiscing by an elderly client be expected to have on her functioning in the hospital?

○ 1. Increase the client's confusion and disorientation.

○ 2. Subject the client to the others' impatient responses.

○ 3. Decrease the client's feelings of isolation and loneliness.

○ 4. Keep the client from participating in therapeutic activities.

The nurse is conducting a home visit to a client with Alzheimer's disease. The client lives with her family in their home.

63. The client's daughter tells the nurse that her mother thinks someone is stealing her things. Which of the following responses by the nurse would be most helpful?

○ 1. "That behavior is typical of people with Alzheimer's and will only get worse."

○ 2. "Your mother has problems with remembering where she puts things, and this may be causing her to think someone is stealing them."

○ 3. "Perhaps your mother is imagining things."

○ 4. "Your mother is having delusions, which are firm, false beliefs."

64. The nurse assesses the client's hair to be dirty and her clothing soiled with an odor of urine. The nurse's best action would be to

○ 1. ask the client when was the last time she bathed and changed her clothes.

○ 2. instruct the client to bathe and put on clean clothing.

○ 3. ask the daughter to bathe her mother.

○ 4. help the client with her bath, allowing her to do as much for herself as she is able.

65. The client is taking tacrine (Cognex), 10 mg qid for 6 weeks. The nurse instructs the daughter

○ 1. to take her mother to the clinic next week for bloodwork.

○ 2. to give her mother an extra dosage if needed at night.

○ 3. to observe her mother for signs of constipation.

○ 4. that the side effects of Cognex are minimal.

The client in the early stage of Alzheimer's disease and his adult son attend an appointment at the community mental health center.

66. While conversing with the nurse, the son states, "I'm tired of hearing about how things were 30 years ago.

Why does Dad always talk about the past?" The nurse judges the son's statement to indicate
- ○ 1. a lack of knowledge regarding the disease process.
- ○ 2. unusual behavior in the father.
- ○ 3. his father's level of anxiety.
- ○ 4. his father's antagonism toward him.

67. The nurse discusses the possibility of the client attending day treatment for clients with Alzheimer's disease. The best rationale the nurse would give for day treatment is that
- ○ 1. the client would have more structure to his day.
- ○ 2. the staff are excellent in the treatment they offer clients.
- ○ 3. the client would benefit from increased social interaction.
- ○ 4. the family would have more time to engage in their daily activities.

A client exhibits confusion and severe memory loss. At 11:30 AM, he tells the nurse that he is going to work and proceeds to walk toward the door.

68. The nurse should take which of the following actions?
- ○ 1. Remind him that he retired from his job 10 years ago.
- ○ 2. Tell him that she'll accompany him for a short walk outdoors.
- ○ 3. Divert his attention toward the dining room where lunch is being served.
- ○ 4. Tell him that he does not have to go to work today.

69. With a client experiencing delirium, the nurse prioritizes interventions to first maintain
- ○ 1. orientation.
- ○ 2. life.
- ○ 3. optimal level of functioning.
- ○ 4. consistency in routine.

Using a Therapeutic Milieu

The nurse is employed in a psychiatric hospital, working toward providing a therapeutic milieu for clients.

70. The primary purpose of managing the milieu on a psychiatric unit is to ensure that the environment will
- ○ 1. help clients meet treatment goals.
- ○ 2. meet the comfort needs of clients and staff.
- ○ 3. allow the staff to observe and evaluate clients.
- ○ 4. facilitate implementation of physicians' orders.

71. For a closed or locked unit, the nurse judges the milieu as therapeutic because priorities are given to
- ○ 1. socialization and self-understanding.
- ○ 2. education and vocation counseling.
- ○ 3. safety, structure, and support.
- ○ 4. developing communication, social, and leisure skills.

72. A client asks the nurse for a medication because he is feeling nervous. In terms of a therapeutic milieu, what would be the nurse's best response to the client's request?
- ○ 1. "Let's sit down and talk about your feelings of nervousness."
- ○ 2. "Why don't you play Ping-Pong with another client?"
- ○ 3. "Try lying down awhile and thinking about something else."
- ○ 4. "I'll call your doctor and get an order for some medication."

73. It is least important that the nurse take steps to set limits for which of the following clients?
- ○ 1. The client who uses the telephone most of the day.
- ○ 2. The client whose behavior is disturbing other clients.
- ○ 3. The client whose attire is offensive to the nursing staff.
- ○ 4. The client whose behavior indicates that she may harm herself.

74. Several adolescents are playing the stereo loudly in a common recreation area, and the adult clients are complaining about the loud music. As a first step in setting limits in this situation, the nurse should set limits
- ○ 1. on permissible volume while the stereo is being used.
- ○ 2. by prohibiting the use of the stereo in the recreation area.
- ○ 3. by turning down the volume while the stereo is on.
- ○ 4. by explaining to the adults that the adolescents need recreational activity.

75. A client diagnosed with a cognitive disorder is showing signs of confusion and a short attention span. Which of the following activities would be best suited for this client? Having the client
- ○ 1. join others going on a field trip.
- ○ 2. become a member in group therapy.
- ○ 3. meet with an assertiveness training group.
- ○ 4. participate in a reality-orientation group.

76. A hyperkinetic 5-year-old child exhibits signs of extreme restlessness, short attention span, and impulsiveness. Which of the following ways that the nurse

could alter the child's milieu would likely be most therapeutic for him?

○ 1. Increase the child's sensory stimulation and activity.

○ 2. Limit the child's opportunities to display anger and frustration.

○ 3. Define behaviors of the child that will be acceptable and those that will be unacceptable.

○ 4. Allow the child freedom to choose activities in which to participate and other children with whom to associate.

77. A 15-year-old male client shows signs of mild intoxication. When questioned, he states that another client gave him beer, and he refuses to name the client. The best course of action to initiate at this time would be to

○ 1. search the client's room for beer.

○ 2. call a community meeting to deal with the problem.

○ 3. try to persuade the client to tell who gave him the beer.

○ 4. call the physician to obtain additional orders.

The nurse treats clients who have dual diagnoses at a community mental health center.

78. Which of the following clients would be included in the nurse's caseload? The client with

○ 1. Axis I Schizophrenia and Alcohol Abuse

○ 2. Axis I Major Depression and Axis II Borderline Personality Disorder

○ 3. Axis I Cocaine Abuse and Axis III Hypertension

○ 4. Axis I Bipolar Disorder and Axis II Dependent Personality Disorder

79. The nurse will conduct a group therapy session on relapse prevention for clients with chronic schizophrenia and alcohol abuse or dependency. In this group, the nurse would use

○ 1. strong confrontation techniques.

○ 2. concrete concepts and simplified material.

○ 3. an unstructured format.

○ 4. a nondirective leadership style.

80. One of the clients in the group session states, "I'm not going to take medicine everyday." The nurse's best response is

○ 1. "Your doctor wants you to take your medication everyday."

○ 2. "Would anyone in group like to discuss this?"

○ 3. "Let's discuss this tomorrow if we have time."

○ 4. "I hear you say that you don't like taking medication daily."

CORRECT ANSWERS AND RATIONALE

The letters in parentheses following the rationale identify the step of the nursing process (A, D, P, I, E); cognitive level (K, C, T, N); and client needs (S, G, L, H). See the Answer Grid for the key.

The Client With Paranoid Schizophrenia

1. 2. When a client refuses to have his belongings checked for valuables or contraband according to hospital policy, the least threatening course of action is to ask him to open his briefcase while he describes its contents. Getting help to take the briefcase away from the client is a threatening maneuver. Inspecting the briefcase while the client is out of his room involves secrecy and is less desirable than an open discussion with the client. Telling the client that he must observe hospital policy to stay is threatening and probably inaccurate as well. (P, T, L)

2. 1. Asking the client who "they" are when he is fearful helps the nurse understand his behavior and is least demanding of the client. The client is unlikely to accept statements that indicate that no one will see the nurse and that there is no reason to be afraid. Asking the client what will happen if someone sees the nurse is also unlikely to be acceptable and validates the client's delusion. (I, T, L)

3. 3. The client's behavior is likely to be reinforced when the nurse takes steps to agree with the false ideas he holds. The nurse's action of moving away from the window as the client requests is less likely to be interpreted as a lack of poise, an effort to humor the client, or an admission of giving in to the client's wishes. (E, N, L)

4. 4. The client's thought process is best defined as a delusion of persecution. A delusion of grandeur involves an exaggerated idea of one's importance or identity. An idea of reference assumes that the remarks and behavior of others apply to oneself. An idea of influence refers to the belief that people or objects have control over one's behavior. (D, C, L)

5. 2. The nursing diagnosis, Alteration in Thought Processes related to increased anxiety, as evidenced by delusional thinking, most accurately reflects this client's problem given the data. Sensory-Perceptual Alteration, Impaired Verbal Communication, and Social Isolation are nursing diagnoses typically present in clients with thought disorders and paranoia. Additional data would be needed to support these diagnoses. (D, N, L)

6. 4. The nurse does not reason, argue, challenge, or try to disprove the delusion. The nurse verbalizes the feeling conveyed by the client or the impact the delusion has on the client. Assure the client he is safe and no harm will come to him. Telling the client that you will find his doctor or that you don't know what the client means ignores the client's needs and conveys nonacceptance of the client as an individual. (I, T, L)

7. 2. To promote a therapeutic relationship with a suspicious client, it is best to set aside periods for conversation at the same time each day. The nurse should be as consistent as possible. It is less satisfactory to use unspecified times or to allow the client to initiate meetings. It is difficult to have meaningful conversations that promote a therapeutic relationship when meetings occur only when the client is agitated, although the nurse may need to intervene at those times as well. (P, T, L)

8. 3. When the client becomes restless during a conversation with the nurse, the first course of action is typically to help him recognize and acknowledge his feelings by sharing observations with him. Other courses of action, such as changing the subject and leaving him, do not encourage him to express anxiety. Walking with the client may be therapeutic as the next action to decrease anxiety. (I, T, L)

9. 2. The nurse intervenes with the client experiencing hallucinations to assist with increasing the client's awareness that the hallucinations are not part of reality but a symptom of illness. The nurse does not ignore the client because the hallucinations can continue and escalate. Sending him to his room ignores the client's need and permits him to engage in his psychosis, increases confusion, and increases withdrawn behavior. Stating that vulgar language is not permissible ignores and dismisses the client. (I, T, L)

10. 4. The client exhibits aggression against his perceived adversary when he names another client as his adversary. The staff will need to watch him carefully for signs of impending violent behavior that may injure others. Crying about a divorce would be appropriate, not pathologic, behavior. A petition to end the curfew hour would be a positive, direct action aimed at a bothersome situation. Declining to attend group therapy needs follow-up but may be due to any number of unknown reasons. (E, N, L)

11. 1. It is generally best to try giving a medication in its liquid form if the patient fights taking it. If he refuses to swallow or expectorates the medication,

the intramuscular route then can be used if ordered by the physician, although that too will probably meet with resistance. (P, T, L)

12. 2. The client's behavior is best defined as akathisia. Dyskinesia is characterized by twitching or involuntary muscular movement. Dystonia is characterized by uncoordinated, spasmodic movements. (D, N, G)

13. 2. The drug of choice for a client experiencing extrapyramidal side effects to haloperidol (Haldol) is benztropine mesylate (Cogentin) because of its anticholinergic properties. Chlordiazepoxide (Librium) is a minor tranquilizer, or antianxiety agent. Imipramine hydrochloride (Tofranil) is an antidepressant. Thioridazine hydrochloride (Mellaril) is a major tranquilizer, or antipsychotic agent. (D, N, G)

14. 3. The nurse is sensitive to the parents' feeling of guilt and lack of knowledge about the etiologies of schizophrenia. The nurse reassures the parents they are not to blame for their daughter's illness and then begins to educate the parents by explaining the biologic theories of the disease in a simple, straightforward manner. (I, N, L)

15. 2. Self-care deficits occur because of alterations in thought resulting in introspection, confusion, and distraction from external reality. Clients need encouragement to do as much for themselves as they are capable of to increase self-esteem and independent functioning. Simple tasks that require concentration and effort may be difficult for the client, especially during the acute phase of illness. Visits from friends should be discussed with the client and the client encouraged to decrease social isolation. Relapse typically occurs with medication noncompliance. Vulnerability to stress, a low threshold for stress, the number of stressors, and the client's lack of adaptive coping behaviors contribute to relapse. (E, N, H)

16. 1. Anxiety, fear, and sleep disturbances contribute to caregiver role strain. The nurse recognizes the mother's feelings of being overwhelmed with issues concerning the management of the client at home. The nurse would help the mother elicit the support of other family members or friends, continue with psychoeducation, and help the family connect with the Alliance for the Mentally Ill for support, reassurance, and education. (D, N, L)

17. 1. The client is voicing paranoid delusions of being followed and of poison being placed in his food. Presence of delusions is described in the area of thought content in the mental status examination. (D, N, L)

18. 3. The nurse uses approaches to assist the client who is suspicious, fearful, and withdrawn to feel a measure of trust, comfort, and security with the nurse on a one-to-one basis. Progression to interact-

ing with peers on an individual basis, attending groups, interacting in groups, and engaging with peers in activities will follow. Attending and interacting in groups and leading or organizing activities usually are too overwhelming for the client and can result in increased anxiety, fear, and withdrawal. (P, N, L)

19. 2. The nurse evaluates the client's wife as needing education or knowledge about paranoid schizophrenia, the course of the illness, and medications. Expecting an absence of delusions by the end of the client's first day of hospitalization is unrealistic. An increase in the client's medication would also be unreasonable because not enough time has elapsed to evaluate the effectiveness of the medication. (E, N, L)

The Client With Other Types of Schizophrenia and Psychotic Disorders

20. 1. It is important to help make the client feel safe and accepted. Helping the client get acquainted with others and giving her information about the program are important but are of lower priority at admission. Providing the client with clean clothes is desirable but less important than conveying feelings of safety and trust. (P, T, L)

21. 3. The best charting describes exactly what the client did and said in a particular situation. Noting that the client was unable to answer questions, was uncooperative, and was disoriented and incoherent do not follow this basic principle of documenting and also are not objective descriptions. (E, N, L)

22. 3. The best approach for a client who has difficulty expressing herself verbally is to use a nondemanding, open-ended statement. When the client is ready to talk, the silences following the statement will give her the opportunity to do so. Asking the client questions, using hand signals, and assuming what the client is experiencing are ineffective for this client. (I, T, L)

23. 3. Punishment and reward are likely to be of little value when a client does the opposite of what she is asked to do. The client simply may not eat if allowed to decide when to go to the dining room. The best course of action is to firmly lead the client to the dining room. This type of positive and firm approach is also needed to help increase the client's socialization. (I, T, L)

24. 2. A client's behavior is best described as regression when it is typical of an earlier stage of development. Fixation means not progressing beyond a given level of development. Substitution means replacing unacceptable ideas with more acceptable ones. Symbolization occurs when one idea or object comes to stand for another. (D, T, L)

25. 4. Showering and dressing self by the end of 1 week is most therapeutic to the client. A client with schizophrenia often appears to be apathetic and lack initiative. These effects are typically related to the ambivalence associated with schizophrenia. The client may tell the nurse that she will shower and dress and be able to explain why she should shower and dress but be unable to do so because of the ambivalence that impedes her ability to initiate and complete self-care. (P, N, L)

26. 3. Initiating therapy with risperidone (Risperdal) typically begins with 0.5 to 1 mg bid. The dosage is increased slowly to minimize the risk of orthostatic hypotension. The dose is slowly increased until the client is taking 3 mg/day, and the client is maintained on this dose for at least 1 week before further adjustments in dosage are made. Recommended dose ranges from 4 to 6 mg/day. (E, N, G)

27. 1. The client's negative symptoms of apathy, flat affect, and social withdrawal should improve. Risperidone is effective in diminishing the positive and negative symptoms of schizophrenia. (E, N, G)

28. 3. The recommended first course of action is to prevent accidents and injuries when a client becomes violent. In this situation, it would be best to call for help to handle the situation safely. Other actions may be taken later, after safety is ensured. (I, T, S)

29. 2. Mandatory weekly white blood cell counts are used to detect developing agranulocytosis, which can be fatal and occurs in 1% to 2% of clients taking clozapine. This medication is also associated with risk of seizures; this risk is dose dependent, meaning that it increases in moderate to high doses (600–900 mg/day). Use of alcohol and over-the-counter medications is contraindicated. Clients should be taught to report lethargy, weakness, fever, sore throat, malaise, mucous membrane ulceration, or other possible signs of infection or influenza-like complaints. (E, N, L)

30. 3. Sialorrhea (excessive salivation) is associated with clozapine therapy. Clients sometimes use paper cups to spit in. (E, N, G)

31. 3. The nurse recognizes the client's cognitive and perceptual disturbances and level of anxiety and acknowledges the client's message in a respectful and neutral manner, while clearly and directly stating the need for medication. Stating, "God helps those who help themselves," challenges the patient. Stating, "God wants you to take your medicine," is deceitful. Stating, "Medicine will help clear your thinking and decrease the voices," will be helpful to the client later when the client is less acutely psychotic and anxious. (I, T, L)

32. 1. The nurse recognizes the client's action to be a result of concrete thinking and instructs the client clearly and directly to put the medication in her mouth and then to swallow it with some water. Clear, step-by-step directions assist the client to process what the nurse is saying. Telling the client to sit in the dayroom and wait for the nurse, asking another staff member to stay with the client, and saying nothing are not helpful and do nothing to assist the client with taking her medication. (I, T, L)

33. 2. Delusional Disorder is marked by nonbizarre delusions with the absence of other characteristic symptoms of the active phase of schizophrenia. Disruptions in social, marital, and occupational functioning in clients with Delusional Disorder are usually less severe than those occurring in clients with Schizophrenia. The statement, "My neighbor is trying to steal my land by moving his fence" is an example of Delusional Disorder, Persecutory Type. The example, "The geezbots (a neologism) from outerspace are following me" is a bizarre delusion and not believable. "My wife is being unfaithful and I have proof" is more specific to Delusional Disorder, Jealous Type. "No one knows but I'm the President's secret top adviser" is more specific to Delusional Disorder, Grandiose Type. (E, N, L)

34. 4. The specific behavior stated as, the client will accurately interpret the behaviors of staff and clients in the milieu, is the expected outcome the nurse would hope the client to achieve. An absence of hostile behavior, expressing own needs assertively, and using adaptive coping behaviors are desirable behaviors but are not specific to the nursing diagnosis of Defensive Coping Secondary to Suspiciousness, as evidenced by the paranoid statements "everyone's talking about me." (P, N, L)

35. 2. Whispering and laughing with another person where the client can see or observe the nurse but not hear the conversation, increases the client's anxiety and suspiciousness. Appropriate actions by the nurse include informing the client of schedule changes, gently informing the client that the nurse does not share the client's interpretation of an event, and inviting the client to participate in leisure activities. These actions decrease anxiety and suspiciousness and help the client to focus on actual or realistic events. (I, T, L)

36. 2. The nurse would expect the client to have exhibited symptoms of both schizophrenia and major depression. The full criteria for both disorders must be met. (D, C, L)

37. 4. Because the client is able to live in an apartment setting, further development of independent functioning and the skills to gain as much independence as he is capable of need to be fostered. The nurse arranges for the client to participate in day treatment, where social skill development, recreational activities, and psychoeducation in a structured environment would be beneficial to the client at this time. (P, N, L)

The Client With Chronic Mental Illness

38. 4. Among the needs of the chronically mentally ill are community-based treatment programs, psychosocial rehabilitation programs, and appropriate employment opportunities. During necessary periods of hospitalization, active treatment, rather than custodial care, is needed. (D, C, L)

39. 3. The nurse's role in a psychosocial rehabilitation program involves teaching the client to live independently by using interpersonal skills and community resources. Insight-oriented psychotherapy is not beneficial for this client population. (P, C, L)

40. 1. Symptom exacerbation is most often related to noncompliance with the prescribed medication regimen. Therefore, obtaining information about the client's compliance is the first priority. Helping the client recognize the symptoms and her ability to manage them and checking with her employer are appropriate, but not the first priority. Hospitalization is not indicated because the client is still working and can talk about the symptoms. (I, T, L)

41. 3. Recognizing the client's feeling and her progress while obtaining more information is the most therapeutic response. Reminding the client of her previous related experience is also appropriate but could be done more therapeutically. To suggest the possibility of a drug holiday when symptoms are recurring is clinically unsound. (I, T, L)

42. 3. The nurse would speak with the client to question her about perceptions or reasons interfering with going to the sheltered workshop. This conveys that the nurse is interested and willing to help the client. Calling the director of the workshop can only be done if the nurse receives the client's permission. If the nurse needs additional information about the client's progress, making an appointment would be a method to assess further problems. Reserving an empty bed is not appropriate until the nurse has assessed the client's needs. (I, T, L)

43. 3. Making an appointment with the client at the mental health center to explore her feelings and behavior acknowledges the client's importance and makes her a partner in resolving the problem. Threatening the client with loss of a position at the workshop, asking for a new assignment for her at the workshop, or changing her program are premature actions. (I, T, L)

44. 3. Psychoeducational groups for families aim to provide education about the biochemical etiology of psychiatric disease to reduce family guilt. These groups also provide information about symptoms and symptom management, medication, family networking, and ways of coping with a mentally ill family member. (D, C, L)

45. 1. This client's ability to care for herself is most relevant to a decision about her disposition. If she is gravely disabled or needs treatment to care for herself, involuntary hospitalization is indicated whether or not she is known to the mental health center. Having monetary resources does not necessarily mean that she will be able to use them to care for herself. (P, N, L)

46. 4. Clients have a right to see visitors regardless of admission status. Involuntary hospitalization requires a psychiatrist state-of-need. Release requires medical or legal approval. Any client admitted involuntarily has the right to legal counsel. (I, T, L)

47. 2. To be committed involuntarily, a client must not only be suffering from a mental illness but must be gravely disabled (unable to care for self or come to harm if discharged) or dangerous to self or others. Having a mental illness alone is not grounds for commitment. Having a supportive family or home and not wanting treatment are not reasons not to pursue involuntary commitment if indicated or necessary to ensure the well-being of the client or another person. (I, T, L)

48. 1. It is most therapeutic to let the client know of the staff's continued concern and to ask her what might be useful to her. Making the point that she did not use the hospital well is not therapeutic on discharge. Offering information and reviewing the client's knowledge of symptoms are both therapeutic responses. (I, T, L)

49. 1. The psychotropic drugs used to treat chronic mental illness are more appropriate for the teaching plan than are a variety of psychotropic drug categories. Teaching should be focused on the needs and interests of the target audience. Such topics as interventions for common side effects of psychotropic drugs, the role of medication in treating chronic mental illness, and the effects of using common street drugs with psychotropic medication should be included in the teaching program. (P, T, L)

50. 1. Chronically mentally ill young adults are between 18 and 35 years of age. Due to deinstitutionalization, they did not experience long periods of hospitalization in which to learn the chronic client role and accompanying decreased self-expectations so commonly seen in older chronically mentally ill clients. Substance abuse is common in this client population. (D, C, L)

The Client With a Cognitive Disorder

51. 3. When admitting an elderly client, especially one who is confused and disoriented, it is best to give the client extra time in which to gain an understanding of what is happening to her. This will help her to get her bearings and adjust to a new environment. In this situation, it would be less desirable to leave the client alone, medicate her, or try to orient her to the new environment. (I, T, L)

52. 2. Multiple sclerosis is a progressive chronic disease; its course cannot be reversed, although clients may experience periodic remissions. Cerebral abscess, syphilitic meningitis, and electrolyte imbalance are treatable, and cure is possible. (D, C, L)

53. 1. People of all ages need to sense future well-being. They must have hope for things to come and believe in growth and change to live life to its fullest. Health personnel need to foster this feeling of hopefulness and subscribe to it to help clients attain well-being, even when the prognosis appears poor. (P, T, L)

54. 2. Basic symptomatology demonstrates that clients with chronic cognitive disorders experience defects in memory, orientation, and intellectual functions, such as judgment and discrimination. Loss of other abilities is less typical. (D, N, L)

55. 1. Because of the client's short-term memory impairment, the nurse gently corrects the client by stating her name and who she is. This approach decreases anxiety, embarrassment, and shame and maintains the client's self-esteem. (I, T, L)

56. 4. To promote reality orientation, the nurse should be as specific as possible when addressing a confused and disoriented client. Such comments as indicating what day it is, where the client is, and the nurse's name can help. Asking the client questions about her environment is likely to be challenging and may decrease the client's self-esteem. Stereotyped comments give the client no basic information; nor is it helpful when the nurse provides mostly irrelevant information. (I, T, L)

57. 2. When caring for a client with cognitive impairment, it may be necessary to have two people accompany her when she ambulates, place her favorite things in safekeeping, and give medications in a liquid form to be sure she swallows them. However, it is most essential to remove objects in the client's path of ambulation to help prevent falls. (P, T, S)

58. 3. A client with insomnia is more likely to sleep well if she feels tired at bedtime, which is likely if she had enough daily exercise so that she is comfortably tired at night. Having the client take a daily afternoon nap is likely to interfere with night-time sleep. Offering the client tea at bedtime is unlikely to promote sleep, especially if the tea contains caffeine,

which may lead to further wakefulness. Sedatives should be used only as a last resort because they are likely to be habit forming. (P, T, L)

59. 3. The best procedure for helping the client to remain independent and observe good hygiene habits is to encourage her to do as much self-care as she is capable of doing. For this client, it would be inappropriate to accept her poor personal hygiene habits. It would be impractical and unrealistic to expect the client to start taking care of all her hygiene needs. To do all of the client's hygienic care would cause further dependence, and it would be dishonest to care for the client while letting her think she did it herself. (I, T, L)

60. 1. The most likely reason for a nurse's discomfort with elderly clients is that she has not examined her own fears and conflicts about aging. Until she does, it is unlikely that she will feel comfortable with elderly clients. (E, N, L)

61. 4. A will is an important legal document, and it is best to have one prepared with the help of an attorney. It would be unwise to help the client because a nurse is not a lawyer. Asking the client to delay preparing the will just avoids the problem. It is also not helpful to seek out another nurse to help the client prepare a will. (I, T, L)

62. 3. Reminiscing can help reduce depression in an elderly client and lessens feelings of isolation and loneliness. (D, C, L)

63. 2. The best response explains that cognitive deficits and memory loss lead the client to forget where she placed something and may lead to accusations of someone stealing her possessions. These are not delusions or her imagination but a reaction to not being able to remember. Stating that the behavior is typical of someone with Alzheimer's disease dismisses the daughter, is not helpful, and does not increase the daughter's knowledge about the disease. (I, T, L)

64. 4. The best action would be for the nurse to help the client bathe and dress, allowing the client to do as much for herself as she is able, to foster independence. Instructing the client to do her activities of daily living is not appropriate or helpful. Asking the daughter to bathe her mother fosters dependence on the daughter. Asking the client when she bathed last is futile because the client may not remember and because it may embarrass the client and decrease her self-esteem. (I, T, L)

65. 1. There are serious side effects of tacrine, and the most serious is liver toxicity. Elevations in serum aminotransferase levels occur simultaneously, and these levels must be closely monitored weekly for at least the first 18 weeks of treatment. Then monitoring may be decreased to every 3 months. Increased dosage necessitates monitoring for at least 6 weeks. (I, T, G)

66. 1. The son's statements regarding his father's recalling of past events is typical in the early stage of Alzheimer's disease, when recent memory is impaired. Reminiscing is a positive experience for the client that brings forth familiar feelings and allows the client to engage in social interaction. (E, N, L)

67. 3. The best rationale for day treatment for clients with Alzheimer's disease is the enhancement of social interactions. More daily structure, excellent staff, and allowing the caregivers more time for themselves are all positive but focus less on the client's needs. (I, T, L)

68. 3. The client who is a fantasy or reminiscent wanderer can be helped most by diverting his attention toward an activity to relieve boredom or tension. Reminding the client with severe memory loss that he retired from his job 10 years ago will not help him and may increase his frustration. Telling the client that the nurse will accompany him for a short walk outdoors reflects poor judgment by the nurse and may compromise the client's safety. Telling the client that he does not have to work today can further confuse the client and reinforce his fantasy and disorientation. (I, T, L)

69. 2. Nursing interventions that maintain life are a priority for the client with delirium. Facilitating orientation, optimal functioning, and consistency in daily routine are of less importance whether caring for a client with delirium or a client with dementia. Maintaining an optimal level of functioning is the primary goal for a client with dementia. (P, T, L)

Using a Therapeutic Milieu

70. 1. A therapeutic milieu is an environment that helps clients meet treatment goals. Meeting the comfort needs of clients and staff, allowing staff to observe and evaluate clients, and facilitating the implementation of physicians' orders are significant but are not the primary purposes of managing the milieu. (D, C, L)

71. 3. Clients on a closed or locked inpatient psychiatric unit are typically acutely ill. Providing safety, structure, and support are immediate priorities in the therapeutic milieu for clients with cognitive impairment and inability to handle stress. For clients who are less acutely ill, socialization, self-understanding, education, vocational counseling, and developing leisure, social, and communication skills are important. As clients improve, they become better organized in their thinking and more capable of tolerating stress. They would then be more apt to

benefit from additional groups and therapies. (E, N, L)

72. 1. The nurse should take the time to listen to the client to discover more about his feelings before making an assessment or intervening. Calling the physician is an intervention made without complete data. Giving advice by suggesting that the client rest or play a game with another client is not therapeutic in this situation. (I, T, L)

73. 3. The nurse should judge the client's behavior in relation to the milieu and clarify the behavior's effect on the milieu, not on personal values held by staff members. Overusing the telephone, behavior that disturbs other clients, and behavior that may harm the client are situations requiring a degree of limit setting. (E, N, L)

74. 1. The nurse should state the limits clearly to a client who is disturbing others. The limits should be objective and fair and should reflect the situation at hand. The client should be included in decision making when possible, but the nurse is ultimately responsible. (P, T, L)

75. 4. Because the client has confusion and a short attention span and lacks concentration, a reality-orientation group is recommended to help her maintain an optimal level of functioning. Entering group therapy, going on a field trip, and meeting with an assertiveness training group are likely to be too stressful or stimulating to the client and may increase her frustration and decrease her sense of accomplishment. (P, T, L)

76. 3. Children need to know what behaviors are acceptable and what behaviors are unacceptable. They feel more secure when boundaries are clear and when policies concerning their behavior are consistently enforced. Increasing sensory stimulation and activity, limiting opportunities to display anger and frustration, and allowing freedom to choose activities would tend to increase stress and frustration for the hyperkinetic child. (P, T, L)

77. 2. The milieu should be used to increase peer support and handle confrontation when necessary. For adolescents, peer pressure is generally more effective in changing behavior than the staff's influence. Searching the client's room and trying to persuade a client who was involved to tell on his friends are authoritarian actions and may increase mistrust of the staff. Calling a physician is not necessary at this time. (I, T, L)

78. 1. Clients with dual diagnoses refers to the presence of at least one psychiatric disorder in addition to a substance abuse or dependency problem. The psychiatric disorder can be a mental illness or a personality disorder. Clients with a mental illness on

Axis I and a personality disorder on Axis II are referred to as having *multiple diagnoses* but not dual diagnoses. (D, C, L)

79. 2. The nurse would use concrete concepts and simplified material when conducting a psychoeducational group for clients with chronic schizophrenia and alcohol abuse or dependency. Most of these clients experience difficulties in concentration and memory. Groups should be structured with simplified material and concrete concepts. Handouts and simple homework assignments may be helpful for the clients to review and apply concepts. Strong confrontation techniques, an unstructured format, and a nondirective leadership style are inappropriate and not helpful for these clients. (P, N, L)

80. 4. The nurse accepts the client's statement so that the client feels heard and understood. The nurse demonstrates openness toward hearing nonacceptable attitudes to foster further sharing among the clients. The statements, "would anyone anyone like to discuss this," "let's discuss this tomorrow if we have time," and "your doctor wants you to take medicine everyday" are neither helpful nor therapeutic. The client is ignored and dismissed, which can lead to increased anxiety, decreased self-esteem, and anger toward the nurse and other clients. (I, N, L)

THE NURSING CARE OF CLIENTS WITH PSYCHIATRIC DISORDERS AND MENTAL HEALTH PROBLEMS

TEST 2: Schizophrenia and Other Psychoses, Cognitive Disorders, and Using a Therapeutic Milieu

Directions: Use this answer grid to determine areas of strength or need for further study.

NURSING PROCESS

A = Assessment
D = Analysis, nursing diagnosis
P = Planning
I = Implementation
E = Evaluation

COGNITIVE LEVEL

K = Knowledge
C = Comprehension
T = Application
N = Analysis

CLIENT NEEDS

S = Safe, effective care environment
G = Physiologic integrity
L = Psychosocial integrity
H = Health promotion and maintenance

Question #	Answer #	Nursing Process					Cognitive Level				Client Needs			
		A	D	P	I	E	K	C	T	N	S	G	L	H
1	2			P					T				L	
2	1				I				T				L	
3	3					E				N			L	
4	4		D					C					L	
5	2		D							N			L	
6	4				I				T				L	
7	2			P					T				L	
8	3				I				T				L	
9	2				I				T				L	
10	4					E				N			L	
11	1			P					T				L	
12	2		D							N		G		
13	2		D							N		G		
14	3				I					N			L	
15	2					E				N				H
16	1		D							N			L	
17	1		D							N			L	
18	3			P						N			L	
19	2					E				N			L	
20	1			P					T				L	
21	3					E				N			L	
22	3				I				T				L	
23	3				I				T				L	
24	2		D						T				L	

ANSWER GRID: 1

NURSING PROCESS

A = Assessment
D = Analysis, nursing diagnosis
P = Planning
I = Implementation
E = Evaluation

COGNITIVE LEVEL

K = Knowledge
C = Comprehension
T = Application
N = Analysis

CLIENT NEEDS

S = Safe, effective care environment
G = Physiologic integrity
L = Psychosocial integrity
H = Health promotion and maintenance

Question #	Answer #	A	D	P	I	E	K	C	T	N	S	G	L	H
25	4			P						N			L	
26	3					E				N		G		
27	1					E				N		G		
28	3				I				T		S			
29	2					E				N			L	
30	3					E				N		G		
31	3				I				T				L	
32	1				I				T				L	
33	2					E				N			L	
34	4			P						N			L	
35	2				I				T				L	
36	2		D					C					L	
37	4			P						N			L	
38	4		D					C					L	
39	3			P				C					L	
40	1				I				T				L	
41	3				I				T				L	
42	3				I				T				L	
43	3				I				T				L	
44	3		D					C					L	
45	1			P						N			L	
46	4				I				T				L	
47	2				I				T				L	
48	1				I				T				L	
49	1			P					T				L	
50	1		D					C					L	
51	3				I				T				L	
52	2		D					C					L	
53	1			P					T				L	
54	2		D							N			L	

NURSING PROCESS

A = Assessment
D = Analysis, nursing diagnosis
P = Planning
I = Implementation
E = Evaluation

COGNITIVE LEVEL

K = Knowledge
C = Comprehension
T = Application
N = Analysis

CLIENT NEEDS

S = Safe, effective care environment
G = Physiologic integrity
L = Psychosocial integrity
H = Health promotion and maintenance

Question #	Answer #	Nursing Process					Cognitive Level				Client Needs			
		A	D	P	I	E	K	C	T	N	S	G	L	H
55	1				I				T				L	
56	4				I				T				L	
57	2			P					T		S			
58	3			P					T				L	
59	3				I				T				L	
60	1					E				N			L	
61	4				I				T				L	
62	3		D					C					L	
63	2				I				T				L	
64	4				I				T				L	
65	1				I				T			G		
66	1					E				N			L	
67	3				I				T				L	
68	3				I				T				L	
69	2			P					T				L	
70	1		D					C					L	
71	3					E				N			L	
72	1				I				T				L	
73	3					E				N			L	
74	1			P					T				L	
75	4			P					T				L	
76	3			P					T				L	
77	2				I				T				L	
78	1		D					C					L	
79	2			P						N			L	
80	4				I					N			L	
Number Correct														
Number Possible	80	0	16	19	31	14	0	10	42	28	2	6	71	1

NURSING PROCESS

A = Assessment
D = Analysis, nursing diagnosis
P = Planning
I = Implementation
E = Evaluation

COGNITIVE LEVEL

K = Knowledge
C = Comprehension
T = Application
N = Analysis

CLIENT NEEDS

S = Safe, effective care environment
G = Physiologic integrity
L = Psychosocial integrity
H = Health promotion and maintenance

		Nursing Process					Cognitive Level				Client Needs			
Question #	Answer #	A	D	P	I	E	K	C	T	N	S	G	L	H
Percentage Correct														

Score Calculation: To determine your **Percentage Correct,** divide the **Number Correct** by the **Number Possible.**

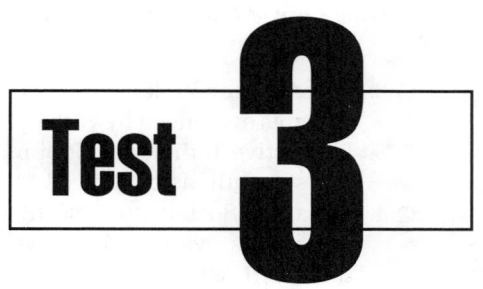

Personality Disorders, Substance-Related Disorders, and Eating Disorders

- **The Client With a Personality Disorder**
- **The Client With Maladaptive Behavioral Patterns**
- **The Client With an Alcohol-Related Disorder**
- **The Client With an Opioid-Related Disorder**
- **The Client With a Sedative-, Hypnotic-, or Anxiolytic-Related Disorder**
- **The Client With an Eating Disorder**
- **Correct Answers and Rationale**

Select the one best answer, and indicate your choice by filling in the circle in front of the option.

The Client With a Personality Disorder

A client is readmitted to the hospital psychiatric unit. His history of impulsive acts and aggressive behavior toward others, including his wife, has resulted in problems with the police. He has been unable to hold a job for longer than 2 months and feels no remorse about using others for personal gain.

1. The client is called a *manipulator* by a nurse because in the past, he played staff members against each other, resulting in angry feelings among the staff. When the staff analyzes the nurse's comment, they correctly judge that labeling the client as a manipulator is most likely to
   - ○ 1. prevent staff from expecting too much of the client.
   - ○ 2. prevent staff from seeing the client as he really is.

   - ○ 3. help staff find ways to prevent the client from mocking them.
   - ○ 4. help staff identify approaches for appropriate therapy for the client.

2. An attitude by the nurse that would most likely foster a therapeutic relationship between the nurse and the client who tries to manipulate people is
   - ○ 1. sympathy.
   - ○ 2. aloofness.
   - ○ 3. strictness.
   - ○ 4. consistency.

3. The client makes derogatory comments toward the nurse when the nurse does not allow him to eat breakfast in his room. He states, "You're inadequate and don't know what you're doing. The evening nurse always lets me eat in my room. In fact, the nurse brings me my supper tray and gets me what I want." Based on this information, which nursing diagnosis would be most appropriate for this client?
   - ○ 1. Self Esteem Disturbance related to dependency needs, as evidenced by attempts to manipulate staff.

53

○ 2. Potential for Violence related to antisocial character, as evidenced by verbal threats to the nurse.

○ 3. Ineffective Individual Coping related to lack of ego strength, as evidenced by impulsiveness.

○ 4. Impaired Social Interaction related to low self-esteem, as evidenced by dysfunctional interactions with wife.

4. To decrease the client's manipulation of staff, the nurse would include which of the following measures in the plan?

○ 1. Convey an accepting attitude toward the client regardless of his behavior.

○ 2. Ignore the client's derogatory comments and use diversional activities.

○ 3. Explain the consequences of manipulative behavior and maintain staff consistency.

○ 4. Consistently give the client negative feedback about his behavior and tell him what he should do.

5. Because the client has a potential for violence and aggressive behavior, which short-term goal would be most appropriate for the nurse to include in the plan of care? The client will

○ 1. not harm others while on the unit.

○ 2. discuss feelings of anger with the nurse in 1 week.

○ 3. ask the nurse for medication when upset.

○ 4. verbalize reasons for his anger to the nurse in 1 week.

A 16-year-old client is readmitted to the psychiatric hospital's adolescent unit. She recently ran away from home for the fifth time this year and, while hitchhiking in a state of drug-induced euphoria on a freeway, was picked up by the police. She is accompanied to the unit by her juvenile worker.

6. The nurse recognizes that it is difficult to maintain control in the relationship with this client. Which of the following actions would be best for the nurse to take when feeling outmaneuvered by this client?

○ 1. Seek help from the other staff members.

○ 2. Request to be assigned to a different client.

○ 3. Discuss feelings of frustration with the client.

○ 4. Focus attention on the client's nonadaptive behavior.

7. In the course of their conversation, the client tells the nurse bitterly, "My parents are mean. They don't care about me at all." Which of the following responses by the nurse would be the least therapeutic?

○ 1. "You feel that your parents don't care about you."

○ 2. "What would be a sign to you that your parents cared?"

○ 3. "I'm sure your parents have your best interests at heart."

○ 4. "Tell me more about your parents being mean and not caring."

8. The client is quick to recognize weakness in others. She targets a 15-year-old withdrawn client to tease and play tricks on. Of the following people, who would probably have the most influence in helping the client change her behavior?

○ 1. Physician.

○ 2. Peer group.

○ 3. Juvenile worker.

○ 4. Religious counselor.

9. When planning the client's nursing care, the nurse should take into account which of the following traits that the client also would be likely to display?

○ 1. Poor judgment.

○ 2. Faulty memory.

○ 3. Low intelligence.

○ 4. Disordered thinking.

A client is in treatment at the day hospital. This is her seventh admission. She has been unable to hold even part-time jobs and has had four abortions in the last 4 years. She is now living with her family after being evicted from her apartment. She complains of feeling empty and lonely, and her arms are scarred from frequent self-mutilation.

10. Which of the following personality disorders does this client exhibit?

○ 1. Antisocial personality disorder.

○ 2. Avoidant personality disorder.

○ 3. Borderline personality disorder.

○ 4. Compulsive personality disorder.

11. Which nursing diagnosis would not apply to this client at this time?

○ 1. High Risk for Self-Mutilation.

○ 2. Identity Disturbance.

○ 3. Self-Esteem Disturbance.

○ 4. Sensory/Perceptual Alteration.

12. The client has become attached to a part-time nurse and frequently refuses to share her history with any other staff member. She tells this nurse that other staff members mistreat her, that she can trust only her, and that she fears for her safety during the nurse's absence. This common defense mechanism is known as

○ 1. reaction formation.

○ 2. splitting.

○ 3. projection.

○ 4. denial.

13. The client repeatedly states that she is not like the other clients and asks the staff for special privileges. She does not follow the rules about using the telephone or watching television. An immediate and major focus of this client's nursing care plan would be to

○ 1. enforce the unit rules consistently.
○ 2. limit the client's contact with others.
○ 3. obtain vocational training for the client.
○ 4. ignore the client's behavior.

14. The client describes her personal history with sadness. Her mother died when she was 2 years old, and she lived with a number of relatives and in foster homes. In planning the client's care, the nurse attempts to promote completion of the developmental task on which the client would most likely have been working when her mother died. According to Erikson, this basic task is the achievement of

○ 1. trust.
○ 2. independence.
○ 3. safety.
○ 4. autonomy.

15. As the client's discharge date approaches, she asks to stay in the program and makes threats to "do something" to herself if discharged. The staff remains firm on the discharge date. Which of the following interventions would be most important to ensure the client's safety?

○ 1. Request an immediate extension for the client.
○ 2. Ask the client to leave early.
○ 3. Transfer the client to another hospital.
○ 4. Assess the seriousness of the client's threats.

The Client With Maladaptive Behavioral Patterns

A 19-year-old client is admitted to a psychiatric unit. His Axis II diagnosis is Personality Disorder NOS. He is accompanied by his mother and a lawyer, who tells the nurse that he hopes his client will "stay out of mischief until we get the messes straightened out."

16. According to the client's mother, the client "always was a mean little boy, forever playing pranks on people and teasing the small animals in the neighborhood. Now he's just a bigger prankster and less easy to control." In view of the client's history, which of the following courses of action would likely be the most effective for the nursing staff to follow initially?

○ 1. Let the client know the staff has the authority to subdue him if he gets unruly.
○ 2. Keep the client isolated from the other clients until he is better known by the staff.

○ 3. Provide the client with a list of rules while emphasizing that he will have to pay for any damage he causes.
○ 4. Closely observe the client's behavior on the unit to establish a baseline pattern of physical and social functioning.

17. After the client has been on the unit for a few days, the nurses notice that he uses his shortness and unattractiveness as an excuse for not attending various social functions, such as the weekly dance. Which of the following interventions would be best to undertake first to deal with the client's avoidance of social functions?

○ 1. Tell the client he will need a better excuse than his appearance for not participating.
○ 2. Explain to the client that everyone's cooperation is necessary to make the program a success.
○ 3. Confront the client with the fact that he is using his appearance as an excuse to avoid socializing.
○ 4. Insist that the client come up with some alternative ways to spend the time when he should be socializing.

18. A staff member asks the client after one of his loud belches, "Do you wonder why people find you repulsive?" This comment most likely will make the client feel

○ 1. defensive and defiant.
○ 2. insulted and indignant.
○ 3. ashamed and remorseful.
○ 4. embarrassed and unhappy.

19. The client's past history of cruelty and current crass behavior arouse feelings of anxiety and antagonism in staff and other clients. What is the most likely reason for these responses? The client's behavior is

○ 1. beyond comprehension.
○ 2. viewed as alien to their value system.
○ 3. easily misinterpreted as to its meaning.
○ 4. seen as only too understandable by others.

20. The client attempts to provoke the male nurse by yelling, "Hey nursie, where's your hat and purse?" In relation to being baited by the client, which of the following actions is best for the nurse to take?

○ 1. Ignore the client's kidding to avoid reinforcing it.
○ 2. Smilingly shake his head no at the client to stop his teasing.
○ 3. Use feminine gestures to indicate acceptance of the client's ribbing.
○ 4. Challenge the client to an arm-wrestling match to prove his masculinity.

21. One evening the client takes the nurse aside and whispers, "Don't tell anybody, but I'm going to call in a bomb threat to this hospital tonight." Of the following actions by the nurse, which would best

preserve the client's trust in the nurse and provide the best protection for all concerned parties?
- ○ 1. Warn the client that his telephone privileges will be taken away if he abuses them.
- ○ 2. Offer to disregard the client's plan if he does not go through with it.
- ○ 3. Say nothing to anyone until the client has actually completed the call, then notify the proper authorities.
- ○ 4. Explain to the client that this information will have to be shared immediately with the staff and the physician.

22. Constructive discipline is applied each time the client behaves in a cruel manner. At those times, which of the following ideas is the most basic and most important for the staff to convey to the client?
- ○ 1. The client is accepted although his behavior may not be.
- ○ 2. Everyone must cope with some restrictions on his actions.
- ○ 3. No one would bother with the client if the staff did not care about him.
- ○ 4. If the client cannot control his behavior, then others will have to control it for him.

A client on the inpatient psychiatric unit has a history of impulsive antisocial behaviors. He feels no remorse for any of his actions and is egocentric.

23. In planning care for the client, the nurse considers which of the following principles to be inaccurate?
- ○ 1. Short-term goals should be realistic.
- ○ 2. Long-lasting dysfunctional patterns of behavior are impossible to change during one short-term hospital stay.
- ○ 3. Behavior modification should not be used.
- ○ 4. Explaining to the client the effects of his behavior on others will be helpful.

24. The nurse–client relationship develops so that they are able to delineate and concentrate on a goal to help the client increase his social skills. The nurse is talking with the client about being able to socialize at mealtime without being disruptive. While discussing this topic, it would be best for the nurse to focus the discussion on the client's
- ○ 1. strengths and responsibilities in the situation.
- ○ 2. manipulation and disruption in similar situations.
- ○ 3. explanations concerning his behavior at mealtimes in the past.
- ○ 4. rationalizations of his behavior.

25. In treating the client with antisocial behavior patterns, which of the following outcomes would be unrealistic?
- ○ 1. identify feelings before acting impulsively.

- ○ 2. express sorrow and remorse for his impulsive actions.
- ○ 3. describe how his actions affect others.
- ○ 4. identify impulsive acts that have resulted in problems with others.

26. The client with an Axis II diagnosis of Narcissistic Personality Disorder tells the nurse he can get an executive position with the best company around anytime he wants. The nurse is aware that the client has no further education beyond high school and has only held a series of short-term part-time jobs for the last 2 years. The nurse judges the client's statement to be
- ○ 1. a grandiose delusion.
- ○ 2. a blatant lie.
- ○ 3. overevaluation of self-importance.
- ○ 4. realistic and a positive plan.

27. Which of the following approaches would the nurse specifically use with the client who has a narcissistic personality disorder when discrepancies exist between what the client states and what actually exists?
- ○ 1. Limit setting.
- ○ 2. Supportive confrontation.
- ○ 3. Consistency.
- ○ 4. Rationalization.

The Client With an Alcohol-Related Disorder

A friend accompanies the client to the hospital's substance abuse unit, where he is to be admitted for alcohol withdrawal.

28. The client consumed about 6 ounces of alcohol just before coming to the hospital. Which of the following methods would be best for the nursing staff to use to promote alcohol metabolism in the client's body?
- ○ 1. Give the client black coffee to drink.
- ○ 2. Walk the client around the unit.
- ○ 3. Have the client take a cold shower.
- ○ 4. Provide the client with a restful room to sleep in.

29. Hospital policy requires that the client's belongings be searched for contraband on admission. In view of the client's drinking problem, which of his possessions is most likely to be confiscated by the nursing staff?
- ○ 1. Hair dressing.
- ○ 2. Electric razor.
- ○ 3. Shaving cream.
- ○ 4. Antiseptic mouthwash.

30. While obtaining a nursing history, the nurse questions the client about the amount of alcohol he consumes daily. The nurse can expect the client to likely the question by
○ 1. exaggerating the amount.
○ 2. underestimating the amount.
○ 3. indicating that he does not know the amount.
○ 4. expressing uncertainty about the amount.

31. The most important reason for investigating the amount of alcohol the client has consumed during the 24 to 48 hours before admission is to help determine
○ 1. how far the disease has progressed.
○ 2. the severity of withdrawal.
○ 3. whether the client will experience delirium tremens.
○ 4. whether the client should be considered an alcoholic.

32. Of the following nursing diagnoses, which would the nurse correctly judge to be most important during the early detoxification period?
○ 1. Sleep Pattern Disturbance.
○ 2. Self-Esteem Disturbance.
○ 3. Ineffective Individual Coping.
○ 4. Knowledge Deficit.

33. Which of the following medications is most likely to be prescribed for the client during withdrawal from alcohol to provide sedation and to ease some of the anxiety and discomfort of the withdrawal process?
○ 1. Paraldehyde (Paral).
○ 2. Lorazepam (Ativan).
○ 3. Phenytoin sodium (Dilantin).
○ 4. Temazepam (Restoril).

34. To assess the client's physiologic response and the effectiveness of the medication prescribed specifically for alcohol withdrawal, the nurse would first
○ 1. assess the client's nutritional status.
○ 2. assess the client for tremors in the extremities.
○ 3. monitor the client's vital signs.
○ 4. monitor the client's sleep pattern.

35. The client could not remember the events of the past weekend, although he had receipts in his pockets from several shops where he made purchases on Saturday. This problem illustrates what condition?
○ 1. Blackout.
○ 2. Hangover.
○ 3. Dry drunk syndrome.
○ 4. Alcoholic hallucinosis.

36. After a day of abstinence, the client has coarse tremors of the hands, making it hard for him to feed himself. He asks the nurse low long it will be before this shaking goes away. On which of the following statements should the nurse base the response? The tremors
○ 1. can only be relieved by alcohol intake.

○ 2. usually disappear after about 2 days of abstinence.
○ 3. may persist for several days or even longer after alcohol intake has stopped.
○ 4. are a permanent condition due to irreversible central nervous system damage.

37. The client craves a drink while withdrawing from the alcohol. Which of the following measures is the best way to help him resist the urge to drink?
○ 1. A locked-door policy.
○ 2. A routine search of visitors.
○ 3. One-to-one supervision by the staff.
○ 4. Support from other alcoholic clients.

The nurse works in an outpatient setting with clients engaging in alcohol rehabilitation.

38. The nurse is teaching the client about the disease concept of alcoholism. Which of the following client statements indicates that the client understands the nurse's teaching?
○ 1. "Now that I know I have this disease, it's up to me to decide if I'm going to take that drink."
○ 2. "I can't help it if I drink. I have an illness."
○ 3. "All of my relatives have problems with alcohol, but I'm not as bad as they are."
○ 4. "My children won't be affected by my drinking since I've quit."

39. The client is beginning to participate in the alcohol treatment program. Which nursing approach would be most effective in decreasing his denial about his alcoholism?
○ 1. Give him reading materials about the disease of alcoholism.
○ 2. Point out concrete problems that are a direct consequence of his alcoholism.
○ 3. Explain the physiologic effects of alcohol on the body.
○ 4. Teach him assertiveness techniques.

40. The nurse is teaching members of the client's group how to give each other constructive feedback. Which of the following statements by the nurse best illustrates constructive feedback?
○ 1. "I think you're a real con artist."
○ 2. "You're dominating the conversation."
○ 3. "You interrupted John twice in 4 minutes."
○ 4. "You don't give anyone a chance to finish talking."

41. The client ashamedly tells the nurse that he hit his wife during a recent argument and asks the nurse if she thinks his wife will ever forgive him. Which of the following replies by the nurse would be best in this situation?
○ 1. "Perhaps you could ask her and find out."

○ 2. "That's something you can explore in family therapy."

○ 3. "It would depend on how much she really cares for you."

○ 4. "You seem to have some feelings about hitting your wife."

42. The client's wife meets with the nurse and her husband. She says she has about had it with her husband's foolishness and bad temper. Which of the following organizations would probably be the most helpful to her in obtaining additional assistance and support in coping with her alcoholic spouse?

○ 1. Alateen.

○ 2. Al-Anon.

○ 3. Narcotics Anonymous.

○ 4. Alcoholics Anonymous.

43. The client is started on a regimen of disulfiram (Antabuse). A valuable and expected result of successful disulfiram therapy is that it

○ 1. decreases the need for alcohol.

○ 2. acts to deter alcohol consumption.

○ 3. improves the alcoholic's ability to drink limited amounts of alcohol.

○ 4. creates a nerve block so that the effects of alcohol are not felt.

44. Which statement would indicate to the nurse that the client needs further teaching about disulfiram?

○ 1. "I can drink one or two beers and not get sick while on Antabuse."

○ 2. "I need to stop taking Antabuse for at least 2 weeks before I can drink alcohol without experiencing an alcohol–Antabuse reaction."

○ 3. "A metallic or garlic taste in my mouth is normal when starting on Antabuse."

○ 4. "Reading labels on cough syrup, after-shave lotion, and mouthwash is important because they might contain alcohol."

45. While on disulfiram therapy, the client becomes nauseated and vomits severely. The nurse is justified in judging that the client has most probably

○ 1. developed an allergy to disulfiram.

○ 2. been given an overdose of disulfiram accidentally.

○ 3. been drinking alcohol while on disulfiram therapy.

○ 4. developed gastritis as a result of disulfiram therapy.

46. The client in an outpatient alcohol treatment program states to the nurse, "Why do we need to talk about relapse? I know I'll never drink again." Which of the following responses by the nurse is best?

○ 1. "Anyone can slip. Relapse commonly occurs during the first few months after a treatment program."

○ 2. "Relapse prevention is important in follow-up care."

○ 3. "It's important to talk about relapse prevention since your recovery has only begun."

○ 4. "If you don't continue with follow-up care, you won't hear about relapse prevention."

47. Which of the following client statements indicates an understanding of relapse prevention?

○ 1. "I know I can stay dry if my wife keeps alcohol out of the house."

○ 2. "I'm open to looking at the symptoms of relapse every night so that I'll be able to recognize them in myself."

○ 3. "I'll have my sponsor at AA keep the list of relapse symptoms for me."

○ 4. "If someone tells me I'm about to relapse, I'll do something about it."

A client enters the hospital for treatment of cirrhosis of the liver. She is accompanied by her husband.

48. The client sees no connection between her liver disorder and her alcohol intake. She believes that she drinks very little and that her family is making something out of nothing. Which of the following defense mechanisms is the client using?

○ 1. Denial.

○ 2. Displacement.

○ 3. Rationalization.

○ 4. Reaction formation.

49. Medications for the client include a B-complex vitamin. The client wants to know why she must take this vitamin. What would be the nurse's best response?

○ 1. "Alcoholics are vitamin depleted."

○ 2. "Your daily alcohol consumption causes malnutrition."

○ 3. "The B vitamins help reduce the damaging effects alcohol."

○ 4. "The amount of vitamins in the alcohol you drink is very low."

50. Besides cirrhosis, the client suffers from numbness, itching, and pain in her extremities and is prone to footdrop. This disorder of the nervous system is termed

○ 1. neuralgia.

○ 2. Bell's palsy.

○ 3. neurasthenia.

○ 4. peripheral neuritis.

51. Numbness, itching, and pain in the extremities indicates which of the following nursing diagnoses?

○ 1. Alteration in Comfort.

○ 2. Impaired Skin Integrity.

○ 3. Anxiety.

○ 4. Self-Care Deficit.

52. The client has neurologic damage. As a precautionary measure, the nurse must be especially careful when

○ 1. cleansing the client's skin.

○ 2. massaging the client's feet.

○ 3. turning the client from side to side.

○ 4. applying heat to the client's lower legs.

53. A noncaffeinated beverage is substituted for the client's usual morning coffee. This measure is taken because

○ 1. clients transfer their oral dependency needs symbolically to coffee.

○ 2. regular coffee aggravates tremors and interferes with sleep.

○ 3. clients tend to abuse coffee in the same way they once abused alcohol.

○ 4. regular coffee has a diuretic effect that interferes with hydration.

54. After 5 days in the hospital, the client begins to thrash about in bed, slapping the sheets and yelling, "Go away, bugs, go away!" Which of the following nursing notes best sums up the client's behavior?

○ 1. Restless, disoriented, and hallucinating.

○ 2. Agitated and experiencing visual hallucinations.

○ 3. Fidgety and out of contact with reality.

○ 4. Seeing "bugs" in her bedclothes and slapping at them.

55. When the client thrashes in bed and yells, "Go away, bugs, go away," this behavior indicates which of the following nursing diagnoses?

○ 1. Sensory/Perceptual Alteration.

○ 2. Sleep Pattern Disturbance.

○ 3. Altered Thought Processes.

○ 4. Ineffective Individual Coping.

56. Which of the following measures should be included in the nursing care plan when the client has alcohol withdrawal delirium?

○ 1. Restrain her and keep the room quiet.

○ 2. Touch her before saying anything, and tell her where she is.

○ 3. Have someone stay with her and keep a light on in the room.

○ 4. Tell her she is having nightmares and that she will be better soon.

57. For the client experiencing alcohol withdrawal delirium, which of the following physician orders should the nurse question?

○ 1. Chlordiazepoxide, 25 mg PO qid.

○ 2. Chlordiazepoxide, 100 mg q 4 hours p.r.n., for agitation.

○ 3. Chlorpromazine, 100 mg q 4 hours p.r.n., for agitation.

○ 4. Thiamine, 100 mg IM qd for 3 days.

58. When developing a one-to-one relationship with the client after she is physiologically stable, the nurse should use the first meeting to determine the client's

○ 1. healthy coping mechanisms.

○ 2. most probable reasons for alcohol abuse.

○ 3. knowledge about Alcoholics Anonymous.

○ 4. childhood experiences that predispose to alcoholism.

59. The client's husband tells the nurse that he also drinks heavily in the evenings and would like to stop. The nurse suggests that he attend Alcoholics Anonymous, but he says, "I went to one men's meeting and all they did was swear and brag about how drunk they got." Which of the following responses would be best for the nurse to make?

○ 1. "That's too bad. I can see how you might have been turned off by the experience."

○ 2. "Not everyone finds Alcoholics Anonymous helpful. There are other therapies available."

○ 3. "The Alcoholics Anonymous meetings vary from group to group. Have you thought about attending another group?"

○ 4. "If you really want to stop your drinking, you would go back to Alcoholics Anonymous whether you liked it or not."

60. The client's husband asks the nurse about requirements to become a member of Alcoholics Anonymous. Which reply by the nurse is accurate?

○ 1. "Resolve to abstain from alcohol and to help others to do so."

○ 2. "Admit that you are powerless over alcohol and that you need help."

○ 3. "Analyze the wrongs you have done while drinking and try to make amends for them."

○ 4. "Turn your life over to a higher power and seek to improve contact with that power through meditation."

61. The client is to be discharged from the hospital. What information is likely to be most helpful in her efforts to stop drinking?

○ 1. Dependency on her husband to help her stop drinking.

○ 2. The disease concept of alcoholism.

○ 3. The stages of alcoholism.

○ 4. The importance of perseverance in her efforts to change her behavior.

The Client With an Opioid-Related Disorder

A client is brought to the hospital's emergency room by a friend, who states, "I guess he had some bad junk (heroin) today."

62. In assessing the client, the nurse would likely find which of the following symptoms?
    - ○ 1. Increased heart rate, dilated pupils, and fever.
    - ○ 2. Tremulousness, impaired coordination, increased blood pressure, and ruddy complexion.
    - ○ 3. Decreased respirations, constricted pupils, and pallor.
    - ○ 4. Eye irritation, tinnitus, and irritation of nasal and oral mucosa.
63. The client is in a light coma. Which nursing diagnosis would receive the highest priority?
    - ○ 1. Ineffective Individual Coping.
    - ○ 2. Ineffective Breathing Pattern.
    - ○ 3. Alteration in Nutrition.
    - ○ 4. Self Care Deficit.
64. Which nursing intervention would receive the lowest priority for the client with a heroin overdose?
    - ○ 1. Prepare for cardiopulmonary respiration (CPR).
    - ○ 2. Monitor vital signs.
    - ○ 3. Monitor breathing pattern.
    - ○ 4. Discuss treatment options.
65. After administering naloxone (Narcan), a narcotic antagonist, the nurse should monitor the client carefully for signs of
    - ○ 1. cerebral edema.
    - ○ 2. kidney failure.
    - ○ 3. seizure activity.
    - ○ 4. respiratory depression.

The client is admitted to the chemical dependency unit with heroin dependency. After about 12 hours, he develops signs of heroin withdrawal.

66. Of the following signs and symptoms of opiate withdrawal, which occur late, rather than early, in the course of withdrawal?
    - ○ 1. Vomiting and diarrhea.
    - ○ 2. Yawning and diaphoresis.
    - ○ 3. Lacrimation and rhinorrhea.
    - ○ 4. Restlessness and nervousness.
67. The client has numerous complaints of discomfort while abstaining from heroin. Which of the following nursing orders on the client's care plan would be the least advisable and effective?
    - ○ 1. Be empathetic but firm with the client's complaints.
    - ○ 2. Promise to reevaluate the client's withdrawal plan to ease his discomfort.
    - ○ 3. Prepare the client in advance for minor discomforts that might occur.
    - ○ 4. Inform the client of alternative methods, such as warm baths, for dealing with aches and pains.

68. The client is being tested for the human immunodeficiency virus (HIV). The nursing staff is concerned about possible HIV exposure among other clients on the unit and among themselves. Which of the following precautionary measures is the least important?
    - ○ 1. Strict handwashing procedures.
    - ○ 2. A private room for the client.
    - ○ 3. Wearing gloves when handling body fluids.
    - ○ 4. Increased caution in disposing of needles and syringes.
69. The client starts methadone therapy. Which of the following signs would alert the nurse to acute methadone toxicity?
    - ○ 1. Fever.
    - ○ 2. Colitis.
    - ○ 3. Renal shutdown.
    - ○ 4. Respiratory depression.
70. Which of the following characteristics of methadone contributes most to the drug's potential for abuse?
    - ○ 1. It blunts the craving for heroin.
    - ○ 2. It blocks the pleasurable effects of heroin.
    - ○ 3. It is equally effective at low or high doses.
    - ○ 4. It lessens the severity of withdrawal symptoms.
71. Which of the following measures would be the most feasible to ensure the therapeutic use of methadone and to prevent its abuse?
    - ○ 1. Monitor the client's urine drug levels.
    - ○ 2. Administer the methadone in injection form.
    - ○ 3. Supervise the client when administering liquid methadone.
    - ○ 4. Use methadone only for a hospitalized client.
72. While the client is in chemical dependency rehabilitation, which nursing intervention would be least appropriate?
    - ○ 1. Call Narcotics Anonymous to tell them to expect the client after discharge.
    - ○ 2. Enforce unit policies.
    - ○ 3. Confront the client's inappropriate behaviors.
    - ○ 4. Help the client to express feelings.
73. When discussing Narcotics Anonymous, the nurse should explain that the client needs to
    - ○ 1. stay drug-free one day at a time.
    - ○ 2. be clean of drugs at the meetings.
    - ○ 3. abstain from drugs for the rest of his life.
    - ○ 4. commit a certain amount of time to the organization.
74. The client's eventual success or progress when out of the hospital can probably best be measured by what factor?
    - ○ 1. the kinds of friends he makes.
    - ○ 2. the number of drug-free days he has.
    - ○ 3. the way he gets along with parents.
    - ○ 4. the amount of responsibility his job entails.
75. Which of the following physical disorders is the her-

oin addict least likely to develop as a result of the addiction?

○ 1. Hepatitis.
○ 2. Pneumonia.
○ 3. Tuberculosis.
○ 4. Cholelithiasis.

The Client With a Sedative, Hypnotic, or Anxiolytic–Related Disorder

A client is brought by ambulance to the hospital emergency room after taking an overdose of barbiturates. A male friend arrives a short time later, carrying some of the client's personal belongings.

76. The client went into shock at home and is semicomatose on admission. If death occurs shortly, the cause of death would most likely be

○ 1. kidney failure.
○ 2. cardiac standstill.
○ 3. internal hemorrhaging.
○ 4. respiratory depression.

77. The client's friend reports that the client has been taking about eight "reds" (800 mg of secobarbital [Seconal]) daily, besides drinking more alcohol than usual. The client's friend asks anxiously, "Do you think she will live?" Which of the following replies would be best for the nurse to make?

○ 1. "We can only wait and see."
○ 2. "Do you know her well?"
○ 3. "She is very ill and may not live."
○ 4. "Her condition is serious. You sound very worried about her."

78. The nurse talks further with the client's friend and tries to determine the nature of their relationship. Which of the following motivations provides the best justification for the nurse's inquiries?

○ 1. To ascertain the friend's capabilities as a source of support for the client.
○ 2. To encourage the friend to realize the seriousness of the client's condition.
○ 3. To determine whether the friend can be trusted with confidential information about the client.
○ 4. To learn whether the client's relationship with the friend may have caused the suicide attempt.

79. Before her hospitalization, the client needed increasingly larger doses of barbiturates to achieve the same euphoric effect she initially realized from their use. From this information, the nurse should plan care that takes into account that the client is likely suffering from drug

○ 1. tolerance.

○ 2. addiction.
○ 3. habituation.
○ 4. dependence.

80. By which of the following symptoms could the client probably have been identified as a chronic user of barbiturates in the days before her hospitalization?

○ 1. Drooling, fainting, and illusions.
○ 2. Sluggishness, ataxia, and irritability.
○ 3. Diaphoresis, twitching, and sneezing.
○ 4. Suspiciousness, tachycardia, and edema.

81. The client's vital signs stabilize, and she later awakens in a confused state. Which of the following nursing measures would be least appropriate while the client is recovering from sedative overdose?

○ 1. Maintain seizure precautions for the client.
○ 2. Close the windows in the vicinity of the client.
○ 3. Use a p.r.n. order for a medication for anxiety and agitation.
○ 4. Use short, complete sentences when speaking to the client.

82. After a dose-response test, the client receives pentobarbital sodium (Nembutal) at a nonintoxicating maintenance level for 2 days and at decreasing doses thereafter. This regimen is prescribed primarily to help prevent possibly fatal

○ 1. psychosis.
○ 2. convulsions.
○ 3. hypotension.
○ 4. hypothermia.

83. During an interaction with the nurse, the client states that her "life has gone down the tubes" since her divorce 6 months ago. After she lost her job and apartment, she "took those pills to sleep and not wake up." From these data, the nurse would give the highest priority to which of the following nursing diagnoses?

○ 1. Self-Esteem Disturbance.
○ 2. Potential for Self-Directed Violence.
○ 3. Ineffective Individual Coping.
○ 4. Sleep Pattern Disturbance.

84. Based on the client's loss of her husband through divorce, the loss of her job and apartment, and her drug dependency, the nurse includes the nursing diagnosis Self Esteem Disturbance on the client's care plan. Based on this information, which of the following short-term goals is appropriate? The client will discuss with the nurse

○ 1. feelings related to her losses.
○ 2. two actions to improve her life.
○ 3. effects of drugs on her life.
○ 4. three strengths that she has.

85. The staff notices that the client spends most of her time with the young adult clients, most of whom have also misused drugs. This group of clients is a dominant force on the unit, keeping the non-drug

users entertained with stories of their "highs." In which of the following ways would staff best deal with this problem?
○ 1. Providing additional recreation.
○ 2. Breaking up drug-oriented discussions.
○ 3. Speaking with the clients individually about their behavior.
○ 4. Bringing up for discussion staff observations of the clients' drug-oriented conversations at the weekly client group meetings.

The nurse is working in a community mental health center. A client with an Axis I diagnosis of Anxiolytic Withdrawal is prescribed prazepam (Centrax) in daily decreasing doses for 3 weeks. She has been taking Centrax for 3 days. The client had been dependent on diazepam (Valium), which she had been taking daily for the last 8 months at a dose of 60 mg.

86. The client states she feels shaky, is having problems sleeping, and does not want to continue with Centrax. She asks the nurse if she can stop taking the Centrax now. The nurse's best response is
○ 1. "You need to continue the Centrax as prescribed to ensure a slow and safe withdrawal."
○ 2. "Because your symptoms of withdrawal are minimal, you can take the Centrax when you feel you need it."
○ 3. "You can discontinue the Centrax because the worse symptoms of withdrawal are over."
○ 4. "I recommend one dose of Centrax at bedtime to help you sleep."

87. The client calls the nurse the following week and states she feels extremely nervous and wants to come to the clinic now because she "can't take it anymore." Which of the following actions by the nurse is best?
○ 1. Instruct the client to take a warm bath.
○ 2. Tell the client to have her neighbor bring her to the clinic immediately.
○ 3. Tell the client to do her relaxation exercises.
○ 4. Speak with the client on the telephone as long as necessary to calm her.

The Client With an Eating Disorder

A client has been referred to a nurse-led group for compulsive overeaters at the mental health clinic by her physician.

88. During the initial interview with the nurse, the client states, "I can't stand myself and the way I look." Which of the following statements by the nurse would be most therapeutic?
○ 1. "All the group members feel the same as you do."
○ 2. "I don't think you look bad at all."
○ 3. "Don't worry. You'll be back in shape soon."
○ 4. "Tell me more about your feelings."

89. It is desirable for group members to use functional roles in the group to obtain the most benefit from the group. In which of the following instances is a group role (versus an individual role) being used by one of the members? The member
○ 1. shows the group the latest pictures of her child.
○ 2. insists that everyone try her favorite reducing diet.
○ 3. makes quiet comments to the person sitting next to her.
○ 4. proposes an alternative task to keep from thinking about food.

90. The group members learn that many people in the American culture have difficulty with weight control because they unconsciously equate food with
○ 1. love and affection.
○ 2. power and control.
○ 3. status and prestige.
○ 4. survival and growth.

91. The client has gained 35 pounds in 7 weeks. Before her admission to the psychiatric unit, she refused to see her friends or to leave her house. Which of the following nursing diagnoses would be most appropriate for this client?
○ 1. Ineffective Individual Coping.
○ 2. Self-Esteem Disturbance.
○ 3. Diversional Activity Deficit.
○ 4. Anxiety.

92. Which of the following nursing interventions would be least appropriate for this client?
○ 1. Invite her to participate in an informal craft activity.
○ 2. Ask the dietitian to meet with her.
○ 3. Tell her to record what she eats throughout the day.
○ 4. Explain to her that obesity can be the result of dysfunctional coping with stress.

An adolescent client is admitted to the psychiatric unit for rapid weight loss associated with anorexia nervosa. She is 5 feet, 2 inches tall and weighs 70 pounds.

93. Physical manifestations most likely to be found during nursing assessment include

○ 1. tachycardia, hypertension, and hyperthyroidism.

○ 2. tachycardia, hypertension, and iron deficiency anemia.

○ 3. hypotension, elevated serum potassium level, and vitamin C deficiency.

○ 4. bradycardia, hypotension, and cold sensitivity.

94. The nurse establishes which of the following nursing diagnoses as being of highest priority for this client?

○ 1. Self-Esteem Disturbance.

○ 2. Ineffective Individual Coping.

○ 3. Altered Nutrition: Less Than Body Requirements.

○ 4. Body Image Disturbance.

95. A behavioral program for weight gain is instituted as part of the nursing care plan. Which of the following nursing interventions would be most specific to attainment of the program goal?

○ 1. Provide emotional support and active listening.

○ 2. Give positive rewards for gradual weight gain.

○ 3. Help the client identify her problematic eating behaviors.

○ 4. Initiate intravenous hyperalimentation.

96. The nurse enters the client's room and finds her doing sit-ups. What would be the nurse's best approach?

○ 1. Wait until she finishes and ask her why she feels the need to exercise.

○ 2. Remind her that if she loses weight, she will lose privileges.

○ 3. Ask her to stop doing the sit-ups and direct her to a quiet activity.

○ 4. Leave the room and allow her to exercise in private.

97. What would be the most appropriate and realistic outcome for the client for this hospitalization?

○ 1. Her weight is stable, and she is willing to begin outpatient group therapy.

○ 2. Her weight is within the normal range, and she no longer feels the need to diet.

○ 3. Her discharge weight is 15% more than her admission weight.

○ 4. Her eating behaviors have changed, and she reports feeling better.

The 17-year-old client with an Axis I diagnosis is hospitalized on the inpatient unit.

98. The client weighs 5 pounds less than her ideal weight for her height. She tells the nurse, "I don't have a problem. I'm not really underweight." The nurse's best response is

○ 1. "Your parents told the physician that you do have a problem."

○ 2. "Even though your weight is almost ideal for your height, purging and using laxatives are harmful to your body."

○ 3. "We'll find out if you do have a problem while you're here."

○ 4. "It's often difficult to acknowledge our imperfections."

99. The client goes to the bathroom and purges after lunch. Which of the following nursing orders would be included in the client's care plan?

○ 1. Observe the client for 2 hours after each meal.

○ 2. Institute a one-to-one observation for the next 24 hours.

○ 3. Tell the client to write about her feelings when she has the urge to purge.

○ 4. Inform the client that an extra snack will be needed after each purging incident.

100. The client's mother has brought the client's drawing supplies at her daughter's request. The nurse judges the client's request

○ 1. as being insignificant.

○ 2. as a negative behavior.

○ 3. as a positive behavior.

○ 4. as manipulation.

CORRECT ANSWERS AND RATIONALE

The letters in parentheses following the rationale identify the step of the nursing process (A, D, P, I, E); cognitive level (K, C, T, N); and client needs (S, G, L, H). See the Answer Grid for the key.

The Client With a Personality Disorder

1. 2. Labels may cause staff to make assumptions about the client, discount the client's point of view, and cause the client to live up to the label in a self-fulfilling prophecy. (E, N, L)

2. 4. It is most important that the nurse maintain a consistent approach when dealing with the client who manipulates others. The nurse should set limits on the client's behavior and then consistently enforce these limits to help prevent manipulation. Strictness for its own sake is not appropriate with this client, nor is sympathy or aloofness. (P, N, L)

3. 1. The client's statements to the nurse reflect an attempt to manipulate the nurse to fulfill his desires and are related to his dependency needs. This behavior reflects the client's low self-esteem and is an attempt to assert his superiority and deny his true feelings about himself. The client is not verbally threatening the nurse or acting impulsively. There is no evidence of dysfunctional interactions with his wife, although this may be a problem. (D, N, L)

4. 3. The client must be aware of the outcomes or consequences of his behavior. Explanations must be clear and concise and conveyed in a matter-of-fact manner. Consistency of approach from the entire staff in following through will help decrease manipulation. Accepting all behaviors or ignoring them is not helpful or safe for the client and others on the unit. Accepting the client but not his behaviors guards against the client feeling rejected and increases his sense of worth. Giving negative feedback and telling him what he should do can be threatening to the client with low self-esteem and may only increase his manipulative behavior. (P, T, L)

5. 2. Discussing angry feelings with the nurse will help the client identify his feelings, express them appropriately, and decrease his anxiety. Not harming others is desirable but is a more long-term goal and does not help the client to learn how to handle his feelings appropriately. Asking the nurse for medication is not helpful and just allows the client to avoid dealing with his feelings. Medication may be needed when the client cannot control his behavior or calm down. Antianxiety agents are not usually prescribed for clients with antisocial personality disorder because these clients often have problems with alcohol or drugs. Verbalizing reasons for his anger implies that the client needs to justify his feelings and helps him displace his feelings onto others without looking at himself and his role in a situation. (P, N, L)

6. 1. When a nurse is having problems dealing with a client, it is best to admit to the need for help and seek the assistance of other staff who can help. (I, T, L)

7. 3. When the client makes a derogatory comment about her parents, a good technique is to help the client discuss her feelings in more detail and to be more specific about her sweeping conclusion. It would be least therapeutic to state that her parents have her best interests at heart because this accuses the client of being unfeeling or wrong about her parents. (I, T, L)

8. 2. Most teenagers respond best to their peers and less well to people of authority, such as physicians, juvenile workers, and religious counselors. (E, N, L)

9. 1. The person with antisocial characteristics frequently uses extremely poor judgment. The person has an intact memory and is a clever rather than a disordered thinker. (D, N, L)

10. 3. This client's primary diagnosis is borderline personality disorder, characterized by impulsive, often self-mutilating behavior and unstable, intense personal relationships. Antisocial personality disorder is characterized by failure to accept social norms, which often results in unlawful behavior. The avoidant personality demonstrates social withdrawal and hypersensitivity to criticism. The compulsive personality is preoccupied with details and rules, to the exclusion of other life activities. (E, N, L)

11. 4. Sensory/Perceptual Alteration is the least appropriate nursing diagnosis for this client. There is no evidence to support disordered thinking, hallucinations, or delusions. During periods of extreme stress, the client with a borderline personality disorder may experience transient psychotic symptoms. (D, N, L)

12. 2. *Splitting* refers to a primitive defense mechanism, as well as learned behavior, in which manipulation becomes an adaptive style. *Reaction formation* is a defense in which negative feelings are replaced with positive ones. *Projection* involves attributing one's own negative traits to someone else. *Denial* is a defense mechanism used to resolve emo-

tional conflict and allay anxiety by disavowing thoughts or external realities that are consciously intolerable. (D, C, L)

13. 1. Consistent enforcement of unit rules will help the borderline client control her behavior. Ignoring the behavior leads to an increase in the behavior to evoke a response from the staff. If the client assumes control of the behavior, the client has little opportunity to learn increased responsibility for the behavior. Although vocational plans will be important for discharge planning, they are not an immediate priority. (P, T, L)

14. 4. The achievement of autonomy is the basic task of 2-year-olds. Developing a sense of trust is a task for infants; becoming independent more appropriately describes adolescent tasks. Safety is not a developmental task. (D, N, L)

15. 4. Assessment is an ongoing process throughout treatment. Any suicidal statement must be assessed. Extending the hospital stay would encourage dependency and manipulation. Early discharge is not indicated and may be seen as a punitive staff response to a client threat. Transfer without careful assessment of need would also encourage dependency. (I, T, L)

The Client With Maladaptive Behavioral Patterns

16. 4. The best initial course of action when admitting a client is to observe him to get to know him and to establish baseline information. This is part of the assessment phase of the nursing process. Isolating a client is not recommended unless there is a very good reason for it. An example would be the very active, combative client who is dangerous to himself and others. Interventions such as telling the client that the staff has authority to subdue him or providing the client with rules he must follow threaten the client and likely will promote trouble. (A, T, L)

17. 3. The antisocial client needs to be confronted by his behavior to learn what is expected of him and how to achieve what is expected. An intervention that indicates the client needs a better excuse than he is using to avoid a social function encourages the use of excuses and belittles the client. The client is unlikely to cooperate when he is told that he should try to make a social event successful. Having the client use an activity other than the one he has planned avoids dealing with a problem and is not a good first action. (I, T, L)

18. 1. When the nurse asks the client if he understands why others find him repulsive, the client is likely to feel defensive and defiant. The question is belittling, and a natural tendency is to counterattack the threat to the self-image. Because the person with an antiso-

cial personality is egocentric and unconcerned about his effect on others, he is unlikely to feel ashamed, remorseful, or embarrassed. (E, N, L)

19. 2. Society tends to stigmatize those who deviate from the dominant value system. Therefore, the client's behavior is a source of anxiety because it is alien to the staffs' and other clients' value systems. (E, N, L)

20. 1. This client is trying to provoke the nurse into a reaction when he taunts him. Behavior that is reinforced will continue. Behavior that is not reinforced tends to become extinguished. Hence, ignoring the client's comment is the best course of action. The other responses would tend to reinforce the client's behavior. (I, T, L)

21. 4. When this client says that he plans to make a bomb threat to the hospital, the possible results are too serious to risk bargaining with the client. The best course of action, and the one most likely to promote trust, is to tell the client honestly what must be done about the bomb threat. It is possible that the client is also asking to be stopped and that he is indirectly pleading for help. (I, T, L)

22. 1. The most basic and important idea to convey to the client is that, as a person, he is accepted, although his behavior may not be. (P, T, L)

23. 3. Behavior modification can be helpful to the client when positive reinforcements are used to reinforce desired behaviors. Realistic short-term goals are important as first steps to changing long-lasting maladaptive patterns of behavior. (P, T, L)

24. 1. The best approach here is to capitalize on the client's strengths and his responsibilities in a given situation. Clients such as this one are skillful at placing the blame or focus on others. The interaction should be oriented in the present and have a positive focus. (I, T, L)

25. 2. The client with an antisocial personality disorder does not feel guilt, sorrow, or remorse for his actions. It would be unrealistic for the nurse to expect the client to acquire these traits. Immediate gratification without regard for the rights of others and hasty decisions often result because of his inability to tolerate frustration. (D, N, L)

26. 3. The nurse judges the client's statement as overevaluation of self-importance. The grandiosity of someone with a narcissistic personality disorder is not a delusion but rather is usually based somewhat in reality, although it can be distorted, embellished, or convoluted. (E, N, L)

27. 2. The nurse would specifically use supportive confrontation with the client to point out discrepancies between what the client states and what actually exists to increase responsibility for self. Limit setting and consistency in approach are also used by staff in treating these clients. Rationalization is typically used by the client to blame others, make excuses, and provide alibis for self-centered behaviors. (I, T, L)

The Client With an Alcohol-Related Disorder

28. 4. The rate of alcohol metabolism is not influenced by drinking black coffee, walking around the unit, or taking a cold shower. Alcohol is destroyed and oxidized in the body at a slow, steady rate. Therefore, it would be best to have the client sleep off the effects of the alcohol. (I, T, L)

29. 4. Antiseptic mouthwashes often contain alcohol and should be taken from clients entering a substance abuse unit, unless labeling clearly indicates that the product does not contain alcohol. Such personal care items as hair dressing and shaving cream do not contain alcohol. An electric razor should present no problem for a client being admitted for the treatment of alcoholism as long as it is in good working order. (I, N, L)

30. 2. The alcoholic usually underestimates the amount of alcohol consumed. He may be unaware of how much he really drinks or may fail to admit, even to himself, how much he really consumes. (D, T, L)

31. 2. The amount of alcohol consumed in the last 24 to 48 hours helps determine how much medication the client needs to relieve withdrawal symptoms when a client is admitted for the treatment of alcoholism. It will not help determine how far the disease has progressed or whether the client should be considered an alcoholic. It is difficult to predict delirium tremens during withdrawal, but if the client has had them previously, he may likely have them again. (E, N, L)

32. 1. Alcoholism disrupts sleeping and eating habits. Most alcoholics are undernourished and in need of extra nourishment and rest. Self-Esteem Disturbance, Ineffective Individual Coping, and Knowledge Deficit reflect potential client problems that the nurse would include in the plan of care when the client's physiologic status has stabilized and alcohol detoxification nears completion. (E, N, L)

33. 2. Antianxiety agents such as lorazepam (Ativan) and chlordiazepoxide (Librium) are commonly used to ease symptoms during alcohol withdrawal. The anticonvulsant phenytoin sodium (Dilantin) does not relieve anxiety, nor does paraldehyde (Paral), which is used primarily for its hypnotic and sedative effects. Temazepam (Restoril) is a sedative-hypnotic not used for alcohol withdrawal. (E, N, L)

34. 3. Monitoring vital signs provides information regarding the client's physiologic status during alcohol withdrawal and his physiologic response to the

antianxiety agent used during detoxification. Vital signs reflect the degree of central nervous system irritability, indicating the effectiveness of the medication in easing withdrawal symptoms. Assessments of the client's nutritional status, sleep pattern, and presence of tremors are less immediate and indirect means of assessing physiologic status during alcohol detoxification. (I, N, L)

35. 1. A client is said to be suffering from a blackout when he cannot recall what he has been doing while under the influence of alcohol. Common symptoms of a hangover, including headaches and gastrointestinal distress, typically follow heavy alcohol consumption. In dry drunk syndrome, a person has not been drinking but acts grandiose and impatient and uses many defense mechanisms. Alcohol hallucinosis occurs after ending or reducing heavy drinking and is marked by auditory hallucinations. (D, C, L)

36. 3. The client with alcoholism may experience tremors for several days or even longer after alcohol intake has stopped. (I, T, L)

37. 4. Group support has proved more successful than individual attention from the staff in influencing positive behavior in alcoholics. Locked doors do not help clients change behavior or develop their own controls. Searching visitors is impractical and externally oriented. (I, T, L)

38. 1. The development of alcoholism is influenced by biologic, sociocultural, and environmental factors. The biologic theories of alcoholism clearly identify genetic factors as a major influence on the development of alcoholism in some people. The disease concept of alcoholism permits the individual with the disease to not feel guilty about causing the illness. However, the responsibility of using alcohol is still up to the individual, who alone decides whether to take that drink of alcohol. Children of alcoholic parents are more likely to become alcoholics than are the children of nonalcoholic parents, even if raised in an alcohol-free environment. (E, N, L)

39. 2. The nurse would discuss concrete problems that are directly due to the client's alcoholism to confront the client and increase his awareness of how alcohol has gotten him into trouble. Providing the client with reading material about the disease of alcoholism, explaining the physiologic effects of alcohol, and teaching assertiveness techniques are all important interventions for the client in alcohol rehabilitation but less effective in decreasing denial. (I, T, L)

40. 3. A nurse using group therapy with clients is giving constructive feedback to the group by describing specifically what was seen and heard in an objective rather than judgmental manner. The nurse is following this principle in telling a client how often he has interrupted the group within a set period of time. (I, T, L)

41. 4. The client is feeling remorse about hitting his wife. Here, it is best to make a comment that will help him focus on his feelings and ventilate them. Reflecting what the client has said is a good technique to accomplish these goals. Comments that give advice to the client or hedge the issue are less satisfactory. (I, T, L)

42. 2. Al-Anon is for the mates of alcoholics. Alateen is for the children of alcoholics. Alcoholics Anonymous is for the alcoholic. Narcotics Anonymous is for the abuser of narcotic substances. (P, C, L)

43. 2. Disulfiram (Antabuse) helps curb the impulsiveness of the problem drinker. Any disulfiram in the body reacts with the alcohol to produce marked discomfort. (D, C, L)

44. 1. Any amount of alcohol consumed while taking disulfiram can cause an alcohol–disulfiram reaction. The reaction experienced is in proportion to the amount of alcohol ingested. The alcohol–disulfiram reaction can begin 5 to 10 minutes after alcohol is ingested. Symptoms can be mild, as in flushing, throbbing in head and neck, nausea, and diaphoresis. Other symptoms include vomiting, respiratory difficulty, hypotension, vertigo, syncope, and confusion. Severe reactions involve respiratory depression, convulsions, coma, and even death. (E, N, L)

45. 3. Nausea with severe vomiting is common when the client drinks alcohol. Other typical signs and symptoms of an alcohol–disulfiram reaction include vasodilation in the upper body, palpitations, hyperventilation, headache, and dyspnea. Severe reaction can be life-threatening. (D, N, L)

46. 1. The client's statement "I know I'll never drink again" reflects overconfidence, one of the symptoms of relapse. The nurse reminds the client that anyone can slip, that anyone is vulnerable to start drinking again, and that relapse often occurs during the first few months after treatment. The statements, "relapse prevention is important in follow-up care" and "it's important since your recovery has just begun," are true statements but incomplete in the information given the client. The statement, "if you don't continue with follow-up treatment, you won't hear about relapse prevention," is not helpful. (I, N, L)

47. 2. The client statement of being open to looking at the list of relapse symptoms every night indicates willingness to be responsible for one's own actions and sobriety. The statements, "I know I can stay dry if my wife keeps alcohol out of the house," "I'll have my sponsor at AA keep the list of relapse symptoms for me," and "if someone tells me I'm about to re-lapse, I'll do something about it," place the responsibility for the client's sobriety on someone else rather than himself. The only person responsible for the client's sobriety is himself. (E, N, L)

48. 1. The person using *denial* as a defense mechanism refuses to acknowledge an aspect of reality. This client is using denial when she refuses to acknowledge that she has a problem with alcohol. *Displacement* involves transferring a feeling to a more acceptable substitute object. *Rationalization* involves substituting one reason for a behavior for the real reason motivating the behavior. *Reaction formation* is when an opposite attitude takes the place of the real attitudes or impulses that the client harbors. (D, C, L)

49. 3. Because the client is in denial regarding her problem with alcohol, it is helpful if confrontation can be avoided during the first few days of withdrawal. This response gives accurate information with minimal confrontation. (I, T, L)

50. 4. Typical symptoms of peripheral neuritis include numbness, itching, and pain in the extremities and a predisposition to footdrop. Neurasthenia is neurotic behavior in which the main pattern is motor and mental fatigue. Neuralgia refers to severe pain along the course of a nerve. Bell's palsy is a type of facial paralysis involving the seventh cranial nerve. (D, C, L)

51. 1. Alteration in Comfort is the correct answer because the client with peripheral neuritis experiences pain, itching, and numbness of the extremities. Impaired Skin Integrity, Anxiety, and Self-Care Deficit are problems that could result if appropriate nursing and medical interventions are not instituted. (D, N, S)

52. 4. Clients often require help to keep their skin clean. Massaging the feet may be important in some instances, and turning from side to side is an essential nursing measure for many clients. However, a client with neurologic disorders is likely to have sensory changes. Therefore, it is particularly important to guard against burns because the client may not feel heat on the skin. (I, T, G)

53. 2. Regular coffee contains caffeine, which acts as a psychomotor stimulant. Hence, serving coffee to the alcoholic client may add to her tremors and wakefulness. (E, N, L)

54. 4. Nursing notes most helpful to others are those that describe exactly what the client did and said. Technical terms used to describe behavior may be misinterpreted by others. (E, N, L)

55. 1. The client is experiencing Sensory/Perceptual Alteration related to alcohol withdrawal, as evidenced by stating, "Go away, bugs." The client's thrashing reflects her agitation. Visual hallucinations, disorientation, and agitation are symptoms of delirium tremens. (D, N, L)

56. 3. The client with alcohol withdrawal delirium should not be left unattended. Unintentional suicide is a possibility when the client attempts to get away from hallucinations. Shadows created by dim lights are likely to cause illusions. Such measures as restraining the client, touching her before saying anything, and telling her where she is would likely add to her agitation. Explaining that she is having a nightmare and that she will soon be better are untruthful statements that offer false assurance. (P, T, L)

57. 3. The nurse should question the order for chlorpromazine (Thorazine), 100 mg q 4 hours p.r.n, for agitation. Chlorpromazine is a major tranquilizer and antipsychotic that decreases the seizure threshold. During alcohol withdrawal, central nervous system irritability is present, and seizures can occur at this time. The nurse would question this drug order because of the increased risk of seizure. (D, N, L)

58. 1. In early one-to-one helping relationships with this client, focusing on the positive aspects and on healthy coping mechanisms likely would help increase the client's self-esteem. Seeking out reasons for alcohol abuse and delving into childhood experiences that predispose to alcoholism describe more traditional mental health therapies that have not proved successful. An alcoholic should have a good understanding of Alcoholics Anonymous, but this should not be the focus in early meetings with this client. (P, T, L)

59. 3. It would be best for the nurse to support Alcoholics Anonymous without threatening the client's husband and encourage him not to judge the group on the basis of one meeting. Offering sympathy and making judgments about the meeting are not recommended. Because this is the first meeting with the man, it would be inappropriate to suggest that he give up on Alcoholics Anonymous and look at other therapies. (I, T, L)

60. 2. Alcoholics Anonymous requires that the alcoholic admit that he is powerless over alcohol and that he needs help. Eligibility for membership in Alcoholics Anonymous does not require that the applicant resolve to abstain from drinking, help others to do so, analyze the wrongs he has done, make amends for wrongs committed, or turn his life over to a higher power. (I, T, L)

61. 4. Information about the importance of continued efforts to change her behavior takes into account the fact that alcohol dependence is a difficult problem but that the client can conquer it. This approach is nonjudgmental and places the responsibility not to drink on the client. (E, N, L)

The Client With an Opioid-Related Disorder

62. 3. Common signs of heroin overdose are respiratory depression, pale or cyanotic skin and lips, pinpoint pupils, shock, cardiac arrhythmias, and convulsions. Death may occur from respiratory depression and pulmonary edema. Increased heart rate, dilated pupils, and increased temperature may indicate stimulant abuse. Tremulousness, impaired coordination, increased blood pressure, and a ruddy complexion may indicate alcohol intoxication. Eye irritation, double vision, tinnitus, and irritated mucous membranes could indicate inhalant intoxication. (A, N, L)

63. 2. The client's ineffective breathing pattern should receive the highest priority. Respiratory depression occurs with heroin overdose owing to central nervous system depression. (D, N, L)

64. 4. The nurse monitors vital signs and breathing pattern, and prepares for emergency intervention like cardiopulmonary resuscitation. Discussing treatment modalities for chemical dependency while the client is physically unstable would be an inappropriate action. (I, T, L)

65. 4. After administering naloxone (Narcan), the nurse should monitor the client's respiratory status carefully. The drug is short-acting, and the client may fall back into a coma with respiratory depression again after its effects wear off. (I, T, L)

66. 1. Vomiting and diarrhea are usually late, rather than early, signs of heroin withdrawal. (A, C, L)

67. 2. When a client complains of discomfort while abstaining from heroin, it would be least desirable for the nurse to promise to reevaluate the client's withdrawal plan for easing the client's discomforts. Better courses of action for this client include being empathetic but firm and explaining alternative methods, such as warm baths, to deal with discomfort. Also, it would be important to prepare the client in advance for the discomfort that likely will occur as heroin is withdrawn. (I, T, L)

68. 2. A private room is not indicated unless necessitated by the presence of another infection. Protection from HIV infection includes wearing gloves before touching mucous membranes and blood or other body fluids. Needles should not be broken or recapped; rather, the syringe and needle should be placed in a puncture-resistant container. Handwashing is the foundation of infection control. (I, T, L)

69. 4. A common sign of methadone toxicity is respiratory depression. Fever, colitis, and renal shutdown are not associated with methadone toxicity. (A, T, L)

70. 3. Methadone is equally effective at low or high

doses. The danger is that clients may take small doses and sell the excess to drug abusers. (E, N, L)

71. 3. The best way to keep methadone out of the illicit drug market is to administer the liquid form under direct supervision. (I, T, L)

72. 1. Calling Narcotics Anonymous to tell them to expect the client is inappropriate and unnecessary because it increases the client's dependency on the nurse. It is the client's responsibility to make arrangements for attending meetings. Enforcing unit policies and confronting inappropriate behaviors like manipulation and use of defense mechanisms such as projection are part of the nurse's role in drug rehabilitation. Helping the client to express feelings appropriately through the use of assertiveness techniques teaches the client appropriate interpersonal skills. (I, T, L)

73. 1. Narcotics Anonymous suggests that a person plan only one day at a time. It is too frightening and unrealistic for the client to agree to be clean of drugs at Narcotics Anonymous meetings and to abstain from drugs the rest of his life. Members do not have to commit a certain amount of time to the organization, although members free of drug use for a certain period often voluntarily work with the organization. (I, T, L)

74. 2. The best judgment concerning progress is based on the number of drug-free days the client has. The longer one is free of drugs, the better the prognosis. The kinds of friends the client has, the way he gets along with parents, and the degree of responsibility his job requires could influence his success, but judgments concerning success are best based on the number of days that he is drug free. (D, N, L)

75. 4. The heroin addict is least likely to develop cholelithiasis as a result of drug abuse. Drug addicts are prone to such disorders as hepatitis, pneumonia, and tuberculosis, primarily owing to poor sanitation and an unhealthful lifestyle. (D, C, L)

The Client With a Sedative-, Hypnotic-, or Anxiolytic-Related Disorder

76. 4. The most likely cause of death from barbiturate overdose is respiratory failure. Cardiac arrest is not common. Circulatory depression may occur. (D, N, L)

77. 4. When a friend asks if a seriously ill client will live, it is best for the nurse to respond by explaining the seriousness of the client's condition and acknowledging the friend's concern. This type of comment does not offer false hope. It is stereotypical to say that one can only wait and see if the client dies, while offering no support. By asking the friend to describe his relationship with the client, the nurse

is not focusing on the problem. Simply to say that the client is very ill and may not live is harsh and nonsupportive. (I, T, L)

78. 1. In this situation, the nurse should focus on the client and her needs for support. The nurse inquires about the relationship between the friend and the client to learn whether the friend is a source of support for the client. The focus of attention at this time is not centered on the seriousness of the client's condition. It is irrelevant at this time to attempt to learn whether the relationship may be a factor in the client's suicide attempt and whether the friend can be trusted with confidential information. (A, N, L)

79. 1. *Tolerance* for a drug occurs when a client requires increasingly large doses to obtain the desired effect. *Addiction* is the highest degree of physical and psychological dependence, and withdrawal is accompanied by severe physical symptoms. Drug *dependence* occurs when the person cannot keep drug intake under control and finds it hard to function without its effects. *Habituation* is defined as a mild degree of dependence. (D, T, L)

80. 2. Typical signs and symptoms of barbiturate abuse include sluggishness, difficulty walking, and irritability. Judgment and understanding are impaired, and speech is slurred and confused. The client acts drunk as from alcohol but does not have the odor of alcohol on her breath. (A, C, L)

81. 3. For the client who is confused when she begins to awaken after taking a large dose of barbiturates, the nurse should plan to maintain seizure precautions, close windows, and speak to her in short, complete sentences. Giving a medication for anxiety and agitation would be inappropriate because it could add to the depressant effects of the barbiturates that the client took. (I, N, L)

82. 2. Generalized convulsions may occur on the second or third day of withdrawal from barbiturates. Without treatment, as described in this item, the convulsions may be fatal. Postural hypotension and psychoses are possibilities but are unlikely to be fatal; they are unrelated to the pentobarbital sodium regimen. Hyperthermia, rather than hypothermia, occurs during withdrawal. (D, C, L)

83. 2. The nurse would give the highest priority to the nursing diagnosis Potential for Self-Directed Violence. Self-Esteem Disturbance, Ineffective Individual Coping, and Sleep Pattern Disturbance are all possible nursing diagnoses but not as important as the client's suicide attempt. (D, N, L)

84. 1. The most appropriate short-term goal is for the client to discuss feelings related to her losses. The nurse would help the client identify and verbalize her feelings instead of turning them inward or internalizing them. (P, N, L)

85. 4. This situation points out how a group of clients can have an undesirable influence on another client. It would probably be best for a nurse who becomes aware of such a situation to discuss her observations with the group at one of their regular therapy sessions. The problem involves all of the clients in the group, and discussing it with them gives all members an opportunity to offer suggestions. It will likely be futile to try to break up the group's drug-oriented discussions. Providing additional recreation and speaking to clients on an individual basis do not approach the problem in a direct manner. (I, T, L)

86. 1. The nurse instructs the client to continue taking prazepam (Centrax) as prescribed to ensure a safe, slow tapering and withdrawal from diazepam (Valium). The length of time a substance has been taken and the higher the dosages used, the more likely the occurrence of severe symptoms of withdrawal. For substances that have a longer half-life, like diazepam, withdrawal symptoms peak in the second week of withdrawal. (I, T, G)

87. 2. To respond accurately and responsibly to the client's needs, the nurse would tell the client to come to the clinic immediately, where further physiologic and mental status examinations can take place. There could be many causes for the client's increased anxiety and call for help. (I, T, L)

The Client With an Eating Disorder

88. 4. The nurse would want to hear more about the client's feelings to assess for potential underlying causes of the eating disorder and to assess the overeating as a maladaptive response. Telling the client that all the group members feel the same, to not worry because she'll be back in shape soon, or that she doesn't look so bad minimizes and ignores the client's feelings and focuses on the weight problem. (I, T, L)

89. 4. A member of the group is assuming a functional role when she proposes an alternate task to keep from thinking about food. She acts in the role of a contributor to the group. Showing pictures of children, insisting that everyone try a favorite reducing diet, and making comments to another group member are examples of individual role behavior that are irrelevant to the group task. Showing pictures of one's child in a group is an example of a "blocker." The person who insists that everyone try her recipe is a special-interest pleader. The person making comments to another group member is withdrawing from the group. (A, N, L)

90. 1. Through the ages, communication has occurred around food. Honor is extended through food, and punishment is given by withholding food. Food is commonly recognized as giving comfort because it often serves this purpose during childhood. Hence, in our culture, food is often equated with love and affection. (D, C, L)

91. 2. Based on the data, the most appropriate nursing diagnosis is Self-Esteem Disturbance related to weight gain, as evidenced by withdrawal. (D, T, L)

92. 3. Telling the client who is withdrawn and an overeater to record what she eats throughout the day focuses her attention on her eating problem and will probably decrease her self-esteem and increase her withdrawal. It is more beneficial to invite the client to an informal craft activity where socialization can occur, which may have a positive effect on the client's self-esteem. Asking the dietitian to meet with the client and discussing overeating as a maladaptive response to stress are therapeutic in that the client can learn important information about nutrition and stress and coping. (I, T, L)

93. 4. Bradycardia, hypotension, and cold sensitivity reflect the slowed metabolism that occurs with severe weight loss. Tachycardia and hypertension reflect increased metabolic rate, which is inconsistent with anorexia nervosa. Hyperthyroidism and elevated serum potassium are atypical with anorexia. Vitamin C deficiency and anemia may occur, but they are not hallmark symptoms of the disorder. (A, C, L)

94. 3. The nursing diagnosis Altered Nutrition: Less Than Body Requirements receives the highest priority at this time. Self-starvation is life-threatening, and gradual weight gain is a priority. Self-Esteem Disturbance, Ineffective Individual Coping, and Body Image Disturbance may be applicable to the client with anorexia nervosa but are of less importance than self-starvation. (D, N, L)

95. 2. Behavioral programs involve rewards and punishments to elicit specific behavioral responses. Emotional support and listening are general interventions not specific to the program goal. Identifying problematic eating behaviors is a general intervention related to behavioral programs but is not specific to a behavioral program for weight gain. Hyperalimentation may be used as a last resort but is a physiologic, not a behavioral, intervention. Rapid weight gain is psychologically intolerable and physically dangerous for the client. (I, T, L)

96. 3. The primary goal with severe anorexia is to promote weight gain through behavior modification. This involves actively monitoring and interrupting undesirable behaviors, even against the client's protests. Waiting for the client to finish exercising may be polite but exacerbates weight loss as more calories are burned. Threatening future loss of privileges does not motivate a client who is in the middle of a compulsion. Active intervention is required to prevent continued weight loss. (I, T, L)

97. 1. The goal of hospitalization for anorexia is to stabilize the client's weight and facilitate entry into outpatient care. Weight gain in the hospital may not be sustained unless the client receives follow-up help for the underlying problem. Most clients do not achieve a normal weight in the hospital and require continued follow-up. The urge to diet can continue for years after hospitalization. A change in eating behaviors does not address the central issue of dangerous weight loss and psychiatric disturbance. (E, N, L)

98. 2. The nurse acknowledges the client's perception and does not challenge the client and her expression of feeling. Telling the client that purging and the use of laxatives are harmful behaviors is honest and accurate information. Stating, "Your parents told the physician that you do have a problem," places blame on the parents for the client's hospitalization, which may foster angry feelings in the client. Stating, "We'll find out if you have a problem while you're here," is trite and instills blame toward the client for not being perfect and guilt for being less than perfect. It also belittles the client. (I, T, L)

99. 1. The nurse will use the therapeutic intervention of observing the client for 2 hours after each meal to decrease purging behaviors. Instituting a one-to-one observation for 24 hours is not necessary in this situation. Telling the client that an extra snack will be needed after purging is abusive and punishes the client. (P, T, G)

100. 3. The client's request for her drawing supplies is a positive step because the client is showing interest in an area of her life that has probably been neglected. The client's action promotes self-esteem, increases feelings of control, and minimizes dysfunctional behaviors. (E, N, L)

THE NURSING CARE OF CLIENTS WITH PSYCHIATRIC DISORDERS AND MENTAL HEALTH PROBLEMS

TEST 3: Personality Disorders, Substance-Related Disorders, and Eating Disorders

Directions: Use this answer grid to determine areas of strength or need for further study.

NURSING PROCESS

A = Assessment
D = Analysis, nursing diagnosis
P = Planning
I = Implementation
E = Evaluation

COGNITIVE LEVEL

K = Knowledge
C = Comprehension
T = Application
N = Analysis

CLIENT NEEDS

S = Safe, effective care environment
G = Physiologic integrity
L = Psychosocial integrity
H = Health promotion and maintenance

Question #	Answer #	A	D	P	I	E	K	C	T	N	S	G	L	H
1	2					E				N			L	
2	4			P						N			L	
3	1		D							N			L	
4	3			P					T				L	
5	2			P						N			L	
6	1				I				T				L	
7	3				I				T				L	
8	2					E				N			L	
9	1		D							N			L	
10	3					E				N			L	
11	4		D							N			L	
12	2		D					C					L	
13	1			P					T				L	
14	4		D							N			L	
15	4				I				T				L	
16	4	A							T				L	
17	3				I				T				L	
18	1					E				N			L	
19	2					E				N			L	
20	1				I				T				L	
21	4				I				T				L	
22	1			P					T				L	
23	3			P					T				L	
24	1				I				T				L	

ANSWER GRID: 1

NURSING PROCESS

A = Assessment
D = Analysis, nursing diagnosis
P = Planning
I = Implementation
E = Evaluation

COGNITIVE LEVEL

K = Knowledge
C = Comprehension
T = Application
N = Analysis

CLIENT NEEDS

S = Safe, effective care environment
G = Physiologic integrity
L = Psychosocial integrity
H = Health promotion and maintenance

Question #	Answer #	A	D	P	I	E	K	C	T	N	S	G	L	H
25	2		D							N			L	
26	3					E				N			L	
27	2				I				T				L	
28	4				I				T				L	
29	4				I					N			L	
30	2		D						T				L	
31	2					E				N			L	
32	1					E				N			L	
33	2					E				N			L	
34	3				I					N			L	
35	1		D					C					L	
36	3				I				T				L	
37	4				I				T				L	
38	1					E				N			L	
39	2				I				T				L	
40	3				I				T				L	
41	4				I				T				L	
42	2			P				C					L	
43	2		D					C					L	
44	1					E				N			L	
45	3		D							N			L	
46	1				I					N			L	
47	2					E				N			L	
48	1		D					C					L	
49	3				I				T				L	
50	4		D					C					L	
51	1		D							N	S			
52	4				I				T			G		
53	2					E				N			L	
54	4					E				N			L	

NURSING PROCESS

A = Assessment
D = Analysis, nursing diagnosis
P = Planning
I = Implementation
E = Evaluation

COGNITIVE LEVEL

K = Knowledge
C = Comprehension
T = Application
N = Analysis

CLIENT NEEDS

S = Safe, effective care environment
G = Physiologic integrity
L = Psychosocial integrity
H = Health promotion and maintenance

Question #	Answer #	Nursing Process					Cognitive Level				Client Needs			
		A	D	P	I	E	K	C	T	N	S	G	L	H
55	1		D							N			L	
56	3			P					T				L	
57	3		D							N			L	
58	1			P					T				L	
59	3				I				T				L	
60	2				I				T				L	
61	4					E				N			L	
62	3	A								N			L	
63	2		D							N			L	
64	4				I				T				L	
65	4				I				T				L	
66	1	A						C					L	
67	2				I				T				L	
68	2				I				T				L	
69	4	A							T				L	
70	3					E				N			L	
71	3				I				T				L	
72	1				I				T				L	
73	1				I				T				L	
74	2		D							N			L	
75	4		D					C					L	
76	4		D							N			L	
77	4				I				T				L	
78	1	A								N			L	
79	1		D						T				L	
80	2	A						C					L	
81	3				I					N			L	
82	2		D					C					L	
83	2		D							N			L	
84	1			P						N			L	

ANSWER GRID: 3

NURSING PROCESS

A = Assessment
D = Analysis, nursing diagnosis
P = Planning
I = Implementation
E = Evaluation

COGNITIVE LEVEL

K = Knowledge
C = Comprehension
T = Application
N = Analysis

CLIENT NEEDS

S = Safe, effective care environment
G = Physiologic integrity
L = Psychosocial integrity
H = Health promotion and maintenance

Question #	Answer #	Nursing Process					Cognitive Level				Client Needs			
		A	D	P	I	E	K	C	T	N	S	G	L	H
85	4				I				T				L	
86	1				I				T			G		
87	2				I				T				L	
88	4				I				T				L	
89	4	A								N			L	
90	1		D					C					L	
91	2		D						T				L	
92	3				I				T				L	
93	4	A						C					L	
94	3		D							N			L	
95	2				I				T				L	
96	3				I				T				L	
97	1					E				N			L	
98	2				I				T				L	
99	1			P					T			G		
100	3					E				N			L	
Number Correct														
Number Possible	100	8	25	11	38	18	0	12	46	42	1	3	96	0
Percentage Correct														

Score Calculation: To determine your **Percentage Correct,** divide the **Number Correct** by the **Number Possible.**

ANSWER GRID: 4

Anxiety, Anger, Abuse, and Terminal Illness

- The Client With an Anxiety Disorder
- The Client With an Obsessive-Compulsive Disorder
- The Client With a Somatoform Disorder
- The Client With Problems Expressing Anger
- The Client With Family Abuse and Violence
- The Client With a Psychophysiologic Disorder
- The Client With a Terminal Illness
- Correct Answers and Rationale

Select the one best answer, and indicate your choice by filling in the circle in front of the option.

The Client With an Anxiety Disorder

A client is brought to the hospital emergency room by his brother. The client is perspiring profusely, breathing rapidly, and complaining of dizziness and palpitations. Problems of a cardiovascular nature are ruled out. The client's diagnosis is tentatively listed as Panic Attack.

1. The emergency room nurse observes that the client is hyperventilating. Which of the following measures would be best to try first to ease the symptoms caused by hyperventilation?
   - ○ 1. Have the client breathe into a paper bag.
   - ○ 2. Instruct the client to put his head between his knees.
   - ○ 3. Give the client a low concentration of oxygen by nasal cannula.
   - ○ 4. Tell the client to take several deep, slow breaths and exhale normally.
2. Which of the following nursing actions would be inappropriate on the client's admission to the unit?
   - ○ 1. Support the client's attempts to discuss feelings.
   - ○ 2. Respect the client's personal space.
   - ○ 3. Reassure the client of his safety.
   - ○ 4. Confront the client's dysfunctional coping behaviors.
3. The client often jumps when spoken to and complains of feeling uneasy. He says, "It's as though something bad is going to happen." Which of the

following nursing actions would be of least benefit to the client?
   - ○ 1. Being physically present.
   - ○ 2. Being technically competent.
   - ○ 3. Conveying optimistic verbalizations.
   - ○ 4. Communicating a respectful attitude.
4. During a conversation with the client, the nurse observes the client shaking his leg and tapping his fingers on the table next to him. The nurse's best statement is,
   - ○ 1. "I see that you're anxious. I'll be back later when you're calmer."
   - ○ 2. "I noticed that your leg is shaking and you're tapping your fingers on the table. How are you feeling now?"
   - ○ 3. "I'll get you something to help you feel less anxious."
   - ○ 4. "I know that you feel anxious. Let's discuss something more pleasant."
5. The nursing diagnosis for the client is Social Isolation related to severe anxiety, as evidenced by withdrawal into his room. An appropriate long-term goal related to this nursing diagnosis is that the client will
   - ○ 1. attend group meetings with a staff member by discharge.
   - ○ 2. initiate interactions with the nurse when feeling anxious.
   - ○ 3. express two adaptive methods of coping with anxiety.
   - ○ 4. participate in milieu activities by discharge.

6. In working with the client with an anxiety disorder, the ultimate nursing goal is to
   ○ 1. reduce the client's anxiety to a manageable level.
   ○ 2. help the client decrease denial and avoidance about his feelings and link feelings with behaviors.
   ○ 3. assist the client with problem solving and developing adaptive coping behaviors.
   ○ 4. use supportive confrontation when the client avoids painful issues.

7. The client seldom experiences feelings of panic and has been participating in groups. He tells the nurse, "I still have problems falling asleep without tossing and turning." Of the following nursing actions, which would be most helpful to the client?
   ○ 1. Teach him relaxation exercises.
   ○ 2. Tell him to ask his physician for medication.
   ○ 3. Recommend that he watch television until he gets sleepy.
   ○ 4. Advise him to ride the exercise bicycle for 10 minutes before retiring for the night.

8. The client is taking alprazolam (Xanax) to treat moderate to severe anxiety. Xanax will help the client to
   ○ 1. focus less on somatic symptoms of anxiety.
   ○ 2. deny problems with symptoms of anxiety.
   ○ 3. avoid feelings of anxiety.
   ○ 4. maintain hypersensitivity to stimuli.

9. While the client is taking alprazolam (Xanax), he should be taught to avoid ingesting
   ○ 1. chocolate.
   ○ 2. cheese.
   ○ 3. alcohol.
   ○ 4. shellfish.

The nurse works at a community mental health center.

10. The client with an Axis I diagnosis of Post-Traumatic Stress Disorder tells the nurse he wishes that he had been on the airplane that crashed and killed his wife and children a month ago. The nurse assesses the client's statement to be
    ○ 1. suicidal ideation
    ○ 2. survivor guilt.
    ○ 3. dysfunctional grieving.
    ○ 4. numbing of responsiveness.

11. The client states, "You don't know what I've been through. What can you do?" The nurse's best response is
    ○ 1. "I need to refer you to a survivor's group where you'll feel more comfortable."

○ 2. "Perhaps you'll feel better if you can become interested in a hobby once again."
   ○ 3. "I'd like to help you if you'll let me."
   ○ 4. "I haven't been through what you have, but I'll be better able to understand if you tell me more about it."

12. The client has been taking buspirone (BuSpar) for 2 days as prescribed. Which client statement indicates a need for further teaching?
    ○ 1. "I can take BuSpar as I need it when I'm anxious."
    ○ 2. "I may not feel better for 7 to 10 days."
    ○ 3. "I can't become physically dependent on BuSpar."
    ○ 4. "I need to take BuSpar with food."

A week ago, a tornado destroyed the client's home and seriously injured her husband. The client has been walking around the hospital in a daze without any outward display of emotions.

13. The client is being admitted to the stress unit with the diagnosis of Acute Stress Disorder. The client tells the nurse in a matter-of-fact manner that her husband is paraplegic, "but that's better than total paralysis." Which protective mechanism is the client exhibiting?
    ○ 1. Suppression.
    ○ 2. Rationalization.
    ○ 3. Denial.
    ○ 4. Intellectualization.

14. The client tells the nurse she feels like she's going crazy. The nurse initially
    ○ 1. explains the effects of stress on the mind and body.
    ○ 2. assures the client her feelings and behaviors are typical reactions to serious trauma.
    ○ 3. reassures the client that her symptoms are temporary.
    ○ 4. acknowledges the unfairness of the client's situation.

15. On discharge, the client is referred to the outpatient clinic for follow-up. Which of the following hospital-learned abilities is probably most important for the continued alleviation of anxiety symptoms? The client
    ○ 1. recognizes when she is feeling anxious.
    ○ 2. understands the reasons for her anxiety.
    ○ 3. can use methods to reduce anxiety.
    ○ 4. can describe the situations preceding her feelings of anxiety.

The Client With an Obsessive-Compulsive Disorder

The client arrives late for an appointment with the nurse at the outpatient clinic. During the interview, he fidgets restlessly, has trouble remembering what topic is being discussed, and says he thinks he is going crazy.

16. Which of the following statements by the nurse would best deal with the client's feelings about "going crazy"?
   ○ 1. "I see that this concerns you, but what does 'crazy' mean to you?"
   ○ 2. "Most people feel that way occasionally. You're no different from anyone else."
   ○ 3. "I don't know enough about you to judge. Why don't you tell me more about yourself?"
   ○ 4. "You sound perfectly sane to me. Maybe your perception of the word 'crazy' is different from mine."

17. The client reveals that he was late for his appointment because of "my dumb habit. I have to take off my socks and put them back on 41 times! I can't stop until I do it just right." The nurse judges correctly that the client's behavior most likely represents an effort to
   ○ 1. relieve his anxiety.
   ○ 2. control his thoughts.
   ○ 3. gain attention from others.
   ○ 4. express hostility.

18. A decision is made not to hospitalize the client. Of the following abilities the client has demonstrated, the one that probably most influenced the decision not to hospitalize him is his ability to
   ○ 1. hold a job.
   ○ 2. relate to his peers.
   ○ 3. perform activities of daily living.
   ○ 4. behave in an outwardly normal manner.

The nurse works at a psychiatric day-care facility.

19. The client with obsessive-compulsive disorder eats slowly and is always the last to finish lunch, which makes it difficult for the group to start a 1 PM outing. Which of the following approaches would be the best plan of action for this problem?
   ○ 1. Change the time of the outing to accommodate the client.
   ○ 2. Arrange for the client to start eating earlier than the others.
   ○ 3. Plan to go without the client so that he will have ample time for his lunch.
   ○ 4. Inform the client that he will have to eat faster so that the group can leave on time.

20. The client wants to take up a hobby and asks the day-care nurse for some suggestions. From a therapeutic standpoint, which of the following activities would be the most desirable for the client?
   ○ 1. Swimming.
   ○ 2. Solo flying.
   ○ 3. Drama club.
   ○ 4. Photography.

A client tells the nurse that he checks all lights to be sure they are off 26 times before he can leave his house. He knows his behavior is senseless but he can't stop. He rarely sees his friends anymore because they are fed up with his being late every time they plan to get together. Besides, he "really is too busy to see them" because of "all the things going on at work."

21. Which of the following nursing diagnoses would be least appropriate for this client?
   ○ 1. Fear.
   ○ 2. Diversional Activity Deficit.
   ○ 3. Social Isolation.
   ○ 4. Powerlessness.

22. In considering the client's immediate needs, which of the following client outcomes is unrealistic at this time? The client will
   ○ 1. increase expression of feelings.
   ○ 2. connect feelings with behavior.
   ○ 3. use two adaptive coping behaviors to deal with anxiety.
   ○ 4. make a decision about one of his problems.

23. The client reports that before he leaves home to go anywhere, he counts the money in his wallet as many as 12 times. The best explanation for the client's motives when performing this particular ritual is that he is attempting to
   ○ 1. channel excessive sexual energy into an appropriate habit.
   ○ 2. compensate for not having enough money to spend as a child.
   ○ 3. avoid the embarrassment of having a shortage of funds on hand.
   ○ 4. channel emotions unacceptable to him with an acceptable activity.

24. Which of the following actions would be best for the nurse to take when the nurse observes the client in a ritualistic pattern of behavior?

○ 1. Isolate the client so that he will not disturb others.
○ 2. Observe the client closely for marked changes in behavior.
○ 3. Remind the client that he can control his behavior if he wishes.
○ 4. Enable the client to continue so that he will not become more agitated.

25. Which of the following qualities is most important for the nurse interacting with obsessive-compulsive clients?
○ 1. Patience.
○ 2. Compassion.
○ 3. Friendliness.
○ 4. Self-confidence.

26. The client has been taking clomipramine (Anafranil) for his obsessive-compulsive disorder. He tells the nurse, "I'm not really better, and I've been taking the medication faithfully for the past week just like it says on this prescription bottle." Which of the following actions would the nurse do first?
○ 1. Tell the client to stop taking the medication, and call the physician.
○ 2. Tell the client to continue taking the medication as prescribed because it takes 5 to 10 weeks for a full therapeutic effect.
○ 3. Encourage the client to call his physician in 1 week and to continue taking his medication.
○ 4. Ask the client if he has resumed smoking cigarettes.

27. Which of the following methods of treatment would initially be least helpful to a client with obsessive-compulsive disorder?
○ 1. Relaxation exercises.
○ 2. Thought stopping.
○ 3. Meditation.
○ 4. Exposure therapy.

The Client With a Somatoform Disorder

The client with an Axis I diagnosis of Pain Disorder is angry and demanding and focuses on the head pain she's experiencing.

28. At 11 AM, the client demands that the nurse call the physician for more pain medication because she's still in pain after the 9 AM analgesic. The best nursing action is to
○ 1. call the physician as the client requests.

○ 2. suggest the client lie down because she has to wait 4 hours for the next dosage.
○ 3. inform the client that the physician will be in later and to talk to her about it.
○ 4. inform the client that the nurse cannot give her additional medication at this time, and invite the client to participate in a card game.

29. A nursing diagnosis for the client with Pain Disorder is Anxiety: severe secondary to dependency as evidenced by inability to care for self. The nurse will support the client to do as much self-care as she can. The purpose of the nurse's action is to
○ 1. maintain secondary gain.
○ 2. decrease secondary gain.
○ 3. increase primary gain.
○ 4. ignore primary gain.

30. The nursing assistant tells the nurse that the client is not in the dining room for lunch. The nurse instructs the nursing assistant to
○ 1. take the client a lunch tray, and have the client eat in her room.
○ 2. tell the client she'll need to wait until supper to eat if she misses lunch.
○ 3. invite the client to lunch, and accompany her to the dining room.
○ 4. inform the client she has 10 minutes to get to the dining room for lunch.

The client with Conversion Disorder has a paralyzed arm.

31. While assisting the client with self-care, which of the following approaches would the nurse employ? The nurse would
○ 1. use a matter-of-fact, caring attitude.
○ 2. use a strong confrontational approach.
○ 3. interact minimally with the client.
○ 4. ignore the client's negative comments.

32. A nurse states, "I would just tell the client her arm is paralyzed because she had an affair and neglected her baby's care to the point where the baby had to be hospitalized for dehydration." Which of the following statements by the head nurse is best?
○ 1. "Ignore the client's behaviors and treat her with respect."
○ 2. "Pushing insight will increase the client's anxiety and the need for physical symptoms."
○ 3. "Pushing awareness will be helpful and further the client's recovery."
○ 4. "We'll meet with the client and confront her with her behavior."

The nurse works in an outpatient clinic at the community hospital.

33. The physician refers a client with Somatization Disorder to the clinic because of problems with nausea. The client tells the nurse that the nausea began when his wife asked him for a divorce. The nurse
○ 1. asks the client to describe his problem with nausea.
○ 2. directs the client to describe his feelings about his impending divorce.
○ 3. allows the client to talk about the many physicians he has seen and the medications he has taken.
○ 4. informs the client about a new medication for nausea.

34. Which of the following treatment modalities would be least helpful for the client?
○ 1. Outpatient group psychotherapy.
○ 2. Individual therapy.
○ 3. Relaxation exercises.
○ 4. Assertiveness training.

The Client With Problems Expressing Anger

A client is admitted to the psychiatric hospital for evaluation after numerous incidents of threatening, angry outbursts and two episodes of hitting a coworker at the grocery store where he works. The client is very anxious and tells the nurse who admits him, "I didn't mean to hit him. He made me so mad that I just couldn't help it. I hope I don't hit anyone here."

35. Which of the following responses by the nurse is best?
○ 1. "You'd better not hit anyone here, even if you do get mad."
○ 2. "Tell me more about what happened."
○ 3. "It sounds like you were angry. When you feel angry here, talk to the staff about it instead of hitting."
○ 4. "I'm sure you didn't mean to hit him and that it won't happen here."

36. Which of the following is the most important initial action the nurse should take to ensure a safe environment?
○ 1. Let other clients know that he has a history of hitting others so that they will not provoke him.
○ 2. Put him in a private room and limit his time out of the room to when staff can be with him.
○ 3. Tell him that hitting others is not acceptable behavior, and ask him to let a staff member know when he begins feeling angry so they can talk.
○ 4. Obtain an order for a medication to decrease his anxiety.

37. The client rushes out of the day room, where he has been watching television with other clients. He is hyperventilating, flushed, and his fists are clenched. He states to the nurse, "That bastard! He's just like Tom. I almost hit him." Which of the following would be the nurse's best response?
○ 1. "You're angry and you did well to leave the situation. Let's walk up and down the hall while you tell me about it."
○ 2. "Even if you're angry, you can't use that language here."
○ 3. "I'm glad you left the situation. Why don't you go to your room and calm down. I'll come in soon to talk."
○ 4. "I can see you're angry. Let me get you some Ativan to help you calm down. Then we'll talk about what happened."

38. Based on the client's potential for violence toward others and inability to cope with anger, which short-term goal would be most helpful? The client will
○ 1. acknowledge his angry feelings.
○ 2. describe situations that provoke angry feelings.
○ 3. list how he's handled his anger in the past.
○ 4. verbalize his feelings in an appropriate manner.

39. In developing a nursing care plan for the client, the staff decides to take an educational approach. Which of the following steps would be least helpful?
○ 1. assisting the client to recognize anger.
○ 2. identifying all the important people in the client's life with whom he is angry.
○ 3. identifying alternative ways to express anger.
○ 4. practicing expressing anger.

40. In talking about discharge with his nurse, the client says, "It's been easy not to get mad and hit people here because the staff won't let me. It's not the same at work." What would be the nurse's most effective response?
○ 1. "We have helped, but you're the one who decided not to hit when you were angry. You can do that at work, too."
○ 2. "Lots of people feel this way. You're just worried about leaving the hospital. You've learned so much that you won't have any problems at work."
○ 3. "You sound worried about going back to work. The things you've learned here can help at work, too. Let's talk about what you learned and how you can use it."
○ 4. "It's hard to leave the hospital, but you're better and need to get back to work. You'll be okay, I know."

The client is admitted to the hospital because of threatening, aggressive behavior toward his family.

41. Which of the following factors is most important for the nurse to consider when assessing the angry client's potential for violence?
    ○ 1. The time of day and level of activity on the unit.
    ○ 2. The attitude of the staff toward the angry client.
    ○ 3. The staff-to-client ratio.
    ○ 4. The client's past history of violent behavior.

42. In the first group meeting after the client is admitted, another client sits near the nurse and says loudly, "I'm sitting here because I'm afraid of Ted. He's so big, and I heard him talk about hitting people." Which of the following responses by the nurse would be the most therapeutic?
    ○ 1. "Everyone is here for different problems. You know you don't have to worry. We'll keep you safe."
    ○ 2. "Ted is new to the group. Since he doesn't know anyone here, let's go around and introduce ourselves."
    ○ 3. "You don't know Ted yet. Once you get to know him, I'm sure you won't be afraid."
    ○ 4. "It can be frightening to have new people on the unit. The purpose of this group is for people to get to know each other so we can talk together about things like being afraid."

43. A female client in the group states, "My doctor tells me I need to get mad more and not let people tell me what to do. Maybe she thinks I should be more like Ted." To respond appropriately to this client, it is most important that the nurse understand that
    ○ 1. denial of anger and the inability to be assertive can be as serious a problem as the aggressive expression of anger.
    ○ 2. it is appropriate for the client to deny her anger because assertive behavior in women is not culturally acceptable.
    ○ 3. because clients frequently distort what they are told by physicians, it is unlikely that the client has been told what she reports.
    ○ 4. because both clients are about the same age, the female client is trying to help Ted feel accepted by the group.

44. The client's face is flushed, and he is swearing, yelling, and pushing chairs around in the milieu. The nurse judges the client to be in which phase of the assault cycle?
    ○ 1. Triggering.
    ○ 2. Escalation.
    ○ 3. Crisis.
    ○ 4. Aggressive.

45. The client loses self-control and throws chairs against the wall. The nurse would
    ○ 1. ask the client to go to the quiet area to talk about his behavior.
    ○ 2. direct the client to the quiet room, give an oral tranquilizer, prepare for a show of determination.
    ○ 3. process the incident with the client and discuss alternative behaviors.
    ○ 4. use involuntary seclusion, restraints, or an intramuscular tranquilizer.

46. The nurse judges that the client is ready to be released from seclusion and restraints when the client
    ○ 1. is adequately sedated.
    ○ 2. struggles less against the restraints.
    ○ 3. stops swearing and yelling.
    ○ 4. shows signs of self-control.

47. The treatment team recommends that the client take an assertiveness training course offered in the hospital. Which of the following behaviors indicates that the client is becoming more assertive?
    ○ 1. He begins to arrive late for unit activities.
    ○ 2. He asks the nurse to call his employer about his insurance.
    ○ 3. He tells his roommate that dirty clothing on the floor bothers him and asks him to put them away.
    ○ 4. He follows the nurse's advice and asks his doctor about being passive-aggressive.

48. Which of the following physiologic responses would be least likely to occur when a client is angry?
    ○ 1. Increased respiratory rate.
    ○ 2. Decreased blood pressure.
    ○ 3. Increased muscle tension.
    ○ 4. Decreased peristalsis.

49. Which of the following psychological responses to anger is least common in psychiatric clients?
    ○ 1. Decreased self-esteem.
    ○ 2. Feelings of invulnerability.
    ○ 3. Fear of retaliation.
    ○ 4. Feelings of guilt.

50. Indirect expression of anger is more common than direct expression. Which of the following client behaviors is most likely to be an indirect expression of anger?
    ○ 1. Responding sarcastically to an invitation to join a unit activity.
    ○ 2. Refusing to take medication.
    ○ 3. Cursing at the physician.
    ○ 4. Shouting at another client.

The Client With Family Abuse and Violence

The client, a married homemaker, has been referred to the mental health center because she is depressed.

51. Seeing the client for the first time, the nurse notices bruises on her upper arms and asks about them. After denying any problems, the client starts to cry

and says, "He didn't really mean to hurt me, but I hate the kids to see. I'm so worried about them." During the interview, it would be most important for the nurse to determine

  ○ 1. the type and extent of abuse in the family.

  ○ 2. the potential of immediate danger to the client and her children.

  ○ 3. the resources available to the client.

  ○ 4. whether the client wants to be separated from her husband.

52. The client describes her husband as a good man who works hard and provides well for his family. She does not work outside the home and states that she is proud to be a wife and mother just like her own mother. The family pattern that the client describes best illustrates which characteristic of abusive families?

  ○ 1. Tight, impermeable boundaries.

  ○ 2. Unbalanced power ratio.

  ○ 3. Role stereotyping.

  ○ 4. Dysfunctional feeling tone.

53. The client agrees to meet with the nurse the following week. Before the nurse terminates the meeting with the client, which nursing action is most important?

  ○ 1. Give the client the telephone numbers of a shelter or a safe house and the crisis line.

  ○ 2. Advise the client to leave her husband.

  ○ 3. Tell the client not to do anything that could upset her husband.

  ○ 4. Ask the client what she could do to de-escalate the situation at home.

54. As the nurse learns more about the client and her family, which of the following characteristics is the nurse least likely to find to be true about the abuser?

  ○ 1. Between episodes of abuse, he has a warm, empathetic relationship with his wife.

  ○ 2. He grew up in an abusive family.

  ○ 3. He is a college graduate and has a stable work history.

  ○ 4. He abuses alcohol.

55. In planning care for the client, which of the following measures would be least helpful?

  ○ 1. Being compassionate and empathetic.

  ○ 2. Teaching the client about abuse and the cycle of violence.

  ○ 3. Explaining to the client her personal and legal rights.

  ○ 4. Sharing feelings of frustration with the client.

56. The nurse discusses the client and her family in a staff meeting. Which of the following statements made by other staff members is likely to be most helpful to the nurse in developing a treatment plan?

  ○ 1. "This client sounds like a lot of women I know

who don't want to change. You can try family therapy, if the husband will come."

  ○ 2. "Have you thought about suggesting that she attend the group for women in abusive families?"

  ○ 3. "I think the police should be notified in case he hits her again and she wants to call them."

  ○ 4. "Have you thought about calling the client's mother to find out what she knows about the family?"

57. In assessing the client's methods of coping, which method would the nurse least expect to find her using?

  ○ 1. Assertiveness.

  ○ 2. Self-blame.

  ○ 3. Alcohol abuse.

  ○ 4. Suicidal thoughts.

58. During the third session with the nurse, the client states, "I don't know what to do anymore. He doesn't want me to go anywhere while he's at work, not even to visit my friends." Which of the following nursing diagnoses would the nurse formulate in respect to this information?

  ○ 1. Violence related to abusive husband, as evidenced by victim's statement of being battered.

  ○ 2. Self-Esteem Disturbance related to victimization, as evidenced by not being able to leave the house.

  ○ 3. Powerlessness related to abusive husband, as evidenced by inability to make decisions.

  ○ 4. Ineffective Individual Coping related to victimization, as evidenced by crying.

59. As the nurse develops a treatment plan for the client, which of the following factors would be least important to consider?

  ○ 1. The abuser's refusal to be involved in treatment.

  ○ 2. The client's coping skills.

  ○ 3. The recent promotion of the client's husband.

  ○ 4. The birthday party for the client's child next week.

60. The client tells the nurse that her 8-year-old daughter refuses to go to school because she is afraid her mother will not be home when she returns. Which of the following is the most therapeutic response for the nurse to make?

  ○ 1. "She must be feeling insecure right now. Let her stay home with you for a few days to reassure her."

  ○ 2. "Children often feel responsible for trouble in the family. Have you talked with her about what she's afraid might happen?"

  ○ 3. "You know she's too young to be home alone after school. If you can't be there, you should find someone else to meet her so she won't be afraid."

  ○ 4. "She's aware of the trouble in the family and is worried about what might happen. Would you like to have her talk to the child therapist here? I think it would be helpful."

61. After months of treatment, the client tells the nurse that she has decided to stop treatment. There has been no abuse during this time, and she feels better able to cope with the needs of her husband and children. In discussing this decision with the client, it would be most important for the nurse to
   ○ 1. tell the client that this is a bad decision that she will regret.
   ○ 2. find out more about the client's decision.
   ○ 3. warn the client that abuse often stops when one partner is in treatment, only to begin again later.
   ○ 4. remind the client of her duty to protect the children by continuing treatment.

A third-grade child is referred to the mental health clinic by the school nurse because he is fearful, anxious, and socially isolated.

62. After meeting with the client, the nurse talks with his mother, who says, "It's that school nurse again. She's done nothing but try to make trouble for our family since my son started school. And now you're in on it." Which of the following responses by the nurse is least likely to help her develop a relationship with this family?
   ○ 1. "The school nurse is concerned about your son and is only doing her job. Does this bother you?"
   ○ 2. "We see a number of children who go to your son's school. He isn't the only one, if you're worried about that."
   ○ 3. "You sound pretty angry with the school nurse. Can you tell me what has happened?"
   ○ 4. "It sounds like you've had some bad experiences with the school. Let me tell you why your son was referred, and then you can tell me about your concerns."

63. The client's mother tells the nurse that last year was a very bad time for the family. Her husband was unemployed, and she worked a second job to help. Twice during the year, she slapped her son repeatedly when he refused to obey. She says it has not happened again and that the family is "back to normal." After assessing the family, the nurse decides that the child is not at risk for abuse. Which of the following observations would least support this decision?
   ○ 1. The parents have a caring and supportive relationship.
   ○ 2. The client has not talked about violence during his visits.

○ 3. The infrequent episodes were limited to a time of intense family stress.
○ 4. The parents have a defensive attitude toward the school nurse.

The Client With a Psychophysiologic Disorder

A client is admitted to the hospital with a diagnosis of chronic ulcerative colitis. He reports frequent bouts of diarrhea that have caused him to lose 10 pounds in the last month.

64. Because this is the client's fourth admission to the hospital in the last 9 months, he is familiar to the nurse caring for him. Which of the following remarks by the nurse on admission would be most beneficial to the client?
   ○ 1. "It's nice to see you again. Did you get lonesome for us on the outside?"
   ○ 2. "I thought we had seen the last of you for a while. What are you doing back?"
   ○ 3. "It's been 2 months since you were last here. What do you think about being back in the hospital?"
   ○ 4. "I see you have your old room again. No need to explain things to you because you're such an old pro."

65. The client becomes tense and nauseated when he hears the cart containing meal trays approaching. Which of the following practices would be best to prevent the premeal buildup of tension that the client experiences?
   ○ 1. Reroute the meal cart so that the client will not be disturbed by it.
   ○ 2. Order a special early tray for the client to let him finish eating before the meal cart comes.
   ○ 3. Turn on the client's television or radio before meals to mask the noise of the approaching meal cart.
   ○ 4. Arrange for someone to keep the client engaged in a relaxing activity or conversation before mealtimes.

66. The client should be involved in suitable activities in his room while his illness is being treated. These activities should be chosen based on which of the following attributes?
   ○ 1. The activity is conducive to rest and relaxation.
   ○ 2. The activity enhances improvement of social skills.
   ○ 3. The activity includes insight and self-awareness experiences.
   ○ 4. The activity involves manual dexterity rather than intellectual processes.

67. The physician recommends that the client have a partial bowel resection and an ileostomy. Later, the client says to the nurse, "That doctor of mine surely likes to play big. I'll bet the more he can cut, the better he likes it." Which of the following replies by the nurse would be most therapeutic?

○ 1. "You sound upset. We can talk about it if you'd like."

○ 2. "What do you mean by that?"

○ 3. "Aren't you being a bit hard on him? He's trying to help you."

○ 4. "Does that remark have something to do with the operation he wants you to have, by any chance?"

68. The client becomes increasingly morose and irritable after thinking more about his physician's recommendations. He is rude to his visitors and pushes nurses away when they attempt to give him medications and treatments. Which of the following nursing interventions would be best when the client has a hostile outburst?

○ 1. Offer the client positive reinforcement each time he cooperates.

○ 2. Encourage the client to discuss his immediate concerns and feelings.

○ 3. Continue with the assigned tasks and duties as though nothing has happened.

○ 4. Encourage the client to direct his anger at staff members who can handle his angry outbursts.

69. Arrangements are made for a member of the ileostomy club to meet with the client. Which of the following aims illustrates the chief purpose for having a representative from the club visit the client preoperatively?

○ 1. To let the client know that he has resources in the community to help him.

○ 2. To provide support for the physician's plan of therapy for the client.

○ 3. To show the client support and provide realistic information on the ileostomy.

○ 4. To convince the client that he will not be disfigured and can lead a full life.

A client is transferred to the medical unit from intensive care after suffering a myocardial infarction 5 days ago.

70. The client states to the nurse, "My secretary should be here by now. I don't have time to lie around here and do nothing. I've never had time to relax, and I don't plan on starting now." Based on this initial information, which of the following nursing diagnoses would the nurse judge to be inappropriate?

○ 1. Ineffective Individual Coping.

○ 2. Knowledge Deficit.

○ 3. Powerlessness.

○ 4. Anxiety.

71. The client further states to the nurse, "Please hand me the telephone. I need to check on what's keeping my secretary. She should have been here 30 minutes ago." Which of the following responses by the nurse would be most therapeutic?

○ 1. "Perhaps she's delayed by traffic. Give her 15 more minutes."

○ 2. "You've just had a myocardial infarction. Let's talk about what that means."

○ 3. "You really don't care about the fact that you're sick, do you?"

○ 4. "Do you realize you've just had a myocardial infarction?"

72. The nurse would judge which client statement as a lack of understanding of his illness and ability to make changes in his lifestyle?

○ 1. "I told my secretary to bring my airline ticket to me before I'm discharged tomorrow so I don't miss my meeting."

○ 2. "These relaxation tapes sound okay; I'll see if they help me."

○ 3. "No more working 10 hours a day for me unless it's an emergency situation."

○ 4. "I talked with my wife yesterday about working on a new budget together."

73. The client refuses to eat lunch and rudely tells the nurse to get out of his room. What would be the nurse's best response?

○ 1. "I'll leave, but you need to eat."

○ 2. "I'll get you something for your pain."

○ 3. "Your anger doesn't bother me. I'll be back later."

○ 4. "You sound angry. What is upsetting you?"

74. The nurse correctly recognizes that an obstacle to the client's therapy is present when the client is

○ 1. closed off emotionally from others.

○ 2. highly intelligent and manipulative.

○ 3. prone to become dependent on the therapist.

○ 4. somewhat willing to tolerate the therapist's suggestions.

75. The most important distinction for the nurse to make between a psychophysiologic disorder, such as ulcerative colitis, and a somatoform disorder, such as conversion disorder, is that a psychophysiologic disorder may be

○ 1. consciously selected by the person.

○ 2. fatal to the person if left untreated.

○ 3. relieved when the mental conflict is arrested.

○ 4. handled by the person with a characteristic attitude of indifference.

76. Certain personality traits are often attributed to clients with ulcerative colitis. Based on this theory, which of the following traits should the nurse expect to see in a client with this disorder?

○ 1. Self-reliance.
○ 2. Decisiveness.
○ 3. Perfectionism.
○ 4. Ambitiousness.

77. One evening the client directs a stream of profanities at the nurse, then abruptly hangs his head and pleads, "Please forgive me. Something just came over me. Why do I say those things?" The nurse should judge that the client is exhibiting what behavior?

○ 1. Punning.
○ 2. Confabulation.
○ 3. Flight of ideas.
○ 4. Emotional lability.

A client with peptic ulcers takes little responsibility for her self-care.

78. To minimize secondary gains, the nurse would be least likely to include which of the following measures in this client's care plan?

○ 1. Giving the client simple choices.
○ 2. Having consistent expectations of what the client can do.
○ 3. Spending additional time with the client when she complains of body aches.
○ 4. Recognizing the client when she does something for herself.

79. The nurse correctly judges that the dynamics underlying the client's passivity regarding self-care center around

○ 1. the need to be perfect.
○ 2. identity problems.
○ 3. dependency needs.
○ 4. mistrust of the nurse's abilities.

80. Of the following possible effects of chronic invalidism on the client's family, the most detrimental to their interrelationships would most probably be that the illness may make family members feel

○ 1. guilty and dominated.
○ 2. put upon and overworked.
○ 3. superior and self-sufficient.
○ 4. sympathetic and concerned.

The Client With a Terminal Illness

The client, who is dying from acquired immunodeficiency syndrome (AIDS), is admitted to the inpatient psychiatric unit because he attempted suicide. His close friend recently died from AIDS.

81. The client states to the nurse, "What's the use of living? My time is running out." What is the nurse's best response?

○ 1. "Let's talk about making some good use of that time."
○ 2. "Don't give up. There could be a cure for AIDS tomorrow."
○ 3. "You're in a lot of pain. What are you feeling?"
○ 4. "Life is precious and worth living."

82. One of the staff members says to the nurse, "Why are we carrying out suicide precautions? It's pointless and a waste of time." The nurse should

○ 1. assign the staff member to other clients.
○ 2. ask the psychiatric clinical nurse specialist to meet with the staff member.
○ 3. agree with the staff member and discontinue suicide precautions.
○ 4. call for a multidisciplinary staff meeting.

83. The client begins to talk about his feelings related to his illness and the loss of his friend. He begins to cry. What would be the nurse's best response?

○ 1. Give the client some tissue, and tell him it is okay for him to cry.
○ 2. Tell the client to stop crying and that everything will be okay.
○ 3. Busy herself with sorting the client's mail.
○ 4. Change the subject.

84. One of the client's visitors tells the nurse, "I wish we would have taken that trip to Europe last year. We just kept putting it off, and now I'm furious that we didn't go." Which of the following stages of adaptation to dying is the client's friend most likely experiencing?

○ 1. Anger.
○ 2. Denial.
○ 3. Bargaining.
○ 4. Depression.

85. The nurse who usually is most effective when caring for the client and helping his friend deal with death is one who

○ 1. has contemplated her own death and mortality.
○ 2. attends continuing education classes on death and dying.
○ 3. can provide compassionate and physical care while remaining distant emotionally.
○ 4. views dying people as distinct populations of people in need of comfort.

86. Which of the following philosophies would most likely help the client and his family best cope during the final stages of the client's illness?

○ 1. Live each day as it comes as fully as possible.
○ 2. Relive the pleasant memories of days gone by.
○ 3. Expect the worst and be grateful when it does not happen.
○ 4. Plan ahead for the remaining good times that will be spent together.

A 13-year-old boy is admitted to the hospital for the third time. His illness is diagnosed as acute lymphatic leukemia. The liaison psychiatric nurse is asked by the team leader to help the nursing staff work more effectively with this terminally ill child and his family.

87. One of the nurses says to the liaison nurse, "Whenever I go to the client's room, I feel that I have to smile and act happy even though I want to cry when I see him." Which of the following responses by the liaison nurse would be best in this situation?
○ 1. "Call me when you feel that way. We can talk it over at the time."
○ 2. "Try not to show emotion, such as crying. You'll upset the client."
○ 3. "Keep smiling. The client and his parents need all the support they can get."
○ 4. "Tell the client that you feel bad because he is ill. If it seems appropriate, you can cry too."

88. Because the client is increasingly prone to outbursts concerning his treatments, which of the following approaches by the nurse would likely be most helpful in gaining his cooperation?
○ 1. Tell him how the treatment can be expected to help him each time.
○ 2. Describe the probable effect on his body that missing a treatment would have.
○ 3. Ask him to be a good boy and to not make the treatment any harder for himself or the staff.
○ 4. Promise to give him a back rub every 2 hours if he does not make a fuss about the treatment.

89. The client suspects that he will not live. However, others talk about only pleasant matters with him and maintain a persistently cheerful facade around him. What will the client most likely feel as a result of such behavior?
○ 1. Relief.
○ 2. Isolation.
○ 3. Hopefulness.
○ 4. Independence.

90. Most authorities would agree that the client's parents should be told as much about the client's disease and prognosis as
○ 1. they wish to know.

○ 2. the nurse believes they can understand.
○ 3. the physician can tell them.
○ 4. their clergyman thinks is advisable for them to know.

91. The liaison nurse suggests that some recreational diversion be planned for the client. In particular, these recreational activities should
○ 1. be of a nonviolent nature.
○ 2. stimulate the imagination.
○ 3. require some physical effort.
○ 4. be geared to early adolescent interests.

92. The client's sister asks the nurse, "Can you check my blood? When my brother got the measles, so did I. And I think I have this, too." Which action by the nurse would be inappropriate?
○ 1. Asking the client's physician to take a sample of the sister's blood.
○ 2. Explaining that leukemia is not a communicable disease.
○ 3. Discussing the sister's concern with her parents.
○ 4. Telling the sister's parents about a group for siblings of clients with terminal illness.

93. When talking with the nurse, the client's 15-year-old brother says, "We used to play pretty rough games together. Maybe some of the bruises he got when I tackled him caused this." What would be the nurse's most helpful response?
○ 1. "Don't feel guilty. You didn't cause your brother's illness."
○ 2. "I can see you're worried about this. Let's talk about how people get leukemia."
○ 3. "Here is some information about leukemia for you to read. You'll see you didn't cause it."
○ 4. "Lot's of people worry about things like this. It isn't your fault."

94. During the nursing shift report, the team leader lists tasks and routines completed for the terminally ill client. Which of the following kinds of behavior is the nurse most likely demonstrating when she emphasizes the technical aspects of caring for a dying client?
○ 1. Tactful behavior.
○ 2. Efficient behavior.
○ 3. Objective behavior.
○ 4. Defensive behavior.

CORRECT ANSWERS AND RATIONALE

The letters in parentheses following the rationale identify the step of the nursing process (A, D, P, I, E); cognitive level (K, C, T, N); and client needs (S, G, L, H). See the Answer Grid for the key.

The Client With an Anxiety Disorder

1. 1. The best way to ease symptoms caused by hyperventilation is to have the client breathe into a paper bag. Having the client put his head between his knees, giving him low concentrations of oxygen, and having him take deep, slow breaths and exhale normally will not alleviate symptoms of hyperventilation. (I, T, G)

2. 4. Supporting the client in his attempts to discuss feelings, respecting personal space, and reassuring him about his safety promote a therapeutic nurse–client relationship and prevent escalation of anxiety. Confronting dysfunctional coping behaviors or defense mechanisms will most likely be viewed as a threat and increase anxiety. (I, T, L)

3. 3. Making optimistic statements avoids the client's feelings and offers little help when he feels uneasy. Being present, demonstrating competence, and respecting how the client feels are helpful for an anxious client. (I, T, L)

4. 2. The nurse helps the client to recognize that he is feeling anxious by pointing out his behaviors to him. The nurse then attempts to help the client recognize his anxiety and describes his feelings to help him connect behaviors with feelings. Telling the client that she will be back later or will get something to help him feel less anxious and changing the subject are not helpful to the client. The client wants to avoid or ignore his anxiety, which will not help him to deal with his feelings. (I, T, L)

5. 4. An appropriate long-term goal for the client who withdraws into his room because of severe anxiety is that the client will participate in milieu activities by discharge. Attending group with a staff member is a short-term goal related to the problem of Social Isolation. Initiating interactions with the nurse when anxious does not relate to Social Isolation and would be an appropriate outcome to be expected earlier during the client's hospitalization. Expressing two adaptive methods of coping with anxiety does not relate to the problem of Social Isolation but would be an appropriate outcome related to the nursing diagnosis Ineffective Individual Coping. (P, T, L)

6. 3. Problem solving and building adaptive coping behaviors to deal with anxiety is the nurse's ultimate goal when working with the client who has an anxiety disorder or an unmanageable anxiety level (severe or panic level). Reducing the client's anxiety to a manageable level, helping the client decrease denial and avoidance about feelings, and linking behaviors with feelings are important goals that are more immediate and short-term. Supportive confrontation is used when the client avoids painful issues that he needs to deal with during his recovery. Supportive confrontation is used by the nurse for a client experiencing mild to moderate anxiety, not during severe and panic levels. (P, T, L)

7. 1. Relaxation exercises would be most helpful because they provide the client with an adaptive mechanism to manage stress and produce a physiologic response opposite that of anxiety. The relaxation response decreases pulse rate, blood pressure, and respiration rate. Telling the client to ask his physician for medication avoids the problem and implies that the client is incapable of managing his behavior adaptively. Recommending that the client watch television avoids the client's needs and may not be helpful in dealing with his anxiety. Advising the client to ride the exercise bicycle at bedtime will produce a physiologic response opposite to that of relaxation by increasing pulse, respirations, and blood pressure. (I, T, L)

8. 1. Alprazolam (Xanax) is a benzodiazepine used on a short-term or temporary basis to treat psychological and somatic symptoms of anxiety and as an adjunct to other treatments. Physical and psychological dependence can occur as well as tolerance. (D, C, G)

9. 3. Using alcohol or any central nervous system depressant when taking benzodiazepines is contraindicated because of additive effects. (P, C, G)

10. 2. With post-traumatic stress disorder, the client experiences survivor guilt or feelings of guilt related to being alive. The client's statement does not indicate suicidal ideation. Dysfunctional grieving is inaccurate because the accident occurred only a month ago. Numbing of responsiveness pertains to having a restricted affect, a limitation in the range of feelings, a feeling of detachment from others and the external world, and hopelessness or lack of expectations about the future. (D, N, L)

11. 4. The nurse is nonjudgmental, is supportive, and conveys honesty and empathy to the client. Telling

the client he'll feel more comfortable in a survivor's group dismisses the client. However, a survivor's group may be needed later. Stating that the client should become interested in a hobby is not helpful. Stating, "I'd like to help you if you'll let me," may alienate the client. (I, T, L)

12. 1. Buspirone (Buspar), a nonbenzodiazepine anxiolytic, is not administered on an as-needed basis because it has a delayed onset of therapeutic action. Therapeutic effects may be experienced in 7 to 10 days, with full effects not occurring for 3 to 4 weeks. This drug is not known to cause physical or psychological dependence. (E, N, G)

13. 4. The client is exhibiting *intellectualization,* which is using logical explanations without feelings or an affective component. *Suppression* is the voluntary exclusion from awareness of feelings, ideas, or situations that are anxiety provoking. *Rationalization* is an attempt to make or prove that one's feelings or behaviors are justifiable. *Denial* is an unconscious refusal to admit an unacceptable idea or behavior. (D, N, L)

14. 2. The nurse initially assures the client that her feelings and behaviors are typical reactions to serious trauma to help decrease anxiety and maintain self-esteem. Explaining the effects of stress on the body may be helpful later. Telling the client that her symptoms are temporary is less helpful. Acknowledging the unfairness of the client's situation does nothing to address the client's needs at this time. (I, T, L)

15. 3. The client with anxiety may be able to learn to recognize when she is feeling anxious, understand the reasons for her anxiety, and be able to describe situations that preceded her feelings of anxiety. However, she is likely to continue to experience symptoms unless she has also learned to use her behaviors to reduce anxiety. (E, N, L)

The Client With an Obsessive-Compulsive Disorder

16. 1. When the client says he thinks he is "going crazy," it is best for the nurse to ask him what "crazy" means to him. Before moving toward consensual validation, the nurse must have a clear idea of what the client means by his words and actions. (I, T, L)

17. 1. The client exhibiting obsessive-compulsive behavior is attempting to control his anxiety. The compulsive component of the behavior is performed to relieve or bind anxiety. Obsessive-compulsive disorder is an anxiety-related disorder. (D, C, L)

18. 3. A client able to take care of his basic nutritional needs is probably not sufficiently incapacitated by his illness to require hospitalization. The ability to

behave normally is of lesser importance in this decision, depending on the client's family's or significant others' tolerance of the behavior. The client's abilities to hold a job and relate to his peers may be considered in making the decision but are not valid criteria for hospitalization. (D, N, L)

19. 2. Letting the client eat earlier meets his needs for more time and also the group's need to depart for the outing on time. It also protects the client from being resented by others and lets him be included in the group activity. Changing the time of an activity to meet the needs of one client is undesirable and may be impractical as well. (P, T, L)

20. 3. Drama clubs are good for their social and self-expressive qualities. This client needs outlets that are creative and oriented toward others. Swimming, solo flying, and photography are hobbies with few social qualities. (P, N, L)

21. 1. Diversional Activity Deficit, Social Isolation, and Powerlessness are appropriate nursing diagnoses for this client. There are no data to support the problem of fear for the client in this situation. Data supporting Powerlessness include the statement, "I know it's senseless. I can't stop." Being too busy at work to see friends and rarely seeing friends anymore support Diversional Activity Deficit and Social Isolation. (D, N, L)

22. 4. Clients with obsessive-compulsive disorder are typically rigid and controlled in their thinking and behavior. They find it difficult to be introspective and to express or even recognize their feelings. Increasing identification and expression of feelings and connecting feelings with behaviors may prove helpful. Learning and using adaptive coping behaviors when anxious would be appropriate for the client. The primary gain experienced by the client with obsessive-compulsive disorder is relief of anxiety. Learning how to manage anxiety decreases the need for obsessions and compulsions. Problem identification and decision making would be neither helpful to the client at this time nor realistic. (P, N, L)

23. 4. The dynamics of compulsive activity involve a defense against anxiety by persistently doing something to bind or reduce anxiety. This behavior occurs each time threatening thoughts occur. Judgment that the client counts money repeatedly to compensate for not having enough money to spend as a child or to avoid the embarrassment of running short of money is based on insufficient data and represents an oversimplification of the client's problem. (D, N, L)

24. 4. It is best to accept compulsive behavior in a comparatively permissive manner. The client may become increasingly anxious if the ritualistic activity is denied him. Isolating the client, observing him for marked changes in behavior, and reminding him that he can control his behavior if he wishes are unwarranted or inappropriate measures in this situation. (I, T, L)

25. 1. Although compassion, friendliness, and self-confidence may be desirable to some degree in caring for a client with an obsessive-compulsive disorder, it is considered most important that the nurse demonstrate patience. It takes the client a long time to complete necessary tasks. Unless nurses are patient, they can easily become frustrated, upset, or angry. The obsessive-compulsive client cannot be hurried. (D, C, L)

26. 2. It takes 5 to 10 weeks of clomipramine (Anafranil) therapy to derive full therapeutic effect for clients with obsessive-compulsive disorder. Asking the client if he has resumed smoking is appropriate because smoking increases the metabolism of clomipramine, necessitating a dosage adjustment to achieve therapeutic effect—but it would not be the first statement to make to this client. (I, T, L)

27. 3. Relaxation exercises, thought stopping, and exposure therapy are potentially therapeutic and beneficial for a client with obsessive-compulsive disorder. Meditation would not be helpful for the client because of increased anxiety, which interferes with concentration, thinking, and focusing. After obsessions and compulsions decrease, the client may find meditation helpful and calming. (P, N, L)

The Client With a Somatoform Disorder

28. 4. The nurse informs the client in a matter-of-fact manner that the nurse cannot give her additional pain medication at this time and invites the client to participate in a card game to decrease rumination about pain by directing the client's attention to a milieu activity. By telling the client the nurse will call the physician as requested, the nurse is manipulated to do what the client demands. Suggesting the client lie down or talk to the physician about it ignores the client's needs and is not helpful. (I, T, L)

29. 2. The nurse supports the client to do as much self-care as she is capable of to decrease secondary gain that reinforces the sick role and to increase independent functioning. Primary gain refers to the symptoms of the illness that reduce the client's anxiety. (I, T, L)

30. 3. The nurse instructs the nursing assistant to invite the client to lunch and accompany her to the dining room to decrease manipulation, secondary gain, dependency, and reinforcement of negative behavior while increasing self-esteem. Taking the client a lunch tray and allowing her to eat in her room reinforces negative behaviors and secondary gain. Telling the client she'll need to wait until supper to eat if she misses lunch and informing the client she has 10 minutes to get to the dining room challenge the client and may increase feelings of anger and the need for physical complaints. (I, T, L)

31. 1. The nurse uses a matter-of-fact, caring approach to decrease secondary gain and to decrease focusing on physical symptoms. Using a strong confrontational approach may anger the client, reinforcing the need for physical symptoms. Minimally interacting with the client and ignoring the client's negative comments are not therapeutic and ignore the client's needs. The client with a somatoform disorder like conversion disorder needs to identify and describe feelings to increase verbalization of feelings, even negative ones, and thus to decrease the need for bodily symptoms. (P, N, L)

32. 2. Pushing insight or awareness into conflicts or problems increases anxiety and the need for physical symptoms to handle or take care of the anxiety. Telling the nurse to ignore the client and treat her with respect is not helpful to the nurse or client. (I, T, L)

33. 2. The nurse helps the client to focus on his feelings about his impending divorce to decrease anxiety and focus on physical ailments. The client with a somatoform disorder typically has problems with identifying, describing, and dealing with feelings. Internalizing feelings leads to increased anxiety and the need for protective mechanisms. (I, T, L)

34. 2. Individual therapy would be least helpful to the client with somatization disorder. Relaxation exercises, assertiveness training, and outpatient group psychotherapy are helpful because they focus on the client's psychosocial needs and not on the illness itself. (P, T, L)

The Client With Problems Expressing Anger

35. 3. Describing acceptable behavior to the client focuses on the immediate problem. Asking the client to explain what happened is a therapeutic statement likely to elicit assessment data, but it is less focused on the client's immediate problem. Threatening statements do not elicit further information and are not therapeutic. (I, T, L)

36. 3. The nurse clearly addresses behavioral expectations and provides alternatives for the client. Isolating the client and making others responsible for the client's behavior are inappropriate because they do not include the client in managing his behavior. Medication may be helpful but does not involve the client in responsibility for his behavior. (I, T, L)

37. 1. The nurse acknowledges and labels the client's emotion and acknowledges his appropriate behavior. Recognizing the client's physiologic arousal, the nurse suggests an activity and stays with him. Setting limits on the client's language does not acknowledge his control. Offering the client medication suggests that he cannot control his behavior. (I, T, L)

38. 4. Verbalizing feelings, especially feelings of anger, in an appropriate manner is an adaptive method of coping and reduces the chance of the client acting out his feelings toward others. Acknowledging feelings of anger and describing situations that precipitate angry feelings are important outcomes in helping the client reach his goal of appropriately verbalizing his feelings but are not ends in themselves. Asking the client to list how he has handled anger in the past is helpful if the nurse discusses coping methods with the client. Based on this client's history, this would not be helpful because the nurse and client are aware of the client's aggression toward others. (P, T, L)

39. 2. Identifying people with whom the client is angry is not important to the overall plan. Helping the client recognize anger, identifying alternative ways to express anger, and practicing the expression of anger are all steps in the process of teaching the client to recognize and respond appropriately to anger. (P, T, L)

40. 3. The nurse acknowledges the client's concern and provides an opportunity to review his progress and to prepare for the work situation. Option 1 is therapeutic but does not review the client's progress or prepare him for the work situation. Options 2 and 4 provide false reassurance. (I, T, L)

41. 4. Violent behavior is more likely when there is a demand for high activity, when there is inadequate staffing, and when the staff feels hopeless about a client. However, the client's past history of violent behavior is the most accurate predictive factor. (A, T, L)

42. 4. This response acknowledges the client's feelings and helps the group accept a new member. The nurse's response should acknowledge the client's fear and address the purpose of the group but should not provide false reassurance. (I, T, L)

43. 1. Both denial of anger with passive, unassertive behavior and the aggressive expression of anger are dysfunctional behavior patterns. Gender-based stereotypes of assertive behavior are not conducive to mental health. Options 3 and 4 are unwarranted assumptions based on inadequate data. (E, N, L)

44. 2. The escalation phase of the assault cycle involves agitation, swearing, screaming, demanding, and provocative behaviors with loss of reasoning ability. Some behaviors in the triggering phase involves muscle tension, irritability, restlessness, perspiration, and changes in breathing and voice quality. The crisis phase involves loss of self-control, hitting, scratching, kicking, and throwing things. Aggressive is not a phase of the assault cycle. (E, N, S)

45. 4. The client is in the crisis phase of the assault cycle and the nurse uses involuntary seclusion, restraints, or an intramuscular tranquilizer. It is too late to ask the client to go to a quiet area to talk because the client's behavior is past the triggering phase. Directing the client to a quiet room, giving an oral tranquilizer, and preparing for a show of determination are nursing interventions used in the escalation phase. Processing the incident with the client and discussing alternative behaviors are interventions used in the postcrisis phase. (I, N, S)

46. 4. The client is ready to be released from restraints when he shows signs of self-control, decreased anxiety and agitation, reality orientation, mood stabilization, increased attention span, and judgment. Adequate sedation, struggling less against restraints, and not swearing and yelling are not adequate signs of being calm and in control. (E, N, S)

47. 3. By requesting that the roommate respect his rights, the client is asserting himself. Arriving late is often passive resistance; asking the nurse to call is dependent behavior. Asking the doctor is more assertive, but the client relies on the nurse's direction to do so. (E, N, L)

48. 2. Blood pressure, as well as respiratory rate and muscle tension, increase in anger owing to the autonomic nervous system response to epinephrine secretion. Peristalsis decreases. (A, C, L)

49. 2. Fear of retaliation, guilt, and decreased self-esteem are common psychological responses to feelings of anger. Although anger may provide an initial feeling of strength and invulnerability, this is rarely a sustained response. (E, N, L)

50. 1. Sarcasm is frequently used to express anger indirectly. Refusing medication, cursing, and shouting are more direct expressions of angry, negative feelings. (E, N, L)

The Client With Family Abuse and Violence

51. 2. The safety of the client and her children is the immediate concern. If there is immediate danger, action must be taken to protect them. The level of abuse in the family, the client's plans, and the available resources are also important considerations in developing a treatment plan but are not the most important concerns. (A, N, L)

52. 3. Impermeable boundaries, unbalanced power ratio, and dysfunctional feeling tone are all common in abusive families. However, the traditional and rigid gender roles described by the client are examples of role stereotyping. (D, N, L)

53. 1. The nurse would provide the client with resources or support systems to turn to when the next battering incident occurs. It is inappropriate to advise the client to leave her husband. The client should not be pushed or coerced into leaving her husband until she is ready. Telling the client not to do anything to upset her husband and asking her what she could do to de-escalate the situation at home place blame for the violence on the client. (I, T, L)

54. 1. Lack of empathy characterizes relationships in abusive families. It is more likely that the relationship is built around the abuser's need for power and control. A history of family violence and low self-esteem are common among abusers. The idea that only poorly educated, poorly employed men are abusive is a myth. Most alcohol abusers batter their partners, regardless of whether they are drinking at the time. (D, N, L)

55. 4. Sharing feelings of frustration with the client is inappropriate. The nurse's feelings of frustration are not unusual, and she needs to discuss these feelings with a clinical supervisor to better understand and deal with them. (P, T, L)

56. 2. Group therapy with women with similar problems may help the client reduce her isolation and sense of shame. The idea that abuse victims do not want to change is inaccurate and leads to feelings of hopelessness among professionals. Contacting other people about the client and family without the client's consent violates confidentiality. (I, T, L)

57. 1. Self-blame, substance abuse, and suicidal thoughts and attempts are possible dysfunctional coping methods used by abuse victims. The nurse would least likely find assertiveness in the victim. The victim is usually compliant with the spouse and feels guilt, shame, and some responsibility for the battering. (A, C, L)

58. 3. The data here best support the nursing diagnosis of Powerlessness related to abusive husband, as evidenced by inability to make decisions. (D, T, L)

59. 4. Although any event in a family can contribute to an abusive episode, the birthday party is less important to treatment planning than the husband's promotion, a potential major stressor. His refusal of treatment and the client's coping skills are both important in treatment planning. (P, N, L)

60. 4. It is important that the nurse address the family problem and include the client in making decisions about her daughter. Allowing the child to remain at home and having someone else at home to meet her ignores the basic family problem. Asking the client to talk to her daughter is appropriate but is not a sufficient intervention in this situation. (I, T, L)

61. 2. The nurse needs more information about the client's decision before deciding what intervention is most appropriate. Judgmental responses could make it difficult for the client to return for treatment should she want to do so. (I, T, L)

62. 1. Defending the school nurse puts the client's mother on the defensive and stifles communication. All the other responses address, either directly or indirectly, the mother's concerns and ask for her view of the situation. This approach is important in building a relationship with the family. (I, T, L)

63. 4. A strong defensive reaction by parents to an appropriate concern by a teacher or other professional may indicate family problems. A caring, supportive relationship among family members and infrequent episodes of abuse during a time of intense family stress are not characteristic of abusive families. (E, N, L)

The Client With a Psychophysiologic Disorder

64. 3. When this client returns to the hospital for the fourth time in 9 months, it is best for the nurse to acknowledge his readmission and give him an opportunity to express his feelings. Telling the client it is nice to see him and asking him if he had become lonesome serve little purpose except as social comments. Telling the client that she thought she had seen the last of him and asking him what he is doing back in the hospital could be interpreted as being rude and challenging. The nurse is making an assumption when she states that the client will not need to be oriented to the hospital because of previous admissions. (I, T, L)

65. 4. Using people for therapeutic interventions is usually more helpful than manipulating the environment, as is the case when a client becomes upset when he hears meal trays approaching. Tension is less likely to develop when a client is interpersonally involved than when the time element in relation to eating has been altered. (P, T, L)

66. 1. Activity within physical limits is desirable. However, the emphasis of treatment lies in providing rest and freedom from emotional stress to the greatest extent possible for a client suffering with a psychophysiologic disorder. This goal is best met when activities that promote rest and relaxation are chosen for the client. The goal is less well met by activities that promote improvement of social skills, insight and self-awareness, and manual rather than intellectual dexterity. (D, T, L)

67. 2. Here, when the client seems to be questioning his physician's goals, it is best for the nurse to present an open statement and ask the client what he means. This technique helps the client express his feelings. It is less therapeutic to tell the client that he sounds upset, that he is being hard on his physician, or that his remark apparently has something to do with the surgery he is about to undergo. (I, T, L)

68. 2. When this client has hostile outbursts, it is best for the nurse to help him express his feelings. This serves as a release valve for the client. Other actions by the nurse are less therapeutic than helping the client express himself. (I, T, L)

69. 3. Preoperative visits and talks with clients who have made successful adjustments to ileostomies are helpful and may tend to make the client less fearful of the operation and its consequences. (D, C, L)

70. 3. The nurse would consider the diagnoses Ineffective Individual Coping, Knowledge Deficit, and Anxiety when working with a client with a psychophysiologic disorder. Powerlessness would not be appropriate because the client projects an image of a person who works hard, does not take time to relax, and is usually in charge and productive. (D, N, L)

71. 2. The nurse presents reality to the client about his condition to help decrease his denial about his physical status. The nurse conveys that she is concerned about him and willing to help him understand his illness. Stating that the secretary could be delayed by traffic is not appropriate and shows poor judgment. Options 3 and 4 are responses that are belittling to the client, may cause the client to become defensive, and convey the nurse's frustration. (I, T, L)

72. 1. Leaving the hospital and immediately flying to a meeting indicates poor judgment by the client and little understanding of what he needs to change regarding his lifestyle. Expressing a willingness to try relaxation tapes, not working 10 hours a day, and working on a new budget with his wife shows that the client understands some of the changes he needs to make to decrease his stress and lead a more healthy lifestyle. (E, N, L)

73. 4. The best response is one that directly expresses the nurse's observations to the client and offers the client the opportunity to vent openly and talk about her feelings or concerns to decrease somatization or the need to express feelings through physical symptoms. Leaving, offering to provide pain medication, and stating that anger does not bother the nurse ignore the client's needs and do not help the client. (I, T, L)

74. 1. Clients with psychophysiologic disorders tend to close themselves off emotionally from others and do not reveal their feelings easily. These characteristics are often an obstacle in therapy. These clients may expect the therapist to help them without having to disclose feelings. (E, T, L)

75. 2. Psychophysiologic disorders, if untreated, may prove fatal. Clients with psychophysiologic disorders do not select the physical ailment they suffer from, do not find relief from physical symptoms when a mental conflict is arrested, and do not handle the symptoms with an attitude of indifference. (D, C, L)

76. 3. Clients with ulcerative colitis commonly have a personality trait described as obsessive-compulsive. Behaviors such as perfectionism, conformity, rigidity, being emotionally on guard, and obstinacy are typical. (A, C, L)

77. 4. This client directs profanities at the nurse and then is sorry for his behavior. This type of behavior illustrates *emotional lability,* which is a readily changeable or unstable emotional affect. *Punning* is using a word when it can have two or more meanings, or a play on words. *Confabulation* involves replacing memory loss by fantasy to hide confusion; it is unconscious behavior. *Flight of ideas* refers to a rapid succession of verbal expressions that jump from one topic to another and are only superficially related. (D, T, L)

78. 3. The nurse would minimize the time she spends with the client when she engages in complaining behavior to decrease somatization and the secondary gain of getting attention. Giving the client simple choices encourages independent decision making and responsibility for herself. Being consistent in expectations of the client decreases manipulation of the nurse. Giving recognition when the client does something for herself rewards the client for appropriate, responsible behavior. (I, T, L)

79. 3. Clients with peptic ulcers are thought to be dependent or overly independent and ambitious, depending on factors in the client's life. Perfectionism, identity problems, and mistrust of staff's abilities are not specific to clients with peptic ulcers. (D, N, L)

80. 1. When a family member has been chronically ill, feelings of guilt and domination tend to cause the greatest amount of intrapsychic conflict in the family's interrelationships. These feelings are not easy to express and communicate openly. Hence, feelings of guilt and domination tend to have the most negative and destructive effect on interrelationships in terms of behavioral symptoms. (D, C, L)

The Client With a Terminal Illness

81. 3. The nurse recognizes the client's pain, hopelessness, and sense of loss related to his condition and the loss of his friend and encourages him to express his feelings. Giving the client permission to talk about his feelings of sadness, loss, and hopelessness and listening to him is an important nursing intervention for the dying client. "Let's talk about making good use of the time you have left," "Don't give up," and "Life is worth living" are statements that ignore the client's needs and inhibit his expression of feelings. (I, T, L)

82. 4. The nurse would call for a multidisciplinary staff meeting because she recognizes the need for staff members to share their feelings of anger, frustration, and grief. Because nurses focus on saving human lives, any feelings of hopelessness regarding a dying client can interfere with the client's care and management. Assigning the staff member to other clients and calling the clinical nurse specialist to deal with the staff member ignore the entire staff's needs and does nothing to help the immediate situation. The psychiatric clinical nurse specialist would be included in the staff meeting to help the entire staff deal with their feelings. Agreeing with the staff member and discontinuing suicide precautions is highly inappropriate. (I, T, L)

83. 1. The nurse would give the client a tissue and tell him it's okay to cry to convey her acceptance and empathy. The client needs understanding and encouragement to talk about his feelings. He needs to know that it is natural and normal to have tremendous feelings of loss and sadness and needs the nurse to help him cope with intense feelings. Telling the client to stop crying, busying oneself in the client's room, and changing the subject are not helpful to the client because they ignore his needs and inhibit the expression of emotion. (I, T, L)

84. 1. The client's friend appears to be experiencing anger in this situation, much of which stems from feelings of guilt. During the stage of denial, the friend is more likely to deny the client's diagnosis and prognosis. During the stage of bargaining, the friend tends to offer to do certain things in exchange for more time before the client dies. In the stage of depression, the friend is likely to make few or no comments and act dejected. (D, T, L)

85. 1. It is best to examine one's own feelings about death and dying before caring for the terminally ill client. Many authorities consider self-examination of one's own finiteness essential before one can successfully meet the needs of a dying client. (E, N, L)

86. 1. It is best when supporting the friend or family of a terminally ill client to focus on the present. This can be accomplished by living each day to its fullest. Friends and families also want to know what to expect and want someone to listen to them as they express grief over death. (D, C, L)

87. 4. Clients often sense a nurse's feelings. Therefore, when the nurse becomes emotionally upset while caring for the terminally ill child, it is best for her to share her emotions with the child when it seems appropriate. It is also acceptable to cry. Trying not to show emotion and trying to smile regardless of how one feels are inappropriate responses. It is of little help to the client or the nurse who is upset if the nurse waits until a later time when she can speak to someone about the situation. (I, T, L)

88. 1. Here, the best course of action when the client has outbursts concerning his treatments is to tell him how the treatment can be expected to help him. Describing the effect on his body if he misses a treatment is a negative approach and may be threatening to the client. The client is likely to feel angry if told to be a "good boy" during treatments. Offering to give the client a back rub if he does not fuss does not give him the information to which he is entitled. (I, T, L)

89. 2. Children are aware of and show anxieties about death at an earlier age than was once thought, and they recognize false cheerfulness. They tend to experience isolation and loneliness when those around them are trying to hide or mask the truth. They are then left to face the realities of death alone. (D, N, L)

90. 1. Most authorities recommend that the parents of an ill child, including a child who is terminally ill, should be told as much as they wish to know. The nurse can determine this by talking with the parents and child. (P, C, L)

91. 4. Recreational activities selected for this 13-year-old client should be geared to the client's interests. Activities that are physical in nature are likely to be too strenuous for a terminally ill child. Activities of a nonviolent nature and those that stimulate the child's imagination are satisfactory, but the first criterion should be that the activity be appropriate for the client's age level. (P, C, L)

92. 1. Taking a blood sample is an unnecessary, invasive procedure that would not directly address the child's fear. Providing an age-appropriate explanation and alerting the parents to the sibling's concern and the resources available to assist siblings with the terminal illness are all appropriate interventions. (I, T, L)

93. 2. A response that acknowledges the brother's concern and provides him with information is most helpful. Providing reassurance without addressing the expressed concern and providing information without acknowledging the expressed concern are not as helpful as acknowledgment plus information. (I, T, L)

94. 4. The nurse caring for a terminally ill client who reports only tasks and routines completed for the client is probably behaving defensively. It is likely that this nurse has not come to grips with death and dying. (A, T, L)

THE NURSING CARE OF CLIENTS WITH PSYCHIATRIC DISORDERS AND MENTAL HEALTH PROBLEMS

TEST 4: Anxiety, Anger, Abuse, and Terminal Illness

Directions: Use this answer grid to determine areas of strength or need for further study.

NURSING PROCESS	COGNITIVE LEVEL	CLIENT NEEDS
A = Assessment	K = Knowledge	S = Safe, effective care environment
D = Analysis, nursing diagnosis	C = Comprehension	G = Physiologic integrity
P = Planning	T = Application	L = Psychosocial integrity
I = Implementation	N = Analysis	H = Health promotion and maintenance
E = Evaluation		

Question #	Answer #	A	D	P	I	E	K	C	T	N	S	G	L	H
1	1				I				T			G		
2	4				I				T				L	
3	3				I				T				L	
4	2				I				T				L	
5	4			P					T				L	
6	3			P					T				L	
7	1				I				T				L	
8	1		D					C				G		
9	3			P				C				G		
10	2		D							N			L	
11	4				I				T				L	
12	1					E				N		G		
13	4		D							N			L	
14	2				I				T				L	
15	3					E				N			L	
16	1				I				T				L	
17	1		D					C					L	
18	3		D							N			L	
19	2			P					T				L	
20	3			P						N			L	
21	1		D							N			L	
22	4			P						N			L	
23	4		D							N			L	
24	4				I				T				L	

ANSWER GRID: 1

NURSING PROCESS

A = Assessment
D = Analysis, nursing diagnosis
P = Planning
I   = Implementation
E = Evaluation

COGNITIVE LEVEL

K = Knowledge
C = Comprehension
T = Application
N = Analysis

CLIENT NEEDS

S = Safe, effective care environment
G = Physiologic integrity
L = Psychosocial integrity
H = Health promotion and maintenance

Question #	Answer #	Nursing Process					Cognitive Level				Client Needs			
		A	D	P	I	E	K	C	T	N	S	G	L	H
25	1		D					C					L	
26	2				I				T				L	
27	3			P						N			L	
28	4				I				T				L	
29	2				I				T				L	
30	3				I				T				L	
31	1			P						N			L	
32	2				I				T				L	
33	2				I				T				L	
34	2			P					T				L	
35	3				I				T				L	
36	3				I				T				L	
37	1				I				T				L	
38	4			P					T				L	
39	2			P					T				L	
40	3				I				T				L	
41	4	A							T				L	
42	4				I				T				L	
43	1					E				N			L	
44	2					E				N	S			
45	4				I					N	S			
46	4					E				N	S			
47	3					E				N			L	
48	2	A						C					L	
49	2					E				N			L	
50	1					E				N			L	
51	2	A								N			L	
52	3		D							N			L	
53	1				I				T				L	
54	1		D							N			L	

ANSWER GRID: 2

NURSING PROCESS

A = Assessment
D = Analysis, nursing diagnosis
P = Planning
I = Implementation
E = Evaluation

COGNITIVE LEVEL

K = Knowledge
C = Comprehension
T = Application
N = Analysis

CLIENT NEEDS

S = Safe, effective care environment
G = Physiologic integrity
L = Psychosocial integrity
H = Health promotion and maintenance

Question #	Answer #	Nursing Process					Cognitive Level				Client Needs			
		A	D	P	I	E	K	C	T	N	S	G	L	H
55	4			P					T				L	
56	2				I				T				L	
57	1	A						C					L	
58	3		D						T				L	
59	4			P						N			L	
60	4				I				T				L	
61	2				I				T				L	
62	1				I				T				L	
63	4					E				N			L	
64	3				I				T				L	
65	4			P					T				L	
66	1		D						T				L	
67	2				I				T				L	
68	2				I				T				L	
69	3		D					C					L	
70	3		D							N			L	
71	2				I				T				L	
72	1					E				N			L	
73	4				I				T				L	
74	1					E			T				L	
75	2		D					C					L	
76	3	A						C					L	
77	4		D						T				L	
78	3				I				T				L	
79	3		D							N			L	
80	1		D					C					L	
81	3				I				T				L	
82	4				I				T				L	
83	1				I				T				L	
84	1		D						T				L	

ANSWER GRID: 3

NURSING PROCESS

A = Assessment
D = Analysis, nursing diagnosis
P = Planning
I = Implementation
E = Evaluation

COGNITIVE LEVEL

K = Knowledge
C = Comprehension
T = Application
N = Analysis

CLIENT NEEDS

S = Safe, effective care environment
G = Physiologic integrity
L = Psychosocial integrity
H = Health promotion and maintenance

Question #	Answer #	Nursing Process					Cognitive Level				Client Needs			
		A	D	P	I	E	K	C	T	N	S	G	L	H
85	1					E				N			L	
86	1		D						C					L	
87	4				I				T				L	
88	1				I				T				L	
89	2		D							N			L	
90	1			P				C					L	
91	4			P				C					L	
92	1				I				T				L	
93	2				I				T				L	
94	4	A							T				L	
Number Correct														
Number Possible	94	6	21	16	39	12	0	13	53	28	3	4	87	0
Percentage Correct														

Score Calculation: To determine your **Percentage Correct,** divide the **Number Correct** by the **Number Possible.**

BIBLIOGRAPHY

American Psychiatric Association. (1994). *Diagnostic and statistical manual of mental disorders.* (4th ed.). Washington, DC: Author.

Barry, P. (1996). *Psychosocial nursing: Care of physically ill patients and their families.* (3rd ed.). Philadelphia: JB Lippincott.

Fortinash, K., and Holoday-Worret, P. (1996). *Psychiatric mental health nursing.* St. Louis: CV Mosby.

Fortinash, K., and Holoday-Worret, P. (1995). *Psychiatric nursing care plans.* (2nd ed.). St. Louis: CV Mosby.

Johnson, B. (1995). *Child, adolescent and family psychiatric nursing.* Philadelphia: JB Lippincott.

Keltner, N., and Folks, D. (1993). *Psychotropic drugs.* St. Louis: CV Mosby.

Keltner, N., Schwecke, L., and Bostrom, C. (1995). *Psychiatric nursing.* (2nd ed.). St. Louis: CV Mosby.

Stuart, G., and Sundeen, S. (1995). *Principles and practice of psychiatric nursing.* (5th ed.). St. Louis: CV Mosby.

Townsend, M.C. (1990). *Drug guide for psychiatric nursing.* Philadelphia: FA Davis.

Part II

The Nursing Care of the Childbearing Family and Their Neonate

Antepartum Care

Test 1

- **The Preconception Client**
- **The Pregnant Client Receiving Prenatal Care**
- **The Pregnant Client in Childbirth Preparation Classes**
- **The Pregnant Client With Risk Factors**
- **Correct Answers and Rationale**

Select the one best answer, and indicate your choice by filling in the circle in front of the option.

The Preconception Client

An 18-year-old nulligravida visits a family planning clinic. The client states that she and her fiancee are planning their wedding and that she doesn't want to become pregnant for at least 1 year.

1. The nurse plans to provide preconception counseling to the client. Before beginning to counsel the client, the nurse should *first*
- 1. have the client and her partner undergo a complete physical examination.
- 2. obtain a sexual history from the client in a private setting.
- 3. ask the client to return to the clinic with her fiancee in 1 week.
- 4. determine if the client has a history of genetic abnormalities.

2. The nurse has instructed the client how to perform a breast self-examination. The nurse determines that the client has understood the instruction when she says,
- 1. "I should perform breast self-examination about 2 days after the onset of menstruation."
- 2. "It's important that I perform breast self-examination on the same day each month."
- 3. "If I notice that one of my breasts is larger than the other, I shouldn't worry."
- 4. "If there is some discharge from my nipples, I should avoid squeezing them."

3. The nurse formulates a nursing diagnosis of Knowledge Deficit related to ovulation and fertility management related to lack of information. Which of the following statements would be important to include in the client's teaching plan?
- 1. The ovum survives for 72 hours after ovulation.

- 2. The basal body temperature falls at least 0.2°F after ovulation.
- 3. Most women can tell they have ovulated by the unusual pain that accompanies ovulation.
- 4. Ovulation usually occurs on day 14, plus or minus 2 days, before the onset of the next menstrual period.

4. After instructing the client about conception and fertilization, the nurse determines that the client understands the instruction when the client says,
- 1. "Under ideal conditions, sperm can reach the ovum in 1 to 5 minutes."
- 2. "To avoid pregnancy using the abstinence method, I should abstain from intercourse during the last 14 days of my menstrual cycle."
- 3. "In a healthy male, sperm usually remain viable for 24 hours."
- 4. "The ovum contains 21 pairs of chromosomes after fertilization."

5. The client expresses a desire to learn more about the symptothermal method of family planning. The nurse should instruct the client that this method
- 1. has a 50% failure rate during the first year of use.
- 2. requires careful monitoring of cervical mucous changes.
- 3. depends on abstinence during the first 7 days of the menstrual cycle.
- 4. needs the use of a diaphragm with spermicide for greater effectiveness.

6. The nurse instructs the client about oral contraceptive agents. The nurse determines that the client understands the instruction when the client says,
- 1. "Despite the effectiveness of this method, about 25% of women discontinue oral contraceptives after 1 year."
- 2. "Only a few minor side effects are associated with oral contraceptives."

○ 3. "Oral contraceptives work by inhibiting ovulation and changing the consistency of cervical mucus."

○ 4. "Effectiveness of oral contraceptives can be increased if the basal body temperature is closely monitored."

7. While discussing anatomy and physiology of the reproductive cycle, the client asks the nurse, "Where is the ovum fertilized?" The best response by the nurse is to instruct the client that fertilization normally occurs in the

○ 1. vagina.

○ 2. uterus.

○ 3. cervix.

○ 4. fallopian tube.

A 35-year-old multigravida visits the family planning clinic 2 months after the delivery of her fourth child. The client is still breast-feeding her neonate.

8. The client tells the nurse that she and her husband have been using natural family planning methods but are considering using condoms. The nurse should instruct the client that

○ 1. natural skin condoms protect against sexually transmitted diseases.

○ 2. the typical failure rate for condoms is 25%.

○ 3. condoms lubricated with a spermicide offer added protection against pregnancy.

○ 4. the major complaint of condom users is that the condom increases penile gland sensitivity.

9. The client inquires about using a diaphragm for contraception. In planning the teaching for this client, the nurse should include which of the following?

○ 1. Douching with an acidic solution after intercourse is recommended.

○ 2. A large percentage of women who used diaphragms develop toxic shock syndrome.

○ 3. The diaphragm should be washed in a weak solution of bleach and water.

○ 4. The diaphragm should be left in place for at least 8 hours after intercourse.

10. The client tells the nurse, "My husband has considered having a vasectomy. Can you tell me about the procedure?" The nurse should explain that a commonly used procedure for a vasectomy involves clamping or excising the

○ 1. epididymis.

○ 2. seminiferous tubules.

○ 3. seminal vesicles.

○ 4. ductus deferens.

11. The client asks the nurse for information about female sterilization. After giving instruction, the nurse determines that the client understands the instruction when she says,

○ 1. "Female sterilization usually involves ligation of the fallopian tubes through a small abdominal incision."

○ 2. "Reversal of a tubal ligation is easily done and can result in a pregnancy success rate of 90%."

○ 3. "With bilateral tubal ligation, there is a decreased risk of ectopic pregnancy."

○ 4. "Both ovaries are usually removed during the tubal ligation procedure."

12. The client tells the nurse that she often experiences orgasms during sexual intercourse. The nurse should explain to the client that the *primary* anatomic female structure involved in sexual arousal and orgasm is the

○ 1. vaginal wall.

○ 2. clitoris.

○ 3. mons pubis.

○ 4. cervix.

A female client and her husband visit the fertility clinic and tell the nurse that they have been married for 4 years and have been unable to conceive. After complete physical examinations, the husband is found to have a mildly low sperm count.

13. Based on the assessment data, a priority nursing diagnosis for this couple is

○ 1. Grief related to inability to conceive.

○ 2. Knowledge deficit related to fertility treatments.

○ 3. Ineffective family coping related to infertility.

○ 4. Anxiety related to decreased spermatogenesis.

14. The client asks the nurse, "What causes infertility in a female?" The nurse should explain to the client that a common factor in female infertility is

○ 1. absence of an ovary.

○ 2. overproduction of prolactin.

○ 3. ovarian dysfunction.

○ 4. obstructed Bartholin's gland or duct.

15. An appropriate goal for this couple would be that by the end of the first visit, the couple will

○ 1. choose an appropriate method of treatment.

○ 2. acknowledge the fact that only half of infertile couples achieve a pregnancy.

○ 3. discuss alternative methods of treatment, such as adoption.

○ 4. describe each of the potential treatment modalities.

16. The couple asks the nurse to explain some of the treatments for infertility. Which of the following would be important for the nurse to include in the couple's teaching plan?

○ 1. During artificial insemination, sperm is inseminated at the time of ovulation through the cervix.

○ 2. In vitro fertilization involves the direct transfer of fertilized ova into the fallopian tubes.

○ 3. Gamete intrafallopian transfer (GIFT) requires the use of estrogen to support the endometrium for implantation.

○ 4. Human menopausal gonadotropin is a drug that decreases the level of prolactin in women.

17. The client is given a prescription by the physician for clomiphene citrate (Clomid). The nurse should explain to the client that one of the potential side effects of this medication is

○ 1. multiple pregnancies.

○ 2. an increase in spontaneous abortions.

○ 3. an increase in fibrocystic breast disease.

○ 4. an increase in congenital anomalies.

18. The client is scheduled for in vitro fertilization. After instruction about the procedure, the nurse determines that the client understands the instruction when she says,

○ 1. "The success rate of this procedure is about 50%."

○ 2. "After the procedure, I'll need to have a series of estrogen injections."

○ 3. "After the ova are fertilized, three or four embryos are transferred through the cervix."

○ 4. "Multiple gestation rates are lower with this procedure than with the GIFT procedure."

A 20-year-old client visits the Ob-Gyn clinic because she has missed one menstrual period and suspects she is pregnant.

19. An immunoassay test is performed to determine if pregnancy has occurred. The nurse should instruct the client that this test is

○ 1. highly accurate within 8 to 10 days after conception.

○ 2. identical to an over-the-counter home pregnancy test.

○ 3. a positive sign of pregnancy.

○ 4. more accurate if blood serum is used for the test.

20. After instructing the client about the immunoassay test, the nurse determines that the client understands the instruction when she says that the test analyzes maternal urine for

○ 1. progestin.

○ 2. prolactin.

○ 3. luteinizing hormone.

○ 4. human chorionic gonadotrophin.

21. Besides amenorrhea, the client tells the nurse that she has experienced nausea and vomiting, urinary frequency, and fatigue. The nurse determines that the client has been experiencing signs of pregnancy considered

○ 1. presumptive.

○ 2. probable.

○ 3. positive.

○ 4. physiologic.

22. The client tells the nurse that her mother had a friend who died from hemorrhage during a vaginal delivery. The nurse's best response is to

○ 1. review how modern technology has resulted in a low maternal mortality rate.

○ 2. recommend to the client that she not concern herself with what happened in the past.

○ 3. reassure the client that a discussion of possible complications of pregnancy and maternal mortality can be done at a later time.

○ 4. gather additional data about the client's concerns about pregnancy, labor, and delivery.

23. The client tells the nurse that she is single, unemployed, and has just returned to college on a full-time basis. She isn't sure that she wants a baby right now because her college career would be interrupted. A priority nursing diagnosis for this client is

○ 1. Knowledge Deficit related to health care benefits available.

○ 2. Fear related to lack of information about first-trimester changes.

○ 3. High Risk for Altered Nutrition related to socio-economic status.

○ 4. Anxiety related to financial impact of child-bearing.

24. The client's pregnancy test is negative. She tells the nurse that she would like to use the basal body temperature method for family planning. After giving instruction, the nurse determines that the client understands the instruction when she says,

○ 1. "When the temperature remains elevated for 7 days, ovulation has occurred."

○ 2. "I should take my temperature every evening before going to bed."

○ 3. "Since this method is not very effective, I should use other forms of contraception in addition to checking the temperature."

○ 4. "It's important to take my temperature at about the same time every morning before arising."

25. The nurse plans to instruct the client about cervical mucous changes that occur throughout the menstrual cycle. Which of the following would be important to include in the teaching plan?

○ 1. Two to 4 days after menstrual flow has stopped, cervical mucus is abundant and clear.

○ 2. During ovulation, the cervix does not produce mucus; thus, the area is dry.

○ 3. As ovulation approaches, cervical mucus is abundant and clear.

○ 4. Immediately after ovulation, cervical mucus disappears until the menstrual flow resumes.

The Pregnant Client Receiving Prenatal Care

A 24-year-old nulligravida schedules an appointment at the prenatal clinic because she has missed two menstrual periods and feels tired all the time. The client suspects she is pregnant.

26. From the initial interview, the nurse learns that the first day of the client's last menstrual period was May 15. According to Nägele's rule, the nurse determines that the client's estimated date of birth is

○ 1. January 8.

○ 2. February 8.

○ 3. February 22.

○ 4. August 22.

27. The nurse practitioner determines that the client is about 10 weeks' pregnant. The client asks the nurse when she will be able to hear the fetal heart rate. The best response by the nurse is to instruct the client that the fetal heart rate can be heard with a Doppler when the gestation is as early as

○ 1. 6 weeks.

○ 2. 10 weeks.

○ 3. 14 weeks.

○ 4. 18 weeks.

28. The client states, "Is it really true? I can't believe I'm going to have a baby!" What is the nurse's best response?

○ 1. "Would you like some pamphlets on the childbirth experience?"

○ 2. "Yes it is true. How does that make you feel?"

○ 3. "You shouldn't have doubts now. Your pregnancy has been confirmed."

○ 4. "It's important for new mothers to accept the pregnancy in the first trimester."

29. The client says, "If I'm going to have all of these discomforts, I'm not sure I want to be pregnant!" The nurse evaluates the client's statement as an indication of

○ 1. normal ambivalence.

○ 2. rejection of the pregnancy.

○ 3. evidence of maternal role attainment.

○ 4. rejection of the fetus.

30. The nurse formulates a nursing diagnosis for this client. What is the priority diagnosis at this time?

○ 1. Impaired Social Interaction related to pregnancy confirmation.

○ 2. Altered Sexuality Patterns related to fear of miscarriage.

○ 3. Ineffective Family Coping: Compromised related to pregnancy discomforts.

○ 4. Altered Nutrition related to increased demands of pregnancy during the first trimester.

A client and her husband are seen in the antepartum clinic. The client had a positive pregnancy test and is now about 11 weeks' pregnant.

31. The client's husband tells the nurse that he has been experiencing nausea and vomiting and fatigue along with his wife. The nurse determines that the client's husband is experiencing

○ 1. couvade syndrome.

○ 2. mittelschmerz.

○ 3. ptyalism.

○ 4. fantasies.

32. The client tells the nurse that she has been vomiting after breakfast nearly every morning. Which of the following measures should the nurse suggest to help the client cope with early morning nausea and vomiting?

○ 1. Drink fluids only during mealtime.

○ 2. Drink only warm liquids for breakfast.

○ 3. Eat dry, unsalted crackers before arising in the morning.

○ 4. Drink a carbonated beverage before bedtime.

33. The client asks the nurse if sexual activity should change during pregnancy if no complications exist. The nurse should instruct the client that

○ 1. the couple should practice coitus interruptus during pregnancy.

○ 2. sexual desire may change, but intercourse does not hurt the baby during an uncomplicated pregnancy.

○ 3. it is best to avoid sexual intercourse until the client is at least 16 weeks' pregnant.

○ 4. the couple should not have sexual intercourse during the last trimester of pregnancy.

34. The client asks the nurse if she can continue to have a glass of wine with dinner during the first trimester. Which of the following statements is the best response by the nurse?

○ 1. "You should limit drinking to beer and wine."

○ 2. "You should abstain from drinking alcoholic beverages."

○ 3. "Drink no more than 1 ounce of liquor per day."

○ 4. "The effects of alcohol during pregnancy are unknown."

35. The client tells the nurse that she has had increased vaginal secretions since becoming pregnant. The nurse should instruct the client that increased acidity and vaginal secretions
○ 1. are a result of decreased glycogen stores.
○ 2. may indicate a sexually transmitted disease.
○ 3. help prevent expulsion of the mucous plug.
○ 4. control the growth of pathologic bacteria.

36. The nurse has instructed the client about desired weight gain during pregnancy. The nurse's teaching is considered effective when the client says,
○ 1. "A maximum weight gain of about 20 pounds (9 kg) is recommended."
○ 2. "The total amount of weight gain is more important than the pattern of weight gain."
○ 3. "A weight gain of about 12 pounds (5.5 kg) each trimester is recommended."
○ 4. "Weight gain varies, but a range of 25 to 35 pounds (11.4 to 16 kg) is usually considered normal."

A 34-year-old nullipara is seen in the prenatal clinic for her first visit. Pregnancy is confirmed, and the client is about 8 weeks' pregnant.

37. The nurse explains to the client that she will need to take vitamins with iron during her pregnancy. The nurse suggests that the absorption of supplemental iron can be increased by taking it with
○ 1. milk.
○ 2. grape juice.
○ 3. hot chocolate.
○ 4. orange juice.

38. The nurse instructs the client about the need for increased folic acid in her diet. The nurse should instruct the client that she should eat more
○ 1. spinach.
○ 2. bananas.
○ 3. carrots.
○ 4. yogurt.

39. The nurse instructs the client about the importance of sufficient vitamin A in her diet. The nurse knows that the instructions have been effective when the client indicates that she should include
○ 1. beans and nuts.
○ 2. mushrooms and melons.
○ 3. spinach and squash.
○ 4. citrus fruits and tomatoes.

40. The nurse plans to instruct the client to include foods rich in riboflavin in her meal planning. An appropriate goal for the client is that every day she will eat two servings of
○ 1. fresh fruit.
○ 2. prunes.
○ 3. whole wheat bread.
○ 4. green leafy vegetables.

41. The client asks the nurse why vitamin C intake is so important during pregnancy. What is the nurse's best response?
○ 1. "Vitamin C is required to promote blood clot and collagen formation."
○ 2. "Supplemental vitamin C in large doses can prevent the fetus from developing neural tube defects."
○ 3. "Eating moderate amounts of foods high in vitamin C can help metabolize fats."
○ 4. "Studies have shown that vitamin C helps the growth of fetal bones."

42. The nurse plans to instruct the client to increase her intake of magnesium because magnesium
○ 1. prevents demineralization of the mother's bones.
○ 2. aids the synthesis of proteins, nucleic acids, and fats.
○ 3. functions as a coenzyme in amino acid production.
○ 4. synthesizes DNA and RNA in the fetus.

43. The physician schedules the client for a chorionic villi sampling test. After instructing the client about the procedure, the nurse considers the teaching effective when the client says,
○ 1. "The procedure requires the use of a needle that is inserted into the uterus."
○ 2. "I can't have anything to eat or drink after midnight on the day of the procedure."
○ 3. "The procedure involves the insertion of a catheter into my uterus."
○ 4. "I need to drink 32 to 40 ounces of fluid 1 hour before the procedure."

A 34-year-old multigravida who has received regular prenatal care for all of her previous pregnancies visits the prenatal clinic at 16 weeks' gestation.

44. The client tells the nurse that she has already felt the baby move. The nurse interprets this as
○ 1. unusual because quickening is not usually felt until 20 weeks' gestation for multiparous clients.
○ 2. normal because most multiparous clients experience quickening by 10 weeks' gestation.
○ 3. evidence that the client's estimated date of delivery is probably incorrect.
○ 4. normal because multiparous clients can experi-

ence quickening between 14 and 20 weeks' gestation.

45. An important assessment for the nurse to make for the pregnant client in the second trimester is whether or not the client desires
   ○ 1. alpha-fetoprotein (AFP) testing.
   ○ 2. her husband in the delivery area.
   ○ 3. to quit working after the baby is born.
   ○ 4. medication to alleviate heartburn.

46. The nurse plans to perform Leopold's maneuvers to examine the client's abdomen. To help make the client feel more comfortable and make the results more accurate, the nurse should have the client
   ○ 1. drink a few sips of water.
   ○ 2. lie on her right side.
   ○ 3. breathe deeply for 1 minute.
   ○ 4. empty her bladder.

47. The client asks the nurse, "What should I do about this brown discoloration across my nose and cheeks?" The nurse should instruct the client that the discoloration
   ○ 1. is a potential indicator of melanoma.
   ○ 2. is related to dilated capillaries.
   ○ 3. will fade if specially prescribed cosmetics are used.
   ○ 4. usually fades after delivery.

A 36-year-old primigravida is seen in the nurse midwife's office at 22 weeks' gestation for a routine visit. The client has had no complications to date.

48. The nurse plans to perform a fundal height assessment on the client to
   ○ 1. determine uterine activity.
   ○ 2. identify the need for an amniocentesis.
   ○ 3. assess the location of the placenta.
   ○ 4. estimate the gestational age.

49. While the client is lying supine on the examination table, she tells the nurse that she is feeling dizzy. After observing that the client is pale and perspiring freely, the nurse should
   ○ 1. turn the client onto her left side.
   ○ 2. obtain the client's pulse.
   ○ 3. assess the client for vaginal spotting.
   ○ 4. lower the client's head between her knees.

50. The client is scheduled for amniocentesis. The nurse explains to the client that one of the risks of amniocentesis is
   ○ 1. rupture of the membranes.
   ○ 2. premature labor.
   ○ 3. fetal death.
   ○ 4. malformation of fetal organs.

51. The client tells the nurse midwife that she and her husband wish to drive to visit relatives who live several hundred miles away. The nurse should make which of the following recommendations concerning automobile travel? Automobile travel during pregnancy should
   ○ 1. be avoided during the last half of pregnancy.
   ○ 2. be limited to a maximum of 3 hours.
   ○ 3. include frequent rest periods.
   ○ 4. be allowed if someone else is driving the car.

52. When the client complains of leg cramps, the nurse midwife suggests which exercise to relieve the cramps?
   ○ 1. Elevate the legs periodically during the day.
   ○ 2. Alternately flex and extend the legs.
   ○ 3. Push upward on the toes and downward on the knees.
   ○ 4. Lie prone in bed with the legs extended.

53. The client tells the nurse that she has been experiencing occasional heartburn. Which preventive measure should the nurse suggest?
   ○ 1. Eat smaller and more frequent meals.
   ○ 2. Take a pinch of baking soda with water after meals.
   ○ 3. Decrease fluid intake to three glasses daily.
   ○ 4. Take 2 tablespoons of Gelusil 3 times per day.

A 15-year-old client is seen in the prenatal clinic with her mother. The client is at about 16 weeks' gestation with her first pregnancy.

54. The client tells the nurse that she has been experiencing an occasional sharp pain from the fundus to her pubic bone on the left side. The nurse determines that the client is most likely experiencing
   ○ 1. appendicitis.
   ○ 2. preterm labor.
   ○ 3. round ligament pain.
   ○ 4. fetal movement.

55. The physician orders AFP screening for the client. In planning instruction for the client about the test, the nurse should stress that AFP studies
   ○ 1. are usually very accurate until 28 weeks' gestation.
   ○ 2. require a freshly voided maternal urine specimen.
   ○ 3. with elevated levels are associated with sickle cell anemia.
   ○ 4. with elevated levels are associated with neural tube defects.

56. The client tells the nurse that she has been having discomfort from her hemorrhoids. After giving in-

struction about strategies to decrease the discomfort, the nurse determines that the client needs *further* instruction when she says she should
○ 1. avoid straining to have a bowel movement.
○ 2. change positions frequently during the day.
○ 3. discontinue iron supplements if they have been prescribed.
○ 4. use warm sitz baths frequently during the day.

57. The nurse reinforces the client's need for continued prenatal care throughout the pregnancy. Continued prenatal care is important because adolescents
○ 1. are especially at risk for pregnancy-induced hypertension.
○ 2. usually lack support systems and need the support from health care providers.
○ 3. need additional instruction related to nutrition.
○ 4. rarely have the father of the baby involved in the pregnancy, especially in the second trimester.

58. The client weighs 100 pounds and has only gained 5 pounds since becoming pregnant. She states, "I haven't had any appetite." What is the most appropriate nursing diagnosis for this client?
○ 1. Knowledge Deficit about fetal development as evidenced by lack of sufficient weight gain.
○ 2. Noncompliance with diet related to fear of body image changes.
○ 3. Altered Nutrition, Less Than Body Requirements related to lack of appetite.
○ 4. Altered Growth and Development related to poor appetite.

59. The nurse plans to instruct the client about breast changes that occur during pregnancy. The nurse plans to instruct the client that
○ 1. growth of the milk ducts is greatest during the first 12 weeks of gestation.
○ 2. enlargement of the breasts indicates adequate levels of progesterone.
○ 3. colostrum is usually secreted during the second half of pregnancy.
○ 4. darkening of the areola occurs during the last month of pregnancy.

60. The nurse plans to discuss various diagnostic tests to determine fetal well-being. Which of the following should be included in the teaching plan?
○ 1. Fetal biophysical profile involves assessing breathing movements, body movements, tone, amniotic fluid volume, and fetal heart rate reactivity.
○ 2. A reactive nonstress test is an ominous sign and requires further evaluation with fetal echocardiography.
○ 3. Contraction stress testing is performed on most pregnant women and can be initiated as early as 16 weeks' gestation.

○ 4. A lecithin-to-sphingomyelin ratio of 2:1 indicates fetal kidney maturation.

61. The nurse plans to teach the client how to do Kegel exercises several times a day. The nurse should explain that the primary purpose of these exercises is to
○ 1. prevent vulvar edema.
○ 2. relieve lower back discomfort.
○ 3. strengthen the perineal muscles.
○ 4. strengthen the abdominal muscles.

A pregnant 25-year-old client visits the clinic during her third trimester. The client began receiving prenatal care at 10 weeks' gestation.

62. The client tells the nurse, "I've been having strange dreams about the baby. Last week I dreamed he was covered with hair." The best response by the nurse is
○ 1. "Dreams like this are very unusual. Tell me more."
○ 2. "Often when a mother has these dreams, she is very frightened about becoming a parent."
○ 3. "Dreams about the baby late in pregnancy means labor is about to begin."
○ 4. "It's not uncommon to have dreams and fantasies about the baby, especially in the last trimester."

63. The client reports frequent constipation. To help relieve constipation, the nurse should instruct the client to
○ 1. use glycerin suppositories as needed.
○ 2. eat four pieces of fruit daily.
○ 3. avoid highly seasoned foods.
○ 4. use a mild laxative, such as milk of magnesia, as needed.

64. The client tells the nurse that she has been experiencing insomnia for the last 2 weeks. The nurse should advise the client to
○ 1. drink a small glass of wine with dinner.
○ 2. exercise for 30 minutes before bedtime.
○ 3. practice relaxation techniques before bedtime.
○ 4. drink a cup of hot chocolate after supper.

65. The client has been instructed about edema, which can occur during the third trimester. The nurse determines that the client needs *further* instruction when the client says,
○ 1. "Swelling of my feet and ankles is normal."
○ 2. "I should continue to drink 6 to 8 glasses of water a day."
○ 3. "It's important to avoid prolonged standing."
○ 4. "Swelling in the hands and face is normal."

The Pregnant Client in Childbirth Preparation Classes

A primigravida and her husband are interested in childbirth preparation classes offered in the community. They have their physician's support for delivery in a birthing center. The client is about 8 weeks' pregnant.

66. The couple asks when they should begin the preparation for childbirth classes that discuss nutrition during pregnancy. The best response by the nurse would be to suggest that the couple start attending
    - ○ 1. as soon as the client experiences lightening.
    - ○ 2. after the client has scheduled a visit with the dietitian.
    - ○ 3. during the first trimester of pregnancy.
    - ○ 4. in the early second trimester.

67. The pregnant client asks the nurse if she can continue to go swimming twice per week. After giving instruction about swimming and bathing, the nurse determines that the client needs *further* instruction when she says,
    - ○ 1. "I can continue to swim as long as my membranes aren't ruptured."
    - ○ 2. "I can relax in a hot tub after swimming in the pool."
    - ○ 3. "I can take a bath daily but should be careful not to fall."
    - ○ 4. "I should avoid sitting in a sauna for prolonged periods."

68. The client reports a history of varicose veins. The nurse instructs the client about strategies to promote comfort. The nurse determines that the client understands the instruction when the client says,
    - ○ 1. "Lying down with my feet elevated should help."
    - ○ 2. "Support hose can be put on just before bedtime."
    - ○ 3. "Restricting milk intake may provide some relief."
    - ○ 4. "I should avoid wearing supportive pantyhose."

Ten couples are enrolled in an early preparation for childbirth class, which will be taught during a 6-week period by a registered nurse.

69. During one of the classes, the nurse plans to discuss the endocrine changes that normally occur during pregnancy. Which of the following should be included in the nurse's teaching plan?
    - ○ 1. Thyroid enlargement and an increase in basal metabolic rate is normal.

- ○ 2. Human placental lactogen maintains the corpus luteum.
- ○ 3. The adrenal glands become enlarged throughout the pregnancy.
- ○ 4. Estrogen helps enlarge the breasts and enhance milk production.

70. The nurse plans instruction on anatomy and physiology of pregnancy and fetal development. Which of the following would be appropriate to include in the teaching plan? By the end of the third month (9 to 12 weeks), the fetus has developed
    - ○ 1. fine, downy hair.
    - ○ 2. brown fat.
    - ○ 3. external genitalia.
    - ○ 4. air ducts and alveoli.

71. One of the participants tells the nurse that there is a history of twins in her family. The nurse should instruct the client that
    - ○ 1. monozygotic twins frequently occur as a result of becoming pregnant within 1 month of stopping oral contraception.
    - ○ 2. monozygotic twins occur by chance regardless of race or heredity.
    - ○ 3. dizygotic twins occur less often in women who have been pregnant numerous times.
    - ○ 4. dizygotic twins occur more often in adolescents who are pregnant.

Six couples all having their first child are enrolled in a childbirth preparation class during the third trimester. The classes last 6 weeks and are taught by a registered nurse.

72. The nurse is planning a 2-hour childbirth preparation class focused on labor and delivery. Included in the plan will be the normal sequence of maneuvers the fetus goes through during labor and delivery when the head is the presenting part. The nurse plans to instruct the group that the first maneuver that the fetus goes through is
    - ○ 1. engagement.
    - ○ 2. flexion.
    - ○ 3. descent.
    - ○ 4. internal rotation.

73. A client in the class asks how much blood will be lost during an uncomplicated delivery. What is the nurse's best response?
    - ○ 1. "The maximum blood loss considered within normal limits is 500 mL."
    - ○ 2. "The minimum blood loss considered within normal limits is 1000 mL."
    - ○ 3. "Most women lose more amniotic fluid and little blood during delivery."

○ 4. "It would be very unusual if you lost more than 200 mL of blood during the delivery."

74. After giving instruction about the amniotic fluid and sac during the preparation for childbirth class, the nurse knows that a client needs *further* instruction by which statement?
○ 1. "The amniotic fluid helps to dilate the cervix."
○ 2. "The fetus is protected from injury by the amniotic fluid."
○ 3. "Fetal nutrition is provided by the amniotic fluid."
○ 4. "The fetus is kept at an even temperature by the amniotic fluid and sac."

75. As the nurse evaluates all causes of pain during labor, she decides to teach the class participants that the primary cause of pain in the first stage of labor is
○ 1. distention of the upper uterine segment.
○ 2. status of the amnionic membranes.
○ 3. stretching of the perineum.
○ 4. dilatation and effacement of the cervix.

76. During the class, one of the participants asks the nurse, "How will I know if I am really in labor?" The best response by the nurse is that with true labor
○ 1. contractions are mainly abdominal.
○ 2. vaginal mucus is clear.
○ 3. the fetus becomes more active.
○ 4. there is cervical dilation and effacement.

77. The nurse has instructed the class participants about methods to cope with discomforts of the first stage of labor. The nurse determines that one of the pregnant clients needs *further* instruction when she says that she has been practicing
○ 1. effleurage.
○ 2. progressive relaxation.
○ 3. guided imagery.
○ 4. rapid breathing techniques.

78. After the first class session, a pregnant client tells the nurse that she has had some vaginal discharge and local itching. The nurse's best action is to advise the client to
○ 1. schedule an appointment at the clinic for an examination.
○ 2. administer a vinegar douche under low pressure.
○ 3. prepare for imminent labor and delivery.
○ 4. use an over-the-counter cream for yeast infections.

The nurse is responsible for teaching preparation for childbirth classes to a group of pregnant adolescents. Most of the clients are not married, but several have brought their boyfriends to the class.

79. One client asks the nurse, "How does the baby breathe inside of me?" The nurse should instruct the client that circulation of oxygenated blood is accomplished by the
○ 1. umbilical vein.
○ 2. pulmonary artery.
○ 3. foramen ovale.
○ 4. fetal lungs.

80. The nurse has instructed the group about the functions of the placenta. After giving the instruction, the nurse knows that a client needs *further* instruction when she says that the hormones produced by the placenta include
○ 1. testosterone.
○ 2. estrogen.
○ 3. progesterone.
○ 4. human chorionic gonadotrophin.

81. The nurse plans to instruct the group about the placenta and the umbilical cord. Which of the following should be included in the teaching plan?
○ 1. The highest oxygen content is found in the umbilical vein.
○ 2. About 25% of umbilical cords have only two vessels.
○ 3. A velamentous insertion exists when the cord inserts centrally at the placenta.
○ 4. A nuchal cord usually occurs when the cord is abnormally short.

82. The nurse plans to discuss physiologic changes that normally occur during pregnancy. Which of the following would be important for the nurse to include in the teaching plan?
○ 1. Hyperventilation and metabolic acidosis may occur.
○ 2. There is greater susceptibility to urinary tract infections.
○ 3. Hemoglobin levels increase owing to increased blood volume.
○ 4. Cardiac output and stroke volume decrease.

83. The nurse plans to emphasize the need for continued prenatal care and well-baby care after delivery. Which of the following should be included in the teaching plan?
○ 1. The infant mortality rate is defined as the number of infant deaths under age 1 year per 1,000 live births.
○ 2. Perinatal mortality rate is the number of deaths of infants under the age of 12 months per 1,000 live births.
○ 3. Neonatal mortality rate is the number of infant deaths under age 12 months per 1,000 live births.
○ 4. The maternal mortality rate has been steadily increasing in the United States during the past 20 years.

The nurse is responsible for a 2-hour presentation on the anatomy and physiology of pregnancy for 25 nursing students.

84. The nurse plans to instruct the group about the development of the placenta. Which of the following should be included in the teaching plan?
○ 1. The placenta is formed by the fusion of chorionic villi and the decidua basalis.
○ 2. The weight of a term placenta is 1,000 to 1,500 g.
○ 3. In the male fetus, human placental lactogen promotes synthesis of testosterone.
○ 4. Viruses are not able to cross the placental barrier.

85. A student asks how the obstetric conjugate of the pelvis is measured. The nurse should instruct the student that the obstetric conjugate is usually measured by
○ 1. using diagnostic fetal pelvimetry.
○ 2. subtracting 1.5 cm from the diagonal conjugate.
○ 3. measuring the diameter of the pelvic inlet.
○ 4. adding 1.5 cm to the transverse diameter.

86. During the presentation, the nurse discusses the risks of adolescent pregnancy. The nurse determines that one of the students needs *further* instruction when the student says that adolescents are at greater risk for
○ 1. lack of prenatal care.
○ 2. low-birth-weight infants.
○ 3. cephalopelvic disproportion.
○ 4. congenital anomalies.

87. After describing the pelvic changes that occur during pregnancy, the nurse determines that a student understands the instruction when the student states that the uterus receives its blood supply directly from the uterine artery and the
○ 1. iliac artery.
○ 2. hypogastric artery.
○ 3. pulmonary artery.
○ 4. ovarian artery.

The Pregnant Client With Risk Factors

A primigravida is admitted to the hospital at 12 weeks' gestation. She has abdominal cramping and bright red vaginal spotting. Her cervix is not dilated.

88. Based on the client's symptoms, the nurse determines that the client is most likely experiencing an abortion termed
○ 1. missed.
○ 2. threatened.
○ 3. inevitable.
○ 4. complete.

89. After the client passes some of the products of conception, she returns to the hospital for a dilation and curettage (D & C). The nurse anticipates that the client will most likely express feelings of
○ 1. guilt.
○ 2. ambivalence.
○ 3. relief.
○ 4. fear.

90. The nurse administers hydroxyzine (Vistaril) as ordered, primarily to
○ 1. counteract nausea.
○ 2. reduce discomfort.
○ 3. decrease urinary retention.
○ 4. promote uterine contractility.

91. Postoperatively, the nurse finds the client crying. Which of the following comments by the nurse would be best in this situation?
○ 1. "Are you having a great deal of pain?"
○ 2. "Often spontaneous abortion means a defective fetus."
○ 3. "I'm sorry you lost your baby."
○ 4. "You can always try again to get pregnant."

92. The nurse determines that the client is Rh negative. Analysis of the client's blood indicates that she is unsensitized. The nurse administers human anti-D globulin (RhoGAM) before the client is discharged from the hospital to prevent the client from
○ 1. becoming Rh positive.
○ 2. Rh-positive sensitivity.
○ 3. an antibody response to Rh-negative blood.
○ 4. future pregnancies with an Rh-positive fetus.

A client visits the emergency room and tells the nurse that she suspects that she is pregnant but has been having a small amount of bleeding and has pain in the lower abdomen.

93. The nurse notifies the physician because the client is most likely experiencing
○ 1. gestational trophoblastic disease.
○ 2. complete abortion.
○ 3. ectopic pregnancy.
○ 4. incompetent cervix.

94. While caring for this client, the nurse should plan to
○ 1. witness an informed consent for surgery.
○ 2. administer ordered intravenous platelets.
○ 3. monitor the client for uterine contractions.
○ 4. assess the client's discharge for a brownish discoloration.

CORRECT ANSWERS AND RATIONALE

The letters in parentheses following the rationale identify the step of the nursing process (A, D, P, I, E), cognitive level (K, C, T, N), and client needs (S, G, L, H). See the Answer Grid for the key.

The Preconception Client

1. 2. When acting as a sexuality counselor, the nurse should begin by obtaining a sexual history from the client. Obtaining a history is part of the assessment phase of the nursing process. Only after the nurse has collected necessary information can the data be analyzed and plans formulated, implemented, and evaluated. Although a complete physical examination, including a Pap smear, is often warranted, this can be done later. There is no need to include the client's sexual partner at this time, nor any need to discuss a history of genetic abnormalities until after the sexual history has been obtained. (I, T, H)

2. 4. The nurse determines that the client has understood the instructions when the client indicates that she should not squeeze her nipples if there is a discharge. If the client notices a discharge, or bleeding she should notify her physician or health care provider, as this may be symptomatic of underlying disease. Ideally, breast self-examination should be performed about a week following the onset of menses. The client should perform breast self-examination on the same day of each month only if the client has stopped menstruating (e.g. menopause). The client's breasts should mirror each other. If one breast is larger than the other, there may be underlying disease, such as a tumor. (E, T, H)

3. 4. Ovulation usually occurs on day 14, plus or minus 2 days, before the onset of the next menstrual cycle. Stated another way, the menstrual period begins about 2 weeks after ovulation. Ovulation does not usually occur during the menstrual period when the endometrium is being shed. The ovum survives for about 12 to 24 hours after ovulation. The basal body temperature rises 0.5° to 1.0°F when ovulation occurs. Clients can be taught to determine when ovulation occurs (eg, cervical mucous changes, basal body temperature changes). Although some women consistently experience some pelvic discomfort during ovulation (mittelschmerz), severe or unusual pain is rare. (P, N, H)

4. 1. Sperm can reach the ovum in only 1 to 5 minutes under ideal conditions. This is an important point to make with a client seeking information related to contraception. Many people believe that the time interval is much longer and that they can wait to take steps to prevent conception until after intercourse, which is usually too late. Using the abstinence method, the couple should abstain from intercourse until 3 days after ovulation has occurred. In a healthy male, sperm remain viable for about 48 to 72 hours. (E, N, H)

5. 2. Natural methods of fertility management depend on knowing when ovulation occurs. Regular menstrual cycles can vary by 1 or 2 days in either direction. The calendar method, basal body temperature method, cervical mucous method, and symptothermal method are all natural methods of fertility management. The symptothermal method requires daily basal body temperature assessments plus close monitoring of cervical mucous changes. Although some record keeping is necessary, it is not extensive. Failure rates depend on the accuracy of determining when ovulation has occurred. Typically, the failure rates are between 10% and 20%. The method relies on abstinence during the period of ovulation. Although a diaphragm with spermicide may increase the effectiveness of this method, most clients who choose natural methods are not interested in chemical or barrier types of family planning methods. (I, N, H)

6. 1. Oral contraceptive agents inhibit ovulation by suppressing follicle-stimulating hormone and luteinizing hormone. Despite the effectiveness of this method, about 5% of users discontinue this method after 1 year, primarily owing to unwanted side effects. Among the many side effects of oral contraceptives are nausea, vomiting, fluid retention, increased vaginal discharge, chloasma, headaches, weight gain, thromboembolic disorders, hepatic adenoma, and possible hypertension. A history of thromboembolic disease is an absolute contraindication to using oral contraceptive agents. It is not necessary to use the basal body temperature method because ovulation does not occur when the medication is taken properly. (E, N, H)

7. 4. The ovum is normally fertilized in the fallopian tube. Although there have been reports of fertilization outside of the fallopian tube, this is not a normal occurrence. (I, T, H)

8. 3. Adding spermicide offers additional protection against pregnancy. Natural skin condoms do not offer the same protection against sexually transmitted diseases as latex condoms. The typical failure rate for condoms is about 12%. Condom users generally report that glans sensitivity is decreased. (I, T, H)

9. 4. A diaphragm should be left in place for at least

8 hours after intercourse. More spermicidal cream or jelly should be used if intercourse is repeated during this period. The client should be instructed to remove the diaphragm at least once every 24 hours. Cases of toxic shock syndrome are infrequent, but clients should be instructed in the danger signs: fever, diarrhea, rash, vomiting, and muscle aches. A client cannot obtain a diaphragm without a prescription. Each woman must be fitted individually by a skilled practitioner. Douching with an acidic solution is not recommended. The diaphragm should be washed in warm, soapy water after use. (P, N, H)

10. 4. In vasectomy, a common procedure for male sterilization, the ductus deferens (vas deferens) is cut and tied. Coagulation may also be used to create an obstruction in the vas deferens. (I, N, H)

11. 1. Female sterilization involves ligation or cauterization of the fallopian tubes through a small abdominal incision. Reversal of a tubal ligation is not easily done, and the pregnancy success rate after reversal is about 30%. With a bilateral tubal ligation, there is a slightly greater risk for ectopic pregnancy. The ovaries are not generally removed during a tubal ligation. (E, N, H)

12. 2. Although the vaginal wall and cervix may be sensitive structures, the primary anatomic female structure involved in sexual arousal is the clitoris. Composed of erectile tissue, the clitoris is especially sensitive to foreplay and movements of the shaft of the penis against its surface. (I, T, H)

13. 1. The diagnosis of infertility is a crisis for most couples. The appropriate nursing diagnosis is Grief related to inability to conceive. The situation does not indicate how much knowledge about infertility treatments the couple may have. There is no evidence to suggest ineffective family coping or anxiety related to decreased spermatogenesis. (D, N, L)

14. 3. A common factor in female infertility is ovarian dysfunction. Other common factors include blocked fallopian tubes and cervical factors. Less frequent causes include endometriosis, vaginitis, polycystic ovaries, and overproduction of prolactin. The causes of infertility can be determined in about 80% to 90% of couples investigated. (I, T, G)

15. 4. By the end of the first visit, the couple should be able to identify potential treatment modalities. They should consider all the various treatments before selecting one. The first visit is not the appropriate time to decide on treatment. The couple may desire information about alternatives, but there are not enough data to suggest that a specific treatment modality may not be successful. The success rate for achieving a pregnancy depends on both the cause and the effectiveness of the treatment, and in some cases may only be as high as 30%. (P, N, H)

16. 1. During artificial insemination, sperm is inseminated during ovulation through the cervix. In vitro fertilization requires the harvesting of several ova from the female ovary; these ova are then fertilized outside the body with sperm in a special culture. The fertilized ova are then transferred through the cervix with a special catheter. GIFT requires the use of progesterone to support the endometrium for implantation. Human menopausal gonadotrophin is a drug that increases the level of prolactin. (P, T, G)

17. 1. Clomiphene citrate (Clomid) is a fertility drug that induces ovulation in women desiring pregnancy. One of the most common disadvantages of the drug is multiple gestation (twins, triplets, or more). There is no evidence that the drug increases spontaneous abortions, fibrocystic breast disease, or increased congenital anomalies. (I, T, G)

18. 3. After the ova are fertilized, three or four embryos are transferred through the cervix through a special catheter. The success rate of this procedure is only about 20%. Estrogen injections are not required with in vitro fertilization. Multiple pregnancy rates are comparable to those resulting from GIFT procedures. (E, T, G)

19. 1. The immunoassay pregnancy test is highly accurate within 8 to 10 days after conception. It uses an antiserum with specificity for the β-subunit of human chorionic gonadotrophin in blood plasma. Over-the-counter or home pregnancy tests are performed on urine and use the hemagglutination-inhibition method. A positive pregnancy test is a probable sign of pregnancy. Certain conditions other than pregnancy, such as choriocarcinoma, can cause elevated human chorionic gonadotrophin levels. The immunoassay pregnancy test is used on both blood and urine. (I, T, H)

20. 4. Human chorionic gonadotrophin is the hormone used in most pregnancy tests. Estrogen stimulates uterine development during pregnancy. Luteinizing hormone stimulates ovulation. Follicle-stimulating hormone is involved in follicle maturation during the menstrual cycle. Progestin and prolactin are not used to detect pregnancy. (E, T, H)

21. 1. Amenorrhea, urinary frequency, breast tenderness, nausea, vomiting, and fatigue are considered presumptive or subjective changes of pregnancy. Probable or objective signs of pregnancy include Goodell's sign (softening of the cervix), Chadwick's sign (discoloration of the mucous membranes of the cervix, vagina, and vulva), and Hegar's sign (softening of the isthmus of the uterus). Other probable signs include enlargement of the abdomen, uterine souffle, and Braxton-Hicks contractions. Positive or diagnostic signs of pregnancy include detection of the fetal heartbeat, detection of fetal movements by a trained examiner, and ultrasound identification of a fetus. (D, N, H)

22. 4. The client's concerns about death during childbirth provided the nurse with an opportunity to gather additional data. Telling the client not to concern herself about what has happened in the past is not useful. Postponing the client's need for a discussion about complications of pregnancy may further increase the client's anxiety. Maternal death does occur, even with modern technology. Leading causes of maternal mortality in the United States include embolism, pregnancy-induced hypertension, hemorrhage, ectopic pregnancy, and infection. (I, T, L)

23. 4. The most appropriate priority diagnosis from the data available is Anxiety related to the financial impact of childbearing. The client has stated that she is unemployed. The nurse does not know whether the client is pregnant, so Knowledge Deficit is not appropriate. From the available data, it is not clear whether the client is at high risk for altered nutrition, nor has the client expressed fear related to first-trimester changes. (D, N, L)

24. 4. The client using the basal body temperature method should take her temperature for 5 minutes every morning on awakening, before arising or starting any activity. It is important that the client take her temperature at about the same time every morning, and the temperature should be recorded on a graph. At this time, temperature is least likely to be influenced by other factors. A slight drop in body temperature before ovulation occurs in some but not all women. The client's temperature may have numerous fluctuations if taken before bedtime. A woman cannot determine exactly when ovulation occurs until it has actually happened. Depending on the client's motivation and the ability to perform the procedure correctly, this can be an effective fertility management method, but it is one of the least reliable methods. Generally, clients who choose this method do not wish to use other chemical or barrier methods for a variety of reasons. (E, N, H)

25. 3. As ovulation approaches, cervical mucus is abundant and clear, resembling raw egg white. Changes in the cervical mucus are related to the influences of estrogen and progesterone. During the luteal phase of the cycle, the cervical mucus is thick and sticky, making it difficult for sperm to pass. (P, T, H)

The Pregnant Client Receiving Prenatal Care

26. 3. When using Nägele's rule to determine the estimated due date, count back 3 calendar months from the first day of the last menstrual period and add 7 days. This means the client's due date is February 22. Measurement of fundal height and ultrasonography are also used to determine gestational age. (A, N, H)

27. 2. With a Doppler device, the fetal heart rate can be heard as early as 10 to 12 weeks' gestation. With a fetoscope, the fetal heart rate can be heard between 17 and 20 weeks' gestation. (I, T, H)

28. 2. This client is expressing a feeling of surprise about having a baby. The nurse responds to the client's feeling by explaining that such feelings are normal and experienced by many women early in pregnancy. Studies have shown that a common reaction to pregnancy is summarized as, "someday, but not now." Fathers must also come to terms with the pregnancy. The nurse practitioner's confirmation of the pregnancy is something the client already suspects. Offering a pamphlet on pregnancy does not respond to the client's feelings. By the end of the first trimester, most new mothers have accepted the pregnancy, although culture may play a role in openly accepting the pregnancy. (I, N, L)

29. 1. Women normally experience ambivalence when pregnancy is confirmed, even if the pregnancy was planned. Although the client's culture may play a role in openly accepting the pregnancy, most new mothers who have initially been ambivalent accept the reality by the end of the first trimester. Ambivalence may be expressed throughout the pregnancy; this is believed to be related to the amount of physical discomforts. (I, N, L)

30. 4. The client at 10 weeks' gestation has a definite need for appropriate nutrition to meet the needs of the growing fetus. The priority nursing diagnosis at this time relates to nutrition and the necessary health teaching. Pregnancy places additional demands on the body, and adequate nutrition is important for fetal well-being. No data are presented to suggest impaired social interaction, ineffective family coping, or altered sexuality patterns. (D, N, H)

31. 1. Couvade syndrome is one in which the expectant father experiences some of the discomforts of pregnancy along with the pregnant woman as a means of identifying with the pregnancy. The expectant father is not experiencing mittelschmerz, which is the term for the lower abdominal discomfort felt by some women during ovulation. There are no data to suggest that the symptoms are related to fantasies. Ptyalism is an oral craving for substances such as clay or starch that some pregnant clients experience. (D, N, H)

32. 3. Eating a dry high-carbohydrate food, such as crackers or dry toast, before arising in the morning often relieves the early morning nausea and vomiting that many pregnant women experience. Eating high-fat foods tend to exacerbate the condition for many women. Fluids should be taken frequently between meals. A carbonated beverage at bedtime has not been successful. (I, N, H)

33. 2. It is generally agreed that couples need not change their pattern of sexual activity during pregnancy unless complications arise. Some women find intercourse uncomfortable during the first and third trimesters owing to the common discomforts of pregnancy. During the third trimester, the couple should consider coital positions other than male superior, such as side-by-side, female superior, and vaginal rear entry. Intercourse is contraindicated when bleeding or ruptured membrane occurs. After 32 weeks' gestation, women with a history of preterm labor should be advised of the possible risks of coitus. (I, T, H)

34. 2. There is no definitive answer as to how much alcohol can be safely consumed by a pregnant woman. Therefore, it is recommended that pregnant clients be taught to abstain from drinking alcohol during pregnancy. Maternal alcohol use may result in fetal alcohol syndrome, marked by mild to moderate mental retardation, physical growth retardation, central nervous system disorders, and feeding difficulties. (P, N, H)

35. 4. Increased vaginal secretions during pregnancy are related to secretion of estrogen. Lactic acid production results in an acidic environment, which helps control the growth of pathologic bacteria. The glycogen-rich environment fosters the development of yeast (*Candida albicans*) infection. Any itching or burning should be promptly reported to a health professional. (I, T, H)

36. 4. The National Academy of Sciences Institute of Medicine recommends that women gain between 25 and 35 pounds (11.4 to 16 kg) during pregnancy. These guidelines were developed to decrease the risk of intrauterine growth retardation. It is believed that the pattern of weight gain is as important as the total amount of weight gained. (I, N, H)

37. 4. Absorption of supplemental iron and nonmeat sources of iron is enhanced by combining them with meat or a good source of vitamin C. Gastrointestinal upset is more likely when iron is taken on an empty stomach. The pregnant woman who experiences gastrointestinal upset should be taught to take iron tablets with meals to decrease adverse gastrointestinal symptoms; however, iron absorption is reduced by 40% to 50% if tablets are taken with meals. (I, N, G)

38. 1. Green leafy vegetables, such as asparagus, spinach, brussel sprouts, and broccoli, are rich sources of folic acid. A well-balanced diet must include whole grains, dairy products, and fresh fruits; however, these foods are not rich in folic acid. (P, N, G)

39. 3. Spinach, squash, and other yellow vegetables are rich sources of vitamin A. (E, T, H)

40. 4. Green leafy vegetables, milk, eggs, veal, beef, and cheddar cheese are rich sources of riboflavin. (P, T, H)

41. 1. Vitamin C is required to promote blood clot and collagen formation. Vitamin C deficiency has been associated with premature rupture of the membranes and pregnancy-induced hypertension. High doses of vitamin C are not recommended. Neonates exposed to excessive doses of vitamin C have developed symptoms of scurvy after birth. High doses of vitamin C do not prevent the fetus from becoming infected. Vitamin C does not help to metabolize carbohydrates, although thiamine is a coenzyme in carbohydrate metabolism. Vitamin C does not affect placental growth. (I, N, G)

42. 2. Magnesium aids in the synthesis of protein, nucleic acids, proteins, and fats. It does not affect demineralization of the mother's bones, aid in synthesis of DNA or RNA, or function as a coenzyme in amino acid production. (I, T, H)

43. 3. Chorionic villi sampling can be performed between 8 and 12 weeks' gestation and involves the insertion of a catheter into the uterus to obtain a sample from the villi. It is a useful diagnostic test to determine trisomy 13, translocations, and sickle cell anemia. There are no food or fluid restrictions. Ideally, the client should empty the bladder before the procedure. (E, N, G)

44. 4. Although some women may perceive quickening between 14 and 20 weeks' gestation, most multiparous women experience it at about 17.5 weeks' gestation. It is not unusual or abnormal for a client at 8 weeks' gestation not to experience quickening. (D, N, G)

45. 1. AFP testing is generally performed between 16 and 18 weeks' gestation to detect neural tube defects such as anencephaly and spina bifida. Assessment of whether the client desires her husband in the delivery area or whether she plans to work after the delivery is not essential. Generally, heartburn medication is not necessary unless the client has indicated this is a problem. (A, T, H)

46. 4. The client should empty her bladder before the nurse palpates the abdomen to perform Leopold's maneuvers. This increases the client's comfort and makes palpation more accurate. The client should be lying in a supine position with the head slightly elevated for greater comfort and with the knees drawn up slightly. The client does not need to breathe deeply or take sips of water before the procedure. (I, T, H)

47. 4. Discoloration on the face that commonly appears during pregnancy, called *chloasma,* usually fades after delivery and is of no clinical significance. The client bothered by her appearance may be able to decrease its prominence with ordinary makeup. No treatment is necessary for this condition. It is not related to melanoma or dilated capillaries. (I, T, G)

48. 4. Assessment of fundal height is a gross estimate of gestational age. By 20 weeks' gestation, the height of the fundus should be at the level of the umbilicus. If the fundal height measurement deviates significantly, further evaluation may be necessary. Fundal height that is significantly different than the estimated gestational age may indicate multiple pregnancy or fetal growth retardation. (I, T, G)

49. 1. The most common reason a pregnant client may feel dizzy, become pale, and perspire freely when lying supine is pressure on the vena cava from the enlarging uterus. The condition is often referred to as *vena cava syndrome* or *supine hypotensive syndrome.* It can be alleviated by turning the client onto her left side. Measuring the client's blood pressure, pulse, and respirations may be performed once the client is positioned on her left side. The symptoms are not related to vaginal spotting. Lowering the client's head is not as helpful as positioning her on her left side. (I, N, G)

50. 2. One of the primary risks of amniocentesis is stimulation of the uterus and subsequent preterm labor. If performed by a skilled practitioner, there is generally little risk to the fetus or rupture of the membranes. (I, T, G)

51. 3. Automobile travel is not contraindicated during pregnancy unless the client develops complications. The client traveling by automobile should be advised to take intermittent rest periods of 10 to 15 minutes every 2 hours. This stimulates the circulation, which becomes sluggish during long periods of sitting. There is no reason why the client cannot drive, if no complications exist. (I, N, H)

52. 3. Leg cramps are thought to result from excessive amounts of phosphorus absorbed from milk products. Pushing up on the toes and down on the knees is an effective measure to relieve leg cramps. Keeping the legs warm and elevating them are good preventive measures. Sitting will not relieve cramps, nor will lying with the legs extended. Lying prone in the bed is not considered helpful. (I, T, G)

53. 1. Heartburn can occur at any time during pregnancy. Contributing factors include stress, tension, worry, fatigue, caffeine, and smoking. Eating smaller and more frequent meals may help prevent heartburn. The client should be advised to avoid fatty foods, sodium bicarbonate antacids (eg, Alka-Seltzer), baking soda, and Bicitra (sodium citrate), which are high in sodium. Increasing fluid intake may help by diluting gastric juices. Occasional heartburn can be reduced by taking calcium carbonate (eg, Tums). If the heartburn is excessive, the client may need further evaluation to rule out other gastrointestinal disorders. (I, T, H)

54. 3. The client is most likely experiencing round ligament pain. Appendicitis usually causes pain on the right side of the abdomen. Preterm labor at 16 weeks is not common. Generally, fetal movement may be felt between 14 and 20 weeks' gestation, but for a primigravida this fluttering feeling usually is not painful and typically is not felt until about 20 weeks' gestation. (D, N, G)

55. 4. AFP levels are usually highest at 15 weeks' gestation. The client's blood is used for the sample, and the test is typically performed at 16 to 18 weeks' gestation. The test is not accurate after this time. Elevated levels are associated with neural tube defects, such as spina bifida, anencephaly, and encephalocele. (I, T, G)

56. 3. The client needs further instruction when she says that discontinuing iron supplements will alleviate hemorrhoids. Warm sitz baths are helpful in providing relief from the discomfort of hemorrhoids. The client should avoid straining, increase fluid and fiber in the diet, and avoid prolonged standing or sitting positions. (E, T, H)

57. 1. The most significant medical complication in pregnant adolescents is pregnancy-induced hypertension. Prenatal care is often the most critical factor influencing pregnancy outcome. Other risks for adolescents include low-birth-weight infants, preterm labor, iron deficiency anemia, and cephalopelvic disproportion. Generally, all first-time mothers need instruction related to nutrition. Adolescent mothers have better nutrition when they attend group classes and are subject to peer pressure. There is no evidence that most adolescents lack support systems. Adolescent fathers may abandon the mothers at any time during the pregnancy; however, some adolescent fathers are supportive throughout the pregnancy. (D, N, H)

58. 3. The most appropriate nursing diagnosis for this client is Altered Nutrition, Less Than Body Requirements related to lack of appetite. She has gained only 1 pound and states that she has no appetite. It is important that the nurse gather additional data to determine the reason for the client's poor appetite. There are no data to support Knowledge Deficit or Noncompliance. Although the pregnant adolescent may be experiencing Altered Growth and Development related to the pregnancy, this is not the priority diagnosis. (D, N, H)

59. 3. Colostrum is usually secreted during the second

half of pregnancy in preparation for breast-feeding. Growth of the milk ducts is greatest in the last trimester, and enlargement of the breasts is usually due to estrogen. Darkening of the areola can occur early in pregnancy. (P, T, H)

60. 1. The fetal biophysical profile includes fetal breathing movements, fetal body movements, tone, amnionic fluid volume, and fetal heart rate reactivity. A reactive nonstress test is a sign of fetal well-being and does not require further evaluation. Contraction stress testing or oxytocin challenge testing should be performed only on women at risk. The contraction stress test is rarely performed before 28 weeks' gestation because of the possibility of initiating labor. A lecithin-to-sphingomyelin ratio performed on amnionic fluid that has a ratio of 2 : 1 indicates fetal lung maturity. (P, N, G)

61. 3. The purpose of Kegel exercises is to strengthen the perineal muscles in preparation for the labor process. There is no evidence to suggest that these exercises prevent vulvar edema, relieve lower back discomfort, or strengthen the abdominal muscles. (I, T, H)

62. 4. During the third trimester, it is not uncommon for clients to have dreams or fantasies about the baby. Sometimes, the dreams are about infants who are malformed or, in this example, covered with hair. There is no evidence to suggest that the client is fearful about becoming a parent. (I, N, L)

63. 2. Measures to relieve constipation include drinking a glass of hot water in the morning, increasing bulk and roughage in the diet, increasing fluid intake, and exercising regularly. It is best not to suggest laxatives or suppositories because a client may become dependent on them. Laxatives should be used only when diet, fluid intake, and exercise do not relieve the problem and after consultation with the nurse or physician. The physician may order glycerin suppositories if the constipation is unrelieved by other measures. (I, N, G)

64. 3. Insomnia in the latter part of pregnancy is not uncommon because the client has difficulty getting into a position of comfort and there is frequent nocturia. The nurse should advise the client to practice relaxation techniques, avoid caffeine products, and exercise during the day but not immediately before bedtime. (I, T, H)

65. 4. Swelling of the hands and face, particularly during the last trimester, may be indicative of pregnancy-induced hypertension. If the client experiences swelling in the face or hands or has any visual disturbances, these should be promptly reported. Swelling of the feet and ankles is a common discomfort of pregnancy. The client should elevate her feet whenever possible and avoid prolonged standing or

sitting. The client should continue to drink 6 to 8 glasses of a noncaffeinated beverage or water daily. (E, N, G)

The Pregnant Client in Childbirth Preparation Classes

66. 3. Early pregnancy classes are appropriate for clients seeking early obstetric care. These classes focus on maternal nutrition, minor discomforts of pregnancy, and newborn nutrition. Most clients make the decision to breast-feed or bottle-feed by the 6th month of pregnancy. Toward the end of the second trimester or the beginning of the third trimester, couples are usually psychologically ready for termination of the pregnancy and are ready for classes dealing with labor and delivery, newborn care, and postpartum care. Lightening occurs about 1 to 2 weeks before the beginning of labor, and the couple should attend childbirth classes before this time. Although clients often have a visit with a dietitian early in pregnancy, there is no need for this to occur before the couple takes childbirth classes. (I, N, H)

67. 2. Relaxing in a hot tub or a sauna can cause damage to the fetus due to temperature extremes, so these activities should be avoided. Swimming and tub bathing are allowed as long as the client's membranes are not ruptured. During the last trimester of pregnancy, the client's center of gravity has shifted; therefore, the nurse should emphasize safety during tub bathing. (E, N, G)

68. 1. The enlarging uterus exerts pressure on blood vessels carrying blood to and from the lower part of the body, especially the extremities, and predisposes to varicosities. Prevention and management of varicosities includes avoiding anything that places constriction on the legs or thighs, such as round garters or knee-high hose. Supportive hose or elastic stockings may be helpful but should be worn as soon as awakening in the morning. Lying down with feet elevated several times a day can also promote venous return. Increased maternal blood volume and constricted blood vessel walls in the extremities do not cause leg varicosities. Restriction of milk intake has no effect on varicosities. (E, N, G)

69. 1. Thyroid enlargement and increased basal body metabolism are common occurrences during pregnancy. Human placental lactogen does not maintain the corpus luteum; it enhances milk production. The adrenal glands should not become enlarged during pregnancy. Progesterone, not estrogen, helps to enlarge the breasts. (P, T, H)

70. 3. At this period of fetal development, external genitalia are identifiable. Fine, downy hair, brown fat, and air ducts and alveoli develop later in the gestational period. (P, T, G)

71. 2. Monozygotic twinning is independent of race, age, parity, or heredity. Dizygotic twinning, or the fertilization of more than one ova during conception, is correlated with increased parity, becoming pregnant within 1 month of stopping oral contraception, and infertility treatments. Adolescents do not have a higher rate of twinning. (I, T, H)

72. 3. If the head is the presenting part, the normal maneuvers during labor and delivery are descent, flexion, internal rotation, extension, external rotation, and expulsion. These maneuvers occur as the fetal head passes through the maternal pelvis. (P, N, H)

73. 1. In a normal delivery and for the first 24 hours after delivery, a total blood loss not exceeding 500 mL is considered normal. (I, N, H)

74. 3. Amnionic fluid does not provide the fetus with nutrition, but it does help dilate the cervix, protect the fetus from injury, and keep the fetus at an even temperature. (E, N, H)

75. 4. Pain during the first stage of labor is primarily due to dilation of the cervix, hypoxia of the uterine muscle cells during contraction, stretching of the lower uterine segment, and pressure on adjacent structures. A client's perceptions of pain and her cultural background can influence pain. During the second stage of labor, pain is thought to be due to hypoxia of the contracting uterine muscle cells, distention of the perineum and vagina, and pressure on the adjacent structures. (I, N, H)

76. 4. In true labor, the cervix dilates and effaces. In false labor, contractions are generally abdominal, there is clear vaginal mucus with no bloody show, and the fetus becomes somewhat more active or fetal activity remains unchanged. (I, T, G)

77. 4. Hyperventilation and rapid breathing techniques are not recommended during pregnancy, unless the client is in the second stage of labor. Progressive relaxation, guided imagery, and effleurage are all appropriate techniques to practice before labor begins. Hyperventilation causes maternal respiratory alkalosis, resulting in reduced placental oxygen exchange for the fetus. For this reason, rapid breathing in labor is no longer advocated. (E, T, G)

78. 1. Increased vaginal discharge is normal during pregnancy, but local itching is associated with infections, such as those due to *Trichomonas vaginalis* or *Candida albicans.* The client's symptoms must be further assessed by a health professional because the client may need treatment. Douches are not commonly prescribed during pregnancy. These symptoms are not associated with onset of labor. The client may have a serious sexually transmitted

disease; therefore, over-the-counter medications are not advised until the client has been evaluated. (I, N, G)

79. 1. The umbilical cord normally consists of two arteries and one vein. Oxygen and other nutrients are carried to the fetal circulation by the umbilical vein. The oxygen-poor blood is pumped back to the placenta by the fetal heart through two umbilical arteries. A single umbilical artery is sometimes associated with congenital anomalies. (I, T, H)

80. 1. The placenta does not produce testosterone. Human placental lactogen, human chorionic gonadotrophin, and progesterone are three of the hormones produced by the placenta during pregnancy. (P, N, H)

81. 1. Oxygenated blood flows through the umbilical vein to the fetus. Blood leaving the fetus to return to the placenta flows through the two umbilical arteries. About 1% of umbilical cords have only one artery. A velamentous cord does not insert centrally into the placenta. A nuchal cord exists when the cord is wrapped around the fetus' neck and often is longer than normal. (P, T, H)

82. 2. During pregnancy, urinary stasis and urinary tract infections are more common. Hyperventilation and metabolic acidosis are not common during pregnancy. Hemoglobin levels usually decrease, and cardiac output and stroke volume increase, in the pregnant client. (P, T, H)

83. 1. Infant mortality rate is defined as the number of deaths of infants under age 1 year per 1,000 live births. The perinatal mortality rate includes all stillborn infants with a gestational age of 28 weeks' or more plus all neonatal deaths under 7 days per 1,000 of this population. The neonatal mortality rate is the number of deaths of infants under age 28 days per 1,000 live births. An estimated one third of pregnant clients do not receive prenatal care. Maternal mortality in the United States has been steadily decreasing. (P, N, H)

84. 1. The placenta is formed by fusion of the chorionic villi and the decidua basalis. The weight of a term placenta is 400 to 600 g, or about one sixth of the weight of the newborn. Larger molecules have more difficulty, with the exception of immune γ-globulin G (IgG). Many viruses, such as rubella, chickenpox, mumps, measles, cytomegalic inclusion disease, and *Treponema pallidum,* may cross the placenta and infect the fetus. Human placental lactogen does not affect testosterone production. (P, N, H)

85. 2. The obstetric conjugate can be estimated by subtracting 1.5 cm from the diagonal conjugate, which can be measured during a pelvic examination. Fetal pelvimetry is not typically used. (I, T, G)

86. 4. Adolescents are at greater risk for lack of prenatal care, low-birth-weight infants, and cephalopelvic disproportion. Congenital anomalies are not more frequent in adolescents. (E, N, H)

87. 4. The uterus receives its blood supply from the uterine and ovarian arteries. The ovarian artery is a branch of the aorta. It enters the broad ligament and supplies the ovary with blood; its main stem makes its way to the upper margin of the uterus. (E, N, H)

The Pregnant Client With Risk Factors

88. 2. In a threatened abortion, there is vaginal bleeding or spotting. The cervix is not dilated, and abdominal cramping may occur. An inevitable abortion is characterized by more bleeding and cramping than a threatened abortion; the cervix is dilating, and termination of the pregnancy cannot be prevented. In an incomplete abortion, some but not all of the products of conception have been expelled; usually, the placenta remains. In a missed abortion, the fetus is dead but has not been expelled from the uterus. (D, N, G)

89. 1. A frequent feeling expressed by clients after a spontaneous abortion is guilt. Ambivalence, relief, and fear are not common reactions. (P, N, L)

90. 2. Hydroxyzine (Vistaril) has a tranquilizing effect and also decreases nausea and vomiting. It does not decrease fluid retention, cause uterine contractions, or control hemorrhage. (D, N, G)

91. 3. After a spontaneous abortion, the client and family members can be expected to suffer from grief for several months or longer. The acute phase of grieving lasts about 6 weeks. When offering support, a simple statement such as, "I'm sorry you lost your baby," is appropriate. Therapeutic communication techniques help the client and family understand the meaning of the loss, move less stressfully through the grief process, and share feelings. Asking why the client is crying suggests that the nurse sees no need for the client's sorrow. Offering the client an analgesic is not appropriate. Telling the client that she can get pregnant again is not therapeutic. This is not the appropriate time to discuss fetal malformations. (I, N, L)

92. 2. Rh sensitization can be prevented by human anti-D globulin, which clears the maternal circulation of Rh-positive cells before sensitization can occur, thereby blocking maternal antibody production. (D, N, G)

93. 3. The client's symptoms indicate a probable ectopic pregnancy, which can be confirmed by ultrasound. The symptoms described are not associated with gestational trophoblastic disease, complete abortion, or incompetent cervix. (D, N, G)

94. 1. The client will most likely need surgery to remove the tube where the pregnancy has occurred, and the nurse is usually responsible for witnessing the surgical consent form. Intravenous therapy may be started. There is scant vaginal bleeding with no discoloration. The client is not having uterine contractions. (I, N, G)

THE NURSING CARE OF THE CHILDBEARING FAMILY AND THEIR NEONATE

TEST 1: Antepartum Care

Directions: Use this answer grid to determine areas of strength or need for further study.

NURSING PROCESS

A = Assessment
D = Analysis, nursing diagnosis
P = Planning
I = Implementation
E = Evaluation

COGNITIVE LEVEL

K = Knowledge
C = Comprehension
T = Application
N = Analysis

CLIENT NEEDS

S = Safe, effective care environment
G = Physiologic integrity
L = Psychosocial integrity
H = Health promotion and maintenance

Question #	Answer #	Nursing Process					Cognitive Level				Client Needs			
		A	**D**	**P**	**I**	**E**	**K**	**C**	**T**	**N**	**S**	**G**	**L**	**H**
1	2				I				T					H
2	4					E			T					H
3	4			P						N				H
4	1					E				N				H
5	2				I					N				H
6	1					E				N				H
7	4				I				T					H
8	3				I				T					H
9	4			P						N				H
10	4				I					N				H
11	1					E				N				H
12	2				I				T					H
13	1		D							N			L	
14	3				I				T			G		
15	4			P						N				H
16	1			P					T			G		
17	1				I				T			G		
18	3					E			T			G		
19	1				I				T					H
20	4					E			T					H
21	1		D							N				H
22	4				I				T				L	
23	4		D							N			L	
24	4					E				N				H
25	3			P					T					H

NURSING PROCESS

A = Assessment
D = Analysis, nursing diagnosis
P = Planning
I = Implementation
E = Evaluation

COGNITIVE LEVEL

K = Knowledge
C = Comprehension
T = Application
N = Analysis

CLIENT NEEDS

S = Safe, effective care environment
G = Physiologic integrity
L = Psychosocial integrity
H = Health promotion and maintenance

Question #	Answer #	Nursing Process					Cognitive Level				Client Needs			
		A	D	P	I	E	K	C	T	N	S	G	L	H
26	3	A								N				H
27	2				I				T					H
28	2				I					N			L	
29	1				I					N			L	
30	4		D							N				H
31	1		D							N				H
32	3				I					N				H
33	2				I				T					H
34	2			P						N				H
35	4				I				T					H
36	4				I					N				H
37	4				I					N		G		
38	1			P						N		G		
39	3					E			T					H
40	4			P					T					H
41	1				I					N		G		
42	2				I				T					H
43	3					E				N		G		
44	4		D							N		G		
45	1	A							T					H
46	4				I				T					H
47	4				I				T			G		
48	4				I				T			G		
49	1				I					N		G		
50	2				I				T			G		
51	3				I					N				H
52	3				I				T			G		
53	1				I				T					H
54	3		D							N		G		
55	4				I				T			G		

ANSWER GRID: 2

NURSING PROCESS

A = Assessment
D = Analysis, nursing diagnosis
P = Planning
I = Implementation
E = Evaluation

COGNITIVE LEVEL

K = Knowledge
C = Comprehension
T = Application
N = Analysis

CLIENT NEEDS

S = Safe, effective care environment
G = Physiologic integrity
L = Psychosocial integrity
H = Health promotion and maintenance

Question #	Answer #	Nursing Process					Cognitive Level				Client Needs			
		A	D	P	I	E	K	C	T	N	S	G	L	H
56	3					E			T					H
57	1		D							N				H
58	3		D							N				H
59	3			P					T					H
60	1			P						N		G		
61	3				I				T					H
62	4				I					N			L	
63	2				I					N		G		
64	3				I				T					H
65	4					E				N		G		
66	3				I					N				H
67	2					E				N		G		
68	1					E				N		G		
69	1			P					T					H
70	3			P					T			G		
71	2				I				T					H
72	3			P						N				H
73	1				I					N				H
74	3					E				N				H
75	4				I					N				H
76	4				I					N				H
77	4				I					N		G		
78	4					E			T			G		
79	1				I					N		G		
80	1				I				T					H
81	1			P					T					H
82	2			P					T					H
83	1			P						N				H
84	1			P						N				H
85	2				I				T			G		

ANSWER GRID: 3

NURSING PROCESS

A = Assessment
D = Analysis, nursing diagnosis
P = Planning
I = Implementation
E = Evaluation

COGNITIVE LEVEL

K = Knowledge
C = Comprehension
T = Application
N = Analysis

CLIENT NEEDS

S = Safe, effective care environment
G = Physiologic integrity
L = Psychosocial integrity
H = Health promotion and maintenance

Question #	Answer #	Nursing Process					Cognitive Level				Client Needs			
		A	D	P	I	E	K	C	T	N	S	G	L	H
86	4					E				N				H
87	4					E				N				H
88	2		D							N		G		
89	1			P						N			L	
90	2		D							N		G		
91	3				I					N			L	
92	2		D							N		G		
93	3		D							N		G		
94	1				I					N		G		
Number Correct														
Number Possible	94	2	13	19	43	17	0	0	40	54	0	31	8	55
Percentage Correct														

Score Calculation: To determine your **Percentage Correct,** divide the **Number Correct** by the **Number Possible.**

ANSWER GRID: 4

Complications of Pregnancy

- **The Client With Pregnancy-Induced Hypertension**
- **The Pregnant Client With a Hypertensive Disorder**
- **The Pregnant Client With Third-Trimester Bleeding**
- **The Pregnant Client With Preterm Labor**
- **The Pregnant Client With Diabetes Mellitus**
- **The Client With an Ectopic Pregnancy**
- **The Client With Hyperemesis Gravidarum**
- **The Pregnant Client With a Hydatidiform Mole**
- **The Pregnant Client With Premature Rupture of the Membranes**
- **Correct Answers and Rationale**

Select the one best answer, and indicate your choice by filling in the circle in front of the option.

The Client With Pregnancy-Induced Hypertension

A 16-year-old unmarried client visits the prenatal clinic at 32 weeks' gestation. The client is 5 feet, 2 inches tall and weighed 120 pounds before the pregnancy. The client now weighs 140 pounds. She has been receiving care at the clinic and is being carefully monitored for early signs of pregnancy-induced hypertension (PIH).

1. The nurse assesses the client for possible risk factors for PIH. Which of the following would be most important for the nurse to assess?
- ○ 1. Proteinuria.
- ○ 2. Small-for-gestational-age fetus.
- ○ 3. ABO incompatibility.
- ○ 4. Fluid intake.

2. The client's baseline blood pressure at her initial visit at 12 weeks' gestation was 110/70 mm Hg. During an assessment at 32 weeks' gestation, which of the following data indicate mild PIH?
- ○ 1. Blood pressure of 160/110 mm Hg on two separate occasions.
- ○ 2. Proteinuria, more than 5 g in 24 hours.

- ○ 3. Elevated serum creatinine.
- ○ 4. Swelling of fingers and ankles.

3. A priority nursing diagnosis for this client is
- ○ 1. Noncompliance related to poor nutrition and lack of exercise during pregnancy.
- ○ 2. Fluid Volume Deficit related to fluid shift from intravascular to extravascular space.
- ○ 3. High Risk for Injury related to cerebral vasospasm.
- ○ 4. High Risk for Injury to fetus related to altered sensorium of mother.

4. The nurse assesses the client for additional symptoms of PIH. Which of the following symptoms would further confirm the diagnosis of PIH?
- ○ 1. Mild headache after reading.
- ○ 2. History of urinary tract infection.
- ○ 3. Frequent voiding in large amounts.
- ○ 4. Mild edema in hands and face.

5. The nurse plans to instruct the client in care while the client is at home. Which of the following is an appropriate goal for the client? The client will
- ○ 1. return to the prenatal clinic in 2 weeks.
- ○ 2. exhibit decreased edema after 1 week of a low-protein, low-salt diet.

○ 3. rest on the left side during the day, with bathroom privileges.

○ 4. immediately report adverse reactions from oral calcium carbonate medication.

6. The nurse teaches the client about how PIH affects the growing fetus. The nurse realizes that the client needs *further* instruction when she says that PIH can lead to

○ 1. anencephaly.

○ 2. low-birth-weight infant.

○ 3. fetal hydrops.

○ 4. intrauterine growth retardation.

A 21-year-old primigravida is diagnosed with mild PIH at 36 weeks' gestation. She is being treated at home and has a home care nurse visit twice weekly.

7. The nurse instructs the client to keep a record of fetal movement patterns at home. The nurse determines that the instructions are effective when the client says that she will count the number of times the baby moves during a

○ 1. 30-minute period three times a day.

○ 2. 45-minute period after lunch each day.

○ 3. 12-hour period each day.

○ 4. 24-hour period each week.

8. The nurse plans to instruct the client about nutritional needs of clients with mild PIH. The teaching plan includes instructing the client about eating a

○ 1. high-residue diet.

○ 2. low-sodium diet.

○ 3. regular diet.

○ 4. high-protein diet.

9. The nurse discusses various theories about the causes of PIH. After giving the instruction, the nurse determines that the client needs *further* instruction when she says that PIH may be caused by

○ 1. iron deficiency anemia.

○ 2. an as yet to be identified toxin.

○ 3. impaired vascular invasion of the uterine lining.

○ 4. an autoimmune response.

10. The client states that she frequently ingests laundry starch. The nurse should assess the client for symptoms of

○ 1. muscle spasms.

○ 2. lactose intolerance.

○ 3. diabetes mellitus.

○ 4. anemia.

11. The client tells the nurse that she doesn't like milk. The nurse should instruct the client that an 8-ounce glass of milk is equal to

○ 1. 2 tablespoons of Parmesan cheese.

○ 2. ½ cup of a milkshake.

○ 3. 1½ to 2 slices of presliced American cheese.

○ 4. ½ cup of cottage cheese.

12. The client tells the nurse that she eats fruits and vegetables but isn't very fond of them. The nurse should instruct the client that one serving of vegetables is equivalent to

○ 1. one fourth of a cantaloupe.

○ 2. 3 ounces of vegetable juice cocktail.

○ 3. 3 tomatoes.

○ 4. 1 raw apricot.

A 26-year-old primigravida visits the prenatal clinic for her regular visit at 34 weeks' gestation. She is diagnosed with mild PIH.

13. The client tells the nurse she takes mineral oil for occasional constipation. The nurse should instruct the client to

○ 1. take the mineral oil with fruit juice to increase the action of the mineral oil.

○ 2. avoid mineral oil because it interferes with the absorption of fat-soluble vitamins.

○ 3. avoid mineral oil because it can lead to vitamin C deficiency in pregnant clients.

○ 4. use the mineral oil only once a week to prevent constipation.

14. When the client complains of flatulence, the nurse can instruct her to

○ 1. decrease the number of meals eaten each day.

○ 2. avoid eating foods such as cauliflower.

○ 3. drink carbonated beverages several times a day.

○ 4. drink a teaspoon of bicarbonate of soda in water as necessary.

15. The client asks the nurse what causes heartburn. The nurse should explain that heartburn during pregnancy is usually due to

○ 1. increased peristaltic action.

○ 2. displacement of the stomach by the diaphragm.

○ 3. decreased secretion of hydrochloric acid.

○ 4. backflow of stomach contents into the esophagus.

16. The nurse asks the client how often the baby has moved today. She replies that she hasn't counted the baby's movements today, but that yesterday the baby moved six times during a 12-hour period. The nurse determines that

○ 1. the client requires follow-up evaluation by a physician.

○ 2. the baby is showing signs of polyhydramnios.

○ 3. the baby could be experiencing fetal lung maturation.

○ 4. the baby is moving an adequate number of times.

17. One week after her prenatal visit, the client calls the nurse and says she has had a continuous headache

for 2 days. She says she is nauseated and does not want to take aspirin. Which of the following responses by the nurse is most appropriate?

○ 1. "Take two acetaminophen tablets. They aren't as likely to upset your stomach."
○ 2. "I think the doctor should see you today. Can you come to the clinic this morning?"
○ 3. "Have you tried lying down in a darkened room?"
○ 4. "I'll ask the doctor to have a prescription for a safe, but strong analgesic phoned in to your pharmacy."

A 17-year-old primigravida at 38 weeks' gestation is scheduled for admission to the hospital with a diagnosis of severe PIH.

18. In reviewing the client's prenatal records, which of the following data would be most indicative of the client's diagnosis of severe PIH?

○ 1. Polyuria.
○ 2. Urine specific gravity of 1.04.
○ 3. Proteinuria, less than 2 g in 24 hours.
○ 4. Weight gain of 0.5 lb in 1 week.

19. In planning for the client's admission, the nurse should prepare the client's room by obtaining

○ 1. sterile perineal pads.
○ 2. padding for the side rails.
○ 3. amnioinfusion equipment.
○ 4. a portable ultrasound machine.

20. Two hours after admission, the physician orders 5% dextrose in Ringer's solution and magnesium sulfate intravenously. Before administering the magnesium sulfate, the most important assessment for the nurse to make is the

○ 1. fetal heart rate variability.
○ 2. maternal urinary output.
○ 3. fetal position.
○ 4. maternal respiratory rate.

21. The nurse monitors the client during magnesium sulfate administration. If the client develops magnesium toxicity, the nurse should plan to obtain the drug

○ 1. calcium gluconate.
○ 2. diazepam.
○ 3. phenytoin.
○ 4. furosemide.

22. The nurse assesses the client receiving magnesium sulfate for symptoms of hypermagnesemia. An important sign for the nurse to note first is

○ 1. cool skin temperature.
○ 2. rapid pulse rate.
○ 3. tingling in the toes.
○ 4. decreased deep tendon reflexes.

A 28-year-old multigravida at 37 weeks' gestation arrives at the hospital in an ambulance. She is taken to the labor area with a diagnosis of severe PIH. On admission, her blood pressure is 160/104 mm Hg, and her reflexes are +3 with no clonus.

23. The client asks the nurse, "What is the cure for my high blood pressure?" The nurse should instruct the client that the primary "cure " is

○ 1. strict, isolated bed rest.
○ 2. delivery of the fetus.
○ 3. sedation with magnesium sulfate.
○ 4. sedation with phenobarbital.

24. In planning for the client's care, the nurse formulates which of the following priority goals?

○ 1. The client will not develop seizures during the first 48 hours.
○ 2. The client will exhibit decreased generalized edema within 12 hours.
○ 3. The client will have decreased nausea and vomiting within 4 hours.
○ 4. The client will be sedated and have decreased reflex excitability within 48 hours.

25. A continuous intravenous infusion of 5% dextrose in Ringer's solution is administered. Which of the following signs should the nurse report immediately?

○ 1. Respiratory rate of 16 breaths/minute.
○ 2. Blood pressure of 150/96 mm Hg.
○ 3. Moist rales in lung fields.
○ 4. Urinary output exceeding intake.

26. The nurse formulates a nursing diagnosis for the client. The most appropriate diagnosis at this time is

○ 1. High Risk for Injury related to possibility of continued convulsions.
○ 2. Knowledge Deficit related to signs and symptoms of PIH.
○ 3. Hypertensive Crisis related to toxicity of magnesium sulfate.
○ 4. Altered Self Concept related to hospitalization.

A 16-year-old unmarried primigravida at about 35 weeks' gestation is admitted to the hospital's labor unit in early active labor, accompanied by her mother. The client has been seen in the prenatal clinic twice weekly for the last 2 weeks for mild PIH and possible HELLP syndrome.

27. While caring for this client, the nurse plans to notify the physician immediately if the client has

○ 1. +2 reflexes with no clonus.

○ 2. proteinuria.

○ 3. platelet count of 80,000/μL.

○ 4. clear to whitish vaginal discharge.

28. The client's blood pressure climbs to 164/110 mm Hg. Which of the following symptoms would suggest to the nurse that the client may be about to convulse?

○ 1. Increased fetal movements.

○ 2. Decreased temperature.

○ 3. Epigastric pain.

○ 4. Urine output of 40 mL/hour.

29. If the client begins to convulse due to eclampsia, the nurse's first action is to

○ 1. pad the side rails with pillows.

○ 2. place a pillow under the left buttock.

○ 3. insert a padded tongue blade into the mouth.

○ 4. suction the mouth and nasopharynx to keep the airway open.

30. Fifteen minutes after an eclamptic seizure, the nurse should assess the client for

○ 1. bradycardia.

○ 2. facial flushing.

○ 3. pretibial edema.

○ 4. uterine contractions.

31. If the client begins to exhibit symptoms of labor after the eclamptic seizure, the nurse plans to assess the client for

○ 1. ruptured membranes.

○ 2. placenta previa.

○ 3. uterine atony.

○ 4. abruptio placenta.

The Pregnant Client With a Hypertensive Disorder

An obese 36-year-old multigravida visits the prenatal clinic for the first time at 12 weeks' gestation. She was diagnosed with chronic hypertension before the pregnancy and is taking methyldopa (Aldomet) daily.

32. When counseling the client about diet during pregnancy, the nurse realizes that the client needs *further* instruction when she says,

○ 1. "I should reduce my caloric intake to 1200 calories."

○ 2. "A high-protein diet is recommended."

○ 3. "I shouldn't use salt when I am cooking."

○ 4. "I need to eat more protein and fiber each day."

33. The client's blood pressure is 160/110 mm Hg. The client asks the nurse what medication will most likely be given for hypertension. The nurse's best response is that the antihypertensive drug of choice during pregnancy is

○ 1. phenobarbital.

○ 2. diazepam.

○ 3. methyldopa.

○ 4. magnesium sulfate.

34. After instructing the client about the need for frequent prenatal visits, the nurse determines that the instructions have been effective when the client says,

○ 1. "I may develop rheumatic heart disease because of my high blood pressure."

○ 2. "I need to be monitored closely because I may have a small-for-gestational-age infant."

○ 3. "It's possible that I will have a large infant and may need a cesarean section."

○ 4. "I may develop placenta previa, so I need to keep my clinic appointments."

The Pregnant Client With Third-Trimester Bleeding

A 28-year-old multigravida at 32 weeks' gestation is admitted to the hospital because of vaginal bleeding.

35. In planning the client's care, one of the first actions the nurse lists in the nursing care plan is to

○ 1. perform a sterile vaginal examination.

○ 2. provide perineal pads.

○ 3. witness a consent for cesarean section.

○ 4. check the fetal heart rate and maternal blood pressure.

36. The nurse assesses the client for symptoms of abruptio placenta, noting especially

○ 1. excessive vaginal bleeding.

○ 2. abdominal rigidity.

○ 3. tetanic uterine contractions.

○ 4. preterm rupture of the membranes.

37. While collecting data about the client's lifestyle, which of the following factors might lead the nurse to suspect a medical diagnosis of abruptio placenta?

○ 1. History of cocaine use.

○ 2. History of placenta accreta.

○ 3. Previous low transverse cesarean delivery.

○ 4. Obesity.

38. If the client develops symptoms of disseminated intravascular coagulation (DIC), the nurse should plan to administer ordered

○ 1. intravenous Ringer's lactate solution.

○ 2. intravenous platelets.

○ 3. intravenous dextrose solution.

○ 4. intravenous packed red blood cells.

A 34-year-old multigravida at 34 weeks' gestation is admitted to the hospital with moderate vaginal bleeding.

39. The nurse assesses the client for symptoms of placenta previa, noting especially

X ○ 1. painless vaginal bleeding.
○ 2. uterine tetany.
○ 3. intermittent pain with spotting.
○ 4. dull lower abdominal pain.

40. The client is diagnosed with partial placenta previa. In explaining the diagnosis, the nurse tells the client that the usual treatment for partial placenta previa is

○ 1. bed rest.
○ 2. administration of platelets.
○ 3. immediate cesarean section delivery.
○ 4. induction of labor with oxytocin.

41. After giving instruction about the cause of the vaginal bleeding, the nurse determines that the teaching has been effective when the client says that the bleeding results from

○ 1. poor clotting factors.
○ 2. altered platelet levels.
○ 3. a large-for-gestational-age fetus.
○ 4. exposure of maternal blood sinuses.

42. The nurse formulates a nursing diagnosis for the client soon after admission. Which of the following nursing diagnoses is most appropriate at this time?

○ 1. Hemorrhagic Disorder related to vaginal bleeding.
○ 2. Fear related to unknown outcome of fetus.
○ 3. Potential for Fetal Demise related to placenta previa.
○ 4. Potential for Shock related to vaginal bleeding.

43. The physician orders whole blood replacement for the client. Before administering the intravenous blood product, the nurse should *first*

○ 1. validate client information and the blood product with another nurse.
○ 2. check the vital signs, then transfuse over 5 to 6 hours.
○ 3. ask the client if she has ever had any allergies.
○ 4. administer 100 mL of 0.9% NaCl solution intravenously.

44. The client begins to have excessive vaginal bleeding soon after admission, and an emergency cesarean section is planned. In planning care for the client, the nurse should *first* plan to

○ 1. shave the abdomen and perineal area.
○ 2. ask family members to wait in the waiting room.
○ 3. check the status of the fetus.
○ 4. be certain that replacement blood is available.

45. After the cesarean section delivery, the client tells the recovery room nurse "I feel like such a failure. None of my other deliveries were like this." The nurse should explain to the client that

○ 1. she will most likely have postpartum depression.
○ 2. maternal infant bonding is likely to be difficult.

○ 3. this type of delivery was necessary to save the baby's life.
○ 4. her feelings of loss and grief are normal reactions.

46. After the cesarean section delivery, the nurse assesses the client for possible uterine atony by

○ 1. checking the abdominal dressing every 15 minutes for 1 hour.
○ 2. supporting the incision and palpating the fundus every 15 minutes for 1 hour.
○ 3. observing the amount of lochia immediately after delivery.
○ 4. palpating the uterus to determine the frequency of uterine contractions.

The Pregnant Client With Preterm Labor

A 28-year-old multigravida at 30 weeks' gestation is admitted to a perinatal center with contractions of moderate intensity occurring every 3 to 4 minutes. The client, who has previously delivered two nonviable fetuses, is crying on admission. She is accompanied by her husband.

47. The client asks the nurse, "What causes preterm labor?" After giving instruction about various factors that place a client at risk for preterm labor, the nurse determines that the client needs *further* instruction when she says that preterm labor is often associated with

X ○ 1. age under 25 years.
○ 2. polyhydramnios.
○ 3. poor pregnancy weight gain.
○ 4. multifetal gestation.

48. The client is a candidate for therapy with terbutaline (Brethine). Which of the following would be most important for the nurse to assess before beginning terbutaline therapy?

X ○ 1. Intensity of uterine contractions.
○ 2. Deep tendon reflexes.
○ 3. Estimated fetal size.
○ 4. Maternal heart rate.

49. After gathering initial assessment data, the nurse formulates a nursing diagnosis for the client. The most appropriate nursing diagnosis at this time is

○ 1. Pain related to intense uterine ischemia and contractions.
○ 2. Altered Nutrition: Less Than Body Requirements related to bed rest.
○ 3. Risk for Preterm Delivery related to frequent uterine contractions.
○ 4. Fear related to unknown outcome of labor and possible preterm delivery.

50. While administering intravenous terbutaline, the

nurse assesses the client for which common side effect?

○ 1. Decreased respirations.
○ 2. Hypotension.
○ 3. Oliguria.
○ 4. Tachycardia.

51. The nurse monitors the client's laboratory studies during terbutaline therapy. The nurse explains to the client that an increase in blood plasma volume is confirmed by

○ 1. decreased hemoglobin level.
○ 2. glycosuria.
○ 3. decreased weight gain.
○ 4. increased serum calcium levels.

52. The external electronic monitor is used to monitor the fetal heart rate. If the fetus is in left occipitoanterior position, the nurse should place the ultrasound transducer (cardiotransducer)

○ 1. near the symphysis pubis.
○ 2. 2 inches above the symphysis pubis.
○ 3. over the fetal back.
○ 4. near the client's umbilicus.

A 34-year-old multigravida at 36 weeks' gestation is admitted to the hospital with an admission diagnosis of preterm labor. The client has experienced one infant death due to preterm birth at 28 weeks' gestation.

53. On admission to the antenatal unit, the nurse determines that the fetal heart rate is 140 beats/minute. The nurse should

○ 1. administer oxygen by mask at 8 L.
○ 2. notify the client's physician.
○ 3. continue to monitor the client and fetus.
○ 4. check the fetal heart rate again in 10 minutes.

54. An ultrasound is scheduled for the client before an amniocentesis. After teaching the client about the purpose of the ultrasound, the nurse determines that the client needs *further* instruction when she says that the ultrasound is done to

○ 1. locate the placenta.
○ 2. identify congenital abnormalities.
○ 3. determine where to insert the needle.
○ 4. locate a pool of amniotic fluid.

55. The client has been ordered to receive betamethasone (Celestone). The nurse should explain to the client that betamethasone is given to

○ 1. enhance fetal lung maturity.
○ 2. counter the effects of tocolytic therapy.
○ 3. treat pyelonephritis.
○ 4. decrease the production of neonatal surfactant.

56. The nurse formulates a nursing diagnosis for the client. The most appropriate diagnosis for a client undergoing antenatal testing is

○ 1. Pain related to abnormal uterine contractions.
○ 2. Anxiety related to diagnostic tests for fetal well-being.
○ 3. Ineffective Family Coping related to hospitalization.
○ 4. Knowledge Deficit related to consequences of having a low-birth-weight infant.

57. To instruct the client about the shake test to be performed on the amniotic fluid, the nurse should plan to explain that the shake test evaluates the maturity of the fetal

○ 1. kidneys.
○ 2. urinary tract.
○ 3. cardiovascular system.
○ 4. pulmonary system.

58. After teaching the client about potential complications of amniocentesis that must be reported immediately, the nurse determines that the client understands the instruction when she says that she should immediately report

○ 1. dizziness.
○ 2. vaginal bleeding.
○ 3. urinary retention.
○ 4. irregular, painless uterine tightness.

The Pregnant Client With Diabetes Mellitus

A 27-year-old primigravida at 34 weeks' gestation is seen in the high-risk prenatal clinic. She has insulin-dependent diabetes.

59. A nonstress test is performed, and the results are documented as reactive. The nurse tells the client that the test results indicate

○ 1. fetal well-being.
○ 2. a need for a contraction stress test.
○ 3. a need for continuous oxygen therapy.
○ 4. evidence of fetal anomalies.

60. A contraction stress test is scheduled for the client at 36 weeks' gestation. After explaining the purpose of the test, the nurse determines that the client understands the instruction when she states that the test is done to detect

○ 1. cardiac anomalies.
○ 2. uteroplacental sufficiency.
○ 3. kidney anomalies.
○ 4. amniotic fluid abnormalities.

61. The client states that the contraction stress test performed 1 week ago was suspicious. The nurse determines that the fetal heart rate pattern showed

○ 1. no late decelerations.

○ 2. frequent accelerations.
○ 3. inconsistent late decelerations.
○ 4. no accelerations.

62. The client is scheduled for a fetal biophysical profile. The nurse plans to explain to the client that this test
○ 1. can determine fetal lung maturity.
○ 2. is an uncomfortable, invasive procedure.
○ 3. requires the client to have an empty bladder.
○ 4. is noninvasive and uses real-time ultrasound.

A 30-year-old multigravida at 8 weeks' gestation is receiving prenatal care in a maternity clinic. She has had insulin-dependent diabetes since she was 20 years of age.

63. The nurse discusses the importance of keeping blood glucose levels near normal throughout the pregnancy. The nurse explains to the client that during the first trimester of pregnancy, her insulin needs
○ 1. will increase.
○ 2. will decrease.
○ 3. will remain constant.
○ 4. cannot be predicted.

64. After explaining the complications of pregnancy that occur with diabetes, the nurse determines that the client needs *further* instruction when she says that one complication is
○ 1. *Candida albicans* infection.
○ 2. multifetal pregnancy.
○ 3. ketoacidosis.
○ 4. PIH.

65. When planning to teach the client how to monitor glucose control and insulin dosage at home, the nurse should explain that the goal of medical management is to maintain blood plasma glucose levels at
○ 1. 40 to 60 mg/dL between 2 and 4 AM.
○ 2. 60 to 80 mg/dL before meals and snacks.
○ 3. 90 to 110 mg/dL before meals and snacks.
○ 4. 140 to 160 mg/dL 1 hour after meals.

66. The client reports that she participated in strenuous aerobic exercise before becoming pregnant. She asks the nurse if she can continue exercising. What is the nurse's best response?
○ 1. "You probably should discontinue strenuous exercise while pregnant."
○ 2. "It is important that you avoid overexertion while you are pregnant."
○ 3. "You can continue exercising while pregnant, but you should eat a carbohydrate or protein snack before exercising."

○ 4. "It's probably a good idea to check your blood sugar before beginning any exercise program."

67. After teaching about symptoms of hyperglycemia and hypoglycemia, the nurse determines that the client understands the instruction when she says that hyperglycemia may be manifested by
○ 1. dehydration.
○ 2. insomnia.
○ 3. weakness.
○ 4. nervousness.

68. At 37 weeks' gestation, the client is admitted to the hospital for induction of labor. The nurse should explain to the client that she is being induced before term to prevent
○ 1. congenital anomalies.
○ 2. perinatal asphyxia.
○ 3. stillbirth.
○ 4. maternal hemorrhage.

69. The physician estimates that the fetus weighs at least 10 pounds. The client asks the nurse, "What causes the baby to be so large?" The nurse should explain that fetal macrosomia is usually related to
○ 1. genetic history of large infants.
○ 2. fetal anomalies.
○ 3. maternal hyperglycemia.
○ 4. fetal hypoglycemia

70. The client plans to breast-feed her neonate and asks the nurse about insulin needs during the postpartum period. The nurse should instruct the client that during the postpartum period, insulin requirements for breast-feeding mothers
○ 1. fall significantly.
○ 2. usually increase.
○ 3. depend on the length of the labor and delivery process.
○ 4. need constant adjustment.

The Client With an Ectopic Pregnancy

A 24-year-old client is admitted to the hospital. It is suspected that she is pregnant, with gestation occurring outside the uterus.

71. Because the client is suspected of having an ectopic pregnancy, on admission it is particularly important for the nurse to assess the client's
○ 1. sexual patterns.
○ 2. use of a diaphragm.
○ 3. type of oral contraceptives.
○ 4. date of last menstrual period.

72. Ultrasonography confirms that the client has an ectopic pregnancy. The nurse explains that in an ec-

topic pregnancy, implantation of the fertilized ovum most commonly occurs in the
○ 1. intrauterine lining.
○ 2. ovary.
○ 3. fallopian tube.
○ 4. peritoneal cavity.

73. The nurse formulates a nursing diagnosis for the client soon after admission. The most appropriate diagnosis for the client is
○ 1. Anticipatory Grieving related to the loss of the pregnancy.
○ 2. Fear related to the outcome of possible surgery.
○ 3. High Risk for Maladaptive Coping related to ectopic pregnancy.
○ 4. High Risk for Infection related to pelvic inflammatory disease.

74. The nurse assesses the client for symptoms of a tubal rupture, noting especially
○ 1. uncontrollable nausea and vomiting.
○ 2. falling hematocrit and hemoglobin levels.
○ 3. slow, bounding pulse with rate of 70 beats/minute.
○ 4. marked abdominal distention.

75. The client is scheduled for emergency surgery. Before surgery, the nurse assesses the client's blood pressure and
○ 1. uterine cramping.
○ 2. skin turgor.
○ 3. vaginal discharge.
○ 4. pulse rate.

A 36-year-old client is admitted to the hospital with possible ruptured ectopic pregnancy.

76. For which of the following procedures should the nurse plan to prepare the client soon after admission?
○ 1. Dilation and curettage.
○ 2. Culdocentesis.
○ 3. Evacuation of the uterus.
○ 4. Oophorectomy.

77. After admission, it is most important for the nurse to assess the client's health history for
○ 1. urinary tract infection.
○ 2. incompetent cervix.
○ 3. history of fraternal twins.
○ 4. pelvic inflammatory disease.

78. After surgery, the nurse instructs the client about potential complications. The nurse determines that the client needs *further* instruction when she states that a potential complication is
○ 1. pain.

○ 2. dizziness.
○ 3. fever.
○ 4. bleeding.

The Client With Hyperemesis Gravidarum

A multiparous client thought to be at 14 weeks' gestation (based on uterine size) visits the prenatal clinic and reports that she is experiencing such severe morning sickness that "she has not been able to keep anything down for a week."

79. Due to the client's excessive vomiting, the nurse assesses the client's urinalysis results for
○ 1. white blood cells.
○ 2. albumin.
○ 3. glucose.
○ 4. acetone.

80. Because the client states she has been vomiting for 1 week, the nurse should assess for symptoms of
○ 1. hypercalcemia.
○ 2. hyponatremia.
○ 3. hypokalemia.
○ 4. hyperglycemia.

81. The nurse explains to the client that hyperemesis gravidarum is thought to be related to high levels of the hormone
○ 1. progesterone.
○ 2. estrogen.
○ 3. somatotropin.
○ 4. aldosterone.

82. The client is admitted to the hospital for further evaluation and treatment. The nurse caring for this client should further assess the client for
○ 1. abdominal pain.
○ 2. leaking amniotic fluid.
○ 3. pinkish vaginal discharge.
○ 4. dehydration.

83. The client will receive intravenous therapy and asks the nurse when she will be able to eat again. The nurse explains that oral intake of food and fluids will most likely be
○ 1. withheld indefinitely until alkalosis is corrected.
○ 2. given in small quantities whenever desired.
○ 3. given as clear liquids after 24 hours if vomiting subsides.
○ 4. withheld until hyperalimentation replace lost electrolytes.

The Pregnant Client With a Hydatidiform Mole

A 38-year-old client at about 14 weeks' gestation is admitted to the hospital with a diagnosis of complete hydatidiform mole.

84. Soon after admission, the nurse should assess the client for symptoms of
○ 1. PIH.
○ 2. diabetes mellitus.
○ 3. hyperthyroidism.
○ 4. polycythemia.

85. After a dilation and curettage to evacuate the molar pregnancy, it is especially important that the nurse assess for
○ 1. urinary tract infection.
○ 2. hemorrhage.
○ 3. abdominal distention.
○ 4. chorioamnionitis.

86. After explaining the need for follow-up care after evacuation of the mole, the nurse determines that the client understands the instruction when she says that she is at risk for developing
○ 1. ectopic pregnancy.
○ 2. choriocarcinoma.
○ 3. multifetal pregnancies.
○ 4. pelvic inflammatory disease.

The Pregnant Client With Premature Rupture of the Membranes

A 26-year-old multigravida at 30 weeks' gestation is admitted to the hospital with premature rupture of the membranes.

87. After admission, it is particularly important for the nurse to assess for symptoms of

○ 1. foul-smelling amniotic fluid.
○ 2. uterine prolapse.
○ 3. small-for-gestational-age fetus.
○ 4. tetanic uterine contractions.

88. The client begins to have contractions every 10 minutes. The physician orders intravenous magnesium sulfate. The nurse explains to the client that the primary purpose of magnesium sulfate is to
○ 1. provide sedation.
○ 2. combat hypomagnesemia.
○ 3. improve uteroplacental function.
○ 4. inhibit contractions.

89. After 48 hours, the client's contractions stop. She is to be discharged with home monitoring. After teaching the client about preterm labor symptoms, the nurse determines that she needs *further* instruction when she says,
○ 1. "I should call the doctor if my contractions occur every hour for 6 hours."
○ 2. "If I start having contractions, I should empty my bladder."
○ 3. "I should report contractions occurring every 10 minutes for an hour."
○ 4. "I should lie in bed on my left side if contractions begin."

90. The client is readmitted at 34 weeks' gestation in active labor. The physician orders intramuscular administration of betamethasone (Celestone). After administration, the nurse plans to assess the client for symptoms of
○ 1. hypoglycemia.
○ 2. infection.
○ 3. urinary frequency.
○ 4. decreased skin turgor.

CORRECT ANSWERS AND RATIONALE

The letters in parentheses following the rationale identify the step of the nursing process (A, D, P, I, E), cognitive level (K, C, T, N), and client needs (S, G, L, H). See the Answer Grid for the key.

The Client With Pregnancy-Induced Hypertension

1. 1. The most important assessment is checking the urine for proteinuria. Proteinuria, even in the absence of an elevated blood pressure, is indicative of PIH. PIH occurs more often in primigravidas, adolescents, women of lower socioeconomic status, primigravidas older than 35 years, women with family histories of PIH, and women with additional complications, such as multiple gestation, diabetes mellitus, Rh incompatibility, and hydatidiform mole. ABO incompatibility, upper socioeconomic status, and unmarried status are not risk factors. (A, N, G)

2. 4. Generalized edema, with swelling of the face, hands, fingers, and ankles, often occurs with mild PIH. Blood pressure readings of 160 mm Hg systolic and 100 mm Hg diastolic, proteinuria, and oliguria (urine output less than 400 mL in 24 hours) are signs of severe PIH. (D, N, G)

3. 2. Based on the information provided, the most appropriate nursing diagnosis is Fluid Volume Deficit related to fluid shift from intravascular to extravascular space. There are no data to suggest Noncompliance or High Risk for Injury, either to the client or the fetus. The potential for these diagnoses exists, however, particularly if the client indicates a knowledge deficit or if her condition deteriorates. (D, N, G)

4. 4. The diagnosis of mild PIH is further confirmed if the client exhibits mild edema in the hands and face. Mild headache after reading, history of a urinary tract infection, and voiding frequently in large amounts are not related to PIH. (D, N, G)

5. 3. The client with mild PIH is often treated at home. Restricting activities is of primary importance, and bed rest for most of the day is recommended. The left lateral recumbent position is recommended to decrease pressure on the vena cava, which increases venous return, circulatory volume, and renal and placental perfusion. A decrease in angiotensin II improves renal blood flow, lowers blood pressure, and increases diuresis. The client should be monitored twice weekly. Her diet needs to be well balanced, with ample protein. If magnesium sulfate is necessary, as in severe PIH, the drug is usually adminis-

tered intravenously, and the client is carefully monitored in the hospital setting because she may convulse. (P, N, G)

6. 1. Congenital anomalies such as anencephaly are not associated with hypertensive disease. Such conditions as stillbirth, prematurity, intrauterine growth retardation, and fetal hydrops are associated with PIH. (E, N, G)

7. 3. Numerous methods have been proposed to record the maternal perceptions of fetal movement. A commonly used method is the Cardiff count-to-10 method. The client begins counting fetal movements at a specified time (eg, 8 AM) and notes the time when the tenth movement is felt. If 10 movements are not felt in a 12-hour period, the client should notify the health care provider. Another method involves monitoring the fetal movements over 1 hour. The client should report if fewer than three movements are felt. (E, N, G)

8. 3. The client should be placed on a regular diet with no caloric modifications. The client should be taught to avoid using salt while cooking, but the client does not need a low salt diet. It is preferable to eat raw fruits and vegetables when possible. (P, N, G)

9. 1. Although the exact cause of PIH is not yet known, several theories have been proposed. These include an as yet to be defined toxin, impaired vascular invasion of the uterine lining, and an autoimmune response. Iron deficiency can lead to anemia, but this has not been linked to PIH. (E, C, G)

10. 4. All pregnant clients should be screened for pica, or the ingestion of nonfood substances, such as clay, dirt, or laundry starch. Screening the client for anemia is important because clients who practice pica commonly are anemic. Muscle spasms, lactose intolerance, and diabetes mellitus are not usually associated with eating starch. (A, N, G)

11. 3. An 8-ounce glass of milk is the equivalent of 1½ to 2 slices of presliced American cheese. (I, T, H)

12. 1. One serving of a vegetable or fruit is equivalent to one fourth of a cantaloupe. The client would need 6 ounces of a vegetable juice cocktail, two tomatoes, or two raw apricots to have one serving. (I, T, H)

13. 2. The client should be advised to avoid taking mineral oil because it interferes with absorption of fat-soluble vitamins from the intestinal tract. Harsh laxatives are contraindicated. If dietary measures and increased fluid intake do not prevent constipation and a mild laxative is indicated, the client should contact the physician or other health care provider.

A stool softener or a mild laxative, such as milk of magnesia, may be prescribed. Mineral oil does not lead to vitamin C deficiency in pregnant clients. (I, T, G)

14. 2. Flatulence is an annoying and fairly common discomfort of pregnancy. Suggestions to help overcome it include avoiding large meals, chewing food well, and avoiding gas-producing foods, such as carbonated beverages and cauliflower. Bicarbonate of soda should be avoided during pregnancy because of the potential for electrolyte imbalance owing to its high sodium content. (I, N, H)

15. 4. Heartburn is caused by stomach contents entering the distal end of the esophagus, producing a burning sensation. (I, N, H)

16. 1. Fewer than 10 fetal movements in a 12-hour period is not reassuring and should be reported to the physician. Fetal lung maturation is not associated with the number of fetal movements. (D, N, G)

17. 2. A client with PIH complaining of a continuous headache for 2 days should be seen by a health care provider immediately. Continuous headache is a symptom of severe PIH, and immediate care is recommended. (I, N, G)

18. 2. Signs of severe PIH include blood pressure of 160/110 mm Hg or greater measured at two different times at least 6 hours apart, oliguria, proteinuria of 5 g or greater in 24 hours, and a urine specific gravity of 1.04 or greater. (D, N, H)

19. 2. The client with severe PIH may develop eclampsia, characterized by convulsions. It would be best to place this client in a quiet room and pad the side rails with thick padding. This helps decrease the potential for injury if a convulsion occurs. In many hospitals, the client is admitted to the labor area, where she and the fetus can be closely monitored. (P, N, G)

20. 4. A central nervous system depressant used as an anticonvulsant for severe PIH, magnesium sulfate may depress respirations to a dangerously low and even life-threatening level. This drug should not be administered without first consulting the physician if the client's respiratory rate is below 12 to 14 breaths/minute. Although fetal heart rate and maternal temperature and pulse are important to assess during the treatment, respiratory rate is the most important vital sign to assess before administering magnesium sulfate. (I, N, G)

21. 1. The antidote for magnesium sulfate is calcium, commonly administered as calcium gluconate. It should be readily available when magnesium sulfate is being administered. Diazepam (Valium), phenytoin sodium (Dilantin), and furosemide (Lasix) are not antidotes for magnesium sulfate. (I, N, G)

22. 4. Typical signs of hypermagnesemia include de-

creased deep tendon reflexes, a flushing of the skin, lethargy progressing to coma with increasing toxicity, and impaired respiration. The nurse should check the client's patellar, biceps, and radial reflexes regularly during magnesium sulfate therapy. Hyperactivity and tingling in the fingers are common symptoms of hypocalcemia. A rapid pulse rate commonly occurs in hypomagnesemia. (A, N, G)

23. 2. The only known cure for PIH is delivery of the fetus. Early diagnosis and careful management are used to control the disorder. Medical treatment for severe PIH includes bed rest, a regular moderate sodium diet, restoration of fluid and electrolyte balance, sedation, and antihypertensive medications. Medical treatment for eclampsia includes steps to control convulsions, correct hypoxia and acidosis, lower blood pressure, and stabilize the client for delivery. (I, N, G)

24. 1. The highest priority for a client with severe PIH is to prevent seizures and deliver the infant safely. Efforts to decrease edema, reduce blood pressure, increase urine output, limit kidney damage, and maintain sedation are desirable but are not as important as preventing convulsions. (P, N, G)

25. 3. When assessing a client receiving an intravenous infusion, the nurse should promptly report moist rales in the lung fields, which indicate fluid overload and pulmonary edema. Urinary output exceeding intake is not likely in the client with PIH; oliguria is more common. Urine output greater than intake is desirable because the client typically retains excess fluids. Respiratory rate of 16 breaths/minute is normal, and a blood pressure of 150/96 mm Hg is typical for a client with severe PIH. (I, N, G)

26. 1. The best nursing diagnosis at this time is High Risk for Injury related to possibility of convulsions. The client has severe PIH with elevated blood pressure. There are no data to suggest Knowledge Deficit or Altered Self Concept. *Hypertensive crisis* is a medical term. (D, N, G)

27. 3. HELLP syndrome involves hemolysis, elevated liver enzymes, and low platelet count (below 100,000 μL). This syndrome is sometimes associated with severe PIH. Women with HELLP syndrome and their offspring have high morbidity and mortality rates and should be cared for in a tertiary care center. Symptoms include anemia, pallor, fatigue, anorexia, and dyspnea. Signs of liver dysfunction include nausea and vomiting, right upper quadrant pain, jaundice, and malaise. Signs of disseminated intravascular coagulation (DIC)—epistaxis, hematuria, petechiae, bleeding gums, and gastrointestinal tract bleeding—should be reported immediately. Reflexes of +2 are normal, proteinuria is to be expected, and a clear to whitish discharge may be normal. (D, N, G)

28. 3. Epigastric pain or acute right upper quadrant pain is associated with an impending convulsion. Increased fetal movements are unlikely in a client receiving a central nervous system depressant. Decreased temperature and urine output of 40 mL/hour have no relationship to an impending convulsion. (D, N, G)

29. 4. During a convulsion, it is most important to keep an open airway. The side rails should have already been padded. Once the client begins to convulse, the nurse needs to monitor the client continuously. If the client is thrashing around in the bed, placing a pillow under her left buttock will not help. Insertion of a padded tongue blade is not recommended. (I, T, G)

30. 4. After an eclamptic seizure, the client often falls into a deep sleep or coma. The nurse must continually monitor the client for signs of impending labor because the client will not be able to verbalize that contractions are occurring. (A, N, G)

31. 4. After an eclamptic seizure, the nurse should assess the client for signs of abruptio placenta, a potential complication. (A, N, G)

The Pregnant Client With a Hypertensive Disorder

32. 1. Pregnancy is not the time for clients to begin a diet. Clients with chronic hypertension should have adequate protein intake. Protein intake of 1.5 g/kg of body weight is recommended for a client with proteinuria. Meat and beans are good sources of protein. (E, N, H)

33. 3. Methyldopa (Aldomet) is the antihypertensive drug of choice for pregnant clients with chronic hypertension. There is a risk of fetal depression with phenobarbital and diazepam (Valium). Magnesium sulfate is not usually prescribed for chronic hypertension. (I, N, G)

34. 2. Women with chronic hypertension during pregnancy are at risk for such complications as preeclampsia (about 25%), abruptio placenta, and intrauterine growth retardation, resulting in a small-for-gestational-age infant. These clients do not have a greater risk for large fetuses, heart disease, or placenta previa. Factors associated with placenta previa include multiparity and advanced maternal age. (E, N, G)

The Pregnant Client With Third-Trimester Bleeding

35. 4. When a client is admitted with bleeding in the third trimester of pregnancy, the nurse should first assess fetal heart rate and maternal blood pressure.

Vaginal examination and an enema are contraindicated for this client because excessive vaginal bleeding may occur if placenta previa is present. The client's bleeding is carefully monitored, and chux are commonly used, not perineal pads. At this point, a cesarean section delivery has not been planned, so witnessing a consent is not warranted. (I, N, G)

36. 2. The most typical symptom of abruptio placenta is a rigid or boardlike uterus. Pain is common, and there may be scant visible bleeding. Tetanic uterine contractions are contractions that are excessively strong and last longer than 90 seconds. The membranes do not ordinarily rupture. (A, N, G)

37. 1. The true cause of abruptio placenta is unknown. Possible contributing factors include excessive intrauterine pressure caused by hydramnios or multiple pregnancy, cigarette smoking, alcohol ingestion, trauma, increased maternal age and parity, cocaine abuse, and amniotomy. A previous low transverse cesarean section delivery is associated with increased risk of placenta previa. History of placenta accreta or obesity is not associated with abruptio placenta. (D, N, G)

38. 2. Treatment of DIC includes treatment of the causative factor and replacement of maternal coagulation factors and support of physiologic functions. Replacement of depleted coagulation factors is usually done with whole blood infusion, fresh-frozen plasma, or platelets. (P, N, G)

39. 1. The most common symptom of placenta previa is painless vaginal bleeding. With placenta previa, the placenta is abnormally implanted and covers a portion or all of the cervical os. (I, N, G)

40. 1. Treatment of partial placenta previa includes bed rest, hydration, and careful monitoring of bleeding. Vaginal birth is the preferred method of delivery. A double setup is the procedure used to detect placenta previa. Immediate cesarean section is not warranted, and induction of labor should be initiated with caution and only if delivery is indicated. (P, N, G)

41. 4. Bleeding precipitated by placenta previa results from exposure of the maternal sinuses when placental villi are torn from the uterine wall as the lower uterine segment contracts and dilates in the later weeks of pregnancy. Bleeding is not initiated because of premature labor, a heavy bloody show, or a large-for-gestational-age fetus. (E, N, G)

42. 2. The most appropriate diagnosis at this time is Fear related to concern for own personal status and the outcome of the fetus. The client is only at 32 weeks' gestation, and delivery would produce a preterm infant. There are no data to suggest Potential for Fetal Demise, although this is a possible diagnosis for future care. Shock and hemorrhage are medical diagnoses. (D, N, G)

43. 1. The nurse should use extreme caution when administering blood replacement therapy. The nurse should validate the client information and the blood product with another nurse. The client can be asked if she has ever had a reaction to a blood product, but a general question about allergies may not elicit the response that the client has had a blood reaction. (P, T, G)

44. 4. Before any type of major surgery, the nurse should be certain that blood replacement therapy is available. Shaving the abdomen, inserting a Foley catheter, and checking the status of the fetus should all be performed, but these are not a priority at this time. Family members can be supportive and should be allowed to stay with the client if the client desires. (P, T, G)

45. 4. Feelings of loss, grief, and guilt are normal after a cesarean section delivery, particularly if it was not planned. The nurse should support the client, listen with empathy, and allow the client time to grieve. There is no evidence that the client will have postpartum depression. Maternal infant bonding may be delayed owing to neonatal complications or maternal pain and subsequent medications, but it should not be difficult. Telling the client that this type of delivery was necessary to save the infant's life is not helpful. (I, T, L)

46. 2. Uterine atony is the relaxation of the uterus and can result in postpartum hemorrhage and possible death. Every postpartum client, regardless of the type of delivery, is at risk for uterine atony and hemorrhage. Even though an abdominal incision and abdominal dressing are present, the nurse should palpate the fundus gently while supporting the incision every 15 minutes for at least 1 hour. This should be done more frequently if bleeding is moderate or severe. The nurse should also observe and note any bleeding on the abdominal incision dressings, but this is not an accurate measure of uterine atony. The nurse should note the amount of lochia immediately after delivery and during the recovery period, usually about 2 hours, but internal bleeding may be concealed. (I, N, G)

The Pregnant Client With Preterm Labor

47. 1. Age under 19 or over 40 years has been associated with preterm labor. Although the exact cause of preterm labor has not been determined, various risk factors are associated with this condition. Some factors associated with preterm labor include polyhydramnios, poor pregnancy weight gain, multifetal gestation, prior preterm delivery, cervical incompe-

tence, reproductive tract infection, renal disease, and chronic hypertension. (E, T, H)

48. 4. Pharmaceutical agents, such as terbutaline, to suppress labor are ordinarily contraindicated for a client with a heart rate greater than 130 beats/minute or any cardiac arrhythmias. The frequency of uterine contractions is an important assessment, but the intensity of the contractions should not be a primary factor in determining if terbutaline therapy is warranted. Estimated size of the fetus should be investigated but does not contraindicate the use of terbutaline. Terbutaline does not affect deep tendon reflexes, although magnesium sulfate may depress reflexes. (A, N, G)

49. 4. For this client, who is crying on admission and has lost two fetuses in the past, the most appropriate diagnosis is Fear related to outcome of labor and possible preterm birth. No evidence in this situation suggests Pain related to uterine ischemia, or Altered Nutrition. Risk for preterm delivery is a medical diagnosis. (D, N, L)

50. 4. Tachycardia is a common side effect of terbutaline therapy. If the client's pulse rate is 130 beats/minute, the nurse should contact the physician before administering the next dose of medication. The client should also be carefully monitored for dyspnea or other symptoms of pulmonary edema. Other side effects include premature ventricular contractions, increased stroke volume, increased blood pressure, palpitations, tremors, nausea and vomiting, and shortness of breath. Other adverse effects include hyperglycemia, metabolic acidosis, and anemia. (A, T, G)

51. 1. Decreased hemoglobin levels are an indicator of an increase in blood plasma volume. Glycosuria, decreased weight gain, and increased serum calcium levels are not indicators of increased blood plasma volume. Increased blood plasma volume causes a type of blood dilution that decreases hemoglobin and hematocrit levels. (I, T, G)

52. 3. As the uterus contracts, the abdominal wall rises and, when external monitoring is used, presses against the transducer. This movement is transmitted into an electrical current, which is then recorded. With the fetus in the left occipitoanterior position, the cardiotransducer should be placed at the top of the fundus, over the fetal back, where uterine displacement during contractions is greatest. (I, N, G)

53. 3. Fetal heart rate is normally between 120 and 160 beats/minute. The nurse should continue to monitor the client and fetus. This is not an abnormal reading, so there is no need to notify the physician. There is no indication that fetal heart rate needs to be checked again in 5 minutes. (I, N, G)

54. 4. Before amniocentesis, an ultrasound is valuable in locating the placenta, locating a pool of amniotic fluid, and showing the physician where to insert the needle. Assessing gestational age by measuring the biparietal diameter of the fetus is not a prerequisite to performing amniocentesis. Late in pregnancy, biparietal diameter may be difficult to measure because of fetal position or engagement. (E, T, G)

55. 1. Betamethasone therapy is indicated when the fetal lungs indicate immaturity. The fetus must be between 28 and 34 weeks' gestation and delivery must be delayed for 24 to 48 hours for the drug to achieve a therapeutic effect. (I, T, G)

56. 2. For this client, who has experienced two stillbirths, the most appropriate diagnosis is Anxiety related to diagnostic tests for fetal well-being. There is minimal pain with most antepartal diagnostic tests. There is no indication that the client is demonstrating Ineffective Family Coping or Knowledge Deficit related to consequences of a preterm birth. (D, N, L)

57. 4. The shake test helps determine the maturity of the fetal pulmonary system. The test is based on the fact that surfactant foams when mixed with ethanol. The more stable the foam, the more mature the fetal pulmonary system. Although the shake test is inexpensive and provides rapid results, problems have been noted with its reliability. False-negative results can occur. For this reason, the lecithin-to-sphingomyelin ratio is usually performed in conjunction with the shake test. (P, N, S)

58. 2. After amniocentesis, the client should promptly report vaginal discharge or bleeding or a decrease in fetal movement. Nausea, urinary frequency, and irregular painless uterine tightness (Braxton-Hicks contractions) are not complications of amniocentesis. (E, N, G)

The Pregnant Client With Diabetes Mellitus

59. 1. A nonstress test that is reactive indicates fetal heart rate accelerations and well-being. The nonstress test is considered reactive when two or more fetal heart rate accelerations occur, along with fetal movement, during a 10- to 20-minute period. The baseline fetal heart rate should be in the normal range of 120 to 160 beats/minute. Each acceleration should have a duration of 15 seconds, and the acceleration should have an amplitude greater than 15 beats/minute. Based on a reactive nonstress test, there is no indication for a contraction stress test; however, contraction stress tests are often scheduled for insulin-dependent diabetic clients in the latter part of pregnancy. The client does not need continuous monitoring. The nonstress test does not detect fetal anomalies; however, cardiac abnormalities may be suspected if the fetal heart rate is abnormal. (I, N, G)

60. 2. The contraction stress test is performed on high-risk clients, such as insulin-dependent diabetic clients. The test subjects the fetus to uterine contractions, during which fetal heart rate is monitored. Contractions compress the arteries to the placenta. A fetus with adequate oxygen reserve can tolerate transient oxygen reductions, and the fetal heart rate remains normal. The test is performed either by nipple stimulation, which releases oxytocin from the maternal posterior pituitary gland, or by intravenous oxytocin administration. The test is not performed to detect cardiac anomalies, kidney anomalies, or amniotic fluid volume. (E, N, G)

61. 3. A suspicious contraction stress test indicates inconsistent late deceleration patterns, and further evaluation is necessary. A negative contraction stress test indicates no fetal heart rate decelerations and is considered normal. A positive contraction stress test indicates fetal compromise. An absence of fetal heart rate accelerations is considered a nonreactive positive contraction stress test. (D, N, G)

62. 4. The fetal biophysical profile assesses five parameters: fetal heart rate reactivity, fetal breathing movements, gross fetal body movements, fetal tone, and amniotic fluid volume. Fetal heart rate reactivity is determined by a nonstress test; the other four parameters are determined by ultrasound scanning. The test is noninvasive, and results are available as soon as it is completed and interpreted. The procedure is not uncomfortable and does not require that the client have an empty bladder before the test. (P, N, S)

63. 2. During the first trimester, it is not unusual for insulin needs to decrease, often as a result of nausea and vomiting. Progressive insulin resistance is characteristic of pregnancy, particularly the second half of pregnancy. It is not unusual for insulin needs to increase by as much as four times the nonpregnant dose. This resistance is due to the production of human placental lactogen, also called *human chorionic somatotropin*, by the placenta. This hormone and, to a lesser degree, estrogen and progesterone are insulin antagonists. (I, N, G)

64. 2. Pregnant diabetic clients are not at greater risk for multifetal pregnancy unless they have undergone fertility treatments. The pregnant diabetic client is at higher risk for complications, such as infection, polyhydramnios, and ketoacidosis, than the pregnant nondiabetic client. Infants of diabetic mothers may be larger than average and have a greater incidence of congenital anomalies. (E, N, G)

65. 2. The goal is to maintain blood plasma glucose levels to 60 to 80 mg/dL before meals and snacks. (P, T, G)

66. 3. Although pregnancy is not an optimum time to begin vigorous exercise, a well-controlled diabetic client who has regularly engaged in exercise may continue to do so. She should be reminded to eat a carbohydrate or protein snack before exercising to prevent hypoglycemia. The fetus is well protected in the amniotic sac, and exercise is not harmful. If the client's blood glucose levels are within normal limits, there is no reason to check the blood glucose again before exercising. (I, N, G)

67. 1. Dehydration, polyuria, fatigue, and drowsiness are manifestations of hyperglycemia. Hyperglycemia is a medical emergency and requires immediate action to prevent maternal and fetal mortality. Hypoglycemia is the most common cause of coma in clients with diabetes. Nervousness is an early sign of hypoglycemia. (E, N, G)

68. 3. Diabetic clients may experience unanticipated stillbirth as a result of premature aging of the placenta. Therefore, these clients are frequently induced before term. (I, N, G)

69. 3. Maternal hyperglycemia has been implicated in fetal macrosomia. Maternal hyperglycemia causes fetal hyperglycemia and results in a large infant. (I, T, G)

70. 1. During the postpartum period, insulin needs fall significantly. If the client breast-feeds, lower blood glucose levels decrease the insulin requirements. The length of the client's labor does not influence insulin needs. (I, N, H)

The Client With an Ectopic Pregnancy

71. 4. It may be important to obtain information from a client with suspected ectopic pregnancy concerning when she last had intercourse, whether she is taking birth control pills, and whether she has been pregnant previously. However, it is of particular importance to determine if she has had amenorrhea and the date of her last normal menstrual period. Such information helps establish an accurate diagnosis. Usually, the client with an ectopic pregnancy has missed a menstrual period or two and often suspects or knows she is pregnant. If the client's menstrual cycle is irregular, she may be unaware she is pregnant. (A, N, G)

72. 3. An ectopic pregnancy is defined as any gestation located outside the uterus. About 95% of ectopic pregnancies occur in the fallopian tube. (I, N, G)

73. 1. The most appropriate nursing diagnosis for this client is Anticipatory Grieving related to the loss of the pregnancy. This is a crisis for the client, and she needs emotional support. There are no data to suggest the diagnoses Fear, Maladaptive Coping, or Infection. (D, N, L)

74. 2. Falling hematocrit and hemoglobin levels are indicators of shock. Other common symptoms of tubal rupture are severe abdominal pain and referred shoulder pain. The pain is knifelike in quality and occurs in a lower abdominal quadrant. Slight vaginal bleeding, often described as spotting, also is common. Vomiting and abdominal distention are not associated with tubal rupture in ectopic pregnancy. (A, N, G)

75. 4. Fallopian tube rupture is an emergency situation because of extensive bleeding into the peritoneal cavity. Shock soon develops if precautionary measures are not taken. The nurse readying a client for surgery should be especially careful to monitor blood pressure and pulse rate for signs of impending shock. The nurse should be prepared to administer fluids, blood, or plasma expanders as necessary through an intravenous line that should already be in place. (A, N, G)

76. 2. Symptoms of ruptured ectopic pregnancy are not always obvious. If bleeding into the pelvic cavity is extensive, then vaginal examination causes intense pain, and blood is detected in the cul-de-sac of Douglas. Culdocentesis validates the diagnosis. Aspiration of nonclotting blood is indicative of ectopic pregnancy. Laparoscopy, ultrasound, and laparotomy also confirm the diagnosis. Dilation and curettage is not indicated for ruptured ectopic pregnancy. The uterus is not evacuated because the pregnancy is located outside the uterus. Oophorectomy (removal of the ovaries) is usually not performed, although a salpingectomy (removal of the tube) or salpinostomy (removal of the conceptus) is often performed to prevent further bleeding. (P, N, S)

77. 4. Anything that causes a narrowing or constriction in the fallopian tubes so that a fertilized ovum cannot be properly transported to the uterus for implantation predisposes to an ectopic pregnancy. Pelvic inflammatory disease is the most common cause of constricted or narrow tubes. Developmental defects are other possible causes. The incidence of ectopic pregnancy has increased dramatically during the past several years. (A, N, G)

78. 2. The client should not experience dizziness. Symptoms that the client should report include pain, bleeding, and temperature elevation. (E, N, G)

The Client With Hyperemesis Gravidarum

79. 4. Combustion cannot be completed when fat is burned in the body in the absence of carbohydrates. Improper fat metabolism results in acetone and diabetic acid in the urine from the starvation this client is experiencing. All pregnant clients have their urine tested for protein and glucose; based on this client's symptoms, her urine should also be screened for acetone. (I, N, G)

80. 3. Gastrointestinal secretion losses from excessive vomiting, diarrhea, and excessive perspiration can result in hypokalemia and acidosis if precautionary measures are not taken. (A, N, G)

81. 2. Although the cause of hyperemesis is still unclear, it is thought to be related to high estrogen levels or to trophoblastic activity or gonadotrophin production. Hyperemesis is also associated with infectious conditions, such as hepatitis or encephalitis, intestinal obstruction, peptic ulcer, and hydatidiform mole. (I, N, H)

82. 4. Based on this client's history of hyperemesis gravidarum, it is particularly important for the nurse to assess for additional signs and symptoms of dehydration. Common signs and symptoms of dehydration include scanty urine output, lassitude, and fever. The client should not experience abdominal pain or bright-red bleeding. With hydatidiform mole, any vaginal bleeding is usually brownish or prune-colored. The client should not have any yellowish vaginal discharge. (A, N, G)

83. 3. Usually the client remains NPO for at least 24 hours with intravenous therapy. If the client is not vomiting after 24 hours, she may be offered clear liquids. If she tolerates liquids, dry toast, crackers, or cereal may be given every 2 to 3 hours. Hyperalimentation is started only if other measures fail. (I, N, G)

The Pregnant Client With a Hydatidiform Mole

84. 1. Hydatidiform mole is suspected when the following symptoms are present: brownish or prune-colored vaginal bleeding, anemia, absence of fetal heart rate, passage of hydropic vessels, uterine enlargement greater than expected for gestational age, elevated human chorionic gonadotrophin (hCG) levels, and PIH. (A, N, G)

85. 2. After dilation and curettage for evacuation of the mole, the nurse should assess the client's vital signs and monitor for signs of hemorrhage. The client should not experience abdominal distention, and the PIH is usually resolved after evacuation. Symptoms of infection are important to assess, but chorioamnionitis is an inflammation of the amniotic fluid membranes. With complete mole, no embryonic or fetal tissue or membranes are present. (A, N, G)

86. 2. A client who has had a hydatidiform mole removed should have regular checkups to rule out the presence of choriocarcinoma, which may compli-

cate the client's clinical picture. The client's hCG levels are monitored for 1 to 2 years. During this time, she should be advised not to become pregnant because this will be reflected in rising hCG levels. Severe anemia, invasion of the mole, and polyps in the fallopian tubes are not associated with hydatidiform mole. (E, N, G)

The Pregnant Client With Premature Rupture of the Membranes

87. 1. It is particularly important that the nurse assess for symptoms of infection, particularly urinary tract infection. Although the cause of premature rupture of the membranes is unknown, it has been associated with incompetent cervix, infection, trauma, and multiple pregnancies. The client should be assessed for a small-for-gestational-age fetus and anemia, but these are not related to premature rupture of membranes. Uterine prolapse is not associated with premature rupture of the membranes. (A, N, G)

88. 4. The primary purpose of the magnesium sulfate is to inhibit uterine contractions. Compared with intravenous ritodrine, magnesium sulfate causes fewer side effects. In some institutions, prostaglandin synthesis inhibitors, such as indomethacin (Indocin), are being investigated. The client may experience a sedative effect from magnesium sulfate. This drug is not given to combat hypomagnesemia, and it does not improve the fetal pulmonary system. (I, N, G)

89. 1. The client should report contractions occurring every 10 minutes or less for 1 hour, or if fluid leakage occurs. If the client experiences preterm labor symptoms for more than 15 minutes, she should empty her bladder, rest on the left side, palpate for uterine contractions, and call the health care provider. It is not necessary for the client to call the health care provider if she experiences contractions every hour for 6 hours, but she should monitor the contraction pattern to determine increasing frequency. (E, N, H)

90. 2. Maternal side effects of betamethasone (Celestone, Soluspan) include increased risk of infection, initiation of lactation, gastrointestinal bleeding, weight gain, edema, and pulmonary edema when used concurrently with tocolytic agents. Hypoglycemia may occur in the neonate but not in the mother. Urinary frequency and decreased skin turgor are not considered side effects of betamethasone. (P, N, G)

THE NURSING CARE OF THE CHILDBEARING FAMILY AND THEIR NEONATE

TEST 2: Complications of Pregnancy

Directions: Use this answer grid to determine areas of strength or need for further study.

NURSING PROCESS

A = Assessment
D = Analysis, nursing diagnosis
P = Planning
I = Implementation
E = Evaluation

COGNITIVE LEVEL

K = Knowledge
C = Comprehension
T = Application
N = Analysis

CLIENT NEEDS

S = Safe, effective care environment
G = Physiologic integrity
L = Psychosocial integrity
H = Health promotion and maintenance

Question #	Answer #	Nursing Process					Cognitive Level				Client Needs			
		A	**D**	**P**	**I**	**E**	**K**	**C**	**T**	**N**	**S**	**G**	**L**	**H**
1	1	A								N		G		
2	4		D							N		G		
3	2		D							N		G		
4	4		D							N		G		
5	3			P						N		G		
6	1					E				N		G		
7	3					E				N		G		
8	3			P						N		G		
9	1					E		C				G		
10	4	A								N		G		
11	3				I				T					H
12	1				I				T			G		
13	2				I				T			G		
14	2				I					N				H
15	4				I					N				H
16	1		D							N		G		
17	2				I					N		G		
18	2		D							N				H
19	2			P						N		G		
20	4				I					N		G		
21	1				I					N		G		
22	4	A								N		G		
23	2				I					N		G		
24	1			P						N		G		
25	3				I					N		G		

NURSING PROCESS

A = Assessment
D = Analysis, nursing diagnosis
P = Planning
I = Implementation
E = Evaluation

COGNITIVE LEVEL

K = Knowledge
C = Comprehension
T = Application
N = Analysis

CLIENT NEEDS

S = Safe, effective care environment
G = Physiologic integrity
L = Psychosocial integrity
H = Health promotion and maintenance

Question #	Answer #	Nursing Process					Cognitive Level				Client Needs			
		A	D	P	I	E	K	C	T	N	S	G	L	H
26	1		D							N		G		
27	3		D							N		G		
28	3		D							N		G		
29	4				I				T			G		
30	4	A								N		G		
31	4	A								N		G		
32	1					E				N				H
33	3				I					N		G		
34	2					E				N		G		
35	4				I					N		G		
36	2	A								N		G		
37	1		D							N		G		
38	2			P						N		G		
39	1				I					N		G		
40	1			P						N		G		
41	4					E				N		G		
42	2		D							N		G		
43	1			P					T			G		
44	4			P					T			G		
45	4				I				T				L	
46	2				I					N		G		
47	1					E			T					H
48	4	A								N		G		
49	4		D							N			L	
50	4	A							T			G		
51	1				I				T			G		
52	3				I					N		G		
53	3				I					N		G		
54	4					E			T			G		
55	1				I				T			G		

ANSWER GRID: 2

NURSING PROCESS

A = Assessment
D = Analysis, nursing diagnosis
P = Planning
I = Implementation
E = Evaluation

COGNITIVE LEVEL

K = Knowledge
C = Comprehension
T = Application
N = Analysis

CLIENT NEEDS

S = Safe, effective care environment
G = Physiologic integrity
L = Psychosocial integrity
H = Health promotion and maintenance

Question #	Answer #	Nursing Process					Cognitive Level				Client Needs			
		A	D	P	I	E	K	C	T	N	S	G	L	H
56	2		D							N			L	
57	4			P						N	S			
58	2					E				N		G		
59	1				I					N		G		
60	2					E				N		G		
61	3		D							N		G		
62	4			P						N	S			
63	2				I					N		G		
64	2					E				N		G		
65	2			P					T			G		
66	3				I					N		G		
67	1					E				N		G		
68	3				I					N		G		
69	3				I				T			G		
70	1				I					N				H
71	4	A								N		G		
72	3				I					N		G		
73	1		D							N			L	
74	2	A								N		G		
75	4	A								N		G		
76	2			P						N	S			
77	4	A								N		G		
78	2					E				N		G		
79	4				I					N		G		
80	3	A								N		G		
81	2				I					N				H
82	4	A								N		G		
83	3				I					N		G		
84	1	A								N		G		
85	2	A								N		G		

NURSING PROCESS

A = Assessment
D = Analysis, nursing diagnosis
P = Planning
I = Implementation
E = Evaluation

COGNITIVE LEVEL

K = Knowledge
C = Comprehension
T = Application
N = Analysis

CLIENT NEEDS

S = Safe, effective care environment
G = Physiologic integrity
L = Psychosocial integrity
H = Health promotion and maintenance

Question #	Answer #	A	D	P	I	E	K	C	T	N	S	G	L	H
86	2					E				N		G		
87	1	A								N		G		
88	4				I					N		G		
89	1					E				N				H
90	2			P						N		G		
Number Correct														
Number Possible	90	17	14	13	31	15	0	1	14	75	3	73	4	10
Percentage Correct														

Score Calculation: To determine your **Percentage Correct,** divide the **Number Correct** by the **Number Possible.**

ANSWER GRID: 4

The Birth Experience

- **The Primigravida in Labor**
- **The Multigravida in Labor**
- **The Intrapartal Client With Risk Factors**
- **Correct Answers and Rationale**

Select the one best answer, and indicate your choice by filling in the circle in front of the option.

The Primigravida in Labor

A 20-year-old obese primigravida at 40 weeks' gestation is admitted to the birthing center in the first stage of labor.

1. The client is admitted to the birthing center with contractions lasting 50 seconds and occurring every 3 to 4 minutes. The client's cervix is dilated 5 cm and is 75% effaced. In assessing the client's emotional status, the nurse anticipates that she will be
   - ○ 1. serious.
   - ○ 2. fearful.
   - ○ 3. joyful.
   - ○ 4. panicky.

2. The client is to have intermittent fetal heart rate monitoring. When the client asks the nurse how often the fetal heart rate pattern will be monitored, the nurse's best response is to explain that the fetal heart rate pattern will be monitored every
   - ○ 1. 15 minutes during the transition phase.
   - ○ 2. 30 minutes during the active phase.
   - ○ 3. 60 minutes during the active phase.
   - ○ 4. 2 hours in the latent phase.

3. The nurse performs a Nitrazine paper test and notifies the physician of probable rupture of membranes if the Nitrazine paper is
   - ○ 1. blue.
   - ○ 2. green.
   - ○ 3. pink.
   - ○ 4. yellow.

4. The client says, "The doctor said the baby is at +1 station. What does that mean?" After providing instruction, the nurse determines that teaching has been effective when the client states that the fetal presenting part is located
   - ○ 1. 1 cm above the ischial spines.
   - ○ 2. 1 cm below the ischial spines.
   - ○ 3. 1 fingerbreadth above the ischial spines.
   - ○ 4. 1 fingerbreadth below the ischial spines.

5. When the cervix is 6 cm dilated, the client receives a continuous lumbar epidural block. After administration of this anesthesia, it is most important for the nurse to assess the
   - ○ 1. fetal heart rate.
   - ○ 2. amniotic fluid color.
   - ○ 3. level of anesthesia.
   - ○ 4. level of consciousness.

6. While caring for this obese client in labor, the nurse plans to monitor the client for signs of
   - ○ 1. hypertonic reflexes.
   - ○ 2. decreased uterine resting tone.
   - ○ 3. soft tissue dystocia.
   - ○ 4. increased nausea and vomiting.

7. The client delivers a viable male neonate who is given a score of 9 at 5 minutes on the Apgar rating system. The nurse determines that the neonate's physical condition is
   - ○ 1. good.
   - ○ 2. fair.
   - ○ 3. poor.
   - ○ 4. critical.

A 32-year-old primigravida at 39 weeks' gestation is admitted to the hospital in active labor. The client's husband accompanies her to the labor area.

8. The nurse performs Leopold's maneuvers. When the client asks what these maneuvers are for, the nurse's best response is to explain that they help determine
   - ○ 1. fetal presentation.
   - ○ 2. a multifetal pregnancy.

○ 3. estimated gestational age.

○ 4. intensity of contractions.

9. The client's husband coaches her with breathing and relaxation techniques as they were taught in childbirth preparation classes. When the client reaches the transition phase of labor, she screams out, "I can't do this anymore!" The nurse should suggest to the client's husband that he

○ 1. allow the nurse to take over the coaching.

○ 2. ask his wife if she wants anesthesia.

○ 3. tell his wife that it will be over soon.

○ 4. maintain direct eye contact and breathe with her.

10. The nurse formulates a nursing diagnosis for the client in the transitional phase of labor. The most appropriate diagnosis is

○ 1. Altered Urinary Elimination Patterns related to physiologic changes of labor.

○ 2. Dizziness related to hyperventilation.

○ 3. Ineffective Family Coping related to lack of confidence.

○ 4. Pain related to increasing frequency and intensity of uterine contractions.

11. The client delivers a viable neonate. The physician orders oxytocin intravenously after delivery of the placenta. Which of the following data would indicate that the placenta is about to be delivered?

○ 1. The abdominal wall relaxes noticeably.

○ 2. The cord lengthens outside the vagina.

○ 3. There is decreased vaginal bleeding.

○ 4. The uterus cannot be palpated.

12. While the client holds and looks at her neonate, she begins to cry. The nurse correctly interprets this behavior as indicating that the client is

○ 1. disappointed in the baby's appearance.

○ 2. grieving over the loss of the pregnancy.

○ 3. experiencing a normal response to the birth.

○ 4. a candidate for postpartum depression.

13. The client plans to breast-feed the neonate. The nurse plans to assist the client to breast-feed

○ 1. during the neonate's first period of reactivity.

○ 2. in about 2 hours, after the baby has been evaluated.

○ 3. in about 4 hours, after the baby has had some sleep.

○ 4. after the neonate's first period of reactivity.

A 15-year-old primigravida arrives at the birthing unit in early labor. On admission, the client's cervix is 2 cm dilated and 50% effaced, and contractions are occurring every 5 to 6 minutes, with membranes intact.

14. After admission, the nurse instructs the client that the most effective position for dilating the cervix is

○ 1. right lateral recumbent.

○ 2. left lateral recumbent.

○ 3. standing.

○ 4. sitting in a comfortable chair.

15. The nurse plans to instruct the client in active relaxation techniques to help her cope with the pain of contractions. The nurse should plan to instruct the client to

○ 1. relax uninvolved body muscles during uterine contractions.

○ 2. be in a deep, meditative, sleeplike state.

○ 3. alter the position of the client frequently.

○ 4. breathe rapidly and deeply between contractions.

16. The client asks the nurse what *effleurage* means. The nurse's best response is to explain that effleurage is a type of massage involving

○ 1. deep kneading of superficial muscles.

○ 2. secure grasping of muscular tissues.

○ 3. light stroking of the skin surface.

○ 4. prolonged pressure on specific sites.

17. Soon after the client arrives, the nurse observes moderately increased bloody vaginal discharge (show). The nurse's best action is to

○ 1. check fetal descent by performing Leopold's maneuvers.

○ 2. perform a vaginal examination to determine cervical dilation.

○ 3. check for rupture of the membranes with a sterile speculum.

○ 4. notify the physician of possible abruption of the placenta.

18. The client asks the nurse why she can have only fluids while in labor. After providing an explanation, the nurse determines that the teaching has been effective from which client statement?

○ 1. "Intravenous fluids will be started if I get hungry."

○ 2. "The digestive process is normally slow during labor."

○ 3. "Most clients don't get hungry during labor."

○ 4. "Eating solid foods during labor is unnecessary."

19. Because the client is only 15 years old, the nurse caring for the client during the labor process assesses the client for signs of

○ 1. uterine tetany.

○ 2. cephalopelvic disproportion.

○ 3. rapid second stage of labor.

○ 4. early deceleration pattern.

A 19-year-old primigravida at 38 weeks' gestation is admitted to the hospital in active labor that began 8 hours ago. Her mother accompanies her to the labor unit.

20. On admission, the client is breathing rapidly and complains of feeling dizzy and lightheaded. The client's cervix is 5 cm dilated. The nurse determines that she is most likely experiencing effects of
    ○ 1. rapid cervical dilation.
    ○ 2. elevated blood pressure.
    ○ 3. hyperventilation.
    ○ 4. excitement about the labor process.

21. When the client's cervix is 7 cm dilated and the presenting part is at +1 station, the client tells the nurse, "I need to push!" The nurse should
    ○ 1. place the client in a lithotomy position.
    ○ 2. increase the rate of intravenous fluids.
    ○ 3. instruct the client to use a pant–blow pattern of breathing.
    ○ 4. tell the client to push only when absolutely necessary.

22. For the client in this phase of labor, the nurse's primary action should be to provide
    ○ 1. ice chips.
    ○ 2. extra blankets.
    ○ 3. frequent mouth rinsing.
    ○ 4. encouragement and support.

23. To determine if the client is completely dilated, the nurse performs a vaginal examination. To assess the suture most readily felt, the nurse would determine the position of the cranial suture termed
    ○ 1. sagittal.
    ○ 2. transverse.
    ○ 3. coronal.
    ○ 4. biparietal.

24. The nurse tells the client that she is beginning the second stage of labor. The nurse realizes that the client understands the second stage of labor from which of the following statements?
    ○ 1. "I'm going to have a higher blood pressure."
    ○ 2. "My membranes are likely to have a foul odor."
    ○ 3. "My contractions are going to be less painful."
    ○ 4. "I should try to push with each contraction."

25. After delivery of a viable neonate, the client makes comments to her mother about the baby. Which of the following comments should the nurse interpret as a possible sign of potential maternal–infant bonding problems?
    ○ 1. "She's got my funny looking nose."
    ○ 2. "I think I'll let my mother give her the first feeding."
    ○ 3. "She's a lot smaller than I expected her to be."
    ○ 4. "I want to buy her frilly dresses to wear."

A 23-year-old primigravida at 40 weeks' gestation is admitted to the birthing unit in the active labor. Assessment reveals that her cervix is 3 cm dilated and 100% effaced, and contractions are occurring ever 4 minutes. She is accompanied by her husband.

26. The nurse plans to instruct the client about the gate control theory of pain. Which of the following statements would be appropriate for the nurse to include in the teaching plan?
    ○ 1. The gating mechanism is located at the pain site.
    ○ 2. Pain is a matter of perception.
    ○ 3. Shallow chest breathing can open the gate.
    ○ 4. The gating mechanism is in the spinal cord.

27. The nurse explains that according to the gate control theory of pain, a closed gate means that the client should experience
    ○ 1. no pain.
    ○ 2. sharp pain.
    ○ 3. light pain.
    ○ 4. reduced pain.

28. After 12 hours of experiencing regular contractions, the nurse determines that the client is still in the latent stage of labor. The nurse plans to observe the client closely for signs of
    ○ 1. exhaustion.
    ○ 2. hypotension.
    ○ 3. fluid overload.
    ○ 4. bradycardia.

29. The client's labor is progressing, but her cervix is still only 5 cm dilated and 100% effaced. She appears relaxed, although she is aware of labor contractions. At this time, the nurse suggests to the client's husband that he can be of most assistance by
    ○ 1. keeping a record of her contraction pattern.
    ○ 2. encouraging her to rest between contractions.
    ○ 3. suggesting that she receive an epidural anesthetic.
    ○ 4. suggesting that she practice rapid, shallow breathing.

30. The client's cervix is 6 cm dilated, and she is starting to feel considerable discomfort during contractions. The nurse suggests that the client change from slow chest breathing to
    ○ 1. shallow abdominal breathing.
    ○ 2. deep chest breathing.
    ○ 3. rapid pant–blow breathing.
    ○ 4. rapid chest breathing.

A 16-year-old primigravida is admitted to the hospital in active labor. She is at 37 weeks' gestation, and her cervix is 7 cm dilated with the presenting part at −1 station. She has had only one prenatal visit.

31. Soon after admission, the nurse determines that the

client is hyperventilating. The nurse's most appropriate action is to have the client breathe

- ○ 1. several whiffs of oxygen through a nasal cannula.
- ○ 2. into a paper bag.
- ○ 3. quickly, then hold her breath.
- ○ 4. with forceful inspiration.

32. Due to the hyperventilation, the nurse should assess the client for signs and symptoms of

- ○ 1. metabolic alkalosis.
- ○ 2. metabolic acidosis.
- ○ 3. respiratory alkalosis.
- ○ 4. respiratory acidosis.

33. The client complains of severe back pain during labor. The nurse should instruct the client that her severe back pain is most likely due to the fetal occiput being in a position termed

- ○ 1. oblique.
- ○ 2. transverse.
- ○ 3. posterior.
- ○ 4. asynclitic.

34. In planning care for the client experiencing severe back pain while in labor, the nurse should plan to

- ○ 1. provide firm pressure to the sacral area.
- ○ 2. prepare the client for a cesarean section.
- ○ 3. prepare for a precipitate delivery.
- ○ 4. maintain the client in a side-lying position.

35. Based on the client's symptoms, the most appropriate nursing diagnosis is

- ○ 1. Anxiety related to lack of support and adolescence.
- ○ 2. Knowledge Deficit related to lack of prenatal care.
- ○ 3. Alteration in Normal Physiologic Process related to failure of fetus to descend.
- ○ 4. High Risk for Injury related to lack of control during transition.

The Multigravida in Labor

A 31-year-old multigravida at 39 weeks' gestation is admitted to the hospital in active labor.

36. While the nurse begins the admission process, the amniotic membranes rupture spontaneously. The client's cervix is 5 cm dilated and the presenting part is at 0 station. The nurse should *first*

- ○ 1. perform a vaginal examination to determine dilation.
- ○ 2. auscultate the client's blood pressure.
- ○ 3. note the color, amount, and odor of the amniotic fluid.
- ○ 4. prepare the client for imminent delivery.

37. An intravenous solution of lactated Ringer's is

started, and a continuous epidural anesthetic is administered to the client. During the first hour after administration of the anesthetic, the nurse plans to monitor the client for

- ○ 1. respiratory depression.
- ○ 2. diaphoresis.
- ○ 3. urinary frequency.
- ○ 4. tremors.

38. The client's contractions and fetal heart rate are monitored with external electronic equipment. The nurse determines that there is a variable deceleration pattern on the fetal heart rate. The nurse should *first*

- ○ 1. notify the anesthesiologist.
- ○ 2. change the client's position.
- ○ 3. administer oxygen at 2 liters by mask.
- ○ 4. prepare the client for a cesarean section.

39. The client's cervix is 10 cm dilated, and she begins to push. The nurse notes early decelerations of the fetal heart rate and determines that the early deceleration pattern is most likely due to

- ○ 1. cord compression.
- ○ 2. fetal bradycardia.
- ○ 3. fetal head compression.
- ○ 4. inadequate uteroplacental perfusion.

40. The client delivers a viable neonate. About 15 minutes after delivery, she complains of a chill. The nurse should

- ○ 1. assess the client's temperature.
- ○ 2. increase the rate of intravenous fluids.
- ○ 3. provide the client with a warm blanket.
- ○ 4. assess the amount of blood loss.

41. After delivery, the nurse formulates a nursing diagnosis. The most appropriate diagnosis at this time is

- ○ 1. Pain related to exhaustive pushing efforts.
- ○ 2. Urinary retention related to epidural anesthesia.
- ○ 3. High Risk for Injury related to epidural anesthesia.
- ○ 4. Fluid Volume deficit related to process of labor.

The Intrapartal Client With Risk Factors

A 39-year-old multiparous client at 39 weeks' gestation is admitted to the hospital in active labor. She has been diagnosed with class II heart disease.

42. When assessing the client after admission to the birthing area, the nurse should *first* assess the

- ○ 1. fetal position and station.
- ○ 2. last food and fluid intake.
- ○ 3. frequency of contractions.
- ○ 4. ability to follow directions.

43. To ensure cardiac emptying and adequate oxygen during labor, the nurse plans to encourage the client to
○ 1. breathe rapidly after a contraction.
○ 2. limit the number of visitors.
○ 3. remain in a side-lying position.
○ 4. request local anesthesia for delivery.

44. Based on the client's medical diagnosis of class II heart disease, during labor the nurse should frequently assess the client for
○ 1. dehydration.
○ 2. nausea and vomiting.
○ 3. bradycardia.
○ 4. tachycardia.

A 22-year-old primigravida at 39 weeks' gestation is admitted to the hospital for induction of labor. The client is a class B, insulin-dependent diabetic. The fetus is in a cephalic position, and the client's cervix is dilated 1 cm.

45. The physician has ordered prostaglandin E₂ gel for the client. The nurse plans to explain to the client that the purpose of the gel is to
○ 1. increase the intensity of uterine contractions.
○ 2. prevent uterine rupture.
○ 3. ripen the cervix.
○ 4. ensure a good fetal outcome.

46. Before prostaglandin E₂ gel is administered to the client, the nurse should *first*
○ 1. assess the frequency of uterine contractions.
○ 2. place the client in a prone position.
○ 3. determine if the membranes have ruptured.
○ 4. prepare the client for an amniotomy.

47. The physician orders intravenous infusion of oxytocin. Before oxytocin induction, the nurse plans to
○ 1. administer a 500 mL bolus of fluid to prevent hypotension.
○ 2. continuously monitor the fetal heart rate and contraction pattern for at least 20 minutes.
○ 3. insert a Foley catheter to determine intake and output accurately.
○ 4. call the anesthesiologist to administer epidural anesthesia.

48. While caring for the pregnant diabetic client in labor, the nurse plans to
○ 1. measure urine output every 4 hours.
○ 2. administer insulin subcutaneously every 4 hours.
○ 3. check reflexes every 2 hours.
○ 4. monitor blood glucose levels every hour.

49. The nurse plans to explain to the client that one of the possible disadvantages of oxytocin induction is

○ 1. urinary frequency.
○ 2. hypoglycemia.
○ 3. preterm birth.
○ 4. neonatal hyperbilirubinemia.

50. The nurse formulates a nursing diagnosis for the client. The most appropriate nursing diagnosis at this time is
○ 1. Fluid Volume Deficit related to oxytocin infusion.
○ 2. Pain related to prolonged labor and uterine ischemia.
○ 3. Fear related to probable need for cesarean section.
○ 4. High Risk for Maternal or Fetal Injury related to uterine hyperstimulation.

51. The fetal presenting part is at −1 station when the membranes are ruptured. Immediately after the membranes are ruptured, the nurse should
○ 1. position the client on her left side.
○ 2. prepare for a cesarean section delivery.
○ 3. determine the client's pulse rate.
○ 4. check for prolapsed umbilical cord.

52. After rupture of the membranes, the nurse observes meconium-stained amniotic fluid. The nurse should plan to
○ 1. increase the rate of the oxytocin infusion.
○ 2. turn the client to a supine position.
○ 3. assess fetal position and presentation.
○ 4. monitor the fetal heart rate continuously.

A 26-year-old primigravida at 40 weeks' gestation is admitted to the hospital's labor unit for induction of labor. The client's membranes rupture spontaneously, and there is evidence of meconium staining.

53. After 1 hour of intravenous oxytocin, the nurse observes late fetal heart rate decelerations. The nurse should
○ 1. inform the client about the cause of the fetal heart rate pattern.
○ 2. prepare the client for an immediate cesarean section.
○ 3. evaluate the contraction pattern for 15 minutes.
○ 4. administer oxygen at 8 to 10 liters by mask.

54. The nurse prepares the client for lumbar epidural anesthesia. Before anesthesia administration, the nurse instructs the client to assume which of the following positions?
○ 1. Sitting.
○ 2. Side-lying.
○ 3. Knee to chest.
○ 4. Supine.

55. The nurse instructs the client about the procedures that will be performed on the neonate immediately after delivery to prevent meconium aspiration. The nurse determines that the instructions have been effective when the client states that the neonate will be
○ 1. suctioned as soon as the head is delivered.
○ 2. intubated immediately after delivery.
○ 3. given oxygen through an airway after delivery.
○ 4. given a drug to dilate the bronchi after delivery.

56. The client has a history of smoking one to two packs of cigarettes daily. In response to a question, the nurse tells the client that due to her smoking, the neonate is likely to have a
○ 1. higher hematocrit.
○ 2. lower hemoglobin.
○ 3. lower birth weight.
○ 4. higher bilirubin level.

57. The nurse plans to instruct the client about pushing during the second stage of labor. Which of the following should be included in the teaching plan? The client should push
○ 1. for at least 1.5 to 2 minutes.
○ 2. when she feels a contraction.
○ 3. with an open glottis.
○ 4. only when she feels the urge.

58. The nurse instructs the client about the purpose of the episiotomy. The nurse determines that the client has understood the instructions when she says that an episiotomy
○ 1. shortens the second stage of labor.
○ 2. enlarges the pelvic inlet.
○ 3. prevents perineal edema.
○ 4. ensures quick delivery of the placenta.

59. The physician determines that forceps are needed to assist in delivery. The nurse explains to the client that outlet forceps are used when the fetal skull
○ 1. is not visible on the perineum.
○ 2. is at a station of +1.
○ 3. is visible at the vaginal opening.
○ 4. has reached the level of the ischial spines.

A multigravida is admitted to the hospital in active labor. The client's and the fetus's conditions have been good since admission. The client has a history of rapid labor.

60. The client calls out to the nurse, "The baby is coming!" The nurse's first action is to
○ 1. inspect the perineum.
○ 2. open the emergency delivery pack.
○ 3. auscultate the fetal heart rate.
○ 4. contact the birth attendant.

61. It appears that delivery is imminent, and the nurse has no help immediately available. The nurse should first
○ 1. have the client push with a contraction.
○ 2. ask the client to hold her breath.
○ 3. prepare a clean area on which to deliver the neonate.
○ 4. lower the head of the bed to a flat position.

62. To help the client remain calm and cooperative during the imminent delivery, the nurse should tell the client
○ 1. "You're right, the baby is coming, so just relax."
○ 2. "Do you want to help me get you through this?"
○ 3. "Your doctor will be here soon."
○ 4. "I'll explain what's happening and guide you as we go along."

63. As the head is being delivered, the nurse should
○ 1. tell the client to push between contractions.
○ 2. check for an umbilical cord around the neonate's neck.
○ 3. apply gentle traction on the neonate's anterior shoulder.
○ 4. try to transfer the client to the delivery room.

64. As the placenta is being delivered, the nurse should not take any action until the nurse has
○ 1. asked the client to push down forcefully.
○ 2. massaged the fundus forcefully.
○ 3. observed for signs of placental separation.
○ 4. reached into the uterus with sterile gloves.

65. Because the client had a precipitous delivery, during the immediate postpartum period, the nurse should monitor the client closely for symptoms of
○ 1. delayed bonding.
○ 2. uterine atony.
○ 3. intrauterine infection.
○ 4. urinary tract infection.

A 30-year-old multigravida at 37 weeks' gestation is admitted to the hospital in early labor. She is pregnant with dizygotic twins.

66. The twins' heart rates are continually monitored with electronic fetal monitoring. After giving instruction about the purpose of the electronic monitoring, the nurse determines that the client needs *further* instruction when she says that an electronic monitor
○ 1. allows assessment of the fetus after analgesia.
○ 2. causes less discomfort for the client.
○ 3. provides a continuous recording of fetal heart rate.

4. allows the nurse to provide care to a greater number of clients.

67. In addition to electronic monitoring, the nurse plans to assess the client during labor more frequently for symptoms of
    ○ 1. urinary tract infection.
    ○ 2. oligohydramnios.
    ○ 3. pregnancy-induced hypertension.
    ○ 4. abdominal distention.

68. While the client is in active labor and the cervix is 5 cm dilated, the nurse observes contractions occurring at a rate of every 7 to 8 minutes in a 30-minute period. The nurse's most appropriate action is to
    ○ 1. note the fetal heart rate patterns.
    ○ 2. notify the physician.
    ○ 3. administer oxygen at 6 liters by mask.
    ○ 4. have the client pant–blow during the contractions.

69. The physician orders oxytocin to be added to the client's intravenous fluids after the delivery. The nurse plans to administer the oxytocin after delivery of the
    ○ 1. first twin.
    ○ 2. first placenta.
    ○ 3. second twin.
    ○ 4. second placenta.

70. During the immediate postpartum period, the client experiences uterine atony. The nurse should *first*
    ○ 1. gently massage the fundus.
    ○ 2. assess the client for infection.
    ○ 3. determine if the uterus has ruptured.
    ○ 4. increase the intravenous fluid rate.

71. The twin neonates require additional hospitalization after the client is discharged. In planning the family's care, an appropriate goal for the nurse to formulate is: The parents will
    ○ 1. discuss how they will cope with twin infants at home.
    ○ 2. participate in care of the twins on a daily basis.
    ○ 3. take turns providing 24-hour observation of the twins.
    ○ 4. identify complications that may occur as the twins develop.

A primigravida is admitted to the hospital's labor and delivery unit in active labor. She is about 10 days post-term.

72. The client desires a bilateral pudendal block anesthetic before delivery. The nurse should explain to the client that this type of anesthesia will relieve discomfort primarily in her
    ○ 1. back.

○ 2. abdomen.
○ 3. fundus.
○ 4. perineum.

73. After the bilateral pudendal block anesthesia, the nurse assesses the fetus for potential side effects of the anesthetic. The nurse should assess the fetus for
    ○ 1. bradycardia.
    ○ 2. decreased movements.
    ○ 3. increased variability.
    ○ 4. meconium-stained fluid.

74. The nurse instructs the client in techniques of pushing to use during the second stage of labor. The nurse determines that the client needs *further* instructions when she says she will need to
    ○ 1. be in a semi-Fowler's position or a position of comfort.
    ○ 2. flex her thighs onto her abdomen before bearing down.
    ○ 3. exert downward pressure as if she were having a bowel movement.
    ○ 4. hold her breath throughout the contraction.

75. The neonate is in good condition. After suctioning to clear the airway after delivery, the nurse should next
    ○ 1. keep the infant warm.
    ○ 2. instill erythromycin in the eyes.
    ○ 3. weigh the infant.
    ○ 4. put identification bracelets on each wrist.

76. After delivery following 20 hours of labor with membranes ruptured for 24 hours, a priority nursing diagnosis for the client is
    ○ 1. Maternal exhaustion related to prolonged second stage of labor.
    ○ 2. Sleep deprivation related to prolonged labor.
    ○ 3. Hypothermia related to cool delivery area.
    ○ 4. High Risk for Infection related to birth trauma.

77. Because the neonate is postmature, the nurse should assess the neonate for symptoms of
    ○ 1. infection.
    ○ 2. hypoglycemia.
    ○ 3. delayed meconium.
    ○ 4. elevated bilirubin.

78. While assessing a post-term neonate, the nurse anticipates that the neonate will have
    ○ 1. a flattened nose.
    ○ 2. small hands and feet.
    ○ 3. a red rash on the abdomen.
    ○ 4. wrinkled, peeling skin.

A primigravida at 39 weeks' gestation is admitted to the hospital in early active labor. Because the fetus has been determined to be large for gestational age, there is question about whether the mother's pelvis is of adequate size for vaginal delivery.

79. After 5 hours of active labor, the client's cervix is dilated 5 cm, with 100% effacement—the same as 2 hours before. Contractions are 4 to 6 minutes apart, lasting 45 seconds. The nurse determines that the client is most likely experiencing
   ○ 1. cephalopelvic disproportion.
   ○ 2. prolonged latent phase.
   ○ 3. prolonged transitional phase.
   ○ 4. hypertonic contraction pattern.

80. An ultrasound is scheduled for the client. The ultrasound reveals that the client has polyhydramnios. Based on this diagnosis, if the client's membranes rupture, the nurse should observe the client for
   ○ 1. prolapsed cord.
   ○ 2. inversion of the uterus.
   ○ 3. meconium-stained fluid.
   ○ 4. signs of infection.

81. The physician elects to perform a cesarean section and has informed the client of possible risks during the procedure. When the nurse asks the client to sign the consent form, the client's husband says, "I'll sign it for her. She's too upset by what is happening to make this decision." The nurse should
   ○ 1. ask the client if this is acceptable to her.
   ○ 2. have the client and her husband both sign the consent form.
   ○ 3. ask the client to sign the consent form.
   ○ 4. ask the doctor to witness the consent form.

82. The nurse plans to prepare the client for the cesarean section. Before transferring the client to the operating suite, the nurse should
   ○ 1. ask the client to empty her bladder.
   ○ 2. remove the client's wedding ring.
   ○ 3. cleanse the abdomen with povidone-iodine (Betadine).
   ○ 4. allow time for the couple to be alone.

A multigravida is admitted to the hospital for a trial labor and possible vaginal birth. She has a history of previous cesarean delivery because of fetal distress.

83. After several hours of active labor, the physician orders nalbuphine (Nubain). The nurse evaluates the drug as effective when the client says
   ○ 1. "I'll be able to get some sleep until after the delivery."
   ○ 2. "The contractions don't seem as painful as before."

   ○ 3. "I don't feel that burning sensation in my stomach anymore."
   ○ 4. "I don't feel the nausea like I did the last time."

84. While monitoring fetal heart rate with internal monitoring equipment, the nurse observes minimal variability and a rate of 120 beats/minute. The nurse should explain to the client that the decreased variability is most likely due to
   ○ 1. maternal sleep.
   ○ 2. fetal malposition.
   ○ 3. small-for-gestational-age fetus.
   ○ 4. effects of analgesic medication.

85. The fetus develops severe bradycardia and fetal distress, and an emergency cesarean section is performed under general anesthesia. After the delivery, the client tells the nurse, "I feel terrible. This is exactly what happened during my last delivery." A priority nursing diagnosis for this client is
   ○ 1. High Risk for Hemorrhage related to previous cesarean section.
   ○ 2. Anxiety related to neonatal outcome.
   ○ 3. Pain related to surgical incision and uterine cramping.
   ○ 4. Low Self-Esteem related to inability to deliver vaginally.

86. A neonatologist is present in the operating room after delivery. The nurse explains to the client that the neonatologist is present because neonates born by cesarean delivery tend to have increased incidence of
   ○ 1. congenital anomalies.
   ○ 2. pulmonary hypertension.
   ○ 3. meconium aspiration syndrome.
   ○ 4. respiratory distress syndrome.

A 28-year-old multigravida with suspected acute pyelonephritis is admitted to the hospital at 28 weeks' gestation.

87. The client's diagnosis is confirmed, and intravenous fluids and antibiotics are started. The nurse has instructed the client about the rationale for the aggressive therapy and determines that the client needs *further* instruction when she says that acute pyelonephritis can lead to
   ○ 1. preterm labor.
   ○ 2. maternal sepsis.
   ○ 3. intrauterine growth retardation.
   ○ 4. central nervous system damage in the fetus.

88. The client's health assessment reveals a chlamydial infection. The nurse explains that if the infection is left untreated, the neonate may have
   ○ 1. conjunctivitis.

○ 2. renal disease.
○ 3. harlequin syndrome.
○ 4. brain damage.

A 34-year-old multigravida at 36 weeks gestation' is admitted to the hospital in active labor. She has been diagnosed with Rh sensitization.

89. The client's contractions and the fetal heart rate are monitored electronically. The nurse detects a sinusoidal pattern of fetal heart rate. The nurse explains to the client that this is usually due to
○ 1. severe fetal anemia.
○ 2. maternal analgesia.
○ 3. congenital anomalies.
○ 4. polyhydramnios.

90. The fetus is in a frank breech presentation. The client's membranes rupture spontaneously, and the nurse documents the color of the fluid as yellowish. The nurse explains to the client that this is usually due to

○ 1. Rh sensitization.
○ 2. abnormal presentation.
○ 3. amniotic fluid embolism.
○ 4. oligohydramnios.

91. After spontaneous rupture of the membranes, if the cord prolapses, the nurse should plan to immediately
○ 1. place the client in a Trendelenburg position.
○ 2. administer oxytocin intravenously.
○ 3. ask the client to begin pushing.
○ 4. cover the cord with sterile towels.

92. The client delivers a viable male neonate by cesarean section. The neonate is scheduled for an immediate exchange transfusion. In planning the neonate's care during the exchange transfusion, the nurse would include which of the following measures?
○ 1. Administer calcium gluconate intramuscularly before the procedure.
○ 2. Monitor the neonate's status before and during the procedure.
○ 3. Administer heparin before the procedure.
○ 4. Keep the phototherapy lights on during the procedure.

CORRECT ANSWERS AND RATIONALE

The letters in parentheses following the rationale identify the step of the nursing process (A, D, P, I, E), cognitive level (K, C, T, N), and client needs (S, G, L, H). See the Answer Grid for the key.

The Primigravida in Labor

1. 1. As labor progresses, the client becomes serious and ready to get down to work. Early in the first stage of labor (1 to 4 cm) when complications are absent and contractions are still not very strong, the client is usually not very uncomfortable. She is usually excited that the delivery day has finally arrived, and she can expect to be happy and eager. As transition approaches, she is likely to become irritable, tired, and sometimes, panicky. (A, C, L)

2. 2. The client can expect to have intermittent fetal monitoring every 30 minutes during the active stage of labor. If complications develop, the client can expect to have more frequent or continuous electronic fetal monitoring. (I, T, G,)

3. 1. The Nitrazine paper test helps determine the pH of fluid. The membranes have likely ruptured if the pH of the fluid is above 6.5 and the Nitrazine paper turns blue-green, blue-gray, or deep blue. Ferning may also be seen under a microscope. If the pH of the fluid is below 6.0, the fluid is most likely vaginal secretions, and the paper turns olive or olive-yellow. (A, C, G)

4. 2. The ischial spines are used as landmarks to determine the descent of the fetal presenting part. The station +1 means that the presenting part is 1 cm below the level of the ischial spines. The station −1 means that the presenting part is 1 cm above the level of the ischial spines. (E, N, H)

5. 1. One complication of regional anesthesia is a decreased fetal heart rate. The anesthetic agent may cause poor muscle tone and fetal hypoxia. Maternal effects of epidural anesthesia include hypotension and slow labor, and may necessitate the need for forceps. The nurse should monitor fetal heart rate patterns, maternal blood pressure, pulse, and respirations every 5 minutes for at least 30 minutes after an epidural anesthetic and should report any drop in fetal heart rate or maternal blood pressure immediately. The person responsible for administering the anesthesia is also responsible for determining the level of anesthesia. Although some clients may sleep after an epidural, the client normally remains conscious while under the influence of regional anesthesia, such as an epidural block. (A, N, G)

6. 3. The obese client is more susceptible to soft tissue dystocia, which can impede the progress of labor. Hypertonic reflexes, nausea and vomiting, and decreased uterine resting tone are not associated with obesity. (A, N, G)

7. 1. An Apgar score of 9 out of a possible score of 10 means that the neonate is in good condition. The Apgar rating system evaluates the neonate on the basis of heart rate, respiratory effort, muscle tone, reflex irritability, and color at 1- and 5-minute intervals after birth. The neonate receives a score between 0 and 10. The higher the score, the better the neonate's condition. A score between 4 and 6 indicates fair condition, and a score between 0 and 3 indicates a need for resuscitation and critical condition. (D, N, G)

8. 1. Leopold's maneuvers assist in identifying fetal presentation and position. The procedure should be performed between contractions and after the client empties her bladder. There are four maneuvers. For the first maneuver, the nurse palpates the upper abdomen with both hands to determine whether the head or the buttocks fills the fundus. For the second maneuver, the nurse places one palm on each side of the abdomen and locates the fetal back. In the third maneuver, the nurse determines what fetal part is located at the inlet by gently grasping the lower portion of the abdomen, just above the symphysis pubis. In the fourth maneuver, the nurse faces the client's feet and attempts to locate the fetal brow, moving the hands down the sides of the uterus toward the pubis. Leopold's maneuvers are often performed before initial auscultation of the fetal heart rate. Although the maneuvers can determine deviations, such as multifetal pregnancy, this is usually confirmed through ultrasound procedures. (D, N, G)

9. 4. The transition stage of labor requires reinforcement of techniques learned during preparation for childbirth classes. It is best when the husband speaks to his wife using direct eye contact and breathes with her when she loses control during the transition stage. This often helps her regain control. The client should be encouraged to focus on one contraction at a time at this point in labor. Telling the husband that he should allow the nurse to take over the coaching is not appropriate. When the client reaches transition, or 8 to 10 cm of dilation, it is usually too late for anesthesia. Telling the client that it will soon be over does not help her gain control. (I, N, H)

10. 4. During transition, contractions are increasing in frequency, duration, and intensity. The most appropriate nursing diagnosis is Pain related to strength and duration of the contractions. There are no data to suggest Altered Urinary Elimination, Dizziness, or Ineffective Family Coping. (D, N, G)

11. 2. The most reliable sign that the placenta has detached from the uterine wall is the cord lengthening outside the vagina. Oxytocin is administered after delivery of the placenta to promote uterine contractions and thereby control postpartum bleeding. (D, N, G)

12. 3. Childbirth is a very emotional experience. An expression of happiness with tears is a normal reaction. (D, N, G)

13. 1. A neonate is active and alert soon after birth, if no complications exist. The American Academy of Pediatrics recommends beginning breast-feeding as soon as possible after delivery, or during the first period of reactivity. A neonate that will be breast-fed should not be given formula by bottle at this time. Many institutions provide sterile water for the initial feeding to assess for esophageal atresia. Because colostrum is not irritating if aspirated and is readily absorbed by the neonate's respiratory system, breast-feeding can be done immediately after birth. (I, N, G)

14. 3. Most authorities suggest that a woman in an early stage of labor should be allowed to walk if she wishes as long as no complications are present. Birthing centers or single-room maternity units allow women considerable latitude without much supervision at this stage of labor. If the client's membranes rupture, however, it would be wise for the nurse to check for potential prolapsed cord. (I, N, G)

15. 1. Childbirth educators use various techniques and methods to prepare parents for labor and delivery. Active relaxation involves relaxing uninvolved muscle groups while contracting a specific group and using chest breathing techniques to lift the diaphragm off the contracting uterus. Breathing rapidly and deeply can lead to hyperventilation and is not recommended. (E, N, H)

16. 3. Light stroking of the skin, or effleurage, is often used with the Lamaze method of childbirth preparation. (I, N, G)

17. 2. Increased bloody show normally occurs when cervical dilation increases. Fetal descent is unrelated to show. Rupture of the fetal membranes results in the escape of amniotic fluid, not bloody show. Abruptio placenta is usually accompanied by boardlike abdominal pain and bleeding, which is frequently concealed. (I, N, G)

18. 2. Recommendations for food and fluid intake during labor vary widely in the literature and in clinical practice. Gastric emptying is slower in pregnancy, and the potential for nausea and vomiting poses a risk for aspiration of stomach contents. Clients are often limited to clear fluids or ice chips. Many institutions have a policy of administering intravenous fluids to prevent dehydration or to have an intravenous line in place, in case the client needs medications or blood replacement. Even without food in the stomach, nausea and vomiting are common late in the first stage of labor. (I, N, G)

19. 2. Because maturation is generally not complete in adolescent clients, there is potential for cephalopelvic disproportion. Uterine tetany, rapid second stage, and early deceleration may occur regardless of the client's age. (A, N, G)

20. 3. When a client is hyperventilating during labor, she is eliminating more carbon dioxide than usual. As a result, she becomes lightheaded or dizzy. Being lightheaded or dizzy is not correlated with rapid cervical dilation, elevated blood pressure, or excitement about the labor process. (D, N, G)

21. 3. Pushing during the first stage of labor when the urge is felt but the cervix is not completely dilated may produce cervical swelling and make labor more difficult. The client should be encouraged to use a pant–blow (or blow–blow) pattern of breathing to help overcome the urge to push. (I, N, G)

22. 4. During the transition phase of the first stage of labor, the client needs encouragement and support. This is a difficult and painful time, when contractions are especially strong. During this phase, the client usually finds it difficult to maintain self-control. Everything else seems secondary to her as she progresses into the second stage of labor and delivery. (I, N, G)

23. 1. The sagittal suture is the most readily felt during a vaginal examination. (A, T, G)

24. 4. The second stage of labor begins with complete cervical dilation and ends with delivery. Show normally is bloody during the first stage of labor, especially when in the transition phase. The membranes often rupture in the second stage of labor, but they may also rupture earlier—in some instances, even before labor begins. The fluid should *not* have a foul odor, which is indicative of an infectious process. Contractions can be strong and painful in the first stage of labor as well as in the second stage. The client's blood pressure should remain within normal limits. (E, N, H)

25. 2. Avoidance, hostility, or low-key (passive) behavior toward the baby may be a cue to potential bonding problems. Expressions of disappointment with the baby's gender may also signal problems with maternal infant bonding. (D, N, L)

26. 4. According to the gate control theory of pain perception, when the endings of small peripheral nerve fibers detect a stimulus, they transmit it to cells in the dorsal horn of the spinal cord. These impulses pass through a network of cells in the spinal cord called the *substantia gelatinosa,* and a synapse occurs that returns the transmission to the peripheral site through a motor nerve. The impulse is then transmitted through the spinal cord to the brain, where the impulse is perceived as pain. Gate control mechanisms in the spinal cord are capable of halting these impulses (closing the gate), so pain is not perceived. (I, N, G)

27. 1. According to the gate control theory of pain, a closed gate means that the client should feel no pain. (I, N, G)

28. 1. If the client is having prolonged labor, the nurse should monitor the client for signs of exhaustion as well as dehydration. (A, N, G)

29. 2. Because the client has had prolonged labor, the client should be encouraged to rest as much as possible. In addition, the client should be encouraged to use appropriate breathing techniques, particularly slow chest breathing. Although the husband or significant other may keep track of the client's contraction pattern, this responsibility is that of the nurse caring for the client. Suggesting that she receive an epidural anesthetic is not appropriate as the client may be desirous of natural childbirth methods. Rapid, shallow breathing is not appropriate for this stage of labor. (I, N, G)

30. 1. The psychoprophylaxis method of childbirth suggests using slow chest breathing until it becomes ineffective during labor contractions, then to switch to shallow abdominal breathing during the peak of a contraction. When transition nears, a pant–blow pattern of breathing is used. (I, T, G)

31. 2. The symptoms of hyperventilation result from excess carbon dioxide elimination from the body. Hence, rebreathing into a paper bag or cupping the hands is beneficial. This increases the carbon dioxide intake during respiration. Taking whiffs of oxygen, holding her breath, and breathing with forceful inspirations will not resolve the dizziness. (I, N, G)

32. 3. The carbon dioxide insufficiency that occurs during hyperventilation will lead to respiratory alkalosis. (A, N, G)

33. 3. When a client complains of severe back pain during labor, the fetus is most likely in an occipitoposterior position. This means that the fetal head presses against the client's sacrum, which causes marked discomfort during contractions. Repositioning the client and providing sacral back rubs may help alleviate the discomfort. Transverse, oblique, and asynclitic occiput positions do not cause pressure on the sacrum. (I, N, G)

34. 1. The client with back pain during labor experiences marked discomfort, more so than when the fetus is in the anterior position. Application of firm pressure to the sacral area can help to alleviate the pain. Severe back pain during labor does not necessarily require a cesarean delivery. The physician may elect to do an episiotomy, but it is not necessarily required. It is unlikely that a primigravida with a fetus in an occipitoposterior position will have a precipitous delivery. A side-lying position is not as effective as rocking on all fours. (P, N, S)

35. 3. The most appropriate nursing diagnosis at this time is Alteration in Physiologic Process related to failure of the fetus to descend. There is no information to indicate the diagnoses Anxiety or High Risk for Injury. Although the client has had no prenatal care, there is no information related to the level of the client's knowledge. (D, N, S)

The Multigravida in Labor

36. 3. The nurse's first action when membranes rupture spontaneously is to check the odor, consistency, and volume of the amniotic fluid. For this client, the fetal head is engaged and at 0 station, so there is little likelihood of cord prolapse. When the fetal head is not engaged, however, checking for cord prolapse is the first priority when the membranes spontaneously rupture. Amniotic fluid is usually straw-colored. Greenish-brown fluid (meconium) indicates that the fetus has suffered a hypoxic event. Yellowish fluid may indicate fetal anemia, hypoxia, or intrauterine infection. All clients have their contractions monitored while in labor. Delivery is not imminent if the client is 5 cm dilated, but multigravidas may progress quickly, especially after rupture of the membranes. After rupture of the membranes, vaginal examinations should be kept to a minimum to decrease the chance of infection. (I, T, G)

37. 1. Respiratory depression, especially during the first hour after administration of the anesthetic, is a potential complication. Diaphoresis, urinary frequency, and tremors are not usually associated with epidural anesthesia. (I, N, G)

38. 2. Variable decelerations usually indicate cord compression. After the membranes rupture, variable decelerations are common. This decreases protection to the cord, particularly as the fetus descends the birth canal. Repositioning the client often helps to correct this fetal heart rate pattern. If repositioning is not successful, the clinician may choose to perform amnioinfusion—infusion of sterile saline solution into the uterus through a sterile catheter. This procedure helps take the pressure off the

cord. Increasing the intravenous fluid rate is not helpful. There is no need to prepare the client for a cesarean delivery at this time. Administering oxygen at 2 liters is not helpful. Then nurse may wish to alert the obstetrician or nurse midwife, but the anesthesiologist is responsible for anesthesia, not the fetus. (I, N, G)

39. 3. Early decelerations are usually due to pressure on the fetal head as the fetus progresses through the birth canal. These decelerations mirror the contraction pattern and are usually benign, unless the pattern occurs in early labor. If this pattern is demonstrated in early labor, it may indicate cephalopelvic disproportion. Variable decelerations are associated with cord compression. Fetal bradycardia may occur as a result of analgesia, and this can occur at any time. Inadequate placental perfusion is associated with late fetal heart rate decelerations. (E, N, G)

40. 3. A chill shortly after delivery is not uncommon. Warm blankets can help provide comfort for the client. The nurse should also explain that the reaction is normal. It has been suggested that the shivering response is caused by a difference in internal and external body temperatures. A different theory proposes that the woman is reacting to fetal cells that have entered the maternal bloodstream through the placental site. It takes time to produce a temperature change after a chill. An analgesic is not indicated. The volume of blood loss is not necessarily related to a chill. (A, N, G)

41. 3. The most appropriate diagnosis at this time is High Risk for Injury related to the effects of the epidural anesthesia. The client may have no sensation in her lower abdomen and legs for several hours after delivery. Care should be taken to avoid injury, and ambulation should be delayed until sensation has returned. There are no data to suggest Pain due to exhaustive pushing or Fluid Volume Deficit. Although urinary retention may occur as a result of epidural anesthesia, the birth attendant usually empties the client's bladder before delivery to avoid injury. (D, N, G)

The Intrapartal Client With Risk Factors

42. 3. When admitting a client to the hospital's labor unit, the nurse needs to obtain certain information about the client promptly to plan care. Particularly with a multigravida, the information should include the frequency, intensity, and duration of labor contractions. In addition, the nurse should determine when the labor began, whether the membranes have ruptured, and the client's estimated delivery date. From this information, the nurse gets a quick overview of the client's status and can then proceed to plan effective care. The fetal position, when the client last had food or fluids, and her ability to follow directions are important but less influential in initial plans for care. (A, N, G)

43. 3. A side-lying or semi-Fowler's position helps to ensure cardiac emptying and adequate oxygenation. In addition, oxygen by mask, analgesics and sedatives, diuretics, prophylactic antibiotics, and digitalis may be warranted. Breathing rapidly during a contraction, limiting the number of visitors, and requesting analgesia or anesthesia do not help the load on the cardiac system. (I, N, G)

44. 4. Pulse rate above 100 beats/minute or respiratory rate above 25 breaths/minute may indicate cardiac decompensation which may result in cardiac arrest. While the nurse should note any signs of significant dehydration, nausea, and vomiting, the client's cardiac status is more important. (A, N, G)

45. 3. Prostaglandin E_2 gel is used to soften and ripen the cervix for induction of labor. (P, T, G)

46. 1. Prostaglandin E_2 gel is contraindicated if the client is having contractions. Although an amniotomy may be performed once the client begins to dilate and the fetal head is engaged, it is not necessary for the nurse to prepare the client for this at this time. (I, T, G)

47. 2. Before beginning intravenous oxytocin infusion, the nurse should obtain a baseline measurement of fetal heart rate. If the fetal heart rate pattern shows fetal distress, the client is not a candidate for induction. Induction of labor with an oxytocic agent carries risks. It is essential that a nurse remain with the client at all times to monitor uterine contractions and fetal heart rate. Even if the client is being monitored with electronic monitoring equipment, a nurse needs to remain at the bedside. Oxytocin administration carries a risk of water intoxication and uterine rupture. The usual protocol is to increase the dosage of the oxytocin in accordance with institutional policy, until a regular contraction pattern is established, at which time the infusion should be maintained at that rate or decreased. The infusion should be discontinued and the physician notified if fetal distress is noted or if contractions occur less than 2 minutes apart or last longer than 60 seconds. The client's cervix is only 1 cm dilated, so it is too early for epidural anesthesia. It is not necessary to administer a bolus of intravenous fluid, nor is it necessary for the client to have a Foley catheter at this time. (I, N, G)

48. 4. Metabolic changes occurring during labor and delivery require close monitoring of the diabetic client's blood glucose level—every hour, during labor. There is no indication that the client's urine output needs to be measured every 4 hours. Insulin, if needed, is usually given intravenously and depends on the client's blood sugar levels. There is no indication that the client's reflexes should be checked every 2 hours. Because pregnant diabetic clients are more prone to pregnancy-induced hypertension, however, any evidence of protein in the urine should be reported. (P, N, G)

49. 4. One of the potential disadvantages of oxytocin induction is neonatal hyperbilirubinemia. Urinary frequency and hypoglycemia are not associated with oxytocin infusion. Ultrasound procedures should be used to estimate gestational age. (I, T, G)

50. 4. The most appropriate diagnosis at this time is High Risk for Maternal or Fetal Injury related to uterine hyperstimulation. Diabetic mothers have a higher incidence of pregnancy-induced hypertension, polyhydramnios, preterm birth, and larger-than-average fetuses and often have decreased placental perfusion. Infants of diabetic mothers may have polycythemia, congenital anomalies, and respiratory distress. There is no information to support the diagnosis of Pain related to prolonged labor. There is no indication that the client will require cesarean delivery at this time. Oxytocin infusion poses a risk of fluid overload, not fluid deficit. (D, N, S)

51. 4. With the fetus at −1 station, the cord may prolapse as amniotic fluid rushes out. The nurse should inspect the perineal area to detect cord prolapse immediately after the amniotomy. The color, amount, and odor of the amniotic fluid should be noted. Fetal heart rate should be monitored. The client's optimal position is on the left side, but this is not a priority at this time. The client is not having a precipitous delivery with the fetal skull at −1 station. Maternal blood pressure should be monitored throughout labor, but this is not a priority at this time, nor is the pulse rate. (I, N, G)

52. 4. A common sign of fetal distress due to an inadequate transfer of oxygen to the fetus is meconium-stained fluid. Because the fetus has suffered hypoxia, close fetal heart rate monitoring is necessary. Increasing the rate of the oxytocin infusion, turning the client to a supine position, and assessing fetal position and presentation are not helpful measures. (P, N, G)

53. 4. Late deceleration of fetal heart rate signals poor placental perfusion. The physician usually writes a standing order for oxygenation of the client if necessary. The oxygen should be administered at 8 to 10 liters by mask to improve fetal hypoxia. The nurse should also stop the oxytocin infusion and report the pattern to the attending clinician. The client should be turned onto her side. If the pattern persists or if decreased variability occurs, then delivery may be indicated. The nurse should provide information about fetal well-being throughout the labor process. Immediate cesarean delivery is not indicated unless the pattern persists. The contraction pattern should be monitored throughout the induction of labor, but the priority here is to oxygenate the compromised fetus. (I, N, G)

54. 2. Lumbar epidural anesthesia is usually administered with the client in a left side-lying position with shoulders parallel and legs slightly flexed. (I, N, G)

55. 1. Aspiration of meconium is best prevented by suctioning the neonate's nasopharynx immediately after the head is delivered and before the shoulders and chest are delivered. As long as the chest is compressed in the vagina, the infant will not inhale and aspirate meconium in the upper respiratory tract. Meconium aspiration blocks the air flow to the alveoli, leading to potentially life-threatening respiratory complications. Based on the information provided, there is no need for intubation, oxygenation, or medication at this time. (E, N, S)

56. 3. Neonates born to mothers who smoke tend to have lower-than-average birth weights. Maternal smoking is not related to higher neonatal hematocrit, below-average hemoglobin, or higher bilirubin levels. Increased respiratory rate may occur if complications arise, such as preterm birth or respiratory distress. (I, N, G)

57. 3. The client should be urged to push with an open glottis to prevent the Valsalva maneuver. Because the client has had an epidural anesthetic, she may not feel the urge to push and needs coaching. (I, T, G)

58. 1. An episiotomy serves several purposes. It shortens the second stage of labor, substitutes a clean surgical incision for a tear, and decreases undue stretching of perineal muscles. An episiotomy helps prevent tearing of the rectum but does not necessarily relieve pressure on the rectum. Although an episiotomy usually helps prevent tearing, this may still occur. An episiotomy does not prevent perineal edema, ensure quick delivery of the placenta, or cause enlargement of the pelvic inlet. (E, T, G)

59. 3. The American College of Obstetricians and Gynecologists has classified forceps applications into three categories: outlet or low, middle, and high. When the fetal skull is on the perineum with the scalp visible at the vaginal opening, this is considered outlet forceps. When the fetal skull is at +2 station or more, this is considered low forceps. Middle and high forceps deliveries are not recommended; cesarean section is the preferred method of delivery in these situations. (I, C, G)

60. 1. When the client says the baby is coming, the nurse should first inspect the perineum and observe for crowning. It is vital in this situation that the nurse validate the client's statement. If the client is not delivering precipitously, the nurse can calm her and use appropriate breathing techniques. Timing contractions is not the priority action. Fetal heart rate is monitored throughout the labor process. The nurse should try to obtain assistance if delivery is imminent but should never leave the client. Delivery may occur before the physician arrives. (I, N, S)

61. 3. The nurse should immediately prepare a clean area for delivery when birth is imminent and no additional help is available. Most hospital labor units have emergency delivery packs with sterile towels, a bulb syringe, and a cord clamp. The nurse should remember to use universal precautions and don a pair of sterile gloves for the delivery. Trying to delay the birth is contraindicated. The nurse should instruct the client to pant or pant–blow to decrease the urge to push. Pushing the head out quickly can cause tearing of the perineum. The head of the bed should be elevated to about 45 degrees, not lowered. The client should assume a position of comfort. (I, N, G)

62. 4. The nurse should remain calm during a precipitous delivery. Explaining to the client what is happening as the birth progresses and how she can assist is likely to help her remain calm and cooperative. Maintaining eye contact is also beneficial. The cliche, "everything is fine," is not appropriate. Saying that the physician will be there soon may not be an accurate statement and is not reassuring if the client is concerned about the delivery. (I, N, L)

63. 2. During a precipitous delivery, the cord may be wrapped around the neonate's neck. It is important to check for the cord and to gently slip it over the neonate's head. The shoulder cannot be delivered until the head is delivered. It is not appropriate to tell the client to push between contractions because this may lead to lacerations. If the head is beginning to emerge, transfer to the delivery room is not necessary. (I, N, G)

64. 3. The best course of action is to wait for a sign of placental separation. Pulling on the cord before the placenta is delivered may cause inversion of the uterus. Signs of placental separation include lengthening of the umbilical cord, a slight gush of dark blood, and a change in the contour of the fundus from discoid to globular. After separation occurs, the client can be asked to bear down. Massaging the fundus is not helpful. (I, N, G)

65. 2. One complication of a precipitous delivery is a boggy fundus, or uterine atony. There is no relationship between a precipitous delivery and delayed bonding, intrauterine infection, or urinary tract infection. (A, T, G)

66. 2. Clients who have either external or internal fetal monitoring have greater discomfort because of the equipment. A major advantage of monitoring fetal heart rate electronically is that it provides for a continuous recording of the heart rate during and between contractions. A fetoscope allows only a sampling of readings and is not as accurate in determining variables in fetal heart rate. The client is less mobile with the monitoring belts in place. (E, N, H)

67. 3. The client should be carefully assessed for symptoms of pregnancy-induced hypertension, which is more common in clients expecting twins. Urinary frequency may occur as the uterus impinges on the bladder, but this is not unusual. Oligohydramnios, abdominal distention (flatus), and urinary tract infection are not typically associated with twin gestations. Anemia is more common than polycythemia. (P, N, G)

68. 2. The nurse should contact the physician because the client is most likely experiencing hypotonic uterine contractions. These contractions tend to be painful but ineffective. The usual treatment is oxytocin augmentation, unless cephalopelvic disproportion exists. The heart rates of both fetuses are continuously monitored. There is no indication that oxygen is necessary. Having the client flex pant–blow may be done in the second stage of labor when she is pushing. (I, N, H)

69. 4. Oxytocin should be administered after delivery of the second placenta and after both twins are delivered safely. (P, T, G)

70. 1. Uterine atony means that the uterus is not firm or boggy because it is not contracting. The nurse should first gently massage the uterus which will contract the uterus and make it firm. Clients with multiple gestation, polyhydramnios, prolonged labor, or large-for-gestational-age fetus are more prone to uterine atony. Puerperal infection and uterine rupture are not associated with uterine atony. Increasing the intravenous fluid rate may be ordered if the client develops symptoms of shock. (I, N, G)

71. 2. It is important that the parents be allowed to touch, hold, and participate in care of the twins whenever they desire. Ideally, this will be on a daily basis, to promote parent–infant bonding. It is not appropriate to discuss how they will cope with twin infants at home until the couple is ready to take the infants home. Having the couple visit the twins to provide care on a 24-hour basis is not warranted, although they should visit and provide care whenever they desire. Identifying complications that may occur is not appropriate. (P, N, H)

72. 4. A bilateral pudendal block is used for vaginal deliveries to relieve pain primarily in the perineum and vagina. It does not relieve discomfort in the abdomen, fundus, or back. Pudendal block anesthesia is adequate for episiotomy and its repair. (I, N, G)

73. 1. The fetus should be assessed for bradycardia, which is a potential complication of pudendal block anesthesia. Decreased movements, increased variability, and meconium-stained fluid are not associated with pudendal anesthesia. Adverse effects on the neonate after pudendal block may also include hypotonia, reduced responsiveness, and seizures. These complications are thought to be related to accidental injection of the fetal scalp. (I, N, G)

74. 4. The client should use exhale breathing while pushing to avoid the adverse physiologic effects of the Valsalva maneuver, which occurs with prolonged breath-holding during pushing. The technique for exhale breathing involves inhaling several deep breaths, holding the breath for 5 to 6 seconds, and exhaling slowly every 5 to 6 seconds through pursed lips while continuing to hold the breath. The Valsalva maneuver can also be avoided by exhaling continuously while pushing. Semi-Fowler's position enhances the effectiveness of the abdominal muscle efforts during pushing, but the client can assume a squatting or side-lying position if desired. The client should flex her thighs and exert downward pressure while pushing. (E, N, H)

75. 1. A neonate in good condition needs to be kept warm. This reduces cold stress and potential respiratory problems. The infant can be evaluated under a radiant warmer or wrapped in dry, warm blankets on the mother's abdomen. A neonate in good condition will eventually need to be weighed and have erythromycin drugs or ointment and identification bracelets, but these are not priorities at this time. (I, N, G)

76. 4. The priority diagnosis is High Risk for Infection related to birth trauma. The client has had a prolonged labor and prolonged ruptured membranes, and infection can be a serious complication. (D, N, G)

77. 2. Postmature neonates frequently have difficulty maintaining adequate glucose reserves. Other common problems include meconium aspiration syndrome, polycythemia, congenital anomalies, seizure activity, and cold stress. These complications are primarily due to a combination of advanced gestational age, placental insufficiency, and continued exposure to amniotic fluid. (I, N, G)

78. 4. A common finding for postmature neonates is wrinkled, peeling skin. There is no relationship between postmaturity and a flattened nose, small hands and feet, or a red rash. (A, T, G)

79. 1. If a client has been in active labor and there is no change in cervical dilation after 2 hours, the nurse should suspect cephalopelvic disproportion. The client is not experiencing a prolonged latent phase (0 to 3 cm dilation), prolonged transitional phase (pushing), or a hypertonic contraction pattern. (D, N, G)

80. 1. Polyhydramnios is a term for excessive amniotic fluid. If the membranes rupture, the volume of fluid and pressure can result in a prolapsed cord. (A, T, G)

81. 3. Preparation for cesarean delivery is similar to preparation for any abdominal surgery. The client must give informed consent. Another person may not sign for the client unless the client is unable to sign the form. If this is the case, only certain designated people can do so legally. The husband does not need to sign the form unless his wife is unable to do so. (I, N, S)

82. 4. If at all possible, the couple should have a few minutes alone so that they can provide support to one another. The client undergoing a cesarean section will often have a Foley catheter, so she does not need to empty her bladder. The wedding ring can be taped in place. Abdominal cleansing will be done in the operating suite. (I, T, L)

83. 2. Nalbuphine (Nubain), a synthetic agonist-antagonist similar to butorphanol and pentazocine, is used for analgesia during labor. Although the client may rest or fall asleep after administration, it is not a sedative. The client should not experience numbness or anesthesia from this drug. The drug is not given to counteract nausea or indigestion (heartburn). (E, N, G)

84. 4. Decreased variability may be seen in various conditions; however, it is most commonly due to analgesic administration. Other factors that can cause decreased variability include anesthesia, deep fetal sleep, anecephaly, prematurity, hypoxia, tachycardia, brain damage, and arrhythmias. Maternal sleep, fetal malposition, and small for gestational age, are not commonly associated with decreased variability. (I, N, G)

85. 4. It is not unusual for clients who undergo an emergency cesarean section to express thoughts of failure. Pain, hemorrhage, and anxiety may all occur, but the priority diagnosis at this time is Low Self-Esteem. (D, N, L)

86. 4. Respiratory distress syndrome is more common in neonates delivered by cesarean section than in those delivered vaginally. Congenital anomalies, pulmonary hypertension, and meconium aspiration are not more common in cesarean delivery. (I, N, G)

87. 4. A client with acute pyelonephritis is susceptible to preterm labor, maternal sepsis, and intrauterine growth retardation. Central nervous system damage is not related. (P, N, G)

88. 1. Conjunctivitis is a common complication of neonates who are born to mothers with untreated chlamydial infections. Untreated chlamydial infections are not associated with renal disease, harlequin syndrome, or brain damage. (I, T, G)

89. 1. An ominous sign, the sinusoidal pattern is usually associated with Rh isoimmunization, severe anemia, and asphyxiation. It can also be attributed to the administration of nalbuphine hydrochloride (Nubain) and intravenous butorphanol tartrate (Stadol). Because no medication has been given to this client, the pattern suggests fetal anemia. Internal fetal monitoring should be instituted and cesarean delivery considered. (I, N, G)

90. 1. Amniotic fluid is normally clear. Yellowish fluid indicates Rh sensitization. The yellowish color is related to fetal anemia and bilirubin. In a breech presentation, it is not uncommon for the amniotic fluid to be greenish owing to meconium expelled by the fetus. Amniotic fluid embolism is not related to the fluid color. This dangerous situation may occur naturally after a difficult labor or from hyperstimulation of the uterus. Amniotic fluid may leak into the maternal circulation. Symptoms include respiratory distress, circulatory collapse, acute hemorrhage, tachycardia, hypotension, chest pain, and cyanosis. Amniotic fluid embolism is a medical emergency, and maternal mortality is high. Polyhydramnios refers to an excessive volume of amniotic fluid. (I, N, G)

91. 1. The first step in cord prolapse is to relieve pressure on the cord. Immediate measures include lowering the client's head by using the Trendelenburg position or knee-to-chest position so that the fetal presenting part will move away from the pelvis, and moving the fetal presenting part off the cord by applying pressure through the vagina with a sterile gloved hand. Oxygen may be administered. Immediate cesarean delivery is usually performed. The nurse should not attempt to replace the cord into the vagina. (P, N, G)

92. 2. Nursing responsibilities during exchange transfusion include assembling the equipment, preparing the neonate and parents, assisting the physician during the procedure, monitoring the neonate's status before and during the procedure, and maintaining careful records. Calcium gluconate is not given before the procedure but may be administered intravenously after each 100 mL of blood infusion, if indicated. The neonate should be in a warm environment, preferably under a radiant warmer, and should be NPO for at least 4 hours before the procedure to prevent possible aspiration. The parents should be kept informed of the neonate's condition. Heparin administration is not performed before the procedure. Phototherapy lights are not necessary during the procedure. (P, N, G)

THE NURSING CARE OF THE CHILDBEARING FAMILY AND THEIR NEONATE

TEST 3: The Birth Experience

Directions: Use this answer grid to determine areas of strength or need for further study.

NURSING PROCESS

A = Assessment
D = Analysis, nursing diagnosis
P = Planning
I = Implementation
E = Evaluation

COGNITIVE LEVEL

K = Knowledge
C = Comprehension
T = Application
N = Analysis

CLIENT NEEDS

S = Safe, effective care environment
G = Physiologic integrity
L = Psychosocial integrity
H = Health promotion and maintenance

Question #	Answer #	A	D	P	I	E	K	C	T	N	S	G	L	H
1	1	A						C					L	
2	2				I				T			G		
3	1	A						C				G		
4	2					E				N				H
5	1	A								N		G		
6	3	A								N		G		
7	1		D							N		G		
8	1		D							N		G		
9	4				I					N				H
10	4		D							N		G		
11	2		D							N		G		
12	3		D							N		G		
13	1				I					N		G		
14	3				I					N		G		
15	1					E				N				H
16	3				I					N		G		
17	2				I					N		G		
18	2				I					N		G		
19	2	A								N		G		
20	3		D							N		G		
21	3				I					N		G		
22	4				I					N		G		
23	1	A							T			G		
24	4					E				N				H
25	2		D							N			L	

NURSING PROCESS

A = Assessment
D = Analysis, nursing diagnosis
P = Planning
I = Implementation
E = Evaluation

COGNITIVE LEVEL

K = Knowledge
C = Comprehension
T = Application
N = Analysis

CLIENT NEEDS

S = Safe, effective care environment
G = Physiologic integrity
L = Psychosocial integrity
H = Health promotion and maintenance

Question #	Answer #	A	D	P	I	E	K	C	T	N	S	G	L	H
26	4				I					N		G		
27	1				I					N		G		
28	1	A								N		G		
29	2				I					N		G		
30	1				I				T			G		
31	2				I					N		G		
32	3	A								N		G		
33	3				I					N		G		
34	1			P						N	S			
35	3		D							N	S			
36	3				I				T			G		
37	1				I					N		G		
38	2				I					N		G		
39	3					E				N		G		
40	3	A								N		G		
41	3		D							N		G		
42	3	A								N		G		
43	3				I					N		G		
44	4	A								N		G		
45	3			P					T			G		
46	1				I				T			G		
47	2				I					N		G		
48	4			P						N		G		
49	4				I				T			G		
50	4		D							N	S			
51	4				I					N		G		
52	4			P						N		G		
53	4				I					N		G		
54	2				I					N		G		
55	1					E				N	S			

ANSWER GRID: 2

163

NURSING PROCESS

A = Assessment
D = Analysis, nursing diagnosis
P = Planning
I = Implementation
E = Evaluation

COGNITIVE LEVEL

K = Knowledge
C = Comprehension
T = Application
N = Analysis

CLIENT NEEDS

S = Safe, effective care environment
G = Physiologic integrity
L = Psychosocial integrity
H = Health promotion and maintenance

Question #	Answer #	Nursing Process					Cognitive Level				Client Needs			
		A	D	P	I	E	K	C	T	N	S	G	L	H
56	3				I					N		G		
57	3				I				T			G		
58	1					E			T			G		
59	3				I			C				G		
60	1				I					N	S			
61	3				I					N		G		
62	4				I					N			L	
63	2				I					N		G		
64	3				I					N		G		
65	2	A							T			G		
66	2					E				N				H
67	3			P						N		G		
68	2				I					N				H
69	4			P					T			G		
70	1				I					N		G		
71	2			P						N				H
72	4				I					N		G		
73	1				I					N		G		
74	4					E				N				H
75	1				I					N		G		
76	4		D							N		G		
77	2				I					N		G		
78	4	A							T			G		
79	1		D							N		G		
80	1	A							T			G		
81	3				I					N	S			
82	4				I				T				L	
83	2					E				N		G		
84	4				I					N		G		
85	4		D							N			L	

ANSWER GRID: 3

NURSING PROCESS

A = Assessment
D = Analysis, nursing diagnosis
P = Planning
I = Implementation
E = Evaluation

COGNITIVE LEVEL

K = Knowledge
C = Comprehension
T = Application
N = Analysis

CLIENT NEEDS

S = Safe, effective care environment
G = Physiologic integrity
L = Psychosocial integrity
H = Health promotion and maintenance

Question #	Answer #	Nursing Process					Cognitive Level				Client Needs			
		A	D	P	I	E	K	C	T	N	S	G	L	H
86	4				I					N		G		
87	4			P						N		G		
88	1				I				T			G		
89	1				I					N		G		
90	1				I					N		G		
91	1			P						N		G		
92	2			P						N		G		
Number Correct														
Number Possible	92	14	13	10	46	8	0	3	15	74	6	73	5	8
Percentage Correct														

Score Calculation: To determine your **Percentage Correct,** divide the **Number Correct** by the **Number Possible.**

ANSWER GRID: 4

Postpartum Care

- The Postpartal Client With a Vaginal Birth
- The Postpartal Client Who Breast-Feeds
- The Postpartal Client Who Bottle Feeds
- The Postpartal Client With a Cesarean Birth
- The Postpartal Client With Complications
- Correct Answers and Rationale

Select the one best answer, and indicate your choice by filling in the circle in front of the option.

The Postpartal Client With a Vaginal Birth

A primipara has delivered her baby, with labor, delivery, recovery, and the postpartum period in the same hospital room. The client had a midline episiotomy and epidural anesthesia.

1. While assessing the client's pulse 30 minutes after the delivery, the nurse determines that the pulse rate is 60 beats/minute. The nurse should
   - ○ 1. explain to the client that this is a normal finding.
   - ○ 2. contact the client's physician about the pulse rate.
   - ○ 3. check the client's record to determine the amount of blood loss.
   - ○ 4. recheck the pulse in 30 minutes, and compare the two readings.

2. When instilling erythromycin ointment into the neonate's eyes, the nurse should explain to the parent that the medication prevents
   - ○ 1. neonatal conjunctivitis.
   - ○ 2. blindness as a result of gonorrhea.
   - ○ 3. blindness as a result of syphilis.
   - ○ 4. strabismus as the neonate matures.

3. The physician orders an intramuscular injection of phytonadione (AquaMEPHYTON) for the neonate. The nurse should explain to the mother that this medication will be injected to prevent
   - ○ 1. hypoglycemia.
   - ○ 2. hyperbilirubinemia.
   - ○ 3. bleeding problems.
   - ○ 4. polycythemia.

4. When the nurse accidentally bumps the bassinet, the neonate throws out its arms, hands opened, and begins to cry. After giving instruction, the nurse de-

termines that the mother understands this reflex when she states that it is the
   - ○ 1. startle reflex.
   - ○ 2. Babinski reflex.
   - ○ 3. extrusion reflex.
   - ○ 4. tonic neck reflex.

5. In response to the nurse's question about how she is feeling, the client replies that she is tired, sore, and hungry. She then begins to relate her birth experience. Based on the assessment data, the nurse determines that the client is in which phase of the postpartal psychological adaptation process?
   - ○ 1. Acting out.
   - ○ 2. Taking in.
   - ○ 3. Taking hold.
   - ○ 4. Letting go.

6. In planning care for the client for the first 12 hours, the nurse should plan for her primary concerns, which will most likely focus on her
   - ○ 1. baby.
   - ○ 2. family.
   - ○ 3. own comfort.
   - ○ 4. husband.

7. Assessing the client 14 hours after delivery, the nurse notes an ecchymotic area to the right of the episiotomy. The nurse should
   - ○ 1. apply an ice bag to the perineum.
   - ○ 2. assess the client's temperature.
   - ○ 3. encourage the client to take a warm sitz bath.
   - ○ 4. contact the physician for further orders.

8. Thirty hours after delivery and before dismissal, the nurse plans to teach the client about infant care. By this time, the client is most likely in which phase of postpartal psychological adaptation?
   - ○ 1. Taking in.
   - ○ 2. Letting go.

○ 3. Taking hold.
○ 4. Giving up.

The nurse is caring for a multipara who has just delivered a viable male neonate vaginally under local anesthesia. The client has a midline episiotomy.

9. One hour after delivery, the client ambulates to the bathroom to void. After the client has voided, the nurse determines that the client's bladder is distended. The nurse should explain to the client that this is most likely due to
   ○ 1. prolonged first stage of labor.
   ○ 2. a urinary tract infection.
   ○ 3. pressure of the uterus on the bladder.
   ○ 4. edema in the lower urinary tract area.

10. During the first hour after delivery, the nurse formulates a nursing diagnosis for the client. An appropriate nursing diagnosis at this time is
    ○ 1. High Risk for Infection related to labor process and episiotomy.
    ○ 2. Fatigue related to multiparity.
    ○ 3. Fluid Volume Deficit related to diaphoresis.
    ○ 4. Urinary Retention related to trauma of delivery.

11. The nurse caring for the client detects a firm fundus, yet on inspection of the perineum, there is a constant trickle of blood. The nurse should assess the client for
    ○ 1. retained placental tissue.
    ○ 2. uterine inversion.
    ○ 3. uterine infection.
    ○ 4. vaginal tears.

12. The client asks the nurse about postpartum exercises. The nurse should instruct the client that the most appropriate exercise to start with on the first postpartum day is to assume a
    ○ 1. sitting position, lie back, and then return to a sitting position.
    ○ 2. prone position, then do push-ups by using the arms to lift the upper body.
    ○ 3. supine position with the knees flexed, then inhale deeply while allowing the abdomen to expand and exhale while contracting the abdominal muscles.
    ○ 4. supine position with the knees flexed, bring the chin onto the chest wall while exhaling, and reach for the knees by lifting the head and shoulders while inhaling.

13. The client tells the nurse, "I think my baby likes to hear me talk to him." The nurse should explain to the client that most neonates
    ○ 1. prefer high-pitched speech with tonal variations.

○ 2. respond to low-pitched speech with a sameness of tone.
○ 3. like cooing sounds rather than words.
○ 4. do not like to be overstimulated.

14. Eight hours after delivery, the client complains to the nurse that when she ambulated to the bathroom after sleeping for 4 hours, her lochia seemed heavier. The nurse should explain to the client that increased lochia on ambulation
    ○ 1. should be reported to the physician.
    ○ 2. is due to lochia pooling in the vaginal vault.
    ○ 3. may be an early sign of postpartum hemorrhage.
    ○ 4. usually indicates retained placental fragments.

The nurse is caring for a primipara who delivered a viable neonate by spontaneous vaginal delivery under local anesthesia.

15. About 4 hours after delivery, the client says she needs to urinate. The nurse should plan to
    ○ 1. catheterize the client and obtain a urine specimen.
    ○ 2. offer her a bedpan for more accurate measurement.
    ○ 3. check her bladder for distention before she voids.
    ○ 4. measure the first few voidings.

16. While the client is taking her first shower after delivery, the nurse should remain nearby to assess her for
    ○ 1. fatigue.
    ○ 2. fainting.
    ○ 3. diuresis.
    ○ 4. hemorrhaging.

17. Twenty-four hours after delivery, the nurse documents that involution is progressing normally after palpating the client's fundus
    ○ 1. slightly below the level of the umbilicus.
    ○ 2. midway between the umbilicus and the symphysis pubis.
    ○ 3. barely above the upper margin of the symphysis pubis.
    ○ 4. slightly above the level of the umbilicus.

18. After teaching the client about lochia, the nurse determines that the client understands the instructions when she says that on the 10th or 11th postpartum day, the lochia should be
    ○ 1. pink.
    ○ 2. white.
    ○ 3. dark red.
    ○ 4. brown.

19. The nurse plans to teach the client to provide visual

stimulation to the neonate. The nurse should plan to explain that this is best accomplished by
- ○ 1. maintaining eye contact with him.
- ○ 2. holding him so he can look at pictures on the wall.
- ○ 3. using brightly colorful wallpaper in the neonate's room.
- ○ 4. moving a brightly colorful rattle in front of his eyes.

20. The client asks the nurse how often she should hold her baby without "spoiling" him. The nurse should instruct her to hold him
- ○ 1. only when he is fussy or crying.
- ○ 2. as much as she desires.
- ○ 3. infrequently to avoid overstimulation.
- ○ 4. before and after the daily bath.

21. The nurse on the night shift finds the client drenched in perspiration. The nurse formulates which of the following nursing diagnoses for the client?
- ○ 1. Postpartal Infection related to birth trauma.
- ○ 2. Ineffective Thermoregulation related to hormonal changes.
- ○ 3. Altered Protection related to effects of analgesia.
- ○ 4. Fluid Volume Excess related to normal postpartal elimination process.

The nurse is caring for an 18-year-old primipara who delivered a viable neonate vaginally under epidural anesthesia.

22. When assessing the client 24 hours after delivery, the nurse determines that the fundus is firm but to the right of midline. Based on this finding, the nurse further assesses for
- ○ 1. uterine inversion.
- ○ 2. paralytic ileus.
- ○ 3. urinary retention.
- ○ 4. perineal hematoma.

23. The client asks the nurse, "How can I tell whether my baby is spitting up or vomiting?" The nurse explains that in contrast to regurgitated material, vomited material is characterized by
- ○ 1. variable amounts.
- ○ 2. a curdled appearance.
- ○ 3. a brownish color.
- ○ 4. usually occurring before a feeding.

24. On the second postpartum day, the client complains to the nurse that she has perineal pain that was unrelieved by ibuprofen 400 mg given 2 hours ago. The nurse should assess the client for
- ○ 1. puerperal infection.
- ○ 2. retained placental fragments.

- ○ 3. history of drug abuse.
- ○ 4. perineal hematoma.

25. While observing the client interact with her neonate, the nurse observes that the client appears hesitant to care for the neonate. The nurse should
- ○ 1. make a referral to the social worker.
- ○ 2. ask the client about her childhood experiences.
- ○ 3. continue to provide praise and support to the client.
- ○ 4. contact the client's family members for support.

26. The client asks the nurse, "Can my baby see?" The nurse should instruct the client that neonates
- ○ 1. can see only moving objects.
- ○ 2. can see within a limited range.
- ○ 3. can see clearly about 2 days after birth.
- ○ 4. can only distinguish light from dark.

27. During a home visit on the fifth postpartum day, the client begins to cry and says that she is worried about her ability to care for her baby adequately. She tells the nurse, "I wish I could just get organized—I need 8 hours of sleep!" The nurse determines that she is experiencing the
- ○ 1. taking-in phase of childbearing and exhibiting typical signs of adaptation.
- ○ 2. postpartum blues phase of childbearing and needs psychological counseling.
- ○ 3. letting-down phase of childbearing and needs help to assume the maternal role.
- ○ 4. taking-hold phase of childbearing and reacting to her feelings of inadequacy in relation to neonatal care.

28. During the home visit, a breast-feeding client asks the nurse what contraception method she and her husband should use until she has her 6-week postpartum examination. The nurse explains that an appropriate contraception method is
- ○ 1. condom with spermicide.
- ○ 2. oral contraceptives.
- ○ 3. calendar method.
- ○ 4. cervical mucous method.

The nurse is caring for a 16-year-old unmarried primipara after a vaginal delivery under epidural block anesthesia. The client's family is supportive, and the client intends to keep the baby. The client's boyfriend stayed with the her during the entire labor and delivery process.

29. About 4 hours after delivery, the client tells the nurse that she needs to void for the first time after the delivery. The nurse should
- ○ 1. ask her to sit on the edge of the bed for a few minutes before ambulating.

2. instruct her to remain flat in bed for 2 more hours.

3. assess for bladder distention before ambulation.

4. provide her with an analgesic before ambulation.

30. While assessing the client, the nurse determines that the client has a positive Homan's sign. The nurse should

1. place a cold pack on the client's perineal area.

2. position the client in a semi-Fowler's position.

3. notify the client's physician.

4. ask the client to ambulate around the room.

31. The client changes her baby's diaper for the first time, and the nurse evaluates her mothering skills. While caring for the adolescent primipara, the nurse should focus on her need for

1. praise and encouragement.

2. detailed written instructions.

3. her family to assist her.

4. peer acceptance.

32. After teaching the client how to care for the neonate's umbilical cord, the nurse determines that the instructions have been effective when the client states that care of the cord area should be done with

1. soap and water.

2. baby wipes.

3. sterile water.

4. alcohol pledgets.

33. The client tells the nurse that she gained 19 pounds during pregnancy and asks how long it will take to return to her normal prepregnant weight. The nurse should explain that this will most likely occur in about

1. 2 weeks.

2. 4 weeks.

3. 6 weeks.

4. 8 weeks.

34. The client tells the nurse that she and her baby will be living with her parents so that she can finish high school and go on to college. The client's boyfriend has been supportive of the client and neonate. Which of the following would be an appropriate nursing diagnosis at this time?

1. Anxiety related to return to high school and peer pressure.

2. Ineffective Individual Coping related to inability to view motherhood realistically.

3. Family Coping, Potential for Growth, related to addition of new family member.

4. Knowledge Deficit related to financial and emotional costs of childrearing.

35. The client is to receive a rubella vaccine during the postpartum period. In planning instructions for the client before the injection, the nurse should include which of the following in the teaching plan?

1. The vaccine prevents a future fetus from developing congenital anomalies.

2. Pregnancy should be avoided for 3 months after the immunization.

3. The client should avoid contact with children who have been diagnosed with rubella.

4. The injection will provide immunity against the 7-day measles.

The Postpartal Client Who Breast-Feeds

A 24-year-old primipara decides to breast-feed her baby. She delivered a viable neonate vaginally and received a local anesthetic for a midline episiotomy.

36. The client says, "I'm worried that I won't be able to breast-feed my baby because my breasts are so small." The nurse should explain to the client that

1. breast milk can be enhanced by occasional formula feeding.

2. the woman's motivation to breast-feed is less important than breast size.

3. because her breasts are small, she will have to feed the baby more often.

4. breast size does not influence the ability to breast-feed.

37. The nurse plans to instruct the client about inverted nipples. Which of the following measures should be included in the teaching plan?

1. At times during the day, leave the brassiere off for a short time.

2. Pat the nipples lightly with a terry cloth towel twice daily.

3. Cutting out a portion of the brassiere can aid a client with inverted nipples.

4. Push the areolar tissues away from the nipples, then grasp the nipples to tease them out of the tissues.

38. The client asks the nurse, "Is it important for my baby to get colostrum?" The nurse should instruct the client that feeding the infant colostrum provides the neonate with

1. more fat than breast milk.

2. vitamin K, which the neonate lacks.

3. sufficient iron stores until breast milk is produced.

4. many important antibodies that the neonate lacks.

39. The nurse plans to instruct the client to avoid taking any medications while breast-feeding unless prescribed by the physician because many drugs have been found to

1. decrease breast milk quality.

○ 2. depress the mother's motivation to breast-feed.

○ 3. be excreted in breast milk to the nursing neonate.

○ 4. interfere with the let-down reflex.

40. If ibuprofen, 200 mg, is prescribed for analgesia, the nurse should instruct the client to take the medication

○ 1. only before bedtime.

○ 2. midway between feedings.

○ 3. immediately after a feeding.

○ 4. when supplemental formula is provided.

41. Before the first feeding, the nurse should instruct the client that for the first few feedings, the mother should allow the neonate to nurse

○ 1. whenever the infant is crying.

○ 2. for only 1 to 2 minutes per side.

○ 3. for at least 7 to 10 minutes per side.

○ 4. for 20 to 30 minutes per side.

42. After the first feeding, the client asks the nurse, "How often should I try to breast-feed?" The nurse should instruct the client to feed the neonate

○ 1. at least every hour for the first 48 hours.

○ 2. every 2 to 3 hours for the first 48 hours.

○ 3. every 4 to 5 hours for the first 5 days after delivery.

○ 4. whenever she desires, until weaning occurs.

A multipara delivered a viable male neonate 12 hours ago. The client plans to breast-feed her baby, although she bottle fed her first two children.

43. The client tells the nurse that she has cramps every time she breast-feeds. The nurse should

○ 1. offer the client a prescribed analgesic.

○ 2. advise the client to breast-feed more often.

○ 3. suggest that the client ambulate frequently during the day.

○ 4. offer the client a prescribed stool softener.

44. When a multipara complains of cramps or afterpains, the nurse explains that these are caused by

○ 1. flatulence following a vaginal delivery.

○ 2. retention of small placental fragments.

○ 3. excessive abdominal distention with pressure on the uterus.

○ 4. release of oxytocin during breast-feeding.

45. The nurse has counseled the client about diet and nutrition during lactation. The nurse determines that the client needs *further* instruction when she says

○ 1. "I need to increase my intake of vitamin D."

○ 2. "I need to drink at least four glasses of fluid daily."

○ 3. "I should get an extra 500 calories per day."

○ 4. "I need to have adequate calcium in my diet."

46. The client asks how breast milk differs from cow's milk. The nurse should instruct the client that breast milk is higher in

○ 1. fat.

○ 2. iron.

○ 3. sodium.

○ 4. calcium.

47. The nurse explains to the client that the primary action that stimulates the neonate to open the mouth and grasp the nipple is to

○ 1. pull down gently on his chin.

○ 2. squeeze both of his cheeks simultaneously.

○ 3. place the nipple into his mouth on top of his tongue.

○ 4. brush his lips lightly with the nipple.

A 25-year-old primipara delivered a viable neonate 2 hours ago. The client plans to breast-feed.

48. The nurse plans to teach the client how to prevent nipple soreness. Which of the following should be included in the teaching plan?

○ 1. Keep plastic liners in the brassiere to keep the nipple drier.

○ 2. Place as much of the areola as possible into the baby's mouth.

○ 3. Pull the nipple out of the baby's mouth smoothly when breast-feeding after 10 minutes of feeding.

○ 4. Remove any remaining milk left on the nipple with a soft washcloth.

49. The nurse teaches the client how to express milk manually, instructing her to use her thumb and forefinger to

○ 1. alternately release and compress each nipple.

○ 2. compress and release the breast at the edge of the areola.

○ 3. slide forward from the edge of the areola toward the end of the nipple.

○ 4. roll the nipple while exerting a gentle pull on areola.

50. After giving instruction about burping the neonate, the nurse determines that the client understands the instructions when she says that babies who are

○ 1. burped frequently eat more.

○ 2. supplemented with formula rarely need to be burped.

○ 3. breast-fed every 3 hours do not need to be burped.

○ 4. breast-fed usually do not swallow as much air as bottle-fed infants.

171

51. The client plans to return to work and asks the nurse about storage of breast milk. After teaching the client how to store breast milk, the nurse determines that she needs *further* instruction when she says that breast milk
    - ○ 1. should be stored in sterile plastic formula bottles.
    - ○ 2. should be labeled with the date, time, and amount.
    - ○ 3. can be safely stored for 48 hours in the refrigerator.
    - ○ 4. kept frozen in the freezer no longer than 1 week.

52. The nurse plans to instruct the client in methods to prevent breast engorgement. Which of the following measures should be included in the nurse's teaching plan?
    - ○ 1. Feed the neonate for only 5 minutes per side on the first day.
    - ○ 2. Wear a supportive brassiere with nipple shields.
    - ○ 3. Breast-feed the neonate frequently.
    - ○ 4. Decrease fluid intake for 24 to 48 hours.

53. The client tells the nurse that she plans to return to work in 6 months and will probably wean her baby then. The client asks the nurse, "How will I stop producing milk when I want to wean the baby?" The nurse should instruct the client that
    - ○ 1. her milk supply will diminish as the baby nurses less.
    - ○ 2. she should request a prescription for a lactation suppressant when she decides to stop breast-feeding.
    - ○ 3. wearing of a tight breast binder usually effectively suppresses lactation.
    - ○ 4. her milk supply naturally diminishes about 6 months after delivery.

54. During a home visit on the third postpartum day, the client tells the nurse that she is aware of a "let-down sensation" in her breasts and asks what causes it. The nurse should explain to the client that the let-down sensation is stimulated by
    - ○ 1. Adrenalin.
    - ○ 2. Estrogen.
    - ○ 3. Prolactin.
    - ○ 4. Oxytocin.

A 19-year-old primipara delivered a viable male neonate 2 hours ago. She has decided to breast-feed, and her 22-year-old husband supports her decision. The neonate has a strong sucking reflex.

55. The client tells the nurse, "My mother breast-fed all of her children, but I'm going to need lots of help with breast-feeding. I'm worried that I won't be able to do this." When assessing the client, the nurse should
    - ○ 1. determine the client's level of motivation to breast-feed.
    - ○ 2. ask the client if she has read any literature about breast-feeding.
    - ○ 3. perform a complete physical examination of the client to determine how much help she will need.
    - ○ 4. assess her body-to-fat ratio before beginning breast-feeding.

56. A priority nursing diagnosis for the client at this time is
    - ○ 1. High Risk for Breast Engorgement related to lack of knowledge about breast-feeding.
    - ○ 2. High Risk for Sore Nipples related to infant's strong suck.
    - ○ 3. Anxiety related to inexperience with breast-feeding.
    - ○ 4. Fear related to lack of motivation about breast-feeding.

57. The client asks the nurse if she should supplement breast-feeding with formula feeding. The nurse should explain to the client that
    - ○ 1. formula supplements tend to interfere with the breast milk supply and should be avoided.
    - ○ 2. to prevent jaundice, water supplements are appropriate.
    - ○ 3. formula supplements can provide nutrients not found in breast milk.
    - ○ 4. the baby must suck more vigorously on a bottle than a breast, so supplements should be avoided.

58. During a home visit on the fourth postpartum day, the client tells the nurse that she has been experiencing breast engorgement. To relieve engorgement, the nurse plans to teach the client that before nursing her baby, the client should
    - ○ 1. apply an ice cube to the nipples.
    - ○ 2. rub her nipples gently with hand cream.
    - ○ 3. express a small amount of breast milk.
    - ○ 4. breast-feed less often for a few days.

59. The client asks the nurse, "What should I do when I want to wean the infant?" The nurse should instruct the client that to wean the infant, the client should
    - ○ 1. wait until she has breast-fed for at least 4 months.
    - ○ 2. eliminate baby's favorite feeding times first.
    - ○ 3. omit the daytime feedings last.
    - ○ 4. eliminate one feeding at a time.

60. A week after the client is discharged, she calls the birthing center and says that she is afraid she is "losing her breast milk. The baby had been nursing every 4 hours, but now she's crying to be fed every 2 hours." The nurse should explain to the client that the neonate's behavior is most likely due to
    - ○ 1. digesting the breast milk too quickly.

○ 2. the mother's fears about the baby's weight gain.

○ 3. not allowing the neonate to suck long enough with each feeding.

○ 4. the neonate's temporary growth spurt, which requires more feedings.

The Postpartal Client Who Bottle Feeds

A 24-year-old client has delivered a healthy neonate in the hospital's birthing center. She plans to bottle feed her neonate.

61. The nurse plans to instruct the client about the number of calories each day per pound of body weight that a neonate requires for normal growth and development. The nurse should explain to the client that the number of calories required per pound of body weight is
○ 1. 30 to 35.
○ 2. 40 to 45.
○ 3. 50 to 55.
○ 4. 60 to 65.

62. When the neonate is 24 hours of age, the client asks the nurse, "Why does my baby spit up the formula after feeding?" The nurse should explain that the regurgitation is thought to result from
○ 1. an immature cardiac sphincter.
○ 2. a defect in the gastrointestinal system.
○ 3. burping the infant too often.
○ 4. feeding the neonate too often.

63. After teaching the client about bottle feeding, the nurse determines that the client needs *further* instruction when she says,
○ 1. "Bottle fed babies up to 6 months of age may gain as much as 1 ounce per day."
○ 2. "Iron-fortified formulas are usually recommended for newborns."
○ 3. "Bottle fed babies will usually regain their birth weight by 10 days of age."
○ 4. "Whole milk is an acceptable alternative to formula once the baby is 4 months old."

64. The client asks the nurse, "What is the best position for the baby after the feeding?" The nurse should instruct the client to position the neonate
○ 1. On the right side.
○ 2. On the left side.
○ 3. Prone without a pillow.
○ 4. Sitting in the mother's lap for 20 minutes.

65. The client asks, "When should I start giving the baby solid foods?" The nurse should instruct the client to introduce solid foods no sooner than
○ 1. 2 months of age.
○ 2. 4 months of age.

○ 3. 8 months of age.
○ 4. 1 year of age.

66. The nurse has instructed the client about burping the neonate who is being formula fed. The nurse determines that the client needs *further* instruction when she says burping should be done
○ 1. after 2 minutes of feeding.
○ 2. in the middle and at the end of the feeding.
○ 3. while the baby is in an upright position.
○ 4. by gently patting the baby's back.

The Postpartal Client With a Cesarean Birth

A 30-year-old multipara has delivered a healthy term female neonate by cesarean section owing to fetal distress. The client has three male children at home.

67. After admission to the postpartal unit, the nurse assesses the client's retention catheter and observes that the client's urine is slightly red-tinged. The nurse should
○ 1. continue to monitor the client's input and output.
○ 2. massage the client's fundus gently.
○ 3. increase the rate of intravenous fluids.
○ 4. contact the client's physician.

68. On the first postpartum day, the client is ordered a full liquid diet as tolerated. Before providing a full liquid breakfast, the nurse should assess the client's
○ 1. thirst.
○ 2. desire to eat.
○ 3. bowel sounds.
○ 4. degree of discomfort.

69. On the second postpartum day, the client complains of gas pains. The nurse should instruct the client to
○ 1. ask the physician for a prescription for simethicone.
○ 2. chew on some ice chips.
○ 3. maintain bed rest.
○ 4. ambulate more often.

70. While changing the neonate's diaper, the client asks the nurse about some red-tinged drainage from the neonate's vagina. The nurse determines that her teaching has been effective when the client says,
○ 1. "It's of no concern because it is such a small amount."
○ 2. "The cause of vaginal bleeding in neonates is usually related to swallowing blood during the delivery."
○ 3. "Sometimes baby girls have a small amount of vaginal bleeding from hormones received from the mother."
○ 4. "Vaginal bleeding in neonates is caused by hem-

orrhagic disease of the newborn, and the doctor should be aware of this."

71. The client asks, "If I get pregnant again, will I need to have a cesarean section?" The nurse should instruct the client that vaginal delivery after a cesarean delivery is
- ○ 1. possible if the client has not had a classic uterine incision.
- ○ 2. possible if the client has a history of rapid labor.
- ○ 3. not possible because the client is a multipara.
- ○ 4. not possible unless the client has had a preterm neonate.

72. The client is a candidate for anti-Rh (D) γ-globulin (RhoGAM). The nurse plans to administer the ordered medication
- ○ 1. within 1 hour after delivery.
- ○ 2. immediately after delivery of the placenta.
- ○ 3. within 72 hours after delivery.
- ○ 4. within 7 days after delivery.

The Postpartal Client With Complications

A 34-year-old multiparous client is admitted to the hospital in active labor. The client delivers a 7 pound, 15 ounce (3, 600 g) neonate vaginally under local anesthesia and has a midline episiotomy.

73. This was the client's fourth pregnancy. The client has one set of twins, and all five children are living. The twins were preterm, while the other three neonates were term. The client has no history of abortion. Using the TPAL method, the nurse documents the client as
- ○ 1. Gravida 4, 3205
- ○ 2. Gravida 5, 3104
- ○ 3. Gravida 4, 4205
- ○ 4. Gravida 5, 5205

74. In developing a plan of care for the client, the nurse reviews her prenatal, labor, and delivery records. Of the following data in the client's record, which requires further assessment by the nurse?
- ○ 1. Perineal laceration.
- ○ 2. Leukocytosis of 16,000/mm.
- ○ 3. Blood loss of 400 mL at delivery.
- ○ 4. Temperature of 37.2 C (99 F) at 1 hour postpartum.

75. The client is diagnosed with a puerperal infection. The nurse explains to the client that the most likely contributor to the infection is
- ○ 1. maternal age over 30 years.
- ○ 2. vaginal manipulation and trauma.
- ○ 3. use of low forceps for delivery.
- ○ 4. antepartal infection before labor.

76. The physician orders intravenous antibiotic therapy with ampicillin sodium (Polycillin). Before administering this drug, the nurse should
- ○ 1. ask the client if she has any drug allergies.
- ○ 2. assess the client's pulse rate.
- ○ 3. place the client in a side-lying position.
- ○ 4. check the client's perineal pad.

77. During intravenous antibiotic therapy for puerperal infection, the nurse should encourage the client to
- ○ 1. ambulate to the bathroom frequently.
- ○ 2. discontinue breast-feeding temporarily.
- ○ 3. maintain a semi-Fowler's position.
- ○ 4. keep visitors to a minimum.

A 39-year-old grand multipara is admitted to the postpartum unit after a cesarean delivery because of fetal distress. The client weighed 305 pounds at her last prenatal visit.

78. The client is diagnosed with thrombophlebitis. The physician orders prophylactic heparin (Panheparin) therapy. After instructing the client about the purpose of the medication, the nurse determines that the client understands the instructions when she says that the drug will
- ○ 1. make her blood clots thinner.
- ○ 2. decrease the lochial flow.
- ○ 3. increase diaphoresis.
- ○ 4. prevent blood clot formation.

79. While the client is receiving heparin, the nurse plans to keep which of the following drugs available to counteract bleeding complications due to heparin overdose?
- ○ 1. Calcium gluconate.
- ○ 2. Protamine sulfate.
- ○ 3. Methergine.
- ○ 4. Nitrofurantoin.

80. The nurse plans to contact the client's physician immediately if the client experiences
- ○ 1. pain in her calf.
- ○ 2. dyspnea.
- ○ 3. bleeding gums.
- ○ 4. bradycardia.

81. The client is to be discharged while on heparin therapy. After teaching her about signs of hemorrhage during heparin therapy, the nurse determines that she needs *further* instruction when she states that symptoms that should be reported include
- ○ 1. epistaxis.
- ○ 2. bleeding gums.
- ○ 3. anorexia.
- ○ 4. petechiae.

A 30-year-old multipara is admitted to the postpartum unit after a vaginal delivery. On the second postpartum day, the client is diagnosed with cystitis, and the physician orders antibiotic therapy.

82. The nurse plans to instruct the client about self-care during treatment. Which of the following measures should be included in the nurse's teaching plan?
- ○ 1. Limit fluid intake to 1 liter daily.
- ○ 2. Empty the bladder every 2 to 4 hours.
- ○ 3. Wash the perineum with povidone-iodine (Betadine) solution after voiding.
- ○ 4. Avoid drinking acidic fruit juices.

83. An appropriate nursing diagnosis for the client at this time is
- ○ 1. Fear related to intravenous therapy.
- ○ 2. Ineffective Family Coping related to prolonged hospitalization.
- ○ 3. Dysuria related to lengthy labor and decreased fluid intake.
- ○ 4. Pain related to dysuria and frequency.

84. The client asks, "Can I still continue to breast-feed my baby?" The nurse should instruct the client that breast-feeding should be
- ○ 1. continued as long as she desires.
- ○ 2. alternated with formula feeding to help her rest.
- ○ 3. discontinued until the antibiotic therapy is stopped.
- ○ 4. modified by manually pumping the breasts.

A 30-year-old multipara is admitted to the postpartum unit after cesarean delivery owing to abruptio placenta. Her neonate weighs 10 pounds, 2 ounces (4,593 g) and is in the special care nursery for observation. The client is receiving intravenous Ringer's lactate solution in her left arm.

85. The client develops symptoms of early postpartum hemorrhage. In planning care for the client, the nurse should plan to
- ○ 1. administer oxytocin intravenously.
- ○ 2. place the client in a side-lying position.
- ○ 3. massage the fundus vigorously every 5 minutes.
- ○ 4. prepare the client for an emergency hysterotomy.

86. The client asks, "Why am I bleeding so much?" The nurse's best response is that the most likely cause of uterine atony is
- ○ 1. trauma during labor.
- ○ 2. oxytocin use after delivery.
- ○ 3. lengthy and prolonged second stage of labor.
- ○ 4. overdistention of the uterus.

87. A priority nursing diagnosis for the client at this time is
- ○ 1. Altered Tissue Perfusion related to excessive uterine bleeding.
- ○ 2. Cardiac System Impaired related to excessive blood loss.
- ○ 3. Anxiety related to emergency measures to control bleeding.
- ○ 4. Potential for Hypertension related to use of oxytocin.

A 26-year-old primipara is seen in the urgent care clinic 2 weeks after she delivered a viable female neonate. The client has been breast-feeding and is diagnosed with infectious mastitis.

88. The client asks, "Can I continue breast-feeding?" The nurse should instruct the client that breast-feeding should be
- ○ 1. continued and the neonate fed frequently.
- ○ 2. continued only if symptoms decrease.
- ○ 3. discontinued until antibiotic therapy is completed.
- ○ 4. discontinued because the breast milk may be contaminated.

89. After teaching the client about treatment of infectious mastitis, the nurse determines that she needs *further* instruction when she says,
- ○ 1. "I can apply heat to the infected area."
- ○ 2. "I should increase my fluid intake."
- ○ 3. "I'll need to take antibiotics for 10 days."
- ○ 4. "I need to avoid analgesics while I'm taking antibiotics."

90. The client expresses anxiety to the nurse because she has a nephew with Down syndrome. After teaching the client about Down syndrome, the nurse determines that the client needs *further* instruction when she says,
- ○ 1. "Down syndrome is an abnormality that can result from an extra chromosome."
- ○ 2. "Down syndrome results in some degree of mental retardation."
- ○ 3. "There is no method available to determine if my baby has Down syndrome."
- ○ 4. "Older mothers are more likely to have a baby with Down syndrome."

A 15-year-old unmarried primipara is being cared for by the nurse in the hospital's birthing center following low forceps delivery of a viable male neonate. The client has a fourth-degree laceration and a midline episiotomy. The neonate is being placed for adoption.

91. The nurse has provided the client with instructions about episiotomy care. The nurse determines that the client understands the teaching when the client says,

○ 1. "I should use cool, sudsy water to clean the episiotomy area."

○ 2. "I should wipe the area from front to back using a blotting motion."

○ 3. "Sitz baths with cold water should be taken before bedtime."

○ 4. "Ice packs should be used after the first 24 hours."

92. Four hours after delivery, the client asks if she can feed her baby. The nurse should tell the client

○ 1. "I'll bring the baby to you for feeding."

○ 2. "I think we should ask your physician if this is a good idea."

○ 3. "It's probably not a good idea for you to feed the baby."

○ 4. "I'll check with the social worker to see if the adopting parents will permit this."

93. Four days after delivery, the client visits the clinic complaining of excessive lochia rubra with clots. The physician orders methylergonovine maleate (Methergine), 0.2 mg intramuscularly. Before administering this drug, the nurse should monitor the client's

○ 1. blood pressure.

○ 2. pulse rate.

○ 3. breath sounds.

○ 4. bowel sounds.

94. The client asks the nurse, "Why did my bleeding start again?" The nurse should instruct the client that this type of postpartum hemorrhage is usually due to

○ 1. uterine atony.

○ 2. cervical lacerations.

○ 3. vaginal lacerations.

○ 4. retained placental fragments.

95. The client says, "I've been crying a lot the last few days. I just feel so depressed sometimes. Why is this?" The nurse's best response is

○ 1. "These feelings often indicate symptoms of postpartum blues and are normal. Do you want to talk about it?"

○ 2. "I think you're probably overreacting to the adoption proceedings. You're doing the best thing for the baby."

○ 3. "It's unusual for mothers to feel depressed, even when they are putting the baby up for adoption. I'll talk to your doctor so you can get a prescription for an antidepressant."

○ 4. "This may be a symptom of a serious mental illness. I think I should tell the doctor about these feelings."

CORRECT ANSWERS AND RATIONALE

The letters in parentheses following the rationale identify the step of the nursing process (A, D, P, I, E), cognitive level (K, C, T, N), and client needs (S, G, L, H). See the Answer Grid for the key.

The Postpartal Client With a Vaginal Birth

1. 1. Bradycardia is a normal physiologic change for 6 to 10 days postpartum. Rates above 100 beats/minute may indicate infection, hemorrhage, or pain; a rapid, thready pulse may indicate shock. (I, N, G)

2. 2. The instillation of erythromycin into the neonate's eyes is a prophylactic for ophthalmia neonatorum, or neonatal blindness from gonorrhea in the mother. Erythromycin is also effective in the prevention of infection from *Chlamydia trachomatis.* (I, T, G)

3. 3. Vitamin K, or AquaMEPHYTON, acts as a preventive measure against neonatal hemorrhagic disease. (I, T, G)

4. 1. The Moro, or startle, reflex occurs when the neonate responds to stimuli by extending the arms, hands open, and then moving the arms in an embracing motion. The Moro reflex should be present at birth but disappears at about age 3 months. The grasping reflex is present when the neonate grasps an object placed in the hand. The Babinski reflex is elicited by stroking the neonate's foot. The tonic neck reflex (or fencing reflex) is demonstrated when the neonate, while lying supine, turns the head to one side. (E, N, H)

5. 2. The client is in the taking-in phase for up to 3 days after birth. During this time, food and sleep are a major focus for the client. In addition, she works through the birth experience to sort out reality from fantasy and to clarify any misunderstandings. The taking-hold phase is the second phase of postpartal psychological adaptation; the letting-go phase is the final phase. (D, N, L)

6. 3. During the taking-in phase of maternal postpartum adjustment, the client's primary concern is with her own needs. This phase usually lasts 1 to 3 days after birth. (P, N, L)

7. 1. During the first 24 hours after delivery, ice packs can be applied to the perineal area to reduce the swelling. Usually, hematomas resolve without further treatment. (I, T, G)

8. 3. Beginning after completion of the taking-in phase, the talking-hold phase lasts about 10 days. During this phase, the client is concerned with her

need to resume control of all facets of her life in a competent manner. At this time, she is ready to learn self-care and infant care skills. The letting-go phase is the final phase of postpartal psychological adaptation. (P, N, L)

9. 4. Urinary retention soon after delivery is usually due to edema and trauma of the lower urinary tract. Edema is commonly present in the area of the lower urinary tract after delivery. This condition often makes it difficult to start voiding. Hyperemia of the bladder mucosa also commonly occurs. The combination of hyperemia and edema predisposes to decreased sensation to void, overdistention of the bladder, and incomplete bladder emptying. Nursing care of the postpartum client should include careful monitoring of the bladder to help prevent urine retention and its associated problems. (I, N, G)

10. 4. The most appropriate nursing diagnosis is Urinary Retention related to the trauma of delivery. The client is not at high risk for infection, although some risk is present. With adequate cleanliness and hygiene, infection can be prevented. There is no indication that the client is experiencing fatigue from a lengthy labor. Typically, during the immediate postpartum period, the client experiences a fluid volume deficit from lack of fluid intake and blood and other fluid loss during delivery. (D, N, G)

11. 4. A constant trickle of blood and a firm fundus are usually indicative of a vaginal tear. Uterine atony indicates a soft or boggy fundus. (A, T, G)

12. 3. After an uncomplicated delivery, postpartum exercises may begin on the first postpartum day with exercises to strengthen the abdominal muscles. This is done in the supine position with the knees flexed, inhaling deeply while allowing the abdomen to expand and then exhaling while contracting the abdominal muscles. Such exercises as reaching for the knees, push-ups, and sit-ups are ordinarily too strenuous for the first postpartum day but may be done later in the postpartum period. Kegel exercises should be done often in the postpartal period to restore perineal and vaginal muscle tone. Increased lochia or pain indicates overactivity; the client should be instructed to decrease activity if this occurs. (I, N, H)

13. 1. Providing stimulation and speaking to neonates is important, and the nurse should encourage the client to do so. Some authorities believe that speech is the most important type of sensory stimulation for a neonate. Neonates respond best to speech with tonal variations and a high-pitched voice. Although cooing can be used, a neonate does respond to words, and these should be used as a stimulus to language development. A neonate can hear all sounds louder than about 55 decibels. (I, N, H)

14. 2. Lochia can be expected to increase when the client first ambulates. Lochia tends to pool in the uterus and vagina when the client is recumbent and flows out when the client arises. If bright red bleeding continues, the client should be put to bed. Massaging the fundus is not indicated because the lochia is normal. (I, N, G)

15. 4. After delivery, the nurse should plan to measure the client's first few voidings to make sure that the client is emptying the bladder. (I, T, G)

16. 2. Clients sometimes feel faint when ambulating for the first time after delivery. This results from the sudden change in blood circulation in the body. Primarily for this reason, the nurse remains nearby while the client takes her first shower after delivery. (I, N, H)

17. 1. The height of the uterus is normally felt slightly below the umbilicus about 24 hours after delivery. Unless complications occur, this client can expect normal progress of involution. Immediately after delivery, however, the top of the fundus normally is midway between the umbilicus and the symphysis pubis. It descends at a rate of about one fingerbreadth each day. It is barely palpable above the upper margin of the symphysis pubis 7 to 10 days after delivery. Although there is individual variation, these are the normal ranges. (I, N, G)

18. 2. The vaginal discharge that normally occurs for 2 to 3 days after delivery, *lochia rubra,* contains mostly blood and is dark red in color. The discharge then becomes more serous and watery, at which time it is called *lochia serosa.* About the 10th day after delivery, the discharge becomes thinner, scanty, and almost without color and is called *lochia alba.* (E, N, G)

19. 1. Neonates like to look at eyes, and eye-to-eye contact is a good way to provide visual stimulation. The parent's eyes are circular, move from side to side, and become larger and smaller; neonates have been observed to fix on them. In general, neonates prefer circular objects of darkness against a white background. (I, N, H)

20. 2. Holding and patting neonates helps them develop trust in caregivers. Tactile stimulation is important and should be encouraged. Holding neonates often is unlikely to spoil them. (I, N, H)

21. 4. Excessive perspiration is common during the puerperium. The most appropriate nursing diagnosis is Fluid Volume Excess related to normal postpartal elimination. There are no data to suggest urinary tract infection, impaired thermoregulation, or altered protection related to effects of anesthesia. (D, N, G)

22. 3. A full bladder is likely to push the uterus to the right of midline, so the nurse should further assess for symptoms of urine retention. When the bladder is empty, it normally is nonpalpable and lies about in the midline. A full bladder can prevent the uterus from contracting properly (uterine atony); hemorrhage can occur. Here, the client's uterus is firm. Deviation of the fundus is not related to retention of blood clots. (A, N, G)

23. 2. Vomited material has been digested and looks like curdled milk, with a sour odor. Vomiting usually occurs between feedings and empties the stomach of its contents. In contrast, regurgitation is undigested material; it does not have a sour odor and occurs during or immediately after feeding. The amount of material is not a reliable guide in distinguishing vomiting from regurgitation. (I, N, H)

24. 4. If the client continues to complain of perineal pain after an analgesic medication has been given, the nurse should inspect the client's perineum for a hematoma. (I, T, G)

25. 3. The new mother may seem hesitant to handle the neonate owing to lack of experience. The role of the nurse is to continue to provide support, praise, and encouragement. A primipara often has concerns about her ability to care for her infant properly during the taking-hold phase. She is working toward independence and autonomy and wants to be able to perform well. She needs emotional support, advice on how to manage, reassurance, and reinforcement of appropriate behavior. The letdown phase, sometimes called the postpartum blues, is characterized by irritability and generally occurs later in the postpartum period. Psychological counseling is rarely necessary. (D, N, G)

26. 2. The neonate has immature oculomotor coordination, an inability to accommodate for distance, and poorly developed eyes, visual nerves, and brain. However, the normal neonate can see clearly within about 9 to 12 inches. (I, N, G)

27. 4. A primipara often has concerns about her ability to care for her infant properly during the taking-hold phase. She is working toward independence and autonomy, and wants to be able to perform well in her new role as mother. She needs emotional support, advice on how to manage, reassurance, and reinforcement of appropriate behavior. The letdown phase generally occurs later in the postpartum period. Psychological counseling is not warranted. (D, N, G)

28. 1. If not contraindicated for moral, cultural, or religious reasons, a condom with spermicide is often recommended for contraception after delivery until the client's 6-week postpartal examination. The diaphragm must be refitted, which is usually done at the 6-week examination. The cervical mucous and calendar methods are not effective because the client is unlikely to be able to determine when ovulation has occurred until her menstrual cycle returns. Although breast-feeding is not considered an effective form of contraception, breast-feeding usually delays the return of both ovulation and menstruation. The length of the delay varies with the duration of lactation and frequency of breast-feeding. Most lactating women resume menstruation within 12 weeks postpartum. Women who are not breast-feeding can use oral contraceptive agents. (I, N, G)

29. 1. Before ambulating the client for the first time, the nurse should ask the client to sit on the edge of the bed for a few minutes. Orthostatic hypotension is a common occurrence in the first few hours after delivery and may even persist longer. The client feels the urge to void, so it is not necessary for the nurse to check for bladder distention at this time. The bladder can be assessed after the client has voided. (I, T, G)

30. 3. A positive Homan's sign is indicative of thrombophlebitis. The nurse should notify the physician and ask the client to remain in bed. Pulmonary embolism is a serious consequence of thrombophlebitis. (I, N, G)

31. 1. The adolescent client may have special needs during the postpartum period. Praise and encouragement of her mothering skills are important for confidence and self-esteem. She does not need prolonged verbal instructions; lengthy explanations may overwhelm the first-time mother. It is not essential that the client's mother assist her; however, the nurse can instruct the client while her mother is present. Special psychological counseling is not necessary. (I, N, H)

32. 4. It is best to care for the neonate's umbilical cord area by cleaning it with pledgets moistened with alcohol. The alcohol promotes drying and helps decrease the risk of infection. Because alcohol is not effective against some bacteria, however, the nurse should continue to assess the neonate's cord for redness or drainage. Sometimes, an antibiotic ointment may be used instead of alcohol. Such agents as baby wipes, sterile water, and soap and water are not as effective as alcohol or an antibiotic ointment. At home, the client can use cotton balls moistened with alcohol. (E, N, H)

33. 2. In most cases, unless complications develop or the client has gained excessive weight during the antepartal period, she can expect to return to pre-

pregnant weight by 6 weeks. Many clients lose 14 to 20 pounds by 2 weeks postpartum. (I, N, H)

34. 3. The most appropriate nursing diagnosis based on the information provided is Family Coping, Potential for Growth, related to addition of new family member. There is no information to support the diagnoses Anxiety, Ineffective Individual Coping to unrealistic expectations, and High Risk for Infection. (D, N, L)

35. 2. After administration of rubella vaccine, the client should be instructed to avoid pregnancy for at least 3 months to prevent toxic effects of the vaccine to the fetus. The vaccine does not protect a future fetus from infection. The vaccine is not given to pregnant clients, even though they are not immune. The injection immunizes the client against the 3-day or German measles, not the 7-day measles. (P, N, G)

The Postpartal Client Who Breast-Feeds

36. 4. Various hormones have a role in lactation. The pituitary hormone prolactin has a central role. Breast size is not important as long as there is glandular tissue to secrete the milk. Various factors can influence milk supply, such as suckling, emptying of the breasts, diet, exercise, rest, level of contentment, and stress. The fat in breast tissue plays no role in milk production. Women with small breasts do not produce less milk. The client's belief in her ability to breast-feed is important. The size of the breast does not influence the neonate's ability to grasp the nipple. The neonate may have difficulty grasping inverted nipples. (I, N, H)

37. 4. The areolar tissues can be pushed in and away from the nipples, then the nipples grasped and pulled out gently. Using a Woolrich breast shield, which pushes the nipples through openings in the shield, also can help overcome inverted nipples. A cut-open brassiere is not effective. Brushing the nipples with a terry cloth towel is not advised because this can cause injury to the delicate breast tissue. (P, N, H)

38. 4. Colostrum contains antibodies that the neonate lacks, such as immunoglobulin A; therefore, it is important for the neonate to receive colostrum. (I, T, H)

39. 3. Various medications can be excreted in the breast milk and affect the nursing neonate. The client should avoid all nonprescribed medications. Some medications can suppress milk production; these may be prescribed for clients who bottle feed. Medications usually do not affect the neonate's appetite or interfere with the milk ejection, or letdown, reflex. (I, N, G)

40. 3. Taking ibuprofen, 200 mg, after breast-feeding

41. 3. The mother should be encouraged to nurse frequently during the first few days after delivery. Breast-feeding for at least 7 to 10 minutes per side is recommended for the let-down reflex to begin. (I, T, H)

42. 2. Soon after delivery, the client should breast-feed every 2 to 3 hours until her milk supply is established. Feeding every 4 to 5 hours is not often enough. The client may only feel like feeding less often, so this is not appropriate. The neonate may be sleepy during the first 24 hours after birth, so his state of hunger or crying is not reliable. (I, N, G)

43. 1. Multiparas tend to experience cramps while breast-feeding more frequently than do primiparas. This is because breast-feeding releases oxytocin, which causes uterine muscles to contract. The uterine muscles tend to be more tonically contracted after delivery in primiparas. An analgesic is most commonly offered to provide relief from discomfort. Breast-feeding more often is not indicated. Ambulation or laxative use is not helpful. (I, N, G)

44. 4. Breast-feeding stimulates the oxytocin secretion, which causes the uterine muscles to contract. These contractions account for the discomfort associated with afterpains. The cramps are not related to blood loss. Afterpains tend to be more common when small placental tags have been retained, when the uterus has been excessively stretched (twins), and with increasing parity. (I, N, H)

45. 2. Drinking at least 8 to 10 glasses of fluid a day is recommended for the breast-feeding client. An increase in vitamin D, an extra 500 calories, and adequate calcium in the diet are appropriate. An inadequate calorie intake can reduce milk volume but should not affect milk quality. (I, N, H)

46. 1. Breast milk is higher in fat content than cow's milk. Thirty to 55% of the calories in breast milk are from fat. The fat composition of breast milk greatly differs from cow's milk. Cow's milk is higher in iron, sodium, calcium, and phosphorous. (I, N, H)

47. 4. Lightly brushing the neonate's lips with the nipple causes the neonate to open the mouth the begin sucking. Such techniques as pulling down on the chin, squeezing the cheek, or placing the nipple directly in the mouth force the mouth open or force the neonate to take the nipple. The neonate should be taught to open the mouth and grasp the nipple on his or her own. The neonate should not be forced to nurse. (I, N, H)

48. 2. Several methods can be used to prevent nipple soreness. Placing as much of the areola as possible into the neonate's mouth is one method. Other methods include changing position with each nursing so that different areas of the nipples receive the greatest stress from nursing and avoiding breast engorgement, which makes it difficult for the neonate to grasp the nipple. In addition, nursing more frequently, so that a ravenous neonate is not sucking vigorously at the beginning of feedings, and feeding on demand to prevent overhunger are helpful. Air-drying the nipples and exposing them to light have also been recommended. Some authorities have suggested using warm tea bags, which contain tannic acid, as compresses to help healing. (P, N, H)

49. 2. The best technique for expressing milk from the breast is alternately compressing and releasing the breast at the edge of the areola. With the thumb on top and two fingers on the bottom of the breast at the edge of the areola, the client pushes in toward her chest and then squeezes her thumb and fingers together while pulling forward on the areola, without sliding her fingers or thumb on her skin. Manipulating the nipples may injure them. (I, N, H)

50. 4. Breast-fed neonates do not swallow as much air as bottle-fed neonates, but they still should be burped. Neonates do not eat more if they are burped frequently. Neonates fed on demand need to be burped. (E, N, H)

51. 4. Breast milk should not be stored in clean glass containers because immunoglobulin tends to stick to glass bottles and the containers should be sterile. The client should use sterile plastic containers labeled with date, time, and amount. Stored breast milk can be safely kept in the refrigerator for 48 hours or in a freezer for 2 months. Frozen breast milk should be thawed in the refrigerator for a few hours, placed under warm tap water, then shaken. (E, N, H)

52. 3. If at all possible, it is better to prevent breast engorgement. The best technique is to empty the breasts regularly and frequently with feedings. Engorgement is less likely when the mother and neonate are together, as in single room maternity care or continuous rooming in, because nursing can be done conveniently to meet the neonate's and mother's needs. Wearing a supportive brassiere does not prevent engorgement. Feeding the neonate for only 5 minutes per side on the first day is not adequate and does not prevent engorgement. Decreasing fluid intake is not advised. (P, N, H)

53. 1. The milk supply diminishes normally as the infant nurses less. Gradual weaning by eliminating one feeding at a time over several weeks is the best recommendation. Medication to suppress lactation is most effective when started as soon after delivery as possible. Mechanical methods of suppressing lactation (a breast binder) are most effective when used as soon after delivery as possible. The milk supply persists beyond 6 months after delivery if the breasts are emptied regularly. (I, N, H)

54. 4. Oxytocin brings on the let-down reflex when milk is carried to the nipples. Prolactin stimulates milk production. Estrogen influences development of female secondary sex characteristics and controls menstruation. Progesterone increases the lobes, lobules, and alveoli of the breasts prenatally. A lactating mother can experience the let-down reflex suddenly when she hears her baby cry or when she anticipates a feeding. Adrenalin may increase if the mother is excited but has no direct influence on breast-feeding. (I, N, G)

55. 1. Successful breast-feeding depends on the client's willingness and motivation to breast-feed. Women who have a strong desire to breast-feed tend to continue breast-feeding longer. They are often more tolerant of the discomforts of breast-feeding and more accepting of the need for frequent feedings. The type of literature is not a significant factor in successful breast-feeding. Physical examination of the client's breasts is not necessary. Although adequate nutrition during lactation is important, even clients who have had poor nutrition can be taught how to improve their diets. Assessing the client's body-to-fat ratio is not important for breast-feeding. (A, N, H)

56. 3. The most appropriate initial nursing diagnosis for this client is Anxiety related to inexperience with breast-feeding. The client is not at higher risk for engorgement than other clients who may have breast-fed before. The client may have a risk for sore nipples, but the nursing diagnosis should involve pain or discomfort, not just simply high risk for sore nipples. There is no evidence that the client is fearful. (D, N, H)

57. 1. Bottle supplements tend to cause a decrease in the breast milk supply and demand for breast-feeding, and should be avoided. Once in a while, if the client is tired, a bottle supplement may be given to the neonate by another caregiver. The husband can become involved in other aspects of the neonate's care besides feeding. Bottle supplements are not appropriate to prevent jaundice, although if neonatal bilirubin level is excessive, some pediatricians recommend temporary discontinuation of breast-feeding, while others recommend increasing the frequency of breast-feeding. Neonates suck less vigorously on a bottle than on the breast. (I, N, G)

58. 3. Various measures may be tried to relieve breast engorgement. Expressing a little milk before nursing, massaging the breasts gently, or taking a warm shower before feeding may all help to improve milk flow. Applying lanolin to the nipples or applying ice does not relieve breast engorgement. (I, N, H)

59. 4. To wean the infant, the client should eliminate one feeding at a time. The client may wish to begin with daytime feedings when the infant is busy. (I, T, H)

60. 4. Neonates normally increase breast-feeding during periods of rapid growth (growth spurts). These can be expected at age 10 to 14 days, 5 to 6 weeks, 2.5 to 3 months, and 4.5 to 6 months. Each growth spurt is usually followed by a regular feeding pattern. (I, N, H)

The Postpartal Client Who Bottle Feeds

61. 3. As a general rule, most neonates require 50 to 55 calories per pound of body weight, or about 117 calories per kilogram of weight, each day. (P, N, H)

62. 1. Initial regurgitation in the neonate may be due to excessive mucus and gastric irritation from foreign substances in the stomach from birth. Later regurgitation is thought to be due to the neonate's immature cardiac sphincter. It represents an overflow of stomach contents and is probably due to feeding the neonate too fast or too much. Regurgitation is normal, but vomiting or forceful fluid expulsion is not. (I, N, G)

63. 4. Neither unmodified cow's milk nor whole milk is an acceptable alternative for newborn nutrition. The American Academy of Pediatrics recommends that infants be given breast milk or formula until 1 year of age. The American Academy of Pediatrics Committee on Nutrition, however, has decreed that cow's milk could be substituted in the second 6 months of life, but *only if* the amount of milk calories does not exceed 65% of total calories and iron is replaced by solid foods. The protein content in cow's milk is too high, is poorly digested, and may cause gastrointestinal tract bleeding. Bottle-fed infants may gain as much as 1 ounce per day up to age 6 months. Iron-fortified formulas are recommended. Bottle-fed neonates may regain their birth weight by 10 days of age. (E, N, H)

64. 1. To aid digestion, the neonate should be placed on the right side after a feeding. Placing the neonate in a prone position has been associated with sudden infant death syndrome. (I, N, H)

65. 2. Pediatricians recommend that neonates be given either breast milk or formula until at least 4 months of age. Giving solid foods too early can lead to food allergies, and the neonate has difficulty digesting solid foods. (I, T, G)

66. 1. Burping (bubbling) the neonate should be done after about 5 minutes of feeding, in the middle of the feeding, and at the end of the feeding. The neonate should be held in an upright position and patted on the back gently. (E, T, G)

The Postpartal Client With a Cesarean Birth

67. 4. Red-tinged urine may indicate that the bladder was accidentally cut during the cesarean section. The nurse should notify the physician as soon as possible about the urine. (I, T, G)

68. 3. Before providing the client with a full liquid lunch, the nurse should first assess for the presence of bowel sounds. Breath sounds, the ability to ambulate, and degree of pain are all important to assess, but not in relation to the client's diet. The client may not desire to eat or have great thirst. (I, N, G)

69. 4. During the first few days postpartum, the accumulation of gas in the intestines may cause discomfort. Measures to decrease gas pain discomfort include increasing activity, doing leg exercises, avoiding carbonated or very hot or cold beverages, avoiding using ice or straws, and maintaining a high-protein liquid diet for the first 24 to 48 hours. A rectal tube may also be used. A gastric or intestinal tube is sometimes used when other measures fail. Maintaining bed rest does not help relieve the discomfort from gas pains. Simethicone tablets may provide some relief, but the nurse should ask the physician for this medication, not the client. (I, N, H)

70. 3. Estrogen is believed to cause slight vaginal bleeding in the female neonate. The condition disappears spontaneously, so there is no need for concern. No treatment is necessary. (E, N, H)

71. 1. Vaginal birth after a previous cesarean delivery can be attempted if the client has not had a classic uterine incision. This type of incision carries a danger of uterine rupture. A physician must be available, and a cesarean delivery must be possible within 30 minutes. A history of rapid labor and having a small-for-gestational-age neonate are not criteria for vaginal birth after cesarean delivery. (I, N, G)

72. 3. For maximum effectiveness, RhoGAM should be administered within 72 hours after delivery. Most Rh-negative clients also receive RhoGAM during the prenatal period at 28 weeks' gestation. (I, N, G)

The Postpartal Client With Complications

73. 1. The TPAL acronym (T, number of term infants; P, number of preterm infants; A, abortions; and L, number of currently living children) is useful for recording a client's obstetric history. This client has had four pregnancies, three term infants, two preterm infants, and no abortions and has five living children. (I, N, G)

74. 1. Localized infection may occur in the perineum at laceration, episiotomy, or abdominal incision sites. During pregnancy and the puerperium, the white blood cell count may be slightly elevated, but leukocytosis is uncommon. Blood loss of 400 mL is within normal limits. Temperature of 99 F 1 hour after delivery is usually due to dehydration. (A, N, G)

75. 2. Vaginal examination during labor results in deposits of pathogens in the cervix and later invasion of the decidua by the pathogens. Vaginal trauma, such as laceration, increases the risk of infection. Maternal age over 30 years, use of low forceps, and antepartal infection before labor do not contribute to puerperal infection. (I, N, G)

76. 1. Before administering ampicillin sodium (Polycillin) intravenously, the nurse should ask the client if she has any drug allergies. Antibiotic therapy can cause adverse side effects such as rash or even anaphylaxis. Assessing the amount of lochia is important for all postpartum clients but not necessary before antibiotic therapy. Placing the client in a side-lying position and checking her pulse rate are not necessary. (I, N, G)

77. 3. The nurse should encourage the client to maintain a semi-Fowler's position, which promotes comfort and facilitates drainage. (I, N, H)

78. 4. Heparin (Panheparin) therapy is ordered to prevent clot formation. A side effect of heparin therapy during the puerperium is increased lochia flow. (E, N, G)

79. 2. Protamine sulfate is a heparin antagonist given intravenously to counteract bleeding complications caused by heparin overdose. Calcium gluconate is not used as a heparin antagonist. Methergine is used to treat late postpartum hemorrhage. Nitrofurantoin is an anti-infective drug. (P, N, G)

80. 2. A major complication of deep vein thrombosis is pulmonary embolism. Signs and symptoms, which may occur suddenly and require immediate treatment, include severe chest pain, apprehension, cough (possibly accompanied by hemoptysis), tachycardia, fever, hypotension, diaphoresis, pallor, shortness of breath, and friction rub. Pain in the calf is common with a diagnosis of thrombophlebitis. Bleeding gums may occur due to the heparin therapy and the mother should be cautioned to use a soft toothbrush. Bradycardia in the postpartum period is normal. (P, N, G)

81. 3. Signs of hemorrhage include hematuria, epistaxis, ecchymosis, and bleeding gums. Anorexia is not symptomatic of hemorrhage. (E, N, G)

82. 2. The client diagnosed with cystitis needs to void every 2 to 4 hours while awake to keep her bladder empty. In addition, she should maintain adequate fluid intake and wear cotton-crotch underwear. (P, N, H)

83. 4. The priority nursing diagnosis is Pain related to dysuria and frequency. There are no data to suggest Fear or Ineffective Family Coping. Dysuria related to lengthy labor is not a nursing diagnosis. (D, N, G)

84. 1. The client can continue to breast-feed as often as she desires. Continuation of breast-feeding is limited only by the client's discomfort or malaise. The antibiotic should be chosen carefully to avoid affecting the neonate through the breast milk. (I, N, G)

85. 1. Early postpartal hemorrhage occurs in the first 24 hours postpartum. Postpartal hemorrhage is defined as blood loss greater than 500 mL. Rapid intravenous oxytocin infusion, oxygen therapy, and gentle fundal massage to contract the uterus are usually effective. If bleeding persists, the nurse inspects the cervix and vagina for lacerations. Severe uncontrolled hemorrhage may necessitate hysterectomy. (P, N, G)

86. 4. The most likely cause of this client's uterine atony is overdistention of the uterus from the 10 pound, 2 ounce (4,593 g) neonate. Trauma during delivery is not a likely cause. Although excessive oxytocin use and lengthy or prolonged labor can contribute to uterine atony, this client had a cesarean section for abruptio placenta; it is not likely that she had a long labor or received excessive oxytocin. Besides a large infant, polyhydramnios and bleeding from abruptio placenta or placenta previa can also contribute to uterine atony during the postpartum period. (I, N, H)

87. 1. The priority nursing diagnosis is Altered Tissue Perfusion related to excessive uterine bleeding. Anxiety may occur but is not the nursing priority in this case. There are no data to suggest that the client's cardiac system is impaired. The client is at risk for shock and hypotension, not hypertension, because of the excessive uterine bleeding. (D, N, G)

88. 1. The client being treated for infectious mastitis should continue to breast-feed often. Treatment also includes bed rest, increased fluid intake, local heat application, analgesics, and antibiotic therapy. Continually emptying the breasts decreases the risk of breast abscess. (I, N, G)

89. 4. There is no reason why this client cannot take mild analgesic medications while on antibiotic therapy. The client should apply heat to the infected area, increase fluid intake, and continue taking the antibiotics for 10 days. (E, N, G)

90. 3. Various methods can determine whether a neonate has Down syndrome. The simian crease and genetic studies can be indicative of this disorder. The degree of mental retardation is difficult to predict in a neonate. Down syndrome is an abnormality that can result in an extra chromosome, and it is one form of mental retardation. Older mothers (over 35 years of age) have a higher incidence of Down syndrome children, but this disorder can occur regardless of the mother's age. (E, N, H)

91. 2. The nurse should instruct the client to cleanse the perineal area with warm, soapy water and wipe from front to back with a blotting motion. Plain cool water is not helpful. Sitz baths taken three or four times a day can help increase circulation to the area. Ice packs are helpful for the first 24 hours. (E, N, H)

92. 1. After birth, the client should make the decision about how much she would like to participate in the neonate's care. Seeing and caring for the neonate often facilitates the grief process. The nurse should be nonjudgmental and allow the client any opportunity to see, hold, and care for the neonate. (I, T, L)

93. 1. Methylergonovine maleate (Methergine) can cause hypertension, so the nurse should monitor the client's blood pressure before and after administration. Assessing pulse, respiration, and temperature is important for all postpartum clients but is not specific to Methergine administration. (I, N, G)

94. 4. The most likely cause of delayed postpartum hemorrhage is retained placental fragments. Uterine atony and vaginal and cervical tears are associated with early postpartum hemorrhage. (I, T, G)

95. 1. The client is most likely experiencing postpartum depression. An estimated 50% to 70% of women experience some degree of postpartum depression, or postpartum blues. Explaining that these feelings are normal and asking if she would like to talk about them can be very helpful, especially since she is placing the baby for adoption. Telling her that she is overreacting, is not helpful. She does not exhibit symptoms of mental illness and does not need medication. (I, N, L)

THE NURSING CARE OF THE CHILDBEARING FAMILY AND THEIR NEONATE

TEST 4: Postpartum Care

Directions: Use this answer grid to determine areas of strength or need for further study.

NURSING PROCESS	COGNITIVE LEVEL	CLIENT NEEDS
A = Assessment	K = Knowledge	S = Safe, effective care environment
D = Analysis, nursing diagnosis	C = Comprehension	G = Physiologic integrity
P = Planning	T = Application	L = Psychosocial integrity
I = Implementation	N = Analysis	H = Health promotion and maintenance
E = Evaluation		

Question #	Answer #	Nursing Process					Cognitive Level				Client Needs			
		A	D	P	I	E	K	C	T	N	S	G	L	H
1	1				I					N		G		
2	2				I				T			G		
3	3				I				T			G		
4	1					E				N				H
5	2		D							N			L	
6	3			P						N			L	
7	1				I				T			G		
8	3			P						N			L	
9	4				I					N		G		
10	4		D							N		G		
11	4	A							T			G		
12	3				I					N				H
13	1				I					N				H
14	2				I					N		G		
15	4				I				T			G		
16	2				I					N				H
17	1				I					N		G		
18	2					E				N		G		
19	1				I					N				H
20	2				I					N				H
21	4		D							N		G		
22	3	A								N		G		
23	2				I					N				H
24	4				I				T			G		
25	3		D							N		G		

ANSWER GRID: 1

184

NURSING PROCESS

A = Assessment
D = Analysis, nursing diagnosis
P = Planning
I = Implementation
E = Evaluation

COGNITIVE LEVEL

K = Knowledge
C = Comprehension
T = Application
N = Analysis

CLIENT NEEDS

S = Safe, effective care environment
G = Physiologic integrity
L = Psychosocial integrity
H = Health promotion and maintenance

Question #	Answer #	Nursing Process					Cognitive Level				Client Needs			
		A	D	P	I	E	K	C	T	N	S	G	L	H
26	2				I					N		G		
27	4		D							N		G		
28	1				I					N		G		
29	1				I				T			G		
30	3				I					N		G		
31	1				I					N				H
32	4					E				N				H
33	2				I					N				H
34	3		D							N			L	
35	2			P						N		G		
36	4				I					N				H
37	4			P						N				H
38	4				I				T					H
39	3				I					N		G		
40	3				I					N		G		
41	3				I				T					H
42	2				I					N		G		
43	1				I					N		G		
44	4				I					N				H
45	2				I					N				H
46	1				I					N				H
47	4				I					N				H
48	2			P						N				H
49	2				I					N				H
50	4					E				N				H
51	4					E				N				H
52	3			P						N				H
53	1				I					N				H
54	4				I					N		G		
55	1	A								N				H

ANSWER GRID: 2

NURSING PROCESS

A = Assessment
D = Analysis, nursing diagnosis
P = Planning
I = Implementation
E = Evaluation

COGNITIVE LEVEL

K = Knowledge
C = Comprehension
T = Application
N = Analysis

CLIENT NEEDS

S = Safe, effective care environment
G = Physiologic integrity
L = Psychosocial integrity
H = Health promotion and maintenance

Question #	Answer #	Nursing Process					Cognitive Level				Client Needs			
		A	D	P	I	E	K	C	T	N	S	G	L	H
56	3		D							N				H
57	1				I					N		G		
58	3				I					N				H
59	4				I				T					H
60	4				I					N				H
61	3			P						N				H
62	1				I					N		G		
63	4					E				N				H
64	1				I					N				H
65	2				I				T			G		
66	1					E			T			G		
67	4				I				T			G		
68	3				I					N		G		
69	4				I					N				H
70	3					E				N				H
71	1				I					N		G		
72	3				I					N		G		
73	1				I					N		G		
74	1	A								N		G		
75	2				I					N		G		
76	1				I					N		G		
77	3				I					N				H
78	4					E				N		G		
79	2			P						N		G		
80	2			P						N		G		
81	3					E				N		G		
82	2			P						N				H
83	4		D							N		G		
84	1				I					N		G		
85	1			P						N		G		

NURSING PROCESS

A = Assessment
D = Analysis, nursing diagnosis
P = Planning
I = Implementation
E = Evaluation

COGNITIVE LEVEL

K = Knowledge
C = Comprehension
T = Application
N = Analysis

CLIENT NEEDS

S = Safe, effective care environment
G = Physiologic integrity
L = Psychosocial integrity
H = Health promotion and maintenance

Question #	Answer #	Nursing Process					Cognitive Level				Client Needs			
		A	D	P	I	E	K	C	T	N	S	G	L	H
86	4				I					N				H
87	1		D							N		G		
88	1				I					N		G		
89	4					E				N		G	L	
90	3					E				N				H
91	2					E				N				H
92	1				I				T				L	
93	1				I					N		G		
94	4				I				T			G		
95	1				I					N			L	
Number Correct														
Number Possible	95	4	9	11	58	13	0	0	15	80	0	50	6	39
Percentage Correct														

Score Calculation: To determine your **Percentage Correct,** divide the **Number Correct** by the **Number Possible.**

ANSWER GRID: 4

The Neonatal Client

- **The Neonatal Client**
- **Physical Assessment of the Neonatal Client**
- **The Post-Term Neonate**
- **The Neonate With Risk Factors**
- **Correct Answers and Rationale**

Select the one best answer, and indicate your choice by filling in the circle in front of the option.

The Neonatal Client

The nurse notes that for almost an hour after birth, the neonate was awake, alert, and startled and cried easily. Respirations rose to 70 breaths/minute, and heart rate on two occasions was 160 beats/minute.

1. After sleeping quietly for about 2 hours, the neonate then awoke with a start, cried, extended and flexed all four extremities, and then choked, gagged, and regurgitated some thick mucus. The nurse should
- ○ 1. call the physician because the neonate appears to be choking.
- ○ 2. change the neonate's position and aspirate mucus as necessary.
- ○ 3. place the neonate under a radiant warmer because these signs suggest chilling.
- ○ 4. wrap the neonate in a blanket and offer glucose water.

2. During the first feeding, the nurse observes the neonate gagging on mucus and becoming cyanotic. The nurse should *first*
- ○ 1. start mouth-to-mouth resuscitation.
- ○ 2. contact the neonatal resuscitation team.
- ○ 3. raise the neonate's head and pat the back gently.
- ○ 4. clear the neonate's airway with suction or gravity.

3. The nurse is able to retract the neonate's foreskin only slightly beyond the urethral opening without using force. Before cleansing the penis, the nurse should
- ○ 1. retract the foreskin as far as it will move back easily.
- ○ 2. use gentle force to retract the foreskin gradually farther each day.
- ○ 3. leave the foreskin in place, and prepare to use cotton balls to help with cleansing.
- ○ 4. report the condition to the physician for possible corrective measures.

4. During a home visit on the third postpartum day, the nurse weighs the neonate. The neonate weighed 9 pounds, 1 ounce at birth. He now weighs 8 pounds, 12 ounces. The nurse instructs the mother to
- ○ 1. continue feeding on demand because the weight loss is within normal limits.
- ○ 2. increase the amount of formula to prevent further weight loss.
- ○ 3. switch to a soy milk formula because the current formula appears inadequate.
- ○ 4. give additional feedings because the weight loss indicates inadequate intake.

5. To assess the neonate for jaundice, the nurse plans to
- ○ 1. blanch the skin on the forehead during a feeding.
- ○ 2. blanch the skin on the buttocks during a diaper change.
- ○ 3. observe the skin in natural daylight.
- ○ 4. observe the skin when the neonate is asleep.

6. The client asks the nurse, "When will this soft spot near the back of his head close?" The nurse should instruct the mother that the neonate's posterior fontanel will normally close by age
- ○ 1. 2 to 3 months.
- ○ 2. 6 to 8 months.
- ○ 3. 10 to 12 months.
- ○ 4. 14 to 16 months.

A viable female neonate is delivered vaginally at 40 weeks' gestation. The neonate has Apgar scores of 9 at 1 minute and 10 at 5 minutes after birth.

7. Immediately after delivery, the nurse keeps the infant under a radiant warmer away from the cooling ducts in the room to prevent heat loss. The nurse should explain to the mother that keeping the infant away from the cooling ducts prevents heat loss by
   ○ 1. evaporation.
   ○ 2. convection.
   ○ 3. conduction.
   ○ 4. radiation.

8. Soon after delivery, the neonate receives an injection of vitamin K. After explaining the purpose of vitamin K, the nurse determines that the mother understands when she says that it is given to the neonate because
   ○ 1. neonates have no gastrointestinal bacteria.
   ○ 2. neonates are susceptible to clotting disorders.
   ○ 3. hemolysis of the fetal red blood cells destroys vitamin K.
   ○ 4. the neonate's liver does not produce sufficient vitamin K.

9. When instructing the mother about the neonate's need for sensory and visual stimulation, the nurse should plan to explain that the most highly developed sense in the neonate is
   ○ 1. taste.
   ○ 2. smell.
   ○ 3. touch.
   ○ 4. vision.

10. The nurse assesses the neonate's cry as infrequent and very high-pitched. The nurse should
    ○ 1. tell the mother that excessive analgesia in labor can cause this type of cry.
    ○ 2. notify the physician because this may indicate a neurologic problem.
    ○ 3. stimulate the neonate to cry and document findings.
    ○ 4. continue to monitor the infant.

11. The nurse notes small, shiny white specks on the neonate's gums and hard palate. The nurse should
    ○ 1. place the neonate in an isolation area.
    ○ 2. try to remove the specks with a wet washcloth.
    ○ 3. try to obtain a sterile specimen on a swab.
    ○ 4. continue to monitor the neonate because these spots are normal.

12. During the initial assessment, the nurse notes that the neonate's hands and feet are bluish. The nurse should
    ○ 1. wrap the neonate in several warm blankets.
    ○ 2. ask the mother to massage the neonate's hands and feet.
    ○ 3. keep the neonate in an isolation incubator for at least 2 hours.
    ○ 4. report the cyanosis to the physician promptly.

Physical Assessment of the Neonatal Client

The nurse is responsible for assessing a male neonate about 12 hours old. The neonate was delivered vaginally.

13. The nurse should plan to assess the neonate's physical condition
    ○ 1. midway between feedings.
    ○ 2. while the infant is awake and crying.
    ○ 3. after the neonate has been NPO for 4 hours.
    ○ 4. at least every hour.

14. During the assessment, the nurse observes a gray pigmented nevi on the neonate's buttocks. The nurse documents this as
    ○ 1. Mongolian spot.
    ○ 2. harlequin's sign.
    ○ 3. port wine stain.
    ○ 4. molar nevi.

15. The nurse notes a swelling on the neonate's scalp that crosses the suture line. The nurse should instruct the mother that this condition is known as
    ○ 1. cephalhematoma.
    ○ 2. caput succedaneum.
    ○ 3. cranial edema.
    ○ 4. normal caput.

16. The nurse plans to assess the neonate's temperature with a disposable digital thermometer. The nurse plans to place the thermometer
    ○ 1. under the neonate's tongue.
    ○ 2. under the neonate's arm.
    ○ 3. into the neonate's rectum.
    ○ 4. into the neonate's ear.

17. The nurse measures the circumference of the neonate's head and chest, then explains to the mother that when the two measurements are compared, the head is normally about
    ○ 1. the same size as the chest.
    ○ 2. 2 cm larger than the chest.
    ○ 3. 3 cm smaller than the chest.
    ○ 4. 4 cm larger than the chest.

18. The nurse has explained to the mother about the causes of the neonate's cranial molding. After giving instruction, the nurse determines that the mother needs *further* instruction when she says,
    ○ 1. "The molding is due to an overriding of the cranial bones."
    ○ 2. "The amount of molding is related to the amount and length of pressure on the head."
    ○ 3. "The molding will usually disappear in a couple of days."
    ○ 4. "The neonate may suffer brain damage if the molding doesn't resolve quickly."

The nurse is responsible for the initial assessment of a term female neonate, about 4 hours old.

19. The nurse documents the neonate's anterior fontanel as normal because it is
○ 1. oval.
○ 2. square.
○ 3. diamond shaped.
○ 4. triangular.

20. While performing a gestational age assessment, the nurse determines that the neonate is at term when the nurse observes the neonate's
○ 1. ear lying flat against the head.
○ 2. absence of rugae in the scrotum.
○ 3. sole creases covering the entire foot.
○ 4. absence of tremors.

21. The nurse plans to perform a complete assessment of the neonate. For which of the following findings should the nurse notify the pediatrician?
○ 1. Red reflex in the eyes.
○ 2. Expiratory grunt.
○ 3. Respiratory rate of 40 breaths/minute.
○ 4. Full breast areola.

22. The nurse instructs the mother about normal reflexes of term neonates. The nurse determines that the mother understands the instructions when she describes the tonic neck reflex as when the neonate
○ 1. steps briskly when placed near a firm surface.
○ 2. pulls both arms and does not move the chin beyond the point of the elbows.
○ 3. turns the head to the left side, extends the left extremities, and flexes the right extremities.
○ 4. turns the head to the left side, and then forward when lifted from the crib.

23. The mother expresses concern when it is discovered that the neonate's eyes are crossed. The nurse explains to the mother that strabismus in a neonate is considered
○ 1. normal because the eyes cannot focus on light at this time.
○ 2. normal because there is lack of eye muscle coordination in neonates.
○ 3. abnormal because this indicates that a neurologic impairment exists.
○ 4. abnormal because most neonates can focus the eyes well.

24. The nurse notes a white, cheese-like substance on the neonate's body creases. The nurse should instruct the mother to
○ 1. remove it with hand lotion.
○ 2. remove it with alcohol and cotton balls.
○ 3. allow it to remain on the skin.
○ 4. brush it off with a dry wash cloth.

A term neonate is to be [   ] days of age. The nurse p[   ] before discharge.

25. The nurse examine[   ] Which of the follo[   ] sessment?
○ 1. Many creases [   ]
○ 2. Frequent snee[   ]
○ 3. A single crease on the palm.
○ 4. Dry, peeling skin.

26. The neonate's mother asks, "When will the soft spot near the front of his head close?" The nurse should explain that the neonate's anterior fontanel will normally close by age
○ 1. 4 to 6 months.
○ 2. 6 to 8 months.
○ 3. 10 to 12 months.
○ 4. 12 to 18 months.

27. Laboratory findings indicate that the neonate's hemoglobin is 16 g/100 mL of blood. The nurse should
○ 1. document this as a normal finding.
○ 2. assess for symptoms of polycythemia.
○ 3. recheck the hemoglobin in 1 hour.
○ 4. assess for skin pallor and anemia.

28. While assessing the neonate's eyes, the nurse notes the following: absence of tears, corneas of unequal size, constriction of the pupils in response to bright light, and presence of a red circle on the pupils on ophthalmoscopic examination. The nurse should notify the physician about the neonate's
○ 1. absence of tears.
○ 2. corneas of unequal size.
○ 3. constriction of pupils.
○ 4. presence of red circle on pupils.

29. After teaching the mother about the neonate's positive Babinski's reflex, the nurse determines that the mother understands the instructions when she says that a positive Babinski's reflex indicates
○ 1. possible partial paralysis.
○ 2. immature central nervous system.
○ 3. possible lower limb defect.
○ 4. possible injury to nerves that innervate the legs.

30. The nurse is planning to obtain a blood sample to screen the neonate for phenylketonuria. The nurse plans to obtain the sample from the neonate's
○ 1. heel.
○ 2. radial artery.
○ 3. scalp vein.
○ 4. brachial artery.

The Post-Term Neonate

The nurse is caring for a neonate delivered by cesarean section at 42 weeks' gestation. The neonate weighed 9

(4.1 kg) and had Apgar scores of 8 at 1
at 5 minutes after birth.

While assessing the neonate, the nurse explains to
the mother that post-term neonates typically have
○ 1. Soft, oily skin.
○ 2. a long, thin body.
○ 3. very few sole creases.
○ 4. abundant lanugo.

32. When the neonate is 2 hours old, the nurse notes
increased respiratory rate and tremors of the hands
and feet. A priority nursing diagnosis is
○ 1. Ineffective Airway Clearance related to post-term
gestational age.
○ 2. Hyperthermia related to large size and use of radiant warmer.
○ 3. Decreased Cardiac Output related to difficult delivery.
○ 4. Altered Nutrition, Less Than Body Requirements
related to depleted glycogen stores.

33. After circumcision, the nurse observes a 2-cm circle
of bright red bleeding on the neonate's diaper. The
nurse should *first*
○ 1. notify the physician immediately.
○ 2. check the diaper and circumcision again in 30
minutes.
○ 3. secure the diaper tightly to apply pressure on the
site.
○ 4. apply gentle pressure to the site with a sterile
gauze pad.

34. The nurse formulates a goal for the neonate before
dismissal. Because of the neonate's postmaturity, a
priority goal is: Before discharge, the neonate will
○ 1. establish a deep respiratory pattern.
○ 2. gain 4 ounces by the time of dismissal.
○ 3. maintain normal temperature.
○ 4. maintain a normal bilirubin level.

35. The nurse makes a home visit to the family when the
neonate is 5 days old. The nurse notes the following:
frequent hiccups; loose, wet stool in diaper; red rash
on face; and dry peeling skin. Which of these findings warrant further assessment?
○ 1. Frequent hiccups.
○ 2. Loose, wet stool in diaper.
○ 3. Red rash on face.
○ 4. Dry, peeling skin.

A male neonate is admitted to the observation nursery
after a vaginal delivery with low forceps. He is post-term
and weighs 9 pounds (4,000 g).

36. During initial assessment, the nurse detects Ortolani's sign. The nurse should
○ 1. determine if the neonate's mother had anesthesia.
○ 2. notify the physician promptly.
○ 3. keep the neonate under the radiant warmer for
2 hours.
○ 4. obtain a blood sample to check for hypoglycemia.

37. After circumcision using a Plastibell, the nurse instructs the neonate's mother to cleanse the circumcision site with
○ 1. alcohol swabs.
○ 2. warm water.
○ 3. povidone-iodine (Betadine) solution.
○ 4. diluted hydrogen peroxide.

38. At 24 hours of age, the nurse observes that the infant
has his eyes closed, is breathing regularly, and has
no sign of eye movements. The nurse determines
that this neonate is most likely in
○ 1. drug withdrawal.
○ 2. first period of reactivity.
○ 3. a state of deep sleep.
○ 4. cardiac distress.

The Neonate With Risk Factors

A male neonate is delivered by cesarean section owing to
placenta previa. He is classified as preterm and appropriate for gestational age of 37 weeks.

39. As soon as the neonate is delivered, the circulating
nurse should *first*
○ 1. stimulate the neonate to cough deeply.
○ 2. aspirate mucus from the mouth with a bulb syringe.
○ 3. begin resuscitation procedures with bag and
mask.
○ 4. hold the infant upright for the mother to view.

40. The neonate is to be given oxygen through a mask
attached to wall oxygen. While administering the
oxygen, the nurse should position the neonate on
the
○ 1. left side, with the neck slightly flexed.
○ 2. back, with the head turned to the left side.
○ 3. abdomen, with the head down.
○ 4. back, with the neck slightly extended.

41. External cardiac massage becomes necessary for the
neonate. The nurse should
○ 1. alternate cardiac massage with ventilation.
○ 2. compress the sternum with the palm of the hand.
○ 3. compress the heart 70 to 80 times/minute.
○ 4. displace the chest wall 1.5 inches.

42. After respirations and heartbeat are established, the

neonate is placed in an oxygen hood in a radiant warmer. While administering oxygen in a hood, the nurse should
- ○ 1. humidify the air being delivered.
- ○ 2. cover the neonate's scalp with a warm cap.
- ○ 3. continue to check the neonate's pulse continuously.
- ○ 4. check the neonate's glucose level.

43. The neonate is to be transferred by ambulance to a level III nursery. To prepare the parents for the transfer, the nurse should plan to
- ○ 1. instruct the parents that the neonate is in critical condition.
- ○ 2. obtain the father's consent for the neonate's transfer.
- ○ 3. allow the parents to touch the neonate before transfer.
- ○ 4. Ask the father if he desires to ride in the ambulance during the transfer.

44. The neonate is diagnosed with respiratory distress syndrome (RDS). The nurse should explain to the parents that this syndrome is caused by an alteration in the body's secretion of
- ○ 1. somatotropin.
- ○ 2. surfactant.
- ○ 3. pituitary hormone.
- ○ 4. progesterone.

45. The nurse evaluates the adequacy of the neonate's oxygen therapy by monitoring
- ○ 1. cyanosis on hands and feet.
- ○ 2. pulse rate continuously.
- ○ 3. arterial blood gas levels.
- ○ 4. the percentage of oxygen received.

A 28-year-old primigravida delivered a viable male neonate at 34 weeks' gestation by cesarean section because of a frank breech presentation. The neonate is admitted to the neonatal intensive care nursery.

46. The neonate is diagnosed with RDS and is given oxygen. The nurse plans to instruct the mother that the neonate is at greater risk for respiratory distress syndrome because the
- ○ 1. client had a breech presentation.
- ○ 2. neonate was preterm.
- ○ 3. client received analgesia during labor.
- ○ 4. neonate had sluggish respiratory efforts after delivery.

47. The mother asks why the neonate's oxygen is humidified. The nurse's best response is that oxygen is humidified to help
- ○ 1. promote expansion of the lungs.

- ○ 2. decrease bacterial growth in the nasopharynx.
- ○ 3. prevent drying of the mucous membranes.
- ○ 4. improve blood circulation in the cardiac system.

48. To prevent heat loss in the neonate from conduction, the nurse should
- ○ 1. dry the neonate with warm sterile towels.
- ○ 2. keep the infant away from air conditioning.
- ○ 3. place the neonate in a radiant warmer.
- ○ 4. warm the stethoscope before using it on the neonate.

49. The neonate is to be fed by a nasal gavage catheter. In planning for this procedure, the nurse should *first* plan to lubricate the catheter with
- ○ 1. normal saline.
- ○ 2. sterile water.
- ○ 3. plain water.
- ○ 4. water-soluble jelly.

50. After a gavage catheter is inserted for the neonate's next feeding, the nurse should
- ○ 1. clamp the catheter for one minute.
- ○ 2. obtain an order for a chest radiograph.
- ○ 3. aspirate stomach contents through the catheter.
- ○ 4. instill about 10 mL of sterile water into the catheter.

A preterm neonate is admitted to the neonatal intensive care nursery at about 30 weeks' gestation and is placed in an oxygenated isolation incubator.

51. The neonate's mother tells the nurse that she was planning to breast-feed the neonate. The nurse should instruct the client that breast-feeding
- ○ 1. is not recommended because the neonate needs increased fat in the diet.
- ○ 2. can be done once the neonate no longer needs oxygen.
- ○ 3. is contraindicated because the neonate needs a high-calorie formula every 2 hours.
- ○ 4. can be given by gavage feedings until the neonate can coordinate sucking and swallowing.

52. The nurse plans to explain care of the neonate to the parents. The nurse should plan to explain to the parents that the neonate will be assessed daily for symptoms of retinopathy of prematurity (ROP) because the neonate is
- ○ 1. at risk because of multiple factors.
- ○ 2. likely to have hypoglycemia.
- ○ 3. alkalotic at birth.
- ○ 4. likely to receive phototherapy.

53. While assisting the neonatologist to assess the neonate for symptoms of ROP, the nurse becomes con-

cerned when the neonatologist says that the neonate has
- ○ 1. sunken orbital sockets.
- ○ 2. strabismus.
- ○ 3. a reaction to bright light.
- ○ 4. constricted retinal vessels.

54. The mother asks the nurse about treatment for complications related to retinopathy of prematurity. The nurse should explain to the mother that treatment may include
- ○ 1. laser therapy.
- ○ 2. continual eye drops.
- ○ 3. frequent testing for glaucoma.
- ○ 4. corneal transplants.

55. Before the neonate's discharge, the mother tells the nurse that she is worried that her 5-year-old daughter will be jealous of the new baby when they get home. After explaining ways to deal with sibling rivalry, the nurse determines that the mother understands the instructions when she says she will
- ○ 1. divide her time equally between the baby and the daughter.
- ○ 2. tell the daughter that the baby is just like one of her dolls.
- ○ 3. let the 5-year-old feed the baby every day.
- ○ 4. allow the 5-year-old undivided attention several times a day.

A neonate is admitted to the neonatal intensive care nursery at about 28 weeks' gestation, weighing 3 pounds, 4 ounces (1,474 g).

56. Soon after admission to the neonatal intensive care unit, the nurse formulates a nursing diagnosis for the neonate. A priority nursing diagnosis at this time is
- ○ 1. Potential for Respiratory Distress Syndrome related to prematurity.
- ○ 2. Altered Nutrition related to preterm gestational age.
- ○ 3. Impaired Gas Exchange related to immature pulmonary vasculature.
- ○ 4. Transient Tachypnea related to immature respiratory system.

57. Three days after admission, the neonatologist plans to assess the neonate for intraventricular hemorrhage (IVF). The nurse should plan to assist the neonatologist with the
- ○ 1. ultrasound scan.
- ○ 2. arterial blood draw.
- ○ 3. gestational age assessment.
- ○ 4. exchange transfusion.

58. The nurse should explain to the parents that signs and symptoms of IVF include
- ○ 1. polycythemia.
- ○ 2. hyperbilirubinemia.
- ○ 3. bulging fontanels.
- ○ 4. hyperactivity.

59. The nurse assesses the neonate daily for symptoms of necrotizing enterocolitis. The nurse should notify the neonatologist if the nurse observes
- ○ 1. 5 mL of gastric residual before gavage feedings.
- ○ 2. jaundice of the face and chest.
- ○ 3. increase in bowel peristalsis.
- ○ 4. abdominal distention.

60. The neonate is diagnosed with bronchopulmonary dysplasia. After teaching the mother about the disease, the nurse determines that she understands the instructions when she says that bronchopulmonary dysplasia
- ○ 1. is an acute disease that can be treated with antibiotics.
- ○ 2. may require permanent ventilation.
- ○ 3. can be cured with the use of bronchodilators.
- ○ 4. can lead to seizures.

61. The neonatologist diagnoses the neonate as having a pneumothorax. The nurse plans to assist the neonatologist to
- ○ 1. place the neonate on a ventilator.
- ○ 2. administer oxygen by endotracheal tube.
- ○ 3. suction the neonate's nares with wall suction.
- ○ 4. insert a chest tube into the neonate.

A neonate is admitted to the neonatal intensive care nursery for observation with a diagnosis of probable meconium aspiration syndrome (MAS). The neonate weighs 10 pounds, 4 ounces and is at 42 weeks' gestation.

62. The neonate has a heart rate of 110 beats/minute and a respiratory rate of 40 breaths/minute with periods of apnea. The nurse should further assess the neonate for
- ○ 1. alkalosis.
- ○ 2. hypoglycemia.
- ○ 3. hyporesonance.
- ○ 4. excessive coughing.

63. Soon after admission, the nurse formulates a nursing diagnosis for the neonate. A priority nursing diagnosis for the neonate is
- ○ 1. Ineffective Breathing Pattern related to respiratory distress.
- ○ 2. Altered Nutrition, More than Body Requirements related to large size.

○ 3. Potential for Pneumothorax related to meconium aspiration syndrome.

○ 4. Ineffective Gas Exchange related to the presence of respiratory distress.

64. The nurse plans care for the neonate diagnosed with MAS. The nurse should plan for

○ 1. insertion of an umbilical arterial line.

○ 2. frequent ultrasound scans.

○ 3. orogastric feedings as soon as possible.

○ 4. detection of symptoms of hyperglycemia.

65. The physician orders intravenous tolazoline (Priscoline) to be given to the neonate. While the drug is being administered, the nurse plans to monitor the neonate's

○ 1. activity pattern.

○ 2. temperature.

○ 3. skin color.

○ 4. blood pressure.

A gravida II, para II has learned that her neonate is diagnosed with hemolytic disease of the newborn. The neonate is admitted to the neonatal intensive care unit soon after delivery.

66. The mother asks the nurse why the neonate has hemolytic disease of the newborn. The nurse explains that the neonate develops the disease when the

○ 1. mother is Rh positive and the father is Rh negative.

○ 2. parents are both Rh negative.

○ 3. the mother is Rh negative and the father is Rh positive.

○ 4. the fetus is Rh negative and the mother is Rh positive.

67. After teaching the client about Rh sensitization, the nurse determines that the client understands why she was not sensitized during her other pregnancy when she says that

○ 1. the other baby probably had a different father.

○ 2. most women today have immunity against the Rh factor.

○ 3. antibodies are not ordinarily formed until after exposure to an antigen.

○ 4. the mother's blood was able to neutralize antibodies formed during the first pregnancy.

68. The nurse teaches the client about the effects of hemolysis due to Rh sensitization on the neonate at delivery. The nurse determines that the client needs *further* instruction when she says that the neonate may have

○ 1. cardiac decompensation.

○ 2. polycythemia.

○ 3. anemia.

○ 4. enlargement of the spleen.

69. The neonate is to receive phototherapy. The nurse should plan to instruct the neonate's mother that during the phototherapy, the neonate's

○ 1. genital area will be covered.

○ 2. temperature will be assessed every 30 minutes.

○ 3. feedings will be given by orogastric tube.

○ 4. parents will not be able to provide any care.

A 30-year-old gravida IV, para III at 30 weeks' gestation is admitted to the hospital for evaluation. The client has experienced three stillbirths due to hemolytic disease of the newborn.

70. An amniocentesis is to be performed to evaluate bilirubin density. In preparing for this procedure, the nurse obtains a specimen container that is

○ 1. dark.

○ 2. clear.

○ 3. clean.

○ 4. heat resistant.

71. Because the client has experienced hemolytic disease of the newborn in previous pregnancies, the nurse should explain to the client that the client will most likely have frequent antibody titers evaluated by withdrawing

○ 1. placental blood.

○ 2. amniotic fluid.

○ 3. fetal blood.

○ 4. maternal blood.

72. The client is to undergo percutaneous umbilical blood sampling (PUBS) to assess fetal hemoglobin and hematocrit. After giving instruction, the nurse determines that the client needs *further* instruction when she says that

○ 1. she will be placed in a supine position in a cylindrical unit.

○ 2. transient fetal bradycardia is common after the procedure.

○ 3. fetal blood transfusion is possible with this procedure.

○ 4. a needle will be inserted into the client's abdomen.

73. After delivery, a direct Coombs' test is performed on the umbilical cord blood. The nurse explains to the client that this test is done to detect

○ 1. degree of anemia in the neonate.

○ 2. electrolyte imbalances in the neonate.

○ 3. antibodies coating the neonate's red blood cells.

○ 4. antigens coating the neonate's red blood cells.

74. The neonate is to receive an exchange transfusion.

After explaining the purpose of the exchange transfusion, the nurse determines that the mother understands when she says that exchange transfusion is done to

○ 1. replenish the neonate's leukocytes.

○ 2. restore the fluid and electrolyte balance.

○ 3. correct the neonate's anemia.

○ 4. replace Rh-negative blood with Rh-positive blood.

75. Before the transfusion, the nurse explains to the mother that treatment of hemolytic disease by exchange transfusion is necessary to prevent damage to the neonate's

○ 1. heart.

○ 2. brain.

○ 3. lungs.

○ 4. pituitary gland.

A neonate is delivered by cesarean section because the mother is a class B insulin-dependent diabetic. The neonate weighs 10 pounds, 1 ounce (4,564 g), is large for gestational age, and is admitted to the neonatal intensive care unit.

76. The nurse formulates a nursing diagnosis for the neonate soon after admission. A priority nursing diagnosis is

○ 1. Potential for Hyperbilirubinemia related to maternal diabetes.

○ 2. High Risk for Hypothermia related to cesarean section delivery.

○ 3. Potential for Hypoglycemia related to cesarean section.

○ 4. Altered Nutrition, Less Than Body Requirements related to increased glucose metabolism.

77. The mother visits the neonate 3 hours after birth. The nurse should explain to the mother that the neonate is being closely monitored for symptoms of hypoglycemia because of

○ 1. an increased use of glucose stores during a difficult labor.

○ 2. an interruption in the supply of maternal glucose and continued high production of insulin by the neonate.

○ 3. a normal response that occurs during transition from intrauterine to extrauterine life.

○ 4. an increase in the urine production, which occurs as a result of decreased glucose stores.

78. In planning care for the neonate of a diabetic mother, the nurse plans to assess the neonate for fracture of the neonate's

○ 1. clavicle.

○ 2. skull.

○ 3. wrist.

○ 4. rib cage.

79. After therapy for hypoglycemia, the nurse observes that the neonate's blood glucose level is 60 mg/dL but that the neonate is still exhibiting jitteriness and tremors. The nurse notifies the physician because these symptoms may indicate

○ 1. galactosemia.

○ 2. biliary duct obstruction.

○ 3. viral infection.

○ 4. hypocalcemia.

80. The neonate's mother asks, "Why is my baby in the neonatal intensive care unit?" The nurse's best response is that neonates of class B diabetic mothers frequently develop

○ 1. anemia.

○ 2. hypertension.

○ 3. hemolytic disease.

○ 4. RDS.

A primigravida at about 36 weeks' gestation is admitted to the hospital's labor and delivery unit in active labor. The client has had no prenatal care and admits to the nurse that she has been using cocaine during the pregnancy.

81. After learning that the client has been using cocaine, the nurse should inform

○ 1. the nursing unit manager so appropriate agencies can be notified.

○ 2. the head of the hospital's security department.

○ 3. the chaplain in case the fetus dies in utero.

○ 4. the physician who will attend the delivery of the infant.

82. After delivery, the neonate is admitted to the intensive care unit, where the nurse observes her closely for symptoms of cocaine withdrawal. The nurse should observe the neonate for

○ 1. postmaturity.

○ 2. high-pitched cry.

○ 3. sluggishness.

○ 4. hypocalcemia.

83. The nurse instructs the mother about likely gastrointestinal symptoms in the neonate. The nurse determines that the instructions have been effective when the mother states that a common symptom is

○ 1. colic.

○ 2. constipation.

○ 3. vomiting.

○ 4. abdominal distention.

84. The nurse plans to instruct the mother to help comfort the neonate when she is fussy by

○ 1. tightly swaddling the neonate.

○ 2. feeding the neonate extra, high-calorie formula.

○ 3. keeping the neonate in a brightly lit environment.

○ 4. touching the neonate only when she is crying.

A neonate born at 36 weeks' gestation is admitted to the neonatal nursery for observation. The neonate's mother is human immunodeficiency virus (HIV) positive and has received no prenatal care.

85. The neonate's mother asks the nurse if her neonate has HIV. The nurse should instruct the mother that

○ 1. more than 80% of neonates born to mothers who are positive for HIV are also positive.

○ 2. an enlarged skull at birth generally means the neonate is HIV positive.

○ 3. only a complete blood serum analysis can determine if the neonate is HIV positive.

○ 4. most neonates are asymptomatic at birth and are usually positive for the HIV antibody.

86. The mother of the neonate tells the nurse that she breast-fed with her last neonate and would like to breast-feed this neonate as soon as possible. The nurse should instruct the mother that breast milk

○ 1. can help prevent the spread of the HIV virus.

○ 2. contains antibodies that can protect the neonate from HIV.

○ 3. can be beneficial for the bonding process.

○ 4. has been found to contain the retrovirus HIV.

87. While caring for the neonate, the nurse prepares to administer an ordered vitamin K intramuscular injection. The nurse plans to *first*

○ 1. wear clean gloves to bathe the baby.

○ 2. perform a gestational age assessment.

○ 3. wash the injection site with povidone-iodine (Betadine) solution.

○ 4. wear sterile gloves before administration of the medication.

A male neonate is delivered at 38 weeks' gestation by cesarean section. The neonate's mother had prolonged rupture of membranes and an oral temperature of 102 F (38.8 C).

88. The nurse plans to observe the neonate closely for symptoms of infection. Which of the following observations suggesting infection should the nurse report to the physician?

○ 1. Leukocytosis.

○ 2. Apical heart rate of 132 beats/minute.

○ 3. Lethargy or extreme irritability.

○ 4. Warm, moist skin.

89. The neonate is diagnosed with sepsis and is to be treated with intravenous antibiotics. The nurse should instruct the parents that because of the neonate's infection, they will

○ 1. need to be cautious around the isolation incubator and equipment.

○ 2. be able to visit the neonate but not touch him.

○ 3. need to wash their hands thoroughly before touching him.

○ 4. be required to avoid the intravenous access site.

90. Later in the day, the neonate's condition deteriorates, and death appears likely within the next few minutes. The parents are Roman Catholic, and they request that the neonate be baptized. The nurse should

○ 1. contact the hospital chaplain to perform the baptism.

○ 2. alert the hospital's director that a neonatal death is imminent.

○ 3. find a health care provider who is Roman Catholic to perform the baptism.

○ 4. baptize the neonate, regardless of the nurse's own religious beliefs.

A female neonate delivered vaginally at term with a cleft lip and cleft palate is admitted to the regular nursery.

91. The first time that the parents visit the neonate in the nursery, the nurse should

○ 1. explain the surgical interventions that will be performed.

○ 2. stress that this defect is not life-threatening.

○ 3. emphasize the neonate's normal characteristics.

○ 4. reassure the parents about the success rate of the surgery.

92. The nurse teaches the parents about appropriate feeding techniques when the neonate is 2 hours of age. The nurse determines that the mother needs *further* instruction when the mother says,

○ 1. "I should clean her with soapy water after feeding."

○ 2. "I should feed her in an upright position."

○ 3. "I need to remember to burp her often."

○ 4. "I may need to use a special nipple for feeding."

93. The nurse formulates a nursing diagnosis for the neonate soon after admission. A priority nursing diagnosis for the neonate is

○ 1. Activity Intolerance related to respiratory distress syndrome.

○ 2. High Risk for Infection related to potential for aspiration during feedings.

○ 3. Dysfunctional Family Coping related to congenital malformation of the neonate.

○ 4. Impaired Skin Integrity related to frequent treatments.

A male neonate born at about 36 weeks' gestation is admitted to the neonatal intensive care nursery with a diagnosis of probable fetal alcohol syndrome (FAS).

94. The mother visits the nursery soon after the neonate is admitted. When instructing the mother about FAS, the nurse plans to instruct the mother that

○ 1. withdrawal symptoms usually do not occur until 7 days after delivery.

○ 2. intrauterine growth retardation is unlikely with this condition.

○ 3. facial deformities associated with FAS can be corrected by plastic surgery.

○ 4. symptoms of withdrawal include tremors, sleeplessness, and seizures.

95. The nurse instructs the mother about long-term outcomes for the neonate with FAS. The nurse should instruct the mother that neonates with FAS

○ 1. are often listless and lethargic.

○ 2. tend to have average IQ scores.

○ 3. tend to be hyperactive with speech disorders.

○ 4. have a 70% mortality rate unless treated.

96. The nurse formulates a nursing diagnosis for the neonate soon after admission. A priority nursing diagnosis is

○ 1. Altered Growth and Development related to poor parenting abilities of the mother.

○ 2. Altered Nutrition, Less Than Body Requirements related to hyperirritability.

○ 3. High Risk for Respiratory Distress related to jitteriness.

○ 4. High Risk for Brain Damage related to FAS.

A neonate is admitted to the intensive care nursery and is diagnosed with gastroschisis. The father of the neonate accompanies the neonate to the nursery.

97. The nurse caring for the neonate plans to *first*

○ 1. weigh the neonate.

○ 2. insert an orogastric tube.

○ 3. prepare for an immediate blood transfusion.

○ 4. cover the abdomen with a moistened sterile gauze.

98. The father of the neonate tells the nurse that his wife planned on breast-feeding the neonate. The nurse should instruct the father that the neonate will

○ 1. remain NPO until after surgery.

○ 2. need to receive iron-fortified formula.

○ 3. receive nourishment by hyperalimentation.

○ 4. be allowed to breast-feed before surgery.

99. The nurse has instructed the father about the major nursing goals for the neonate. The nurse determines that the father needs *further* instruction when he says that one of the goals is to

○ 1. prevent hypothermia.

○ 2. maintain fluid and electrolyte balance.

○ 3. provide adequate nourishment.

○ 4. prevent infection.

100. The parents seem hesitant to touch the neonate because of his appearance. The nurse determines that the parents are most likely in the stage of grief termed

○ 1. denial.

○ 2. shock.

○ 3. fear.

○ 4. anger.

CORRECT ANSWERS AND RATIONALE

The letters in parentheses following the rationale identify the step of the nursing process (A, D, P, I, E); cognitive level (K, C, T, N); and client needs (S, G, L, H). See the Answer Grid for the key.

The Neonatal Client

1. 2. The first period of reactivity begins at birth and lasts about 30 minutes. The neonate then falls asleep for 2 to 4 hours. The neonate then begins the second period of reactivity, which lasts 4 to 6 hours. This neonate's signs and symptoms are normal for the neonate's age. The neonate appears to be regurgitating and choking on mucus, which is common during the second period of reactivity. The recommended procedure in this situation is to change the neonate's position and aspirate mucus as necessary. These symptoms are not indicative of chilling. Placing the neonate in a radiant warmer is not warranted unless the temperature falls. Offering glucose water is not appropriate if the neonate is choking. (I, N, G)

2. 4. If a neonate gags on mucus and becomes cyanotic during the first feeding, the airway is most likely closed. The nurse should clear the airway with gravity (by lowering the infant's head) or suction. Mouth-to-mouth resuscitation and contacting the neonatal resuscitation team are not warranted unless the infant remains cyanotic. Raising the neonate's head and patting the back are not appropriate actions for removing mucus. (I, N, G).

3. 1. For uncircumcised neonates, efforts should not be made to move the foreskin back any farther than it will retract with ease. Adhesions between the prepuce and the glans are common in the neonate. Current opinion is to wait until separation occurs normally as the male grows. By age 3 to 5 years, the foreskin usually is easily retracted. The foreskin should never be forcibly retracted. Leaving the foreskin in place and using cotton balls is not an appropriate way to clean the penis. Notifying the physician is not necessary at this time. (I, T, G)

4. 1. Neonates tend to lose 5% to 15% of their birth weight during the first few days after birth, most likely owing to minimal nutritional intake. If breastfeeding, the breasts are not secreting milk for the first few days. If bottle feeding, the infant's intake varies from one feeding to the next. In addition, the neonate experiences loss of extracellular fluid. This neonate's weight loss falls within a normal range,

and therefore no action is needed at this time. Switching to a soy milk formula and giving extra feedings are not necessary. (I, T, H)

5. 1. Assessing for jaundice in the neonate is an important nursing responsibility. The best technique is to blanch the skin over a bony prominence, such as the forehead, chest, or tip of the nose, by applying pressure to the area and observing the area before the normal skin color returns. Until blood returns to the area, the yellow color of the jaundice is relatively obvious. The nurse may also examine the sclera to assess for jaundice. Appropriate lighting is necessary for an accurate assessment. Simply observing the skin does not provide an accurate assessment of the jaundice. (P, N, H)

6. 1. Normally, the posterior fontanel closes by age 2 to 3 months. (I, N, H)

7. 2. Keeping the neonate away from air conditioning or cooling ducts prevents heat loss by *convection*. *Evaporation* occurs when wet surfaces, such as the neonate's skin, are exposed to air. *Conduction* of heat away from the body may occur when the neonate comes in direct contact with cold surfaces, such as a scale or a cold stethoscope. *Radiation* is the transfer of heat to cooler objects that are not in direct contact with the neonate. (I, T, G)

8. 1. At birth, the neonate's intestines are sterile. Vitamin K is synthesized in the intestines, but food and normal intestinal flora are needed for this process to begin. Bacteria that inhibit the large intestine synthesize vitamin K, which is then absorbed. Vitamin K deficiency often results in a bleeding tendency. Neonates are not normally susceptible to clotting disorders, unless they are diagnosed with hemophilia. Hemolysis of fetal red blood cells does not destroy vitamin K. Administration of vitamin K promotes liver formation of clotting factors II, VII, IX, and X. Drugs taken during pregnancy, such as aspirin or phenytoin sodium (Dilantin), can also interfere with clotting abilities of the neonate after birth. (I, T, G)

9. 3. It is believed that the sense of touch is the most highly developed sense at birth. It is probably for this reason that neonates respond well to touch. (P, N, H)

10. 2. A weak, shrill, or high-pitched cry is not normal and may indicate a neurologic problem, such as increased intracranial pressure, drug (eg, heroin) withdrawal, or hypoglycemia. The neonate's cry should be loud and lusty. The nurse should inform

the physician of this observation so the neonate can be evaluated further. Telling the mother that the cry is due to excessive analgesia in labor is not warranted. Stimulating the neonate to cry is not helpful. Continuing to monitor the infant is a routine nursing responsibility and is helpful if the neonate needs to be treated for a neurologic problem or drug withdrawal. (I, N, G)

11. 4. Small, shiny white specks on the neonate's gums and hard palate are known as Epstein's pearls. They have no special significance and often disappear within a few weeks. White patches on the inside of the mouth may signal thrush due to *Candida albicans* infection, and they warrant further investigation. The neonate does not need isolation, nor does the nurse need to remove these with a wet washcloth. Sending a sterile specimen to the laboratory is not necessary. (I, N, H)

12. 1. Acrocyanosis involves the extremities of the neonate and should be distinguished from central cyanosis, which involves the lips, tongue, and trunk, indicating hypoxia. Bluish hands and feet, or acrocyanosis, is due to the neonate being cold, or poor perfusion of the blood to the periphery of the body. The most appropriate action is to wrap the neonate in a warm blanket or place the neonate under a radiant warmer. The nurse should explain to the mother (and father if present) that this is normal. Massaging the extremities, keeping the neonate in an isolation incubator, and notifying the physician are not appropriate actions. (I, N, G)

Physical Assessment of the Neonatal Client

13. 1. If possible, the nurse should examine a neonate about midway between feedings. The hungry neonate is often fussy and irritable, making physical examination difficult. Manipulation after eating may cause the neonate to regurgitate or vomit. The neonate should not be kept NPO for 4 hours because of the potential for hypoglycemia. Unless the neonate is experiencing complications, the nurse does not need to assess the infant every hour. (P, N, H)

14. 1. Mongolian spots are gray, blue, or black marks that are most frequently found on the sacral area but may also be found on the buttocks, arms, shoulders, or other areas. There is no treatment necessary because these usually fade or disappear during the first few years of life. Harlequin's sign occurs when one side of the body turns a deep red color. It occurs when blood vessels on one side of the body constrict, while those on the other side of the body dilate. The observance of harlequin's sign should be documented and reported. Hemangiomas or vascular tumors are nevi flammeus, or port wine stains, and

do not disappear with time. Molar nevi do not exist. (I, N, H)

15. 2. Caused by pressure on the head during labor, caput succedaneum is an edematous area over the place where the scalp was encircled by the cervix, possibly crossing the suture line. It usually results from a difficult and long labor or vacuum extraction. Cephalohematoma is caused by blood between the bone and the periosteum. Because bleeding is under the periosteum, it cannot cross the suture line, whereas a caput can. Caput succedaneum is usually reabsorbed within 12 hours to a few days after birth, whereas cephalhematoma may take as long as a few weeks or months to disappear. The correct term is caput succedaneum, not cranial edema, and the caput, while not life-threatening, is not normal. (I, N, H)

16. 2. The correct method of assessing a neonate's temperature is to place the thermometer under the neonate's arm for an axillary reading. It is not appropriate to place the thermometer in the neonate's mouth, rectum, or ear because this may result in injury to delicate tissues. (P, T, G)

17. 2. At birth, the neonate's head circumference is about 2 cm larger than the chest circumference. The average normal head circumference is 13 to 14 inches (33 to 35 cm); average normal chest circumference is 12.5 to 14 inches (31 to 35 cm). If the neonate's head has molding, it should be measured again after the molding has been corrected for an accurate measurement. (I, N, H)

18. 4. During vaginal delivery, the cranial bones tend to override when the head accommodates to the size of the mother's birth canal. The amount and length of pressure on the head influences the degree of molding. Molding usually disappears in a few days without any special attention. Molding does not affect the fontanels, and brain damage is unlikely. (E, N, H)

19. 3. The anterior fontanel is normally diamond-shaped and about 2 to 3 cm wide and 3 to 4 cm long. The measurements may be somewhat smaller from the effects of molding. The posterior fontanel is small and triangular. (I, N, H)

20. 3. Sole creases covering the entire foot are indicative of a term neonate. If the neonate's ear is lying flat against the head, if there is an absence of rugae in the scrotum, or if there is absence of tremors, then the neonate is most likely preterm. (A, T, H)

21. 2. An expiratory grunt is significant and should be reported promptly because it may indicate respiratory distress. The presence of a red reflex in the eyes is normal. A respiratory rate of 40 breaths/minute and full breast areola are normal findings. (I, T, G)

22. 3. The tonic neck reflex, also called the *fencing po-*

sition, is present when the neonate turns the head to the left side, extends the left extremities, and flexes the right extremities. This reflex disappears in a matter of months as the neonatal nervous system matures. (E, N, H)

23. 2. Convergent strabismus is common during infancy until about age 6 months because of poor oculomotor coordination. The neonate has peripheral vision and can fixate on close objects for short periods. The neonate can also perceive colors, shapes, and faces. (I, N, H)

24. 3. The white, cheese-like substance on the neonate's body creases is called vernix caseosa. Unless the vernix is stained with meconium, it should be left on the skin because it serves as a protective coating. It disappears within about 24 hours after birth. It does not need to be removed with oil or hand lotion. Brushing the vernix off with a washcloth will be difficult because of its sticky nature. Removing it with alcohol and cotton balls is not necessary, and the alcohol is drying on the skin. (I, N, H)

25. 3. A single crease across the palm (simian crease) is most often associated with chromosomal abnormalities, notably Down syndrome. Many creases across the soles of the feet, frequent sneezing, and dry, peeling skin are normal findings. (A, N, G)

26. 4. Normally, the anterior fontanel closes between ages 12 and 18 months. Premature closure (craniostenosis or premature synostosis) prevents proper growth and expansion of the brain, resulting in mental retardation. Premature closure of the anterior fontanel is usually treated surgically. (I, N, H)

27. 1. Normal neonatal hemoglobin level ranges from 15 to 20 g/mL blood. After birth, the hemoglobin level gradually decreases. The nurse should document this as a normal finding. The neonate does not demonstrate symptoms of polycythemia, and there is no need for the nurse to recheck the hemoglobin in an hour. Assessment for skin pallor and anemia is not warranted at this time. (I, N, G)

28. 2. Corneas of unequal size should be reported because this may indicate congenital glaucoma. An absence of tears is common because the neonate's lacrimal glands are not yet functioning. The neonate's pupils normally constrict when a bright light is focused on them. The finding implies that light perception and visual acuity are present, as they should be after birth. A red circle on the pupils seen when an ophthalmoscope's light is shining onto the retina is a normal finding. Called the red reflex, this indicates that the light is shining onto the retina. Lens opacity may indicate congenital cataracts. Constriction of the pupils is normal. (I, T, G)

29. 2. A positive Babinski's reflex in a neonate is a nor-

mal finding demonstrating the immaturity of the central nervous system in corticospinal pathways. A neonate's muscle coordination is immature, but the Babinski's reflex does not help determine this immaturity. A positive Babinski's reflex does not indicate a defect in the spinal cord or an injury to nerves that innervate the legs. There is no evidence to suggest partial paralysis. A positive Babinski's reflex in an adult indicates disease. (E, N, H)

30. 1. Routine screening for phenylketonuria is done after the neonate has been eating for 48 hours. The heel stick is done to obtain the blood sample. The radial artery, brachial artery, and scalp vein are not appropriate sites. The lateral heel is the best site because it prevents damage to the posterior tibial nerve and artery, plantar artery, and the important longitudinally oriented fat pad of the heel. The nurse should try to select a previously unpunctured site to minimize the risk of infection and scar formation. (I, N, G)

The Post-Term Neonate

31. 2. Post-term neonates are born after the 42nd week of gestation. Typical physical characteristics of post-term neonates include a long, thin body; abundant scalp hair; absence of vernix caseosa; dry, thin, cracked, or peeling skin; long, thin nails; abundant sole creases; and an absence of lanugo. At birth, these neonates tend to look as though they were 1 to 3 weeks old. (I, N, H)

32. 4. Increased respiratory rate and tremors are indicative of hypoglycemia, which frequently affects the post-term neonate because of depleted glycogen stores. There is no indication that the neonate has excessive mucus or an ineffective airway. Decreased cardiac output is not indicated. Lethargy, not tremors, would be indicative of infection or hyperthermia. Typically, the post-term neonate has difficulty maintaining temperature. So hypothermia, not hyperthermia, is usually more of a problem. (D, N, G)

33. 4. If bleeding occurs after circumcision, the nurse should first apply gentle pressure on the area with sterile gauze. Bleeding is not common but requires attention when it occurs. Typically, the neonate's circumcision site is examined every 15 minutes for 1 hour to assess bleeding. Applying pressure with the diaper does not allow the nurse to observe whether bleeding has stopped. The physician needs to be notified when bleeding cannot be stopped by conservative measures because this may be a symptom of hemophilia. (I, N, G)

34. 3. Hypothermia and temperature instability are primary problems in the post-term neonate, so maintaining a normal temperature pattern is an appropriate goal. Post-term neonates have little subcutaneous fat, predisposing them to cold stress. A weight gain of 4 ounces may not be feasible because most neonates lose 5% to 15% of their birth weight during the first few days of life. Polycythemia is common in post-term infants and may take a while to resolve. All infants should be assessed for hyperbilirubinemia, but this is not more common with post-term neonates. All neonates tend to breathe in a shallow manner. (P, T, G)

35. 4. A loose, wet stool in diaper is indicative of diarrhea and needs immediate attention as the infant may quickly become severely dehydrated. Frequent hiccups, gray-blue eyes, and a red rash (newborn rash) are normal and do not warrant treatment. (A, N, G)

36. 2. A positive Ortolani's sign indicates probable dislocated hip. Ortolani's maneuver involves flexing the neonate's knees and hips at right angles and bringing the sides of the knees down to the surface of the examining table. A characteristic click felt or heard indicates a positive Ortolani's sign. The nurse should notify the physician promptly because treatment is needed. The dislocated hip needs to be maintained in a position of flexion and abduction. Methods for this include triple or extra diapers, orthopedic splints, Frejka pillow splint, and hip spica cast. Treatment is usually successful within 3 to 4 months. Determining if the mother had anesthesia, keeping the infant under the radiant warmer, and checking for hypoglycemia are not indicated at this time. (I, N, G)

37. 2. The most commonly recommended procedure is to cleanse the circumcision site with warm water with each diaper change. Other treatments are necessary only if complications develop. Alcohol swabs, povidone-iodine solution, and diluted hydrogen peroxide can cause pain for the infant.(I, N, G)

38. 3. At 24 hours of age, the neonate is most likely in a state of deep sleep. Jitteriness and tremors are associated with drug withdrawal. There is no evidence to suggest cardiac distress. The first period of reactivity occurs in the first 30 minutes after birth. (A, N, G)

The Neonate With Risk Factors

39. 2. The first step after cesarean delivery is to aspirate mucus from the neonate's mouth. If this is not done, the neonate will aspirate mucus when beginning to breathe. Later, the neonate may be stimulated to cry, given oxygen, or placed in a resuscitator if necessary. An open airway is the most important aspect immediately after delivery. Once the airway

has been established, the nurse can wipe the infant with sterile towels while keeping the infant under a radiant warmer. (I, N, G)

40. 4. When being given oxygen by mask with wall oxygen, the neonate should be placed on his back with the neck slightly extended, in the sniffing or neutral position. This position provides the most room for lung expansion and puts the upper respiratory tract in the best position for receiving oxygen. Placing a small rolled towel under the neonate's shoulders helps extend the neck properly. Overextension of the neck will block the airway. (I, N, G)

41. 1. Cardiac massage should be alternated with ventilation. A neonate's sternum should be compressed using two fingers, not the palm of the hand. The chest should be compressed 100 to 120 times/minute. The chest wall should be displaced 0.5 to 0.75 inch (1 to 1.5 cm). (I, N, G)

42. 1. Whenever oxygen is administered, it should be humidified to prevent drying of nasal passages and mucous membranes. Although the oxygen concentration in the hood should be monitored and blood gases measured, checking glucose level is not necessary. A stocking cap is not necessary if the neonate is under a radiant warmer. The pulse should be checked frequently, but not continuously, after the heartbeat has been established. (I, N, G)

43. 3. When a neonate is being transferred to a neonatal care center (level III nursery), the parents should be allowed to see and touch him, if possible, before transfer. The parents should be given the location and telephone number of the unit to which the neonate is being transferred. The parents have signed consent for treatment on admission, and in most states, another consent is not necessary. The parents are already aware of the neonate's condition and should recognize that it is critical if the neonate is being transferred to a neonatal care center. The nurse should not ask the husband if he would like to ride in the ambulance with the neonate during transfer. Most ambulances or transferring equipment, such as helicopters or airplanes, do not allow family members to accompany the ill client. Space in the motor vehicle, helicopter, or plane is limited. In addition, most transferring vehicles do not have insurance to cover family members should an accident occur during transfer. (I, N, L)

44. 2. RDS, previously called *hyaline membrane disease,* is a developmental condition that primarily attacks preterm neonates, although it can also affect term and post-term neonates. When surfactant is decreased, the lung alveoli do not expand properly, leading to RDS. Surfactant contains a group of surface-active phospholipids, of which one component—lecithin—is the most critical for alveolar stability. Surfactant production peaks at about 35 weeks' gestation. Some medical centers have been successful in administering surfactant to the neonate soon after birth. (I, N, G)

45. 3. The best way to determine the adequacy of oxygen therapy is to monitor the neonate's arterial blood gas values that indicate oxygen and carbon dioxide tensions. Cyanosis, a late sign, can validate laboratory findings, but using it without laboratory examination is not a sufficiently reliable indicator of the effectiveness of oxygen therapy. Pulse rate likewise does not serve as a good index. Oxygen administration should be monitored carefully, and only the amount required for physiologic requirements should be given. (E, N, G)

46. 2. RDS is a developmental condition that primarily attacks preterm infants before 35 weeks' gestation. There is little correlation between cesarean section deliveries and RDS. When meconium aspiration has not occurred, there is little correlation between breech presentation and RDS. The neonate's sluggish respiratory activity after delivery is not the likely cause of RDS but may be a sign that the neonate has the condition. Although excessive analgesia can depress the neonate's respiratory condition if given shortly before birth, there is no indication of this. (P, N, G)

47. 3. Oxygen should be humidified before administration to help prevent drying of the mucous membranes in the respiratory tract. Drying impedes the normal functioning of cilia in the respiratory tract and predisposes to mucous membrane irritation. (I, N, G)

48. 4. Because a preterm neonate has poor thermal stability, reducing heat loss is very important. *Conduction* involves the loss of heat to a cooler surface by direct skin contact. Cold stethoscopes, cold hands, and cold scales can all cause heat loss by conduction. Drying the neonate with sterile towels prevents heat loss from *evaporation,* the loss of heat when water is converted to a vapor. Administering warm oxygen and placing the neonate in a radiant warmer or incubator prevents heat loss from *convection,* loss of heat from the warm body surface to cooler air currents. Keeping the neonate away from the walls of an incubator prevents heat loss from radiation. *Radiation* losses occur when heat is transferred from a heated body surface and objects not in direct contact with the body. (I, N, G)

49. 2. The catheter used for gavaging a neonate should be lubricated with sterile water before introduction. If the catheter is inadvertently introduced into the lungs, oil-based lubricants can cause serious damage. Normal saline, plain water, and water-soluble jelly are not recommended. (P, N, G)

50. 3. After inserting a gavage catheter, the nurse should next check that the catheter is in the stomach before instilling nourishment. One way is to aspirate stomach contents. Another method is to inject a few millimeters of air into the catheter while auscultating over the stomach with a stethoscope to listen for the sound of air entering the stomach. In the past, it was common to place the catheter under water. If bubbles appeared at regular intervals coordinated with respirations, the nurse determined that the catheter was in the airway. This latter procedure is no longer recommended. The catheter does not need to be clamped momentarily, nor should 10 mL of sterile water be instilled. Routine chest radiograph for gavage feedings is not recommended, but it may be ordered for other reasons. (I, T, G)

51. 4. Many centers that care for high-risk neonates recommend that the mother pump her breasts, store the milk, and bring it to the center so the neonate can be fed with it, even if the neonate is being fed by gavage. As soon as the neonate has developed a coordinated suck-and-swallow reflex, it can breast-feed. Secretory immunoglobulin A, found in breast milk, is an important immunoglobulin that can provide immunity to the mucosal surfaces of the gastrointestinal tract. It can protect the neonate from enteric infections, such as those caused by *Escherichia coli* and *Shigella* species. Some studies have also shown that breast-fed preterm neonates maintain higher transcutaneous oxygen pressure and body temperature better than bottle-fed neonates. There is some evidence that breast milk can decrease the incidence of necrotizing enterocolitis. (I, N, G)

52. 1. ROP was previously called *retrolental fibroplasia.* In the early acute stages of ROP, the neonate's immature retinal vessels constrict. If vasoconstriction is sustained, vascular closure follows, and irreversible capillary endothelial damage occurs. ROP is associated with multiple risk factors, including excessive oxygen administration, prematurity, and very low birth weight. Hypoglycemia, alkalosis, and phototherapy are not related to ROP. (A, N, G)

53. 4. Constricted retinal vessels may indicate the degree of ROP. Sunken orbital sockets, strabismus, and a reaction to bright light are not related to progressive ROP. (E, N, G)

54. 1. In some medical centers, laser therapy and cryotherapy have been successful in the treatment of ROP. The retina may become detached with this condition. It is not treated with eye drops or corneal transplants. It is not associated with glaucoma. (I, T, G)

55. 4. The most appropriate guideline is to suggest that the mother give some undivided time each day to

her 5-year-old, who may be jealous of the new baby. Dividing time equally between the two children may not be feasible. Ignoring behavior typical of jealousy will not help meet the youngster's needs. Allowing the older child to hold and feed the baby occasionally is unlikely to help overcome jealousy and may result in the child hurting the baby. Telling the 5-year-old that the infant is just like a doll is inappropriate and may also result in injury to the infant. (E, N, L)

56. 3. The priority nursing diagnosis for a preterm neonate is Impaired Gas Exchange related to immature pulmonary vasculature. RDS is a primary problem for preterm neonates and a particular problem for neonates of 28 weeks' gestation. The neonate may have a problem with altered nutrition, but the priority is to establish an airway and adequate respirations. Strict handwashing must be observed because these neonates are susceptible to infection. Potential for respiratory distress syndrome and transient tachypnea are not nursing diagnoses. (D, N, G)

57. 1. Neonates weighing less than 1,500 g or born at less than 34 weeks' gestation are susceptible to IVH. Ultrasound scan or computed tomography can confirm the diagnosis. (I, T, G)

58. 3. A symptom of intraventricular hemorrhage is a bulging fontanel. The most common site of hemorrhage is the periventricular subependymal germinal matrix, where there is rich blood supply and where the capillary walls are thin and fragile. The clinical signs of IVH are variable. Other common manifestations are neurologic signs such as hypotonia, lethargy, temperature instability, nystagmus, apnea, bradycardia, decreased hematocrit, and increasing hypoxia. Seizures also may occur. Treatment is supportive, and outcome is variable. (A, N, G)

59. 4. Signs indicating necrotizing enterocolitis include abdominal distention with gastric retention and vomiting. Other signs may include lethargy, irritability, positive blood culture in stool, apnea, diarrhea, metabolic acidosis, and unstable temperature. Treatment includes maintaining the neonate on NPO status, providing intravenous therapy and total parenteral nutrition, and surgically removing the necrotic bowel. (A, N, G)

60. 2. Bronchopulmonary dysplasia is a chronic illness that may require prolonged hospitalization. The disease typically occurs in compromised very-low-birth weight neonates who require oxygen therapy and assisted ventilation for treatment of RDS. The cause is multifactorial, and the disease has four stages. Stage 1 is clinically similar to RDS—the alveoli collapse and the resultant ischemia leads to necrosis of the surrounding tissues and capillaries. Stage 2 is marked by opacification of lung fields. Stage 3

involves a transition to chronic lung disease. Emphysematous areas are surrounded by collapsed alveoli, with small amounts of air trapped in the interstitium. Stage 4 involves hypertrophy of the smooth muscles surrounding the bronchi and bronchioles, which leads to a narrowing of the airways. The neonate's activities may be limited by the disease. The neonate may require permanent ventilation. (E, N, G)

61. 4. Pneumothorax is an accumulation of air in the thoracic cavity between the parietal and visceral pleurae. A life-threatening situation, it requires immediate removal of the accumulated air. The air is aspirated with a syringe attached to an 18-gauge catheter or 23-gauge butterfly drain and inserted into the second or third intercostal space at the midclavicular line with the neonate in a supine position. Complete resolution of pneumothorax requires a size 10F chest tube connected to continuous negative pressure. The neonate does not need to be placed on a ventilator. Administering oxygen by endotracheal tube and suctioning the neonate's nares are not appropriate actions. (I, N, G)

62. 2. MAS affects small-for-gestational age, term, and post-term neonates that have experienced long labor. Meconium in the lungs allows inhalation but not exhalation. Clinical manifestations of MAS include fetal hypoxia in utero and signs of distress at birth, such as pallor, cyanosis, apnea, slow heart rate, and low Apgar scores (below 6) at 1 and 5 minutes after birth. These neonates often require resuscitative efforts at birth to establish adequate respirations. Staining of the skin, nails, and umbilical cord is common but does not require further assessment. The staining is evidence that hypoxia has occurred in utero and that MAS is possible. Hypoglycemia is common. Hyporesonance, alkalosis, and excessive coughing are not symptoms related to MAS. Treatment for MAS includes oxygen, controlled ventilation, chest physiotherapy, and antibiotics. Bicarbonate may be necessary for severely ill neonates. Mortality rates are high for term and post-term neonates because of the difficulty in maintaining oxygenation. (A, N, G)

63. 4. The priority nursing diagnosis for the neonate with probable MAS is Ineffective Gas Exchange related to respiratory distress. Establishing adequate respirations is the primary goal for these neonates. Ineffective Breathing Pattern related to respiratory distress is not an appropriate nursing diagnosis. Nutrition may be altered, but the priority is adequate oxygenation. Potential for pneumothorax is not a nursing diagnosis. (D, N, G)

64. 1. An umbilical arterial line can be used to monitor arterial blood pressures, blood pH, blood gases, and infusion of intravenous fluids, blood, or medications. Vigorous stimulation of the neonate with MAS should be avoided. Orogastric feeding as soon as possible may not be feasible while the health care team focuses interventions on the establishment of adequate oxygenation. The neonate with MAS frequently experiences hypoglycemia, not hyperglycemia. Frequent ultrasound scans are not indicated at this time. (P, N, G)

65. 4. Tolazoline can cause profound hypotension; therefore, the nurse should monitor the neonate's blood pressure. Plasma expanders are often used with tolazoline to prevent dramatic changes in blood pressure. (I, T, G)

66. 4. When there are Rh problems, most often the mother is Rh negative and the father is Rh positive. About 13% of white Americans, 7% to 8% of African Americans, and 1% of Asian Americans are Rh negative. (I, N, G)

67. 3. The problem of Rh sensitivity arises when the mother's blood develops antibodies when fetal red blood cells enter the maternal circulation. In cases of Rh sensitivity, this usually does not occur until the first pregnancy; hence, hemolytic disease of the newborn is rare in a primigravida. A mismatched blood transfusion in the past or an unrecognized spontaneous abortion could also result in hemolytic disease because the transfusion or abortion would have the same effects on the client. Telling the client that the other baby had a different father is inappropriate. (E, N, G)

68. 2. The Rh-sensitized neonate generally does not have problems related to polycythemia. In general, moderate to severe Rh sensitization can cause anemia, enlarged spleen, and cardiac decompensation. Treatment is done with phototherapy or exchange transfusion with Rh-negative blood. Jaundice is not present at birth because the mother's liver breaks down bilirubin and excretes it. Anemia due to the destruction of red blood cells by antibodies may occur as the severity of hemolytic disease of the neonate increases. Heart failure occurs as the heart decompensates because of the severe anemia. Edema results from the anemia; the severe form is called *hydrops fetalis*. Congestive heart failure may occur. (E, T, G)

69. 1. Genital patches as well as eye patches should remain in place while the neonate is receiving phototherapy; however, they can be removed when the neonate is taken out for feedings. Vital signs should be monitored every 2 hours during phototherapy. Intake and output should be closely monitored as well. The parents are allowed to provide care and either breast-feed or formula feed the neonate. (P, N, G)

70. 1. The optical density of the amniotic fluid is evalu-

ated for bilirubin level with a spectrophotometer. The higher the optical density, the more bilirubin is present in the fluid, indicating that fetal red blood cells are being destroyed. From these findings, the severity of the disease can be estimated. Because light destroys bilirubin, specimens should be kept in a dark area. (P, N, G)

71. 4. For the Rh-negative client who may be pregnant with an Rh-positive fetus, an indirect Coombs' test measures antibodies in the maternal blood. Titers should be performed monthly during the first and second trimesters and biweekly during the third trimester and the week before the due date. If an antibody titer of 1:16 or greater is detected, a Delta optical density analysis is performed on the amniotic fluid. Note that titers cannot reliably identify the fetus at risk. In a severely sensitized client, antibody titers may remain at a high level, whereas the fetus becomes more severely affected. For this reason, fetal assessment should include amniocentesis, amniotic fluid analysis, and ultrasonography. Titers are not performed on placental blood, fetal blood, or amniotic fluid. (A, N, G)

72. 1. PUBS is replacing fetoscopy in major medical centers. This procedure has been used to diagnose hemophilia, hemoglobinopathy, chromosome abnormalities, fetal distress in labor, isoimmune hemolytic disorders, and fetal hemoglobin and hematocrit abnormalities. The client is scanned with a linear-array ultrasound placed in a sterile glove. A 25-gauge spinal needle is inserted into the client's abdomen and into the fetal vein. Fetal blood is aspirated into a syringe containing anticoagulant. Risks include transient fetal bradycardia and potential maternal infection. The client is not be placed in a cylindrical unit; this type of unit is used for magnetic resonance imaging (MRI). Fetal bleeding is not a common problem with PUBS. A cannula containing a trocar is used for fetoscopy. (P, N, G)

73. 3. A direct Coombs' test is done on umbilical cord blood to detect antibodies coating the neonate's red blood cells. The direct Coombs' test does not detect degree of fetal anemia, electrolyte imbalances, or antigens coating the neonate's red blood cells. (I, N, G)

74. 3. The goals of care for this neonate are to reduce the blood concentration of bilirubin and to correct the anemia. The exchange transfusion does not replenish the white blood cells or restore the fluid and electrolyte balance. The neonate's Rh-positive blood is replaced by Rh-negative blood. (E, N, G)

75. 2. The organ most susceptible to damage from uncontrolled hemolytic disease is the brain. Bilirubin crosses the blood–brain barrier and damages the

cells of the central nervous system. This condition is called *kernicterus.* (I, N, G)

76. 4. A priority nursing diagnosis is Altered Nutrition, Less Than Body Requirements related to increased glucose metabolism. The increased glucose metabolism is a result of the hyperinsulinemia. (D, N, G)

77. 2. Glucose crosses the placenta, but insulin does not. Hence, a high maternal blood glucose level causes a high fetal blood glucose level. This causes the fetal pancreas to secrete more insulin. At birth, the neonate loses the maternal glucose source but continues to produce much insulin, which often causes a drop in blood glucose levels, or hypoglycemia. (I, N, G)

78. 1. Infants born to diabetic mothers tend to be larger than average, and this neonate weighs 10 pounds, 1 ounce. Although fractures are more common with vaginal deliveries than cesarean section, fractures still may occur. The most common fractures are fractures of the clavicle and long bones, such as the femur. Skull, wrist, and rib cage fractures are not common. (A, T, G)

79. 4. Tremors occurring after therapy for hypoglycemia are clinical signs of hypocalcemia. At term, diabetic women tend to have higher calcium levels, which can cause secondary hypoparathyroidism in their neonates. Other factors that can contribute to hypocalcemia in neonates include hypophosphatemia from tissue metabolism, vitamin D antagonism from elevated cortisol levels, and decreased serum magnesium levels. Tremors after therapy for hypoglycemia are not related to galactosemia, a viral infection, or biliary duct obstruction. (D, N, G)

80. 4. Neonates born to class B diabetic women suffer from RDS about seven times more often than neonates born to nondiabetic women. This neonate should be closely monitored for symptoms of respiratory distress, such as apnea, expiratory grunting, nasal flaring, tachypnea, and sternal or subcostal breathing. Neonates of diabetic mothers frequently have polycythemia, not anemia. Anemia, hypertension, and hemolytic disease are not associated with neonates of diabetic mothers. (I, N, G)

81. 4. The fetus of a cocaine-addicted mother is at risk for hypoxia, meconium aspiration, and intrauterine growth retardation (IUGR). It is important to notify the physician of the client's cocaine use because this knowledge will influence the care of the client and neonate. The information is used only in relation to the client's care. With the client's consent, it may be shared with other social service or health agencies that become involved with the client's long-term care. Establishing rapport with the client is an important aspect of care. (I, N, G)

82. 2. Signs of cocaine withdrawal in the neonate include a shrill, high-pitched cry, irritability, restlessness, fist-sucking, and seizures. These signs usually appear within 72 hours and persist for several days. (I, N, H)

83. 3. Neonates experiencing cocaine withdrawal have gastrointestinal problems similar to those of adults withdrawing from cocaine. The neonates exhibit poor sucking, vomiting, drooling, diarrhea, regurgitation, and anorexia. In addition, they are difficult to console and difficult to feed. Because of these problems, the neonate withdrawing from cocaine needs to be monitored carefully to prevent dehydration. (E, N, G)

84. 1. A neonate undergoing cocaine withdrawal is irritable, often restless, difficult to console, and often in need of increased activity. It is often helpful to swaddle the neonate tightly with a blanket, offer the neonate a pacifier, and cuddle and rock her. Environmental stimuli should be kept to a minimum. Offering extra nourishment is not advised because overfeeding tends to increase gastrointestinal problems, such as vomiting, regurgitation, and diarrhea. (P, N, H)

85. 4. Most neonates test positive for HIV at birth owing to the mother's antibodies. It make take several months before an accurate diagnosis can be made. It is estimated that 20% to 40% of all HIV-positive mothers deliver HIV-positive infants. (I, T, G)

86. 4. Breast milk has been found to contain the retrovirus HIV, and in general, mothers are discouraged from breast-feeding if they are HIV positive. (I, T, G)

87. 1. The nurse should don a pair of clean gloves and bathe the baby thoroughly before injecting the skin. Sterile gloves are not necessary. (I, T, G)

88. 3. Symptoms of infection in a neonate include subtle behavioral changes, lethargy, irritability, and color changes such as pallor or cyanosis. Other symptoms include temperature instability, poor feeding, gastrointestinal disorders, hyperbilirubinemia, and apnea. An elevated white blood cell count (more than 30,000/mm^3) may be normal during the first 24 hours. Flushed, warm, moist skin is not a typical sign of infection in neonates. (I, N, G)

89. 3. The parents of a neonate with an infection should be allowed to participate in daily care as long as they use good handwashing technique. Restricting parental visits has not been shown to have any effect on the infection rate and may have detrimental effects on the neonate's psychological development. Wearing a gown, a mask, and gloves is not necessary. (I, N, G)

90. 4. Tenets of the Roman Catholic Church hold that it would be acceptable for anyone, regardless of his or her religious beliefs, to baptize a neonate. Local practice may vary, and in some situations the parents may prefer to have a Roman Catholic person perform the rites. (I, N, L)

91. 3. On the initial visit, the parents may be shocked, fearful, and anxious. Nursing care should include spending time with the parents to allow them to express their emotions. The nurse should initially emphasize the neonate's normal characteristics. After the parents have had sufficient time to adjust to the neonate's special needs, surgical interventions can be discussed. Telling the parents that this is not a significant defect or that everything will be all right after the surgery is not helpful. (I, N, L)

92. 1. The neonate with a cleft lip and palate should be fed with a special soft nipple that fills the cleft and facilitates sucking. The neonate must be burped frequently and fed in an upright position. After feeding, the mouth should be cleaned with water. The cleft lip should be cleaned with sterile water to prevent crusting before surgical repair. (E, N, G)

93. 2. The priority nursing diagnosis for the neonate with a cleft lip and palate is High Risk for Infection related to potential aspiration. Feeding difficulties are the primary problem before surgical repair. Activity intolerance may occur, but this is not a primary problem. Restraints are not necessary before surgery. Impaired skin integrity related to immobility is not a problem for this neonate, who is allowed to engage in normal activity without restraint before surgery. There is no evidence of dysfunctional family coping at this time. (D, N, G)

94. 4. The long-term prognosis for neonates with FAS is poor. Symptoms of withdrawal include tremors, sleeplessness, seizures, abdominal distention, hyperactivity, and inconsolable crying. Symptoms of withdrawal often occur within 6 to 12 hours or, at the latest, within the first 3 days of life. Most neonates with FAS are mildly to severely mentally retarded. The neonate is usually growth deficient at birth. (P, N, H)

95. 3. Central nervous system disorders are common in neonates with FAS. Speech and language disorders and hyperactivity are common manifestations of central nervous system dysfunction. Mild to severe mental retardation is common. Feeding problems are common, and delayed growth and development is expected. These neonates feed poorly and often have persistent vomiting until age 6 to 7 months. (I, N, H)

96. 2. The priority nursing diagnosis for the neonate with FAS is Altered Nutrition, Less Than Body Requirements related to hyperirritability. There are no data to suggest that growth and development will be altered because of poor parenting abilities. Restraints are not necessary. The neonate's sleep pattern may be disturbed, but this is not the priority problem. (D, N, G)

97. 4. Gastroschisis is a rare anomaly characterized by the evisceration of abdominal contents through a full-thickness defect in the abdominal wall. Immediate surgery is required. The nurse should first protect the abdominal contents with a sterile gauze moistened with sterile saline. (I, T, G)

98. 1. The neonate is kept NPO and intravenous therapy is initiated before surgery. After surgery, the type of feeding will depend on the neonate's condition. (I, T, G)

99. 3. The goals of care are to maintain fluid and electrolyte balance, prevent infection, and prevent hypothermia. No nourishment is given by mouth until after the surgery. A nasogastric tube may be inserted to prevent the intestines from becoming distended with air. (E, T, G)

100. 2. The physical appearance of the anomaly and the life-threatening nature of the disorder may result in shock to the parents. The parents may hesitate to form a bond with the neonate because of the guarded prognosis. There is no evidence of anger, denial, or fear, although all of these emotions may occur at some point in the grief process. (A, N, L)

THE NURSING CARE OF THE CHILDBEARING FAMILY AND THEIR NEONATE

TEST 5: The Neonatal Client

Directions: Use this answer grid to determine areas of strength or need for further study.

NURSING PROCESS

A = Assessment
D = Analysis, nursing diagnosis
P = Planning
I = Implementation
E = Evaluation

COGNITIVE LEVEL

K = Knowledge
C = Comprehension
T = Application
N = Analysis

CLIENT NEEDS

S = Safe, effective care environment
G = Physiologic integrity
L = Psychosocial integrity
H = Health promotion and maintenance

Question #	Answer #	A	D	P	I	E	K	C	T	N	S	G	L	H
1	2				I					N		G		
2	4				I					N		G		
3	1				I				T			G		
4	1				I				T					H
5	1			P						N				H
6	1				I					N				H
7	2				I				T			G		
8	1				I				T			G		
9	3			P						N				H
10	2				I					N		G		
11	4				I					N				H
12	1				I					N		G		
13	1			P						N				H
14	1				I					N				H
15	2				I					N				H
16	2			P					T			G		
17	2				I					N				H
18	4					E				N				H
19	3				I					N				H
20	3	A							T					H
21	2				I				T			G		
22	3					E				N				H
23	2				I					N				H
24	3				I					N				H
25	3	A								N		G		

NURSING PROCESS

A = Assessment
D = Analysis, nursing diagnosis
P = Planning
I = Implementation
E = Evaluation

COGNITIVE LEVEL

K = Knowledge
C = Comprehension
T = Application
N = Analysis

CLIENT NEEDS

S = Safe, effective care environment
G = Physiologic integrity
L = Psychosocial integrity
H = Health promotion and maintenance

Question #	Answer #	Nursing Process					Cognitive Level				Client Needs			
		A	D	P	I	E	K	C	T	N	S	G	L	H
26	4				I					N				H
27	1				I					N		G		
28	2				I				T			G		
29	2					E				N				H
30	1				I					N		G		
31	2				I					N				H
32	4		D							N		G		
33	4				I					N		G		
34	3			P					T			G		
35	4	A								N		G		
36	2				I					N		G		
37	2				I					N		G		
38	3	A								N		G		
39	2				I					N		G		
40	4				I					N		G		
41	1				I					N		G		
42	1				I					N		G		
43	3				I					N			L	
44	2				I					N		G		
45	3					E				N		G		
46	2			P						N		G		
47	3				I					N		G		
48	4				I					N		G		
49	2			P						N		G		
50	3				I				T			G		
51	4				I					N		G		
52	1	A								N		G		
53	4					E				N		G		
54	1				I				T			G		
55	4					E				N			L	

NURSING PROCESS

A = Assessment
D = Analysis, nursing diagnosis
P = Planning
I = Implementation
E = Evaluation

COGNITIVE LEVEL

K = Knowledge
C = Comprehension
T = Application
N = Analysis

CLIENT NEEDS

S = Safe, effective care environment
G = Physiologic integrity
L = Psychosocial integrity
H = Health promotion and maintenance

Question #	Answer #	A	D	P	I	E	K	C	T	N	S	G	L	H
56	3		D							N		G		
57	1				I				T			G		
58	3	A								N		G		
59	4	A								N		G		
60	2					E				N		G		
61	4				I					N		G		
62	2	A								N		G		
63	4		D							N		G		
64	1			P						N		G		
65	4				I				T			G		
66	4				I					N		G		
67	3					E				N		G		
68	2					E			T			G		
69	1			P						N		G		
70	1			P						N		G		
71	4	A								N		G		
72	1			P						N		G		
73	3				I					N		G		
74	3					E				N		G		
75	2				I					N		G		
76	4		D							N		G		
77	2				I					N		G		
78	1	A							T			G		
79	4		D							N		G		
80	4				I					N		G		
81	4				I					N		G		
82	2				I					N				H
83	3					E				N		G		
84	1			P						N				H
85	4				I				T			G		

ANSWER GRID: 3

NURSING PROCESS

A = Assessment
D = Analysis, nursing diagnosis
P = Planning
I = Implementation
E = Evaluation

COGNITIVE LEVEL

K = Knowledge
C = Comprehension
T = Application
N = Analysis

CLIENT NEEDS

S = Safe, effective care environment
G = Physiologic integrity
L = Psychosocial integrity
H = Health promotion and maintenance

Question #	Answer #	Nursing Process					Cognitive Level				Client Needs			
		A	D	P	I	E	K	C	T	N	S	G	L	H
86	4				I				T			G		
87	1				I				T			G		
88	3				I					N		G		
89	3				I					N		G		
90	4				I					N			L	
91	3				I					N			L	
92	1					E				N		G		
93	2		D							N		G		
94	4			P						N				H
95	3				I					N				H
96	2		D							N		G		
97	4				I				T			G		
98	1				I				T			G		
99	3					E				T		G		
100	2	A								N			L	
Number Correct														
Number Possible	100	11	7	13	56	13	0	0	21	79	0	72	5	22
Percentage Correct														

Score Calculation: To determine your **Percentage Correct,** divide the **Number Correct** by the **Number Possible.**

ANSWER GRID: 4

Bibliography

Gorrie, T.M., McKinney, E.S., and Murray, S.S. (1994). *Foundations of maternal newborn nursing*. Philadelphia: WB Saunders.

May, K.A., and Mahlmeister, L.R. (1994). *Maternal and neonatal nursing*. Philadelphia: Lippincott-Raven.

Pilliteri, A. (1992). *Maternal and child health nursing: Care of the childbearing and childrearing family*. Philadelphia: JB Lippincott.

Reeder, S.J., Martin, L.L., and Koniak-Griffin, D. (1996). *Maternity nursing: Family, newborn, and women's health care*. Philadelphia: Lippincott-Raven.

Part III

Nursing Care of Children

Health Promotion

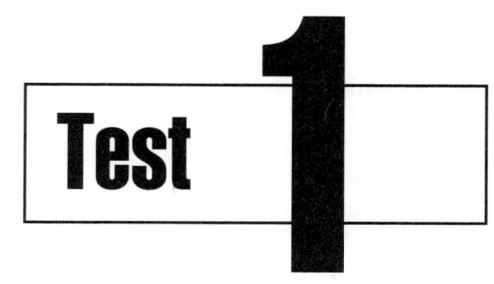

- **Health Promotion of the Infant and Family**
- **Health Promotion of the Toddler and Family**
- **Health Promotion of the Preschooler and Family**
- **Health Promotion of the School-Aged Child and Family**
- **Health Promotion of the Adolescent and Family**
- **Meetings to Discuss Common Childhood and Adolescent Health Problems**
- **Correct Answers and Rationale**

Select the one best answer, and indicate your choice by filling in the circle in front of the option.

Health Promotion of the Infant and Family

A nurse works in a children's clinic and helps with care for well and ill children of various ages.

1. A mother asks the nurse when she should wean her 4-month-old infant from breast-feeding and begin using a cup. The nurse should explain that the infant will show a readiness to be weaned by
   ○ 1. taking solid foods well.
   ○ 2. sleeping through the night.
   ○ 3. shortening the nursing time.
   ○ 4. eating on a regular schedule.

2. The mother says that the infant's physician recommends certain foods, but the infant refuses to eat them after breast-feeding. The nurse should suggest that the mother alter the feeding plan by
   ○ 1. offering dessert followed by vegetables and meat.
   ○ 2. offering breast milk as long as the infant refuses to eat solid foods.
   ○ 3. mixing pureed food with some breast milk and feeding it to the infant through a large-holed nipple.
   ○ 4. allowing the infant to nurse for a few minutes and then offering solid foods.

3. Which of the following abilities would the nurse expect this 4-month-old infant to perform?
   ○ 1. Sit up with support.
   ○ 2. Pick up a small O-shaped cereal with finger and thumb.
   ○ 3. Reach for a toy.
   ○ 4. Say mama or dada.

4. The nurse plans to administer the Denver Developmental Screening Test (DDST) to a 5-month-old infant. The nurse explains to the parent what the test measures. The nurse would evaluate the teaching as effective when the parent states, "This test is designed to measures my infant's
   ○ 1. intelligence quotient."
   ○ 2. emotional development."
   ○ 3. social and physical abilities."
   ○ 4. potential for future development."

5. In addition to immunizing for diphtheria, pertussis, and tetanus (DPT) during the first 6 months of life, the nurse should administer which other immunization?
   ○ 1. Mumps.
   ○ 2. Measles.
   ○ 3. Tuberculosis.
   ○ 4. Hepatitis.

6. A 5-month-old infant's mother asks the nurse, "What about a smallpox vaccination?" The nurse should explain that the current recommendation concerning smallpox immunization is that the vaccination is
   ○ 1. no longer necessary.
   ○ 2. given at age 2 years.
   ○ 3. delayed until starting school.
   ○ 4. postponed until adolescence.

7. When discussing a 7-month-old infant's motor skill development with the mother, the nurse should ex-

plain that by age 7 months, an infant most likely will be able to

○ 1. walk with support.

○ 2. eat with a spoon.

○ 3. stand while holding onto furniture.

○ 4. sit alone using the hands for support.

8. A parent brings a 1-month-old infant to the clinic for a checkup. Which of the following developmental achievements would the nurse assess?

○ 1. Smiling and laughing out loud.

○ 2. Rolling from back to side.

○ 3. Holding a rattle briefly.

○ 4. Turning the head from side to side.

9. A normal healthy infant is brought to the clinic for the first immunization against polio. The nurse should administer Sabin's vaccine by what route?

○ 1. Oral route.

○ 2. Intramuscular route.

○ 3. Subcutaneous route.

○ 4. Intradermal route.

10. The nurse teaches the parent about the normal reaction that an infant may experience 12 to 24 hours after DPT immunization. The nurse evaluates the teaching as effective when the parent asks,

○ 1. "Will the lethargy make it harder to breast-feed?"

○ 2. "How much Tylenol can I give for the fever?"

○ 3. "Can you give Imodium to an infant?"

○ 4. "What kind of nose spray can I use for congestion?"

11. The nurse notes that an infant stares at an object placed in her hand and takes it to her mouth, coos and gurgles when talked to, and sustains part of her own weight when held in a standing position. The nurse correctly assesses this infant's age as

○ 1. 1 month.

○ 2. 4 months.

○ 3. 7 months.

○ 4. 9 months.

12. An infant's parent says, "The soft spot near the front of my child's head is still big. When will it close?" The nurse's correct response would be at

○ 1. 2 to 4 months.

○ 2. 5 to 8 months.

○ 3. 9 to 11 months.

○ 4. 12 to 18 months.

13. The nurse notes a parent propping a bottle for a 2-month-old child in the waiting room. The nurse explains the dangers of propping bottles. The nurse evaluates that the parent understands the teaching when the parent states,

○ 1. "I didn't know it would cause my baby to gain too much weight."

○ 2. "I can see how it might cause choking, but how does it cause dental caries?"

○ 3. "So, because I prop the bottle, I might have trouble weaning?"

○ 4. "I will stop propping the bottle so my child will sleep through the night."

14. A mother states that she thinks her 9-month-old "is developing slowly." When assessing the infant's development, the nurse is also concerned because the child is not

○ 1. vocalizing single syllables.

○ 2. standing alone.

○ 3. putting an arm through a sleeve while being dressed.

○ 4. drinking from a cup with little spilling.

15. The mother of a 9-month-old asks about adding new foods to his diet. The child is being breast-fed and takes formula and cereal when at the sitter's. The nurse should teach the mother to

○ 1. mix new foods with formula or breast milk.

○ 2. mix new foods with more familiar foods.

○ 3. offer new foods one at a time.

○ 4. offer new foods after formula or breast milk has been offered.

Health Promotion of the Toddler and Family

16. A mother brings her 18-month-old to the clinic because the child "eats ashes, crayons, and paper." The nurse would first gather information about whether the toddler is

○ 1. cutting large teeth.

○ 2. experiencing a growth spurt.

○ 3. experiencing changes in the home environment.

○ 4. eating a soft, low-roughage diet.

17. Lack of the ability to do which of the following tasks would be of concern in an 18-month-old?

○ 1. Copy a circle.

○ 2. Pull toys.

○ 3. Play tag with other children.

○ 4. Build a tower of eight blocks.

18. A mother brings her normally developed 3-year-old child to the clinic for a checkup. The nurse would not expect that the child could

○ 1. ride a tricycle.

○ 2. tie shoelaces.

○ 3. string large beads.

○ 4. use blunt scissors.

19. The nurse might use which of the following nursing diagnoses in teaching the mother of a toddler?

○ 1. Activity Intolerance.

○ 2. High Risk for Injury.

○ 3. Alteration in Growth and Development.

○ 4. Impaired Mobility.

20. A 2-year-old child is brought to the clinic by her parents because she constantly pulls at her ears. The toddler is uncooperative when the nurse tries to look in her ears. Which of the following actions would be best for the nurse to try first?

○ 1. Ask another nurse to assist.
○ 2. Allow a parent to assist.
○ 3. Wait until the child calms down.
○ 4. Restrain the child's arms.

21. Ear drops, instilled twice a day, are prescribed for a toddler. When observing the parent instilling the drops, the nurse decides the teaching concerning how to position the ear lobe when instilling drops is effective when the parent pulls the toddler's ear lobe
○ 1. up and forward.
○ 2. up and backward.
○ 3. down and forward.
○ 4. down and backward.

22. A mother tells the nurse that she is using a potty seat but she is still having problems toilet-training her 2-year-old child. The nurse would tell the mother to
○ 1. offer more praise.
○ 2. use a potty chair.
○ 3. focus attention on the "accidents" that occur during training.
○ 4. defer training until the child is developmentally ready.

23. A 2½-year-old child is brought with his 2-month-old sibling to the clinic by their father, who explains that the older child says "no" whenever asked to do something. The nurse would explain that the negativism demonstrated by toddlers is frequently an expression of
○ 1. a pursuit of autonomy.
○ 2. a need to expend excess energy.
○ 3. separation anxiety.
○ 4. sibling rivalry.

24. The father also expresses a concern about the older child's fear of the dark. The nurse would explain to the father which concept of Piaget's cognitive development as the basis for the child's fear of darkness?
○ 1. Reversibility.
○ 2. Animism.
○ 3. Conservation of matter.
○ 4. Object permanence.

25. A parent reports that his 2-year-old child often falls when running. The nurse determines that this may be linked to the fact that a toddler's vision is
○ 1. near-sighted.
○ 2. far-sighted.
○ 3. binocular.
○ 4. nonaccommodative.

26. A mother brings her 2-year-old child to the clinic because of her concerns about the child's nutritional status. She tells the nurse that for the last week the child has refused to eat anything except animal crackers and peanut butter and jelly sandwiches. Which of the following measures would be most appropriate for the nurse to suggest?

○ 1. Give the child a small reward if he eats extra food.
○ 2. Consult a physician because the child's behavior will lead to nutritional deficiency.
○ 3. Do not worry about the child's behavior because food fads usually last only a short time.
○ 4. Insist that the child eat small portions of the family's meal to maintain adequate nutrition.

27. The nurse assesses the child's teeth during the physical examination and teaches the mother to
○ 1. make sure the child brushes his teeth after every meal and at bedtime.
○ 2. give the child a small, soft-bristle toothbrush to use.
○ 3. floss the child's teeth using dental floss.
○ 4. add a fluoride supplement to the child's milk three times a day.

28. The mother asks the nurse for advice about discipline for her 2-year-old. The nurse would suggest that the mother first use
○ 1. structured interactions.
○ 2. spanking.
○ 3. reasoning.
○ 4. scolding.

29. When a nurse assesses for pain in a toddler, which of the following techniques would be most effective?
○ 1. Ask them about the pain.
○ 2. Observe them for restlessness.
○ 3. Use a numeric pain scale.
○ 4. Assess for an increase in blood pressure and pulse rate.

30. A parent of a 15-month-old toddler and the nurse are planning a daily diet for the child. The amount of milk in the plan should be
○ 1. no more than 1 cup.
○ 2. 2 to 3 cups.
○ 3. 5 to 6 cups.
○ 4. 7 to 8 cups.

Health Promotion of the Preschooler and Family

A mother brings her 4-year-old child to the pediatrician's office for an annual checkup.

31. The mother expresses concern that her child may be hyperactive. She describes the child as always in motion, constantly dropping and spilling things. Which nursing intervention would be most appropriate at this time?
○ 1. Determine if there have been any changes at home.
○ 2. Explain that this is not unusual behavior.
○ 3. Explore the possibility that the child is being abused.

○ 4. Suggest that the child be seen by a pediatric neurologist.

32. Which of the following activities would the nurse recommend to the mother to help channel the child's energy?
○ 1. Participate in parallel play.
○ 2. Play a game like *Simon Says*.
○ 3. Ride a bicycle.
○ 4. String large beads.

33. The mother reports that her child creates a scene every night at bedtime. The nurse and the mother decide that the best course of action would be to
○ 1. allow the child to stay up later one or two nights a week.
○ 2. establish a set bedtime and follow a routine.
○ 3. encourage active play before bedtime.
○ 4. give the child a cookie if bedtime is pleasant.

The nurse is having a conversation with several of the parents of preschoolers who attend a well-child clinic.

34. The mother of a 4-year-old asks about dental care for her child. She says that she helps brush the child's teeth daily, and the teeth look healthy. The mother asks when she should take the child to see a dentist. The should respond
○ 1. "Because you help brush her teeth, there's no need to see a dentist now."
○ 2. "It would have been ideal to have begun dental appointments before now, but it's not too late."
○ 3. "Your child doesn't need to see the dentist until she starts school."
○ 4. "A dental checkup is a good idea, even if no noticeable problems are present."

35. Another mother says that she will be glad to let her child brush her teeth without help, but at what age should this begin? The nurse should respond, "At
○ 1. 3 years."
○ 2. 5 years."
○ 3. 7 years."
○ 4. 9 years."

36. The mother tells the nurse that her 4½-year-old child "doesn't seem to know the difference between right and wrong." In assessing this child, the nurse would explain to the mother that this is typical of which level of moral development as described by Kohlberg?
○ 1. Autonomous.
○ 2. Conventional.
○ 3. Preconventional.
○ 4. Moralistic.

37. One mother tells the nurse that her other child, a 4-year-old boy, has developed some strange eating habits, including not finishing meals and eating the same food for several days in a row. She would like to develop a plan to correct this situation. In developing such a plan, the nurse and mother should consider
○ 1. deciding on a good reward for finishing the meal.
○ 2. allowing him to make some decisions about the foods he eats.
○ 3. having only the foods served at meal times available to the child.
○ 4. not allowing him to leave the table until he has eaten the food.

The nurse is seeing a 5-year-old child in the clinic for a preschool physical.

38. Because both parents are near-sighted, the mother is concerned that her 4-year-old may be near-sighted. She says that he likes to look at books and knows most of the alphabet. What assessment technique should the nurse use to evaluate the child's visual acuity?
○ 1. Cross-over test.
○ 2. Allen picture cards.
○ 3. Snellen alphabet chart.
○ 4. Ishihara plates.

39. After having a blood sample drawn, a child insists that the site be covered with a Band-Aid. When the mother tries to remove the Band-Aid before leaving the office, the child screams that all the blood will come out. This behavior indicates
○ 1. fear of injury.
○ 2. fear of compromised body integrity.
○ 3. fear of pain.
○ 4. fear of loss of control.

40. Which nursing intervention would best help prepare a preschool-aged child for an injection?
○ 1. Have an older child explain that shots do not hurt.
○ 2. Help the child to imagine they are in a different place.
○ 3. Give the child a play syringe and a Band-Aid so the child can give a doll injections.
○ 4. Give the child a pounding board to encourage expressions of anger.

Several employees at a flower shop have preschool-aged children. At lunch one day, they decide it would be helpful to meet with a pediatric nurse. An employee arranges for a pediatric nurse specialist to meet with them to discuss their children.

41. A mother at the meeting says that her 5-year-old seems prone to minor accidents like skinning his elbows and knees and falling off his scooter. The nurse would base further assessment of this child on the knowledge that childhood accidents are more likely to occur when the family
- ○ 1. consists of only one child.
- ○ 2. has limited formal education.
- ○ 3. is experiencing changes.
- ○ 4. lives in the suburbs.

42. The nurse knows that one of the most effective strategies that parents can use to teach 4-year-olds about safety is to
- ○ 1. discuss with them potential dangers to avoid.
- ○ 2. provide good examples of safe behavior.
- ○ 3. show them pictures of children who have been involved in accidents.
- ○ 4. tell them they are bad when they do something dangerous.

43. A mother in the group asks how preschoolers perceive illness. The nurse should explain that they generally regard it as
- ○ 1. a necessary part of life.
- ○ 2. a test of self-worth.
- ○ 3. punishment for wrong doing.
- ○ 4. the will of God.

44. A father in the group asks if his 5-year-old son should have the Denver Developmental Screening Test. Before answering, the nurse would need additional information about the
- ○ 1. father's understanding of the test.
- ○ 2. child's intelligence quotient.
- ○ 3. child's developmental level.
- ○ 4. child's previous test experience.

Health Promotion of the School-Aged Child and Family

A 9-year-old girl is brought to the pediatrician's office for a camp physical. She has no history of significant health problems.

45. When the nurse asks the child and mother about the child's best friend, the nurse is assessing
- ○ 1. language development.
- ○ 2. motor development.
- ○ 3. neurologic development.
- ○ 4. social development.

46. The child proudly tells the nurse that brushing and flossing her teeth is her responsibility. The nurse should realize that the child
- ○ 1. is too young to be given this responsibility.
- ○ 2. is most likely capable of this responsibility.
- ○ 3. should have assumed this responsibility much sooner.
- ○ 4. is probably just exaggerating the responsibility.

47. The mother tells the nurse that the child is continually telling jokes and riddles to the point of driving the other family members crazy. The nurse should explain that this behavior is a sign of
- ○ 1. inadequate parental attention.
- ○ 2. mastery of language ambiguities.
- ○ 3. inappropriate peer influence.
- ○ 4. excessive television watching.

48. The mother relates that the child is beginning to identify behaviors that please others as "good" behaviors. The child's behavior is characteristic of which of Kohlberg's levels of moral development?
- ○ 1. Preconventional morality.
- ○ 2. Conventional morality.
- ○ 3. Preautonomous morality.
- ○ 4. Autonomous morality.

49. The mother asks the nurse about the child's apparent need for between-meal snacks, especially after school. The nurse and mother develop a nutritional plan for the child, keeping in mind that the child
- ○ 1. does not need to eat between meals.
- ○ 2. should eat the snacks the mother thinks are appropriate.
- ○ 3. should help prepare own her snacks.
- ○ 4. will instinctively select nutritional snacks.

50. The mother is concerned about the child's compulsion for collecting things. The nurse explains that this behavior is related to the cognitive ability to perform
- ○ 1. concrete operations.
- ○ 2. operational coordination.
- ○ 3. coordination of secondary schemata.
- ○ 4. tertiary circular reactions.

51. When the child's height and weight are compared with standard growth charts, she is found to be in the 85th percentile for height and in the 45th percentile for weight. These findings indicate that the child is
- ○ 1. of average height and weight.
- ○ 2. overweight for height.
- ○ 3. underweight for height.
- ○ 4. of abnormal height.

52. The nurse explained to the mother that according to Erikson's framework of psychosocial development, play as a vehicle of development can help the school-aged child develop a sense of
- ○ 1. initiative.

○ 2. industry.

○ 3. generativity.

○ 4. intimacy.

53. The parents of a 6-year-old child tell the nurse that they are concerned about the child's tonsils. On inspection, the nurse notes that the tonsils are large but not reddened or inflamed. The nurse explains that these findings most likely indicate

○ 1. the need for tonsillectomy.

○ 2. an acute viral infection of the tonsils.

○ 3. a normal increase in lymphoid tissue.

○ 4. a need for an antibiotic.

54. The school nurse is planning a series of safety and accident prevention classes for a group of third graders. What preventive measure should the nurse stress during the first class, knowing the leading cause of accidental injury and death in this age group? The use of

○ 1. flame-retardant clothing.

○ 2. life preservers.

○ 3. protective eyewear.

○ 4. automobile seat belts.

55. The nurse should explain to parents that the immunizations recommended for children between age 4 and 6 years before starting school are

○ 1. diphtheria, tetanus, pertussis, and polio.

○ 2. measles, mumps, rubella, and polio.

○ 3. polio, measles, and pertussis.

○ 4. tetanus, diphtheria, and rubella.

56. The mother of a 10-year-old boy expresses concern that he is overweight. When developing a plan of care with the mother, the nurse should encourage her to

○ 1. eliminate the child's between-meal snacks.

○ 2. eliminate fat from the diet.

○ 3. include the child in meal planning and preparation.

○ 4. limit the child's daily intake to 1200 calories.

Health Promotion of the Adolescent and Family

The school nurse at a high school has the opportunity to counsel many adolescents as they come to talk about various concerns.

57. When planning for the counseling sessions with the adolescents, the nurse must consider their phase of cognitive development. According to Piaget, this phase of development is characterized by the ability to

○ 1. assimilate and accommodate.

○ 2. deal with abstract possibilities.

○ 3. manipulate concrete materials.

○ 4. solve problems of conservation.

58. A 16-year-old girl comes to the school nurse complaining of cramps, backache, and nausea with her periods. The nurse recognizes that the basis for these symptoms is most likely

○ 1. pathologic.

○ 2. physiologic.

○ 3. psychogenic.

○ 4. psychosomatic.

59. The nurse develops a plan with the adolescent to provide relief of dysmenorrhea because it will help her develop

○ 1. positive peer relations.

○ 2. positive self-identity.

○ 3. a sense of autonomy.

○ 4. a sense of independence.

60. The adolescent tells the nurse that she would like to use tampons during her period. An appropriate nursing intervention would be to

○ 1. assess the pattern of her usual menstrual flow.

○ 2. determine if she is sexually active.

○ 3. provide her with information about preventing toxic shock syndrome.

○ 4. refer her to a specialist in adolescent gynecology.

61. The nurse is invited to attend a meeting with several parents. Some parents express frustration with the amount of time their adolescents spend in front of the mirror and the length of time it takes them to get dressed. The nurse should explain that this behavior is

○ 1. an indication of an abnormal narcissism.

○ 2. a method of procrastination.

○ 3. a testing of parents' limit-setting.

○ 4. due to rapid body changes and developing self-concept.

62. One mother asks the school nurse if her 16-year-old son still needs immunizations. The nurse should explain that

○ 1. children older than age 7 years do not need immunizations.

○ 2. adolescents should routinely receive a measles vaccination at age 16 years.

○ 3. the last immunization received is a tetanus booster at age 16 years.

○ 4. adolescents and adults should receive a tetanus diphtheria booster every 10 years.

63. Several high school seniors are referred to the nurse because of suspected alcohol misuse. When the nurse assesses the situation, it would be most important to determine

○ 1. what they know about the legal implications of drinking.

○ 2. the type of alcohol they usually drink.

○ 3. the reasons they choose to use alcohol.

○ 4. when and with whom they use alcohol.

64. Several parents express concerns about the types and large quantities of food their teenagers eat and their refusal to eat foods served at family meals. It would be most appropriate for the nurse to help parents develop a plan to

○ 1. evaluate the adolescent's nutritional intake carefully.

○ 2. inform the adolescent about the adverse effects of fad diets.

○ 3. give the adolescent responsibility for grocery shopping for 1 month.

○ 4. incorporate the adolescent's preferences into meal planning.

65. An 18-year-old senior tells the nurse, "Everyone does it, so it's all right," to justify rule-breaking behavior. The nurse realizes this is an example of which level of moral reasoning as described by Kohlberg?

○ 1. Preconventional.

○ 2. Conventional.

○ 3. Postconventional.

○ 4. Premoralistic.

66. As part of the annual health screening, the nurse visits the eighth-grade physical education classes. The nurse asks each student to bend forward at the waist with the back parallel to the floor and the hands together at midline. The purpose of this is to observe for signs of

○ 1. slipped epiphysis.

○ 2. hip dislocation.

○ 3. idiopathic scoliosis.

○ 4. physical dexterity.

Meetings to Discuss Common Childhood and Adolescent Health Problems

The parents of children attending an elementary school and a high school invite the school nurse to attend Parent–Teacher Association (PTA) meetings to discuss common health problems related to their children.

67. One parent asks about head lice infestation (pediculosis capitis). The nurse discusses the symptoms with the parents. Which of the following symptoms is most common in a child infected with head lice?

○ 1. Itching of the scalp.

○ 2. Scaling of the scalp.

○ 3. Serous weeping on the scalp surface.

○ 4. Pinpoint hemorrhagic spots on the scalp surface.

68. A parent asks, "Can I get head lice too?" The nurse

indicates that adults can also be infested with head lice but that pediculosis is more common among school children primarily because

○ 1. an immunity to pediculosis usually is established by adulthood.

○ 2. children of school age tend to be more neglectful of frequent handwashing.

○ 3. pediculosis is most often spread by close contact with infested children in the classroom.

○ 4. the skin of adults is more capable of resisting the invasion of lice.

69. One parent asks what causes ringworm of the scalp (tinea capitis). The nurse explains that the condition is caused by

○ 1. overexposure to the sun.

○ 2. an infestation with a mite.

○ 3. an infection of the scalp with a fungus.

○ 4. an allergic infection.

70. One mother says that her physician ordered griseofulvin (Grisactin) to treat her child's ringworm of the scalp. The physician said, "It is very important to take the medication exactly as ordered for several weeks." The mother asks why it is so important. The nurse should base a response on the knowledge that

○ 1. a sensitivity to the drug is less likely if it is used over a period of time.

○ 2. fewer side effects occur as the body slowly adjusts to a new substance over time.

○ 3. fewer allergic reactions occur if the drug is maintained at the same level long-term.

○ 4. the growth of the causative organism into new cells is prevented when the drug is used long-term.

71. "How did my children get pinworms?," a mother asks. The nurse should respond by explaining that pinworms are most commonly spread by contaminated

○ 1. food.

○ 2. hands.

○ 3. animals.

○ 4. toilet seats.

72. A parent says that her family will soon be traveling abroad and asks why the drinking water in many regions must be boiled. The nurse would explain that in addition to various types of dysentery, contaminated drinking water is most commonly responsible for the transmission of

○ 1. yellow fever.

○ 2. brucellosis.

○ 3. poliomyelitis.

○ 4. typhoid fever.

73. A mother says one of her children has chicken pox and asks about care measures. The nurse focuses her answer on preventing

○ 1. dehydration.

○ 2. malnutrition.

○ 3. skin infection.

○ 4. respiratory infection.

74. Which of the following home regimens should the nurse suggest to relieve itching in children with chicken pox? Applying

○ 1. generous amounts of fine baby powder.

○ 2. a paste of baking soda and water.

○ 3. terry cloth towels moistened with hydrogen peroxide.

○ 4. cool compresses moistened with a weak salt solution.

75. A mother says that a physician described her child as having 20/60 vision and asks the nurse what this means. The nurse should explain that the child

○ 1. has lost about one third of her visual acuity.

○ 2. sees at 60 feet what she should see at 20 feet.

○ 3. sees at 20 feet what she should see at 60 feet.

○ 4. has about three times better visual acuity than average.

76. A parent says that her child has hemophilia and she worries whenever the child has a bump or cut. The nurse should explain that after the area is cleansed, the wound should be cared for by applying

○ 1. gentle pressure.

○ 2. warm, moist compresses.

○ 3. a tourniquet above the injured area.

○ 4. A wet-to-dry dressing.

77. The nurse should also tell this mother to avoid giving her hemophilic child which of the following over-the-counter medications?

○ 1. Acetylsalicylic acid.

○ 2. Magnesium hydroxide.

○ 3. Acetaminophen.

○ 4. Poly-Vi-Sol.

78. Some parents ask the school nurse how they can best prepare their children to start school. The nurse should assist the parents to plan to

○ 1. have an older sibling tell the child about school.

○ 2. orient the child to the school's physical environment.

○ 3. offer to stay with the child for the first few days of school.

○ 4. discuss school with the child if he or she asks asks about it.

79. The nurse should explain that the most common cause for the unhappiness some children experience when first entering school is

○ 1. feelings of insecurity.

○ 2. social isolation.

○ 3. emotional maladjustment.

○ 4. poor language development.

80. Some parents ask about food requirements for school children. The nurse explains that compared with the food requirements of preschoolers and adolescents, the food requirements of school-aged children are not as great because they have a lower

○ 1. growth rate.

○ 2. metabolic rate.

○ 3. level of activity.

○ 4. hormonal secretion rate.

81. The nurse discusses the eating habits of school-aged children, explaining to the parents that these habits are most influenced by

○ 1. food preferences of their peers.

○ 2. the smell and appearance of the foods offered to them.

○ 3. the atmosphere and examples provided by parents at mealtimes.

○ 4. parental encouragement to eat nutritious foods.

82. The nurse discusses adolescent behavior with the parents, explaining that according to Erikson, the central problem of adolescence is establishing a sense of

○ 1. identity.

○ 2. industry.

○ 3. initiative.

○ 4. intimacy.

83. Which of the following statements would be best for the nurse to use when describing the onset of adolescence in boys and girls? "The onset of adolescence occurs

○ 1. at the same age for both boys and girls."

○ 2. 1 to 2 years earlier in boys than in girls."

○ 3. 1 to 2 years earlier in girls than in boys."

○ 4. 3 to 4 years later in boys than in girls."

84. In discussing safety issues with parents of adolescents, the nurse would use which of the following nursing diagnoses?

○ 1. Ineffective Family Coping.

○ 2. Altered Health Maintenance.

○ 3. Risk for Injury.

○ 4. Risk for Violence.

85. Parents report that their 15-year-old son is moody and rude. The nurse develops a plan with the parents that includes

○ 1. limiting involvement in nonschool activities.

○ 2. discussing their feelings with him.

○ 3. obtaining family counseling.

○ 4. talking to other parents of adolescents.

86. Several parents express concern about problems that acne creates in their children and ask the nurse how a teenager with acne should cleanse affected areas. The nurse suggests that the parents plan a regimen of care with their adolescents that includes cleaning the skin with

○ 1. witch hazel.

○ 2. soap and water.

○ 3. hydrogen peroxide.

○ 4. lotions and creams.

87. A parent asks the nurse what precautions should be taken to prevent the spread of mononucleosis. The nurse should advise the parents to
○ 1. take no particular precautionary measures.
○ 2. boil the child's eating utensils before they are reused.
○ 3. wash the child's linens separately in hot, soapy water.
○ 4. wear masks when providing direct personal care.

88. Another parent asks how you would know if a child developed mononucleosis. The nurse should explain that in addition to fatigue, the most typical symptom of mononucleosis is
○ 1. liver tenderness.
○ 2. enlarged lymph glands.
○ 3. persistent nonproductive cough.
○ 4. generalized skin rash resembling a blush.

89. The subject of sexually transmitted diseases (STDs) and their control is discussed at one meeting. The nurse correctly explains that community health measures designed to control STDs are most often directed toward
○ 1. mass screening for STDs.
○ 2. locating the sources of STDs.
○ 3. treating people who have STDs.
○ 4. isolating people suspected of having STDs.

90. A parent asks why it is recommended that adolescent girls not routinely be given measles vaccine. The nurse answers that the most important reason why girls after the age of puberty are usually not given rubella vaccine is that
○ 1. if the girl is pregnant, risks to the fetus are high.
○ 2. the chance of contracting the disease is much lower after puberty than before it.
○ 3. dangers associated with a strong reaction to the vaccine are increased after puberty.
○ 4. changes occurring in the immunologic system may affect the rhythm of the menstrual cycle.

CORRECT ANSWERS AND RATIONALE

The letters in parentheses following the rationale identify the step of the nursing process (A, D, P, I, E), cognitive level (K, C, T, N), and client needs (S, G, L, H). See the Answer Grid for the key.

Health Promotion of the Infant and Family

1. 3. Readiness for weaning is an individual matter but is usually indicated when an infant begins to decrease the time spent nursing. The infant is then showing independence and will soon be ready to take a cup and learn a new skill. The infant ready for weaning may also demonstrate an ability to take solid foods well, sleep through the night, and eat on a regular schedule, but these behaviors are not necessarily evidence of readiness for weaning. (I, T, H)

2. 4. It is typical for an infant just starting on solid foods to spit them out because the infant does not know how to swallow them. Also, the infant is hungry and is accustomed to having milk to satisfy that hunger. It is generally recommended that an infant be given some milk first and then offered solids. An infant who takes all the milk first will have no interest in the solids. Offering dessert before vegetables and meat, mixing pureed foods with cow's or breast milk, or continuing with breast milk only and delaying offering solid foods are not appropriate approaches. (I, T, H)

3. 1. A 4-month-old infant should be able to sit with support from a person holding the infant lightly in the area of the hips or lower chest. A 4-month-old does not have a fine pincer grasp, does not reach for a toy, and does not say any recognizable syllables like mama or dada. (A, K, H)

4. 3. The Denver Developmental Screening Test (DDST) measures a child's social and physical abilities. It is not designed to measure intelligence or emotional development, nor does it necessarily predict future development. (E, T, H)

5. 4. The American Academy of Pediatrics has developed recommended guidelines for immunization of children (*Report of the Committee on Infectious Diseases,* 1994). A series of three injections of diphtheria, pertussis, and tetanus (DPT) and a series of three injections of *Haemophilus influenzae* vaccine are recommended during the first year of life. In addition, the infant should receive three immunizations for hepatitis B. Poliomyelitis protection is administered twice during the first year—unless the disease is prevalent in the area where the child lives, in which case another dose may be given. Measles, mumps, and rubella vaccine and *Haemophilus influenzae* vaccine administration are recommended when the child reaches age 15 months. (I, T, H)

6. 1. Routine vaccination for smallpox is no longer recommended. The dangers and incidence of complications after vaccination have been determined to be greater than the risk of contracting the disease because there have been no reported cases worldwide for several years. (I, T, H)

7. 4. By age 6 months, an infant can sit alone, leaning forward on the hands for support. The ability to sit follows progressive head control and straightening of the back. At 11 months, an infant can walk while holding onto furniture; by 12 months, an infant can walk with one hand held. At about 18 months, an infant can eat successfully with a spoon. (I, C, H)

8. 4. A 1-month-old infant is able to lift the head and turn it from side to side when lying prone. (The full-term infant with no abnormalities or complications probably has been able to do this since birth.) Smiling and laughing aloud are expected behaviors for a 2- to 3-month-old infant. Holding a rattle for a brief time and rolling from the back to the side are characteristic behaviors of a 4-month-old infant. (A, K, H)

9. 1. Sabin's polio vaccine is given by oral route. Salk's vaccine is given by deep injection into the largest muscle available if a killed viral vaccine is needed. A killed virus is given to immunocompromised children. (I, T, S)

10. 2. Mild fever 12 to 24 hours after administration of a DPT vaccine is common in an infant. The mother should be taught to give the infant acetaminophen for the fever. Fever above 102 F (measured rectally) should be reported to the physician. An infant with a fever tends to be restless rather than lethargic. Diarrhea (for which loperamide [Imodium] is given in adults, not infants) and nasal congestion are not associated with the DPT vaccine. (E, N, H)

11. 2. Typical behaviors of a 4-month-old infant include holding the head erect when sitting, staring at an object placed in the hand, taking the object to the mouth, cooing and gurgling, and sustaining part of her body weight when in a standing position. (D, N, H)

12. 4. The anterior fontanel usually closes between age 12 and 18 months. The small posterior fontanel usually closes by age 3 months. (I, K, H)

13. 2. Many mothers prop a bottle of formula or fruit juice at bedtime for their infants. The infant then awakens periodically to take more formula or juice, constantly bathing the teeth with high-carbohydrate liquid. The practice has been noted to predispose infants to dental caries. There is also the chance of choking on the fluids dripping from the hole in the nipple if the child falls asleep while the nipple is still in the mouth. Propping a bottle does not necessarily lead to obesity, an abnormally prolonged use of a bottle, or nighttime feedings. (E, N, S)

14. 1. Normally, a 9-month-old infant should have been voicing single syllables since around 6 months of age. A 9-month-old would not be expected to be able to perform such activities as standing alone, putting an arm through a sleeve, or drinking from a cup with little spilling. (A, N, H)

15. 3. Infants should be offered new foods one at a time. This gives the infant the chance to become gradually familiar with a variety of food tastes and textures and also helps identify any allergies or adverse reactions to a specific food. Mixing new foods with formula, breast milk, or other familiar foods would make it impossible to detect allergic or other unfavorable reactions satisfactorily. This practice may also cause the infant to refuse familiar foods. If a new food is offered after the infant's appetite is satisfied with formula or breast milk, then the infant is not likely to eat the new food. (I, T, H)

Health Promotion of the Toddler and Family

16. 3. It is important to determine if the child is experiencing any change in the home environment that could cause anxiety, which is relieved through oral gratification. A craving to eat nonfood substances is known as *pica*. Nutritional deficiencies, especially iron deficiency, were once thought to cause pica, but research has not substantiated this theory. Unlikely causes of pica include teething, growth spurts, and a low-roughage diet. (A, N, H)

17. 2. Pulling toys is a typical task of a normally developed 18-month-old child. Copying a circle and building a tower of eight or more blocks are typical behaviors of a 3-year-old. Playing tag with other children requires cooperative play and the ability to follow rules; this behavior develops at about age 5 years. (A, K, H)

18. 2. Tying shoelaces is not expected of a 3-year-old child because it requires motor skills that remain underdeveloped until the end of the preschool years. A 3-year-old can ride a tricycle, string large beads, and use blunt scissors with one hand. (A, K, H)

19. 2. The most appropriate nursing diagnosis here would be High Risk for Injury. A normal toddler would not have Activity Intolerance, Altered Growth and Development, or Impaired Mobility. Safety issues are part of anticipatory guidance with parents of toddlers. (D, N, S)

20. 2. Parents can be asked to assist when their child becomes uncooperative during a procedure. The child's poor cooperation is commonly due to fright, and he or she will feel more secure with a parent present. Other methods may be necessary, but obtaining a parent's assistance is the recommended first action. (P, T, G)

21. 4. In a child, under the age of three the ear lobe is pulled back and down, because the auditory canals are almost straight in children. In an adult, the ear lobe is pulled up and backward because the auditory canals are directed inward, forward, and down. (E, T, S)

22. 4. The most common reason for failed toilet-training is that the child is simply not developmentally ready for training. Even with appropriate rewards and proper equipment, the child who is not ready for training will not be able to learn voluntary control. "Accidents" during training should be ignored. They are usually caused by the child's incomplete sphincter control and to poor recognition of the impending need to defecate until it is too late to get to the potty chair. (I, T, H)

23. 1. According to Erikson, the developmental task of toddlerhood is acquiring a sense of autonomy while overcoming a sense of doubt and shame. Characteristics of negativism and ritualism are typical of behaviors in this quest for autonomy. The toddler often does the opposite of what others request. Hyperactivity, separation anxiety, and sibling rivalry are behaviors that may be demonstrated by the toddler, but they do not explain a toddler's negativism. (D, C, H)

24. 2. The concept of animism, in which the child attributes the quality of conscious thought to inanimate objects, is a peculiarity of preconceptual thought. The preconceptual phase of cognitive development, which is a part of the preoperational stage, lasts from age 2 to 4 years, according to Piaget's theory. Children in Piaget's concrete operational stage (school age) comprehend the concept of reversibility (an act can be undone by performing an opposite act). Reversibility allows mental action to replace physical action. School-aged children also understand the concept of conservation (things remain the same even when their form and shape change). Object permanence, a milestone of the sensorimotor period of Piaget's theory, is demonstrated at age 6

to 9 months when the infant reaches for a hidden object. (I, C, H)

25. 2. Until age 7 years, children are normally hyperopic or farsighted. Because of accommodative ability, however, children usually see objects at close range. Myopia, or near-sightedness, is the ability to see objects at close range but not at a distance. Binocular vision (seeing with both eyes in stereo) assists in depth perception, so would tend to make the child less clumsy. There is no such thing as nonaccommodative vision. (D, C, H)

26. 3. Food preferences and appetite are changeable during the toddler years. A child may enjoy one food for several days in a row and suddenly refuse to eat it again for days. Attempts to alter such food fads are met with resentment and obstinacy. It is best to accept such extremes and offer small portions of other foods. Offering rewards and insisting that the child eat small portions of the family's meal are not appropriate nutritional strategies. Consulting a physician is unnecessary because food fads are normal and usually temporary. (P, T, G)

27. 3. A parent should clean and floss the toddler's teeth. A toddler does not have the cognitive or motor skills needed for effective cleaning. The parent should brush the toddler's teeth after every meal and at bedtime, using a small toothbrush with soft, rounded nylon bristles that are short and uniform in length. A fluoride supplement is needed only if the child ingests minimal amounts of tap water or the family has well water. (I, C, H)

28. 1. Structuring interactions with 3-year-olds helps minimize unacceptable behavior. This approach involves setting clear and reasonable rules and calling attention to unacceptable behavior as soon as it occurs. Physical punishment (spanking) does cause a dramatic decrease in a behavior but has serious negative effects. However, slapping a child's hand is effective when the child refuses to listen to verbal commands. Reasoning is more appropriate for older children, especially when moral issues are involved. Reasoning combined with scolding often takes the form of shame or criticism. Unfortunately, children take such remarks seriously, believing that they are "bad." (I, T, H)

29. 2. Toddlers usually express pain through such behaviors as restlessness, facial grimaces, irritability, and crying. It is not particularly helpful to ask toddlers about pain; they may not understand or may be unable to describe the nature and location of pain. (A, T, G)

30. 2. Toddlers at this age need 2 to 3 cups of milk per day; 1 cup of milk does not provide enough calcium. More than 3 cups may take the place of other nutrients that are just as important. (I, K, H)

Health Promotion of the Preschooler and Family

31. 2. Preschool-aged children have been described as powerhouses of gross motor activity who seem to have endless energy. A limitation of their motor ability is that in moving as quickly as they do, they are not always able to judge distances, nor are they able to estimate the amount of strength and balance needed for activities. As a result, they have frequent mishaps. (P, T, H)

32. 2. A game such as *Simon Says,* which requires the preschooler to use a variety of motor skills, can help channel activity and meet developmental needs. Parallel play and stringing large beads are appropriate for a younger child. Although the preschooler can ride a tricycle well, riding a bicycle requires more skill in balance than a 4-year-old is likely to have. (P, T, H)

33. 2. Bedtime is often a problem with preschoolers. Recommendations for reducing conflicts at bedtime include establishing a set bedtime; having a dependable routine, such as story reading; and conveying the expectation that the child will comply. Excitement just before bedtime and the misuse of food should be avoided. (P, T, H)

34. 4. Routine dental examinations should begin when a child is young, before any obvious problems develop. Dental caries can occur before age 2 years. Teeth should be brushed after meals and at bedtime. Reprimanding the mother for not taking the child to the dentist is not helpful. (P, T, H)

35. 3. Children under age 7 years do not have the manual dexterity needed for tooth brushing; thus, parents should help with this. (I, T, H)

36. 3. The preconventional level of Kohlberg's stages of moral development is typical of the preschool-aged child. Stage I behaviors of this preconventional level have a punishment–obedience orientation. Conventional morality pertains to children aged 7 to 12 years. Autonomous and moralistic are not stages of moral development as described by Kohlberg. (A, T, H)

37. 2. Allowing a child to make some decisions about the foods he eats and not insisting that he finish meals can avoid power struggles. Refusing to finish meals and to eat certain foods is normal behavior for a preschool-aged child. It is important to avoid tension at mealtime and to avoid confrontation about food, which can be used as a weapon, a bribe, or a pacifier. (P, T, G)

38. 2. Allen picture cards are used to test visual acuity in children who are not proficient with the alphabet. The Snellen alphabet chart is commonly used by age 8 or 9 years. Ishihara plates are used to test for color-

blindness. The cover and cross-over test is used to rule out strabismus. (A, T, H)

39. 2. The preschool-aged child does not have an accurate concept of skin integrity and can view medical and surgical treatments as hostile invasions that can destroy or damage the body. The child does not understand that exsanguination will not occur from an injection site. The other fears are unrelated to this behavior. (D, C, H)

40. 3. Allowing the preschool-aged child to give play injections can help prepare the child to receive an injection. Giving play injections after the experience and using a pounding board after the experience can help the child feel in control again. Preschool-aged children know that injections hurt. Imagery is appropriate with an older child during an injection. (P, T, L)

41. 3. Family changes and stresses (such as moving, having company, taking vacations, or adding new members) can distract parental attention and contribute to accidents. Only children tend to receive more attention than children with siblings. The environment of lower socioeconomic families is more conducive to childhood accidents. (A, T, H)

42. 2. Young children tend to imitate what they see, and parents teach by example, whether intentionally or not. Parents should know where their child plays and should discuss safety with him or her. Even a child who knows safety measures may forget them while playing with friends. A child should not be labeled "bad" or "good" based on behavior; it is the behavior that is undesirable, not the child. As a child matures, parental interventions aimed at preventing accidents progress from protection to education. (I, T, H)

43. 3. Preschool-aged children may view illness as punishment for their fantasies. At this age children do not have the cognitive ability to separate fantasies from reality and may expect to be punished for their "evil thoughts." The other options require a higher level of cognition than preschoolers possess. (I, T, H)

44. 1. The father's knowledge and understanding of the test must be assessed, as well as the reason for asking the question. The DDST is used to evaluate development in children from age 1 month to 6 years. Gathering information about the other options is premature. The child's intelligence quotient (IQ) is not relevant to the father's question since the DDST does not measure IQ. (A, C, H)

Health Promotion of the School-Aged Child and Family

45. 4. During the school-aged years, the child learns to socialize with children the same age. The "best friend" stage, which occurs around age 9 or 10 years, is very important in providing a foundation for self-esteem and later relationships. (A, C, H)

46. 2. Children are capable of mastering the skills required for flossing when they reach age 9. By age 9 or 10, many children are able to assume responsibility for personal hygiene. (I, T, H)

47. 2. School-aged children delight in riddles and jokes. Mastery of the ambiguities of language and of sentence structure allows the school-aged child to manipulate words, and telling riddles and jokes is a way of practicing this skill. (I, T, H)

48. 2. Behaviors characteristic of Kohlberg's conventional level of moral development (level 2) are those related to expectations of others and the desire to conform to social expectations. In stage 3 of the conventional level of moral reasoning, good behaviors are seen as those that are approved by others. The other two levels of moral development are preconventional (level 2) and postconventional (level 3). Preconventional morality pertains to children up to age 7 years; postconventional morality pertains to older children, adolescents, and adults. (I, C, H)

49. 3. Snacks are necessary for school-aged children; they should help prepare their own snacks. School-aged children are in a stage of cognitive development in which they can learn to categorize or classify and can also learn cause and effect. By preparing their own snacks, school-aged children can learn the basics of nutrition (for example, what carbohydrates are and what happens when they are eaten). (P, T, G)

50. 1. The school-aged child (age 7 to 11 years) who has achieved the cognitive abilities required to master concrete operations often collects various objects when learning to manipulate and classify these objects. Coordination of secondary schemata and tertiary circular reactions are part of the sensorimotor phase of cognitive development (up to age 2 years). Formal operations do not emerge until later (age 11 to 15 years). The term *operational coordination* is not one used in describing the developmental progress of cognitive ability. (I, T, H)

51. 1. The values of height and weight percentiles are usually similar for an individual child. Marked discrepancies identify overweight or underweight children. Measurements between the 5th and 95th percentiles are considered normal. (D, T, H)

52. 2. According to Erikson, industry versus inferiority is the theme of psychosocial development during middle and late childhood. The challenge is mastering skills to create and complete projects; this is often done through play. Sense of initiative is the theme of the preschool-aged child. Sense of identity is the theme of early adolescence, and sense of intimacy and solidarity is the theme of late adolescence and young adulthood. (P, K, H)

53. 3. Lymphoid tissue develops rapidly in relative size until age 10 to 11 years. Lymphoid hyperplasia in the form of enlarged tonsils is normal until age 6 to 7 years, after which the tissue slowly atrophies. Enlarged tonsils are not surgically removed unless they become abscessed or compromise physiologic functioning. (D, N, G)

54. 4. Motor vehicle accidents are the most common cause of accidental injury and death in children between ages 1 and 12 years. Measures that prevent accidents involving motor vehicles, bicycles, or motorized bikes should be emphasized. Other major causes of accidental injury and death in school-aged children are drowning, burns, and firearms. Accidents in children up to age 1 year involve falls, poisoning, and burns. (I, T, H)

55. 1. Boosters of diphtheria, tetanus, and pertussis (DPT) and oral polio vaccine (OPV) are the immunizations recommended for children between ages 4 and 6 years before entering school. The recommended ages for measles, mumps, and rubella (MMR) immunizations are 15 months and 12 years. These recommendations are made by the American Academy of Pediatrics, Committee on Infectious Diseases (1994). (I, T, H)

56. 3. Children ages 9 to 10 years can assume increasing responsibility for their health, and helping in meal preparation is an opportunity to learn about nutrition. The school-aged child's food intake cannot be continually monitored by parents owing to the child's expanding world. Physical activity should be encouraged. A school-aged child requires about 2400 calories per day. (P, T, H)

Health Promotion of the Adolescent and Family

57. 2. The ability to deal with abstract possibilities develops in adolescents, but not all adolescents develop this ability. Assimilation and accommodation are characteristics of the sensorimotor development of infants. Problems of conservation are part of concrete operations learned by children between ages 4 and 7 years. (P, K, H)

58. 2. The basis for these symptoms is most likely physiologic. There are two types of dysmenorrhea: primary and secondary. Primary is the most common type and is believed to be caused by an increased level of prostaglandins. The increased level produces uterine hyperactivity and contractions. About 80% of females who take prostaglandin inhibitors, such as ibuprofen (Motrin), experience relief of symptoms. (I, N, H)

59. 2. Relieving dysmenorrhea in adolescence is crucial for the female's development of positive self-identity, of which positive body image and sexual identity are parts. Menstruation should not be viewed as painful and debilitating. Sense of autonomy, according to Erikson, is the developmental task of toddlers that, if successfully mastered, leads to a sense of self-control. (P, T, H)

60. 3. About 95% of cases of toxic shock syndrome occur during menses, and a relationship between tampon use and development of toxic shock syndrome has been identified. Most adolescent females can use tampons safely if they change them frequently. (I, T, H)

61. 4. Adolescence is a time of integrating physical changes into the self-concept, and most teenagers spend much time worrying about their personal appearance. (I, T, H)

62. 4. The American Academy of Pediatrics, Committee on Infectious Diseases (1994) recommends routine immunization with a combined tetanus toxoid and diphtheria toxoid booster every 10 years for adolescents and adults. Measles vaccines are to be repeated at the end of grade school or on entering junior high school (11 to 14 years of age). In addition, Measles vaccination should not be routinely given to adolescent girls because of the possible effects on a fetus if the girl is pregnant. (I, T, H)

63. 3. Information about why adolescents choose to use alcohol or other drugs can be used to determine whether they are becoming responsible users or problem users. A person may use alcohol out of simple curiosity or as a means of escape. (A, T, L)

64. 4. It is important to prevent food intake from becoming the center of an independence–dependence struggle. Nursing responsibilities include helping parents realize that adolescents require a high caloric intake and need to make individual decisions. Adolescents are subject to peer pressure, which often supersedes family pressure. Responsibility for grocery shopping for a month may encourage independence but does not ensure adequate nutritional status. (P, T, H)

65. 2. Stage 3 behaviors of Kohlberg's conventional level of moral reasoning focus on the approval of others. Moral dilemmas are solved by the group standard, with an emphasis on conformity. Adolescents usually function at this level of moral development. Children up to age 2 years function at the preconventional level; older adolescents and adults function at the postconventional level. (D, C, H)

66. 3. When bending forward, a person who has idiopathic scoliosis has an obvious rib hump. The two sides of the back at the hips, ribs, or shoulders are not level. Slipped epiphysis is characterized by continuous or intermittent hip pain and a tendency of the leg to rotate externally. Congenital hip dislocation is an abnormality of the hip joint at birth. (A, T, H)

Meetings to Discuss Common Childhood and Adolescent Health Problems

67. 1. The most common characteristic of head lice infestation (pediculosis capitis) is severe itching. Itching also occurs when lice infest other parts of the body. Scratch marks are almost always found when lice are present. The head is the most common site of lice infestation. (A, T, G)

68. 3. Lice are spread by personal contact and contact with infested clothing, bed and bathroom linens, and combs and brushes. Lice are more common in school-aged children than in adults because of the close contact in school and the common practice of sharing possessions. Children may be more neglectful of handwashing than adults, but lice are not commonly spread by hand contact. Adults do not have an immunity to lice, nor is their skin resistant to lice. (I, T, G)

69. 3. Ringworm of the scalp is caused by a fungus of the dermatophyte group of the species. (I, T, G)

70. 4. Griseofulvin (Grisactin) is an antifungal agent that acts by binding to the keratin that is deposited in the skin, hair, and nails as they grow. This keratin is then resistant to the fungus. But as the keratin is normally shed, the fungus then enters new uninfected cells unless drug therapy continues. Long-term administration does not prevent sensitivity or allergic reactions. (I, T, G)

71. 2. The adult pinworm emerges from the rectum and colon at night onto the perianal area to lay its eggs. Itching and scratching introduces the eggs to the hands, from where they can easily reinfect the child or infect others. Nightclothes and bed linens can also be sources of infection. The eggs can also be transmitted by dust in the home. Transmission through food and water supplies is possible but rare. (I, K, G)

72. 4. Water is the usual vehicle for spreading typhoid fever. Yellow fever is spread through insect bites. Brucellosis (undulant fever) is spread by cow's milk. Poliomyelitis is most probably spread through respiratory secretions. (I, K, G)

73. 3. The care of a child with chicken pox focuses primarily on preventing infection in the lesions. The lesions cause severe itching, and organisms are ordinarily introduced into the lesion through scratching. (I, T, G)

74. 2. A paste of baking soda and water often helps relieve the itching associated with chicken pox. Calamine lotion can be used also. Baby powder, a terry-cloth towel moistened with hydrogen peroxide, or a cool compress is unlikely to relieve itching. (I, T, G)

75. 3. A child with 20/60 vision sees at 20 feet what others with 20/20 vision see at 60 feet. 20/200 is considered the boundary of legal blindness. (I, K, G)

76. 1. In children with hemophilia, an inherited bleeding disorder, a bump, bruise, or cut can cause serious bleeding. After the injured area is cleansed, gentle pressure should be applied over the area to allow clot formation to help stop the bleeding. In addition, the area should be immobilized and elevated. Cold applications are often used to promote vasoconstriction and help control the bleeding. Warmth and moisture do not help promote coagulation. A tourniquet should not be used because of the high risk of tissue hypoxia and resulting necrosis. (I, T, G)

77. 1. Acetylsalicylic acid (aspirin) inhibits platelet aggregation, prolongs bleeding time, and inhibits prothrombin synthesis. It is therefore contraindicated for a child with hemophilia. Acetaminophen (Tylenol) is the recommended alternative for analgesic and antipyretic purposes. Magnesium hydroxide (Milk of Magnesia) and multiple vitamin capsules have no effect on bleeding and are not contraindicated for patients with hemophilia. (I, T, G)

78. 2. To help prepare a child to enter school, it is generally recommended that the child be taken to school to become orientated to the physical surroundings. Older siblings are likely to criticize the younger child, and staying with the child for a few days is not advised. The child may ask questions out of fear, and therefore good preparation probably cannot be accomplished through discussions. (I, T, H)

79. 1. The child entering school is moving into a new environment after having experienced security at home. Unhappiness is a normal response to the lost sense of security, with resulting feelings of insecurity. Stronger-than-usual bonds between the child and other members of the family, especially parents, are characteristic of the child with school phobia. Such factors as social isolation, emotional maladjustment, and poor language development suggest psychosocial disturbances and should not be playing a role among normal children who seem unhappy about entering school. (I, T, L)

80. 1. Children between ages 6 and 12 years have a slower growth rate than do younger children and adolescents. As a result, their food requirements are comparatively less. (I, K, H)

81. 3. Children are most likely to be influenced by examples and the atmosphere provided by their parents, although at times they may be influenced by their peers. Coaxing and badgering a child to eat most likely will aggravate poor eating habits. (I, T, H)

82. 1. According to Erikson's theory, the central problem confronting adolescents is establishing a sense of identity. The core problem of young adulthood is concerned with intimacy. School-aged children are concerned mainly with industry; preschool children, with initiative. (I, K, H)

83. 3. Girls experience the onset of adolescence about 1 to 2 years earlier than boys. The reason for this is not understood. (I, K, H)

84. 3. Because the risk for injury is high for children, safety issues should be discussed whenever possible. Nursing diagnoses related to coping and health maintenance are not appropriate here. Although violence is a major cause of death and disability in adolescents, this diagnosis is related to actual violent behavior and is not appropriate for preventive teaching of parents. (D, T, H)

85. 2. Mood swings and rudeness are not abnormal for adolescents. Parents should first discuss their feelings with their adolescent. Family counseling is not indicated as a first intervention. Restricting activities may make the situation worse. Talking to other parents of adolescents may or may not be helpful. (P, T, H)

86. 2. Acne is a disorder of the pilosebaceous follicles (hair follicles and sebaceous gland complex). During adolescence, the secretions of the sebaceous glands increase with alterations of the follicular lining so that the ducts of the sebaceous glands become occluded with accumulated sebum. Bacteria in the fol-

licle then causes an infection. Frequent washing of affected areas with soap and water is recommended to act as a mild peeling agent and reduce secondary infection. Witch hazel is an astringent that can be used after cleansing the skin thoroughly. Lotions and creams aggravate the condition by adding more oily substances to the already oily skin. Hydrogen peroxide is a poor cleansing agent for skin with acne. (I, T, G)

87. 1. The cause of infectious mononucleosis is thought to be the Epstein-Barr virus. No precautionary measures are recommended for patients with mononucleosis. The virus is believed to be spread only by direct intimate contact. (I, T, G)

88. 2. Mononucleosis usually has an insidious onset, with fatigue and the inability to maintain usual activity levels as the most common symptoms. The lymph nodes are typically enlarged, and the spleen also may be enlarged. Fever and a sore throat often accompany mononucleosis. (I, T, G)

89. 2. Public health measures used to control STDs are most often directed toward locating the sources of infection. For a person diagnosed with an STD, an important nursing responsibility is to identify all the person's sexual contacts and urge them to get treatment. Although STDs are prevalent, mass screening is impractical. Isolating patients after they have therapy is unnecessary. Sex education has been found to be an important strategy in the control of STDs. (I, T, S)

90. 1. After receiving the rubella vaccine, the person develops a mild form of the disease, stimulating the body to develop an immunity. Administration to a pregnant woman early in pregnancy puts the fetus at risk for deformity or spontaneous abortion. Some authorities recommend withholding the immunization for rubella after puberty because a woman does not always know when she is pregnant, and the fetus will be placed in jeopardy. (I, T, H)

NURSING CARE OF CHILDREN

TEST 1: Health Promotion

Directions: Use this answer grid to determine areas of strength or need for further study.

NURSING PROCESS

A = Assessment
D = Analysis, nursing diagnosis
P = Planning
I = Implementation
E = Evaluation

COGNITIVE LEVEL

K = Knowledge
C = Comprehension
T = Application
N = Analysis

CLIENT NEEDS

S = Safe, effective care environment
G = Physiologic integrity
L = Psychosocial integrity
H = Health promotion and maintenance

Question #	Answer #	Nursing Process					Cognitive Level				Client Needs			
		A	D	P	I	E	K	C	T	N	S	G	L	H
1	3				I				T					H
2	4				I				T					H
3	1	A					K							H
4	3					E			T					H
5	4				I				T					H
6	1				I				T					H
7	4				I			C						H
8	4	A					K							H
9	1				I				T		S			
10	2					E				N				H
11	2		D							N				H
12	4				I		K							H
13	2					E				N	S			
14	1	A								N				H
15	3				I				T					H
16	3	A								N				H
17	2	A					K							H
18	2	A					K							H
19	2		D							N	S			
20	2			P					T			G		
21	4					E			T		S			
22	4				I				T					H
23	1		D					C						H
24	2				I			C						H
25	2		D					C						H

NURSING PROCESS

A = Assessment
D = Analysis, nursing diagnosis
P = Planning
I = Implementation
E = Evaluation

COGNITIVE LEVEL

K = Knowledge
C = Comprehension
T = Application
N = Analysis

CLIENT NEEDS

S = Safe, effective care environment
G = Physiologic integrity
L = Psychosocial integrity
H = Health promotion and maintenance

Question #	Answer #	Nursing Process					Cognitive Level				Client Needs			
		A	D	P	I	E	K	C	T	N	S	G	L	H
26	3			P					T			G		
27	3				I			C						H
28	1				I				T					H
29	2	A							T			G		
30	2				I		K							H
31	2			P					T					H
32	2			P					T					H
33	2			P					T					H
34	4			P					T					H
35	3				I				T					H
36	3	A							T					H
37	2			P					T			G		
38	2	A							T					H
39	2		D					C						H
40	3			P					T				L	
41	3	A							T					H
42	2				I				T					H
43	3				I				T					H
44	1	A						C						H
45	4	A						C						H
46	2				I				T					H
47	2				I				T					H
48	2				I			C						H
49	3			P					T			G		
50	1				I				T					H
51	1		D						T					H
52	2			P			K							H
53	3		D							N		G		
54	4				I				T					H
55	1				I				T					H

ANSWER GRID: 2

NURSING PROCESS

A = Assessment
D = Analysis, nursing diagnosis
P = Planning
I = Implementation
E = Evaluation

COGNITIVE LEVEL

K = Knowledge
C = Comprehension
T = Application
N = Analysis

CLIENT NEEDS

S = Safe, effective care environment
G = Physiologic integrity
L = Psychosocial integrity
H = Health promotion and maintenance

Question #	Answer #	Nursing Process					Cognitive Level				Client Needs			
		A	D	P	I	E	K	C	T	N	S	G	L	H
56	3			P					T					H
57	2			P			K							H
58	2				I					N				H
59	2			P					T					H
60	3				I				T					H
61	4				I				T					H
62	4				I				T					H
63	3	A							T				L	
64	4			P					T					H
65	2		D					C						H
66	3	A							T					H
67	1	A							T			G		
68	3				I				T			G		
69	3				I				T			G		
70	4				I				T			G		
71	2				I		K					G		
72	4				I		K					G		
73	3				I				T			G		
74	2				I				T			G		
75	3				I		K					G		
76	1				I				T			G		
77	1				I				T			G		
78	2				I				T					H
79	1				I				T				L	
80	1				I		K							H
81	3				I				T					H
82	1				I		K							H
83	3				I		K							H
84	3		D						T					H
85	2			P					T					H

ANSWER GRID: 3

NURSING PROCESS

A = Assessment
D = Analysis, nursing diagnosis
P = Planning
I = Implementation
E = Evaluation

COGNITIVE LEVEL

K = Knowledge
C = Comprehension
T = Application
N = Analysis

CLIENT NEEDS

S = Safe, effective care environment
G = Physiologic integrity
L = Psychosocial integrity
H = Health promotion and maintenance

Question #	Answer #	A	D	P	I	E	K	C	T	N	S	G	L	H
86	2				I				T			G		
87	1				I				T			G		
88	2				I				T			G		
89	2				I				T		S			
90	1				I				T					H
Number Correct														
Number Possible	90	15	9	15	47	4	14	10	58	8	5	20	3	62
Percentage Correct														

Score Calculation: To determine your **Percentage Correct,** divide the **Number Correct** by the **Number Possible.**

The Child With Respiratory Health Problems

- **The Client With Tonsillitis**
- **The Client With Chronic Otitis Media**
- **The Client With Foreign Body Aspiration**
- **The Client With Asthma**
- **The Client With Cystic Fibrosis and Bronchopneumonia**
- **The Client With Sudden Infant Death Syndrome**
- **The Client Requiring Cardiopulmonary Resuscitation**
- **Correct Answers and Rationale**

Select the one best answer, and indicate your choice by filling in the circle in front of the option.

The Client With Tonsillitis

A 4-year-old child is admitted to the pediatric unit for a tonsillectomy and adenoidectomy. The parents plan to stay as often as possible. The child's growth and development are normal.

1. The child asks the nurse if it will hurt to have the tonsils and adenoids out. Which of the following responses would be best for the nurse to make?
   - 1. "It won't hurt because we put you to sleep."
   - 2. "It won't hurt because you're so big."
   - 3. "It will hurt because of the incisions made in the throat."
   - 4. "It will hurt, but we have medicine to help you feel better."
2. Preoperatively, the nurse discusses with the child and parents the plan of care that will be implemented when the child returns from the recovery room. Which of the following interventions should the nurse emphasize? The child
   - 1. should cough frequently.
   - 2. can have acetylsalicylic acid for pain, as needed.
   - 3. can have ice cream right after surgery.
   - 4. can have sips of clear liquids when awake.
3. Which of the following would the nurse identify as a priority nursing diagnosis preoperatively?

- 1. Anxiety.
- 2. Altered Parenting.
- 3. Pain.
- 4. Altered Nutrition.

4. Which of the following is an expected outcome related to the nursing diagnosis of High Risk for Injury related to surgical procedure? The child
   - 1. is able to tell about the surgery and recovery.
   - 2. is NPO for the designated period of time preoperatively.
   - 3. and family demonstrate an understanding of the procedure.
   - 4. is not left alone.
5. The nurse explains to the parents that after surgery and a brief stay in the recovery room, their child will return to the room and be positioned to prevent aspiration. The nurse will place the child in which of the following positions?
   - 1. Trendelenburg.
   - 2. Supine.
   - 3. Prone.
   - 4. Lithotomy.
6. After the child finally awakens, the mother asks the nurse for something for her child to eat or drink. Which of the following would be best for the child *initially*?
   - 1. A yellow popsicle.

○ 2. Chocolate milk.

○ 3. Red Kool-Aid.

○ 4. Vanilla pudding.

7. The nurse monitors the child frequently for signs and symptoms of hemorrhage. Which of the following would be an early indication of hemorrhage?

○ 1. Drooling of bright red secretions.

○ 2. A pulse rate of 95 beats/minute.

○ 3. Vomiting of 25 mL of dark brown emesis.

○ 4. A blood pressure of 90/55 mm Hg.

8. The nurse concludes that the parents understand the discharge instructions when they state that medical attention should be sought for which of the following occurrences?

○ 1. Low-grade fever.

○ 2. Frequent swallowing.

○ 3. Slight ear pain.

○ 4. Objectionable mouth odor.

9. The nurse judges that the parents understand what to feed their child the day after discharge when the mother says, "For dinner the first night, I will fix his favorite:

○ 1. meat loaf, french fries, and corn."

○ 2. pork and noodle casserole."

○ 3. cream of chicken soup and orange sherbet."

○ 4. hot dog and potato chips."

10. The nurse teaches the parents that the possibility of postoperative hemorrhage is greatest within

○ 1. 2 to 3 days after surgery.

○ 2. 4 to 5 days after surgery.

○ 3. 6 to 7 days after surgery.

○ 4. 9 to 10 days after surgery.

The Client With Chronic Otitis Media

A 13-month-old child is being seen in the pediatric day-surgery unit for preoperative evaluation for a bilateral tympanotomy tube insertion. In the past 7 months, the child has had multiple ear infections that have not responded to antibiotic therapy.

11. The nurse judges that the mother understands why children are prone to develop otitis media when she states that the key anatomic difference between adults and children is the

○ 1. nasopharynx.

○ 2. eustachian tubes.

○ 3. ear canals.

○ 4. tympanic membranes.

12. The nurse would determine whether the parents took which of the following measures to help prevent recurrent otitis media?

○ 1. Cleansed the child's ear canals with hydrogen peroxide.

○ 2. Administered continuous small-dose antibiotic therapy.

○ 3. Instilled ear drops regularly to prevent accumulation of cerumen.

○ 4. Held the child upright for bottle feedings.

13. The nurse is assessing the child. The parents report that the child has a runny nose, fever, and cough and is irritable. He is constantly rubbing his ears. The nurse would expect to see a tympanic membrane that is

○ 1. bulging and red.

○ 2. clear and inverted.

○ 3. pearly gray.

○ 4. scarred.

14. The child is being sent home with a prescription for co-trimoxazole. The nurse teaches the mother about the drug. The nurse would know more teaching was needed if the mother stated,

○ 1. "I will watch to see that he is wetting his diapers as usual."

○ 2. "I should give the suspension with food."

○ 3. "If he gets a sunburn-type rash, I will not give him another dose until speaking with the physician."

○ 4. "I will make sure he drinks a lot of extra fluids."

15. The nurse instructs the parents to bring their child to the office for a recheck after the child completes a course of antibiotic therapy. The purpose of the recheck is to

○ 1. determine if the ear infection has affected the child's hearing.

○ 2. make certain all the antibiotic has been taken.

○ 3. verify that the infection has completely cleared.

○ 4. obtain a prescription for another course of antibiotics.

16. When approaching this toddler for the first time, the nurse should

○ 1. talk to the mother first so the toddler can get used to the new person.

○ 2. hold the toddler so the toddler becomes more comfortable.

○ 3. walk over to and pick the toddler up right away so the mother can relax.

○ 4. pick up the toddler and take the child to the play area so the mother can rest.

After the acute infection has resolved, the child is scheduled for placement of tympanotomy tubes.

17. The nurse should teach the parents that the purpose of the tubes is to

○ 1. allow transport of antibiotic solution into the middle ear.

○ 2. assist in the shrinking of the mucosal lining of the middle ear.

○ 3. increase pressure in the middle ear.

○ 4. allow ventilation of the middle ear.

18. A goal of postoperative nursing care is to facilitate drainage from the right ear. Which of the following interventions would be most likely to accomplish this goal?

○ 1. Apply warm compresses to the right ear.

○ 2. Position the child lying on the right side.

○ 3. Apply a gauze pressure dressing to the right ear.

○ 4. Apply cold compresses to the left ear.

19. Two interventions included in the child's postoperative nursing care plan are to apply external heat or cool compresses and to offer liquid or soft foods to keep the child from chewing. Which of the following nursing diagnoses do these interventions address?

○ 1. Hyperthermia related to infectious process.

○ 2. Potential for Impaired Skin Integrity related to ear drainage.

○ 3. Pain related to the inflammatory process.

○ 4. Anxiety related to unfamiliarity with the situation.

20. Before the client's discharge from the day surgery center, the parents ask, "What will happen to the tubes in my child's ears?" The nurse should explain that the tubes will

○ 1. dissolve in about 1 year.

○ 2. probably fall out in about 6 months.

○ 3. remain permanently in place.

○ 4. be removed in about 6 months.

21. The nurse also should teach the parents which of the following before their child is discharged?

○ 1. If the child's head will be getting wet, place plugs in the ear canals beforehand.

○ 2. Have the child use a nose plug when swimming.

○ 3. Administer an antibiotic while the tubes are in place.

○ 4. Disregard any drainage from the ear after 1 week.

22. Ear drops are ordered for the child at home. The nurse teaches the child's parents to instill them. Which of the following statements indicates that the child's father has understood the teaching? "I'll gently pull the earlobe

○ 1. up and forward."

○ 2. up and backward."

○ 3. down and out."

○ 4. down and backward."

23. Which of the following techniques is best for the nurse to use in evaluating the parents' ability to administer ear drops correctly?

○ 1. Observe the parents instilling the drops in the child's ear.

○ 2. Listen to the parents as they describe the procedure.

○ 3. Ask the parents to list the steps in the procedure.

○ 4. Ask the parents if they have read the handout on the procedure.

The Client With Foreign Body Aspiration

A 2-year-old child is brought to the emergency department with coughing, shortness of breath, and fever. The parents tell the nurse that the child choked on a peanut about 1 week ago. They thought that he had coughed it out and had forgotten about the incident until he began to cough and became short of breath. The mother asks the nurse if her child's shortness of breath and fever could be related to aspiration of the peanut.

24. The nurse would choose which of the following as the priority nursing diagnosis?

○ 1. Ineffective Breathing Pattern.

○ 2. High Risk for Injury.

○ 3. Altered Parenting.

○ 4. Altered Health Maintenance.

25. The mother tells the nurse that her pediatrician said that peanuts are one of the worst things a child can aspirate and asks why this is so. The nurse should explain that the main reason is because peanuts

○ 1. swell when wet.

○ 2. contain a fixed oil.

○ 3. decompose when wet.

○ 4. contain sodium.

26. The nurse plans to discuss with the parents other foods that are easily aspirated. Which of the following foods are most likely to be aspirated?

○ 1. Popcorn.

○ 2. Raw vegetables.

○ 3. Round candy.

○ 4. Crackers.

27. A goal for a client after bronchoscopy treatment is to stay quiet. Which of the following nursing interventions would help accomplish this goal in this client?

○ 1. Have the parents stay at the bedside.

○ 2. Allow the child to go to the playroom.

○ 3. Have the child play with another child in the room.

○ 4. Turn the television set on to cartoons.

28. The child begins to fuss and cry when the parents attempt to leave the hospital for an hour. As the nurse tries to take the child out of the crib, the child pushes the nurse away. The nurse explains to the parents that their child is experiencing what stage of separation anxiety?

○ 1. Protest.
○ 2. Despair.
○ 3. Regression.
○ 4. Detachment.

29. To help the client's parents best manage the separation anxiety, the nurse would suggest that they
○ 1. Leave while the child is sleeping.
○ 2. Bring the child's favorite toys from home.
○ 3. Tell the child that they are leaving and when they will return.
○ 4. Shorten their visits.

30. After bronchoscopy, which of the following parameters would be *most important* for the nurse to assess when the child returns to the room?
○ 1. Cardiac rate.
○ 2. Respiratory quality.
○ 3. Sputum color.
○ 4. Pulse deficit.

31. Before the child is discharged, the nurse teaches the parents the three signs that indicate a child is truly choking and needs immediate life-saving interventions. The nurse knows that the parents understand the teaching when they state that a child is choking when he cannot speak, turns blue, and
○ 1. vomits.
○ 2. gasps.
○ 3. gags.
○ 4. collapses.

32. The nurse teaches the parents about cardiopulmonary resuscitation for their child. The nurse would teach the parents
○ 1. to cover the child's nose and mouth with their own mouth when giving breaths.
○ 2. how to locate the brachial artery to check for a pulse.
○ 3. to place the fingers for compression on an imaginary line between the child's nipples.
○ 4. give one breath for every 5 compressions.

The Client With Asthma

A 10-year-old with bronchial asthma is brought to the hospital's emergency room by the mother. The child has a history of attacks that are triggered by exposure to cold, smoke, and nuts. The nurse notes that the child's respiratory rate is 36 breaths/minute, the pulse rate is 160 beats/minute, and the child appears restless and anxious.

33. The nurse would be most concerned about the child's
○ 1. expiratory phase being longer than the inspiratory phase.
○ 2. loose cough.

○ 3. absence of wheezing.
○ 4. prolonged expiratory phase.

34. After the acute attack is over, the nurse would teach the mother to expect which of the following signs and symptoms to alert her to her child's asthma attack?
○ 1. Thin, copious mucous secretions.
○ 2. Tight productive cough.
○ 3. Whistling sound on expiration.
○ 4. Fever of 99.4°F.

35. Which of the following manifestations would the nurse identify as most closely related to the child's blood pH of 7.46, bicarbonate of 21, and a PCO_2 of 33 mm Hg?
○ 1. Greatly diminished breath sounds.
○ 2. A tingling sensation in the fingertips.
○ 3. Heart rate of 68 beats/minute.
○ 4. No urination for several hours.

36. The child is admitted to the hospital. The mother stays with the child for several hours, but then leaves to attend to her other children. The child continues to experience respiratory distress. The nurse makes a diagnosis of Anxiety related to respiratory distress. The diagnosis is based on which of the following findings? The child
○ 1. complains of an inability to get comfortable.
○ 2. frequently asks for someone to stay in the room.
○ 3. is unable to remember his exact address.
○ 4. verbalizes a feeling of tightness in his chest.

37. The child is to receive methylprednisolone (Solu-Medrol) intravenously. During the infusion, the nurse should plan to monitor the child for
○ 1. hypertension.
○ 2. hypotension.
○ 3. flushing of the skin.
○ 4. seizures.

38. The nurse is to give 1 mg/kg methylprednisolone (Solu-Medrol). The child weighs 73¼ pounds. The medication is mixed so that 1 mL delivers 40 mg. How many milliliters of the medication should the nurse give?
○ 1. 0.18 mL
○ 2. 0.83 mL
○ 3. 1.75 mL
○ 4. 3.85 mL

39. The child continues to have a heart rate of 160 beats/minute, to have a respiratory rate of 36 breaths/minute, and to be restless and anxious. The child is given an albuterol (Ventolin) updraft. Which of the following would indicate that the updraft has been effective? The child has
○ 1. a pulse oximeter reading of 95%.
○ 2. a nonproductive cough.
○ 3. wheezing.
○ 4. an increase in peak expiratory flow rate.

40. The child is switched to prednisone by mouth. The

dose is to be given one time per day. The nurse teaches the parents to
○ 1. administer the dose before bedtime to minimize side effects.
○ 2. give the medication according to the child's response.
○ 3. give the dose with meals to prevent gastric irritation.
○ 4. make sure the pill is given intact to maintain the enteric coating.

41. The mother tells the nurse that she does not understand why her child had another attack. He was not around any of the things that trigger his asthma. The nurse explains to the mother that asthma attacks may be triggered by various mechanisms, including certain food allergies, and states that which of the following foods would most likely be responsible for such an allergic reaction?
○ 1. Whitefish.
○ 2. Tossed salad.
○ 3. Hamburger patty.
○ 4. Fudge brownies.

42. The mother expresses concern that the child's 2-month-old sibling may also have food allergies. When discussing feeding techniques for the infant, the nurse should suggest that the mother
○ 1. give only rice cereal to the child.
○ 2. use only apple juice as a supplementary fluid.
○ 3. introduce new foods to the infant one at a time.
○ 4. discontinue formula feedings when the infant begins to eat baby food.

43. The mother asks the nurse what measures she can take to help prevent her child's asthma attacks. Which of the following suggestions by the nurse would be most appropriate?
○ 1. Cover the child's mattress with a sheepskin pad.
○ 2. Use an aerosol spray disinfectant in the child's bedroom.
○ 3. Clean showers and tile areas with an antimold agent.
○ 4. Have the child sleep with the window open.

44. The nurse would also assess this child for allergic rhinitis, inspecting the child for which of the following to support this diagnosis?
○ 1. Nasal crease.
○ 2. Abdominal pain.
○ 3. Fever.
○ 4. Mouth breathing.

45. The child is taught to use a peak expiratory flow meter. The parents are taught to assist the child and are taught the reasons for using the meter. The nurse would know that further teaching is necessary when the father states,
○ 1. "If there is no increase in flow after he gets his

bronchodilator, we should give another treatment."
○ 2. "Now we have a way of predicting when he is getting worse."
○ 3. "This meter will help to monitor our child's condition, so changes can be made in therapy."
○ 4. "The meter readings will help us determine if there are any other things that trigger his attacks besides nuts, smoke, and cold."

46. The mother tells the nurse that the child wants a pet. Which of the following pets should the nurse tell the mother is most appropriate?
○ 1. Cat.
○ 2. Fish.
○ 3. Gerbil.
○ 4. Canary.

47. The nurse discusses the use of cromolyn sodium (Aarane) with the mother. The nurse should teach the mother that the medication will be ineffective if it is administered when the child is
○ 1. exposed to cold.
○ 2. having an asthmatic attack.
○ 3. being readied for bed.
○ 4. about to engage in strenuous exercise.

48. Which of the following statements best reflects the family's positive adjustment to the child's disorder?
○ 1. "We try to keep him happy at all costs, if not he has an asthma attack."
○ 2. "We keep our child away from other children, to cut down on infections."
○ 3. "Although our child's disease is serious, we try not to let it be the focus of our family."
○ 4. "I'm afraid when my child gets older, he won't be able to care for himself like I do."

49. The mother states that the child wants to participate in sports and asks the nurse to suggest appropriate activities. The nurse should teach the mother that
○ 1. physical activities are inappropriate for asthmatic children.
○ 2. asthmatic children should be excluded from team sports.
○ 3. vigorous physical exercise frequently precipitates an asthmatic episode.
○ 4. most asthmatic children can participate in sports if the asthma is controlled.

The Client With Cystic Fibrosis and Bronchopneumonia

A 3-year-old child is admitted to the hospital with bronchopneumonia. This child also has cystic fibrosis.

50. The nurse would assess for which of the following signs and symptoms to help provide pertinent diagnostic data?

○ 1. Weight loss and stringy stools.

○ 2. Cough and fever.

○ 3. Constipation and distended abdomen.

○ 4. Dysuria and rash.

51. The child is to receive ampicillin four times in every 24-hour period. The nurse should schedule the medication to be given

○ 1. at 9 AM, 1 PM, 5 PM, and 9 PM.

○ 2. during mealtime and with an evening snack.

○ 3. so each dose is about 4 hours apart.

○ 4. after consulting with the mother about the best hours for home administration on an every 6-hour schedule.

52. The child is to have postural drainage. The nurse should plan to carry out postural drainage shortly

○ 1. after meals.

○ 2. before meals.

○ 3. after rest periods.

○ 4. before inhalation treatments.

53. The nurse determines that the child's mother understands about the pancreatic enzymes her child receives when she says they

○ 1. should be taken 1 hour before meals.

○ 2. can be sprinkled on food.

○ 3. are only needed when the child is sick.

○ 4. should be taken 30 minutes after meals.

54. The nurse assesses the type of diet that the child was on before admission. This child should be on a

○ 1. low-fat, low-protein diet.

○ 2. moderate-fat, high-protein diet.

○ 3. low-protein, low-carbohydrate diet.

○ 4. high-carbohydrate, high-fat diet.

55. The nurse asks the mother what type of stools her child had before the diagnosis of cystic fibrosis was made. The mother most likely would answer

○ 1. hard and almost odorless.

○ 2. bulky and foul-smelling.

○ 3. watery, with an ammonia odor.

○ 4. firm with a fruity odor.

56. The nurse plans recreational therapy for the child. Which of the following toys would provide the child with the most support while hospitalized?

○ 1. A jigsaw puzzle.

○ 2. The child's favorite doll.

○ 3. A fuzzy stuffed animal.

○ 4. Scissors, paper, and paste.

57. The nurse knows the parents understand the effects of hot weather when they state that hot weather is hazardous for their child because a child with cystic fibrosis has

○ 1. poor ability to concentrate urine.

○ 2. little skin pigment to prevent sunburn.

○ 3. a poorly functioning temperature control center.

○ 4. abnormally high salt loss through perspiration.

58. The nurse judges that the parents understand the nature of cystic fibrosis when they state that the disease is characterized by

○ 1. an abnormality in the body's mucus-secreting glands.

○ 2. the formation of fibrous cysts in various body organs.

○ 3. the failure of the pancreatic ducts to develop properly.

○ 4. a reaction to the formation of antibodies against streptococcus.

59. Which of the following is an expected client outcome related to the nursing diagnosis of Ineffective Breathing Pattern related to an infection? The client will

○ 1. exhibit no manifestations of respiratory distress.

○ 2. have no symptoms of fever, such as chills.

○ 3. be able to engage in normal activities for age.

○ 4. be able to tolerate food without vomiting.

60. The parents ask the nurse what activities their child can become involved in as he becomes older. The nurse should advise such activities as

○ 1. swimming and bowling.

○ 2. football and track.

○ 3. baseball and soccer.

○ 4. basketball and golf.

61. The parents express concerns about how the disease was transmitted to their child. The nurse would explain that

○ 1. a disease carrier also has the disease.

○ 2. two parents who are carriers may produce a child who has the disease.

○ 3. a disease carrier and an affected person will never have children with the disease.

○ 4. a disease carrier and an affected person will have a child with the disease.

62. The nurse refers the parents to the local chapter of the National Cystic Fibrosis Foundation. The Foundation has been especially beneficial for parents of children with cystic fibrosis by helping them

○ 1. find tutors to educate their children at home.

○ 2. obtain genetic counseling.

○ 3. meet with other parents of children with cystic fibrosis for mutual support.

○ 4. obtain financial assistance to purchase medications for their children.

63. The child is discharged with home intravenous ampicillin therapy. The home care nurse judges that the mother needs further teaching about how to properly administer intravenous antibiotics at home after observing that the mother

○ 1. allows the antibiotic to run into the child's vein for 30 minutes.

○ 2. flushes the venous access port with heparin 20 minutes after the antibiotic is administered.

○ 3. stops the infusion when the area around the insertion site becomes hard and reddened.
○ 4. calls the nurse because the antibiotic will not infuse.

The Client With Sudden Infant Death Syndrome

A 3-month-old infant is brought into the emergency room by the parents. The infant is not breathing, and a tentative diagnosis of sudden infant death syndrome (SIDS) is made.

64. What would be the best action for the nurse to take in regard to the parents?
○ 1. Offer to telephone their spiritual advisor.
○ 2. Tell them that the doctor will talk with them soon.
○ 3. Ask another client to sit with them.
○ 4. Accompany them to a private area and stay with them.
65. The emergency room nurse obtains a brief history of events occurring before and after the parents found their infant. Which of the following questions would be most appropriate for the nurse to ask the parents?
○ 1. "Was the infant wrapped in a blanket?"
○ 2. "Was the infant lying on his stomach?"
○ 3. "What did the infant look like when you found him?"
○ 4. "When had you last checked the infant?"
66. The parents have been told that the infant has died. Which of the following interventions is most important to include in the plan of care to assist the parents with their grieving process?
○ 1. Reassure them that the infant's death was not their fault.
○ 2. Provide an opportunity for them to see the infant.
○ 3. Ask them if they would like to call their religious advisor.
○ 4. Give them a package containing the infant's clothing.
67. Before the parents leave the hospital, the nurse asks the parents what they understand about the cause of SIDS. The nurse evaluates their understanding as correct when the parents state, "The cause is
○ 1. unknown."
○ 2. apnea."
○ 3. infection."
○ 4. cardiac dysrhythmias."
68. Which of the following should the nurse write on the parents' care plan as an expected client outcome

related to the nursing diagnosis of Anticipatory Grieving related to their child's death? The parents will
○ 1. keep to themselves until 3 months after the baby's death.
○ 2. be able to discuss their feelings with each other.
○ 3. immerse themselves in work and outside activities.
○ 4. act as if nothing has happened.
69. The community health nurse makes plans to visit the family at home. When should the nurse visit the parents?
○ 1. A few days after the funeral.
○ 2. Two weeks after the funeral.
○ 3. As soon as the parents are ready to talk.
○ 4. As soon after the infant's death as possible.
70. The community health nurse develops nursing goals for the visits with the parents. The primary goal for the second visit would be to help them
○ 1. express their feelings.
○ 2. gain an understanding of the disease.
○ 3. assess the impact of the infant's death on their other children.
○ 4. deal with issues such as having other children.

The Client Requiring Cardiopulmonary Resuscitation

The nurse prepares to discharge a 5-year-old child from the 1-day surgery unit. The nurse leaves the room to get supplies, then, on returning, finds that the child is not breathing.

71. Which of the following priority nursing measures should the nurse initiate first?
○ 1. Clear the airway.
○ 2. Begin mouth-to-mouth resuscitation.
○ 3. Initiate oxygen therapy.
○ 4. Start chest compressions.
72. Continuing cardiopulmonary resuscitation (CPR), the nurse palpates for a pulse. Which of the following sites is best for checking the pulse during CPR in a 5-year-old child?
○ 1. Femoral.
○ 2. Carotid.
○ 3. Radial.
○ 4. Brachial.
73. Which of the following rescue breathing rates should the nurse administer during CPR for a 5-year-old?
○ 1. 10 breaths/minute.
○ 2. 12 breaths/minute.

○ 3. 15 breaths/minute.

○ 4. 30 breaths/minute.

74. The client is pulseless, and the nurse begins chest compressions. Because effective chest compressions depend on proper technique, the nurse should apply pressure

○ 1. on the lower sternum with the heel of one hand.

○ 2. midway on the sternum with the tips of two fingers.

○ 3. over the apex of the heart with the heel of one hand.

○ 4. on the upper sternum with the heels of both hands.

75. The nurse would plan to administer which of the following rates of external chest compression to a 5-year-old child?

○ 1. 50 to 70 compressions/minute.

○ 2. 60 to 80 compressions/minute.

○ 3. 70 to 80 compressions/minute.

○ 4. 80 to 100 compressions/minute.

76. When providing chest compressions, the nurse should compress the child's chest to a depth of

○ 1. 1 to 1.5 inches.

○ 2. 1.5 to 2 inches.

○ 3. 2 to 2.5 inches.

○ 4. 2.5 to 3 inches.

77. The nurse would know that compressions are effective when the child's

○ 1. skin begins to mottle.

○ 2. pupils dilate.

○ 3. pulse is palpable.

○ 4. skin is cool and dry.

78. A nurse walks into the room just as a 10-month-old infant places a catheter plug in his mouth and starts to choke; the nurse attempts to clear the airway. What should the nurse do next after opening the infant's mouth?

○ 1. Use blind finger sweeps.

○ 2. Deliver four back blows.

○ 3. Apply four subdiaphragmatic abdominal thrusts.

○ 4. Attempt to visualize the object.

79. In which of the following positions should the nurse place an infant to deliver back blows?

○ 1. Face up, with the head lower than the trunk.

○ 2. Face down, with the head lower than the trunk.

○ 3. Face to one side, with the head lower than the trunk.

○ 4. Face up, with the head supported above the trunk.

80. What is the appropriate technique for delivering back blows to an infant?

○ 1. With the palm of the hand.

○ 2. With the heel of the hand.

○ 3. With the fingertips.

○ 4. With the entire hand.

81. Suddenly the infant begins to cry. What would be the nurse's most appropriate action?

○ 1. Deliver four chest thrusts.

○ 2. Deliver four back blows.

○ 3. Finger-sweep the mouth.

○ 4. Observe the infant closely.

82. When performing mouth-to-mouth breathing for the infant, the nurse should tilt the infant's head back slightly to

○ 1. prevent airway obstruction.

○ 2. minimize gastric distention.

○ 3. prevent excessive pressure on the neck.

○ 4. inhibit extensor posturing.

CORRECT ANSWERS AND RATIONALE

The letters in parentheses following the rationale identify the step of the nursing process (A, D, P, I, E), cognitive level (K, C, T, N), and client needs (S, G, L, H). See the Answer Grid for the key.

The Client With Tonsillitis

1. 4. Preschool-aged children are fearful of physical injury. Truthful but simple explanations will minimize distorted fears and reduce anxiety. A detailed explanation may be beyond the child's understanding and add to these fears. (I, T, G)

2. 4. Once the child is alert, he may have sips of clear liquids. Eating enhances the blood supply to the throat, which promotes rapid healing. However, the child should start with clear fluids. Coughing is discouraged because it can cause bleeding. Acetylsalicylic acid is contraindicated because it promotes bleeding. Talking is not restricted. (I, T, G)

3. 1. A 4-year-old child is aware of what is happening and would be anxious in a new environment when he is not sure of what may happen, or what is expected of him. The parents would be anxious about how the child will tolerate the surgery and concerned about any complications that may occur. The child will not be in any pain during the preoperative period. (D, T, G)

4. 2. The expected outcome for High Risk for Injury related to surgical procedure would be that the child remains NPO for the designated period of time before surgery. The other outcomes are related to a nursing diagnosis of Anxiety or Fear related to separation from support system and to unfamiliar environment.(P, N, L)

5. 3. Placing the child in a prone or a side-lying position facilitates drainage of secretions and helps prevent aspiration. The Trendelenburg position is contraindicated because it decreases effective lung volumes. The supine position is contraindicated owing to the risk of aspiration. The lithotomy position is used for a pelvic examination. (I, T, G)

6. 1. The nurse must consider both the color and consistency of foods and fluids given initially. Red or brown foods and fluids should be avoided so that if vomiting occurs, fresh or old blood can be distinguished from the ingested liquids. Ice cream and pudding are not offered until the child can retain clear liquids. (I, T, G)

7. 1. Drooling of bright red blood indicates hemorrhage. Children tend to avoid swallowing after surgery because of discomfort. Therefore, they drool. Frequent swallowing would also be an indication of hemorrhage because the child attempts to clear the airway of blood by swallowing. It is not unusual for the secretions to be slightly blood-tinged owing to the small amount of oozing after surgery, but bright red secretions indicate bleeding. A pulse rate of 95 beats/minute and blood pressure of 90/55 mm Hg are within the normal range for a 4-year-old child. A small amount of blood that is partially digested, and therefore dark brown, is often present in postoperative emesis because of the surgical procedure. (A, N, G)

8. 2. The physician should be notified of any sign of bleeding. Frequent swallowing indicates that the child is probably swallowing bloody drainage from the tonsilar beds. It is expected that the child will have a low-grade fever and objectionable mouth odor owing to the presence of some old blood after this surgical procedure. Pain from the surgical site is often referred to the ear. (E, N, G)

9. 3. Liquids and soft foods are better tolerated by the child during the first few days after surgery while the throat is sore. Children do not chew their food thoroughly, and solid foods are therefore difficult to swallow. Foods that have sharp edges, such as pieces of potato chips, are contraindicated. (E, N, G)

10. 3. Hemorrhage might occur about 1 week after surgery as the tissue where the tonsils were starts to loosen. (I, T, G)

The Client With Chronic Otitis Media

11. 2. In infants and young children, the eustachian tubes are short and lie in a relatively horizontal position. This anatomic position favors the development of otitis media because it is easy for materials from the nasopharynx to enter the tubes. Bacteria may be present in the nasopharynx, but this does not affect middle ear function. An intact tympanic membrane prevents bacteria from entering the middle ear from the external ear canal. The tympanic membrane changes appearance with an ear infection, but its structure does not predispose infants and young children to ear infection. (E, T, G)

12. 4. Sitting or holding a child upright for formula feedings helps prevent pooling of formula in the pharyngeal growth. When the vacuum in the middle ear opens into the pharyngeal cavity, formula (along with bacteria) is drawn into the middle ear. Clean-

sing the ears will not reduce the incidence of otitis media because the pathogenic bacteria are in the nasopharynx. Continuous low-dose antibiotic therapy is used only in cases of recurrent otitis media. Accumulation of cerumen does not effect inner ear infections. It does make it difficult to visualize the tympanic membrane. (E, T, G)

13. 1. A bulging, bright red tympanic membrane (because of increased middle ear pressure) usually indicates otitis media. Other characteristic findings are rhinorrhea, fever, cough, irritability, pulling at the ears, earache, vomiting, and diarrhea. A reddened, nonbulging tympanic membrane may indicate otitis media if the membrane has ruptured. A pearly gray tympanic is normal. A clear, inverted membrane may indicate that there is a blockage of the eustachian tubes. A scarred tympanic membrane indicates that the membrane has burst due to pressure, but this condition would have occurred earlier if scar tissue has formed. (A, N, G)

14. 2. Co-timoxazole (Bactrim) should be given on an empty stomach to promote absorption. The child should be monitored for decreased urinary function or Steven-Johnson syndrome, which causes a sunburn-type rash. The child needs to drink extra fluids when taking a sulfa-type antibiotic. (E, N, H)

15. 3. Because ear infections are sometimes difficult to treat, it is important to determine whether the antibiotic has resolved the infection. If the client is not rechecked, it will be difficult to determine if another infection is a continuation of a previous infection or a separate infection. Studies may be done to determine if an infection has impaired the child's hearing, but they are not done after each course of antibiotics. A visit to the physician's office cannot validate that all the medication was taken. If the infection is resolved with one course of antibiotics, another course will not be prescribed. (I, T, G)

16. 1. Toddlers should be approached slowly. They are wary of strangers and need time to get used to someone they do not know. The best approach is to ignore them initially but to focus on talking to the parents. (I, C, L)

17. 4. Tympanostomy tubes allow ventilation of the middle ear and facilitate drainage of fluid by maintaining the patency of the eustachian tube. The pressure-equalizing tubes do not distribute medication into the ear. Decongestants may be used to shrink mucous membranes and improve eustachian tube function. (I, T, G)

18. 2. Positioning the child on the affected side will promote drainage from the middle ear by gravity. Application of heat may facilitate drainage of exudate from the ear, but only if the child is lying on the affected side. Application of an ice bag may help reduce pressure and edema. A gauze dressing is not applied after surgery, although a loose wick may be inserted in the external ear canal to absorb drainage. (P, T, G)

19. 3. Application of external heat or cool compresses and the avoidance of chewing address the management of pain or discomfort. Approaches for the nursing diagnosis Potential for Impaired Skin Integrity include keeping the skin around the ear clean and dry, cleansing with hydrogen peroxide, and protecting the skin with a protective coating. Interventions for the diagnosis of Hyperthermia include removing bedclothes and extra clothing, reducing environmental temperature, and encouraging fluids. Interventions for Anxiety related to unfamiliarity with the situation are to teach the child about procedures at a developmentally appropriate level, involve parents in care, and orient the child to his surroundings. (P, T, G)

20. 2. The tympanostomy tubes usually remain in place for about 6 months. The tiny tubes are made of a polyurethane material that does not change in structure or composition while in the ear. The tubes are spontaneously ejected from the ear. Parents should be told about the tubes' appearance so they can observe them if they fall out. (I, T, G)

21. 1. Placing ear plugs in the ears will prevent water from entering the middle ear through the tympanoplasty tube. Using a nose plug when swimming increases pressure in the middle ear. It is not necessary to administer antibiotics continuously to a child with a tympanostomy tube. Drainage from the ear may be a sign of middle ear infection and should be reported to the health care provider. (I, T, S)

22. 4. For children age 3 years and younger, the external auditory canal is straightened by gently pulling the earlobe down and backward. For the older child and adult, the earlobe is gently pulled up and backward. (E, T, G)

23. 1. Return demonstrations are the best way to evaluate a person's ability to perform a skill. This technique enables the teacher to observe not only the learner's sequencing of steps of the procedure but also the learner's ability to perform the skill. (E, T, G)

The Client With Foreign Body Aspiration

24. 1. For a child who has shortness of breath, cough, and fever, the priority nursing diagnosis would be Ineffective Breathing Pattern, which requires immediate intervention. This diagnosis would be the basis for planning and implementing nursing care. (D, N, G)

25. 1. Peanuts swell and become soft when moistened

with bronchial secretions, making them difficult to remove. Because peanuts contain a fixed oil, they can cause lipoid pneumonia, but this is not why they are so dangerous when aspirated. Peanuts do begin to decompose when wet, and they do contain calcium, but neither of these factors makes them particularly dangerous when aspirated. (I, T, G)

26. 3. Spherical or cylindric objects are more likely to be aspirated and plug the airway than objects with other shapes. The size, shape, and consistency of foods are important factors in their ability to cause obstruction. (I, T, G)

27. 1. A 2-year-old child is difficult to keep quiet. The parents have a better chance of doing this because they know their child well. Encouraging the parents to stay with the child will help keep the child quiet. A 2-year-old's attention span is short, so watching television would keep the child quiet for only a short time. A 2-year-old does engage in parallel play but does not know how to play with others. Going to the playroom may encourage the child to be active. (P, T, H)

28. 1. Young children have specific reactions to separation and hospitalization. In the protest stage, the toddler physically and verbally attacks anyone who attempts to provide care. In the despair stage, the toddler becomes withdrawn and obviously depressed. Denial or detachment occurs if the toddler's stay in the hospital without the parent is prolonged because the toddler settles in to the hospital life and denies the parents' existence. Regression is a return to a developmentally earlier phase owing to stress or crisis. (I, T, G)

29. 2. Bringing a child's favorite toys, security blanket, or familiar objects from home can make the transition from home to hospital less stressful. Leaving without explaining may decrease the child's trust in the parents. The parents should tell their toddler when they are leaving and when they will return, not by time but in relation to the child's usual activities (e.g., by bedtime); 2-year-olds have a limited sense of time. Short parental visits do not satisfy a toddler's overwhelming need for comfort. (I, T, G)

30. 2. After bronchoscopy, the child should be observed for signs and symptoms of respiratory distress. Laryngeal edema may occur and cause airway obstruction. Signs and symptoms of respiratory distress include tachypnea, increased stridor and retractions, and tachycardia. The sputum may be bloody after bronchoscopy. A change in pulse pressure is not associated with bronchoscopy but rather with intracranial pressure and shock. Pulse deficit is associated with some dysrhythmias. Assessing cardiac rate and rhythm is important but not the most important assessment step. (A, T, G)

31. 4. The three signs indicating that a child is truly choking and requires immediate life-saving interventions are inability to speak, blue color (cyanosis), and collapse. (E, T, G)

32. 4. In 2-year-old child, the ratio of breaths to compressions is 1:5. The nose should be pinched shut and the mouth of the rescuer should make a seal over the child's mouth. The carotid pulse is palpated in a child older than 1 year. Compressions on the child 1 to 8 years of age are applied to the lower sternum two finger breadths above the sternal notch. (I, C, G)

The Client With Asthma

33. 3. Knowing that this child is having an asthma attack, the nurse would expect to hear wheezing and note some shortness of breath and prolonged expiratory phase. During an asthma attack, the cough usually is dry and sounds tight. The absence of wheezing would indicate that the child is not moving air well through the lungs and will become hypoxic. (A, C, G)

34. 3. The wheezing sound heard during an asthma attack sounds like a whistle. During an asthma attack, secretions are thick and not usually expelled until the bronchioles are more relaxed. The pulse rate is elevated, and urine production is increased because of the increased renal circulation. The expiratory phase is normally longer than the inspiratory phase. (I, N, G)

35. 2. In respiratory alkalosis, the alkalinity of the body fluids results in a decrease in the ionization of calcium. A low level of circulating ionized calcium increases the excitability of nerve and muscle tissue. This is manifested by paresthesia (numbness and tingling) of the digits, upper lip, and earlobes. In mild asthma with respiratory alkalosis, breath sounds are typically loud with expiratory wheezing. The pulse rate is elevated, and urine production is increased because of the increased renal circulation. (I, T, G)

36. 2. A 10-year-old should be able to tolerate being alone. Asking for someone to be in the room indicates a degree of psychological distress at this age. The inability to get comfortable is characteristic of child with a diagnosis of Pain. Tightness in the chest occurs as a result of bronchial spasms and indicates a diagnosis of Ineffective Airway Clearance. Inability to answer questions correctly may reflect a state of anoxia or lack of knowledge. (D, N, L)

37. 1. A serious side effect of intravenous administration of methylprednisolone is hypertension. This side effect occurs more often when the infusion is given too rapidly. Seizures occur if an infusion of ampicillin is given too rapidly. Flushing of the skin is not related to methylprednisolone infusion. (I, K, S)

38. 2. The child weighs 33.3 kg (73¼ pounds divided by 2.2 equals 33.29 kg).

$$1 \text{ mg/kg} = 1 \times 33.3 = 33.3 \text{ mg.}$$

$$40 \text{ mg}/33.3 \text{ mg} = 1 \text{ mL}/x \text{ mL.}$$

$$40 \text{ mg} \times x \text{ mL} = 33.3 \text{ mg} \times 1 \text{ mL.}$$

$$x \text{ mL} = 33.3/40.$$

$$x = 0.83 \text{ mL.}$$

(I, T, S)

39. 4. The best indicator of the effectiveness of the albuterol is an increase in peak expiratory flow rate. The updraft may have the effect of increasing wheezing by opening the airways enough so that air can travel through the bronchioles that have excess mucous productions, resulting in the Venturi effect and wheezing. Because this child is still in respiratory distress, some wheezing would be expected. In fact, the presence of wheezing in a child with asthma who is in acute distress may indicate an improvement. As the airways open, the child should begin to have a productive cough. The pulse oximeter reading is meaningless unless there are previous readings for comparison. (E, N, G)

40. 3. Prednisone causes severe gastric upset; therefore, it should be given with food. The drug must be given as ordered and not titrated to response. Abrupt cessation of the drug if it has been given over a long period can cause serious side effects. It is recommended that the daily dose be given in the morning before 9 AM because if given at this time the medication will suppress adrenal cortex activity less, which may reduce the risk of HPA-axis suppression. The pills are not enteric coated and may be crushed. (I, T, G)

41. 4. In asthma, the airways react to certain external and internal stimuli, including allergens, infections, exercise, and emotions. Food allergens commonly associated with asthma include wheat, egg white, dairy products, citrus fruits, corn, and chocolate. (I, T, G)

42. 3. When introducing solid foods to infants, only one new food should be added at a time so that if an allergic reaction occurs, the food allergen can be easily identified. In the absence of evidence of allergy, all foods are appropriate except mixed foods, which should be avoided to facilitate allergen identification. Infant formula is a major source of nutrition for the first year and should not be eliminated when solids are introduced. Rice cereal is usually recommended as the starter cereal, but other cereals, such as oatmeal, are also recommended. (I, T, H)

43. 3. Inhaled irritants and allergens are a common trigger for asthmatic episodes. Exposure to mold is one such allergen. In addition, frequent cleaning decreases the amount of inhalable allergens available to the asthmatic child. Wool fibers (from sheepskin), aerosols, and open windows are all potential sources of respiratory irritants. (I, T, G)

44. 1. Allergic reaction to inhaled particles generally causes a nasal crease from frequent nose rubbing. Allergic shiners are dark circles under the eyes caused by nasal congestion. Fever and abdominal pain are unrelated to allergic rhinitis. Mouth breathing usually occurs when the child has enlarged tonsils or adenoids.(A, C, G)

45. 1. Although the meter does assist in evaluating the effectiveness of a treatment, repeating the dose is not recommended unless prescribed by a physician. Bronchodilators have serious side effects, and the child would need to be monitored closely if several treatments in a row were given. The peak expiratory flow meter is used to monitor the asthma and assist in making decisions about increasing or decreasing therapy. It is also used to follow trends for diurnal variations that predict instability of asthma and need for increased therapy. It assists in early detection of exacerbation of the asthma because decreases in the peek expiratory flow rate may indicate a worsening condition. It can also be used to identify triggers of asthma. (E, N, S)

46. 2. Pets are discouraged when trying to allergy-proof a home for a child with bronchial asthma, unless the pets are kept outside. Pets with hair or feathers are especially likely to trigger asthma attacks. A fish would be a satisfactory pet for this child, but the parents should be taught to keep the fish tank clean to prevent it from harboring mold. (I, T, G)

47. 2. Cromolyn sodium is used as a prophylactic agent to help prevent bronchial asthmatic attacks. The drug is not an antiinflammatory, bronchodilator, or antihistamine agent. Therefore, it is of no use during an asthma attack. The drug inhibits histamine release and acts locally to prevent the release of mediator substances from mast (connective tissue) cells after exposure to allergens. (I, T, G)

48. 3. Developing a positive family life requires placing the child's illness in its proper perspective. Some parents tend to overprotect the child with a chronic illness. This overprotectiveness may cause a child to have an exaggerated feeling of importance or later, as an adolescent, to rebel against the overprotectiveness. Children with asthma need to be treated as normally as possible within the scope of the limitations imposed by the illness. (I, T, G)

49. 4. Physical activities are beneficial to asthmatic children. Most of these children can engage in school and sports activities with minimal difficulty if the asthma is kept in check. (I, T, G)

The Client With Cystic Fibrosis and Bronchopneumonia

50. 2. Classic signs of pneumonia include fever and cough. Weight loss may occur in a child with cystic fibrosis because of the energy expenditure needed to fight the infection. Rash, constipation, and dysuria are not associated with pneumonia. Vomiting may occur, especially if the child is coughing frequently and has a lot of mucus. (A, C, G)

51. 4. It is important to give some antibiotics, like ampicillin, spaced at equal intervals over a 24-hour period to help maintain therapeutic levels of the medication in the bloodstream. If a medication is to be given four times in each 24-hour period, it should be given every 6 hours. It is important to consult with the caregiver about the best times within the prescribed schedule to give the medication. This action gives the mother some control, and the regimen is more likely to be followed. (I, N, S)

52. 2. Postural drainage is generally recommended before meals, to avoid the possibility of vomiting or regurgitating food. The need for rest periods is not as important a factor in scheduling postural drainage. Inhalation treatments are usually given before postural drainage. (I, T, G)

53. 2. One problem associated with cystic fibrosis is poor digestion and absorption of foods, especially fats. Pancreatic enzymes can help improve digestion and absorption of nutrients. They are given with meals and can be sprinkled on food. (E, N, G)

54. 2. Cystic fibrosis affects the exocrine glands. Mucus is thick and tenacious, sticking to the walls of the pancreatic and bile ducts and eventually causing obstruction. Because of the difficulty with digestion and absorption, a moderate-fat, high-protein, high-calorie diet is indicated. (A, K, G)

55. 2. In children with cystic fibrosis, poor digestion and absorption of foods, especially fats, results in frequent bowel movements with bulky, foul-smelling stools. The stools also contain abnormally large quantities of fat, which is called *steatorrhea*. (A, T, G)

56. 2. The child's favorite doll would be a good choice of toys. The doll provides support and is a familiar toy. In view of the child's lung pathology, a fuzzy stuffed animal would not be advised because of its potential as a reservoir for dust and bacteria. Scissors, paper, and paste are not appropriate for a 3-year-old unless the child is supervised. A jigsaw puz-zle is not particularly appropriate for an ill 3-year-old child. (I, T, G)

57. 4. One characteristic of cystic fibrosis is the excessive loss of salt through perspiration. Salt supplements are almost always necessary during warm weather or any other time the child perspires more than usual. The absence of sweat glands, little skin pigment, and a poorly functioning temperature control center are conditions unrelated to cystic fibrosis. (I, T, G)

58. 1. Cystic fibrosis is characterized by a dysfunction in the body's mucus-producing exocrine glands. The mucus secretions are thick and sticky rather than thin and slippery. The mucus obstructs various passages in the body, especially in the bronchi, bronchioles, and pancreatic ducts. Mucus plugs in the pancreatic ducts can prevent pancreatic digestive enzymes from reaching the small intestine, resulting in poor digestion and poor absorption of various food nutrients. (E, K, G)

59. 1. This is the client outcome that deals directly with the nursing diagnosis Ineffective Breathing Pattern. The child may have vomiting and activity intolerance, but these problems are not directly related to respiratory symptoms. (P, N, G)

60. 1. Swimming and bowling are the best physical activities for a child with cystic fibrosis. They are non-contact sports yet can be team sports. Swimming is excellent because it coordinates breathing and movement of all muscle groups. Bowling is a low-energy-output game that still requires skill. The other sports listed require much energy expenditure, which may become increasingly difficult as the child gets older. (I, C, G)

61. 2. Cystic fibrosis is the most common inherited disease in children. It is inherited as an autosomal recessive trait, meaning the child inherits the defective genes from both parents. The chances are one in four for each of this couple's pregnancies. (P, C, G)

62. 3. An important function of the National Cystic Fibrosis Foundation is to put parents of children with cystic fibrosis in touch with each other. Other parents are often able to offer support and help. In some instances, the Foundation gives parents financial assistance for equipment required for home care of their child with cystic fibrosis (but not for medications). The Foundation does not obtain tutors for children or provide genetic counseling for parents. (I, T, G)

63. 2. Although ampicillin can be given as a slow intravenous push, to decrease inflammation of the vein, it is infused over 30 minutes. Heparin or saline should be infused as soon as the antibiotic infusion is finished, so the access remains patent. The infusion should be stopped if there is any question about whether the fluid is entering a vein or subcutaneous tissue. If the intravenous access is not allowing infusion of the medication, the nurse should be called. (E, N, S)

The Client With Sudden Infant Death Syndrome

64. 4. The most important nursing intervention would be to reach out to the anxious parents and stay with them while the infant is being evaluated. (I, T, L)

65. 3. A sensitive approach to the parents can help minimize their guilt and prevent later emotional disturbances. The nurse should never ask any questions that imply parental neglect, wrongdoing, or abuse. (I, T, L)

66. 2. The parents should be given the opportunity to say their final farewells to their infant. This last contact helps them focus on the reality of the infant's death. Reassuring them that they are not at fault does not focus on the reality of death. The presence of their pastor may be helpful but enabling them to see their child would be more important. For some parents, clothes may be too painful a reminder of their child's death, and they may not wish to take them home. (I, T, L)

67. 1. One of the main techniques used in crisis intervention in the hospital includes helping parents begin to gain an intellectual understanding of SIDS. Numerous theories have been proposed, but no specific cause of SIDS has been identified. Evidence suggests that infants with SIDS have chronic hypoxia, possibly from prolonged periodic apnea. (E, T, G)

68. 2. The parents need to discuss their feelings with each other to begin the healing process. Avoiding discussing their feelings causes each one to become isolated and to grieve without support. Working long hours is detrimental to the grieving process; there is no time to come to terms with what has occurred. Acting as if nothing has happened is avoiding the issue. (D, T, L)

69. 4. The nurse should visit as soon after the death as possible. The parents need expert counseling to deal not only with the death of their child but also with a sudden, unexpected, and unexplained tragedy. (I, T, L)

70. 1. The goal of the second visit is to help the parents express their feelings. Gaining an understanding of the disease is a goal of the first visit. Although it is important to assess the impact of SIDS on siblings, this is not the primary goal for the second visit, although plans must be flexible. Parents are unable to deal with decisions such as having other children during the second visit; this should be discussed later. (P, T, L)

The Client Requiring Cardiopulmonary Resuscitation

71. 1. When breathlessness is determined, the priority nursing action is to clear the airway. This action alone may reestablish spontaneous respiration. If the client does not begin breathing, mouth-to-mouth resuscitation is begun. Oxygen therapy would not be initiated at this time. Chest compressions are begun only after the client is determined to be pulseless. (I, T, G)

72. 2. Checking the carotid artery pulse in a child during CPR provides information about perfusion of the brain. The brachial pulse is checked in an infant because the infant's short and often fat neck makes it difficult to palpate the carotid pulse. The femoral and radial arteries might indicate perfusion to the peripheral body sites, but the critical need is for adequate circulation to the brain. (I, T, G)

73. 3. The rescue breathing rate for a child is one every 4 seconds, or 15 times per minute. Rescue breaths should be delivered slowly at a volume that makes the chest rise and fall. (I, T, G)

74. 1. The chest is compressed with the heel of one hand positioned on the lower sternum, two finger breadths above the sternal notch. Fingertips are used to compress the sternum in infants, and the heel of two hands is used in adult CPR. (I, T, G)

75. 4. Chest compressions should be delivered at a rate of 80 to 100 times per minute for a 5-year-old child. This rate approximates the resting minimum pulse, which allows for adequate brain perfusion. A rate less than 80 per minute does not provide adequate brain perfusion for a 5-year-old child. (I, T, G)

76. 1. In a 5-year-old child, the chest is compressed to a depth of 1 to 1.5 inches. This depth forces blood out of the heart into the vital organs (lungs and brain). Deeper compressions could damage the liver, lungs, or other underlying structures. Shallower compressions would not provide adequate circulation to the vital organs. (I, T, G)

77. 3. Signs of recovery from cardiopulmonary arrest include palpable peripheral pulses, the disappearance of mottling and cyanosis, the return of pupils to normal size, and warm dry skin. To determine if the victim of cardiopulmonary arrest has resumed spontaneous breathing and circulation, chest compressions must be stopped for 5 seconds at the end of the first minute and every few minutes thereafter. (E, T, G)

78. 4. After opening the infant's mouth, the nurse attempts to find and remove the object. The nurse should attempt to remove only a visible object; blind finger sweeps are not appropriate in infants and children because the foreign body may be pushed back into the airway. If the nurse cannot see the foreign body, mechanical force—back blows and chest thrusts—should be used in an attempt to dislodge the object. Subdiaphragmatic abdominal thrusts are not used for infants age 1 year or younger because of the risk of injury to abdominal organs. (I, T, G)

79. 2. The infant is placed face down, straddled over the nurse's arm with the head lower than the trunk and the head supported. This position, together with the back blows, facilitates dislodgement and removal of a foreign object and minimizes aspiration if vomiting occurs. (I, T, G)

80. 2. Back blows are delivered rapidly and forcefully with the heel of the hand between the infant's shoulder blades. Slowly delivered back blows are less

likely to dislodge the object. Using the heel of the hand allows more force to be applied, increasing the likelihood of loosening the object. (I, T, G)

81. 4. Crying indicates that the airway obstruction has been relieved, and the infant needs close observation. Delivering chest or back blows could jeopardize a patent airway. Blind finger sweeps are contraindicated in infants. (I, T, G)

82. 1. Tilting the head slightly prevents the tongue from obstructing the airway. Gastric distention interferes with diaphragmatic excursion, which occurs when breaths are delivered too rapidly. Tilting the head back as far as possible will probably result in airway obstruction as the narrow flexible trachea is bent. Excessive pressure on the neck does not directly affect an obstructed airway. Extensor posturing indicates brain damage and is not related to airway obstruction. (I, T, G)

NURSING CARE OF CHILDREN

TEST 2: The Child With Respiratory Health Problems

Directions: Use this answer grid to determine areas of strength or need for further study.

NURSING PROCESS

A = Assessment
D = Analysis, nursing diagnosis
P = Planning
I = Implementation
E = Evaluation

COGNITIVE LEVEL

K = Knowledge
C = Comprehension
T = Application
N = Analysis

CLIENT NEEDS

S = Safe, effective care environment
G = Physiologic integrity
L = Psychosocial integrity
H = Health promotion and maintenance

Question #	Answer #	A	D	P	I	E	K	C	T	N	S	G	L	H
1	4				I				T			G		
2	4				I				T			G		
3	1		D						T			G		
4	2			P						N			L	
5	3				I				T			G		
6	1				I				T			G		
7	1	A								N		G		
8	2					E				N		G		
9	3					E				N		G		
10	3				I				T			G		
11	2					E			T			G		
12	4					E			T			G		
13	1	A								N		G		
14	2					E				N				H
15	3				I				T			G		
16	1				I			C					L	
17	4				I				T			G		
18	2			P					T			G		
19	3			P					T			G		
20	2				I				T			G		
21	1				I				T		S			
22	4					E			T			G		
23	1					E			T			G		
24	1		D							N		G		
25	1				I				T			G		

ANSWER GRID: 1

NURSING PROCESS

A = Assessment
D = Analysis, nursing diagnosis
P = Planning
I = Implementation
E = Evaluation

COGNITIVE LEVEL

K = Knowledge
C = Comprehension
T = Application
N = Analysis

CLIENT NEEDS

S = Safe, effective care environment
G = Physiologic integrity
L = Psychosocial integrity
H = Health promotion and maintenance

Question #	Answer #	Nursing Process					Cognitive Level				Client Needs			
		A	D	P	I	E	K	C	T	N	S	G	L	H
26	3				I				T			G		
27	1			P					T					H
28	1				I				T			G		
29	2				I				T			G		
30	2	A							T			G		
31	4					E			T			G		
32	4				I			C				G		
33	3	A						C				G		
34	3				I					N		G		
35	2				I				T			G		
36	2		D							N			L	
37	1				I		K				S			
38	2				I				T		S			
39	4					E				N		G		
40	3				I				T			G		
41	4				I				T			G		
42	3				I				T					H
43	3				I				T			G		
44	1	A						C				G		
45	1					E				N	S			
46	2				I				T			G		
47	2				I				T			G		
48	3				I				T			G		
49	4				I				T			G		
50	2	A						C				G		
51	4				I					N	S			
52	2				I				T			G		
53	2					E				N		G		
54	2	A					K					G		
55	2	A							T			G		

NURSING PROCESS

A = Assessment
D = Analysis, nursing diagnosis
P = Planning
I = Implementation
E = Evaluation

COGNITIVE LEVEL

K = Knowledge
C = Comprehension
T = Application
N = Analysis

CLIENT NEEDS

S = Safe, effective care environment
G = Physiologic integrity
L = Psychosocial integrity
H = Health promotion and maintenance

Question #	Answer #	A	D	P	I	E	K	C	T	N	S	G	L	H
56	2				I				T			G		
57	4				I				T			G		
58	1					E	K					G		
59	1			P						N		G		
60	1				I			C				G		
61	2			P				C				G		
62	3				I				T			G		
63	2					E				N	S			
64	4				I				T				L	
65	3				I				T				L	
66	2				I				T				L	
67	1					E			T			G		
68	2		D						T				L	
69	4				I				T				L	
70	1			P					T				L	
71	1				I				T			G		
72	2				I				T			G		
73	3				I				T			G		
74	1				I				T			G		
75	4				I				T			G		
76	1				I				T			G		
77	3					E			T			G		
78	4				I				T			G		
79	2				I				T			G		
80	2				I				T			G		
81	4				I				T			G		
82	1				I				T			G		
Number Correct														
Number Possible	82	8	4	7	48	15	3	7	57	15	6	64	9	3

NURSING PROCESS

A = Assessment
D = Analysis, nursing diagnosis
P = Planning
I = Implementation
E = Evaluation

COGNITIVE LEVEL

K = Knowledge
C = Comprehension
T = Application
N = Analysis

CLIENT NEEDS

S = Safe, effective care environment
G = Physiologic integrity
L = Psychosocial integrity
H = Health promotion and maintenance

Question #	Answer #	Nursing Process					Cognitive Level				Client Needs			
		A	D	P	I	E	K	C	T	N	S	G	L	H
Percentage Correct														

Score Calculation: To determine your **Percentage Correct,** divide the **Number Correct** by the **Number Possible.**

The Child With Cardiovascular Health Problems

- **The Client With a Ventricular Septal Defect**
- **The Client With Tetralogy of Fallot**
- **The Client With Down Syndrome**
- **The Client With Rheumatic Fever**
- **The Client With Sickle Cell Anemia**
- **The Client With Iron-Deficiency Anemia**
- **The Client With Hemophilia**
- **The Client With Leukemia**
- **Correct Answers and Rationale**

Select the one best answer, and indicate your choice by filling in the circle in front of the option.

The Client With a Ventricular Septal Defect

A 4-year-old child is admitted for a cardiac catheterization. He was born with a ventricular septal defect that has never been repaired. He is accompanied by both of his parents.

1. When providing care for this child before the cardiac catheterization, the nurse would designate which of the following nursing diagnosis as priority?
   - ○ 1. Pain.
   - ○ 2. Knowledge Deficit.
   - ○ 3. Noncompliance.
   - ○ 4. Altered Cardiac Output.
2. Which of the following should be included as the nurse teaches this child about the cardiac catheterization?
   - ○ 1. A plastic model of the heart.
   - ○ 2. A catheter that will be inserted into the artery.
   - ○ 3. Both parents.
   - ○ 4. Other children undergoing a catheterization.
3. In planning care, the nurse considers the child's stage of development and explains to the parents that a 3-year-old child is most likely resolving Erikson's stage of
   - ○ 1. autonomy versus shame and doubt.

   - ○ 2. identity versus role diffusion.
   - ○ 3. initiative versus guilt.
   - ○ 4. industry versus guilt.
4. The child is scheduled for a cardiac catheterization tomorrow. The nurse's plan of care should be to tell the parents that this procedure usually involves the use of
   - ○ 1. ultra-high-frequency sound waves.
   - ○ 2. a catheter placed in the right femoral vein.
   - ○ 3. a cutdown procedure to place a catheter.
   - ○ 4. general anesthesia.
5. The nurse considers the client's need for psychological preparation for cardiac catheterization. The nurse should base interventions on the fact that
   - ○ 1. protecting a preschooler from learning about unpleasant occurrences decreases anxiety considerably.
   - ○ 2. preschoolers are unable to understand the procedure.
   - ○ 3. little psychological preparation can be given to preschoolers.
   - ○ 4. preparation is a joint responsibility of the physician, parents, and nurse.
6. After the catheterization is performed, the child is returned to the room with a pressure dressing and an intravenous line in place. He is slightly drowsy.

The nurse should give highest priority to which of the following postprocedure assessments?

○ 1. Assessing for a gag reflex.

○ 2. Checking for pulses above the catheterization site.

○ 3. Checking the temperature of the right leg.

○ 4. Comparing color in the right and left legs.

7. When preparing the child's parents for his discharge, the nurse should tell them that

○ 1. the child's activities should be limited for 3 weeks.

○ 2. the child should be given sponge baths until the stitches are removed.

○ 3. antibiotics should be given before the child receives any dental work.

○ 4. the pressure dressing should remain in place until the first postprocedural visit with the physician.

The Client With Tetralogy of Fallot

A 6-year-old child is admitted to the hospital for heart surgery to repair tetralogy of Fallot. The nurse observes that the child is cyanotic at admission.

8. The nurse judges that the parents understand this disorder when they explain that one of the underlying causes of their child's cyanosis is

○ 1. constriction of the aorta.

○ 2. stenosis of the mitral valve.

○ 3. stenosis of the pulmonary artery.

○ 4. the aorta receiving blood directly from the vena cava.

9. When teaching the parents about the echocardiogram that their child will undergo, the nurse should explain that the primary reason for this procedure is to determine

○ 1. cardiac structure.

○ 2. pressure of the blood in the heart.

○ 3. the amount of blood entering the heart.

○ 4. various sounds made by each heartbeat.

10. The child asks the nurse if the cardiac catheterization will hurt. Which of the following statements offers the nurse the best guide for responding to the child's question?

○ 1. The medication used to numb the insertion site will sting.

○ 2. Momentary sharp pain will usually occur when the catheter enters the heart.

○ 3. It is usual for a 6-year-old to feel discomfort during the procedure.

○ 4. It is a painless procedure, although a tingling sensation may be felt in the extremities.

11. The child becomes upset when blood is drawn, and he starts to cry and thrash around. The child's color becomes blue, and his respiratory rate increases to 44 breaths/minute. The nurse should initially

○ 1. ask for a sedation order for this child.

○ 2. assess for an irregular heartbeat.

○ 3. explain to the child that it will only hurt for a short time.

○ 4. place the child in a knee-to-chest position.

12. The nurse teaches the child coughing and deep-breathing exercises before corrective heart surgery. Of the following teaching and learning principles to take into account when teaching the client, which should assume *first* priority?

○ 1. Arranging the order of information to be taught to the child in a logical sequence.

○ 2. Arranging to use actual equipment for demonstrations.

○ 3. Building the teaching on the child's current level of knowledge.

○ 4. Presenting the information to be taught in order from simplest to most complex.

13. When planning care for this client before corrective heart surgery, the nurse would choose which of the following as the priority nursing diagnosis?

○ 1. Ineffective Family Coping.

○ 2. Pain.

○ 3. Knowledge Deficit.

○ 4. Impaired Gas Exchange.

14. After corrective heart surgery is done, the nurse monitors the child for low cardiac output. Which of the following findings would indicate low cardiac output?

○ 1. Cool extremities, bounding pulses, and mottled skin.

○ 2. Altered level of consciousness, cool extremities, and thready pulse.

○ 3. Capillary refill of 2 seconds and blood pressure of 96/67 mm Hg.

○ 4. Altered level of consciousness, warm extremities, and pallor.

15. The nurse plans to teach the parents about the digoxin prescribed for their child. Which of the following would the nurse tell the parents?

○ 1. Digoxin should be given with at least a full glass of water.

○ 2. Digoxin is absorbed better when taken 1 hour before eating.

○ 3. Signs of digoxin toxicity include increased heart rate and loss of appetite.

○ 4. If the child vomits 30 minutes after taking the medication, the dose should be repeated.

16. The nurse should teach the mother that digoxin (Lanoxin)

○ 1. should be kept in the refrigerator.

○ 2. can be kept in the child's bedroom for easy administration.

○ 3. should be locked up with the key kept out of reach.

○ 4. should be kept somewhere the family gathers so a dose is not forgotten.

17. The nurse should plan to teach the parents that the child will have to

○ 1. receive antibiotics before any invasive procedures.

○ 2. drink at least 10 glasses of water per day before the next appointment.

○ 3. take frequent naps for the first 4 weeks at home.

○ 4. restrict ingestion of bananas and citrus fruits.

18. The nurse should teach the parents that when the child returns to the pediatric unit after corrective surgery, he will be

○ 1. on a 2-g to 3-g per day sodium diet.

○ 2. allowed no physical activity.

○ 3. allowed only a few visitors.

○ 4. assigned to an isolation room.

19. The parents express concern that their child wants to be held more frequently than usual postoperatively. Which of the following best describes this behavioral response to stress?

○ 1. Repression.

○ 2. Depression.

○ 3. Regression.

○ 4. Discomfort.

20. The mother asks the nurse why her child has clubbed fingers. The nurse should explain that the clubbing is due to

○ 1. anemia.

○ 2. peripheral hypoxia.

○ 3. delayed physical growth.

○ 4. destruction of bone marrow.

21. The nurse should anticipate that when the child goes home, the parents will most likely have a concern about

○ 1. allowing the child to lead a normal, active life.

○ 2. persuading the child to get enough rest.

○ 3. having the child develop postoperative complications.

○ 4. having the child out of school for a month.

22. The child's 3-year-old sibling has become quiet and shy and demonstrates more than the usual amount of sexual curiosity, according to the mother. These behaviors reflect

○ 1. usual behavior for a 3 year old.

○ 2. a need for more attention.

○ 3. exposure to a sexual experience.

○ 4. an indication of depression.

The Client With Down Syndrome

A community health nurse has been visiting a home regularly to supervise the personal care of a severely retarded child who is 10 years of age. The child's mother has a back ailment of recent origin that prevents her from assuming responsibility for the child's care.

23. After talking with the parents, the nurse would determine that the goal for care of this child is to

○ 1. encourage self-care skills in the child.

○ 2. teach the child something new each day.

○ 3. encourage more lenient behavior limits for the child.

○ 4. set strict behavior limits for the child.

24. The child's disability was apparent at birth, and her development was slow. Which of the following behaviors is least characteristic of a delay in early development common to mentally retarded children?

○ 1. Delay in the use of expressive language.

○ 2. Poor response to verbal commands.

○ 3. Starting to walk at age 20 months.

○ 4. Being able to sit up at age 6 months.

25. Which of the following would be a priority nursing diagnosis for this child?

○ 1. Self-Care Deficit.

○ 2. Knowledge Deficit.

○ 3. Altered Nutrition.

○ 4. Impaired Physical Mobility.

26. The client has an intelligence quotient (IQ) of about 40. The type of environment and interdisciplinary program most likely to benefit this child would be best described as

○ 1. custodial.

○ 2. institutional.

○ 3. habit training.

○ 4. sheltered workshop.

27. The nurse discusses with the parents how to best raise their child's IQ. Which of the following means would be most appropriate?

○ 1. Serving hearty, nutritious meals.

○ 2. Giving vasodilator medications as prescribed.

○ 3. Letting the child play with more able children.

○ 4. Providing stimulating, nonthreatening life experiences.

28. The nurse would instruct the parents that which of the following signs are potentially indicative of a physical problem commonly associated with Down syndrome?

○ 1. Weight loss.

○ 2. Irregular heart rate.

○ 3. Rapid respirations.

○ 4. Increased blood pressure.

29. A primary goal of the nurse working with this child's parents is to increase their sense of

○ 1. affection for the child.

○ 2. responsibility for their child's welfare.

○ 3. understanding of their child's disability.

○ 4. confidence in their abilities to care for their child.

30. When discussing plans for genetic counseling for the mother's other daughter, the nurse should teach the mother that the primary role of the genetic team working with a family is to
    ○ 1. provide the parents with the facts about the risks of birth defects.
    ○ 2. report to the parents the findings of chromosome analysis of the amniotic cells.
    ○ 3. prepare the parents psychologically for the birth of a defective child.
    ○ 4. prescribe birth control or abortion measures for the parents as needed.

31. The nurse mentions that a group meeting for mothers of retarded children is to be held soon. "Not retarded!," blazes the client's mother, "Exceptional." When responding to this outburst, which of the following replies by the nurse would be best?
    ○ 1. "*Retarded* is the accepted term."
    ○ 2. "I'm sorry if I offended you by my thoughtless remark."
    ○ 3. "No matter what it's called, the condition is still the same, isn't it?"
    ○ 4. "I'd like to hear more of your thoughts and feelings on that."

32. In relation to teaching goals, the mother's expressed desire for her child is that she be able to dress herself independently. This would be best written in the nursing care plan as a
    ○ 1. single attainable goal.
    ○ 2. goal that may be postponed.
    ○ 3. series of small, short steps.
    ○ 4. part of the overall larger goal of optimal functioning.

33. Sometimes, the child seems deliberately to do things that cause her mother to become displeased and upset. The nurse should explain to the mother that the child tends to act this way to
    ○ 1. exhibit independence.
    ○ 2. get attention from the mother.
    ○ 3. express anger toward the mother.
    ○ 4. relieve boredom.

34. The community health nurse observes the family at mealtime and notes that the child is messy and eats noisily. Which of the following approaches that the nurse could recommend to decrease the child's undesirable eating habits would provide the most positive reinforcement for her desirable table manners?
    ○ 1. Praising the child when she chews quietly.
    ○ 2. Scolding the child when she smacks her lips.
    ○ 3. Ignoring the child when she plays with her food.
    ○ 4. Making the child leave the table after she makes any mess.

The Client With Rheumatic Fever

A 7-year-old child is admitted to the hospital with the medical diagnosis of acute rheumatic fever.

35. When obtaining a health history from the child's mother, the nurse should ask questions to determine if the child was recently ill with
    ○ 1. the measles.
    ○ 2. the mumps.
    ○ 3. a sore throat.
    ○ 4. influenza virus.

36. On initial assessment, the nurse determines that the physician should be contacted, based on which of the following signs?
    ○ 1. Heart rate of 150 beats/minute.
    ○ 2. Swollen and painful knee joints.
    ○ 3. Twitching in the extremities.
    ○ 4. Red rash on the trunk.

37. The nurse and mother should work on a plan to
    ○ 1. allow either the mother or the father to stay at the child's bedside.
    ○ 2. allow the child to have long periods of rest.
    ○ 3. allow the child to participate in activities that will not cause fatigue.
    ○ 4. encourage the child to eat a high-protein diet.

38. The nurse plans to develop a nursing care plan for the child and family. Which of the following nursing diagnoses would be a priority for this child?
    ○ 1. Altered Comfort.
    ○ 2. Altered Fluid Volume.
    ○ 3. Altered Nutrition.
    ○ 4. Altered Tissue Perfusion.

39. Which of the following laboratory blood findings would confirm that the child likely has had a streptococcal infection?
    ○ 1. High leukocyte count.
    ○ 2. Low hemoglobin count.
    ○ 3. Elevated antibody level.
    ○ 4. Low erythrocyte sedimentation rate.

40. The nurse determines that the parents understand that their child will need to receive long-term antibiotic therapy when they state,
    ○ 1. "It will prevent further streptococcal infections."
    ○ 2. "It will protect against further joint damage."
    ○ 3. "The inflammation will subside more quickly."
    ○ 4. "The inflammation will be reduced with future attacks."

41. Activity is sharply restricted during the acute phase of the child's illness. Which of the following outcomes indicate this activity restriction has been effective?
    ○ 1. There is no permanent injury to joints.

○ 2. The resting heart rate is between 60 and 100 beats/minute.

○ 3. The choreic movements are decreased.

○ 4. The subcutaneous nodules over the joints disappear.

42. During the acute phase of the illness, it would be least desirable to interest the child in which of the following diversional activities?

○ 1. Reading a book to the father.

○ 2. Playing with a doll with the nurse.

○ 3. Watching the television with a sibling.

○ 4. Playing checkers with a roommate.

43. Which of the following initial physical findings are indicative of carditis?

○ 1. Heart murmur.

○ 2. Low blood pressure.

○ 3. Irregular pulse.

○ 4. Pain over the anterior chest wall.

44. The physician prescribes digoxin (Lanoxin) for the child. The nurse teaches the child's mother that the primary reason for giving this drug is that it helps

○ 1. relax the walls of the heart's arteries.

○ 2. improve the strength of the heartbeat.

○ 3. prevent irregularities in ventricular contractions.

○ 4. decrease inflammation of the heart wall.

45. The child's daily digoxin (Lanoxin) dose is 0.15 mg PO. The digoxin is available in liquid form at a concentration of 0.05 mg/mL. How much of the medication should the nurse administer at each dose?

○ 1. 0.2 mL.

○ 2. 0.5 mL.

○ 3. 3.0 mL.

○ 4. 5.0 mL.

46. The child's daytime heart rate is 120 beats/minute. The nursing care plan specifies that the child's pulse be assessed several times through the night. The nurse teaches the mother that the primary reason for obtaining a sleeping pulse rate is to ensure that the elevation in the child's pulse rate is not due to

○ 1. the morning dose of digitalis.

○ 2. normal activity during waking hours.

○ 3. being in a warmer environment during the day than at night.

○ 4. having various nurses obtain the pulse rate during day and evening hours.

47. The child is to receive 10 grains of acetylsalicylic acid (aspirin) every 4 hours. The nurse would administer the metric equivalent, which would be

○ 1. 0.065 g.

○ 2. 0.65 g.

○ 3. 6.5 g.

○ 4. 65 g.

48. Which of the following signs or symptoms should lead the nurse to suspect that the child is experiencing early salicylate toxicity?

○ 1. Chest pain.

○ 2. Pink-colored urine.

○ 3. Slow pulse rate.

○ 4. Dizziness.

49. Which of the following measures would the nurse use to help minimize any joint pain the child is experiencing?

○ 1. Massaging the affected joints.

○ 2. Applying ice to the affected joints.

○ 3. Limiting movement of the affected joints.

○ 4. Encouraging progressive weight bearing.

50. Which of these other nursing measures would be appropriate to help alleviate joint pain?

○ 1. Maintaining the joints in an extended position.

○ 2. Applying gentle traction to the child's affected joints.

○ 3. Supporting the child's body in proper alignment with rolled pillows.

○ 4. Using a bed cradle to remove the weight of bed linens on the child's joints.

51. If the child develops chorea-like movements, which of the following eating utensils would the nurse suggest the parents not allow the child to use?

○ 1. Fork.

○ 2. Spoon.

○ 3. Plastic cup.

○ 4. Drinking straw.

52. When discussing long-term care for the child with the parents, the nurse should teach them that a necessary part of this long-term care is

○ 1. physical therapy.

○ 2. antibiotic therapy.

○ 3. psychological therapy.

○ 4. antiinflammatory therapy.

53. The parents express concern that their other children will develop rheumatic fever. What would be the nurse's best response?

○ 1. "This disease is usually not contagious."

○ 2. "Your other children are just as likely to develop rheumatic fever."

○ 3. "There is medicine available to prevent this; check with your doctor."

○ 4. "Your other children are all girls, so there is no need to worry."

The Client With Sickle Cell Anemia

A 1-year-old child is admitted to the hospital with sickle cell crisis. He is the second child to have sickle cell disease in a family of five children.

54. When preparing for the child's admission, the nurse should anticipate and prepare for therapy that most likely will include
○ 1. parenteral iron therapy.
○ 2. exchange transfusion.
○ 3. intravenous fluid therapy.
○ 4. fast-acting anticoagulant therapy.

55. The nurse would explain to the parents that the local tissue damage the child is likely to show at admission is due to
○ 1. an autoimmune reaction complicated by hypoxia.
○ 2. lack of oxygen in the red blood cells.
○ 3. circulatory obstruction.
○ 4. high serum bilirubin levels and adrenocortical imbalance.

56. The nurse notes that the child prefers a side-lying position with the knees sharply flexed. The child's positioning should cause the nurse to further assess for evidence of
○ 1. nausea.
○ 2. backache.
○ 3. abdominal pain.
○ 4. emotional regression.

57. The sickle cell crisis subsides, and the child is to be discharged. The nurse reminds the parents to seek prompt health care if their child develops
○ 1. headaches and nausea.
○ 2. fatigue and lassitude.
○ 3. skin rash and itching.
○ 4. sore throat and fever.

58. The nurse reviews with the parents how to care for their child at home. The nurse determines that the parents understand the basic principles of care when they state that they are
○ 1. keeping the child with them at all times.
○ 2. restricting the child's fluids at night.
○ 3. encouraging their child to drink as much fluid as possible.
○ 4. not allowing their child to play with other children.

59. Which of the following explanations would the nurse offer when the mother asks why her affected children's hemoglobin was normal at birth and then developed the S hemoglobin?
○ 1. "The placenta bars passage of the hemoglobin S from the mother to the fetus."
○ 2. "The red bone marrow does not begin to produce hemoglobin S until several months after birth."
○ 3. "Antibodies transmitted from the mother to the fetus provide the newborn with temporary immunity."
○ 4. "The newborn has a high concentration of fetal hemoglobin in the blood for some time after birth."

60. The parents ask about the chances of sickle cell disease occurring in future children. The nurse should respond to this question based on knowledge that both parents are carriers and therefore the risk of one of their children having the disease is
○ 1. 1 in 4, in the total number of their children.
○ 2. 1 in 4, with each pregnancy.
○ 3. 1 in 2, in the total number of their children.
○ 4. 1 in 2 with each pregnancy.

61. The nurse would identify which of the following as the priority nursing diagnosis during the crisis?
○ 1. Ineffective Coping.
○ 2. Altered Cardiac Output.
○ 3. Pain.
○ 4. Fluid Volume Deficit.

The Client With Iron-Deficiency Anemia

An 11-month-old infant is brought to an outpatient pediatric clinic by her mother. She is very pale, and the mother explains that she drinks more than a quart of cow's milk daily, eats very few solids, and sleeps excessively.

62. The mother asks the nurse what she could have done to prevent the iron-deficiency anemia. The nurse should teach the mother that it is helpful to introduce solid foods into the infant's diet at age
○ 1. 1 to 2 months.
○ 2. 5 to 6 months.
○ 3. 8 to 10 months.
○ 4. 10 to 12 months.

63. The infant's diet needs to be modified. The nurse teaches the mother about diet modifications. The nurse evaluates the teaching as initially effective when the mother states, "I will try to change my baby's diet so that there is an
○ 1. equal amount of iron-rich solids and milk."
○ 2. increased intake of iron-rich solids and decreased milk intake."
○ 3. elimination of all milk products."
○ 4. increased amount of iron-rich solids and the same amount of milk."

64. The nurse teaches the mother about iron-rich foods that are most appropriate for an 11-month-old infant. The mother's selection of which of the following foods would indicate that she understands the teaching?
○ 1. Eggs, fortified cereals, meats, and green vegetables.
○ 2. Fruits, cereals, milk, and yellow vegetables.
○ 3. Eggs, fruits, milk, and mixed vegetables.
○ 4. Juices, fruits, fortified cereals, and milk.

65. The mother asks the nurse if the anemia has anything to do with her child's frequent infections. The nurse should teach the mother that

- ○ 1. little is known about iron-deficiency anemia and its relationship to infection in children.
- ○ 2. children with iron-deficiency anemia are more susceptible to infection than are other children.
- ○ 3. children with iron-deficiency anemia are less susceptible to infection than are other children.
- ○ 4. children with iron-deficiency anemia are no more susceptible to infection than are other children.

66. The infant is started on iron therapy. The nurse plans to teach the mother how to administer the iron drops. Which of the following instructions would be most appropriate?
- ○ 1. Mix the iron drops in the child's milk.
- ○ 2. Put the iron drops in the child's mouth, then follow with juice.
- ○ 3. Put the iron drops in the child's mouth, then follow with milk.
- ○ 4. Mix the iron drops in the child's bedtime water bottle.

The Client With Hemophilia

A neonate has prolonged bleeding following a circumcision and is suspected of having hemophilia A (classic hemophilia).

67. The physician has ordered several laboratory tests to help diagnose the bleeding disorder. The nurse would explain to the parents that which test would most likely be abnormal in a neonate with hemophilia?
- ○ 1. Bleeding time.
- ○ 2. Platelet count.
- ○ 3. Clot retraction test.
- ○ 4. Partial thromboplastin time.

68. Which information that the nurse notes in the neonate's family history would help support the diagnosis of hemophilia?
- ○ 1. A brother and sister who are healthy.
- ○ 2. The ethnic background of the family is Italian and German.
- ○ 3. A maternal brother who experienced prolonged bleeding after surgery.
- ○ 4. The paternal grandmother died from chronic lymphocytic leukemia.

69. A diagnosis of hemophilia A is confirmed. As the child enters the second half of infancy, the nurse should teach the parents to
- ○ 1. administer one half of a children's aspirin for a temperature higher than 101°F.

- ○ 2. sew thick padding into the elbows and knees of the child's clothing.
- ○ 3. check the color of the child's urine every day.
- ○ 4. expect the eruption of the primary teeth to produce moderate to severe bleeding.

70. The nurse plans to teach the neonate's parents to recognize hemarthrosis, explaining that an early sign of hemarthrosis is
- ○ 1. the child's reluctance to move a body part.
- ○ 2. a cool, pale, clammy extremity.
- ○ 3. ecchymosis formation around a joint.
- ○ 4. instability of a long bone on passive movement.

71. The neonate's mother tells the nurse that she is planning to do home teaching when the child reaches school age. She does not want her child in school because the teacher will not watch him as well as she would. The mother's comments represent what common parental reaction to a child's chronic illness?
- ○ 1. Overprotection.
- ○ 2. Devotion.
- ○ 3. Mistrust.
- ○ 4. Insecurity.

72. The neonate experiences bleeding in the elbow, necessitating a trip to the emergency department. A lyophilized concentrate of factor VIII is administered intravenously. Besides monitoring the infusion, which of the following nursing interventions would be appropriate to minimize bleeding in the affected area?
- ○ 1. Apply constant pressure to the elbow.
- ○ 2. Keep the elbow below the level of the heart.
- ○ 3. Place a warm, moist pack on the elbow.
- ○ 4. Elevate the elbow and apply ice.

73. Because of the risks associated with administration of factor VIII concentrate, the nurse would teach the neonate's family to recognize and report
- ○ 1. yellowing of the skin.
- ○ 2. constipation.
- ○ 3. abdominal distention.
- ○ 4. puffiness around the eyes.

74. The mother tells the nurse she will be afraid to allow her child to be very active because of the danger of injury and bleeding. The nurse explains that physical fitness is important for children with hemophilia and that one ideal activity for them is
- ○ 1. snow skiing.
- ○ 2. swimming.
- ○ 3. basketball.
- ○ 4. gymnastics.

75. Which of the following nursing diagnoses would the nurse implement as part of this client's long-term care?
- ○ 1. Knowledge Deficit.
- ○ 2. Potential for Injury.

○ 3. Self-Esteem Disturbance.
○ 4. Altered Health Maintenance

76. The parents attend a support group for parents of children with hemophilia. They are concerned because several of the families have had older children who have died from acquired immunodeficiency syndrome (AIDS). They ask the nurse how these children got the AIDS virus. The nurse knows that the most likely route of transmission of AIDS to these children was
○ 1. contamination of the factor VIII replacement received during bleeding episodes.
○ 2. casual contact with a child who tested positive for human immunodeficiency virus (HIV).
○ 3. use of a contaminated needle to obtain a blood sample.
○ 4. exposure of the children to children with AIDS who attend the same hematology clinic.

77. A parent of a child with AIDS asks the nurse how to look for signs and symptoms of infection. The nurse responds that they need to be especially alert for which of the following?
○ 1. Erythema around the infected area.
○ 2. Rectal temperature higher than 100.5 F.
○ 3. Tenderness of the infected area.
○ 4. Warmth of the infected area.

The Client With Leukemia

An acutely ill 10-year-old girl is hospitalized with an upper respiratory infection and right otitis media. She is diagnosed with leukemia.

78. The nurse teaches the parents about leukemia. Which of the following descriptions given by the mother best indicates that she understands the nature of leukemia?
○ 1. The disease is infectious in nature and characterized by increased white blood cell production.
○ 2. The disease is neoplastic in nature and characterized by a proliferation of immature white blood cells.
○ 3. The disease is inflammatory in nature and characterized by enlargement of the lymph nodes.
○ 4. The disease is autoimmune in nature and characterized by increased circulating antibodies in the bloodstream.

79. Laboratory findings show that the child is anemic. The nurse explains to the parents that the anemia most likely has resulted from blood loss and
○ 1. inadequate dietary folic acid intake.
○ 2. decreased red blood cell production.

○ 3. increased destruction of red blood cells by lymphocytes.
○ 4. progressive replacement of the bone marrow with scar tissue.

80. Which of the following statements would the nurse use to describe to the parents why their child was prone to infections?
○ 1. Play activities were too strenuous.
○ 2. Vitamin C intake has been inadequate over a period of time.
○ 3. The number of red blood cells were inadequate for carrying oxygen for tissue nourishment.
○ 4. Immature white blood cells are incapable of handling an infectious process.

81. The nurse notes that the child has petechiae; that her gums, lips, and nose bleed easily; and that she has bruises on various parts of her body. Which of the following laboratory test results would be consistent with these findings?
○ 1. Platelet count of 80×10^3
○ 2. Serum calcium level of 5 mg/dL.
○ 3. Fibrinogen level of 75 mg/dL.
○ 4. Partial prothromboplastin time of 60 seconds.

82. Which of the following measures should be kept to a minimum, when possible, because the child is prone to bruise and bleed easily?
○ 1. Administering stool softeners.
○ 2. Changing the position in bed.
○ 3. Having visitors.
○ 4. Administering drugs intramuscularly.

83. Which of the following measures would be contraindicated when the nurse assists the child with oral hygiene?
○ 1. Applying petroleum jelly to the lips.
○ 2. Cleaning the teeth with a toothbrush.
○ 3. Swabbing the mouth with moistened cotton swabs.
○ 4. Rinsing the mouth with a nonirritating mouthwash.

84. The nurse observes that an area in the child's mouth is bleeding. Which of the following items would the nurse use because it is most effective for promoting homeostasis over the lesion?
○ 1. Karaya gum.
○ 2. A cotton ball imbedded with petroleum jelly.
○ 3. A nonsticking gauze sponge.
○ 4. A dry tea bag.

85. Which of the following beverages would the nurse plan to give the child when she feels nauseated?
○ 1. Orange juice.
○ 2. Weak tea.
○ 3. Plain water.
○ 4. A carbonated beverage.

86. The nurse should question the order if which drug is prescribed for the child to help relieve discomfort?

○ 1. Acetaminophen.
○ 2. Acetophenetidin.
○ 3. Ibuprofen.
○ 4. Propoxyphene hydrochloride.

87. The child is scheduled for a bone marrow aspiration. The nurse evaluates the teaching concerning the site of puncture as successful when the child points to the
○ 1. right lateral side of the right wrist.
○ 2. middle of the chest.
○ 3. distal end of the thigh.
○ 4. back of the hip bone.

88. Which of the following nursing diagnosis would the nurse identify as a priority in dealing with this newly diagnosed leukemic child and family?
○ 1. Potential for Injury.
○ 2. Altered Comfort.
○ 3. Altered Nutrition.
○ 4. Anticipatory Grieving.

89. Mercaptopurine (Purinethol), 75 mg/day, is prescribed. Mercaptopurine is packaged in 50-mg tablets for oral administration. How many tablets should the nurse give the child each day?
○ 1. One half of one tablet.
○ 2. 1 and one half tablets.
○ 3. 2 tablets.
○ 4. 2 and one half tablets.

90. Which of the following signs and symptoms would suggest to the nurse that the client is experiencing mercaptopurine toxicity?
○ 1. Nausea, vomiting, and diarrhea.
○ 2. Skin rash, constipation, and polyuria.
○ 3. Dry mouth, blurred vision, and headache.
○ 4. Drowsiness, malaise, and low blood pressure.

91. The child is receiving mercaptopurine and methotrexate. The nurse explains to the child's mother that these drugs
○ 1. selectively destroy malignant cells, thereby slowing tumor growth.
○ 2. create a hormonal imbalance within the body that acts to suppress tumor growth.
○ 3. damage deoxyribonucleic acid (DNA) within cell nuclei, which in turn disrupts cell growth and division.
○ 4. imitate nutrients essential for malignant cell growth, thus preventing those cells from using natural nutrients.

92. The child has an absolute neutrophil count of 400. The nurse should
○ 1. restrict only staff and visitors with active infection.
○ 2. place the child in strict isolation.
○ 3. consult with the physician about administering an antiemetic.
○ 4. increase fluid intake.

93. Allopurinol is prescribed. Which of the following nursing measures should be carried out for a client taking allopurinol?
○ 1. Encouraging a high fluid intake.
○ 2. Omitting carbonated fluids.
○ 3. Giving foods high in potassium.
○ 4. Limiting foods high in natural sugar.

94. The nurse should question the order for methotrexate if the physician has not also ordered
○ 1. the child to be kept in a state of fasting.
○ 2. a white blood cell count.
○ 3. an radiographic examination of the spinal canal.
○ 4. collection of a specimen for urinalysis.

95. The physician orders methotrexate to be given by intrathecal injection. The nurse should prepare the child for an injection into the
○ 1. bone marrow of the hip.
○ 2. femoral artery.
○ 3. subdural space.
○ 4. spinal canal.

96. The child's absolute neutrophil count is now 900. The nurse would teach the mother that
○ 1. the child should wear a mask when in contact with others.
○ 2. the child should stay away from crowds.
○ 3. anyone who has direct contact with the child should wear a gown and mask.
○ 4. the child should not eat raw fruits and vegetables.

97. The child fails to respond to therapy. Which of the following statements offers the nurse the best guide in making plans to assist the parents in dealing with their child's imminent death?
○ 1. Knowing that the prognosis is poor helps prepare relatives for the death of children.
○ 2. Relatives are especially grieved when a child does well at first but then declines rapidly.
○ 3. Trust in health personnel is most often destroyed by a death that is considered untimely.
○ 4. It is more difficult for relatives to accept the death of a 10-year-old than the death of a younger child whose family membership has been short.

98. Authorities generally agree that to help others deal with death, a nurse first must have
○ 1. experienced the death of a loved one.
○ 2. developed a belief that accepts life after death.
○ 3. taken a course that examined how best to deal with death and grieving.
○ 4. worked out a personal philosophy of life and death.

99. Which of the following nursing diagnoses would be a priority for the family at this time?
○ 1. Ineffective Family Coping.
○ 2. Altered Parenting.
○ 3. Fear.
○ 4. Grieving.

100. Which of the following courses of action would be most appropriate for the nurse when planning to meet the child's emotional needs during the last days of life?
- ○ 1. Restrict visitors to the parents so as not to over-tax the child.
- ○ 2. Answer the child's questions about the illness and imminent death honestly.
- ○ 3. Concentrate nursing efforts on meeting the child's physical needs to help keep her mind on other things.
- ○ 4. Encourage the child to play quietly with a room-mate to replace thoughts of sadness with thoughts of pleasurable things.

101. After the child dies, the mother asks the nurse, "What if we had brought her in when she first complained of an earache?" Which of the following would be the nurse's best response to the mother?
- ○ 1. Explain that nothing could have helped the child.
- ○ 2. Provide comfort by saying that the child is no longer suffering with an incurable illness.
- ○ 3. Reassure the mother that all possible care was given.
- ○ 4. Explain that infections are often the result of leukemia rather than the cause of it.

CORRECT ANSWERS AND RATIONALE

The letters in parentheses following the rationale identify the step of the nursing process (A, D, P, I, E), cognitive level (K, C, T, N), and client needs (S, G, L, H). See the Answer Grid for the key.

The Client With a Ventricular Septal Defect

1. 2. The child and family would need to know what the cardiac catheterization is, what to expect, and what care will be provided. Alteration in Comfort might be a consideration after the catheterization. There is no evidence that the child or family is noncompliant. Altered Cardiac Output is not the priority problem here. (D, N, G)

2. 3. Preschoolers are able to understand information that is individualized to their level. Including a plastic model of the heart and a catheter as part of the preoperative preparation may be helpful. The other family members will understand the heart model and catheter better than the preschooler. The most important aspect of teaching a preschooler is to have the family members there for support. (P, T, S)

3. 3. Erikson maintains that the chief psychosocial task of the preschool period is acquiring a sense of initiative. The child's activities center around energetic learning and seeking accomplishment and satisfaction in these activities. The conflict of guilt arises when the child oversteps the limits of abilities and behaves or acts inappropriately. Autonomy versus shame and doubt is the psychosocial task of toddlers. Identity versus identity diffusion is the task of early adolescents, and industry versus inferiority is the task of school-aged children. (P, C, L)

4. 2. In children, cardiac catheterization usually involves a right-sided approach because septal defects permit entry into the left side of the heart. The catheter is usually inserted into the femoral vein through a percutaneous puncture; a cutdown procedure is rarely used. The catheterization is usually performed under local anesthesia with sedation. Echocardiography involves the use of ultra-high-frequency sound waves. (P, T, G)

5. 4. Preparation is the joint responsibility of the physician, parents, and nurse. Overprotecting a preschooler can increase anxiety rather than decrease it. Preschoolers are ready to understand information that is individualized to their level. Little psychological preparation can be given to infants and toddlers. (I, T, L)

6. 4. The involved and uninvolved extremities should be compared in terms of color, temperature, pedal pulses, and capillary filling time. Vital signs, including blood pressure, are checked as often as every 15 minutes after the procedure to detect dysrhythmias and hypotension. Pulses, especially those below the catheterization site, are checked for equality and symmetry. Fluids should be encouraged after the procedure; the dye used during the catheterization procedure causes osmotic diuresis. (P, T, G)

7. 3. Antibiotics are suggested for children with heart defects before dental work is done to reduce the risk of bacterial infection. Activities are not restricted. Stitches are not necessary with a percutaneous approach. The pressure dressing will be removed before the child is discharged, allowing showering or bathing as usual. (P, T, G)

The Client With Tetralogy of Fallot

8. 3. The three congenital defects associated with tetralogy of Fallot are (1) stenosis of the pulmonary artery, (2) interventricular septal defect, and (3) deviation of the aorta. A possible fourth defect is hypertrophy of the right ventricle, which occurs as an adaptive mechanism to help overcome the effects of the three congenital defects. When pulmonary stenosis is severe, the child is cyanotic because insufficient blood reaches the lungs for good oxygenation. (E, N, G)

9. 1. An echocardiogram records the structure of the heart muscle and provides a graphic presentation of the heart working. It does not provide information about the pressure of the blood in the heart. Cardiac catheterization is used to measure the pressure in the heart chambers and major vessels and to measure the amount of blood entering the heart. Auscultation with a stethoscope is required to detect the various sounds made with each heartbeat. A phonocardiogram provides a graphic presentation of heart sounds. (P, T, G)

10. 1. The nurse's best response when a child asks if cardiac catheterization is painful is to explain that the child will feel a little stinging when the numbing medicine is inserted into the area around the introduction site of the catheter. There may also be a feeling of pressure when the catheter is introduced. The child's trust in the nurse will be quickly lost if the nurse is untruthful. Most children are sedated and feel little during the procedure. (I, T, S)

11. 4. Flexing the legs reduces venous flow of blood

from the lower extremities and reduces the volume of blood being shunted through the interventricular septal defect and the overriding aorta in the child with tetralogy of Fallot. As a result, the blood then entering the systemic circulation has a higher oxygen content, and dyspnea is reduced. Flexing the legs also increases vascular resistance and pressure in the left ventricle. An infant will often assume a knee-to-chest position in a crib, or the mother learns to put the infant over her shoulder while holding the child in a knee-to-chest position to relieve dyspnea. (I, T, G)

12. 3. Before planning any teaching program for a child or an adult, the nurse's first step is to assess the child to determine what is already known. Even a 5-year-old child has some understanding of a condition present since birth. The child's interest will soon be lost if familiar material is repeated too often, however. Such techniques as placing information in a logical sequence, presenting the material in a progression from simple to complex, and using actual equipment for demonstrations are recommended but should be used after obtaining baseline information about what the child already knows. (P, C, S)

13. 3. When planning care for this child, Knowledge Deficit would be the priority nursing diagnosis. The child would need to be prepared for what occurs before and after surgery. There is no evidence of Ineffective Family Coping or Altered Comfort before surgery. The child has been cyanotic since birth, so Impaired Gas Exchange would not be a priority diagnosis. (D, N, G)

14. 2. Clinical signs of low cardiac output and poor tissue perfusion include pale, cool extremities; cyanosis; weak, thready pulses; delayed capillary refill; and altered consciousness. (A, K, G)

15. 2. Taking digoxin 1 hour before meals or 2 hours after meals results in better drug absorption. Signs of digoxin toxicity include decreased heart rate. A digoxin dose is not repeated if the child vomits 30 minutes after ingestion. There would be no way to ascertain how much of the dose had been absorbed. (I, T, G)

16. 3. Digoxin should be kept locked up out of the reach of children. It is toxic and can be harmful, perhaps even fatal, if an overdose is taken. (I, T, G)

17. 1. Parents whose children have undergone open heart surgery with a patch as part of the correction are at risk for infections and should receive information on subacute bacterial endocarditis (SBE) precautions. SBE precautions include receiving an antibiotic before any invasive procedure. Having the child drink a large amount of fluid before a follow-up appointment is not necessary, nor is taking frequent

naps. Children will gear their rest schedule to their activities. In this situation, there are no data to indicate that the child has a high serum potassium concentration; therefore, restricting foods that are high in potassium such as bananas and citrus fruits would not be appropriate. (I, T, G)

18. 1. Because of the hemodynamic changes that occur with repair of the ventricular septal defect and pulmonary valvular stenosis, transient congestive heart failure may develop, and thus a sodium-restricted diet is used. The child will not be on bed rest and should be encouraged to walk in the halls of the unit. The child can be placed in a room with other children who are not contagious. Visitors are not restricted unless the pediatric unit has restrictive visiting. (I, T, G)

19. 3. *Regression* is defined as the act of moving backward. In psychology, the term is used to describe a person who reverts to an earlier stage of behavior or emotion. *Depression* is characterized by feelings of sadness, gloom, and dispiritedness. *Repression* is a defense mechanism by which an unacceptable or painful experience is put out of the conscious mind. *Discomfort* is a negative feeling state. (D, K, L)

20. 2. The child with persistent hypoxia will eventually experience tissue changes in the body because of the low oxygen content of the blood (hypoxemia). Clubbing of the fingers is one common finding. It apparently results from tissue fibrosis and hypertrophy from the hypoxemia and from an increase in capillaries in the area, which occurs as the body attempts to improve blood supplies. The child may be small for his or her chronologic age, but clubbing does not result from slow physical growth. Clubbing of the fingers is also associated with polycythemia, but polycythemia is not a component of tetralogy of Fallot. Destruction of the bone marrow is not related to a cyanotic heart malformation. Instead, bone marrow is actively producing erythrocytes to compensate for the chronic hypoxia. (P, C, G)

21. 1. Most parents find it especially difficult to allow a child who was unable to be normally active before corrective heart surgery to lead a normal and active life after surgery. These parents are less likely to be apprehensive about persuading the child of the need for rest, about the child developing postoperative complications, and about the child's siblings treating the child as a handicapped person. (P, C, L)

22. 2. The central psychosocial task for the preschool-aged child is to develop a sense of initiative versus guilt, according to Erikson's theory. Any environmental change may affect a child. In this situation, the sibling is likely feeling less attention from the mother and is attempting to resolve the conflict with inappropriate behavior. (D, T, L)

The Client With Down Syndrome

23. 1. The goal in working with mentally retarded children is to train them to be as independent as possible, focusing on developmental skills. The child may not be capable of learning something new every day, but needs to repeat what has been taught previously. The parents need to be strict and consistent when setting limits on behavior. (P, T, G)

24. 4. Being able to sit up at age 6 months is a typical developmental skill of a normal infant that could be expected to be delayed in a mentally retarded infant. Mentally retarded children tend to not use expressive language and to not respond to verbal commands at a level appropriate to their chronologic age. Walking, which normally occurs at about age 1 year, is almost always delayed in mentally retarded children. (A, K, G)

25. 1. Self-Care Deficit would be the priority diagnosis for this child. The nurse should guide the family toward helping the child become as independent as possible. The child has a knowledge deficit inherent in her medical diagnosis of mental retardation, but this would not be a priority diagnosis. There are no data to support an alteration in nutritional status. The child is developmentally delayed but has no physical impairment. (D, N, G)

26. 3. With advances in the care of the mentally retarded, it has been found that most people with IQs between about 35 and 50 can learn to take care of their hygienic needs, use acceptable social manners, and manage speech and other simple means of communication. People with IQs between about 50 and 75 are educable. Custodial care is required for the severely and profoundly retarded, those with IQs below about 35. Whether to institutionalize a child is dependent on multiple factors, only one of which is IQ. (A, K, G)

27. 4. Nonthreatening experiences that are stimulating and interesting to the child have been observed to help raise IQ. Such practices as serving nutritious meals, structuring the environment, and letting the child play with more able children have not been demonstrated to increase intelligence. (P, T, G)

28. 3. It is especially important to observe the nature of the child's respirations because children with Down syndrome are prone to develop respiratory infections. (P, T, G)

29. 4. The parents must continue to work daily with their retarded child when the nurse is not there. Instructions and counseling are directed toward increasing their ability to care for the child confidently. A sense of liking for, responsibility for, and understanding of the child tends to grow as this primary goal is accomplished. (P, T, L)

30. 1. The primary aim of genetic counseling is to inform couples of birth defect risks. Reporting results of chromosome analysis of amniotic cells and preparing a couple psychologically for the birth of a defective child are secondary. A decision about birth control methods should be left to the couple. (P, T, L)

31. 4. To respond to a mother who becomes angry when someone calls her child retarded instead of exceptional, the nurse should give the mother a chance to explore her feelings on the subject because she is upset. Trying to use logic, defending the comment, or apologizing are not effective ways to handle the situation. Asking "why" questions may cause the mother to become defensive and does not encourage exploration of feelings. (P, T, L)

32. 3. Goals for a mentally retarded child should be simple and attainable. It is best to break down skills, such as dressing oneself, into many small steps and have the child repeat each step with slowly advancing variations. A series of small, short-term goals would be most appropriate. (P, T, S)

33. 2. The most likely explanation why this mentally retarded child tends to do things deliberately that displease her mother is that she is seeking attention from the mother. Often, the child's need for attention is greater than her fear of being punished and is worth risking the mother's displeasure. (I, C, L)

34. 1. Often, the best reinforcement for desired behavior in children is reward or praise, as described in this situation. Such techniques as scolding the child, ignoring the child, or making the child leave the table when misbehaving do not help reinforce desired behavior. (I, N, H)

The Client With Rheumatic Fever

35. 3. Rheumatic fever is an inflammatory collagen disease that typically follows an infection by group A β-hemolytic streptococci. The infection ordinarily occurs in the throat. Rheumatic fever generally follows infection with streptococci within about 2 weeks. It is believed that the disease involves an autoimmune or allergic response to the organism. Mumps, measles, and viral influenza are caused by viruses and do not predispose to rheumatic fever. (A, T, G)

36. 1. A heart rate of 150 beats/minute is very high for a 7-year-old child and may indicate carditis. Red, swollen joints, red rash, and twitching or chorea are all findings indicative of rheumatic fever. These signs do not require immediate physician notification. (A, N, G)

37. 2. The nurse would encourage and plan to provide long periods of rest for the child with carditis to allow the heart to rest. With carditis, the client will be on bed rest, which will curtail many types of activities. There is no reason to encourage the child to eat as much as possible; in fact, overeating should be discouraged because it taxes the heart muscle. The parents should be made to feel as if they can come and go as they need to. The child is not in critical condition, so the parents do not need to be encouraged to stay at the bedside. (P, T, S)

38. 1. A nursing diagnosis should state a health problem derived from existing evidence about the client and from sound nursing knowledge. The health problem should be amenable to nursing care and should serve as a basis for planning and carrying out client-centered nursing care. Promoting comfort is a nursing responsibility and can serve as a basis for planning and carrying out nursing care. Based on the information given about this client, it is less likely for the child to have impaired fluid volume, tissue perfusion, or nutrition. (D, N, G)

39. 3. Exactly why rheumatic fever follows a streptococcal infection is not known, but it is theorized that an antigen–antibody response occurs to an M protein present in certain strains of streptococci. The antibodies developed by the body attack certain tissues, such as in the heart and joints. Antistreptolysin O (ASO) titer findings show elevated or rising antibody levels. This blood finding is the most reliable evidence indicating a streptococcal infection. (A, K, G)

40. 1. Long-term treatment for rheumatic fever involves monthly penicillin injections to prevent subsequent streptococcal infections, which can cause further heart damage. The inflammation subsides with bed rest and aspirin or steroids. There is no indication that inflammation subsides with fewer side effects while the child receives long-term antibiotic therapy. (E, N, G)

41. 2. Every effort is made to reduce the work of the heart during the acute phase of rheumatic fever when the heart is inflamed. A resting heart rate of between 60 and 100 beats/minute is normal for a 7-year-old. Bed rest with limited activity is recommended to help prevent heart failure. Rheumatic fever is among the leading causes of heart failure and death in children between 5 and 15 years of age. The chorea associated with rheumatic fever is self-limiting and usually disappears in 1 to 3 months. There is no permanent damage to joints associated with rheumatic fever. Subcutaneous nodules that occur over joint surfaces also resolve over time with no treatment. (E, K, G)

42. 4. School-aged children enjoy board games and are commonly intense about following rules. Their play can often become emotional. Adequate rest is of ut-most importance during the acute stage of rheumatic fever. Therefore, playing a game with another child probably would be too strenuous. Such diversional activities as reading a book, playing with a doll, and watching television would be more satisfactory. (P, C, G)

43. 1. In rheumatic fever, the connective tissue of the heart is inflamed. Signs of carditis indicate inflammation severe enough to compromise heart function. The most common signs of carditis include heart murmurs, tachycardia during rest, cardiac enlargement, and changes in the electrical conductivity of the heart. Heart murmurs are present in about 75% of all clients during the first week of carditis and in 85% of clients by the third week. Low blood pressure, an irregular pulse rate, and pain over the anterior chest wall are not related to the inflammatory process of rheumatic fever. (A, T, S)

44. 2. Digitalis preparations, such as digoxin (Lanoxin), act to improve and strengthen the heartbeat. They increase cardiac output by increasing the strength of the heart's contraction and by decreasing the heart rate. Digitalis is not used to relax artery walls, prevent irregularities in ventricular contractions, or eliminate dissociation of ventricular and atrial rhythms. (I, T, G)

45. 3. The following calculation shows how to determine the correct amount of medication when 0.15 mg of a drug is prescribed for each dose and the preparation on hand contains 0.05 mg/mL:

$$0.15 \text{ mg}/x \text{ mL} = 0.05 \text{ mg}/1 \text{ mL}$$
$$0.05x = 0.15$$
$$x = 0.15/0.05$$
$$x = 3 \text{ mL}$$

The correct dosage will be contained in 3 mL of the drug in solution. (I, T, S)

46. 2. An above-average pulse rate that is out of proportion to the degree of activity is an early sign of cardiac failure in a client with rheumatic fever. The sleeping pulse is used to determine whether mild tachycardia continues during sleep (inactivity) or whether it is the result of daytime activity. Digitalis lowers the heart rate. (I, T, G)

47. 2. Ten grains of a drug are equivalent to 0.65 g. (I, T, S)

48. 4. Signs and symptoms of early salicylate toxicity include tinnitus, disturbances in hearing and vision, and dizziness. Salicylate toxicity may cause nausea, vomiting, diarrhea, and bleeding from mucous membranes from long-term use. Chest pain, pink-colored urine, and a slow pulse rate are not associated with salicylate toxicity. (A, N, S)

49. 3. In rheumatic fever, the joints—especially the knees, ankles, elbows, and wrists—are painful, swollen, red, and hot to the touch. Pain is typically minimized by limiting movement of the affected joints. Exercise should be avoided, contrary to usual recommendations for clients with other forms of arthritis. Despite joint involvement in rheumatic fever, permanent deformities do not occur. Massaging the joints and applying ice likely will not relieve pain. (I, T, G)

50. 4. For a child with arthritis associated with rheumatic fever, the joints are generally so tender that even the weight of bed linens can cause pain. Using a bed cradle is recommended to help remove the weight of the linens on painful joints. Supporting the body in good alignment, and changing the client's position are recommended, but these nursing measures are not likely to relieve pain. Applying traction to the joints is not recommended. Traction is usually used to relieve muscle spasms, and these are not associated with rheumatic fever. (I, T, G)

51. 1. For a child with chorea-like movements, safety is of prime importance. Feeding the child may be difficult. Forks should be avoided because of the danger of injury to the mouth and face with the tines. (P, T, S)

52. 2. A child who has had rheumatic fever is likely to develop the illness again after a future streptococcal infection. Therefore, it is advised that such a child receive antibiotic prophylaxis for at least 5 years and sometimes even longer after the acute attack to prevent recurrence. (I, T, G)

53. 1. Usually, other children in the family do not get rheumatic fever. There is no medicine to give the children as prophylactic therapy. They have been exposed to their sibling's streptococcal infection. If the other children do not have a streptococcal infection at this time, they probably will not develop it now. Girls are also at risk for developing rheumatic fever. (I, T, G)

The Client With Sickle Cell Anemia

54. 3. A major therapeutic consideration during a sickle cell crisis is increasing the transport and availability of oxygen to the body's tissues. Ways to do this include administering a high volume of intravenous fluid and electrolytes to help compensate for the acidosis resulting from hypoxemia associated with sickle cell crisis. The fluids also help overcome the dehydration with which the patient usually suffers. Rest and analgesics are common components of therapy for sickle cell crisis. Anticoagulants have been suggested, but they are not included in the general treatment of crisis. Exchange transfusions are used only in certain situations. Iron therapy is contraindicated for this condition. (P, T, G)

55. 3. Characteristic sickle cells tend to cause "log jams" in capillaries. This results in poor circulation to local tissues, leading to ischemia and necrosis. The basic defect in sickle cell disease is an abnormality in the structure of the red blood cells. The erythrocytes are sickle-shaped, rough in texture, and rigid. (I, T, G)

56. 3. Alerted by the child's self-positioning on the side with the knees sharply flexed, the nurse should assess for further evidence of abdominal pain. Regression is common in acutely ill hospitalized children, but insufficient data are given in this item to confirm regression to early infancy. Nausea usually causes an infant to refuse nourishment. A backache would most probably cause an infant to lie supine to relieve discomfort. (A, C, G)

57. 4. Children with sickle cell disease are prone to develop infections as a result of the necrosis of areas within the body and a generalized less-than-optimal health status. The child is often anoretic, gains weight slowly, and exhibits malaise and irritability. Specific signs of infection are sore throat and fever. Fatigue, lassitude, headaches, and nausea could be prodromal signs of infection but could also be signs of other illnesses. Skin rash and itching usually do not indicate an infection but may be a contact dermatitis. The exception would be varicella; therefore, an assessment should include questions about recent contact with infected people. An infection in a child with sickle cell disease often brings on a crisis and should be treated promptly. (I, T, G)

58. 3. Because sickle cells tend to "log jam" in capillaries, it is important that the child receive adequate fluids. The fluids increase the blood volume and help prevent the "log jam" action. Children with a chronic illness need to be around other children for normal growth and development. This child should not be around anyone with an active infection, however. The parents need to allow the child some independence for normal development. Keeping the child with them at all times will overprotect that child and make the child dependent. (E, T, H)

59. 4. Sickle cell disease is an inherited disease that is present at birth. However, 60% to 80% of a newborn's hemoglobin is fetal hemoglobin, which has a structure different from hemoglobin S or A. Sickle cell symptoms generally occur about 4 months after birth. Some hemoglobin S is produced by the fetus near term. The fetus produces all its own hemoglobin from the earliest production in the first trimester. Passive immunity conferred by maternal antibodies is not related to sickle cell disease, but this transmission of antibodies is important to protect the infant from various infections during early infancy. (I, T, G)

60. 2. Sickle cell disease is an autosomal recessive mendelian disorder. Therefore, if both parents have the trait, there is a 1 in 4 chance that any child will have the disease and a 1 in 2 chance that a child will have the trait. (I, T, G)

61. 3. Pain is a priority problem that nurses can do something about. Promoting comfort is a nursing responsibility and serves as a basis for planning and carrying out nursing care. Fluid volume deficit is also a problem that the nurse can treat, with intravenous fluids and electrolytes. There is no information here to indicate that ineffective coping is occurring. Altered cardiac output is not a problem with this type of vasoocclusive crisis. (D, T, G)

The Client With Iron-Deficiency Anemia

62. 2. Solids should be introduced at about age 5 to 6 months. Full-term infants use up their prenatal iron stores within 4 to 6 months after birth. Cow's milk contains insufficient iron. (I, C, G)

63. 2. Intake of iron-rich solids needs to be increased, and intake of milk needs to be decreased to 1 quart per day. It is impossible to obtain the needed iron from milk alone, but milk does contain essential minerals and vitamins. Decreasing milk intake will increase the child's hunger for and tolerance of solids. Near-exclusive intake of iron-rich solids can cause constipation and inadequate absorption of essential nutrients. (E, T, H)

64. 1. Relatively high amounts of iron are contained in eggs, iron-fortified cereals, meats, and green vegetables. Fruits, nonfortified cereals, milk, yellow vegetables, and juices contain less iron. (E, N, G)

65. 2. Children with iron-deficiency anemia are more susceptible to infection because of marked decreases in bone marrow functioning with microcytosis. (I, C, G)

66. 2. Iron drops are better absorbed when mixed with fruit juice or followed by fruit juice. Milk tends to decrease iron absorption. Medication should not be mixed in a bottle of fluids. If the child does not drink all the bottle, it is not known how much of the medication the child actually received. (I, T, G)

The Client With Hemophilia

67. 4. Partial thromboplastin time (PTT) measures the activity of thromboplastin, which is dependent on intrinsic clotting factors. In hemophilia, the intrinsic clotting factor VIII (antihemophilic factor) is deficient, resulting in a prolonged PTT. Bleeding time, tourniquet test, and clot retraction test measure

platelet function, vasoconstriction, and capillary fragility. These are unaffected in people with hemophilia. (I, C, G)

68. 3. Hemophilia A is a genetically transmitted X-linked recessive disorder characterized by a deficiency of plasma factor VIII. A hemophiliac man and a normal woman have normal male children and female children who carry the hemophilia trait. The carrier females pass the abnormal gene to half of their sons. Ethnic background and familial leukemia are unrelated to the development of hemophilia. (A, K, G)

69. 2. As the hemophilic child begins to acquire motor skills, the risk of bleeding increases because of falls and bumps. Such injuries can be minimized by padding vulnerable joints. Aspirin is contraindicated because of its antiplatelet properties. Because genitourinary bleeding is not a typical problem in children with hemophilia, urine testing is not indicated. Tooth eruption does not normally cause bleeding episodes in children with hemophilia. (P, T, G)

70. 1. Bleeding into the joints in the child with hemophilia leads to pain and tenderness, resulting in restricted movement. If the bleeding continues, the area becomes hot, swollen, and immobile. Petechial bleeding is not a problem in hemophilia. (P, T, G)

71. 1. Overprotection is a typical parental reaction to chronic illness. Characteristics include sacrifice of self and family for the child, failure to recognize the child's capabilities and sense of responsibility, placement of overly stringent restrictions on play and peer friendship, and a lack of confidence in other peoples' capabilities. (D, K, G)

72. 4. When a bleeding episode occurs, the affected area should be immobilized and elevated to slow blood flow to the area and promote hemostasis. Pressure should be applied to the area for 10 to 15 minutes to promote clot formation. Cold packs promote vasoconstriction; warm packs promote vasodilation and bleeding. (I, C, G)

73. 1. Because factor VIII concentrate is derived from large pools of human plasma, the risk of hepatitis is always present. Clinical manifestations of hepatitis include yellowing of the skin, mucous membranes, and sclera. (P, T, G)

74. 2. Swimming is an ideal activity for a child with hemophilia. Many noncontact sports and physical activities that do not place excessive strain on joints are also appropriate. Such activities strengthen the muscles surrounding joints and help control bleeding in these areas. Noncontact sports also enhance general mental and physical well-being. (I, T, G)

75. 2. The priority long-term nursing diagnosis for this child would be Potential for Injury. This is always a concern for children with hemophilia. As with all children who have chronic illnesses, there is a potential for self-esteem problems, but there are no data in this item to support this diagnosis. The parents should have a good understanding of the disease process and realize the importance of obtaining regular health care for their child. Pain would be an appropriate diagnosis of the child who has bleeding into a joint, but this would be a transient situation.(D, T, G)

76. 1. The AIDS virus is spread by direct contact with blood or blood products and by sexual contact. Children with hemophilia are at particular risk for AIDS because of the factor VIII concentrate infusions they receive. These concentrates are derived from larger quantities of pooled plasma, exposing recipients to thousands of blood donors. There is no evidence that casual contact between infected and uninfected people transmits the responsible virus. The sterile disposable needles used in all hospitals and clinics to perform venipunctures are not a source of AIDS transmission. (I, C, G)

77. 2. Fever is a cardinal manifestation of infection in people with AIDS. Because the major physiologic alteration in AIDS is generalized immune system dysfunction, typical indicators of the body's response to infection, such as erythema, warmth, and tenderness, may be absent. (I, T, G)

The Client With Leukemia

78. 2. Leukemia is a neoplastic disorder of blood-forming tissues characterized by a proliferation of immature white blood cells. Leukemia is not an infectious, inflammatory, or allergic disease. (E, N, G)

79. 2. The anemia seen in leukemia is caused by the bone marrow's overproduction of immature white blood cells at the expense of producing red blood cells and platelets. In this client, anemia is not caused by an inadequate intake of iron but rather by insufficient red blood cells. The bone marrow is not scarred. (I, C, G)

80. 4. In leukemia, normal white blood cells are decreased (that is, they fail to mature); hence, a child with leukemia is subject to infection. The major morbidity and mortality factor associated with leukemia is infection due to the presence of granulocytopenia. (I, C, G)

81. 1. Megakaryocytes, from which platelets derive, are decreased in leukemia. Platelet counts are low, and the child is subject to easy bruising and bleeding. Low serum calcium, faulty thrombin production, or insufficient fibrinogen concentration are not related to bleeding and bruising in a child with leukemia. (A, C, G)

82. 4. All treatments should be performed gently when caring for a child with leukemia, who is prone to bruising and bleeding. When there is a choice, injections should be avoided or limited. Such measures as administering a stool softener, changing the position in bed, and offering food at frequent intervals are indicated and need not be curtailed because of the increased risk of bleeding. (I, T, S)

83. 2. The oral mucous membranes are easily damaged and are often ulcerated in clients with leukemia. It is better to provide oral hygiene without using a toothbrush, which can easily damage sensitive oral mucosa. Applying petrolatum jelly to the lips, swabbing the mouth with moistened cotton swabs, and rinsing the mouth with a nonirritating mouthwash are appropriate oral care measures for a child with leukemia. (I, T, G)

84. 4. A dry tea bag placed on the bleeding area can be effective to control bleeding from lesions on the oral mucosa. The tannic acid in the tea apparently helps control bleeding. (I, T, G)

85. 4. Carbonated beverages ordinarily are best tolerated when the child feels nauseated. Many children find cola drinks especially easy to tolerate, but non-cola beverages are also recommended. (P, T, G)

86. 3. Ibuprofen prolongs bleeding time. This drug is contraindicated in clients with leukemia. Nonnarcotic drugs other than ibuprofen or aspirin, such as acetaminophen (Tylenol), may be prescribed to control pain; narcotic analgesics may be required when pain is severe. (I, T, G)

87. 4. Although bone marrow specimens may be obtained from various sites, the most commonly used site in children is the posterior iliac crest. The area is close to the body's surface but removed from vital organs. The area is large, so specimens can be easily obtained. For infants, the proximal tibia and the posterior iliac crest are used. (E, C, G)

88. 4. The newly diagnosed child and parents are overwhelmed when first informed of the diagnosis. The family and child go through the beginning stages of grieving in anticipation of what may occur. The child may have some discomfort, some changes in nutritional status, and increased potential for injury, but these would not be priority diagnoses. (D, N, L)

89. 2. The nurse determines the number of 50-mg tablets of a drug to give when the client is to receive 75 mg of the drug for each dosage by using ratios, as follows:

$$1 \text{ tablet}/50 \text{ mg} = x \text{ tablets}/75 \text{ mg}$$

$$50x = 75$$

$$x = 75/50$$

$$x = 1.5 \text{ tablets}$$

(I, T, S)

90. 1. Toxic doses of mercaptopurine most likely produce anorexia, nausea, vomiting, and diarrhea. This drug tends to cause bone marrow suppression; thus, blood counts are especially important. Some of the other signs described in this scenario may be present but are not characteristic of mercaptopurine toxicity. (A, K, S)

91. 4. Antimetabolites have chemical structures resembling those of substances used normally for cell growth and metabolism. These drugs keep cancer cells from using natural nutrients in metabolic processes and therefore interfere with the cellular growth and development of cancer cells. (I, C, G)

92. 1. With a low absolute neutrophil count, the child will have difficulty fighting off an infection, so staff and visitors are restricted to those without an active infection. The child will be in protective isolation, not strict isolation. Low neutrophil counts do not increase the likelihood of vomiting; therefore, an antiemetic is not needed. (P, T, S)

93. 1. Destruction of malignant cells during chemotherapy produces large amounts of uric acid. The client's kidneys may not be able to eliminate the uric acid, and tubular obstruction from the crystals could result in renal failure and uremia. Allopurinol (Zyloprim) interrupts the process of purine degradation to reduce uric acid buildup. The client should be encouraged to increase fluid intake to further assist in eliminating uric acid. (P, C, G)

94. 2. Methotrexate is not highly toxic in low doses but may cause severe leukopenia at higher doses. It is customary and recommended for blood tests to be done before therapy to provide a baseline from which to study the effects of the drug on white blood cell levels. (I, T, G)

95. 4. Methotrexate is administered intrathecally when it is injected into the spinal canal. This route is also called the *intraspinal route,* and the technique is the same as that for a lumbar puncture. The intraosseous route involves injecting a drug in bone tissue. The intraarterial route involves injection into an artery. (I, C, S)

96. 2. The child should avoid crowds because of the risk of exposure to infection. Siblings and others should stay away from the child if they have an active infection. The child's absolute neutrophil count is high enough so that a mask, gown, and isolation are not necessary. (I, N, G)

97. 2. It has been found that parents are more grieved when optimism is followed by defeat. The nurse should recognize this when planning various ways to help the parents of a dying child. It is not necessarily true that knowing about a poor prognosis for years helps prepare parents for a child's death, that trust in health personnel is destroyed when a death is untimely, or that it is more difficult for parents to accept the death of an older child than a younger child. (P, T, L)

98. 4. Nurses caring for terminally ill clients are better prepared to do so when they have worked out a personal philosophy of death. Although other experiences, such as having lost a loved one to death, taking classes in caring for dying clients and grieving, and developing a personal belief in a supreme being and a life hereafter may be helpful in assisting the nurse in thinking about death, most important are the nurse's own feelings about life and death. (P, K, L)

99. 4. Because this family is waiting for the child to die, the most appropriate nursing diagnosis would be Grieving. Families grieve at the time of diagnosis, as well as during the illness, as the child is dying, and after death has occurred. This is a normal process and does not indicate Ineffective Family Coping, Altered Parenting, or Fear. (D, N, L)

100. 2. Most clients, even children, are aware when death appears imminent. The best policy is to answer the child's questions honestly. This helps the child tend to feel less isolated and alone. Such actions as restricting visitors, concentrating on efforts to make the child think of something other than death, and encouraging the child to replace thoughts of sadness with thoughts of pleasurable things are not recommended and tend to increase the dying child's fear, isolation, and feelings of loss of control. (P, T, L)

101. 4. Just as with the child, it is best to answer relatives honestly when they ask questions about their loved one's condition. The nurse answers the questions honestly when explaining that infections are often the result of leukemia rather than a cause of it. It is less satisfactory to tell parents that everything possible has been done for their child, that the child is no longer suffering from the illness, and that nothing could have helped the child. (I, C, L)

NURSING CARE OF CHILDREN

TEST 3: The Child With Cardiovascular Health Problems

Directions: Use this answer grid to determine areas of strength or need for further study.

NURSING PROCESS

A = Assessment
D = Analysis, nursing diagnosis
P = Planning
I = Implementation
E = Evaluation

COGNITIVE LEVEL

K = Knowledge
C = Comprehension
T = Application
N = Analysis

CLIENT NEEDS

S = Safe, effective care environment
G = Physiologic integrity
L = Psychosocial integrity
H = Health promotion and maintenance

Question #	Answer #	A	D	P	I	E	K	C	T	N	S	G	L	H
1	2		D							N		G		
2	3			P					T		S			
3	3			P				C					L	
4	2			P					T			G		
5	4				I				T				L	
6	4			P					T			G		
7	3			P					T			G		
8	3					E				N		G		
9	1			P					T			G		
10	1				I				T		S			
11	4				I				T			G		
12	3			P				C			S			
13	3		D							N		G		
14	2	A					K					G		
15	2				I				T			G		
16	3				I				T			G		
17	1				I				T			G		
18	1				I				T			G		
19	3		D				K						L	
20	2			P				C				G		
21	1			P				C					L	
22	2		D						T				L	
23	1			P					T			G		
24	4	A					K					G		
25	1		D							N		G		

NURSING PROCESS

A = Assessment
D = Analysis, nursing diagnosis
P = Planning
I = Implementation
E = Evaluation

COGNITIVE LEVEL

K = Knowledge
C = Comprehension
T = Application
N = Analysis

CLIENT NEEDS

S = Safe, effective care environment
G = Physiologic integrity
L = Psychosocial integrity
H = Health promotion and maintenance

Question #	Answer #	Nursing Process					Cognitive Level				Client Needs			
		A	D	P	I	E	K	C	T	N	S	G	L	H
26	3	A					K					G		
27	4			P					T			G		
28	3			P					T			G		
29	4			P					T				L	
30	1			P					T				L	
31	4			P					T				L	
32	3			P					T		S			
33	2				I			C					L	
34	1				I					N				H
35	3	A							T			G		
36	1	A								N		G		
37	2			P					T		S			
38	1		D							N		G		
39	3	A					K					G		
40	1					E				N		G		
41	2					E	K					G		
42	4			P				C				G		
43	1	A							T		S			
44	2				I				T			G		
45	3				I				T		S			
46	2				I				T			G		
47	2				I				T		S			
48	4	A								N	S			
49	3				I				T			G		
50	4				I				T			G		
51	1			P					T		S			
52	2				I				T			G		
53	1				I				T			G		
54	3			P					T			G		
55	3				I				T			G		

ANSWER GRID: 2

274

NURSING PROCESS

A = Assessment
D = Analysis, nursing diagnosis
P = Planning
I = Implementation
E = Evaluation

COGNITIVE LEVEL

K = Knowledge
C = Comprehension
T = Application
N = Analysis

CLIENT NEEDS

S = Safe, effective care environment
G = Physiologic integrity
L = Psychosocial integrity
H = Health promotion and maintenance

Question #	Answer #	Nursing Process					Cognitive Level				Client Needs			
		A	D	P	I	E	K	C	T	N	S	G	L	H
56	3	A						C				G		
57	4				I				T			G		
58	3					E			T					H
59	4				I				T			G		
60	2				I				T			G		
61	3		D						T			G		
62	2				I			C				G		
63	2					E			T					H
64	1					E				N		G		
65	2				I			C				G		
66	2				I				T			G		
67	4				I			C				G		
68	3	A					K					G		
69	2			P					T			G		
70	1			P					T			G		
71	1		D				K					G		
72	4				I			C				G		
73	1			P					T			G		
74	2				I				T			G		
75	2		D						T			G		
76	1				I			C				G		
77	2				I				T			G		
78	2					E				N		G		
79	2				I			C				G		
80	4				I			C				G		
81	1	A						C				G		
82	4				I				T		S			
83	2				I				T			G		
84	4				I				T			G		
85	4			P					T			G		

ANSWER GRID: 3

NURSING PROCESS

A = Assessment
D = Analysis, nursing diagnosis
P = Planning
I = Implementation
E = Evaluation

COGNITIVE LEVEL

K = Knowledge
C = Comprehension
T = Application
N = Analysis

CLIENT NEEDS

S = Safe, effective care environment
G = Physiologic integrity
L = Psychosocial integrity
H = Health promotion and maintenance

Question #	Answer #	A	D	P	I	E	K	C	T	N	S	G	L	H
86	3				I				T			G		
87	4					E		C				G		
88	4		D							N			L	
89	2				I				T		S			
90	1	A					K				S			
91	4				I			C				G		
92	1			P					T		S			
93	1			P				C				G		
94	2				I				T			G		
95	4				I			C			S			
96	2				I					N		G		
97	2			P					T				L	
98	4			P			K						L	
99	4		D							N			L	
100	2			P					T				L	
101	4				I			C					L	
Number Correct														
Number Possible	101	12	11	29	41	8	10	20	57	14	15	68	15	3
Percentage Correct														

Score Calculation: To determine your **Percentage Correct,** divide the **Number Correct** by the **Number Possible.**

ANSWER GRID: 4

276

The Child With Health Problems of the Upper Gastrointestinal Tract

- **The Client With Cleft Lip and Palate**
- **The Client With a Tracheoesophageal Fistula**
- **The Client With Imperforate Anus**
- **The Client With Pyloric Stenosis**
- **The Client With Intussusception**
- **The Client With Inguinal Hernia**
- **The Client With Hirschsprung's Disease**
- **Correct Answers and Rationale**

Select the one best answer, and indicate your choice by filling in the circle in front of the option.

The Client With Cleft Lip and Palate

A neonate born with a cleft lip and palate is transferred from the hospital's newborn nursery to a pediatric unit for care.

1. The parents are shocked when they see their child for the first time. Which of the following nursing actions would most help the parents accept their infant's anomaly?
   - ○ 1. Encourage the parents to visit more often.
   - ○ 2. Reassure them that surgery will correct the defect.
   - ○ 3. Show them pictures of babies before and after corrective surgery.
   - ○ 4. Allow them to complete their grieving process before seeing the infant again.
2. Which of the following goals would the nurse identify as a priority for the infant?
   - ○ 1. Maintaining skin integrity in the oral cavity.
   - ○ 2. Using techniques to minimize crying.
   - ○ 3. Altering the usual method of feeding.
   - ○ 4. Preventing the infant from putting fingers in the mouth.
3. Which of the following measures would the nurse use to help the infant retain feedings?

- ○ 1. Bubble the infant at frequent intervals.
- ○ 2. Feed only small amounts at one time.
- ○ 3. Place the end of the nipple far to the back of the infant's tongue.
- ○ 4. Hold the infant in a lying position while feeding.

4. The nurse would identify which of the following as a priority nursing diagnosis for the infant or family?
   - ○ 1. Ineffective Breathing Pattern.
   - ○ 2. Anticipatory Grieving.
   - ○ 3. Ineffective Family Coping.
   - ○ 4. Anxiety.
5. The infant has surgery to repair the cleft lip. The nurse observes that the infant is having difficulty breathing postoperatively. Which of the following measures would be most helpful in bringing relief?
   - ○ 1. Raising the infant's head.
   - ○ 2. Turning the infant onto the abdomen.
   - ○ 3. Administering oxygen per mask.
   - ○ 4. Exerting downward pressure on the infant's chin.
6. Which of the following methods would the nurse use to feed an infant after surgical repair of cleft lip?
   - ○ 1. Gastric gavage.
   - ○ 2. Intravenous fluids.
   - ○ 3. A rubber-tipped medicine dropper.
   - ○ 4. A bottle with a lamb's nipple.

7. Which of the following nursing diagnoses would the nurse identify as a priority after surgical repair?
   ○ 1. Pain.
   ○ 2. High Risk for Infection.
   ○ 3. Impaired Physical Mobility.
   ○ 4. Altered Parenting.

8. To keep the surgical suture line clean and free of debris, the nurse should remove formula and drainage with cotton-tipped applicators moistened with
   ○ 1. mouth wash.
   ○ 2. distilled water.
   ○ 3. mild antiseptic solution.
   ○ 4. half-strength hydrogen peroxide.

9. The nurse teaches the parents about the use of elbow restraints at home. The teaching is evaluated as successful when the parents state,
   ○ 1. "We will leave them on all the time, except when we check the skin under the restraints for redness."
   ○ 2. "We will keep them on all day, but leave them off when the child is asleep."
   ○ 3. "After we get home, we won't have to use the restraints because our child does not suck on his hands or fingers."
   ○ 4. "We will leave them on all the time until the next doctor's visit."

10. The parents ask the nurse when their infant's cleft palate likely will be repaired. The nurse should base the response on knowledge that first repair of a cleft palate is usually done
    ○ 1. before the eruption of teeth.
    ○ 2. when the child weighs at least 10 kg.
    ○ 3. before the development of speech.
    ○ 4. after the child learns to drink from a cup.

11. The child is eventually admitted to the hospital for repair of the cleft palate. Which of the following eating utensils would be most appropriate for the child on the second day after the surgery? A
    ○ 1. cup.
    ○ 2. drinking tube.
    ○ 3. rubber-tipped Asepto syringe.
    ○ 4. large-holed nipple.

12. Which of the following types of restraints would be best for the nurse to use for the child in the immediate postoperative period after cleft palate repair?
    ○ 1. Safety jacket.
    ○ 2. Elbow restraints.
    ○ 3. Wrist restraints.
    ○ 4. Body restraints.

13. In which of the following positions would the nurse place the child to irrigate the mouth after cleft palate repair?
    ○ 1. On the back with the head turned to the side.
    ○ 2. In low Fowler's position with the head straight.
    ○ 3. In a sitting position with the head tilted forward.

○ 4. In Trendelenburg position with the head tilted back.

14. Which of the following activities by the mother would offer the most support to the child during the first few days after surgery?
    ○ 1. Holding and cuddling the child.
    ○ 2. Helping the child play with some of toys.
    ○ 3. Reading some of the child's favorite stories.
    ○ 4. Staying at the bedside and holding the child's hand.

15. The nurse teaches the mother that after the child has had the cleft palate surgery, there is a chance that her child may have which of the following problems?
    ○ 1. Weight loss.
    ○ 2. Difficulty swallowing.
    ○ 3. Lack of a strong self-concept.
    ○ 4. Speech defect.

The Client With Tracheoesophageal Fistula

Several hours after birth, assessment reveals that the newborn has a tracheoesophageal fistula.

16. The parents express feelings of guilt about their baby's anomaly. Which of the following approaches by the nurse would best support the parents?
    ○ 1. Help the parents accept their feelings.
    ○ 2. Explain that the parents did nothing to cause the newborn's defect.
    ○ 3. Encourage the parents to concentrate on planning their baby's care.
    ○ 4. Urge the parents to visit their newborn as often as possible during hospitalization.

17. The newborn is admitted to the pediatric surgical unit. In the initial assessment, the nurse can expect to observe which typical sign of a tracheoesophageal fistula (TEF)?
    ○ 1. Continuous drooling.
    ○ 2. Diaphragmatic breathing.
    ○ 3. Bloody emesis.
    ○ 4. Passage of large amounts of frothy meconium.

18. The nurse reports that the newborn responds to initial feeding attempts with behavior characteristic of TEF. The nurse has not been able to feed the newborn because
    ○ 1. his sucking attempts were too poorly coordinated to be effective.
    ○ 2. he had projectile vomiting after drinking 4 ounces.
    ○ 3. he coughed after several swallows, choked, and became cyanotic.

○ 4. he took about 10 mL of formula, fell asleep, and could not be stimulated to take more formula.

19. The nurse judged that the parents understood their newborn's defect when they said,

○ 1. "The muscle below the stomach is too tight and needs to be loosened."

○ 2. "There is a blind upper pouch and a tube into the trachea from the lower pouch of the esophagus."

○ 3. "There is a lack of certain nerves in the bowel."

○ 4. "The stomach muscles are not there, and part of the stomach and bowel are on the outside."

20. Which of the following nursing diagnoses would the nurse identify as a priority for this newborn?

○ 1. Altered Parenting related to newborn's illness.

○ 2. High Risk for Injury related to aspiration.

○ 3. Ineffective Breathing Pattern related to a weak diaphragm.

○ 4. Altered Nutrition related to poor sucking ability.

21. Before corrective surgery, the newborn is placed on his back in a crib with his head and shoulders elevated. The reasons for this positioning are to

○ 1. reduce cardiac workload, which has been increased by the anomaly.

○ 2. alleviate the pressure of the distended abdominal contents on the diaphragm.

○ 3. enhance pooling of secretions in the bottom of the upper esophageal pouch.

○ 4. allow air to escape from the fistula into the trachea to reduce gastric distention.

22. Which of the following signs should indicate to the nurse that the newborn needs suctioning?

○ 1. Barky cough.

○ 2. Substernal retractions.

○ 3. Decreased activity level.

○ 4. Increased respiratory rate.

23. The newborn is receiving gastrostomy feedings after surgery to correct the TEF. The gastrostomy tube extends from the surface of the abdomen. A pressure clamp is placed on the gastrostomy tube, and a syringe barrel is used to instill formula into the tube. While the newborn is being fed, which of the following techniques should the nurse use to prevent air from entering the stomach after the syringe barrel is attached to the gastrostomy tube? Open the clamp

○ 1. after pouring all the formula into the syringe barrel.

○ 2. before pouring all the formula into the syringe barrel.

○ 3. and continuously pour the formula down the side of the syringe barrel.

○ 4. and allow a small portion of the formula to enter the stomach before pouring additional formula into the syringe barrel.

24. The most appropriate nursing diagnosis for the nurse to identify after surgery is

○ 1. High Risk for Infection.

○ 2. Pain.

○ 3. Altered Bowel Elimination.

○ 4. Impaired Physical Mobility.

25. After feeding the newborn through the gastrostomy tube, the nurse cradles and rocks him for about 15 minutes, primarily to help

○ 1. promote peristalsis.

○ 2. prevent regurgitation of formula.

○ 3. relieve pressure on the surgical repair.

○ 4. associate eating with a pleasurable experience.

26. When the newborn begins receiving oral feedings, the nursing care plan should be based on which of the following principles? Oral feedings

○ 1. are better adjusted to when small, frequent feedings are offered.

○ 2. on a closely followed feeding schedule help the infant accept oral feedings more readily.

○ 3. after intubation are best accepted when offered by the same nurse repeatedly or by the infant's mother.

○ 4. after gastrostomy intubation are best planned in conjunction with observations of the infant's behavior.

27. When preparing for the newborn's discharge from the hospital, the nurse teaches the parents about the need for long-term health care because their child has a high probability of developing

○ 1. speech problems.

○ 2. esophageal stricture.

○ 3. ulcers.

○ 4. recurrent mild diarrhea with dehydration.

28. Which of the following conditions occurring in the mother's pregnancy would have provided a clue that the newborn might have gastrointestinal tract anomaly?

○ 1. Meconium in the amniotic fluid.

○ 2. Low implantation of the placenta.

○ 3. Increased amount of amniotic fluid.

○ 4. Toxemia in the last trimester.

The Client With Imperforate Anus

Nursing assessment of a newborn reveals an imperforate anal membrane. Based on this and other assessment information, a medical diagnosis of imperforate anus is made.

29. The nurse would expect further physical assessment to reveal

○ 1. an absence of meconium stool.

○ 2. abdominal distention.

○ 3. ribbon-like stools.

○ 4. hydrocele.

30. The neonate is to be scheduled for a radiographic examination. The nurse explains to the parents that this examination is done to determine the distance between the anal dimple and the

○ 1. perineum.

○ 2. closed end of the rectum.

○ 3. colon.

○ 4. rectovesical pouch.

31. The nurse establishes which of the following as the priority nursing diagnosis for this newborn?

○ 1. Altered Bowel Elimination.

○ 2. Self-Care Deficit.

○ 3. Body Image Disturbance.

○ 4. Impaired Physical Mobility.

32. The nurse monitors the neonate's urine output for the presence of

○ 1. meconium.

○ 2. blood.

○ 3. bile.

○ 4. acetone.

33. The father observes that the neonate's big toe dorsiflexes and the other toes fan when the nurse gently strokes the sole of the foot. The nurse should explain that this is a normal

○ 1. Tonic foot sign.

○ 2. Plantar reflex.

○ 3. Galant reflex.

○ 4. Babinski reflex.

34. The nurse judges that the parents know what a *low defect* is when the father says that the rectum

○ 1. is below the abdominal rectus muscle.

○ 2. is above the abdominal rectus muscle.

○ 3. has descended through the puborectalis muscle.

○ 4. has ascended through the puborectalis muscle.

35. Before surgery, the neonate is to receive an intramuscular injection of an antibiotic. Which of the following gauges and sizes of needle should be used?

○ 1. 19-gauge, 1.5-inch needle.

○ 2. 20-gauge, 1-inch needle.

○ 3. 23-gauge, 2-inch needle.

○ 4. 25-gauge, ⅝-inch needle.

36. The nurse would select which of the following muscles as the best injection site for this child?

○ 1. Deltoid.

○ 2. Dorsogluteal.

○ 3. Ventrogluteal.

○ 4. Vastus lateralis.

37. After successful surgery, the neonate is returned to the crib with only an intravenous infusion. The mother indicates that she understands her child's prognosis when she states, "Because it was a low anorectal anomaly, my baby

○ 1. will need to wear protective pads or diapers until he reaches maturity."

○ 2. will generally achieve social continence."

○ 3. will probably never be potty trained."

○ 4. has a good chance of being potty trained."

38. A postoperative nursing diagnosis for this neonate would be

○ 1. Altered Parenting.

○ 2. Anticipatory Grieving.

○ 3. Urinary Retention.

○ 4. High Risk for Infection.

39. A postoperative nursing goal is to prevent tension on the perineum. To achieve this goal, the nurse should avoid placing the neonate on his

○ 1. abdomen, with legs pulled up under the body.

○ 2. back, with legs suspended at a 90-degree angle.

○ 3. left side, with hips elevated.

○ 4. right side, with hips elevated.

40. The father asks the nurse how neonates respond to painful stimuli. The nurse's best response would be that neonates

○ 1. cry, and cannot be distracted into stopping.

○ 2. try to roll away.

○ 3. move the whole body.

○ 4. withdraw the affected part.

41. The neonate's anorectal malformation and subsequent surgery are stressors on the parents. A nursing goal would be to facilitate parent–infant bonding. Which of the following interventions would most likely help achieve this goal?

○ 1. Explain to the parents that they can visit at any time.

○ 2. Encourage them to hold their infant.

○ 3. Ask them to help monitor the child's intake and output.

○ 4. Help them plan for their infant's discharge.

The Client With Pyloric Stenosis

A 4-week-old infant is admitted to the hospital with a history of vomiting. The mother explains that initially her daughter seemed to have a problem with regurgitation, then developed nonprojectile vomiting during and after feedings. The vomiting became more forceful until, "one time she vomited across the room."

42. Which of the following serum electrolyte imbalances occur in an infant with persistent vomiting?

○ 1. K^+, 3.2 mEq/L; Cl^-, 92 mEq/L; Na^+, 120 mEq/L.

○ 2. K^+, 3.4 mEq/L; Cl^-, 120 mEq/L; Na^+, 140 mEq/L.

○ 3. K^+, 3.5 mEq/L; Cl^-, 90 mEq/L; Na^+, 145 mEq/L.

○ 4. K$^+$, 5.5 mEq/L; Cl$^-$, 110 mEq/L; Na$^+$, 130 mEq/L.

43. Due to the excessive vomiting in pyloric stenosis, the nurse should assess the child for which of the following acid-base imbalances?
○ 1. Respiratory alkalosis.
○ 2. Respiratory acidosis.
○ 3. Metabolic alkalosis.
○ 4. Metabolic acidosis.

44. A tentative medical diagnosis of hypertrophic pyloric stenosis is made. Given this diagnosis, the nurse would anticipate that the client's vomitus would contain gastric contents,
○ 1. bile, and streaks of blood.
○ 2. mucus, and bile.
○ 3. mucus, and streaks of blood.
○ 4. bile, and stool.

45. The infant's skin is inelastic, and the upper abdomen is distended. To feel the pyloric tumor most easily, the nurse palpates the epigastrium just to the right of the umbilicus
○ 1. just before the infant vomits.
○ 2. while the infant is eating.
○ 3. while the infant is lying on the left side.
○ 4. when the stomach is empty.

46. The most appropriate nursing diagnosis at this time would be
○ 1. Fluid Volume Deficit.
○ 2. Ineffective Airway Clearance.
○ 3. Altered Nutrition.
○ 4. Altered Bowel Elimination.

47. When the infant is admitted to the hospital, the nurse should first
○ 1. weigh the infant.
○ 2. begin an intravenous infusion.
○ 3. switch the child's feedings to oral electrolyte solution.
○ 4. orient the mother to the hospital unit.

48. Which of the following statements by the mother would indicate that she understands pyloric stenosis? "Pyloric stenosis is caused by
○ 1. an enlarged muscle below the stomach sphincter."
○ 2. a telescoping of the large bowel into the smaller bowel."
○ 3. giving the baby more formula than is necessary."
○ 4. the baby's taking the formula too quickly."

49. Before scheduling the infant for surgery, the physician orders the administration of parenteral fluids and electrolytes. Which of the following will need to be added to the intravenous solution in addition to dextrose, water, and sodium chloride for this child?
○ 1. Calcium chloride.
○ 2. Bicarbonate chloride.
○ 3. Potassium chloride.
○ 4. Magnesium chloride.

50. Which of the following should the nurse write on the infant's care plan as an expected client outcome related to the nursing diagnosis Fluid Volume Deficit related to vomiting? The client exhibits no
○ 1. abdominal distention.
○ 2. weight loss.
○ 3. vomiting.
○ 4. increase in respiratory effort.

51. Knowing that the infant is at risk owing to decreased circulating fluid volume, the nurse should assess for which of the following disorders?
○ 1. Inappropriate antidiuretic hormone release.
○ 2. Acute renal failure.
○ 3. Paralytic ileus.
○ 4. Adrenal insufficiency.

52. After undergoing a pyloromyotomy, the infant returns to the room in stable condition. While standing by the crib, the mother says, "Perhaps if I had brought my baby to the hospital sooner, the surgery could have been avoided." What would be the nurse's best response?
○ 1. "Surgery is the most effective treatment for pyloric stenosis."
○ 2. "Try not to worry; your baby will be fine."
○ 3. "Do you feel that this problem indicates that you are not a good mother?"
○ 4. "Do you think that earlier hospitalization could have avoided surgery?"

53. Which of the following is an expected outcome related to the nursing diagnosis Pain related to the surgical procedure? The client
○ 1. exhibits no manifestations of discomfort.
○ 2. has a bowel movement within 2 hours of surgery.
○ 3. has a temperature of 100.0°F measured rectally.
○ 4. retains the first feeding.

54. The nurse instructs the parents about the postoperative feeding schedule. The parents exhibit understanding of these instructions when they state, "If our child does not vomit after surgery, we can start feeding our child in
○ 1. 6 hours."
○ 2. 8 hours."
○ 3. 10 hours."
○ 4. 12 hours."

55. The parents want to be involved in their infant's care postoperatively, and the nurse teaches them proper feeding techniques. The nurse would determine that they understood the teaching if, after a feeding, they positioned the infant in the crib with her head elevated and on her
○ 1. left side.
○ 2. abdomen.
○ 3. right side.
○ 4. back.

56. Immediately after the first feeding, the infant is fussy and restless. The nurse would
    ○ 1. encourage the parents to hold the infant.
    ○ 2. hang a mobile over the infant's crib.
    ○ 3. feed the infant more.
    ○ 4. give the infant a pacifier.

57. The infant's hospitalization and surgery are stressful events for the parents. Which of the following would the nurse correctly interpret as a positive indication of parental coping? They
    ○ 1. tell the nurse they have to get away for a while.
    ○ 2. discuss the infant's care realistically.
    ○ 3. repeatedly ask about whether the child is normal.
    ○ 4. fear that they will disturb the infant.

The Client With Intussusception

A healthy, thriving, 4-month-old boy suddenly experiences episodes of acute abdominal pain. The infant is admitted to the hospital with the diagnosis of intussusception.

58. In an interview with the nurse, the infant's mother describes his behavior before admission. The mother would most likely describe him as crying
    ○ 1. constantly and extending his legs.
    ○ 2. intermittently and drawing his knees to his chest.
    ○ 3. shrilly when ingesting food.
    ○ 4. intermittently when held at a 30-degree angle.

59. The nurse asks the mother several questions during the initial nursing history. Which of the following questions would be most helpful in obtaining pertinent diagnostic data?
    ○ 1. "Did his stool look like currant jelly?"
    ○ 2. "When was the last time he urinated?"
    ○ 3. "Is he eating normally?"
    ○ 4. "Has he vomited?"

60. Which of the following would the nurse identify as a priority nursing diagnosis for this infant?
    ○ 1. Fluid Volume Deficit.
    ○ 2. Altered Bowel Elimination.
    ○ 3. Impaired Skin Integrity.
    ○ 4. Pain.

61. Which of the following is an expected client outcome related to one of the nursing diagnoses made for this child: Pain related to cramping? The client
    ○ 1. exhibits no manifestations of discomfort.
    ○ 2. is very still.
    ○ 3. has a normal bowel movement.
    ○ 4. has not vomited in 3 hours.

62. The infant underwent surgery to reduce the invagination and returns to the room with a nasogastric tube in place. The infant is allowed nothing by mouth and is receiving intravenous fluids. Which of the following parameters would be used to calculate the amount of intravenous fluid and electrolyte solution to be infused over the next 24 hours? Body weight and
    ○ 1. stool output.
    ○ 2. urine output.
    ○ 3. gastric output.
    ○ 4. degree of temperature elevation.

63. A nasogastric tube placed during surgery is no longer freely removing gastric secretions. The nurse should
    ○ 1. aspirate the tube with a syringe.
    ○ 2. irrigate the tube with distilled water.
    ○ 3. increase the level of suction.
    ○ 4. rotate the tube.

64. When fluids by mouth are appropriate for an infant, the nurse most likely would initiate feeding with
    ○ 1. cereal-thickened formula.
    ○ 2. full-strength formula.
    ○ 3. half-strength formula.
    ○ 4. oral electrolyte solution.

65. The infant is at risk for an ileus postoperatively. Which observation would the nurse *not* include in an assessment for this complication?
    ○ 1. Measurement of urine specific gravity.
    ○ 2. Assessment of bowel sounds.
    ○ 3. Characteristics of the first stool.
    ○ 4. Measurement of gastric output.

66. When the infant resumes taking oral feedings after surgery, the parents comment that he seems to suck on the pacifier more since the surgery. Sucking
    ○ 1. provides an outlet for emotional tension.
    ○ 2. indicates readiness to take solid foods.
    ○ 3. indicates intestinal motility.
    ○ 4. is an attempt to get attention from the parents.

67. The nurse teaches the parents at discharge that their infant will
    ○ 1. have a change in the usual home schedule.
    ○ 2. immediately return to the prehospital schedule.
    ○ 3. need more calories at home than what he consumed in the hospital.
    ○ 4. continue experiencing abdominal cramping for a few days.

The Client With Inguinal Hernia

A mother brings her 7-month-old son to the clinic after noticing a swelling in his right groin. The swelling varies in size. It disappears when the infant is resting but appears when he is crying. A tentative diagnosis of inguinal hernia is made.

68. Which of the following assessment findings are most significant?

○ 1. The inguinal swelling is reddened, and the abdomen is distended.

○ 2. The infant is irritable, and a thickened spermatic cord can be palpated on the right side.

○ 3. The inguinal swelling can be reduced, and the infant has a stool in the diaper.

○ 4. The infant's diaper is wet with urine, and the abdomen is nontender.

69. The physician reduces the hernia and schedules the infant for a herniorrhaphy in 2 days. The mother asks the nurse why the surgery is not performed now. The nurse should explain that delaying surgery

○ 1. ensures proper preoperative preparation.

○ 2. ensures the infant will be NPO at least 24 hours before surgery.

○ 3. allows the edema and inflammation in the area to subside.

○ 4. allows the infant to wear a truss for at least 24 hours.

70. The mother is concerned about her infant's surgery. She asks the nurse if her infant would have been scheduled for surgery even if the hernia had been asymptomatic. Which of the following statements offers the best explanation why the surgical repair would be done at this time?

○ 1. An infant is better able to tolerate the physical stress of surgery than an older child.

○ 2. The experience of surgery is less frightening the younger the child is.

○ 3. There is less danger and fewer complications when surgery is an elective procedure rather than an emergency procedure.

○ 4. There is a preference for doing surgery near the genital organs before a child becomes conscious of sexual identity.

71. Which of the following would the nurse identify as a priority nursing diagnosis for this infant and family?

○ 1. Altered Family Processes.

○ 2. Pain.

○ 3. Altered Parenting.

○ 4. Fluid Volume Deficit.

72. The infant is scheduled for a herniorrhaphy tomorrow. A goal should be to prepare the infant psychologically for the surgery. The best method to achieve this goal is to

○ 1. explain preoperative and postoperative procedures to the mother.

○ 2. have the mother stay with the infant.

○ 3. make sure the infant's blanket is there.

○ 4. allow the infant to play with sterile dressings.

73. The infant has undergone an inguinal herniorrhaphy and has been on the day surgery unit for several hours. The mother says the surgeon told her that her child can go home today and asks the nurse when they will be able to leave. The nurse would

tell her that her infant must be fully recovered from the anesthesia and

○ 1. have a cough reflex.

○ 2. have a bowel movement.

○ 3. have a systolic blood pressure reading of 90 mm Hg.

○ 4. retain an oral feeding.

74. The nurse prepares the mother for home care. The nurse would teach the mother

○ 1. to change diapers as soon as they become soiled.

○ 2. how to apply an abdominal binder.

○ 3. to keep the incision covered with a sterile dressing.

○ 4. how to restrain the infant's hands.

75. The mother asks the nurse what to do about bathing her infant. The nurse should tell the mother that the best way to bathe the baby is to

○ 1. cleanse the face and diaper area only for 2 weeks.

○ 2. use sterile sponges and to cleanse the inguinal incision.

○ 3. do daily sponge baths for 1 week.

○ 4. give the infant full tub baths every day.

76. A 15-year-old boy had an inguinal hernia repaired earlier today and is getting ready to go home. The nurse instructs the client about resumption of physical activities. Which of the following statements would indicate that he has understood the instructions?

○ 1. "I can start riding my bike next week."

○ 2. "I have to skip physical education classes for 2 weeks."

○ 3. "I can start wrestling again in 3 weeks."

○ 4. "I can return to my weight-lifting class in 6 weeks."

The Client With Hirschsprung's Disease

A 7-month-old infant is admitted to the hospital with a tentative diagnosis of Hirschsprung's disease.

77. As the nurse is obtaining the infant's initial health history from the parents, which of the following statements made by the mother would most likely result in pertinent diagnostic data? "She

○ 1. is constipated often."

○ 2. sometimes gets colds."

○ 3. sometimes spits up."

○ 4. has a rectal temperature of 99.5 F.

78. During physical assessment, the nurse would be most likely to note that the infant

○ 1. has a scaphoid-shaped abdomen.

○ 2. weighs less than expected for her height and age.

○ 3. has clubbing and cyanosis of the fingers and toes.

○ 4. demonstrates hyperactive deep tendon reflexes.

79. The infant is scheduled for a barium enema to confirm the diagnosis. A primary concern after this procedure is evacuation of barium from the colon. Which of the following indicates that the barium has been adequately evacuated after the procedure?

○ 1. Absence of fecal mass in the lower abdomen.

○ 2. Stools that proceed from clay-colored to brown.

○ 3. Bowel sounds of 30 per minute.

○ 4. Stool guaiac that is negative.

80. The nurse assesses the infant's growth and development. Which behavior would the nurse consider *unusual?*

○ 1. Drinking from a cup and spilling little of the liquid.

○ 2. Raising the chest and upper abdomen off the bed with the hands.

○ 3. Imitating sounds that the nurse makes.

○ 4. Crying loudly in protest when the mother leaves the room.

81. Diagnostic evaluation confirms the medical diagnosis of Congenital Aganglionic Megacolon, and a colostomy is planned. When initially discussing the diagnosis and treatment with the parents, it would be most appropriate for the nurse to

○ 1. assess the adequacy of their coping skills.

○ 2. reassure them that their child will be fine.

○ 3. encourage them to ask questions.

○ 4. give them printed material on the procedure.

82. The nurse judges that the parents understand the diagnosis when the father states,

○ 1. "There is no rectal opening."

○ 2. "The small intestine is not mature."

○ 3. "The nerves to the end of the large colon are missing."

○ 4. "The muscle below the stomach is too tight."

83. Before surgery, the infant is to receive oral neomycin for 3 days. The appropriate pediatric dosage of neomycin sulfate is 10.3 mg/kg q 4 hours. The infant weighs 15 pounds, 6.4 ounces. Which of the following dosages most closely approximates a safe daily dose?

○ 1. 50 mg/day.

○ 2. 150 mg/day.

○ 3. 280 mg/day.

○ 4. 430 mg/day.

84. The nurse anticipates that 24 to 48 hours before surgery, the infant's preoperative preparation will most likely include

○ 1. administration of a tap-water enema.

○ 2. insertion of a gastrostomy tube.

○ 3. restriction of oral intake to clear liquids.

○ 4. preparation of the perineum with povidone-iodine solution (Betadine).

85. Which of the following nursing diagnoses would be the priority diagnosis for this client and family preoperatively?

○ 1. Pain.

○ 2. Altered Bowel Elimination.

○ 3. Fluid Volume Deficit.

○ 4. Altered Parenting.

86. The infant has surgery, and a temporary colostomy is created. The infant's postoperative recovery is uneventful. The nurse prepares the parents for their infant's discharge. Which of the following instructions should the nurse give the parents?

○ 1. Flush the stoma with tap water at least once a day.

○ 2. Allow the diaper to absorb the colostomy drainage.

○ 3. Give the infant plenty of liquids to drink.

○ 4. Expect the stoma to become dusky red within 2 weeks.

87. Which of the mother's questions about the colostomy would indicate that she needs further teaching?

○ 1. "Do you think my child will be able to care for the colostomy by the time he's 9 years old?"

○ 2. "The colostomy will give the intestine time to shrink to its normal size."

○ 3. "The colostomy may include two separate abdominal openings."

○ 4. "Right after the procedure, the stoma will appear big and red."

88. The nurse plans to teach the parents about the appearance of the stoma before discharge. The nurse would teach the parents that the stoma normally will

○ 1. become dark brown in 2 months.

○ 2. stay deep red in color.

○ 3. change to several shades of pink.

○ 4. turn almost purple.

89. The nurse teaches the mother about the types of foods the child will be able to eat with a colostomy. The nurse would advise a

○ 1. high-fiber diet.

○ 2. low-fat diet.

○ 3. decrease in fluid intake.

○ 4. low-residue diet.

90. The child, now age 15 months, has been readmitted to the hospital for colostomy closure. After surgery, the child returns to the pediatric unit with an intravenous line in place. The infusion set delivers 1 mL per 60 drops. A total of 200 mL over the next 3 hours has been ordered. How many drops per minute should the infusion deliver?

○ 1. 14 drops/minute.

○ 2. 21 drops/minute.

○ 3. 67 drops/minute.
○ 4. 83 drops/minute.

91. The child is receiving meperidine hydrochloride (Demerol) postoperatively for pain. Which of the following dosages would be a safe dose for the child (who weighs 30 pounds) to receive every 4 hours?

○ 1. 15 mg/dose.
○ 2. 35 mg/dose.
○ 3. 40 mg/dose.
○ 4. 45 mg/dose.

92. It has been 8 hours since surgery. Which of the following findings would necessitate calling the physician now?

○ 1. An increase of 3 cm in abdominal circumference.
○ 2. A decrease of 1 cm in abdominal circumference.
○ 3. Absence of bowel sounds since surgery.
○ 4. The child's returning appetite.

93. The child will be discharged in 1 or 2 days. When evaluating the parent's knowledge of the overall effects of their child's surgery, the nurse knows that the parents understand when they say,

○ 1. "The abdomen will be large for awhile."
○ 2. "When he is ready, toilet training may be difficult."
○ 3. "We will limit dairy products."
○ 4. "We will give vitamin supplements until adolescence."

CORRECT ANSWERS AND RATIONALE

The letters in parentheses following the rationale identify the step of the nursing process (A, D, P, I, E), cognitive level (K, C, T, N), and client needs (S, G, L, H). See the Answer Grid for the key.

The Client With Cleft Lip and Palate

1. 3. Preoperative and postoperative pictures of babies with cleft palates and lips provide a clear and concrete image of expectations of corrective surgery described by health personnel. Providing these pictures is specific to the parents' behavior because the parents reflect societal values that emphasize an infant's facial appearance and responsive expressiveness. Encouraging the parents to visit more often may make them believe they are currently not visiting enough and could cause unwarranted guilt because there is no evidence they will not visit frequently. Allowing the completion of the grieving process before another interaction between the infant and parents could result in a separation that could last months. (P, T, L)

2. 3. It is important for the infant to have formula before corrective surgery for a cleft lip. Methods for feeding will need to be adjusted to fit the infant's needs. Commonly, a rubber-tipped syringe or medicine dropper is used. Infection or problems with skin integrity in the mouth are uncommon, and minimizing crying is of no particular help. There is no special need to keep the infant's fingers out of the mouth preoperatively, and this may upset the infant even further. (P, T, G)

3. 1. An infant with a cleft palate and lip swallows large amounts of air while being fed and therefore should be bubbled frequently. The soft palate defect allows air to be drawn into the pharynx with each swallow of formula. The stomach will become distended with air, and regurgitation, possibly with aspiration, is likely if the infant is not bubbled frequently. Feeding frequently would not prevent swallowing large amounts of air. A nipple is likely to cause the infant to gag and aspirate. Holding the infant in a lying position during feedings can also produce aspiration and regurgitation of formula. (I, C, G)

4. 2. Parents of an infant with a congenital defect are frequently in a state of shock when the child is first born. The parents go through a period of grieving for the normal child they did not have. (D, N, L)

5. 4. After the repair of a cleft lip, the infant must become accustomed to nasal breathing. If the infant is having difficulty breathing, however, it would be best to open the mouth by exerting downward pressure on the chin. In some instances, an airway is used postoperatively, but when it is not in place, it is best to try pressure on the chin first. Raising the infant's head and turning the infant onto the abdomen are likely to aggravate the situation. Oxygen is not necessary if opening the airway is successful. Using a mask over the child's face may aggravate the problem and could potentially damage the suture line. (I, T, S)

6. 3. A rubber-tipped medicine dropper has been found to be a satisfactory method for feeding an infant who has had surgical repair of a cleft lip. Gastric gavage is ordinarily not used unless complications develop. Intravenous fluids do not supply complete nutrition for the infant. A lamb's nipple may be successful for feeding a child with a cleft palate once the lip is healed; however, the action of making a seal around the nipple would put tension on the suture line. Feeding methods should produce the least tension possible on the sutures to promote effective healing of the cleft lip repair. (I, C, G)

7. 2. After surgery, the most important nursing diagnosis should be High Risk for Infection. Surgery involves an incision, which is at risk for infection. The infant with this type of procedure does have discomfort, which can be relieved with acetaminophen. Pain would be an important nursing diagnosis but not the priority. The infant may be in arm restraints or have the cuff of the sleeve pinned to the diaper or pants. It is important that the infant does not touch the incision line or disrupt the sutures. There is no indication of Altered Parenting. The parents are reacting normally with the first reaction of shock. (D, N, G)

8. 4. Half-strength hydrogen peroxide is recommended for cleansing the suture line after cleft lip repair. The bubbling action of the hydrogen peroxide is effective for removing debris. Normal saline may be the preferred solution in some agencies. (I, T, G)

9. 1. To keep the infant from disturbing the suture line by placing his fingers or other objects in his mouth, either intentionally or accidentally, the restraints should be in place at all times. They should be removed for a short period, however, so that the underlying skin can be checked for any breakdown. Parents should be instructed to manually restrain

the hands and arms while the restraints are removed. (E, T, S)

10. 3. The optimal time for cleft palate repair depends on many factors, but it is best done before speech development and before the child learns faulty speech habits. Such factors as when teeth erupt, how much the child weighs, and when the child learns to drink from a cup are not ordinarily used to determine the time for palate repair. (I, C, G)

11. 1. A cup is the preferred eating utensil after the repair of a cleft palate. At the age when repair is done, the child is ordinarily able to drink from a cup, and using it avoids having to place a utensil in the mouth, which increases the potential for injury to the suture lines. (I, T, G)

12. 2. Recommended restraints for a child who has had palate surgery would be elbow restraints. They minimize the limitation placed on the child but still prevent the child from injuring the repair with fingers and hands. A safety jacket, wrist or body restraints restrict the child unnecessarily. (I, T, S)

13. 3. A sitting position (i.e., with the trunk of the body upright and head tilted forward) is recommended for oral irrigation. This position is best because the child is least likely to choke and aspirate fluid during the irrigation. (I, T, S)

14. 1. The mother should be encouraged to hold and cuddle her child to provide needed emotional support. Such activities as helping the child play with toys, reading stories, and staying with the child would not be contraindicated but do not offer as much emotional support as holding and cuddling. (P, C, L)

15. 4. A speech defect is common after the repair of a cleft palate, and many children require speech therapy after surgery. Such conditions as nutritional inadequacies or difficulty swallowing or in developing a healthy self-concept are uncommon if a child receives adequate care and support. (I, T, G)

The Client With Tracheoesophageal Fistula

16. 1. The parents of children born with defects often have feelings of guilt and ask what they might have done to cause the condition or how they might have avoided it. It is important to allow parents to express their feelings and to accept these feelings as normal reactions. Encouraging parents to begin long-term planning and having them visit their infant as often as possible would generally be of little help when a nurse is offering emotional support to distraught parents, and it could appear to the parents as though they are being "talked out" of their feelings. Explaining that the parents are not at fault would not be appropriate until they have dealt with their feelings of guilt. (P, T, L)

17. 1. Esophageal atresia prevents the passage of swallowed mucus and saliva into the stomach. After fluid has accumulated in the pouch, it flows from the mouth and the infant then drools continuously. The lack of swallowed amniotic fluid prevents the accumulation of normal meconium; lack of stool results. Responsiveness of the infant to stimuli would depend on the overall condition of the infant and is not considered a classic sign of a TEF. Diaphragmatic breathing is not associated with TEF. (A, C, G)

18. 3. The newborn with TEF swallows normally, but the fluids quickly fill the blind pouch. The infant then coughs, chokes, and becomes cyanotic while the fluid returns through the nose and mouth. Poor rooting reflexes and projectile vomiting are typical of infants who have neurologic dysfunctions; these reflexes may also be depressed by medication given to the mother during labor. Falling asleep after taking little formula is characteristic of an infant who becomes exhausted with the exertion of feeding and is often caused by a cardiac anomaly. (E, N, G)

19. 2. Although the term *tracheoesophageal fistula* includes several different structural anomalies, the type of TEF in this item is a blind upper pouch and a fistula from the esophagus into the trachea. A tightened muscle below the stomach and projectile vomiting of normal amounts of formula are characteristic of pyloric stenosis. Aganglionic megacolon is a lack of autonomic parasympathetic ganglion cells in a portion of the lower intestine. (E, T, G)

20. 2. Children with TEF frequently have aspiration pneumonia because the blind pouch fills quickly with fluids. Thus, High Risk for Aspiration is a priority nursing diagnosis, and a nursing activity would be to prevent aspiration by suctioning or positioning. As a result of the aspiration, the newborn may have an Altered Breathing Pattern. There is no evidence here to support the diagnoses Altered Parenting and Altered Nutrition. (D, T, G)

21. 3. Gravity encourages the flow of secretions with pooling in the bottom of the upper pouch when an infant with TEF is placed on the back with the head and shoulders elevated. More effective removal of secretions can be accomplished by positioning a catheter in this pool of secretions. Each breathing cycle forces some air into the stomach, which prevents upward passage of air into the trachea. Although abdominal distention would eventually result from air entering the stomach, this is a much later manifestation of TEF. There is generally no additional cardiac workload and little possibility of cardiac failure unless other anomalies complicate TEF. (I, T, G)

22. 2. Laryngospasm results from the overflow of secretions into the larynx in an infant with TEF. The obstruction to inspiration stimulates the strong contraction of accessory muscles of the thorax to assist the diaphragm in breathing. This produces substernal retractions. A brassy cough is related to a relatively constant laryngeal narrowing, usually due to edema. Decreased activity level and increased respiratory rate are usually due to hypoxia. This is a relatively long-term and constant phenomenon in infants with TEF. The laryngospasm occurring with TEF resolves quickly when secretions are removed from the oropharynx area. (A, C, G)

23. 1. The best way to prevent air from entering the stomach when feeding an infant through a gastrostomy tube is to open the clamp after all the formula has been placed in the syringe barrel. The other techniques allow air to enter the stomach through the gastrostomy tube. (I, K, G)

24. 1. High Risk for Infection would be a priority nursing diagnosis after surgery. With any type of incision, the immediate concern is preventing infection at the site. Pain is also a diagnosis of concern and would be next in order of priority. The infant would be partially restrained to prevent disturbance of the intravenous infusion and nasogastric tube. Bowel elimination should begin in a few days. (D, T, G)

25. 4. Helping meet the psychological needs of an infant being fed through a gastrostomy tube can be accomplished by rocking the infant after a feeding. The infant soon learns to associate eating with a pleasurable experience. Holding and rocking an infant may also help accomplish certain other goals, but these are not primary goals in caring for the infant described here. (I, T, L)

26. 4. It is best to follow a plan of care based on the principle that oral feedings started after an infant or newborn has been fed through a gastrostomy tube are best planned in conjunction with observation of the infant's needs and behavior. When the infant's needs and behavior are overlooked, plans are likely to be unsatisfactory and are more likely to meet the nurse's needs rather than the infant's needs. (P, C, G)

27. 2. Dilation at the anastomosis site is needed during the first years of childhood in about half of the children who have had corrective surgery for TEF. Speech problems are likely if other abnormalities are present to produce them. The larynx and structures of speech are not affected by TEF. Dysphagia and strictures may decrease food intake, and poor weight gain may be noted, but gastric ulcers are not associated with TEF repair. Recurrent mild diarrhea with dehydration should not develop from surgery to correct TEF. (I, C, G)

28. 3. Maternal hydramnios occurs in infants that have a congenital obstruction of the gastrointestinal tract, such as occurs in the presence of a TEF. The fetus normally swallows amniotic fluid and absorbs the fluid from the gastrointestinal tract. Excretion then occurs through the kidneys and placenta. Most fluid absorption occurs in the colon. Absorption cannot occur when the fetus has a gastrointestinal obstruction. Meconium in the amniotic fluid, low implantation of the placenta, and toxemia could occur but are more specifically associated with fetal hypoxia. (A, K, G)

The Client With Imperforate Anus

29. 1. The absence of meconium stool is consistent with a diagnosis of imperforate anus. Abdominal distention is a later sign of imperforate anus. Ribbon-like stools are associated with anal stenosis. Hydrocele is not associated with anorectal malformations. (A, K, G)

30. 2. The purpose of the radiographic examination is to ascertain the distance between the anal dimple and the closed end of the rectum. (I, K, G)

31. 1. With the medical diagnosis of imperforate anus, the priority nursing diagnosis would be Altered Bowel Elimination. The other nursing diagnoses are inappropriate. All infants have self-care deficit, and there is no impaired physical mobility with this defect. At this age, the child would not have body image disturbance.(D, T, G)

32. 1. Passage of meconium in the urine is a sign of rectourinary fistula, in which the rectum and bladder communicate. (A, T, G)

33. 4. A normal Babinski reflex involves dorsiflexion of the big toe and fanning of the other toes. Although normal in infants, this response is abnormal after about age 1 year or when walking begins. A plantar reflex is characterized by flexion of the toes. The tonic foot sign does not exist. A normal Galant reflex is initiated by stroking an infant's back alongside the spine; the hips should move toward the stimulated side. (I, K, H)

34. 3. In a low anorectal anomaly, the rectum has descended normally through the puborectalis muscle. In an intermediate anomaly, the rectum is at or below the level of the puborectalis muscle; in a high anomaly, the rectum ends above the puborectalis muscle. (E, N, G)

35. 4. A 25- to 27-gauge, 0.5- to 1-inch long needle is appropriate for administering an intramuscular injection to an infant. (I, T, S)

36. 4. The vastus lateralis muscle of the thigh is preferred for administering intramuscular injections to infants because there is less danger of injuring nerves, blood vessels, or bony structures. The deltoid muscle is used for intramuscular injections only when other areas are unavailable. The dorsogluteal site is contraindicated for use in children who have not been walking for at least 1 year. The ventrogluteal site is relatively free of major nerves and blood vessels, but the vastus lateralis remains the preferred intramuscular injection site in infants. (I, T, S)

37. 4. Children who have correction as infants for low anorectal anomalies are generally continent. Fecal continence can be expected after successful correction of anal membrane atresia. Children with high anomalies may or may not achieve continence. Therefore, this child will probably be successful at potty training. (E, T, G)

38. 4. High Risk for Infection is an appropriate priority nursing diagnosis when corrective surgery is performed. This diagnosis is amenable to nursing care and should serve as a basis for planning and carrying out client-centered nursing care. Anticipatory Grieving is an important nursing diagnosis but would not be the priority at this particular time. Altered Parenting and Urinary retention may be applicable nursing diagnoses but, again, not priority diagnoses. (D, T, G)

39. 1. When placed on the abdomen, a neonate pulls the legs up under the body, which puts tension on the perineum. Therefore, after surgery, the neonate should be positioned either supine with the legs suspended at a 90-degree angle or on either side with the hips elevated. (P, T, G)

40. 3. The neonate responds to pain with total body movement associated with brief, loud crying that ceases with distraction. After age 6 months, an infant reacts to pain with intense physical resistance and tries to escape by rolling away. A toddler reacts by withdrawing the affected part. (I, T, L)

41. 2. Encouraging the parents to hold their neonate promotes parent–infant bonding. Explaining that the parents can visit anytime will promote bonding only if they do visit with, talk to, and hold the newborn. Asking the parents to help monitor the intake and output at this time may be anxiety-producing and would not facilitate bonding. Helping the parents plan for the infant's discharge involves them in the newborn's care. (P, T, L)

The Client With Pyloric Stenosis

42. 1. These serum electrolyte values in an infant with persistent vomiting reflect hypokalemia, hypochloremia, and hyponatremia. (A, K, G)

43. 3. Metabolic alkalosis occurs because of the excessive loss of potassium, hydrogen, and chloride in the vomitus. Chloride loss leads to a compensatory increase in the number of bicarbonate ions. The bicarbonate side of the carbonic acid–base bicarbonate is increased, and the pH becomes more alkaline. Metabolic acidosis results from severe diarrhea and starvation. Respiratory acidosis is caused by conditions that result in excessive retention of $PaCO_2$. Respiratory alkalosis is caused by conditions that result in loss of $PaCO_2$. (A, K, G)

44. 3. The vomitus of an infant with hypertrophic pyloric stenosis contains gastric contents, mucus, and streaks of blood. The vomitus does not contain bile because the pyloric constriction is proximal to the ampulla of Vater. (A, K, G)

45. 2. The pyloric tumor is most easily palpated when the abdominal muscles are relaxed during a feeding or immediately after vomiting. (A, K, G)

46. 1. Infants with pyloric stenosis usually have some degree of dehydration because of the vomiting of the stomach contents. A nursing priority would be to restore fluid and electrolyte imbalances. Altered Nutrition: Less Than Body Requirements could be applicable but would not be the priority diagnosis. There is no information here to identify Altered Bowel Elimination as the priority diagnosis. A normal infant should be able to protect the airway when vomiting, so a diagnosis of Ineffective Airway Clearance would not apply. (D, T, G)

47. 1. Unless the infant is in hypovolemic shock, obtaining a baseline weight is an important first action. The intravenous fluid rate and amount of electrolytes to be added to the fluid are based on the infant's weight. The weight also helps determine the infant's degree of dehydration. Beginning the intravenous infusion is also important after the weight is obtained. Orientation of the mother could wait until treatment is under way. Because emesis leads to metabolic alkalosis, the child is made NPO. (P, T, G)

48. 1. Pyloric stenosis is hypertrophy of the pylorus muscle distal to the stomach. Telescoping of the bowel is intussusception. Overfeeding or underfeeding cannot cause pyloric stenosis. (E, N, G)

49. 3. The major electrolyte lost during vomiting is potassium. Infants with pyloric stenosis typically have low or low-normal serum potassium levels. The vomiting also causes loss of hydrochloric acid, which leads to metabolic alkalosis, so bicarbonate replacement would not be indicated. Calcium and magnesium usually remain within normal limits in these infants. (E, K, G)

50. 2. An expected client outcome relative to the nursing diagnosis of Fluid Volume Deficit related to vomiting is that the client exhibits no evidence of dehydration, such as weight loss or decreased skin turgor. (P, N, G)

51. 2. Acute renal failure can occur secondary to a decrease in circulating fluid volume because of renal hypoperfusion. Paralytic ileus, adrenal insufficiency, and inappropriate antidiuretic hormone release can result in a fluid volume alterations but do not occur secondary to a decrease in circulating fluid volume, (A, T, G)

52. 4. Restating a mother's response provides the opportunity for clarification and validation. Surgery is the most effective treatment for pyloric stenosis, but this response does not give the mother an opportunity to express her feelings. The nurse should avoid giving premature reassurance and should allow the mother to express her concerns. (I, T, L)

53. 1. An expected client outcome relative to the nursing diagnosis of Pain related to the surgical procedure is that the client will exhibit no evidence of pain, such as total body movement accompanied by crying. (P, N, L)

54. 1. Clear liquids containing glucose and electrolytes are usually prescribed 4 to 6 hours after surgery. If vomiting does not occur, formula or breast milk can be gradually substituted for clear liquids until the infant is taking normal feedings. (E, C, G)

55. 3. Positioning the infant on the right side with the head elevated facilitates passage of food through the pyloric sphincter into the intestine. (E, N, G)

56. 4. Giving the infant a pacifier would help meet the nonnutritive sucking needs and ensure oral gratification. Encouraging the parents to hold the infant and hanging a mobile over the crib do not meet this need. The post pyloromyotomy infant does not need to be fed more. (I, N, G)

57. 2. The fact that the parents can verbalize the infant's care realistically indicates that they are working through their fears and concerns. Without further data, the fact that the parents "have to get away" could be interpreted as ineffective coping. Continuing to ask about the child's general condition even when answers are given does not suggest effective coping, nor does fear of disturbing the infant. (D, N, L)

The Client With Intussusception

58. 2. The infant with intussusception experiences acute episodes of colic-like abdominal pain. Typically, the infant screams and draws the knees to the chest. In between these episodes of acute abdominal pain, the infant appears comfortable and normal. Ingestion of food does not precipitate episodes of pain. Pain that occurs when the infant is positioned

in a reclining position is not associated with intussusception. (A, T, G)

59. 1. Stools in children with intussusception look like currant jelly due to the intestinal inflammation and hemorrhage because of the intestinal obstruction. The other questions relating to urination, fever, and vomiting can also elicit important data, but the currant-jelly stools are diagnostic for intussusception. (A, T, G)

60. 4. Due to the colic-like abdominal pain, Pain would be the priority nursing diagnosis. There are no data to indicate a skin problem or dehydration. Constipation or diarrhea may precede the appearance of currant-jelly stools. (A, C, G)

61. 1. An expected client outcome relative to the nursing diagnosis of Pain related to cramping is that the client exhibits no manifestations of discomfort, such as crying or drawing the legs to the abdomen. Being very still may indicate either a pain state or a state of relaxation.(P, N, G)

62. 3. The volume of parental fluids needed is based on fluid requirements determined according to body weight and, in this situation, gastric output. If these fluids are not replaced with an appropriate intravenous solution, serious fluid and electrolyte imbalances could develop. Urine output is monitored but is not used to calculate maintenance and replacement needs. (A, K, G)

63. 1. To check tube position, the nurse should aspirate the syringe. A return of gastric contents indicates that the end of the tube is in the stomach. Another method is to inject a small amount of air while auscultating with a stethoscope over the epigastric area. The tube is irrigated with normal saline only after the position of the tube is confirmed. The suction level should not be increased; an increased level could damage the mucosa. Rotating the tube could irritate or traumatize the nasal mucosa. (I, C, G)

64. 4. When a child is ready to take fluids by mouth postoperatively, clear liquids are given initially. If clear liquids are tolerated, the concentration and amount of oral feeding are gradually increased. This means advancing to half-strength and then full-strength formula while increasing the amount given with each feeding. (I, C, G)

65. 1. A postoperative ileus is a functional obstruction of the bowel. Assessment of bowel sounds, the first stool, and the amount of gastric output provide information about the return of gastric function. Measurement of urine specific gravity provides information about fluid and electrolyte status. (A, C, G)

66. 1. Sucking provides the infant with a sense of security and comfort. It also is an outlet for releasing tension. The infant should not be discouraged from sucking on the pacifier. Fussiness and irritability after feeding may indicate that the infant's appetite is not satisfied. Sucking is not manipulative in the sense that the infant is seeking parental attention. (D, N, L)

67. 1. Infants who have had an interruption in their normal routine and experiences such as hospitalization and surgery typically manifest behavior changes when discharged. The infant's normal routine has been significantly altered, so it will take time to reestablish another routine. The infant does not need more calories at home than in the hospital. The surgical procedure corrected the problems, so the infant should not continue to have abdominal cramping. (I, T, L)

The Client With Inguinal Hernia

68. 1. A hernia that cannot be reduced, together with abdominal distention, area tenderness, and redness, indicates an incarcerated hernia. An incarcerated hernia can lead to strangulation, necrosis, and gangrene of the bowel. Other findings associated with strangulation include irritability, anorexia, and difficulty in defecation. A palpable thickened spermatic cord on the affected side is diagnostic of inguinal hernia. (A, T, G)

69. 3. If nonoperative reduction is successful, delaying surgery for 2 to 3 days allows the edema and inflammation in the inguinal area to subside. Preoperative preparation is minimal, and the infant is fed until a few hours before surgery to prevent dehydration. Trusses do not prevent incarceration, and there is no reason to use a truss preoperatively. (I, T, G)

70. 3. Inguinal hernia repair is ordinarily done promptly after diagnosis in healthy infants and children. If surgery is delayed, there is a possibility of a partial obstruction when a loop of the bowel protrudes into the inguinal canal. Serious progression with complete obstruction and perhaps strangulation of the bowel requires emergency surgery to prevent gangrene, which could be fatal. The infant does not have a physiologic or psychological advantage over older children. Although performing surgery around the genitals before the preschool years is recommended, the best reason for performing this surgery now would be to avoid having to perform emergency surgery later. (I, T, G)

71. 1. The diagnosis is Altered Family Processes related to the child's surgical procedure. A goal for this nursing diagnosis is that the family will receive adequate support and reassurance. To achieve this goal, the parents need information about the surgical procedure and expected care after surgery. At this time, the child does not have problems with pain or a fluid volume deficit, nor is there any evidence of altered parenting. (D, N, G)

72. 2. The best way to psychologically prepare a 7-month-old child for surgery is to have the primary caretaker stay with the child. Infants in the second 6 months of life commonly develop separation anxiety. Therefore, the priority in this case is to support the child by having the parent present. Teaching the mother what to expect may decrease her anxiety; and although this is also important because infants sense anxiety and distress in parents, the priority in this case is to support the child by having the parent present. Taking a favorite toy or blanket to the operating room provides additional security for the child. Actual play and acting out life experiences are appropriate for preschool-aged children. (P, T, L)

73. 4. Before discharge, the infant must be completely recovered from the anesthesia and take and retain an oral feeding. A normal systolic blood pressure reading for a 7-month-old infant is about 116 mm Hg. (I, T, G)

74. 1. Changing a diaper as soon as it becomes soiled helps prevent wound infection. This is the most common complication after inguinal hernia repair in an infant because of possible contamination of the wound with urine and stool. The surgical wound is unlikely to separate, so an abdominal binder is unnecessary. An infant who is not toilet-trained may or may not have the incision covered with a dressing. A topical spray that protects the wound may be applied. (I, T, G)

75. 3. The incision should be kept as clean and dry as possible. Therefore, daily sponge baths are given for about 1 week postoperatively. Because this type of surgery results in a wound that will heal through primary intention, the skin will heal and cover the wound in about 2 to 3 days. Therefore, it is not necessary to use sterile gauze to cleanse the incision. Clean technique is acceptable. (I, C, G)

76. 3. Activities such as bicycle riding, physical education classes, weight-lifting, and wrestling are contraindicated for about 3 weeks because of possible stress on the incision. (E, N, G)

The Client With Hirschsprung's Disease

77. 1. Infants with Hirschsprung's disease typically have a history of abdominal distention, constipation, periodic diarrhea (when liquid stool leaks around the semiobstructed colon), and failure to thrive. Having an occasional cold and spitting up once in a while are normal for infants. A temperature of 99.5 F measured rectally is considered normal. (A, C, G)

78. 2. Infants with Hirschsprung's disease typically display failure to thrive, with poor weight gain due to malabsorption of nutrients. Clubbing and cyanosis of fingers and toes and hyperactive deep tendon reflexes are not associated with Hirschsprung's disease. The abdomen is usually distended in this disease. (A, N, G)

79. 2. Barium produces white or clay-colored stools. The presence of normal brown-colored stools is an indication that the barium has been evacuated. Presence or absence of a fecal mass does not give definitive information about the passage or retention of barium. Bowel sounds of 30 per second are within normal limits and do not necessarily indicate passage of barium. Guaiac is a test done to determine the presence of occult blood, not barium. (E, N, G)

80. 1. Infants at age 7 months are not capable of drinking from a cup without spilling. At age 6 months, the infant can partially lift his weight on the hands, enjoys imitating sounds, and is developing separation anxiety. (A, T, H)

81. 3. By encouraging parents to ask questions during information-sharing sessions, the nurse can clarify misconceptions and determine their understanding of information. Assessing the adequacy of the parent's coping skills is important but secondary to encouraging them to express their concerns. The questions they ask and their interactions with the nurse may provide clues to the adequacy of their coping skills. The nurse should never give false reassurance to parents. Written materials are appropriate for augmenting the nurse's verbal communication but also are secondary to encouraging questions. (I, N, L)

82. 3. The primary defect in Hirschsprung's disease is an absence of autonomic parasympathetic ganglion cells in the distal portion of the colon. (E, N, G)

83. 4. The dose is calculated first determining the weight in kilograms: 15 pounds, 6.4 ounces is equal to 15.4 pounds; 15.4 pounds divided by 2.2 is equal to 7 kg. Multiplying 10.3 mg by 7 kg equals 72.1 mg. In computing a daily dosage, the dose is multiplied by the number of times it will be given per day (72.1 mg × 6 = 432.6 mg/day). (I, N, S)

84. 3. Dietary intake is limited to clear liquids for 24 to 48 hours before intestinal surgery. A clear liquid diet meets the child's fluid needs and avoids the formation of fecal material in the intestine. Repeated saline enemas are given to empty the bowel. Soap suds enemas are contraindicated for infants, as are tap water enemas. A nasogastric tube may be inserted for gastric decompression. The perineal area is not prepared because it is not involved in this surgery. (P, C, G)

85. 2. Altered Bowel Elimination would be the priority nursing diagnosis in this case. The nursing history information of constipation and occasional diarrhea would lead to this diagnosis. In this situation, it is not likely that the child would have a fluid volume deficit or pain. There are no data to support a diagnosis of Altered Parenting. (D, N, G)

86. 3. Because of decreased fluid reabsorption from the colon, the child with a colostomy benefits from a liberal fluid intake. Tap water flushes of the stoma are contraindicated in infants owing to the absorption of free water and potential for fluid overload. The stoma has a good blood supply and no nerve endings. An appliance should be fitted for stool collection to help prevent skin breakdown. The stoma should always be reddish-pink and moist. A dusky-red stoma may indicate impaired circulation to the area. (I, T, G)

87. 1. The goal of surgery is to remove the aganglionic bowel and to improve functioning of the internal sphincter. A temporary loop or double-barreled colostomy is usually created to rest the bowel. This enables the normal distal bowel to regain its original tone and size. Final corrective surgery is done when the child is age 6 to 12 months or weighs about 10 kg. The colostomy probably will be reversed before the child is old enough to be responsible for its care. A new stoma is swollen and erythematous. (E, N, G)

88. 2. The stoma should remain deep red in color as long as the child has the colostomy. A dark-red to purplish color may indicate impaired circulation to the stoma. (I, T, G)

89. 4. A low residue diet would be recommended for the child with a colostomy. Such a diet causes less bulky stools and facilitates their passage. High-fiber foods, such as fruits and vegetables, should be minimized because they increase the bulk in the stool. A low-fat diet is not indicated, in fact fat is important for brain growth in the first year of life. Although decreasing fluid intake may decrease the number of stools and increase their consistency, because the water usually absorbed through the large intestine is decreased when a colostomy is placed, it is important to maintain fluid intake. Adequate fluid intake is especially important in a child younger than 1 year of age owing to the immaturity of the kidneys and incomplete ability to conserve or eliminate water. (I, T, G)

90. 3. The drop rate is determined as follows:

200 mL fluid/3 hours = 67 mL (rounded from 66.67) fluid/1 hour

67 mL × 60 drops/mL = 4,020 drops

4,020 drops ÷ 60 minutes = 67 drops/minute.

(I, T, S)

91. 1. The dosage for meperidine hydrochloride is 0.5 to 1 mg per pound per dose. This child weighs 30 pounds, so an appropriate dose would be 15 to 30 mg. (I, T, S)

92. 1. Abdominal circumference is measured to monitor for abdominal distention. An increase of 3 cm in 8 hours would require notification of the physician. Absence of bowel sounds would be expected after surgery. Even if the child is hungry, fluids will not be offered until bowel sounds are heard. (A, N, G)

93. 2. Toilet-training is commonly more difficult for children who have undergone surgery for Hirschsprung's disease than it is for other children. This is because of the trauma to the area and the associated psychological implications. Distention is an early sign of infection. Dietary restrictions or vitamin supplementation are usually not required. (E, N, G)

NURSING CARE OF CHILDREN

TEST 4: The Child With Health Problems of the Upper Gastrointestinal Tract

Directions: Use this answer grid to determine areas of strength or need for further study.

NURSING PROCESS

A = Assessment
D = Analysis, nursing diagnosis
P = Planning
I = Implementation
E = Evaluation

COGNITIVE LEVEL

K = Knowledge
C = Comprehension
T = Application
N = Analysis

CLIENT NEEDS

S = Safe, effective care environment
G = Physiologic integrity
L = Psychosocial integrity
H = Health promotion and maintenance

Question #	Answer #	Nursing Process					Cognitive Level				Client Needs			
		A	D	P	I	E	K	C	T	N	S	G	L	H
1	3			P					T				L	
2	3			P					T			G		
3	1				I			C				G		
4	2		D							N			L	
5	4				I				T		S			
6	3				I			C				G		
7	2		D							N		G		
8	4				I				T			G		
9	1					E			T		S			
10	3				I			C				G		
11	1				I				T			G		
12	2				I				T		S			
13	3				I				T		S			
14	1			P				C					L	
15	4				I				T			G		
16	1			P					T				L	
17	1	A						C				G		
18	3					E				N		G		
19	2					E			T			G		
20	2		D						T			G		
21	3				I				T			G		
22	2	A						C				G		
23	1				I		K					G		
24	1		D						T			G		
25	4				I				T				L	

NURSING PROCESS

A = Assessment
D = Analysis, nursing diagnosis
P = Planning
I = Implementation
E = Evaluation

COGNITIVE LEVEL

K = Knowledge
C = Comprehension
T = Application
N = Analysis

CLIENT NEEDS

S = Safe, effective care environment
G = Physiologic integrity
L = Psychosocial integrity
H = Health promotion and maintenance

Question #	Answer #	Nursing Process					Cognitive Level				Client Needs			
		A	D	P	I	E	K	C	T	N	S	G	L	H
26	4			P				C				G		
27	2				I			C				G		
28	3	A					K					G		
29	1	A					K					G		
30	2				I		K					G		
31	1		D						T			G		
32	1	A							T			G		
33	4				I		K							H
34	3					E				N		G		
35	4				I				T		S			
36	4				I				T		S			
37	4					E			T			G		
38	4		D						T			G		
39	1			P					T			G		
40	3				I				T				L	
41	2			P					T				L	
42	1	A					K					G		
43	3	A					K					G		
44	3	A					K					G		
45	2	A					K					G		
46	1		D						T			G		
47	1			P					T			G		
48	1					E				N		G		
49	3					E	K					G		
50	2			P						N		G		
51	2	A							T			G		
52	4				I				T				L	
53	1			P						N			L	
54	1					E		C				G		
55	3					E				N		G		

NURSING PROCESS

A = Assessment
D = Analysis, nursing diagnosis
P = Planning
I = Implementation
E = Evaluation

COGNITIVE LEVEL

K = Knowledge
C = Comprehension
T = Application
N = Analysis

CLIENT NEEDS

S = Safe, effective care environment
G = Physiologic integrity
L = Psychosocial integrity
H = Health promotion and maintenance

Question #	Answer #	A	D	P	I	E	K	C	T	N	S	G	L	H
56	4				I					N		G		
57	2		D							N			L	
58	2	A							T			G		
59	1	A							T			G		
60	4	A						C				G		
61	1			P						N		G		
62	3	A					K					G		
63	1				I			C				G		
64	4				I			C				G		
65	1	A						C				G		
66	1		D							N			L	
67	1				I				T				L	
68	1	A							T			G		
69	3				I				T			G		
70	3				I				T			G		
71	1		D							N		G		
72	2			P					T				L	
73	4				I				T			G		
74	1				I				T.			G		
75	3				I			C				G		
76	3					E				N		G		
77	1	A						C				G		
78	2	A								N		G		
79	2					E				N		G		
80	1	A							T					H
81	3				I					N			L	
82	3					E				N		G		
83	4				I					N	S			
84	3			P				C				G		
85	2		D							N		G		

ANSWER GRID: 3

NURSING PROCESS

A = Assessment
D = Analysis, nursing diagnosis
P = Planning
I = Implementation
E = Evaluation

COGNITIVE LEVEL

K = Knowledge
C = Comprehension
T = Application
N = Analysis

CLIENT NEEDS

S = Safe, effective care environment
G = Physiologic integrity
L = Psychosocial integrity
H = Health promotion and maintenance

Question #	Answer #	Nursing Process					Cognitive Level				Client Needs			
		A	D	P	I	E	K	C	T	N	S	G	L	H
86	3				I				T			G		
87	1					E				N		G		
88	2				I				T			G		
89	4				I				T			G		
90	3				I				T		S			
91	1				I				T		S			
92	1	A								N		G		
93	2					E				N		G		
Number Correct														
Number Possible	93	20	11	13	35	14	11	16	43	23	9	68	14	2
Percentage Correct														

Score Calculation: To determine your **Percentage Correct,** divide the **Number Correct** by the **Number Possible.**

ANSWER GRID: 4

The Child With Health Problems of the Lower Gastrointestinal Tract

- The Client With Diarrhea or Gastroenteritis
- The Client With Appendicitis
- The Client With Ingestion of Toxic Substances
- The Client With Lead Poisoning
- The Client With Celiac Disease
- The Client With Phenylketonuria
- The Client With Colic
- The Client With Obesity
- The Client With Cow's Milk Sensitivity
- Correct Answers and Rationale

Select the one best answer, and indicate your choice by filling in the circle in front of the option.

The Client With Diarrhea or Gastroenteritis

An 11-month-old infant is admitted to the hospital with severe diarrhea.

1. The nurse explains to the infant's mother that diarrhea is best defined on the basis of the stool
- ○ 1. odor.
- ○ 2. amount.
- ○ 3. frequency.
- ○ 4. consistency.

2. The following beds are available for this client. The nurse should assign the infant to a
- ○ 1. four-bed room with postoperative clients.
- ○ 2. two-bed room with an infant who has a respiratory disease.
- ○ 3. two-bed room with no roommate.
- ○ 4. room with other infants younger than 1 year.

3. On admission, the nurse should assess the infant for
- ○ 1. absent bowel sounds.
- ○ 2. pale yellow urine.
- ○ 3. normal skin elasticity.
- ○ 4. depressed fontanel.

4. An intravenous infusion is to be administered through a scalp vein on the infant's head. The nurse should prepare the parents for the procedure by explaining that
- ○ 1. it will be necessary to remove a small amount of hair from the infant's scalp.
- ○ 2. a sedative will be given to the infant to help keep him quiet.
- ○ 3. visiting the infant will be delayed until the infusion has been completed.
- ○ 4. holding the infant will be contraindicated while the infusion is being administered.

5. The nurse would plan to
- ○ 1. monitor the amount of formula taken in an 8-hour period.
- ○ 2. weigh the infant each day.
- ○ 3. check the posterior fontanel every shift.
- ○ 4. monitor skin turgor over the forearm every shift.

6. The infant becomes irritable. Which of the following nursing measures would the nurse implement to comfort this 6-month-old infant?
- ○ 1. Offering a pacifier.
- ○ 2. Placing a mobile above the crib.
- ○ 3. Sitting at the crib side and talking to the infant.
- ○ 4. Turning the television on to cartoons.

7. Which of the following nursing diagnoses would be appropriate for the nurse to identify as a priority diagnosis?
   ○ 1. Pain.
   ○ 2. Altered Bowel Elimination.
   ○ 3. Altered Health Maintenance.
   ○ 4. Altered Urinary Elimination.

8. Which of the following is an expected client outcome related to the nursing diagnosis of Fluid Volume Deficit related to diarrhea? The client
   ○ 1. exhibits moist mucous membranes and normal skin turgor.
   ○ 2. has a normal bowel movement.
   ○ 3. does not have diarrhea for a 4-hour period.
   ○ 4. tolerates the intravenous fluids well.

9. The nurse explains to the father that initially the infant will
   ○ 1. not receive any liquids by mouth.
   ○ 2. receive intravenous antibiotics.
   ○ 3. be placed in a mist tent.
   ○ 4. be fed formula fortified with iron.

10. The nurse teaches the father about the next step of the treatment plan. The nurse would determine that the father understands when he explains that the infant
    ○ 1. will receive clear liquids for 24 hours.
    ○ 2. will be offered formula and juice.
    ○ 3. will have blood drawn daily to test for anemia.
    ○ 4. will be allowed to go to the playroom.

A 2-year-old girl is admitted to the hospital with gastroenteritis. The mother states that the child vomited seven or eight times in the past 24 hours and has large, green, liquid stools.

11. The mother says she cannot stay with the child because she has other children at home. Which response would be best for the nurse to make?
    ○ 1. "You really should stay. Your child is very sick."
    ○ 2. "I understand. You may visit anytime or call to see how your child is doing."
    ○ 3. "It really isn't necessary to stay with your child because we are here to care for her."
    ○ 4. "Is it possible for you to get someone to stay with your children? Your child here needs you because she seems very afraid of us."

12. The nurse is concerned about spreading this child's infection to others. Her best action would be to
    ○ 1. institute universal precautions.
    ○ 2. place the child in a private room.
    ○ 3. use disposable eating utensils.
    ○ 4. double-bag all linens.

13. Which of the following signs would the nurse recognize as an indication of moderate dehydration?
    ○ 1. Vomiting.
    ○ 2. Diaphoresis.
    ○ 3. Absence of tear formation.
    ○ 4. Decreased urine specific gravity.

14. The physician orders 250 mL of intravenous fluids every 4 hours. What rate should be set on the infusion pump?
    ○ 1. 10 mL/hour.
    ○ 2. 25 mL/hour.
    ○ 3. 42 mL/hour.
    ○ 4. 63 mL/hour.

15. The nurse has an order to add 16 mEq of potassium chloride to the intravenous fluid. The potassium chloride bottle has 40 mEq per 20 mL. How much potassium chloride would the nurse add to the intravenous fluid?
    ○ 1. 4 mL.
    ○ 2. 8 mL.
    ○ 3. 13 mL.
    ○ 4. 26 mL.

16. Before adding the potassium chloride to the intravenous fluid, the nurse would determine that the child had
    ○ 1. voided.
    ○ 2. a stool.
    ○ 3. a baseline electrocardiogram.
    ○ 4. a serum calcium level drawn.

17. The nurse determines that the child is experiencing discomfort and notes swelling in the region where the intravenous needle is inserted. These signs are due to the fact that the
    ○ 1. needle has come out of the vein.
    ○ 2. intravenous site has been used too long.
    ○ 3. child is allergic to the plastic in the needle.
    ○ 4. rate of fluid administration is too rapid for the size of the vein.

18. After several hours of intravenous fluid therapy, the nurse suspects that the child may have circulatory overload when there is
    ○ 1. a drop in blood pressure.
    ○ 2. a change to slow, deep respirations.
    ○ 3. auscultation of moist crackles.
    ○ 4. a marked decrease in urine output.

19. A culture reveals that the child's diarrhea is due to *Salmonella bacillus*. The nurse teaches the mother about the course of *S bacillus* enteritis. The nurse evaluates that the mother understands when the mother states,
    ○ 1. "Some people become carriers and stay infectious for a long time."
    ○ 2. "After the acute stage of the disease passes, the organism is usually not still in the stool."
    ○ 3. "The causative organism may live in the body

indefinitely, but in time it will be of no danger to anyone."

○ 4. "If my child continues to have the organism in the stool, there is an antitoxin that is helpful in destroying the organism.

20. The child is started on a soft diet. The nurse helps the mother choose foods for her child. Which of the following foods would be most appropriate?
○ 1. Muffins and eggs.
○ 2. Bananas and rice cereal.
○ 3. Bran cereal and a bagel.
○ 4. Pancakes and sausage.

21. The nurse assesses how the child contracted salmonella diarrhea. Which of the following possible sources would the nurse investigate?
○ 1. A pet dog.
○ 2. A pet canary.
○ 3. Undercooked eggs.
○ 4. Unwashed fruit.

22. The home health nurse visits the family after discharge. The mother tells the nurse that her child answers "No!" and is difficult to manage. The nurse should explain that the most probable explanation for this behavior is that the child is
○ 1. exhibiting beginning leadership skills.
○ 2. demonstrating an inherited personality trait.
○ 3. beginning to act as an individual.
○ 4. showing a typical 2-year-old's lack of interest in everything.

23. The mother says that when the child cannot have things the way she wants, she throws her legs and arms around, screams, and cries. The mother says, "I don't know what to do!" The community health nurse should explain that when a toddler exhibits such behavior, it is probably best for the mother to
○ 1. ignore the behavior.
○ 2. let the child have what she wants occasionally.
○ 3. explain why the child cannot have what she wants.
○ 4. tell the child that she is not being good.

24. The mother asks the nurse why the child has regressed. The nurse should reply that,
○ 1. "Hospitalization is a traumatic experience for children, and it takes them time to return to former behavior."
○ 2. "Hospitalization is a traumatic experience for children, but usually they have no problems when they return home."
○ 3. "After returning home from being hospitalized, children often still feel that they should be the center of attention."
○ 4. "After returning home from being hospitalized, children usually dislike their home surroundings."

25. Which of the following should the home health

nurse suggest the parents do in regard to the regression?
○ 1. Punish the child's unacceptable behavior.
○ 2. Accept the child's behavior as a coping mechanism.
○ 3. Point out to the child how her behavior has changed since hospitalization.
○ 4. Explain to the child that it is now time to grow up.

The Client With Appendicitis

A 14-year-old boy is brought to the emergency department complaining of right lower quadrant pain. The tentative diagnosis is acute appendicitis.

26. When assessing the client, the nurse would expect to find
○ 1. costovertebral angle tenderness.
○ 2. widening pulse pressure.
○ 3. oral temperature of 100°F.
○ 4. gross hematuria.

27. The nurse asks the client several questions during the initial health history. Which of the following questions would be most helpful in eliciting pertinent diagnostic data?
○ 1. "Where did the pain start?"
○ 2. "What did you do for the pain?"
○ 3. "How often do you have a bowel movement?"
○ 4. "What grade are you in?"

28. While in the emergency department, the client complains of severe abdominal pain. The nurse's most appropriate action to help manage the pain would be to obtain an order for
○ 1. a heating pad.
○ 2. a rectal tube.
○ 3. an ice bag.
○ 4. an intravenous narcotic.

29. After assessing the client's abdomen, the nurse documents the findings. Which of the following notations would represent a deviation from normal that could indicate appendicitis?
○ 1. The abdomen appears slightly rounded.
○ 2. Bowel sounds are heard twice in 2 minutes.
○ 3. Tympany is heard in all four quadrants.
○ 4. The patient demonstrates a cremasteric reflex.

30. Which of the client's signs and symptoms would the nurse correctly judge to be unrelated to the transient sympathetic effects caused by the acute abdominal pain?
○ 1. Tachycardia.
○ 2. Chills.

○ 3. Rapid breathing.

○ 4. Dilated pupils.

31. A diagnosis of appendicitis is made. The client is scheduled for an emergency appendectomy and is to be transferred directly from the emergency room to the operating room. Which of the following statements by the client would the nurse consider most significant?

○ 1. "Wow! All of the sudden it doesn't hurt at all."

○ 2. "The pain is around my navel."

○ 3. "I feel like I'm going to throw up."

○ 4. "It hurts when you press on my stomach."

32. During surgery, the client was found to have a ruptured appendix. Postoperatively, the client is to receive gentamicin sulfate (Garamycin) for several days. The nurse would recognize that the adolescent is exhibiting a symptom of gentamicin toxicity when he

○ 1. complains of dizziness.

○ 2. has no appetite.

○ 3. has an increased hemoglobin.

○ 4. is constipated.

33. The client is receiving intravenous fluids at a rate of 95 mL/hour. The drop factor on the infusion pump is 10 drops per mL. How many drops of fluid should be infused each minute?

○ 1. 8 drops.

○ 2. 10 drops.

○ 3. 12 drops.

○ 4. 16 drops.

34. After the client returns from the recovery room, the nurse would *first* assess

○ 1. the dressing on the surgical site.

○ 2. the intravenous fluid infusion site.

○ 3. the functioning of the nasogastric tube.

○ 4. if the client has to urinate.

35. The client returns from surgery alert and oriented. Parenteral fluids are running, and the nasogastric tube is attached to suction. Which of the following nursing measures would be appropriate for the client in the early postoperative period?

○ 1. Irrigate the nasogastric tube every hour.

○ 2. Test the urine for protein.

○ 3. Remove the nasogastric tube when the client is fully alert.

○ 4. Encourage the client to urinate frequently.

36. The client complains of nausea. The nurse would *first*

○ 1. administer an antiemetic.

○ 2. irrigate the nasogastric tube.

○ 3. call the surgeon.

○ 4. take the blood pressure.

37. The nurse recognizes that the most beneficial position for the client in the early postoperative period is

○ 1. semi-Fowler's

○ 2. supine.

○ 3. left lithotomy.

○ 4. prone.

38. Which of the following nursing interventions would most likely be beneficial initially in helping the client's parents deal with the hospitalization?

○ 1. Reassure them that their adolescent will be fine.

○ 2. Assess their current knowledge level before providing information.

○ 3. Encourage them to participate in the client's physical care.

○ 4. Interact with them when they ask for information.

39. Which of the following statements might an adolescent make after this surgery?

○ 1. "Can I have plastic surgery?"

○ 2. "How big will my scar be?"

○ 3. "I don't want to have any pain."

○ 4. "When will I be able to go back to school?"

40. A primary concern of the hospitalized adolescent would be

○ 1. respect for the need for privacy.

○ 2. allowing friends to visit after hours.

○ 3. wearing a hospital gown.

○ 4. the fear of loss of control when in pain.

41. Which of the following client actions would the nurse judge to be a healthy coping behavior?

○ 1. Insisting on wearing a shirt and gym shorts rather than pajamas.

○ 2. Avoiding interacting with other adolescents on the unit.

○ 3. Refusing to fill out the menu, and allowing the nurse to do so.

○ 4. Not taking telephone calls from friends so he can rest.

42. Which approach would likely be most effective in communicating with the adolescent during hospitalization?

○ 1. Provide only essential information.

○ 2. Offer advice and opinions as needed.

○ 3. Use diagrams when explaining procedures.

○ 4. Use age-appropriate jargon when explaining procedures.

The Client With Ingestion of Toxic Substances

A nurse works in the children's unit of a hospital emergency room.

43. The nurse checks the drug supplies in the emergency room to ensure that syrup of ipecac is readily available. This drug is used primarily to

○ 1. induce vomiting.
○ 2. promote diuresis.
○ 3. relieve seizure activity.
○ 4. stimulate the heart rate.

44. A child is brought to the emergency room after ingesting an undetermined amount of drain cleaner. The nurse plans to assist with
○ 1. administering an emetic.
○ 2. performing a tracheostomy.
○ 3. performing gastric lavage.
○ 4. anchoring a Foley catheter.

45. The nurse explains to the parents that after the acute stage following the ingestion of drain cleaner, their child is most likely to develop which complication?
○ 1. Tracheal stenosis.
○ 2. Tracheal varices.
○ 3. Esophageal strictures.
○ 4. Esophageal diverticula.

46. A mother brings her child to the emergency room after the child has taken "some white pills." Which of the following signs should lead the nurse to judge that the pills taken were most probably acetaminophen?
○ 1. Nosebleed.
○ 2. Seizure activity.
○ 3. Nausea and vomiting.
○ 4. Deep, rapid respirations.

47. Knowing a child had ingested a large amount of acetaminophen, the nurse should assess the child for
○ 1. hypertension.
○ 2. frequent urination.
○ 3. right upper quadrant pain.
○ 4. headache.

48. The nurse would prepare the parents for which of the following expected treatments for acetaminophen overdose?
○ 1. Frequent blood draws.
○ 2. Gastric lavage.
○ 3. Tracheostomy.
○ 4. Electrocardiogram.

49. A child has ingested some kerosene. What complication is this child most likely to experience?
○ 1. Uremia.
○ 2. Hepatitis.
○ 3. Carditis.
○ 4. Pneumonitis.

The Client With Lead Poisoning

An 18-month-old child is brought to the urgent care clinic with an upper respiratory infection.

50. Which of the following statements by the mother would indicate to the nurse that the child needs laboratory testing?

○ 1. "My child eats anything, including paint chips."
○ 2. "My child drinks 2 cups of milk every day."
○ 3. "My child has more temper tantrums than other kids."
○ 4. "My child is smaller than other kids the same age."

51. It is determined that the child's blood lead concentration is 17 μg/dL and has been for several months. The nurse would anticipate and prepare the mother for which of the following?
○ 1. No further follow-up is needed.
○ 2. Chelation therapy will start immediately.
○ 3. Environmental investigation should be done.
○ 4. The child will be admitted to the hospital.

52. The nurse would explain to the mother that which of the following complications is most likely to develop if lead poisoning goes untreated?
○ 1. Cirrhosis of the liver.
○ 2. Stunted growth rate.
○ 3. Neurologic changes.
○ 4. Heart failure.

53. The nurse explains to the mother about ways to prevent lead poisoning. Of the following measures, which one has been found to be most effective in preventing lead poisoning?
○ 1. Condemn old housing developments.
○ 2. Educate the public on common sources of lead.
○ 3. Educate the public on the importance of good nutrition.
○ 4. Keep pregnant women out of old homes that are being remodeled.

54. A mother asks the nurse about the outcome for her child with lead poisoning. The nurse would respond:
○ 1. "Many children have brain damage."
○ 2. "Many effects are not reversible when diagnosed early."
○ 3. "Most children become juvenile delinquents."
○ 4. "Most effects are reversible if diagnosed early."

The Client With Celiac Disease

A 6-month-old child is brought to the clinic for suspected celiac disease.

55. Which of the following statements by the mother would support the diagnosis of celiac disease?
○ 1. "His urine seems so dark in color."
○ 2. "His stools are large and smelly."
○ 3. "His belly is so small."
○ 4. "He has never been sick."

56. During assessment, the nurse would most likely note which of the following physical findings?
○ 1. Enlarged liver.
○ 2. Protuberant abdomen.
○ 3. Tender inguinal lymph nodes.
○ 4. Periorbital edema.

57. The nurse teaches the mother about the child's diet. Which of the following foods should not be included in a gluten-free diet?
○ 1. Wheat, oats, rye, and barley.
○ 2. Milk, yogurt, cheese, and butter.
○ 3. Rice, corn, sorghum, and soybeans.
○ 4. Lemons, limes, oranges, and bananas.

58. Which of the following diet plans would be appropriate for this 6-month-old with suspected celiac disease?
○ 1. Cow's milk formula and oatmeal cereal.
○ 2. Cow's milk formula and barley cereal.
○ 3. Breast milk and rice cereal.
○ 4. Breast milk and mixed cereal.

59. The mother asks how long her child will be on a restricted diet. Which of the following would be the the nurse's best response?
○ 1. Until the jejunal biopsy is normal.
○ 2. When the stools are normal in appearance.
○ 3. Only for a few months.
○ 4. Indefinitely.

The Client With Phenylketonuria

A mother brings her 2-year-old child to the physician's office for a routine checkup. The child was diagnosed with phenylketonuria (PKU) as a neonate.

60. For a reliable neonatal screening serum test for phenylketonuria, the infant must have
○ 1. ingested an iron-rich formula.
○ 2. had nothing by mouth for 4 hours before the test.
○ 3. ingested cow's or breast milk for 4 days before the test.
○ 4. ingested a loading dose of glucose water.

61. The child was not screened in the hospital at birth. In screening tests for PKU performed during the first few days of life, false-negative results are most frequently due to the neonate's
○ 1. inadequate fluid intake.
○ 2. low calcium intake.
○ 3. insufficient protein intake.
○ 4. high bilirubin blood level.

62. The goal of care for this child would be to
○ 1. meet the child's nutritional needs for optimal growth.
○ 2. ensure the special diet is started at age 3 weeks.
○ 3. maintain serum phenylalanine level above 12 mg/100 mL.
○ 4. maintain serum phenylalanine level below 2 mg/100 mL.

63. When taking a diet history, the nurse would be concerned if the mother reports feeding her 2-year-old child which of the following?
○ 1. Diet soda.
○ 2. Carrots and celery.
○ 3. Orange juice.
○ 4. Apples and bananas.

64. The mother asks how PKU is transmitted. The nurse would explain that the disorder is transmitted by
○ 1. a translocation gene.
○ 2. a mutation gene.
○ 3. an autosomal recessive gene.
○ 4. a homozygous dominant gene.

65. The client is given Lofenalac, one of several products on the market used to provide an adequate protein intake to a child with PKU. Lofenalac helps maintain low blood levels of what substance?
○ 1. Tyrosine.
○ 2. Dopa.
○ 3. Tryptophan.
○ 4. Phenylalanine.

66. The nurse tells the mother that the child must continue to take Lofenalac
○ 1. until 2 years of age.
○ 2. until 5 years of age.
○ 3. until adolescence.
○ 4. indefinitely.

67. The nurse would request that which of the following people be included in the care of this child?
○ 1. Chaplain.
○ 2. Ophthalmologist.
○ 3. Social worker.
○ 4. Dietitian.

68. Several teaching sessions have been documented in the client's health record. The mother asks the nurse again what caused her child's PKU. Which of the following statements would best explain why the mother keeps asking for information that she has already received?
○ 1. Parents of a chronically ill child often want very detailed explanations about the causes of and treatments for their child's disease.
○ 2. Parents of a chronically ill child often require a long time to work through the grieving process for their child's disease.
○ 3. Parents of a chronically ill child often test a health worker's knowledge about the causes of and treatments for their child's disease.

○ 4. Parents of a chronically ill child often deal with their guilt about possibly causing the child's ill health with impatience and ask challenging questions about their child's disease.

The Client With Colic

A 6-week-old female infant is brought to the health clinic by her parents. The parents state that she has been crying almost constantly since birth and frequently draws her knees up to her abdomen. Colic is suspected.

69. In collecting data about the infant, the nurse would ask the parents some questions. Which of the following would not provide pertinent diagnostic data about colic?
○ 1. The frequency of breast-feeding the infant.
○ 2. The infant's crying pattern.
○ 3. The length of time sleeping.
○ 4. The position of the infant during burping.

70. Which of the following assessment findings would be consistent with a diagnosis of colic?
○ 1. Failure to gain weight.
○ 2. Expulsion of flatus.
○ 3. Soft abdomen.
○ 4. Difficulty with burping.

71. When obtaining information about the infant's problem, the nurse asks the parents to describe the infant's bowel movements. Which of the following descriptions would the nurse expect if the infant does indeed have colic?
○ 1. Soft, yellow stools.
○ 2. Frequent watery stools.
○ 3. Ribbon-like stools.
○ 4. Foul-smelling stools.

72. A diagnosis of colic is made. The mother tells the nurse that the diagnosis upsets her because she knows her infant will continue to have colicky pain. Which of the following responses would be most appropriate for the nurse to make?
○ 1. "I know that your baby's crying upsets you, but she needs your undivided attention for the next few months."
○ 2. "It can be difficult to listen to your baby cry, so try to arrange some free time."
○ 3. "It's distressing to see your baby in pain, but at least she doesn't have an intestinal obstruction."
○ 4. "It will be a difficult 3 months, but she will outgrow the colic by then."

73. Which of the following observations by the nurse while the mother is feeding the infant would indicate that the mother understood the teaching? The mother

○ 1. holds the infant prone while feeding.
○ 2. burps the infant after the feeding.
○ 3. places the infant prone after the feeding.
○ 4. burps the infant during and after the feeding.

74. The mother tells the nurse that it is difficult to make her infant comfortable before falling asleep. The nurse would suggest that the mother
○ 1. place her on her back.
○ 2. place her on her abdomen.
○ 3. leave her in the infant seat.
○ 4. hold her until she falls asleep.

The Client With Obesity

An adolescent boy comes to the clinic for a precollege physical examination. Based on his appearance, the nurse judges him to be overweight.

75. Which of the following methods would give the nurse an accurate assessment of this client's status in regard to his weight?
○ 1. A food intake diary for 1 week.
○ 2. Height and weight growth charts.
○ 3. A 24-hour dietary history.
○ 4. Skin-fold thickness measurements.

76. The client is found to be overweight. He is at greatest risk for
○ 1. lifelong obesity.
○ 2. gastrointestinal problems.
○ 3. orthopedic problems.
○ 4. psychosocial problems.

77. The client tells the nurse that he would like to lose weight and asks the nurse's opinion on how to accomplish his goal. The nurse's most appropriate response would be to suggest that the client
○ 1. exercise more often.
○ 2. severely limit calorie intake.
○ 3. participate in an adolescent weight-reduction program.
○ 4. cut down on sweets and other snacks.

A mother brings her 4-month-old infant to the clinic for a routine checkup. While assessing the infant's nutritional status, the nurse learns that the infant is being fed an 8-ounce bottle five times a day. The nurse realizes that this may be an excessive amount of formula for an infant this age.

78. What other assessment information would support a nursing diagnosis of Altered Nutrition: More Than Body Requirements? The child

○ 1. wears size 9- to 12-month clothes.

○ 2. has a double chin and rolls of fat in the thigh area.

○ 3. when pulled to sit has no head lag.

○ 4. is in the 80th percentile for weight.

79. To decrease the infant's total caloric intake, the nurse should advise the mother to

○ 1. change the feeding from formula to skim milk, and give the same amount as before.

○ 2. decrease the amount of each feeding and add cereal to each bottle.

○ 3. decrease the amount of each feeding to 6 ounces, and use a smaller-holed and firmer nipple.

○ 4. dilute the formula with 4 ounces of water in each bottle.

80. The nurse continues to provide nutritional teaching to the mother, discussing introducing solids into the infant's diet. This teaching plan should include

○ 1. decreasing the amount of formula as solid intake increases.

○ 2. introducing the infant to the taste of foods by mixing them with formula.

○ 3. mixing cereal and fruit in the bottle for the first few times.

○ 4. using a large-bowled spoon during the first several months.

81. The nurse would evaluate the teaching as successful when the mother says

○ 1. "I can't wait to go to the store! They have such a variety of fruits and vegetables for babies."

○ 2. "About 1 month from now I can start her on an Infafeeder."

○ 3. "In 1 to 2 months I can offer my baby rice cereal to start."

○ 4. "Because the baby's tongue will push out the food now, I can just add the fruit and cereal to her bottle."

82. The mother's sister, who is pregnant, has also come to the clinic. The nurse discusses ways to prevent overnourishing her infant, including

○ 1. recognizing clues indicating that a baby is full.

○ 2. establishing a regular feeding schedule.

○ 3. supplementing feedings with sterile water.

○ 4. adding more water than directed when preparing formula.

The Client With Cow's Milk Sensitivity

Parents bring their 1-month-old infant to the hospital because he has had diarrhea and cries excessively. The diarrhea usually occurs after feedings, as does the crying. The infant is not dehydrated, and the mother reports that he is an eager nurser, burps well, and does not spit up much after feedings. Based on these findings, the nurse suspects that the child has a milk allergy.

83. The father says that he has heard of cow's milk allergy but knows nothing about cow's milk sensitivity. The nurse would explain that it is

○ 1. a hereditary disorder of carbohydrate metabolism.

○ 2. an adverse reaction to cow's milk protein.

○ 3. an acquired lactose intolerance.

○ 4. a lifelong allergy.

84. The mother asks about the medical plan of care for her infant. The nurse explains that first an evaluation will be done to determine if the baby has a cow's milk sensitivity or lactose intolerance, and teaches the mother about what lactose intolerance means. The nurse would determine that this teaching was effective when hearing the mother explain to a visitor that lactose intolerance is

○ 1. a lack of something that breaks down lactose.

○ 2. an allergy to lactose.

○ 3. an inability to digest proteins.

○ 4. an inability to digest fats.

85. The infant undergoes a series of tests to differentiate cow's milk sensitivity from lactose intolerance. Which of the following test results would confirm a diagnosis of lactose intolerance?

○ 1. Blood glucose level of 20 mg/dL or less.

○ 2. Positive urine protein.

○ 3. Positive hydrogen breath test.

○ 4. Stool pH of 7.0.

86. If a 2-year-old child were lactose-intolerant, what dairy products could the mother plan to include in the child's diet?

○ 1. Ice cream.

○ 2. Creamed soups.

○ 3. Pudding.

○ 4. Cheese.

87. For the 1-month-old infant, lactose intolerance is ruled out, and the diagnosis of cow's milk sensitivity is confirmed. If the infant is being breast-fed, the nurse should tell the mother to plan to

○ 1. continue to breast-feed but eliminate all milk products from her own diet.

○ 2. discontinue breast-feeding and start feeding a predigested formula.

○ 3. limit breast-feeding to once per day and begin feeding an iron-fortified formula.

○ 4. change to a soy-based formula exclusively and begin solid foods.

88. If the child with cow's milk sensitivity is formula-fed, the nurse should advise the parents to buy

○ 1. at least a 1-month supply of goat's milk–based formula.

○ 2. the same brand of iron-fortified formula as used in the hospital.

○ 3. only a few cans of soy-based formula initially.

○ 4. a 3-day supply of predigested milk substitute.

CORRECT ANSWERS AND RATIONALE

The letters in parentheses following the rationale identify the step of the nursing process (A, D, P, I, E), cognitive level (K, C, T, N), and client needs (S, G, L, H). See the Answer Grid for the key.

The Client With Diarrhea or Gastroenteritis

1. 4. Diarrhea is best defined on the basis of stool consistency, which is ordinarily liquid in nature. The color of diarrheal stools is usually greenish, but stool color is also affected by food and fluid intake. Estimates of the amount of stool can vary widely; therefore, this is not an accurate criterion by which to define diarrhea. The frequency of stools varies also, although stools occur more frequently than normal when diarrhea is present. Odor is not directly related to diarrhea. (A, T, G)

2. 3. A child with diarrhea of undetermined origin should be placed in a room alone until a causative organism can be identified. (P, T, G)

3. 4. A child with severe diarrhea will experience some degree of dehydration. Common signs of dehydration in a child whose fontanel has not closed (younger than 12 to 18 months) would be depressed fontanel, dry mucous membranes, lethargy, hyperactive bowel sounds, dark urine, and sunken eyeballs. (A, C, G)

4. 1. Parents are typically quick to notice changes in their infant's physical appearance. The removal of the infant's hair may be upsetting to them if they have not been told why it is being done. Hair is removed on the scalp at the site of needle insertion for intravenous therapy for better visualization and to provide a smooth surface on which to attach tape to secure the needle. Sedatives are not ordinarily prescribed before intravenous fluid administration. Holding an infant is encouraged to provide comfort. (P, C, L)

5. 2. A child who is dehydrated should be weighed at least once daily to determine if fluid is being restored. Body weight is a good indication of hydration status. Initially, the infant may not be allowed liquids or may be allowed only clear fluids, not formula. The posterior fontanel should close in the second month. Skin turgor is monitored over the abdomen in infants. (A, T, G)

6. 1. An irritable infant receiving nothing by mouth is usually best comforted by providing a pacifier to satisfy sucking needs. Such activities as placing a mobile over the crib, speaking to the infant, and placing the infant with others (unless the infant has an infectious disease) may not necessarily be contraindicated but will not offer the comfort provided by a pacifier. (I, T, L)

7. 2. Given this infant's history of diarrhea, the most likely nursing diagnosis would be Altered Bowel Elimination. Sometimes, cramping will occur and may cause pain, but this (nor any of the others) would not be the priority diagnosis. (D, N, G)

8. 1. The outcome of exhibiting no manifestations of dehydration focuses on the fluid volume deficit. A normal bowel movement, good tolerance of intravenous fluids, and an increasing time interval between bowel movements are all positive signs but they do not specifically address the nursing diagnosis. (P, T, G)

9. 1. Children hospitalized with acute diarrhea and gastroenteritis are usually not allowed fluids by mouth to rest the intestinal track. A mist tent would not be needed for this diagnosis. Clear fluids are the initial feedings. Antibiotics are not indicated. (P, T, G)

10. 1. The usual way to treat diarrhea is to provide clear liquids for 24 hours, after the child is NPO followed by the BRAT diet (bananas, rice cereal, applesauce, and toast). These foods are easily digested and lack bulk, so they do not encourage further diarrhea. In this situation, there is no need to test the infant's blood every day for anemia or to take the infant to the playroom. The infant will remain in a private room until the causative organism can be identified. (E, N, G)

11. 2. The nurse's best course of action would be to support the mother; this is best done by conveying understanding and encouraging the mother to visit or call whenever she wants. Indicating to the mother that she should stay with her ill child seems critical and insensitive. Commenting that the child will be well cared for may suggest that the mother is not needed and may inappropriately direct the mother how to solve her dilemma without sufficient knowledge to warrant the statement. (I, C, L)

12. 1. Universal precautions include good handwashing and use of appropriate protective gear (gowns, gloves, eye protection) when being exposed to body fluids. These actions should protect the nurse and other clients from the pathogen. (I, C, S)

13. 3. The absence of tears is typically found when moderate dehydration is observed. Other typical findings associated with moderate dehydration in-

clude a dry mouth, sunken eyes, poor skin turgor, and an increased pulse rate. Perspiration would be decreased with dehydration because the body is attempting to conserve fluids. The specific gravity of urine increases with decreased output in the presence of dehydration. (A, C, G)

14. 4. The rate set on the pump equals the number of milliliters to be delivered in 1 hour: 250 mL/4 hours is equal to about 63 mL to be infused each hour. (I, C, S)

15. 2.

$$40 \text{ mEq}/20 \text{ mL} = 16 \text{ mEq}/x \text{ mL}$$

$$40x = 320$$

$$x = 320/40$$

$$x = 8 \text{ mL}$$

Thus, 8 mL of potassium chloride will be added to the intravenous fluids. (I, T, S)

16. 1. Potassium chloride is readily excreted in the urine. Before adding potassium chloride to the intravenous fluid, the nurse should ascertain whether the child can void; if not, potassium chloride may build up in the serum and cause hyperkalemia. (E, N, S)

17. 1. Pain and swelling in the area of needle insertion most likely indicate that the needle has come out of the vein. The swelling occurs as the fluid infuses into subcutaneous tissues. Other typical signs of infiltration include skin pallor and coldness around the insertion site. Inflammation is likely if the intravenous site is used too long. Because inert plastic is used for manufacturing intravenous needles, the risk of an allergic reaction is remote. If fluid is administered too rapidly for the size of the vein, the fluid would most probably leak around the needle at the area of assembly onto the tubing. (D, N, S)

18. 3. Typical signs of circulatory overload include moist rales heard when auscultating over the chest wall; elevated blood pressure; engorged neck veins; a wide variation between fluid intake and output, with a higher intake than output; shortness of breath; increased respiratory rate; dyspnea; and cyanosis. (A, N, G)

19. 1. After having *S. bacillus* enteritis, some patients become chronic carriers of the causative organism and remain infectious for a long time as the organism continues to be shed from the body. No antitoxin is available to treat or prevent salmonella infections. (E, C, G)

20. 2. After clear liquids, the foods of choice are bananas, rice cereal, applesauce, and toast. This diet is referred to by the initials BRAT. These foods are easily digested, are low in fat, and are not bulk for-

mers. (Foods high in fat are difficult to digest.) The child is not given high-fiber foods, which will cause more diarrhea. (I, C, G)

21. 3. *Salmonella bacilli* are commonly spread by fowl, eggs, pet turtles, and kittens. (A, C, G)

22. 3. This toddler's behavior is typical for her age as she attempts to be self-assertive as an individual. The negativism reflects the developmental task of establishing autonomy. The toddler is attempting to exert control over her environment. It is too early to assess leadership qualities in a 2-year-old child. Negativism does not show disinterest, nor does it demonstrate an inherited personality characteristic. (D, C, H)

23. 1. Toddlers are busy developing a sense of autonomy. This requires an opportunity to make decisions and express individuality. Temper tantrums occur relatively frequently and are considered normal behavior as toddlers search for autonomy. Ignoring the outbursts is probably the best strategy. However, the mother should intervene in a temper tantrum if the child is likely to injure herself. Allowing the child to have what she wants occasionally, giving her part of what she demands, or expressing disappointment in her behavior would likely add to the problems associated with temper tantrums. (I, C, H)

24. 1. Hospitalization is a traumatic time for a child, and it takes some time to readjust to the home environment. The child may regress at home for a period until she feels comfortable. Children normally do not dislike their home environment; in fact, they usually are anxious to get home to familiar surroundings where they feel safe. (I, C, L)

25. 2. Regression is a method of coping that represents a retreat to an earlier pattern of behavior that preceded the current stresses and discomforts. Conveying acceptance of the child can help increase her feelings of worth and self-esteem, which, in turn, will enhance her ability to cope with stress. Punishing the child and pointing out how her behavior has changed will tend to reinforce the inappropriate behavior. Shaming a child is detrimental and causes self-doubt. (I, C, L)

The Client With Appendicitis

26. 3. The most common manifestations of appendicitis are right lower quadrant pain, localized tenderness, and fever of 99° to 102°F. Other signs of inflammation may be present, including increased pulse and respiratory rates. Costovertebral angle tenderness and hematuria are associated with urologic problems. Widening pulse pressure is seen in increased intracranial pressure. (A, T, G)

27. 1. The pain associated with appendicitis usually be-

gins in the periumbilical area, then progresses to the right lower quadrant. The client's siblings and grade in school may be important information but are not helpful in making this diagnosis. (A, T, G)

28. 3. An ice bag may help relieve pain. A heating pad is contraindicated because heat may increase circulation to the appendix and lead to rupture. Rectal tubes are contraindicated because they stimulate bowel motility and can exacerbate abdominal pain, and would most likely be ineffective because accumulation of gas in the lower bowel is not likely to be causing the adolescent's discomfort. Narcotics may mask symptoms and are not given until a diagnosis is made. (P, T, G)

29. 2. Manifestations of appendicitis include decreased or absent bowel sounds. Normally, bowel sounds are heard every 10 to 30 seconds. The contour of the male adolescent abdomen is normally flat to slightly rounded. Tympany is typically heard over most of the abdomen. Masses should be absent. A cremasteric reflex is normal for males.(A, C, G)

30. 2. Chills are a normal response of the body's immune system to infection and are not a response of the sympathetic nervous system to pain. Tachycardia, increased respiratory rate, and dilated pupils are sympathetic effects. (A, N, G)

31. 1. Sudden relief of pain in a client with appendicitis may indicate that the appendix has ruptured. Rupture relieves the pressure within the appendix but spreads the infection to the peritoneal cavity. Periumbilical pain, vomiting, and abdominal tenderness are common manifestations. (E, N, G)

32. 1. Gentamicin sulfate is a broad-spectrum aminoglycoside antibiotic that can cause nephrotoxicity and ototoxicity. Manifestations of ototoxicity include hearing problems and vestibular disturbances, such as dizziness. Anorexia, increased hemoglobin, and constipation are not side effects of this antibiotic. (A, T, S)

33. 4. Multiplying 95 mL/hour $\times$ 10 (drop factor) equals 950 mL/hour; 950 mL/hour divided by 60 minutes equals 15.8 drops/minute; thus, 16 drops/minute should be infused. (I, T, S)

34. 1. Initial assessment should focus on the surgical site to determine if there is drainage. Then the nurse would assess the intravenous infusion site, assess the nasogastric tube to be sure it is functioning, and finally, determine if the client needs to urinate. (P, T, S)

35. 4. After an appendectomy, the client should be encouraged to void frequently to prevent bladder distention, which could cause strain on the incision. There is no reason to irrigate the nasogastric tube unless it ceases to function, and there is no reason

to test the urine for protein. The nasogastric tube remains in place until peristalsis returns. (I, T, G)

36. 2. The nurse would first ensure that the nasogastric tube is working. If the tube is clogged, it can be irrigated with normal saline. Preparing and administering an antiemetic would take several minutes, and it would not take effect for several more minutes. The physician would not need to be called if irrigating the nasogastric tube relieves nausea. Taking the client's blood pressure has nothing to do with relieving the nausea. (I, T, S)

37. 1. After an appendectomy for a ruptured appendix, assuming the semi-Fowler's or a right side-lying position helps localize the infection. These positions promote drainage from the peritoneal cavity and decrease the incidence of subdiaphragmatic abscess. (I, T, L)

38. 2. Before giving information, it is important for the nurse to assess the learner's current level of knowledge. When dealing with parents of an ill child, the nurse considers their emotional strength and the intensity of the situation and deals with it in an accepting, nonthreatening manner. Parents may feel overwhelmed by the events, and they need time to adjust to the situation. (I, T, L)

39. 2. Typically, an adolescent is concerned about the immediate state of his body and its functioning. The adolescent needs to know if any changes, such as illness, trauma, or surgery, will alter his lifestyle or interfere with his quest for physical perfection. (A, C, L)

40. 4. Fears of the adolescent include body changes and loss of control. The young adolescent is typically concerned about the inability to control body changes and feelings and about embarrassing himself. The typical adolescent is more concerned about being separated from the peer group than from his family and schoolwork and is realistically worried about experiencing pain and loss of control. (A, C, L)

41. 1. Adolescents struggle for independence and identity. Typical concerns include peer acceptance, body changes, and sexuality. Adolescents need to feel in control of situations and to conform with peers. Control and conformity are often manifested in appearance, including clothing, and this carries over into the hospital experience. The adolescent feels best when he is able to look and act as he normally does. Adolescents normally want to interact with peers and seek every opportunity to do so. (E, N, L)

42. 3. Adolescents can comprehend scientific rationale and complexity. They appreciate detailed description and explanations using charts, diagrams, and models. They dislike lectures and unsolicited advice

and opinions. Jargon is a means to establish the identity of the peer group, and an adult's use of adolescent jargon may be viewed as false or dishonest. (P, T, L)

The Client With Ingestion of Toxic Substances

43. 1. Syrup of ipecac is an emetic that exerts its action by direct stimulation of the vomiting center and by producing irritating effects on the stomach mucosa. It is given with one to two glasses of water or fruit juice. If the child does not vomit within 20 minutes after taking syrup of ipecac, a second dose may be administered. Syrup of ipecac should be removed from the stomach by gavage if emesis does not occur because it is cardiotoxic and is likely to produce various dysrhythmias. Most authorities recommend that syrup of ipecac be kept in the home for emergency use, stored safely out of reach of children. (I, K, G)

44. 2. Drain cleaner almost always contains lye, which can burn the mouth, pharynx, and esophagus on ingestion. The nurse should be prepared to assist with a tracheostomy, which may be necessary because of swelling around the area of the larynx. Gastric lavage and emetics would be contraindicated because they may cause perforations in the necrotic mucosa. Anchoring a Foley catheter would be indicated but not as the first intervention. (P, K, G)

45. 3. As the burn from the lye ingestion heals, scar tissue may cause esophageal strictures. This is a more common after effect. Varices and diverticula do not ordinarily occur after lye ingestion. (I, C, G)

46. 3. Acetaminophen is a common drug poisoning agent in children. Symptoms seen in the first 24 hours include nausea and vomiting, anorexia, malaise, and pallor. Nosebleed and deep, rapid respirations are seen in salicylate poisoning. Seizure activity is not commonly seen. (A, N, G)

47. 3. The child would complain of right upper quadrant pain due to hepatic damage not from the drug but from one of its metabolites that is toxic to the liver. The pain is due to the substance glutathione combining with the metabolite to negate its toxic effects. If a child ingests large amounts of acetaminophen, this exceeds the liver's supply of glutathione, which allows the metabolite to cause hepatic necrosis. (A, T, G)

48. 2. Initial management of a child who has ingested a large amount of acetaminophen would include inducing vomiting or gastric lavage with or without following up with activated charcoal. (P, T, G)

49. 4. Chemical pneumonitis is the most common complication of ingestion of hydrocarbons, such as in kerosene. The pneumonitis is due to irritation from the hydrocarbons aspirated into the lungs. (P, C, G)

The Client With Lead Poisoning

50. 1. Pica, or the eating of nonfood substances, is characteristic of children with lead poisoning. Children who eat lead-containing paint chips commonly develop lead poisoning. Drinking 2 cups of milk per day is less than normal, so more nutrition information would need to be obtained. Temper tantrums are characteristic of 18-month-old children as they try to assert themselves. Determining whether the child is smaller than other children the same age requires measuring height and weight and plotting them on growth charts. (E, N, G)

51. 3. The child is considered at moderate risk. Because the blood level concentration has persisted, it will be necessary for environmental investigation and intervention. The child will not have to be chelated at this blood level. (P, T, G)

52. 3. The most serious and irreversible consequence of lead poisoning is mental retardation due to neurologic changes. It can be expected if lead poisoning is long-standing and goes untreated. Lead poisoning also affects the hematologic and renal systems. (I, C, G)

53. 2. Public education about the sources of lead that could cause poisoning has been found to be the most effective measure to prevent lead poisoning. This includes recent efforts to alert the public to lead in certain types of window blinds. Condemning old housing developments has been ineffective because lead paint still exists in many other dwellings. Providing education about good nutrition is not an effective preventive measure. Pregnant women and children should not remain in an older home that is being remodeled because they may breathe in lead in the dust, but this is not the most effective preventive measure. (P, C, G)

54. 4. Most of the pathological effects of lead poisoning are reversible. The most serious are effects on the central nervous system such as brain damage, mental retardation, and behavior changes. (I, T, H)

The Client With Celiac Disease

55. 2. The stools of a child with celiac disease are characteristically malodorous, pale, large (bulky), and soft (loose). Excessive flatus is common, and bouts of diarrhea may occur. (A, C, G)

56. 2. The intestines of a child with celiac disease fill with accumulated undigested food and flatus, causing the characteristic abdominal protrusion. Celiac disease is not ordinarily complicated with poor liver functioning that may cause the liver to enlarge, or with edema around the eyes. Tender inguinal lymph nodes are often associated with an infection, and celiac disease is not an infectious disease. (A, C, G)

57. 1. Damage to intestinal mucosa in celiac disease is caused by gliadin, a part of the protein found in wheat, rye, barley, and oats. Foods containing these grains must be eliminated entirely from the diet of children with celiac disease and of adults with gluten-induced enteropathy (celiac sprue). (I, T, G)

58. 3. The family is not to feed the child foods containing wheat, oats, rye, and barley. Foods containing rice or corn are appropriate. Formula or breast milk does not alter the child's nutritional state. (I, T, G)

59. 4. Most children with celiac disease have a lifelong sensitivity to gluten, which requires that they maintain some type of diet restriction. (I,T,G)

The Client With Phenylketonuria

60. 3. This neonate must have ingested a diet high in phenylalanine, such as cow's or breast milk, for 4 days or more for the serum phenylalanine levels to reach 4 mg/100 mL. (The normal value is below 2 mg/100 mL.) Testing the neonate before that time, excessive vomiting, or poor intake can yield false-negative results. (A, K, G)

61. 3. The result of PKU testing in a neonate will likely be negative even if the neonate has the condition because the neonate is still not receiving either formula or breast milk, both of which are high in phenylalanine content. Insufficient protein intake causes a false-negative result in a screening test because the blood level of phenylalanine is not yet elevated. (A, C, G)

62. 1. The goal of care is to prevent mental retardation. The diet is adjusted to meet the infant's nutritional needs for optimal growth. The diet needs to be started as soon as the infant is diagnosed, ideally within a few days of birth. Serum phenylalanine level should be maintained between 3 and 7 mg/100 mL. Significant brain damage usually occurs if the serum phenylalanine level exceeds 10 to 15 mg/100 mL. If the level drops below 2 mg/100 mL, the body begins to catabolize its protein stores, causing growth retardation. (P, N, G)

63. 1. Foods with low phenylalanine levels include vegetables, fruits, and juices. Foods high in phenylalanine are meats and dairy products, which must be restricted or eliminated. Diet soda is higher in phenylalanine than the fruits listed. (A, K, G)

64. 3. PKU is due to an inborn error of metabolism. It

is an autosomal recessive disorder that inhibits the conversion of phenylalanine to tyrosine. (I, C, G)

65. 4. In PKU, amino acid metabolism is abnormal. Phenylalanine is an amino acid contained in many foods. When the hepatic enzyme phenylalanine hydroxylase is missing, phenylalanine cannot be converted to tyrosine. Dietary treatment is directed toward keeping the phenylalanine blood level within a safe range: about 5 to 9 mg/dL in infants and children. (P, C, G)

66. 4. It is not known how long diet therapy must continue for children with PKU. Many experts suggest continuing diet therapy indefinitely because of academic difficulties and lower intelligence quotients in older children who have stopped the restrictive diet. For females it is necessary to resume the diet before conception to lower the phenylalanine levels in the fetus and prevent complications. (I, C, G)

67. 4. The only treatment for PKU is dietary, so it is necessary to have a dietitian involved once the diagnosis is made. The dietitian should meet periodically with the family to help advise them about food choices as the child grows. (P, T, H)

68. 2. Parents typically grieve about the loss of health in their child afflicted with a chronic disease. Many times, they repeat questions, as though trying to deny what is really happening. This type of behavior represents an attempt to integrate the experience and their feelings with their self-image. Asking for detailed explanations, testing the competence of health workers, and expressing impatience with health workers may explain the parents' behavior, but viewing the behavior as a part of the grieving process is the most plausible explanation. (E, N, L)

The Client With Colic

69. 3. Information on the frequency of feedings, crying pattern, and position for burping all can help verify a diagnosis of colic. Overfeeding may cause discomfort and distention. The colic attack begins abruptly; the cry is loud and continuous and may last for hours. The attack may end when the child is exhausted, or the child may gain some relief after passing a stool or flatus. Holding the infant upright or lying her across the lap may help. (A, K, G)

70. 2. Infants with colic have paroxysmal abdominal pain or cramping caused by the production and accumulation of gas. This causes pain and abdominal distention. They may expel flatus or eructate, but do not vomit. Despite their pain, infants with colic typically tolerate formula well, gain weight, and thrive. (A, C, G)

71. 1. Infants with colic have normal stools, typically soft and yellowish. Abnormal stools may indicate bowel obstruction, malabsorption, or infection. (A, K, G)

72. 2. The nurse needs to provide the parents with support. Parents are stressed and need to be encouraged to get out of the house and arrange for some free time. Comparing colic with other problems is inappropriate; parents have the right to be upset. Although colic usually disappears spontaneously by age 3 months, the nurse should not make any guarantees. (I, T, L)

73. 4. Infants with colic should be burped frequently during and after the feeding. Much of the discomfort of colic appears to be associated with the presence of air in the stomach and intestines. Infants with colic should be held fairly upright while being fed, to help air rise. They should be burped using the shoulder position and placed in an infant seat after feedings. (E, N, G)

74. 2. Infants with colic seem to sleep more comfortably on the abdomen than on the back or side. (P, K, G)

The Client With Obesity

75. 4. Measuring skin-fold thickness with skin-fold calipers is the most common method used to assess obesity. The skin-fold thickness test, which determines the amount of subcutaneous fat, determines obesity more accurately than does a height and weight chart. Assessing dietary intake gives no information about whether a client is overweight. (A, T, H)

76. 1. The most prevalent complication of adolescent obesity is its persistence into adulthood. The odds are 28 to 1 against an obese adolescent becoming a normal-weight adult. Possible gastrointestinal, orthopedic, and psychological problems would be of concern, but these are not as common as the persistence of obesity into adulthood and its associated problems. (A, K, H)

77. 3. Weight loss treatment modalities that include peer involvement have proved to be the most successful approach with obese adolescents. This is because peer support is critical to adolescents, especially with an all-encompassing problem such as obesity. Severe calorie restriction is not recommended because it can result in use of muscle protein for energy in addition to fat. Increasing the amount of exercise is helpful, but this is just one aspect of a weight reduction program. Although decreased ingestion of nonnutritive snacks is helpful in dietary control, there is no evidence that this is a problem for this adolescent. (P, T, H)

78. 2. The obese infant appears fat, with rolls of fat and flabby skin areas. Height and weight tables are used to compare a child's measurements with norms. A difference between height and weight of one stan-

dard deviation is acceptable. Although obesity may cause a delay in motor skills, having no head lag when pulled to a sitting position is not a developmental delay in a 4-month-old. Clothing size is an arbitrary measurement of a child's size. (A, T, H)

79. 3. Six 5-ounce feedings (or 30 ounces) daily is the correct amount for a child this age. Using a firmer and smaller-holed nipple will increase sucking time and help to meet the child's sucking needs. Skim milk is never recommended for infants because it does not provide the essential fatty acids needed for growth and development. Cow's milk provides excessive protein, which increases renal solute loads and water demands. Cereal should never be mixed in formula and given in a bottle; this does not allow the infant to learn to eat from a spoon. Furthermore, this infant would not be able to digest the cereal for another month or two. Diluting the formula to half of its intended calories would result in insufficient caloric intake. (I, N, H)

80. 1. Decreasing the amount of formula as the infant begins to take solids helps prevent excess caloric intake. Mixing the food with formula does not allow the child to become accustomed to new textures. Because of the infant's tendency to push food out with the tongue, it may be helpful to place food at the back of the infant's tongue when feeding. A small bowled spoon is recommended for infants. (P, N, H)

81. 3. Solids are commonly introduced to an infant at about 5 to 6 months of age. Before this age, the infant's gastrointestinal tract is unable to block macromolecules from absorption, which can lead to food-protein allergy. It is recommended that foods be introduced one at a time, starting with rice cereal, which is hypoallergenic. This technique enables ready identification of food allergies. After the introduction of cereal, other foods can be given in any order; a common approach is to start with fruits and vegetables and then introduce meats. Mixing food in a bottle does not allow the infant to learn to eat from a spoon. The use of an Infafeeder also does not allow the infant to learn to eat from a spoon. (E, N, H)

82. 1. Infants generally do not overeat unless they are urged to do so. Parents should watch for clues indicating that the infant is full; for example, stopping sucking and pushing the nipple out of the mouth. Giving a normal-weight infant a regular supplementation of water is unnecessary; the infant's sucking needs can be met by providing a pacifier. A demand schedule, rather than a regulated schedule, allows the infant to regulate intake according to individual needs. Bottle-feeding instead of breast-feeding is more likely to lead to excessive caloric intake. (P, N, H)

The Client With Cow's Milk Sensitivity

83. 2. Cow's milk sensitivity is an adverse local and systemic gastrointestinal reaction to cow's milk protein. This is the most common nutritional allergy in infants. Lactose intolerance involves a deficiency of the enzyme lactase, which is needed for digestion of lactose. Almost all sensitive children can tolerate cow's milk by age 2 years. (I, C, G)

84. 1. Lactose intolerance is caused by the lack of the digestive enzyme lactase. This enzyme, found in intestinal juice, is necessary for the digestion of lactose, the primary carbohydrate in cow's milk. (E, C, G)

85. 1. A lactose intolerance test is used to confirm the diagnosis of lactose intolerance. A blood glucose level of 20 mg/dL or less confirms the diagnosis. In lactose intolerance, fecal pH is less than 6.0 (acidic). A positive hydrogen breath test is associated with, but does not confirm the diagnosis of, lactose intolerance. Hydrogen gas is produced in the intestinal tract of a child who does not digest lactose completely. Urine positive for protein is not associated with lactose intolerance. (A, C, G)

86. 4. Lactose-intolerant people are usually able to tolerate dairy products in which lactose has been fermented, such as yogurt, cheese, and buttermilk. Pudding, ice cream, and creamed soups contain lactose that has not been fermented. (P, T, G)

87. 1. Mothers of children with cow's milk allergy can continue to breast-feed if they eliminate cow's milk from their diet. It is important to encourage mothers to continue to breast-feed because breast milk is usually the least allergenic and most easily digested food for an infant. (P, N, G)

88. 3. Soy protein is the recommended initial milk substitute. Goat's milk is not used because of cross-reactions with cow's milk. If soy milk is not tolerated, then hydrolyzed protein or milk-based formulas may be used. Because the child may be allergic to any formula, it is best not to buy too large a supply until tolerance is verified. (P, N, G)

NURSING CARE OF CHILDREN

TEST 5: The Child With Health Problems of the Lower Gastrointestinal Tract

Directions: Use this answer grid to determine areas of strength or need for further study.

NURSING PROCESS

A = Assessment
D = Analysis, nursing diagnosis
P = Planning
I = Implementation
E = Evaluation

COGNITIVE LEVEL

K = Knowledge
C = Comprehension
T = Application
N = Analysis

CLIENT NEEDS

S = Safe, effective care environment
G = Physiologic integrity
L = Psychosocial integrity
H = Health promotion and maintenance

Question #	Answer #	Nursing Process A	D	P	I	E	Cognitive Level K	C	T	N	Client Needs S	G	L	H
1	4	A							T			G		
2	3			P					T			G		
3	4	A						C				G		
4	1			P				C					L	
5	2	A							T			G		
6	1				I				T				L	
7	2		D							N		G		
8	1			P					T			G		
9	1			P					T			G		
10	1					E				N		G		
11	2				I			C					L	
12	1				I			C			S			
13	3	A						C				G		
14	4				I			C			S			
15	2				I				T		S			
16	1					E				N	S			
17	1		D							N	S			
18	3	A								N		G		
19	1					E		C				G		
20	2				I			C				G		
21	3	A						C				G		
22	3		D					C						H
23	1				I			C						H
24	1				I			C					L	
25	2				I			C					L	

ANSWER GRID: 1

NURSING PROCESS

A = Assessment
D = Analysis, nursing diagnosis
P = Planning
I = Implementation
E = Evaluation

COGNITIVE LEVEL

K = Knowledge
C = Comprehension
T = Application
N = Analysis

CLIENT NEEDS

S = Safe, effective care environment
G = Physiologic integrity
L = Psychosocial integrity
H = Health promotion and maintenance

Question #	Answer #	Nursing Process					Cognitive Level				Client Needs			
		A	D	P	I	E	K	C	T	N	S	G	L	H
26	3	A							T			G		
27	1	A							T			G		
28	3			P					T			G		
29	2	A						C				G		
30	2	A								N		G		
31	1					E				N		G		
32	1	A							T		S			
33	4				I				T		S			
34	1			P					T		S			
35	4				I				T			G		
36	2				I				T		S			
37	1				I				T				L	
38	2				I				T				L	
39	2	A						C					L	
40	4	A						C					L	
41	1					E				N			L	
42	3			P					T				L	
43	1				I		K					G		
44	2			P			K					G		
45	3				I			C				G		
46	3	A								N		G		
47	3	A							T			G		
48	2			P					T			G		
49	4			P				C				G		
50	1					E				N		G		
51	3			P					T			G		
52	3				I			C				G		
53	2			P				C				G		
54	4				I				T					H
55	2	A						C				G		

ANSWER GRID: 2

NURSING PROCESS

A = Assessment
D = Analysis, nursing diagnosis
P = Planning
I = Implementation
E = Evaluation

COGNITIVE LEVEL

K = Knowledge
C = Comprehension
T = Application
N = Analysis

CLIENT NEEDS

S = Safe, effective care environment
G = Physiologic integrity
L = Psychosocial integrity
H = Health promotion and maintenance

Question #	Answer #	Nursing Process					Cognitive Level				Client Needs			
		A	D	P	I	E	K	C	T	N	S	G	L	H
56	2	A						C				G		
57	1				I				T			G		
58	3				I				T			G		
59	4				I				T			G		
60	3	A					K					G		
61	3	A						C				G		
62	1			P						N		G		
63	1	A					K					G		
64	3				I			C				G		
65	4			P				C				G		
66	4				I			C				G		
67	4			P					T					H
68	2					E				N			L	
69	3	A					K					G		
70	2	A						C				G		
71	1	A					K					G		
72	2				I				T				L	
73	4					E				N		G		
74	2			P			K					G		
75	4	A							T					H
76	1	A					K							H
77	3			P					T					H
78	2	A							T					H
79	3				I					N				H
80	1			P						N				H
81	3					E				N				H
82	1			P						N				H
83	2				I			C				G		
84	1					E		C				G		
85	1	A						C				G		

ANSWER GRID: 3

NURSING PROCESS

A = Assessment
D = Analysis, nursing diagnosis
P = Planning
I = Implementation
E = Evaluation

COGNITIVE LEVEL

K = Knowledge
C = Comprehension
T = Application
N = Analysis

CLIENT NEEDS

S = Safe, effective care environment
G = Physiologic integrity
L = Psychosocial integrity
H = Health promotion and maintenance

		Nursing Process					Cognitive Level				Client Needs			
Question #	Answer #	A	D	P	I	E	K	C	T	N	S	G	L	H
86	4			P					T			G		
87	1			P						N		G		
88	3			P						N		G		
Number Correct														
Number Possible	88	27	3	22	26	10	8	30	31	19	9	54	13	12
Percentage Correct														

Score Calculation: To determine your **Percentage Correct,** divide the **Number Correct** by the **Number Possible.**

ANSWER GRID: 4

The Child With Health Problems of the Urinary System

- The Client With Cryptorchidism
- The Client With Hydrocele
- The Client With Hypospadias
- The Client With Urinary Tract Infection
- The Client With Glomerulonephritis
- The Client With Nephrotic Syndrome
- The Client With Acute or Chronic Renal Failure
- Correct Answers and Rationale

Select the one best answer, and indicate your choice by filling in the circle in front of the option.

The Client With Cryptorchidism

A 1-month-old infant is brought to the clinic by his father for a checkup. The father explains that he is concerned because the right side of his son's scrotum seems different. The nurse notes that the infant is circumcised.

1. The father says he is afraid that his son's testicle is missing. The nurse should
   - ○ 1. explain that although the testis should have descended by now, it is not a cause for worry.
   - ○ 2. explain that the testes often do not descend until age 6 months, and examine the child to see if a testis is present.
   - ○ 3. explain that the testis should have been present in the scrotal sac at birth, but surgery can remedy the situation.
   - ○ 4. explain that the testis may descend by 6 weeks of age, and reflect understanding of his concern.
2. While preparing to examine the infant's scrotal sac and testes, the nurse should
   - ○ 1. check for recent urination.
   - ○ 2. give the infant a pacifier.
   - ○ 3. keep the room and the nurse's hands warm.
   - ○ 4. tap lightly on the left inguinal ring.
3. While the nurse is examining the infant, the father

paces around the room shaking his head. Which of the following would be the nurse's best remark at this time?
   - ○ 1. "I'm sure everything will work out for the best, and he'll be fine."
   - ○ 2. "You seem upset; please tell me how you're feeling."
   - ○ 3. "Don't worry; his testes will probably descend on their own."
   - ○ 4. "Would you like to talk with a parent of a child who has the same problem?"
4. Because several other conditions are associated with undescended testes, the nurse should also assess the infant for
   - ○ 1. abnormal lower extremity reflexes.
   - ○ 2. difficulty feeding and a history of frequent emesis.
   - ○ 3. a reducible or nonreducible bulging in the inguinal area.
   - ○ 4. heart murmur and poor weight gain.
5. A diagnosis of undescended testis is confirmed. The father is relieved to learn that surgical intervention will be postponed until the child is 1 to 2 years old. The physician, nurse, and father discuss a nonsurgical treatment consisting of
   - ○ 1. a trial of human chorionic gonadotrophic hormone.

○ 2. a trial of adrenocorticotropic hormone.

○ 3. frequent stimulation of the cremasteric reflex.

○ 4. frequent warm baths.

6. The child fails to respond to nonsurgical treatment, and when he reaches age 14 months, surgery is scheduled. The nurse plans to do preoperative teaching by

○ 1. telling the child that his penis and scrotum will be "fixed."

○ 2. explaining to the parents how the defect will be corrected.

○ 3. telling the child that he will not see any incisions after surgery.

○ 4. using an anatomically correct doll to show the child what will be "fixed" and how it will look.

7. The child returns from surgery, and his postanesthesia recovery period is uneventful. When planning for the child's discharge, the nurse should emphasize which of the following goals to the parents? The child will

○ 1. be free of redness or swelling at the incision site.

○ 2. take clear liquids well within 24 hours.

○ 3. have a normal bowel movement within 24 hours.

○ 4. be ambulatory within 48 hours.

8. The child returns from surgery with traction applied to the testes. The nurse should teach the parents to

○ 1. remove the traction after 24 hours.

○ 2. maintain the traction consistently.

○ 3. increase the traction by one eighth every 12 hours.

○ 4. decrease the traction by one eighth every 6 hours.

9. The client returns to the clinic at the age of 14 years. What anticipatory guidance would the nurse provide to the parents and the adolescent?

○ 1. Discuss the client's sterility.

○ 2. Discuss the client's future plans.

○ 3. Teach the client how to do monthly testicular self-examinations.

○ 4. Teach the parents that the client will need a lot of psychological support.

The Client With Hydrocele

A 2-week-old infant is brought to the clinic by his mother for evaluation of fluid accumulation in the scrotal area.

10. This condition is most likely a result of

○ 1. a blockage in the inguinal canal that allows fluid to accumulate in the epididymis and ductus deferens.

○ 2. a patent processus vaginalis that allows fluid to accumulate in the testicle and peritoneal cavity.

○ 3. a patent processus vaginalis that results in the collection of fluid along the spermatic cord or tunica vaginalis of the testicle.

○ 4. an obliterated processus vaginalis that allows fluid to accumulate in the scrotal sac.

11. A nurse in the neonatal nursery was the first to notice the infant's problem by differentiating between accumulation of fluid and the presence of intestines in the scrotal sac, noting that

○ 1. the bulge could be reduced.

○ 2. the increase in scrotal size was bilateral.

○ 3. the scrotal sac could be transilluminated.

○ 4. the bulge appears during crying.

12. During the clinic visit, the mother states that the infant's scrotum is smaller than when he was born. Which further remark by the mother would indicate to the nurse that she understands why this has happened?

○ 1. "I guess keeping his bottom up has helped."

○ 2. "Massaging his groin area is working."

○ 3. "More time is needed for the fluid to be totally reabsorbed."

○ 4. "Keeping him quiet and in an infant seat has really helped."

13. When he is 1 year old, the child undergoes surgery to correct the hydrocele. Shortly after returning to his room, his mother approaches the nurse and states that her child's scrotum looks swollen and bruised. The nurse's most appropriate response would be

○ 1. "He can have an aspirin; I'll get it right away."

○ 2. "Why don't you wait in his room until I can get there?"

○ 3. "This happens often after this type of surgery. I'll call the doctor and tell him."

○ 4. "This is normal after this type of surgery. Let's look at it together just to be sure."

14. The nurse applies an ice bag to the infant's scrotum. When the mother asks why, the nurse would reply,

○ 1. "It increases the blood flow to the area to increase healing."

○ 2. "It's usually ordered for all this surgeon's clients."

○ 3. "The ice bag will decrease swelling."

○ 4. "The cold stops a reflex that helps keep the testes out of the scrotal sac during healing."

15. The mother says that the surgeon explained that her child may be more susceptible to some problem in the future, but that she was upset at the time and now cannot remember what the surgeon said. The nurse's best reply would be,

○ 1. "I'll call the surgeon if you'd like to speak with him."

○ 2. "An inguinal hernia is associated with this type of condition."

○ 3. "Hydrocele is sometimes associated with sterility."

○ 4. "Your baby might have problems with his bowels."

The Client With Hypospadias

On newborn assessment, a neonate is found to have hypospadias and chordee.

16. The mother asks the nurse to explain what is wrong with her infant. The nurse would reply that
   ○ 1. there is something wrong with his penis, and she should ask the doctor.
   ○ 2. the infant's ureters reflux urine into the kidneys.
   ○ 3. his urine will come out from the top of his penis.
   ○ 4. his urine will come out from under his penis.

17. The child's parents wish to have him circumcised. Which of the following rationales would the nurse discuss with the parents concerning the recommendation to delay circumcision?
   ○ 1. The associated chordee is difficult to remove during circumcision.
   ○ 2. The foreskin is used to repair the deformity surgically.
   ○ 3. The meatus can become stenosed, leading to symptoms of urinary obstruction.
   ○ 4. The infant is too small now to have surgery.

18. When the child is 1 year of age, he is scheduled for surgery to correct the hypospadias and chordee. The nurse would explain to the parents that this is the preferred time for surgical repair because
   ○ 1. the child will experience less pain at this age.
   ○ 2. the child is too young to have developed castration anxiety.
   ○ 3. the surgical experience will not be remembered by the child.
   ○ 4. the repair is easier before the child is toilet trained.

19. After surgical repair of the hypospadias, the child is returned to his room on the pediatric unit with an intravenous line and both a urethral catheter and a suprapubic catheter in place. The nurse explains to the parents that the primary purpose for the suprapubic catheter is to provide an
   ○ 1. accurate measurement of urine output.
   ○ 2. alternate urine elimination route.
   ○ 3. entry port for bladder irrigation.
   ○ 4. easy access for the doctor to observe the surgical site.

20. The nurse would evaluate the preoperative teaching for the parents about the urethral catheter to be successful when the mother states that the catheter in his penis is there to
   ○ 1. decrease pain at the surgical site.
   ○ 2. keep the new urethra from growing together.
   ○ 3. measure his urine correctly.
   ○ 4. prevent bladder spasms.

21. Before the child returns from surgery, the nurse discusses with the parents how the surgical site will appear, explaining that because this is the first of two surgeries, the child's penis will appear swollen and
   ○ 1. very red in color.
   ○ 2. dusky blue at the tip.
   ○ 3. somewhat misshapen.
   ○ 4. pale.

22. A nursing diagnosis for this child is Altered Comfort related to surgical intervention and immobility. An intervention the nurse would carry out in addition to administering an analgesic would be to
   ○ 1. allow him to play with other children.
   ○ 2. ensure his restraints are in place.
   ○ 3. allow his parents to stay at the bedside.
   ○ 4. make sure he sleeps through the night.

23. The nurse should teach the parents to
   ○ 1. assist the child to become familiar with his dressings so he will leave them alone.
   ○ 2. encourage the child to ambulate as soon as possible by using a favorite push toy.
   ○ 3. force fluids, at least 2,500 mL/day, by offering his favorite juices.
   ○ 4. prevent the child from disrupting the catheters by using soft restraints.

24. The nurse encourages the parents to participate in their son's care. Which of the following nursing diagnoses should be of concern to the parents and nurse at this time?
   ○ 1. Altered Self-Concept.
   ○ 2. High Risk for Infection.
   ○ 3. High Risk for Altered Body Temperature.
   ○ 4. Feeding Self-Care Deficit.

25. The physician orders a urinalysis for this child. Which of the following results should the nurse report to the physician?
   ○ 1. Urine specific gravity of 1.017.
   ○ 2. 10 red blood cells per high-powered field.
   ○ 3. 25 white blood cells per high-powered field.
   ○ 4. Urine pH of 6.0.

The Client With Urinary Tract Infection

A 3-year-old girl is brought to the clinic by her mother because she has a fever and is very fussy. Her health history indicates that she has had a urinary tract infection within the past year.

26. To complete the assessment, the nurse should also ask the mother whether the child has recently had
  ○ 1. abdominal pain.
  ○ 2. swollen lymph glands.
  ○ 3. skin rash.
  ○ 4. back pain.

27. The nurse discusses obtaining a urine specimen with the physician. Which of the following would result in the least contamination of the specimen?
  ○ 1. Clean-catch midstream void.
  ○ 2. Straight catheterization.
  ○ 3. Suprapubic bladder aspiration.
  ○ 4. Have the mother bring in a specimen from home.

28. Which of the following results would indicate to the nurse that the child has a probable urinary tract infection? The urine
  ○ 1. is pale and yellow in color.
  ○ 2. is positive for urobilinogen.
  ○ 3. has several white blood cells.
  ○ 4. has a specific gravity of 1.017.

29. The nurse teaches the mother about some measures she can take to help prevent this problem in the future. The nurse would evaluate the teaching as successful when the mother states,
  ○ 1. "She'll like more bubble baths."
  ○ 2. "We'll stop at the store on the way home and buy some of her favorite juice so she'll drink more."
  ○ 3. "We'll try to get her to hold her urine for a longer time."
  ○ 4. "We'll let her soak in the bathtub for 30 minutes every day."

30. The child will be treated with trimethoprim-sulfamethoxazole (Bactrim) for 10 days. What information should the nurse provide to the parents?
  ○ 1. Administer the antibiotic with food.
  ○ 2. Be sure to drink a lot of water with this antibiotic.
  ○ 3. Limit the number of times the child is able to urinate.
  ○ 4. When the child stops complaining of dysuria, start giving the medicine once a day.

31. Several days later, the child's father calls the clinic. He explains, "My wife and I are concerned because our child refuses to obey us concerning the preventions you told us about. She refuses to take her medication unless we buy her a present. We're reluctant to discipline her because she is sick, but we're worried about her behavior." What would be the nurse's best response?
  ○ 1. "I sympathize with your difficulties, but just ignore her behavior for now, and she'll soon return to her old self."
  ○ 2. "I understand that it's hard to discipline your child when she's ill, but she needs the family routines, discipline, and rewards to be kept as normal as possible."

  ○ 3. "I understand that things are difficult for you right now, but she is ill and deserves special treatment."
  ○ 4. "I understand your concern, but this type of behavior happens all the time; she'll get over it when she feels better."

32. The child is found to have vesicoureteral reflux. The nurse explains to the parents that vesicoureteral reflux contributes to the development of urinary infections because it
  ○ 1. prevents complete emptying of the bladder.
  ○ 2. causes urine backflow into the kidney.
  ○ 3. results in painful bladder spasms.
  ○ 4. causes painful urination.

The Client With Glomerulonephritis

An acutely ill 14-year-old boy comes to a health clinic. His mother reports he has periorbital edema in the morning and is not eating.

33. What assessment would the clinic nurse make *first*?
  ○ 1. Ask the mother about fever and skin rashes.
  ○ 2. Ask the client if he has had a sore throat.
  ○ 3. Ask the client if he has had a change in his urine output.
  ○ 4. Ask the mother if he has any allergies.

34. The physician orders a throat culture, which is positive for streptococcal bacteria. The client's mother reports that he is allergic to penicillin, and the physician has ordered amoxicillin. The nurse should
  ○ 1. ask the mother if the child is also allergic to amoxicillin.
  ○ 2. administer amoxicillin; the client's allergy is to penicillin, not amoxicillin.
  ○ 3. substitute erythromycin; it is as effective as amoxicillin.
  ○ 4. notify the physician of the allergy; the order needs to be changed.

35. The client is admitted to the hospital because of decreased urine output and possible diagnosis of acute glomerulonephritis. Which of the following would be the most important nursing intervention for this client?
  ○ 1. Temperature, pulse, and respirations every 4 hours.
  ○ 2. Intake and output every 12 hours.
  ○ 3. Daily weight.
  ○ 4. Daily electrolytes.

36. During admission, the nurse notes that the client has a roller-type elastic bandage from his toes to above the ankle. The mother says that he sprained an ankle playing basketball. Noting that the toes are

swollen and on the cool side, the nurse would suspect that this is because
- ○ 1. the bandage was applied too tightly.
- ○ 2. the bandage had been applied in a figure-eight movement.
- ○ 3. the direction of bandage application was from the ankle down.
- ○ 4. the direction of bandage application was from the toes up.

37. Later, while talking with the nurse alone, the client says that he has had several "wet dreams" during the past couple of weeks, and he is concerned that this has made him ill. When explaining the significance of nocturnal emissions to the client, the nurse should emphasize that they are
- ○ 1. an early symptom of acute glomerulonephritis.
- ○ 2. a normal occurrence in adolescence.
- ○ 3. a positive sign that the young man is producing live sperm.
- ○ 4. a symptom of homosexuality.

38. The client's mouth is dry, and his lips are encrusted with mucus (sordes). The most effective agent to cleanse his mouth would be
- ○ 1. a jelly-type toothpaste.
- ○ 2. a mild, white vinegar solution.
- ○ 3. half-strength hydrogen peroxide.
- ○ 4. full-strength mouthwash.

39. The client's fluid intake is restricted to 1000 mL/day. Which of the following fluids would the nurse consider to be appropriate for the client's condition and effective for preventing excessive thirst?
- ○ 1. Diet cola.
- ○ 2. Ice chips.
- ○ 3. Lemonade.
- ○ 4. Tap water.

40. When the client complains about the food served in the hospital, his mother offers to bring him some food from home. Considering the client's nutritional needs at this time, which of the following would the nurse and mother decide not to offer him?
- ○ 1. Apples and strawberries.
- ○ 2. Pancakes and syrup.
- ○ 3. Buttered noodles.
- ○ 4. Bananas and oranges.

41. The nurse is planning interventions for the nursing diagnosis Diversional Activity Deficit. Based on his growth and development, which of the following activities would be most useful for this client?
- ○ 1. Playing a card game with a boy his same age.
- ○ 2. Putting together a puzzle with his mother.
- ○ 3. Playing video games with an 8-year-old.
- ○ 4. Watching a movie with his younger brother.

42. One of the client's teachers visits him and tells the nurse, "I never worry about him. He always lands on his feet and seems to know where he's going."

This description of the client's personality is characteristic of a teenager who, according to psychologist Erik Erikson,
- ○ 1. has a good relationship with his parents.
- ○ 2. has a sense of identity.
- ○ 3. is of above-average intelligence.
- ○ 4. is emotionally independent from his family.

43. Which of the following would indicate that the client is experiencing a severe complication of acute glomerulonephritis?
- ○ 1. Temperature of 100.2°F (38.8°C).
- ○ 2. Serum sodium of 135 mEq/L.
- ○ 3. Blood pressure of 140/92 mm Hg.
- ○ 4. Weight loss of 2 pounds.

The client's condition worsens on the second morning of hospitalization. His blood pressure is elevated, and he has not voided since 7 PM the previous evening.

44. The appropriate initial nursing action would be to
- ○ 1. assess his neurologic status.
- ○ 2. encourage him to drink more water.
- ○ 3. encourage him to eat a low-sodium breakfast.
- ○ 4. help him to ambulate in the hallway.

45. The nursing care plan should include
- ○ 1. checking urine specific gravity daily.
- ○ 2. checking vital signs every 8 hours.
- ○ 3. keeping a daily calorie count.
- ○ 4. weighing the client daily.

46. The client improves, and the nurse is helping the family plan for his discharge. When developing the plan, the nurse should plan to discuss
- ○ 1. restricting dietary protein.
- ○ 2. monitoring pulse rate and rhythm.
- ○ 3. preventing respiratory infections.
- ○ 4. restricting foods high in potassium.

An older adolescent with a history of losing weight and feeling tired and irritable has been admitted to the hospital. He has been diagnosed with chronic glomerulonephritis.

47. Laboratory data for this adolescent most likely would include
- ○ 1. serum sodium of 133 mEq/L.
- ○ 2. blood urea nitrogen of 7 mg/dL.
- ○ 3. serum potassium of 3.8 mEq/L.
- ○ 4. blood pH of 7.43.

323

48. Which of the following nursing diagnoses would the nurse most likely formulate for this client?
- ○ 1. Chronic Pain.
- ○ 2. Altered Self-Concept.
- ○ 3. Functional Incontinence.
- ○ 4. Anticipatory Grieving.

The Client With Nephrotic Syndrome

A 3-year-old child is hospitalized for observation. He has marked dependent edema and hypoalbuminemia, and his urine is frothy, but he is free from infection.

49. When assessing the child's vital signs, the nurse would expect to observe
- ○ 1. blood pressure of 100/60 mm Hg.
- ○ 2. body temperature of 100.8°F .
- ○ 3. pulse rate of 72 beats/minute.
- ○ 4. respiratory rate of 18 breaths/minute.

50. Urinalysis reveals + 4 for protein, which would indicate
- ○ 1. decreased secretion of aldosterone.
- ○ 2. increased permeability of the glomerular membrane to albumin.
- ○ 3. inhibited tubular reabsorption of sodium and water.
- ○ 4. loss of red blood cells in the urine.

51. The mother reports that the child "has been breathing hard." The child's respiratory rate is 42 breaths/minute, and respirations are shallow. What would be the most appropriate nursing diagnosis?
- ○ 1. Ineffective Breathing Pattern related to accumulation of fluid in the alveoli.
- ○ 2. Ineffective Breathing Pattern related to accumulation of fluid in the abdominal cavity.
- ○ 3. Impaired Gas Exchange related to increased fluid in the pulmonary vascular system.
- ○ 4. Impaired Gas Exchange related to left-sided heart failure.

52. In preparing the child to have blood drawn for tests, the nurse would
- ○ 1. explain the procedure in advance and answer any questions the child asks.
- ○ 2. discuss reasons why the blood needs to be drawn.
- ○ 3. use distraction techniques during the procedure.
- ○ 4. provide verbal explanations about what will occur.

53. When obtaining a health history from the child's mother, the nurse would focus on information concerning which nursing diagnosis?
- ○ 1. Altered Nutrition: More Than Body Requirements.
- ○ 2. Altered Nutrition: Less Than Body Requirements.
- ○ 3. Diversional Activity Deficit.
- ○ 4. Sleep Pattern Disturbance.

54. The parents, nurse, and physician have jointly discussed the child's hospital treatment and care. The nurse would know that the mother had understood the plan when she states,
- ○ 1. "He really likes chips and bologna. I guess we'll have to find something else he'll eat."
- ○ 2. "We'll have to encourage him to drink more fluids. Did you say about 4 liters every day?"
- ○ 3. "We worry about the surgery. Do you think we should do direct donation of blood?"
- ○ 4. "We understand the need for antibiotics. I just wish he could take them by mouth."

55. The parents and the nurse continue to plan for the child's care. In regard to the nursing diagnosis of Fluid Volume Excess, the care plan would include
- ○ 1. limiting visitors to 2 to 3 hours a day.
- ○ 2. observing strict bed rest.
- ○ 3. testing urine specific gravity every shift.
- ○ 4. weighing the child before breakfast.

56. Which of the following nursing measures would help reduce edema in the child's eyelids?
- ○ 1. Apply cool compresses to the child's eyes.
- ○ 2. Elevate the head of the child's bed.
- ○ 3. Apply eye drops every 8 hours.
- ○ 4. Limit the child's television watching.

57. The nurse wishes to evaluate the child's status in relation to fluid retention. Evidence for decreased fluid retention would be
- ○ 1. decreased abdominal girth.
- ○ 2. decreased heart rate.
- ○ 3. increased caloric intake.
- ○ 4. increased respiratory rate.

58. The child is receiving cyclophosphamide (Cytoxan). During therapy, the nurse would monitor the child's blood
- ○ 1. glucose.
- ○ 2. protein.
- ○ 3. sodium.
- ○ 4. white cell count.

59. The child is extremely edematous. Which of the following measures would the nurse take for this child in regard to the nursing diagnosis Impaired Skin Integrity?
- ○ 1. Ambulate every shift while awake.
- ○ 2. Apply lotion on opposing skin surfaces.
- ○ 3. Apply powder to skin folds.
- ○ 4. Separate opposing skin surfaces with soft cloth.

60. The child is started on prednisone. The nurse would explain to the parents that this medication should
- ○ 1. decrease the blood pressure.
- ○ 2. decrease protein in the urine.

○ 3. increase sodium reabsorption.

○ 4. increase hydrostatic pressure.

61. The child responds to treatment and is ready to go home. When helping the family plan for home care, the nurse would instruct the parents to

○ 1. administer pain medication as needed.

○ 2. keep the child away from anyone with an infection.

○ 3. notify the physician of an increase in the child's urine output.

○ 4. administer acetaminophen daily.

The Client With Acute or Chronic Renal Failure

An adolescent girl is admitted to the hospital with acute renal failure. Two weeks ago, she had a catheter inserted through the anterior abdominal wall for peritoneal dialysis.

62. The adolescent asks the nurse to reexplain the advantages of peritoneal dialysis over hemodialysis. The nurse should point out that peritoneal dialysis involves

○ 1. fewer dietary restrictions.

○ 2. less chance of infection.

○ 3. more protein loss.

○ 4. more rapid fluid removal.

63. As the nurse performs the daily catheter exit site care with the adolescent, an important step would be to

○ 1. apply an occlusive dressing after cleansing the site.

○ 2. change the dressing when the peritoneal space is dry.

○ 3. examine the site for signs of infection while cleansing the area.

○ 4. pull on the catheter while cleansing the skin.

64. The nurse plans discharge teaching for the adolescent and the family. The nurse would emphasize that which of the following nutrients should be restricted?

○ 1. Ascorbic acid.

○ 2. Calcium.

○ 3. Magnesium.

○ 4. Phosphorus.

65. The nurse has emphasized to the adolescent the importance of maintaining a positive self-concept. An indicator that the plan is working would be that she

○ 1. complains about headaches, abdominal pain, and nausea.

○ 2. insists on making her own dietary choices even if the foods she chooses are restricted.

○ 3. plans to quit all after-school activities when she returns home.

○ 4. wants to do her own dressing changes and take care of her own medications.

66. For a child with acute renal failure, which of the following diet plans would be appropriate for the nurse to discuss with the family? A diet

○ 1. high in carbohydrate and protein.

○ 2. high in fat and carbohydrate.

○ 3. low in fat and protein.

○ 4. low in carbohydrate and fat.

67. The nurse plans to discuss with the adolescent and her family the psychosocial aspects of going home with a peritoneal dialysis catheter in place. A topic of high priority would be the

○ 1. advantages of limiting social activities for a few months.

○ 2. advisability of not disclosing information about the peritoneal dialysis to people outside the family.

○ 3. possible effect on body image of having an abdominal catheter.

○ 4. importance of relying on her parents to do the dialysis and dressing changes.

A preschool-aged child develops chronic renal failure and has been receiving peritoneal dialysis at home for the past year.

68. During a routine home visit, the public health nurse assesses the child's peritoneal catheter exit site. Which of the following findings would lead the nurse to formulate the nursing diagnosis High Risk for Infection?

○ 1. Dialysate leakage.

○ 2. Granulation tissue.

○ 3. Increased time for drainage.

○ 4. Tissue swelling.

69. After reviewing the signs and symptoms of peritonitis with the child's mother, the nurse would determine that the mother has understood the teaching when she identifies an important sign as

○ 1. cloudy dialysate drainage return.

○ 2. distended abdomen.

○ 3. shortness of breath.

○ 4. weight gain of 3 pounds in 2 days.

70. If peritonitis were suspected, which of the following nursing interventions would be appropriate?

○ 1. Check the blood pressure.

○ 2. Assess for peritoneal leak.

○ 3. Increase the client's fluid intake.

○ 4. Obtain a peritoneal fluid sample for culture and sensitivity.

71. The public health nurse assesses the child for edema. Which of the following findings is associated with edema?
   ○ 1. Absence of pulmonary rales.
   ○ 2. Increased dialysate outflow.
   ○ 3. Normal blood pressure.
   ○ 4. Pallor.

72. The mother tells the public health nurse that she worries about her child's future. She states, "I haven't been able to sleep or eat and have lost 10 pounds during the past month." She has not discussed her concerns with anyone but her husband. Based on this information, the public health nurse would make a tentative nursing diagnosis of
   ○ 1. Altered Parenting.
   ○ 2. Anticipatory Grieving.
   ○ 3. Ineffective Family Coping.
   ○ 4. Social Isolation.

73. During the public health nurse's next visit, the mother says that for the past 2 days it has taken 30 minutes to fill the peritoneal space with dialysate and another 30 minutes to drain the dialysate at the end of a run. The nurse would judge that the
   ○ 1. inflow and drain times are normal.
   ○ 2. inflow and drain times are slower than normal.
   ○ 3. inflow time is normal, but the drain time is slower than normal.
   ○ 4. inflow time is slower than normal, but the drain time is normal.

74. The mother asks what she can do if both inflow and drain times are increased. The nurse would instruct her to
   ○ 1. assess the child for constipation.
   ○ 2. decrease the amount of dialysate infused for each dwell.
   ○ 3. incorporate the increased inflow and drain times into the dialysis schedule.
   ○ 4. monitor the client for shoulder pain during inflow and drain times.

75. The nurse judges that the mother understands the diet restrictions when she reports that she provides a diet
   ○ 1. restricted in sodium and water.
   ○ 2. rich in protein and carbohydrates.
   ○ 3. high in potassium and iron.
   ○ 4. restricted in protein and phosphorus.

A preschool-aged child is admitted to the hospital with an abdominal tumor, which is the most common type of renal cancer in children. The nurse notes that the tumor does not cross the midline. The child has cryptorchidism, which is strongly associated with this type of tumor. Although there is some evidence of genetic inheritance, none of the child's siblings have had this tumor.

76. When assessing the child, the nurse could also expect to find
   ○ 1. hypotension.
   ○ 2. proteinemia.
   ○ 3. pallor.
   ○ 4. petechiae.

77. During assessment, the nurse should keep in mind that it is important to avoid
   ○ 1. measuring the child's chest circumference.
   ○ 2. palpating the child's abdomen.
   ○ 3. placing the child in an upright position.
   ○ 4. measuring the child's occipitofrontal circumference.

78. Once the diagnosis is made, the nurse would prepare the family and child for tests and procedures that will be done preoperatively, including
   ○ 1. barium enema.
   ○ 2. bone scan.
   ○ 3. computed tomography of the abdomen.
   ○ 4. barium swallow.

79. The child is scheduled for a nephrectomy the following morning. In planning preoperative care for the child, the nurse should assign lowest priority to
   ○ 1. allowing the child play time.
   ○ 2. monitoring the child's vital signs frequently.
   ○ 3. providing the child's family with emotional support.
   ○ 4. teaching the parents about the staging of the tumor.

80. The mother tells the nurse that the surgeon has verified that her child has a stage II tumor. The nurse judges that the mother understands staging when she states that the tumor
   ○ 1. has extended beyond the kidney but was completely removed.
   ○ 2. is in the kidney and has spread to the lung, liver, bone, and brain.
   ○ 3. has extended beyond the kidney to the lung and liver.
   ○ 4. is in the kidney and was totally removed.

81. After successful surgery, the child is returned to his room. The nurse should place the child in which position?
   ○ 1. Modified Trendelenburg.
   ○ 2. Sim's.
   ○ 3. Semi-Fowler's.
   ○ 4. Supine.

82. When assisting the family in making plans for the child's treatment protocol, the nurse and the physician would discuss the use of chemotherapy and

○ 1. bone marrow transplantation.
○ 2. hyperbaric oxygen.
○ 3. leukophoresis.
○ 4. radiation therapy.

83. The nurse would continue to assess the child postoperatively for which early sign of a complication of this surgery?
○ 1. increased abdominal distention.
○ 2. elevated blood pressure.
○ 3. increased heart rate.
○ 4. increased urine output.

84. The child is to receive dactinomycin (actinomycin-D) and vincristine. The nurse teaches the parents about side effects of chemotherapy. To evaluate the effectiveness of teaching, the nurse questions them about how many weeks after the initial treatment hair loss usually occurs. Which of the following answers would indicate that they have understood the teaching?
○ 1. 2 weeks.
○ 2. 6 weeks.
○ 3. 8 weeks.
○ 4. 12 weeks.

85. The nurse and parents are planning for the child's discharge. Regarding the prescribed chemotherapy, the nurse should teach the parents to
○ 1. encourage the child to drink plenty of fluids.
○ 2. keep the child out of the sun.
○ 3. monitor the child's heart rate.
○ 4. observe the child for drowsiness.

86. Additional discharge planning should involve identifying interventions that will prevent damage to the child's remaining kidney and
○ 1. minimize pain.
○ 2. prevent dependent edema.
○ 3. prevent urinary tract infection.
○ 4. minimize sodium intake.

CORRECT ANSWERS AND RATIONALE

The letters in parentheses following the rationale identify the step of the nursing process (A, D, P, I, E), cognitive level (K, C, T, N), and client needs (S, G, L, H). See the Answer Grid for the key.

The Client With Cryptorchidism

1. 4. Testes should normally descend by age 6 weeks. Failure to do so may indicate a problem with patency or a hormonal imbalance. By acknowledging the father's concern, the nurse indicates acceptance of his feelings. (I, C, G)

2. 3. A cold environment can cause the testes to retract. Cold and touch stimulate the cremasteric reflex, which causes a normal retraction of the testes toward the body. (A, T, G)

3. 2. The nurse needs more information about the father's perceptions and feelings before providing any information or taking action. It is important that the nurse determine the exact nature of the father's concern rather than making an assumption about it. Telling the father not to worry devalues his concern; the child's testes, in fact, may not descend spontaneously. (A, T, L)

4. 3. An inguinal hernia, hydrocele, or upper urinary tract anomaly may occur on the same side as the undescended testis. One anomaly in a system warrants a more focused assessment of that system. (A, N, G)

5. 1. A trial of human chorionic gonadotrophin may be given to stimulate descent of the affected testis. A trial of adrenocorticotropic hormone will not cause the testis to descend. The cremasteric reflex results in the testis being drawn up. Application of warmth would have little or no effect. (P, T, G)

6. 2. Teaching the parents would be the most appropriate action for the nurse. The child is too young to understand the teaching. (P, N, L)

7. 1. A priority goal at this time would be to prevent infection at the operative site. The child can usually begin to take fluids and solids shortly after surgery and can usually get up as soon as comfort allows. Defecation is not a usual problem after this type of surgery. (P, N, G)

8. 2. In surgery, a rubber band or similar device may be attached by a suture to the testis, then taped to the inner thigh to maintain a moderate, steady tension. This device prevents the testis from ascending. The traction is maintained for 5 to 7 days after surgery. (I, T, G)

9. 3. Removal of a testis would not necessarily make the adolescent sterile. The incidence of testicular cancer is increased in adulthood among children who have had undescended testes. It is important to teach the adolescent the testicular self-examination to be performed monthly. A discussion of his future is a good intervention but not the most important. He should not need a lot of psychological support. (P, T, H)

The Client With Hydrocele

10. 3. A hydrocele is a collection of fluid in the tunica vaginalis of the testicle or along the spermatic cord. (D, K, G)

11. 3. A distended hydrocele can be transilluminated. A hernia, unless incarcerated, can be reduced. Both hydroceles and hernias can enlarge the scrotal sac and can be either unilateral or bilateral. Hernias may be noticed during crying. (A, N, G)

12. 3. Because scrotal size is decreasing, the fluid is being absorbed. Massaging or elevation do not have an effect on fluid reabsorption in hydrocele. (E, N, G)

13. 4. Slight swelling and bruising are normal postoperatively. By assessing the area with the mother, the nurse is conveying acceptance of the mother's concern. Aspirin is not usually prescribed for children because of the link between aspirin and Reye's syndrome. Acetaminophen is commonly administered for fever or pain relief. (P, N, G)

14. 3. Cold application decreases circulation to an area to prevent edema. Cold initiates the cremasteric reflex, which draws the testis up closer to the body. By referring to surgeon's orders, the nurse avoids answering the mother's question and conveys a lack of knowledge about the intervention. (I, N, G)

15. 2. Hydrocele is often associated with inguinal hernia. It is not associated with sterility or bowel problems and has few if any sequelae. (I, C, G)

The Client With Hypospadias

16. 4. In hypospadias, the urethra opens on the ventral surface of the penis or perineum. In congenital chordee, a fibrous band of tissue extends from the scrotum up the penis and pulls it ventrally in an arc; congenital chordee may or may not be associated with hypospadias. In epispadias, the urethra opens

on the dorsal surface of the penis. Urine refluxing into the ureters occurs with vesicoureteral reflux. (A, C, G)

17. 2. The foreskin is often used to reconstruct the urethra. Circumcision involves removal of the end of the prepuce of the penis, whereas removal of the chordee necessitates straightening out the penis. Urethral meatal stenosis, which can occur in circumcised infants, results from meatal ulceration and can lead to symptoms of urinary obstruction. The infant is not too small to have surgery. (P, N, G)

18. 2. The preferred time for surgery is age 6 to 18 months, before the child develops castration and body image anxiety. Pain is different for each client and is not related to the preferred time for repair of the hypospadias or chordee. The child will not remember the experience, but this is not the reason to have surgery now. (I, N, G)

19. 2. An alternate urinary elimination route is important because the surgical site needs to be kept dry, clean, and free from the pressure of a full bladder. Pressure from a full bladder might cause fluid to leak around the urethral catheter or might disrupt the delicate plastic surgery. The bladder is rarely irrigated. Measuring urine output is important but is not the primary purpose of the suprapubic catheter. (I, N, G)

20. 2. The main purpose of the urethral catheter is to maintain patency of the reconstructed urethra. The catheter prevents the new tissue inside the urethra from healing on itself, but it can cause bladder spasms. Recently, stents have been used instead of catheters. Urine output can be measured through the suprapubic catheter. (E, N, G)

21. 3. The penis may appear somewhat misshapen or bumpy because of the intermediate phase of reconstruction. The penis is unlikely to look entirely normal even after reconstruction. Swelling and local bruising would be normal; however, because the blood supply should be adequate, a dusky blue tip may indicate a problem with circulation. The penis may be red but should not be very red in color. (I, C, G)

22. 3. For a 12-month-old infant, the most important comfort measure would be the presence of his parents. He is too young to participate in play with other children. The use of restraints will not make him feel more comfortable. Sleeping through the night would be an indication that the interventions are effective. (I, N, L)

23. 4. The most important consideration in terms of successful outcome of this surgery is the maintenance of the catheters or stents. The child is on strict bed rest postoperatively. A 12-month-old likes to explore his environment but must be prevented from manipulating his dressings through the use of soft restraints. Although increasing fluids is important, 2500 mL/day is an excessive amount for a 12-month-old child. (I, N, S)

24. 2. Preventing infection is something the parent can do through careful handwashing. The child may have an altered temperature, but this condition would be related to infection. Altered self-concept is more important for an older child. The child should be able to maintain whatever skills he had in feeding. (D, N, S)

25. 3. A white blood cell count of 25 per high-powered field indicates urinary tract infection. With normal fluid intake, specific gravity should range from 1.002 to 1.030. Red blood cells are normal in urologic surgery. Normal urine pH is 4.6 to 8. (A, N, G)

The Client With Urinary Tract Infection

26. 1. Abdominal pain frequently accompanies urinary tract infections in young children. Other associated signs and symptoms include decreased appetite, vomiting, fever, and irritability. Flank or back pain is associated with urinary tract infection in older children and adults. Lymphadenopathy is unrelated to urinary tract infection. (A, N, G)

27. 3. Suprapubic bladder aspiration results in the least opportunity for contamination. (A, K, G)

28. 3. Pale and yellow urine indicates that the child is well hydrated. Having several white blood cells may indicate a urinary tract infection. Urine specific gravity is normally 1.002 to 1.030. The presence of urobilinogen is not related. (A, C, G)

29. 2. Increased fluid intake promotes frequent urination, which flushes bacteria out of the urinary tract. Emptying the bladder frequently and at the first urge to void prevents urine stasis and decreases the risk of infection ascending to the kidneys. Bubble baths and long soaks in the tub may result in irritation, which may make urination painful and result in inadequate bladder emptying. Wiping from front to back after defecating and voiding helps prevent urethral contamination. (I, N, H)

30. 2. Trimethoprim-sulfamethoxazole is administered twice a day. It can cause crystals to form in the kidneys if the child does not drink enough water. Mixing unpalatable medications in foods can cause the child to dislike a nutritious food. The child should be allowed to urinate as often as needed to empty out the bladder. Antibiotic therapy should be continued for the full 10 days to eliminate the bacteria. (I, N, S)

31. 2. A 3-year-old needs to have psychosocial development maintained as much as possible during illness.

Family routines and discipline should be kept as normal as possible. (I, N, H)

32. 1. The reason that urinary tract infections are a problem in children with vesicoureteral reflux is that the urine that flows back up the ureter past the incompetent valve drains back into the bladder after the child has finished voiding. It is the incomplete emptying of the bladder that results in stasis of urine and provides a good media for bacterial growth. Vesicoureteral reflex does not cause discomfort or bladder spasms. (I, N, G)

The Client With Glomerulonephritis

33. 3. Oliguria (subnormal urine production) is another symptom of glomerulonephritis. Fever may have been present when the child contacted a strep throat but is usually not present now. Usually children with glomerulonephritis have not had a sore throat and have been mildly ill with upper respiratory symptoms. (A, C, G)

34. 4. People who are allergic to penicillin are also allergic to amoxicillin. The nurse cannot independently change a medication order, although erythromycin is the drug of choice for clients who are allergic to penicillin. (I, T, S)

35. 3. The most important nursing intervention is daily weight. This is the best indication of fluid status. The other interventions are also important. (A, C, H)

36. 3. To facilitate venous drainage of an extremity, it is important to wrap elastic bandages distally to proximally. Edema in the toes, which were not involved in the injury, would indicate poor venous return. The bandage should be wrapped firmly to provide support. A figure-eight application in the ankle area helps keep the bandage in place and is the correct configuration over a flexor joint. (A, N, S)

37. 2. Nocturnal emissions, or wet dreams, occur in about 85% of men. They can occur at any age but usually begin in the teen years. A relatively common misconception is that wet dreams are a sign of sexual disorder or homosexuality. (A, C, G)

38. 3. Half-strength hydrogen peroxide is most often recommended for cleansing the mouth and lips of crusted mucus, or sordes. The foaming action that results when the hydrogen peroxide releases oxygen and the moisture of the solution act to remove the debris. Hydrogen peroxide should not be used for regular and frequent mouth cleansing because repeated exposure to hydrogen peroxide may damage tooth enamel. (I, T, S)

39. 2. Ice chips help moisten the mouth and lips while keeping fluid intake low. Sweet beverages like diet

cola and lemonade tend to increase thirst. Tap water effectively relieves thirst but does not help keep fluid intake low. (I, T, S)

40. 4. During periods of oliguria, foods high in potassium, such as bananas and citrus fruits, are restricted. Strawberries and apples are lower in potassium. High-carbohydrate foods are encouraged to provide calories. (P, N, S)

41. 1. Generally, teenagers enjoy activities with their peers in preference to socializing with their parents or younger people. Clannish peer relationships are common and normal during adolescence. They work to help the teenager develop self-identity. (P, N, L)

42. 2. The teenager who handles and solves daily problems with relative ease and seems to have direction is demonstrating a good sense of self-identity. According to psychologist Erik Erikson, an important aspect of adolescent psychosocial development is developing self-identity. When this does not happen, the adolescent suffers from identity diffusion. An adolescent's success in developing self-identity is not related to intelligence. Although a poor relationship with parents may have an effect on a teenager, the establishment of self-identity is not necessarily affected by such a relationship. The client described here is not demonstrating independence from his family by appearing to develop his self-identity, although teenagers do normally work toward independence from the family. (A, N, L)

43. 3. The elevated blood pressure may indicate hypertension, which is a serious complication of acute glomerulonephritis. The serum sodium level is in the normal range; the temperature is a little elevated. The weight loss is probably from loss of fluid that the client had been retaining. (D, N, L)

44. 1. Neurologic status should be assessed and seizure precautions instituted because hypertensive encephalopathy is a major potential complication of the acute phase of glomerulonephritis. Hypertensive encephalopathy can result in transient loss of vision, hemiparesis, disorientation, and grand mal seizures. A low-sodium diet is encouraged but is not important initially. Bed rest is advocated during the acute phase of glomerulonephritis. Fluids are restricted in clients with oliguria or anuria. (I, N, G)

45. 4. The child should be weighed every day. Urine specific gravity is a measure of hydration status and does not need to be measured daily. Glomerulonephritis causes hematuria and proteinuria. Vital signs need to be assessed more frequently than every 8 hours in a child with an elevated blood pressure. (P, N, G)

46. 3. Infections of all types should be avoided. No diet or fluid restrictions are imposed during convalescence from glomerulonephritis. There is no need for the parents to assess pulse and respiratory rates. (P, N, H)

47. 1. A client with chronic glomerulonephritis is in a permanent salt-losing state, so the sodium level would be on the low end of normal range. Blood urea nitrogen and potassium are usually elevated, and a chronic state of acidosis is usually present. (D, N, G)

48. 4. This adolescent can be expected to be concerned about the loss of kidney function and the result of this loss on his lifestyle. The other diagnoses are unrelated to this disease process. (D, N, L)

The Client With Nephrotic Syndrome

49. 1. In nephrotic syndrome, blood pressure is characteristically normal or slightly low. The other vital signs are likely to be normal unless edema causes respiratory distress and the respirations increase and become labored. The blood pressure reading here is within the normal range for a 3-year-old child. Temperature is elevated, and pulse and respiratory rates are low for a 3-year-old. (D, N, G)

50. 2. Nephrotic syndrome involves altered glomerular permeability, which results in the excretion of large amounts of protein in the urine. Aldosterone secretion is increased, resulting in sodium and water reabsorption. Red blood cells are not lost in the urine. (A, N, G)

51. 2. In nephrotic syndrome, the cause of respiratory distress results from fluid accumulation in the abdominal cavity, which pushes the diaphragm up so that it interferes with adequate chest expansion. There is usually a low vascular fluid volume in nephrotic syndrome, so there is no congestive heart failure or fluid accumulation in the pulmonary vascular bed. (D, N, G)

52. 3. A 3-year-old child will respond best to distraction during the procedure. A 3-year-old is too young for verbal teaching alone. Preparation immediately before the procedure is the preferred method for toddlers. (I, T, L)

53. 2. Diet therapy for a child with nephrotic syndrome includes increasing protein intake to replace albumin lost in the urine. During periods of edema, the child's appetite is poor, so it is important for the nurse to learn about the child's food likes and dislikes. (D, N, G)

54. 1. Sodium intake is restricted in nephrotic syndrome. Potato chips and bologna are high in sodium. Fluid intake is not restricted; however, 4 liters is an excessive amount for a 3-year-old child. Surgical intervention and antibiotic therapy are not part of the treatment plan for nephrotic syndrome. (E, N, G)

55. 4. Daily weight measurements help determine fluid losses and gains. Bed rest and limiting visitors would help ensure that the client gets adequate rest. Urine is tested for protein, not specific gravity, in nephrotic syndrome. (P, N, G)

56. 2. Elevating the head of the bed allows gravity to increase the downward flow of fluids in the body and away from the face. Such measures as limiting television, instilling eye drops, and applying cool compresses may be comforting but will not decrease edema. (I, N, G)

57. 1. Decreased abdominal girth is a sign of reduced fluid in the third spaces and tissues. Although increased caloric intake may indicate decreased intestinal edema, it is not the most accurate indicator of fluid retention. Increased respiratory rate might be an indication of increasing ascites. Heart rate usually stays in the normal range. (E, N, G)

58. 4. Children with nephrotic syndrome who are sensitive to steroids or have frequent relapses are candidates for therapy with cyclophosphamide. Common side effects include decreased white blood cell count, increased susceptibility to infections, cystitis (from bladder irritation when the drug accumulates in the bladder before excretion) and possibly hair loss and sterility. Because a child with nephrotic syndrome is susceptible to infection, it is important to monitor the white blood cell count and take precautions if it is low. (A, N, S)

59. 4. Placing soft cloth between opposing skin surfaces absorbs moisture. Applying lotion or powder to edematous surfaces that touch increases moisture and can lead to maceration. The child with edema is usually maintained on bed rest. (I, T, S)

60. 2. There is little change within the first few days of starting prednisone. Within 7 to 21 days of starting prednisone, diuresis occurs as the urine protein excretion diminishes. (I, T, S)

61. 2. A child in remission from nephrotic syndrome should be protected from infection. Pain is not associated with this disorder. The physician should be notified if urine output decreases. There is no reason to administer acetaminophen daily. (P, T, G)

The Client With Acute or Chronic Renal Failure

62. 1. A client receiving peritoneal dialysis has few dietary restrictions, whereas a client receiving hemodialysis usually has fluid and food restrictions. During peritoneal dialysis, plasma proteins, amino acids, and polypeptides diffuse into the dialysate because of the permeability of the peritoneal membrane. Peritoneal dialysis removes fluid less rapidly than does hemodialysis. Infection is associated with both hemodialysis and peritoneal dialysis. The risk of peritonitis is the major disadvantage of peritoneal dialysis. (I, C, G)

63. 3. Until it heals, the catheter exit site is particularly vulnerable to invasion by pathogenic organisms. Therefore, the site must be monitored for signs of infection. Holding the catheter taut or pulling on it may cause irritation of the skin at the exit site, which could lead to infection. Site care may be done anytime, but the child may experience abdominal discomfort if the peritoneal space is dry during site care. An occlusive dressing is not needed because there is no danger of air being sucked in or out of the peritoneal space. Furthermore, the catheter used is designed with a cuff, so the skin grows around the catheter. (I, T, S)

64. 4. With minimal or absent kidney function, the serum phosphate level rises, and the ionized calcium level falls in response. This causes increased secretion of parathyroid hormone, which releases calcium from the bones. Renal failure results in decreased erythropoietin production, necessitating increased ascorbic acid intake. Magnesium is minimally affected. (P, N, G)

65. 4. Compliance with the medical regimen indicates a positive self-image. Social withdrawal from activities may indicate depression. Diffuse somatic complaints could indicate anxiety. (A, N, L)

66. 2. It may be difficult to provide the calories needed to reduce tissue catabolism, metabolic acidosis, and uremia. If the child is able to tolerate oral foods, concentrated food sources high in carbohydrate and fat but low in protein, potassium, and sodium may be provided. (P, N, G)

67. 3. Body image is an important concern to an adolescent, and the client needs opportunities to discuss feelings about altered body image. Other developmental needs of adolescents are increasing appropriate independence and maintaining social activities. The client may choose to confide in friends for both psychological health and physical safety. (P, N, L)

68. 4. Tissue swelling, pain, redness, and exudate indicate infection. Granulation tissue indicates healing around the exit site. Dialysate leakage is associated with improper catheter function, incomplete healing at the insertion site, or excessive instillation of dialysate. Increased time for drainage may indicate that the tube is kinked. (A, T, G)

69. 1. With peritonitis, large numbers of bacteria, white blood cells, and fibrin cause the dialysate to appear cloudy. Weight gain indicates fluid excess rather than infection. Shortness of breath is associated with fluid excess. Abdominal distention is unrelated to peritonitis. (E, N, S)

70. 4. The nurse notifies the physician so that a change in medical management can be made. A sample of the peritoneal fluid is sent for culture and sensitivity; the results guide the choice of an effective antibiotic agent. The blood pressure should remain normal with peritonitis. Peritonitis can cause an ileus; therefore, fluid intake is not increased. Peritoneal leak can develop owing to sustained hydraulic pressure within the peritoneum. (I, N, S)

71. 4. With edema, pallor can occur owing to hemodilution. Other indications of edema include elevated blood pressure, pulmonary rales, and decreased dialysate outflow. (A, N, G)

72. 2. Anticipatory Grieving refers to the expectation of the loss of a significant relationship. Symptoms of this state include sleeplessness and altered nutritional patterns. Altered Parenting involves a parent's inability to nurture. Ineffective Family Coping refers to the family having difficulty adjusting to the diagnosis and its implications. Social Isolation is marked by interpersonal interaction below the level desired or required for personal integrity. This mother is confiding in the nurse and in her husband. (D, N, L)

73. 2. Normal inflow and drain times are about 10 minutes. (A, T, S)

74. 1. The accumulation of hard stool in the bowel can cause the distended intestine to block the holes of the catheter. Consequently, the dialysate cannot flow freely through the catheter. Decreasing the dialysate infusion and adjusting the dialysis schedule may make the dialysis less effective. Altering fluid, electrolyte, and waste product removal can cause fluid and electrolyte imbalance and elevated blood urea nitrogen and creatinine levels. Shoulder pain can be caused by air in the peritoneal space and diaphragmatic irritation. (P, N, S)

75. 4. Regulation of the diet is the most effective means, besides dialysis, for reducing renal excretion. Dietary phosphorus is restricted, which reduces the protein load on the kidneys. Clients are also given substances to bind phosphorus in the intestines to prevent absorption. Limited protein in the diet should include foods high in essential amino acids. Foods high in fat and carbohydrate are used to increase caloric intake. (E, N, G)

76. 3. Wilms' tumor, or nephroblastoma, is the most common intraabdominal tumor of childhood and the most common type of renal cancer. It is highly malignant. Anemia, which is secondary to hemorrhage within the tumor, causes pallor, anorexia, and lethargy. The most common presenting sign is an abdominal mass. Other signs and symptoms are the result of compression from the tumor mass, metabolic alterations secondary to the tumor, or metastasis. Hypertension occurs occasionally, probably owing to excessive excretion of renin by the tumor. Other common effects of malignancy include weight loss and fever. Petechiae and proteinemia are not associated with Wilms' tumor. (A, N, G)

77. 2. The abdomen of the child with Wilms' tumor should not be palpated because of the danger of disseminating tumor cells. Techniques such as measuring the occipitofrontal circumference, upright positioning, and measuring chest circumference are not necessarily contraindicated; however, the child with Wilms' tumor should always be handled gently and carefully. (A, N, S)

78. 3. Computed tomography scan of the abdomen is done after diagnosis is confirmed to determine the tumor's size and position and its relation to the involved and uninvolved kidney. Upper and lower gastrointestinal series and bone scan are not indicated. (P, N, G)

79. 4. Teaching the parents about staging of Wilms' tumor is done at the time of diagnosis. Preoperative explanations should be kept simple and focus on what the child will experience. Vital signs, including blood pressure, must be monitored frequently because hypertension from excess renin production is possible. Careful bathing and handling are essential to prevent trauma to the tumor. As with all diagnoses of cancer, Wilms' tumor is a shock to the family. The parents may feel guilty for not finding the mass sooner, and with the swiftness of the diagnosis, will need emotional support. Allowing the child play time is important in his adjustment to the hospital and his cancer. (P, N, G)

80. 1. A stage II tumor extends beyond the kidney but is completely resected. The tumor staging is verified during surgery to maximize treatment protocols. The following criteria for staging are commonly used: *stage I:* tumor is limited to the kidney and completely resected; *stage II:* tumor extends beyond the kidney but is completely resected; *stage III:* residual nonhematogenous tumor is confined to the abdomen; *stage IV:* hematogenous metastasis oc-

curs, with deposits beyond stage III (lung, bone and brain, liver); *stage V:* bilateral renal involvement is present at diagnosis. (E, C, G)

81. 3. The child who has undergone abdominal surgery is usually placed in a semi-Fowler's position to facilitate draining of abdominal contents and to promote pulmonary expansion. The Sim's position is likely to be uncomfortable because of the large transabdominal incision. The supine position, without the head elevated, puts the child at increased risk for aspiration. The modified Trendelenburg position is used for clients in shock. (I, T, S)

82. 4. The optimum treatment protocol for Wilms' tumor at stage II is abdominal irradiation and chemotherapy. Postoperative radiotherapy is indicated for all children with Wilms' tumor except those with stage I disease and favorable histology. Chemotherapy is indicated for all stages. (P, C, G)

83. 1. Children who have undergone abdominal surgery are at risk for intestinal obstruction from adynamic ileus. Indications of intestinal obstruction include abdominal distention, decreased or absent bowel sounds, and vomiting. Later signs of intestinal obstruction include tachycardia, fever, hypotension, shock, and decreased urinary output. (A, T, G)

84. 1. Hair loss, or alopecia, does not occur until 2 weeks after the initial chemotherapy treatment. Chemotherapy for Wilms' tumor is begun immediately after surgery. (E, C, G)

85. 1. Dactinomycin and vincristine both cause nausea and vomiting. Oral fluids are encouraged, and antiemetics are given to prevent dehydration. Avoiding sun exposure is not necessary. Drowsiness and monitoring of the heart rate are not associated with either or these drugs. (P, N, S)

86. 3. Because the child only has one kidney, measures should be recommended to prevent urinary tract infection and injury to the remaining kidney. Severe pain and dependent edema are not associated with postoperative Wilms' tumor clients. Dietary sodium is not restricted because function in the remaining kidney is not impaired. (P, N, G)

NURSING CARE OF CHILDREN

TEST 6: The Child With Health Problems of the Urinary System

Directions: Use this answer grid to determine areas of strength or need for further study.

NURSING PROCESS	COGNITIVE LEVEL	CLIENT NEEDS
A = Assessment	K = Knowledge	S = Safe, effective care environment
D = Analysis, nursing diagnosis	C = Comprehension	G = Physiologic integrity
P = Planning	T = Application	L = Psychosocial integrity
I = Implementation	N = Analysis	H = Health promotion and maintenance
E = Evaluation		

Question #	Answer #	A	D	P	I	E	K	C	T	N	S	G	L	H
1	4				I			C				G		
2	3	A							T			G		
3	2	A							T				L	
4	3	A								N		G		
5	1			P					T			G		
6	2			P						N			L	
7	1			P						N		G		
8	2				I				T			G		
9	3			P					T					H
10	3		D				K					G		
11	3	A								N		G		
12	3					E				N		G		
13	4			P						N		G		
14	3				I					N		G		
15	2				I			C				G		
16	4	A						C				G		
17	2			P						N		G		
18	2				I					N		G		
19	2				I					N		G		
20	2					E				N		G		
21	3				I			C				G		
22	3				I					N			L	
23	4				I					N	S			
24	2		D							N	S			
25	3	A								N		G		

ANSWER GRID: 1

NURSING PROCESS

A = Assessment
D = Analysis, nursing diagnosis
P = Planning
I = Implementation
E = Evaluation

COGNITIVE LEVEL

K = Knowledge
C = Comprehension
T = Application
N = Analysis

CLIENT NEEDS

S = Safe, effective care environment
G = Physiologic integrity
L = Psychosocial integrity
H = Health promotion and maintenance

Question #	Answer #	Nursing Process					Cognitive Level				Client Needs			
		A	D	P	I	E	K	C	T	N	S	G	L	H
26	1	A								N		G		
27	3	A					K					G		
28	3	A						C				G		
29	2				I					N				H
30	2				I					N	S			
31	2				I					N				H
32	1				I					N		G		
33	3	A						C				G		
34	4				I				T		S			
35	3	A						C						H
36	3	A								N	S			
37	2	A						C				G		
38	3				I				T		S			
39	2				I				T		S			
40	4			P						N	S			
41	1			P						N			L	
42	2	A								N			L	
43	3		D							N			L	
44	1				I					N		G		
45	4			P						N		G		
46	3			P						N				H
47	1		D							N		G		
48	4		D							N			L	
49	1		D							N		G		
50	2	A								N		G		
51	2		D							N		G		
52	3				I				T				L	
53	2		D							N		G		
54	1					E				N		G		
55	4			P						N		G		

ANSWER GRID: 2

NURSING PROCESS

A = Assessment
D = Analysis, nursing diagnosis
P = Planning
I = Implementation
E = Evaluation

COGNITIVE LEVEL

K = Knowledge
C = Comprehension
T = Application
N = Analysis

CLIENT NEEDS

S = Safe, effective care environment
G = Physiologic integrity
L = Psychosocial integrity
H = Health promotion and maintenance

Question #	Answer #	A	D	P	I	E	K	C	T	N	S	G	L	H
56	2				I					N		G		
57	1					E				N		G		
58	4	A								N	S			
59	4				I				T		S			
60	2				I				T		S			
61	2			P					T			G		
62	1				I			C				G		
63	3				I				T		S			
64	4			P						N		G		
65	4	A								N			L	
66	2			P						N		G		
67	3			P						N			L	
68	4	A							T			G		
69	1					E				N	S			
70	4				I					N	S			
71	4	A								N		G		
72	2		D							N			L	
73	2	A							T		S			
74	1			P						N	S			
75	4					E				N		G		
76	3	A								N		G		
77	2	A								N	S			
78	3			P						N		G		
79	4			P						N		G		
80	1					E		C				G		
81	3				I				T		S			
82	4			P				C				G		
83	1	A							T			G		
84	1					E		C				G		
85	1			P						N	S			

NURSING PROCESS

A = Assessment
D = Analysis, nursing diagnosis
P = Planning
I = Implementation
E = Evaluation

COGNITIVE LEVEL

K = Knowledge
C = Comprehension
T = Application
N = Analysis

CLIENT NEEDS

S = Safe, effective care environment
G = Physiologic integrity
L = Psychosocial integrity
H = Health promotion and maintenance

Question #	Answer #	Nursing Process					Cognitive Level				Client Needs			
		A	D	P	I	E	K	C	T	N	S	G	L	H
86	3			P						N		G		
Number Correct														
Number Possible	86	23	9	21	25	8	2	12	17	55	19	51	11	5
Percentage Correct														

Score Calculation: To determine your **Percentage Correct,** divide the **Number Correct** by the **Number Possible.**

ANSWER GRID: 4

The Child With Neurologic Health Problems

- **The Client With Myelomeningocele**
- **The Client With Hydrocephalus**
- **The Client With a Seizure Disorder**
- **The Client With Meningitis**
- **The Client With Reye's Syndrome**
- **The Client With Near Drowning**
- **The Client With Infectious Polyneuritis (Guillain-Barré Syndrome)**
- **The Client With a Head Injury**
- **The Client With a Brain Tumor**
- **The Client With a Spinal Cord Injury**
- **Correct Answers and Rationale**

Select the one best answer, and indicate your choice by filling in the circle in front of the option.

The Client With Myelomeningocele

A male neonate is admitted to the neonatal unit after delivery and placed in an isolation incubator. He has a 3-cm by 5-cm sac in the lumbar region of his back. The diagnosis is myelomeningocele.

1. When assessing this neonate, the nurse would expect to see
- ○ 1. a cyst containing serosanguineous fluid and fatty tissue located on the spinal column.
- ○ 2. a skin-covered sac containing bits of hair located on the low lumbar or sacral area of the spine.
- ○ 3. a soft sac containing fluid and meninges located on the spine.
- ○ 4. a soft sac containing spinal fluid, meninges, spinal cord, or nerve roots protruding through a bony defect in the spine.

2. Given the clinical manifestations associated with upper lumbar myelomeningocele, which of the following findings would the nurse anticipate when assessing this neonate?

- ○ 1. Minimal movement of the lower extremities and dribbling of urine.
- ○ 2. Minimal movement of the lower extremities and dribbling of urine and feces.
- ○ 3. Paralysis of the lower extremities and rectal prolapse.
- ○ 4. Paralysis of the upper and lower extremities and neurogenic bladder.

3. The family has been informed of the neonate's diagnosis of myelomeningocele. The nurse is planning to have the parents see the neonate as soon as possible. During the parents' first visit, the nurse would plan *initially* to
- ○ 1. emphasize the neonate's normal and positive features.
- ○ 2. encourage the parents to discuss their fears and concerns.
- ○ 3. reinforce the doctor's explanation of the defect.
- ○ 4. have the parents feed the neonate.

4. While discussing a plan of care for the neonate, the mother asks if her baby will be at risk for any other defects. The nurse's answer would be based on the fact the myelomeningocele is frequently associated with

  ○ 1. an abnormal increase in cerebrospinal fluid within the cranial cavity.
  ○ 2. an abnormally small head.
  ○ 3. congenital absence of the cranial vault.
  ○ 4. overriding of the cranial sutures.

5. During the planning session, the parents also ask about their child's future mental ability. The nurse's best response would be

  ○ 1. "About one third are mentally retarded, but it's too early to tell about your child."
  ○ 2. "About two thirds are significantly mentally retarded, and you will know soon if your child is retarded."
  ○ 3. "Your child will probably be of normal intelligence because he is so now."
  ○ 4. "You'll need to talk with the doctor about that later."

6. The neonate is experiencing urine retention with overflow incontinence. The nurse should *first*

  ○ 1. apply gentle pressure to the suprapubic area.
  ○ 2. initiate an intermittent clean catheterization program.
  ○ 3. insert an indwelling urinary catheter.
  ○ 4. collect a urine specimen.

7. The nurse places the infant in an isolation incubator shortly after birth. The nurse judges that this intervention is successful when the neonate's

  ○ 1. arterial PO_2 remains between 94 and 100.
  ○ 2. axillary temperature remains between 97° and 98°F.
  ○ 3. bilirubin level remains stable.
  ○ 4. weight increases by about 1 ounce per day.

8. When planning the nursing care for the neonate before surgical repair of the defect, the nurse should include

  ○ 1. applying thin layers of tincture of benzoin around the defect.
  ○ 2. covering the defect with a dry, nonadherent dressing.
  ○ 3. covering the defect with moist, sterile saline dressings.
  ○ 4. leaving the defect exposed to air.

9. In which of the following positions would the nurse place the neonate with myelomeningocele in the isolation incubator?

  ○ 1. Supine with the hips at 90-degree flexion.
  ○ 2. Supine in the Trendelenburg position with the knees flexed.
  ○ 3. Prone with optimal positioning of the legs.
  ○ 4. Prone with chest and abdomen elevated.

10. The nursing care plan for postsurgical repair should include which of the following nursing diagnoses?

  ○ 1. High Risk for Infection.

  ○ 2. Ineffective Airway Clearance.
  ○ 3. Altered Nutrition: More Than Body Requirements.
  ○ 4. Altered Health Maintenance.

11. To prevent musculoskeletal deformity, the postoperative nursing care plan for a child with myelomeningocele should include maintaining the

  ○ 1. feet in a flexed position.
  ○ 2. hips in an abducted position.
  ○ 3. knees in neutral position.
  ○ 4. legs in the adducted position.

12. During postoperative assessment of the neonate, the nurse would look for which initial signs of hydrocephalus?

  ○ 1. Seizures and vomiting.
  ○ 2. Frontal bossing and sunset eyes.
  ○ 3. Increased head circumference and bulging fontanel.
  ○ 4. Irritability and shrill cry.

13. As the nurse prepares the family for the infant's discharge, which of the following would the nurse judge to be the *most* important?

  ○ 1. Providing a list of available hospital services.
  ○ 2. Scheduling daily home health care.
  ○ 3. Referral to chaplaincy for psychological support.
  ○ 4. Parent's knowledge of daily care of the infant.

14. Which of the following statements by the mother would indicate that the parents understand the nurse's teaching at the time of discharge? "We will

  ○ 1. apply a heating pad to his lower back."
  ○ 2. keep him away from other infants."
  ○ 3. notify the doctor if his urine has a bad smell."
  ○ 4. prevent him from rolling over."

The Client With Hydrocephalus

A parent brings a 6-week-old male infant to the well-baby clinic for a checkup.

15. The nurse weighs the infant and measures his length, weight, and head circumference. The infant's weight and length are in the 50th percentile for his age; his head circumference is at the 95th percentile. The nurse should *first*

  ○ 1. assess motor and sensory function of the legs.
  ○ 2. examine the fontanel and sutures.
  ○ 3. advise the mother to bring him back in 1 month for follow-up.
  ○ 4. obtain a permit for transillumination.

16. The infant is admitted to the hospital and, following diagnostic evaluation, is scheduled to have a ventriculoperitoneal shunt implanted. Preoperatively, the

infant is irritable and lethargic and difficult to feed. To maintain his nutritional status, the nurse would
- ○ 1. feed the infant just before doing any procedures.
- ○ 2. give the infant small, frequent feedings.
- ○ 3. feed the infant in a horizontal position.
- ○ 4. schedule the feedings for every 6 hours.

17. The mother asks the nurse what the long-term outcome will be for her child with hydrocephalus. The nurse judges that the mother understands the explanation when she states,
- ○ 1. "It's too early to predict how he will develop."
- ○ 2. "All children with hydrocephalus have serious problems later."
- ○ 3. "He will be mentally retarded for sure."
- ○ 4. "The doctor will be able to tell me in 3 months."

18. Surgery is to be performed, with a ventroperitoneal shunt inserted on the right side. Immediately after surgery, the nurse would plan to position the infant
- ○ 1. on the right side, with the foot of the crib elevated.
- ○ 2. on the left side, with the head of the crib elevated.
- ○ 3. supine, with the head of the crib elevated.
- ○ 4. supine, with the head of the crib flat.

19. Postoperative nursing care of an infant with a ventriculoperitoneal shunt should also include
- ○ 1. administering narcotics for pain control.
- ○ 2. checking the urine for glucose and protein.
- ○ 3. monitoring for increased temperature.
- ○ 4. testing cerebrospinal fluid leakage for protein.

20. Which of the following nursing interventions is most important postoperatively in an infant with ventriculoperitoneal shunt placement?
- ○ 1. Monitoring intake and output.
- ○ 2. Beginning oral feedings.
- ○ 3. Allowing the infant to rest undisturbed.
- ○ 4. Providing age-appropriate diversional activities.

21. After surgery, the infant is to receive vancomycin prophylactically. The nurse should
- ○ 1. inject the medication into the gluteus maximus.
- ○ 2. monitor the child for arrhythmia.
- ○ 3. give the medication intravenously over 1 hour.
- ○ 4. check the infant's history for an allergy to penicillin.

22. While planning for the infant's discharge, the nurse teaches the parents the signs of an obstructed shunt. The nurse evaluates the teaching as successful when the parents identify which of the following as signaling a blocked shunt?
- ○ 1. Decreased urine output with stable intake.
- ○ 2. Cold, clammy skin with pale lips.
- ○ 3. Elevated temperature and reddened areas around the incision site.
- ○ 4. Irritability and feeding difficulty.

23. The mother asks how much acetaminophen (Tylenol) to give the infant when they are at home. The child has an order for 40 mg every 4 hours for pain. The mother indicates that she will use the infant drops, which comes in a concentration of 80 mg/0.8 mL. The nurse would tell her to give the infant
- ○ 1. one dropperful.
- ○ 2. one half of a dropperful.
- ○ 3. 0.78 mL, using a 1-mL syringe.
- ○ 4. 1.5 mL, using a 3-mL syringe.

The Client With a Seizure Disorder

A girl in second grade experiences a generalized tonic-clonic seizure in the classroom. She has no history of seizure disorders nor of any other chronic health problem.

24. The nurse judges an educational program for teaching about seizures to be effective on learning that the teacher *first*
- ○ 1. asked the other children what happened before the seizure.
- ○ 2. moved the child to the nurse's office.
- ○ 3. ensured the child's safety.
- ○ 4. placed a padded tongue blade between the child's teeth.

25. Immediately after the seizure, the nurse arrives and notices that the child has been incontinent of urine and is difficult to arouse. Based on this information, the nurse would
- ○ 1. ask the teacher if the child has had any urinary problems.
- ○ 2. awaken the child every 3 to 5 minutes to assess mentation.
- ○ 3. perform a complete neurologic check every 3 to 5 minutes.
- ○ 4. place the child in a side-lying position, stay with her, and allow her to sleep.

26. The child is hospitalized for a diagnostic workup. The physician orders valproic acid (Depakote). The nurse plans to teach the parents about the drug, stressing the need to
- ○ 1. pay careful attention to oral hygiene, especially in the gum area.
- ○ 2. discontinue the drug if the child becomes drowsy.
- ○ 3. increase the dose by 5 mg/day if breakthrough seizures occur.
- ○ 4. notify the physician if nausea and vomiting or tremors occur.

27. The nurse tells the mother that as long as the child is taking valproic acid, the child will have to have bloodwork routinely, which will consist of
- ○ 1. serum glutamic-oxaloacetic transaminase (SGOT), platelets, and fibrinogen level.

○ 2. complete blood count and alkaline phosphate level.

○ 3. electrolytes and alkaline phosphate level.

○ 4. cholesterol, lipids, and platelets.

28. The nurse teaches the parents about the side effects of valproic acid. Which of the following side effects would the parents report to their health care provider immediately?

○ 1. Weight gain of 2 pounds in 1 month.

○ 2. Vomiting and decreased appetite.

○ 3. Abdominal pain and jaundice.

○ 4. Fever and malaise.

29. When planning for teaching the child and family about pharmacologic treatment of seizures, the nurse should emphasize that the child

○ 1. should take less medication when side effects occur.

○ 2. should never stop taking the medication abruptly.

○ 3. will need less medication as she grows older.

○ 4. will need to take the medication for the rest of her life.

30. Which of the following statements made by the mother would indicate that she understands her child's medication therapy for seizures? "I should

○ 1. call to refill the prescriptions as soon as the bottles are empty."

○ 2. make sure she takes her medication every other day."

○ 3. not give her any other medications without asking the doctor."

○ 4. not worry about giving her the medication when vomiting."

31. While discussing plans for the child's discharge, the nurse teaches the parents about what actions to take when the child has a seizure. The nurse would judge the teaching as effective when the father states, "We'll

○ 1. restrain her arms and legs so she won't get hurt."

○ 2. tilt her neck forward so that her tongue won't fall back into her throat."

○ 3. try to get her to swallow an extra dose of Depekote."

○ 4. stay with her during the seizure and after it's over."

32. The family and nurse discuss the child's return to school. Based on the nursing goal of promoting the child's growth and development, the nurse would plan to advise the parents that a child with a seizure disorder

○ 1. will need to have her activities limited and will not be able to do as others in her class.

○ 2. has a learning disability and needs tutoring to help her reach her grade level.

○ 3. most frequently has normal intelligence and can attend regular school.

○ 4. suffers from social stigma and should not attend public school.

33. Two years after treatment is started, the child is still having occasional generalized seizures. Her parents want to send her to summer camp and contact the nurse for advice on planning for the camping experience. Which of the following activities would the nurse and family decide the child should avoid?

○ 1. Rock climbing.

○ 2. Hiking.

○ 3. Horseback riding.

○ 4. Tennis.

A toddler experiences a simple generalized seizure that is tentatively diagnosed as a febrile seizure.

34. Which of the following statements from the nursing history would support the medical diagnosis of febrile seizure?

○ 1. The child has had a low-grade fever for several weeks.

○ 2. The family history is negative for convulsions.

○ 3. The seizure resulted in respiratory arrest.

○ 4. The seizure occurred when the child had a respiratory infection.

35. The child is to be sent home on no medication even though he has been receiving phenobarbital while hospitalized. The grandmother questions the mother about this situation while the nurse is present. The nurse would judge that the mother understands some of the teaching about febrile seizures when the mother states, "Children who have a seizure with fever

○ 1. do not usually need long-term seizure medication."

○ 2. need anticonvulsants if they have upper respiratory infections or tonsillitis."

○ 3. need anticonvulsants if the seizure lasted for 30 minutes or longer."

○ 4. need anticonvulsants if the seizure lasted less than 15 minutes."

36. The nurse teaches the parents about methods to lower temperature other than medication. The nurse judges that the teaching was successful when the father states,

○ 1. "We'll add extra blankets if he complains of being cold."

○ 2. "We'll wrap him in a blanket if he starts shivering."

○ 3. "We'll make the bath water cold enough to make him shiver."

○ 4. "We'll use a solution of one half alcohol and water when sponging him."

37. An adolescent girl with a seizure disorder that is controlled with phenytoin and carbamazepine (Tegretol) asks the nurse about someday getting married and having children. After discussing this issue with the client, the nurse judges that the teaching was effective when the client states

○ 1. "I probably shouldn't consider having children until my seizures are cured."

○ 2. "My children won't necessarily have an increased risk of seizure disorder."

○ 3. "When I decide to have children, I'll talk to the doctor about changing my medication."

○ 4. "Women who have seizure disorders commonly have a difficult time conceiving."

38. When administering phenytoin intravenously to a child with status epilepticus, the nurse would give the drug slowly because rapid infusion of intravenous phenytoin can result in

○ 1. increased liver enzyme levels.

○ 2. blood glucose level below 60 mg/dL.

○ 3. bradycardia.

○ 4. increased white blood cell count.

The Client With Meningitis

39. A 4-year-old girl is brought to the hospital by her parents. Her temperature is 39°C. The admitting orders read: Give ibuprofen for temperature 102.5°F or higher; sponge for temperature greater than 104.0°F; and obtain blood cultures for temperature 103°F or higher. Based on these orders, the nurse would

○ 1. do nothing; the temperature is below 102.5°F.

○ 2. give ibuprofen, obtain blood cultures, and sponge the child.

○ 3. give ibuprofen and obtain blood cultures.

○ 4. give ibuprofen.

40. The nurse weighs the child on admission. It is important that the weight is accurate because it will be used to

○ 1. calculate drug doses for the child.

○ 2. estimate the child's edema status.

○ 3. evaluate the child's nutritional status.

○ 4. determine the child's fluid status.

41. The physician performs a lumbar puncture, and the cerebrospinal fluid sample is sent to the laboratory for testing. The nurse should then

○ 1. assess the child for discomfort at the insertion site and administer narcotics as ordered.

○ 2. encourage the parents to hold the child.

○ 3. make sure the child lies flat for at least 8 hours.

○ 4. place a sandbag over the puncture site for 3 hours.

42. An intravenous line is inserted, and the child is to receive 500 mL of solution over 12 hours. The tubing delivers microdrips at 60 drops per milliliter. The nurse should time the drops to be

○ 1. 21 drops/minute.

○ 2. 42 drops/minute.

○ 3. 63 drops/minute.

○ 4. 84 drops/minute.

43. The child is restless and irritable during the acute stage of meningitis. The nurse should

○ 1. limit conversation with the child.

○ 2. keep extraneous noise to a minimum.

○ 3. avoid bathing.

○ 4. perform treatments quickly.

44. The nurse knows that it is important to assess the child with meningitis for signs of increasing intracranial pressure. Along with decreased level of consciousness, the nurse would be concerned by

○ 1. blood pressure of 122/74 mm Hg.

○ 2. pulse of 86 beats/minute.

○ 3. respiratory rate of 24 breaths/minute.

○ 4. temperature of 100.2°F.

45. The nurse would suspect that the child had developed disseminated intravascular coagulation based on which of the following signs?

○ 1. Hemorrhagic skin rash.

○ 2. Edema.

○ 3. Cyanosis.

○ 4. Dyspnea on exertion.

46. The child's cerebrospinal fluid analysis shows pneumococcal meningitis. Which of the following illnesses that can be identified in the child's nursing history would predispose her to this type of meningitis?

○ 1. Bladder infection.

○ 2. Middle ear infection.

○ 3. Fractured clavicle.

○ 4. Septic arthritis.

47. When discontinuing the child's intravenous therapy, the nurse allows her to apply a dressing to the area where the needle is removed. The nurse would base this action on the knowledge that a child this age has a need to

○ 1. trust those caring for her.

○ 2. find diversional activities.

○ 3. protect the image of an intact body.

○ 4. relieve the anxiety of separation from home.

48. The child recuperates, and discharge is planned. She becomes angry when the discharge is delayed. Which of the following play activities would be appropriate?

○ 1. Being read a story.
○ 2. Painting with water colors.
○ 3. Pounding a pegboard.
○ 4. Stacking blocks.

49. A small infant is admitted with a diagnosis of meningitis. While performing an assessment, the nurse notes that the infant is less responsive to stimuli and has bradycardia, slight hypertension, irregular respirations, and a temperature of 103.2 F. The infant's fontanel also seems more tense than at the last assessment. The nurse should first
○ 1. ask another nurse to verify the findings.
○ 2. notify the physician of the findings.
○ 3. raise the head of the bed.
○ 4. administer an antipyretic.

The Client With Reye's Syndrome

A school-aged child is admitted to the pediatric unit. Two days ago, the child developed severe and persistent vomiting and diarrhea and complained of increasing fatigue. Now she is combative. Her pulse and respiratory rates are elevated, and she has a fever.

50. The child's mother tells the nurse all the following facts during history taking. Which fact would the nurse associate with Reye's syndrome? The child
○ 1. was exposed to influenza 6 weeks ago.
○ 2. had an upper respiratory tract infection 1 week ago.
○ 3. had chickenpox 6 months ago.
○ 4. was exposed to streptococcal bacteria 2 weeks ago.

51. The best strategy to decrease the incidence of Reye's syndrome would be to teach parents to
○ 1. use acetaminophen when treating viral symptoms.
○ 2. delay immunizations for children with low-grade fever.
○ 3. keep children away from others who have Reye's syndrome.
○ 4. treat scrapes and bruises by cleansing carefully and applying antibiotic cream.

The Client With Near Drowning

A 15-month-old child is found floating in a neighbor's hot tub and has just been admitted to the pediatric intensive care unit.

52. The nurse caring for the toddler is most concerned about which of the following?

○ 1. Hypothermia.
○ 2. Hypoxia.
○ 3. Body heat loss.
○ 4. Cutaneous capillary paralysis.

53. The nurse would explain to the parents that
○ 1. aspiration occurs in most near drownings.
○ 2. aspiration is rarely a problem in near drownings.
○ 3. it is better to drown in salt water.
○ 4. their toddler did not struggle at all.

54. The nurse plans to assess for which of the following?
○ 1. Respiratory and metabolic acidosis.
○ 2. Respiratory acidosis and metabolic alkalosis.
○ 3. Metabolic acidosis and respiratory alkalosis.
○ 4. Respiratory and metabolic alkalosis.

55. In developing a nursing care plan, which of the following nursing diagnoses would be of *highest priority*?
○ 1. Activity Intolerance.
○ 2. Impaired Mobility.
○ 3. Aspiration.
○ 4. Altered Parenting.

56. The parents tell the nurse that they feel guilty because their child nearly drowned. Which of the following remarks by the nurse would be most appropriate?
○ 1. "I can understand why you feel guilty, but these things happen."
○ 2. "Tell me more about why you feel guilty."
○ 3. "You should not have taken your eyes off of your child."
○ 4. "You really shouldn't feel guilty; you're lucky because your child will be all right."

The Client With Infectious Polyneuritis (Guillain-Barré Syndrome)

A young school-aged child is admitted to the hospital complaining of pain and weakness in the feet and legs for several days. The pain and weakness are symmetric and appear to be progressing from distal to proximal.

57. During the first 2 days of hospitalization, the child develops motor paralysis of the legs. The nurse asks the child to squeeze the nurse's hand and to raise her arms and legs as high as possible off the bed. The purpose of these requests is to
○ 1. assess the child's ability to follow simple commands.
○ 2. evaluate the child's bilateral muscle strength.
○ 3. make a game of the range-of-motion exercises.
○ 4. provide the child with a diversional activity.

58. The nurse asks the child to cough and also assesses the child's speech for decreased volume and clarity. The nurse is assessing for

○ 1. inflammation of the larynx and epiglottis.
○ 2. increased intracranial pressure.
○ 3. involvement of facial and cranial nerves.
○ 4. regression to an earlier developmental phase.

59. The nurse notes that the child is unable to cough and has no gag reflex. In developing a nursing care plan for the child during the acute phase of Guillain-Barré syndrome, the *highest priority* nursing diagnosis would be
○ 1. Potential for Infection.
○ 2. Ineffective Breathing Pattern.
○ 3. Impaired Swallowing.
○ 4. Total Incontinence.

60. The child is transferred to the pediatric intensive care unit, intubated, and placed on mechanical ventilation and a cardiac monitor. The rationale for this level of cardiac assessment is that clients with Guillain-Barré syndrome can experience
○ 1. autonomic dysreflexia.
○ 2. brain stem edema.
○ 3. hyperkalemia.
○ 4. hypoglycemia.

61. While being mechanically ventilated, the child should be
○ 1. maintained in a supine position to prevent unnecessary nerve stimulation.
○ 2. moved to a bedside chair three times a day to prevent orthostatic hypotension.
○ 3. engaged in vigorous passive range-of-motion exercises to prevent loss of muscle function.
○ 4. turned slowly and gently from side to side to prevent respiratory complications.

62. The child is successfully weaned from the ventilator but still requires nasogastric tube feedings. The nurse judges that the child is ready for oral feedings when she
○ 1. can sit up in a chair without help.
○ 2. gags when the nasogastric tube is repositioned.
○ 3. tries to remove the nasogastric tube with her hands.
○ 4. tells her parents that she is hungry.

63. After several weeks, the child is transferred to a general pediatric floor. The parents and nurse would develop a discharge plan that focuses on
○ 1. formulating a rehabilitation plan that includes orthopedic care.
○ 2. finding a nursing home that will take children.
○ 3. limiting contact with peers until she has fully recovered.
○ 4. finding a school for handicapped children in the family's neighborhood.

64. The mother brings her daughter to the clinic for her first visit after being discharged. The nurse judges the mother is following the discharge plan when she states,

○ 1. "She and her sister argue all day."
○ 2. "I have to bribe her to get her to do her exercises."
○ 3. "I take her to the pool where she can exercise with other children."
○ 4. "She sleeps late most mornings and misses her therapy."

The Client With a Head Injury

A school-aged child was hit by a car while riding a bicycle. Unconscious at the scene of the accident, he was brought to the hospital emergency department.

65. On the child's arrival at the hospital, the nurse's *first priority* would be to
○ 1. assess his neurologic status.
○ 2. assess for extremity injuries.
○ 3. establish ventilation.
○ 4. establish intravenous access.

66. The nurse evaluates the child's neurologic status using the Glasgow coma scale. Part of the assessment includes eye opening to stimuli. Lack of response to which of the following stimuli would yield the lowest or least desirable score? Having
○ 1. an intravenous started.
○ 2. his leg moved.
○ 3. his mother stroke his face.
○ 4. the nurse speak to him.

67. The nurse plans to insert a nasogastric tube to
○ 1. administer medications.
○ 2. decompress the stomach.
○ 3. obtain gastric specimens for analysis.
○ 4. provide adequate nutrition.

68. If this child had suffered a basilar skull fracture, the nurse would have
○ 1. asked for the order to be changed to oral gastric tube.
○ 2. attempted to place the tube into the duodenum.
○ 3. tested the gastric aspirate for blood.
○ 4. used extra lubrication when inserting the nasogastric tube.

69. The child is to receive dexamethasone (Decadron) intravenously. The ordered dosage is 7.6 mg, and the drug concentration in the vial is 4 mg/mL. How much should the nurse administer?
○ 1. 0.05 mL.
○ 2. 0.72 mL.
○ 3. 1.9 mL.
○ 4. 3.8 mL.

70. The child's parents ask the nurse if the child is going to be all right. Which of the following responses by the nurse would be most appropriate?

○ 1. "Children usually don't do very well after head injuries like this."

○ 2. "Children usually recover rapidly from head injuries."

○ 3. "It's hard to tell this early, but we'll keep you informed of his progress."

○ 4. "That's something you'll have to talk to the doctor about."

71. The parents ask the nurse why the physician ordered mannitol to be given. The nurse should reply, "Mannitol will

○ 1. help hold fluid in the vascular bed, to prevent shock."

○ 2. help decrease fluid, to decrease swelling in the brain."

○ 3. increase caloric intake, to aid wound healing."

○ 4. fight off bacteria, to prevent infections."

72. The nurse would position the unconscious child

○ 1. prone with hips and knees slightly elevated.

○ 2. lying on his side, with the head of the bed elevated.

○ 3. lying on his back, in the Trendelenburg position.

○ 4. in a semi-Fowler's position, with his arms at his side.

73. The child is coming out of the coma and is restless, irritable, and confused about where he is. The nurse should

○ 1. apply a chest restraint.

○ 2. ask the parents to leave.

○ 3. encourage the parents to stay.

○ 4. restrain the lower extremities.

The Client With a Brain Tumor

A junior high school student has seen the school nurse frequently with complaints of vomiting, headache, and difficulty seeing.

74. The nurse would decide to talk with the child's parents concerning her behavior because these symptoms are typical of

○ 1. acute encephalopathy with sinus inflammation.

○ 2. an abnormal involuntary neuromuscular activity.

○ 3. a psychological aversion to school.

○ 4. a space-occupying lesion in the cranial vault.

75. The child is later admitted to the hospital with the diagnosis of infratentorial brain tumor. During the child's admission to the pediatric unit, the nurse would plan to

○ 1. alleviate the child's anxiety.

○ 2. implement seizure precautions.

○ 3. introduce the child to other clients the same age.

○ 4. prepare the child and parents for diagnostic procedures.

76. A diagnosis of probable cerebellar astrocytoma is made, and surgical removal is scheduled. Preoperatively, the nurse should plan to tell the child and her parents about the

○ 1. child's long-term prognosis

○ 2. child's postoperative appearance.

○ 3. long-term effects of radiation therapy.

○ 4. side effects of the planned chemotherapy.

77. An infratentorial craniotomy is performed, and the diagnosis of cerebellar astrocytoma, stage I, is confirmed. The parents want to know what "stage I" means. The nurse should explain that stage I describes a tumor that

○ 1. has grown rapidly.

○ 2. has metastasized.

○ 3. is localized.

○ 4. is undifferentiated.

78. After the child is admitted to the intensive care unit, the nurse's first action would be to ensure adequate

○ 1. cardiorespiratory function.

○ 2. fluid balance.

○ 3. pain control.

○ 4. infection protection.

79. The nurse positions the child postoperatively so as to prevent undue strain on the sutures. Which position would be best for the child?

○ 1. Prone.

○ 2. Reverse Trendelenburg.

○ 3. Side-lying.

○ 4. Trendelenburg.

80. The intubated child shows signs of decreased level of consciousness, and the physician orders manual hyperventilation to keep the PCO_2 between 25 and 29 mm Hg and the PaO_2 between 80 and 100 mm Hg. The nurse would carry out this order to

○ 1. decrease intracranial pressure.

○ 2. ensure a patent airway.

○ 3. lower the arousal level.

○ 4. produce hypoxia.

81. The nurse notes clear drainage on the child's dressing and on the linen under her head. The nurse would first

○ 1. reinforce the dressing.

○ 2. elevate the head of the bed.

○ 3. test the fluid for glucose.

○ 4. test the fluid for protein.

82. The child does well after infratentorial tumor removal and is transferred back to the pediatric unit. Although she had been told about having her head shaved for surgery, she is very upset. After exploring her feelings, the nurse should

○ 1. ask her if she'd like to wear a hat.

○ 2. assure her that her hair will grow back.

○ 3. explain to her parents that her reaction is normal.

○ 4. suggest that the parents buy her a wig as a surprise.

83. Which of the following statements made by the child's mother would warrant further exploration by the nurse?

○ 1. "After this, I'll never let her out of my sight again."

○ 2. "I hope that she'll be able to go back to school soon."

○ 3. "I wonder how long it will be before she can ride her bike."

○ 4. "Her best friend is anxious to see her, I hope she won't be upset."

The Client With a Spinal Cord Injury

An adolescent male was involved in a motorcycle accident and thrown about 40 feet from his motorcycle. A nurse arriving at the scene of the accident finds that he is alert.

84. The adolescent is unable to move his legs. While waiting for the emergency medical service to arrive, the nurse should

○ 1. flex his knees to relieve stress on his back.

○ 2. leave him as is and stay close by.

○ 3. remove his helmet as soon as possible.

○ 4. assess him for abdominal trauma.

85. The adolescent arrives at the emergency department with a diagnosis of suspected thoracic spinal cord injury. The nurse's *first priority* would be to

○ 1. maintain cardiorespiratory function.

○ 2. provide nutritional support by offering him a snack.

○ 3. prevent fluid and electrolyte imbalance.

○ 4. provide emotional support.

86. In the emergency department, the adolescent remains conscious and is agitated and anxious. The nurse observes that his pulse and respirations are increasing and that his blood pressure is decreasing. The nurse suspects that the adolescent is developing

○ 1. autonomic dysreflexia.

○ 2. increased intracranial pressure.

○ 3. metabolic alkalosis.

○ 4. spinal shock.

87. A diagnosis of a T3 spinal cord injury is made. After insertion of an intravenous line, a nasogastric tube, and a Foley catheter, the adolescent is admitted to the intensive care unit. On noting that his feet and legs are cool to the touch, the nurse should

○ 1. cover his legs with blankets.

○ 2. report the change to the physician immediately.

○ 3. reposition his legs.

○ 4. lay him flat to aid circulation.

88. During routine assessment, the nurse auscultates the adolescent's abdomen. The nurse explains to the parents that this is necessary because clients with spinal cord injury often develop

○ 1. abdominal cramping.

○ 2. hyperactive bowel sounds.

○ 3. paralytic ileus.

○ 4. profuse diarrhea.

89. After observing which of the following findings would the nurse decide that spinal shock was resolving?

○ 1. Atonic urinary bladder.

○ 2. Flaccid paralysis.

○ 3. Hyperactive reflexes.

○ 4. Widened pulse pressure.

90. The adolescent is moved to the rehabilitation unit. The nurse notes that he tends to refuse to cooperate in care and to be hostile. The nurse recognizes this behavior as a

○ 1. stage of grief reaction.

○ 2. phase of adolescent rebellion.

○ 3. reaction to sensory overload.

○ 4. response to too much attention.

91. Adjustment to paraplegia is especially difficult for an adolescent. The nurse would try to help the adolescent adjust to the situation by fostering

○ 1. ego integrity.

○ 2. autonomy.

○ 3. self-definition.

○ 4. industriousness.

92. Three months after the adolescent's injury, he complains of a pounding headache, and the nurse notes that his arms and face are flushed and he is diaphoretic. The nurse should

○ 1. check the patency of the Foley catheter.

○ 2. lower his head.

○ 3. lay him flat.

○ 4. prepare to administer epinephrine.

93. The adolescent is to be discharged to his parent's home and will be living with them. The nurse and family should formulate a short-term goal of

○ 1. being able to leave the house.

○ 2. being able to maneuver independently inside the house.

○ 3. having the activities of daily living met by a health aid.

○ 4. meeting all self-care needs independently.

CORRECT ANSWERS AND RATIONALE

The letters in parentheses following the rationale identify the step of the nursing process (A, D, P, I, E), cognitive level (K, C, T, N), and client needs (S, G, L, H). See the Answer Grid for the key.

The Client With Myelomeningocele

1. 4. A myelomeningocele has three components (bony defect, spinal fluid, and nerve tissue) and protrudes over the vertebrae, usually in the lower back. A meningocele is a soft sac containing only spinal fluid and meninges located anywhere on the spine. A pilonidal cyst is a skin-covered sac containing bits of hair located on the low lumbar or sacral area of the spine. A simple cyst contains serosanguinous fluid and fatty tissue located on any area of the spinal column. (A, C, G)

2. 2. Clinical manifestations of myelomeningocele are related to the anatomic level of the defect and the nerves involved. An upper lumbar (L1 to L2) myelomeningocele is associated with minimal movement of the lower extremities and dribbling of urine and feces. The upper lumbar area of the spinal cord controls leg flexion at the hip and adduction of the thigh. The sacral area of the spinal cord controls foot and toe movement as well as sphincter and perineal muscle contraction. (A, T, G)

3. 1. The parents should see the neonate as soon as possible, and the nurse should emphasize the neonate's normal and positive features. The longer the parents have to wait to see the neonate, the more anxiety they will feel. Because the parents are acutely aware of the deficit, emphasizing the neonate's normal and positive features would be more therapeutic than reinforcing the physician's explanation of the defect. The parents should spend time with or care for the neonate after birth because parent–infant contact is necessary for attachment. The parents cannot feed the neonate before the defect is repaired, but they can fondle and stroke him. Although the parents need to discuss their fears and concerns, the nurse should initially emphasize the neonate's normal and positive features. (P, N, L)

4. 1. Hydrocephalus, excessive cerebrospinal fluid in the cranial cavity, is the most common anomaly associated with myelomeningocele. Microencephaly (abnormally small head) and overriding of the sutures are commonly seen and not associated with myelomeningocele. Anencephaly (congenital absence of the cranial vault) is a different neural tube defect. (I, T, G)

5. 1. About one third of infants with myelomeningocele are mentally retarded, but it is particularly difficult to predict intellectual functioning in neonates. The parents are asking for an answer now and should not be told to talk with the physician later. (I, N, G)

6. 1. Overflow incontinence with constant dribbling is common in neonates with myelomeningocele. Applying gentle pressure to the suprapubic area helps empty the neonate's bladder, thus preventing urinary tract infections. Catheterization is done most frequently when a specimen is urgently needed or when the neonate is unable to void. Intermittent clean catheterization is an appropriate technique for management of urine retention in older infants. Collecting a urine specimen will not help with overflow incontinence. (I, T, S)

7. 2. The nurse places the neonate with myelomeningocele in an isolation incubator shortly after birth to help to maintain his temperature. Because the neonate cannot be bundled in blankets, it may be difficult to prevent cold stress. The isolation incubator can be maintained at higher than room temperature, helping maintain the temperature of a neonate who cannot be dressed or bundled. Another use would be for a neonate receiving phototherapy for hyperbilirubinemia. Although preventing cold stress may prevent problems with oxygenation and energy depletion, in this case the isolation incubator is used to keep the infant warm. (E, N, G)

8. 3. The sac is kept moist by covering it with nonadherent, sterile saline dressings. The dressings will need to be moistened often to prevent them from drying out. The sac is inspected carefully for leaks, abrasions, and signs of infection. (P, N, S)

9. 3. Before surgery, the infant is kept flat in the prone position to decrease tension on the sac. This allows for optimal positioning of the hips, knees, and feet because orthopedic problems are common. The supine position is unacceptable because it causes pressure on the defect. (P, T, S)

10. 1. The infant would be at risk for infection both preoperatively and postoperatively. The infant does not have altered nutrition, nor does he have altered health maintenance at this time. Ineffective airway clearance is not usually a problem for these infants. (D, N, G)

11. 2. Because of the potential for hip dislocation, the neonate's legs should be slightly abducted, hips maintained in slight to moderate abduction, and feet

maintained in a neutral position. The infant's knees are flexed to help maintain the hips in abduction. (P, T, S)

12. 3. In a neonate with open cranial sutures, increasing head circumference is the predominant and earliest sign of increased intracranial pressure. Some neonates may exhibit bulging fontanels without head enlargement. Other early signs and symptoms are frontal bossing or enlargement with depressed eyes and the sunset sign, with the sclera visible above the iris. A brief, shrill cry is a later sign, and seizures are more commonly seen in rapidly progressing hydrocephalus. (A, T, G)

13. 4. The most important nursing intervention for the parents is to know what daily care of the infant will involve. Usually, home health care is not needed. Providing a list of available hospital services may be helpful to the parents but is not the most important intervention. Referral for counseling is more appropriately made at the time of need. (P, N, L)

14. 3. Children with myelomeningocele are prone to urinary tract infections. Because of sensory impairment, the child is unaware of bladder discomfort. Similarly, the child is insensitive to pressure and other sources of tissue damage, such as heat. Activities that encourage body consciousness, such as rolling over, are encouraged. The child needs the stimulation of others and has a competent immune system. (E, N, G)

The Client With Hydrocephalus

15. 2. Head circumference usually parallels the percentile for length. The discrepancy found requires close and immediate attention because it could indicate hydrocephalus, with its potential for brain damage. In an infant, bulging fontanels and widening cranial sutures are signs of increasing intracranial pressure related to increased cerebrospinal fluid in the cranial space. Transillumination is a noninvasive procedure and does not require a permit. (A, N, G)

16. 2. Small, frequent feedings given at times when the infant is relaxed and calm are tolerated best. An infant with hydrocephalus is difficult to feed because of poor sucking, lethargy, and vomiting, which are associated with increased intracranial pressure. Ideally, the infant should be held in a slightly vertical position when feeding. (I, N, S)

17. 1. The outcomes for children with hydrocephalus vary from normal growth and development to delayed motor and cognitive development. The degree of impairment is difficult to predict. The nurse should respond now to the inquiry rather than refer the mother to the physician at a later time. (E, N, G)

18. 4. The infant is positioned flat for at least the first 24 hours after surgery. Positioning on the operative side is avoided because it places pressure on the shunt valve. Elevating the head increases cerebrospinal fluid drainage and reduces intracranial pressure; but rapid reduction in the size of the ventricles may cause subdural hematoma. The infant should be kept off the nonoperative side (side opposite the shunt) to help prevent rapid decompression. Elevating the foot of the bed could increase intracranial pressure. (P, T, G)

19. 3. Monitoring the temperature allows the nurse to assess for infection, the most common hazardous postoperative complication after ventroperitoneal shunt placement. Neither proteinuria nor glycosuria is associated with shunt placement. Pain should be mild postoperatively, and mild analgesics are given. Narcotics are not given because they alter level of consciousness and make assessment of cerebral function difficult. Any fluid leakage is tested for glucose, an indication of cerebrospinal fluid. (I, T, G)

20. 1. Intake and output are carefully monitored to prevent fluid overload. Feedings will be started when the infant is fully awake. The infant will need to be disturbed to check vital signs and reposition. Age-appropriate activities are important but not until the infant is awake and less fussy. (I, T, S)

21. 3. Aminoglycoside antibiotics are usually infused intravenously over ½ to 1 hour. Too-rapid infusion can cause severe hypotension. Intramuscular injections can be given in the vastus lateralis in infants. Arrhythmia is not a common side effect of aminoglycosides. There is no relationship between allergy to penicillin and allergy to aminoglycosides. (I, T, S)

22. 4. In an infant, irritability, tense fontanel, increased head circumference, lethargy, poor sucking, vomiting, and decreased level of consciousness are signs of increased intracranial pressure caused by a blocked shunt. Decreased urine output with stable fluid intake indicates fluid loss from a source other than the kidneys. Cold clammy skin and pale lips are symptoms of shock. Elevated temperature and redness around incisions could indicate infection. (E, N, G)

23. 2. The correct amount is one half of a dropperful, or 0.4 mL. 80 mg = 0.8 mL; 40 mg = 0.4 mL. One dropperful is 0.8 mL; one half of a dropperful is 0.4 mL (I, N, S)

The Client With a Seizure Disorder

24. 3. During a generalized tonic-clonic seizure, the first priority is to protect the client from injury. Although obtaining information about events surrounding the seizure and providing privacy are important considerations, they are not priorities. During a seizure, nothing should be forced into the client's mouth because this can cause severe damage to the teeth and mouth. (E, N, S)

25. 4. It is normal for a child to sleep and be difficult to arouse during the postictal period of a generalized tonic-clonic seizure. During this time, the child should be allowed to sleep until he or she awakens. Sleep and drowsiness do not follow other forms of generalized seizures. Obtaining information about neurologic status is important, but awakening the child every 3 to 5 minutes would not be helpful. Urinary incontinence during a seizure is common. (I, N, G)

26. 4. Common side effects of valproic acid include nausea and vomiting. Another side effect is tremors. If these occur, the physician should be notified. Administering the medication with food can help alleviate some of the nausea and vomiting. The dose for children undergoing treatment for seizures should never be discontinued, increased, or decreased without physician order. (P, T, H)

27. 1. Routine blood work for children taking valproic acid includes SGOT, complete blood count, platelets, and fibrinogen level because side effects of this medication include decreased platelets and fibrinogen level. A serious but relatively rare side effect of this medication is hepatic toxicity. (I, T, S)

28. 3. A toxic effect of valproic acid is liver toxicity, which may present with abdominal pain and jaundice. (I, T, S)

29. 2. The most common cause of status epilepticus is sudden withdrawal of anticonvulsant medication. Some children may be able to discontinue their medication, but only under supervised conditions and after being completely seizure-free on medication for several years. Physical growth, such as during adolescence, frequently necessitates a dosage increase. The physician should be notified of troublesome side effects. (P, N, H)

30. 3. Many medications, including over-the-counter drugs such as antihistamines, central nervous system stimulants, and alcohol, can lower the seizure threshold. To maintain plasma drug levels within the threshold range, anticonvulsants should be taken at least once daily. When a child is unable to take an oral anticonvulsant, the physician should be notified. Prescriptions should be refilled before the bottle is empty to keep from interrupting the medication regimen. (E, N, H)

31. 4. Safety is the primary concern. It is a common misconception that a person swallows the tongue during a seizure. Flexing the neck, however, could obstruct the airway. Trying to restrain the child during a seizure or attempting to have her swallow any-

thing, including medications, can result in further injury or aspiration. (E, N, H)

32. 3. Most children who develop seizures after infancy are intellectually normal. A child with seizure disorders needs the same experiences and opportunities to develop his or her intellectual, emotional, and social abilities as any other child. (P, N, H)

33. 1. A child who has generalized seizures should not participate in activities that are potentially hazardous. Even if accompanied by a responsible adult, the child could be seriously injured if she were to have a seizure while rock climbing. Someone needs to accompany the child for activities in or on the water. (P, N, H)

34. 4. Most febrile seizures occur in the presence of an upper respiratory infection, otitis media, or tonsillitis. There appears to be increased susceptibility to febrile seizures within families. Febrile seizures, which occur during a temperature rise rather than after prolonged fever, occasionally (but not always) result in respiratory difficulties. (A, N, G)

35. 1. The child who is at low risk for recurrence is usually not treated with anticonvulsant drugs because drug side effects frequently outweigh the benefits. Without anticonvulsant therapy, the likelihood that a child will experience a second febrile seizure is 30% to 40%; a third seizure occurs in about 15%. Prophylactic treatment is indicated for children who experience their first febrile seizure before age 18 months of age, have a family history of seizures, and have seizures lasting longer than 15 minutes. (E, T, G)

36. 2. Shivering is the body's defense against rapid temperature decrease; the result is increased body temperature. When caring for a shivering child, the nurse should try to stop the shivering by increasing the room temperature until the shivering stops, and then attempt to lower the temperature more slowly. Alcohol can be absorbed through the skin and is a toxic substance. While attempts are being made to decrease temperature, the child will likely complain of being cold; but as long as the child does not shiver, the treatment can continue. (E, N, H)

37. 3. Phenytoin sodium (Dilantin) is a known teratogenic agent, causing numerous fetal problems, and anticonvulsant requirements usually increase during pregnancy. There is a familial tendency for seizure disorders. Seizures can be controlled, but cannot be cured. Seizure disorders and infertility are not related. (E, N, H)

38. 3. Although phenytoin can produce cardiotoxicity, hepatotoxicity, venous irritation, and hyperglycemia, the most life-threatening side effect during rapid administration is cardiotoxicity. Bradycardia, hypotension, and cardiac arrest (asystole) are possible cardiovascular problems associated with intravenous phenytoin administration. The nurse should monitor the child's vital signs closely during and after intravenous phenytoin administration. (I, T, S)

The Client With Meningitis

39. 4. The nurse would give ibuprofen for a temperature of 102.5°F. To convert degrees Fahrenheit to degrees centigrade, the nurse subtracts 32 from the Fahrenheit temperature and multiplies the result by 5/9, as follows:

$$102.5°F - 32 = 70.5$$

$$70.5 \times 5/9 = 39.2°C$$

To convert centigrade to Fahrenheit, the nurse multiplies the centigrade temperature by 9/5 and adds 32. Using this formula, the conversion is determined as follows:

$$39.2°C \times 9/5 = 70.5$$

$$70.5 + 32 = 102.5°F$$

(I, T, G)

40. 1. There is no standard medication dosage for pediatric patients. Medication dosages are most commonly based on a child's weight or total body surface area. The child described in this situation is weighed mainly to help calculate medication dosage. Weighing can also be done to help determine fluid needs, but in this case, nutritional needs are not an immediate concern. A child with meningitis is not typically assessed for edema. (A, N, G)

41. 2. The child needs to be comforted after an invasive procedure by people she trusts. There is little discomfort at the insertion site after the lumbar puncture. Narcotics would not be the drugs of choice because they hinder assessment of neurologic status. Applying a small bandage after applying pressure for a short time is usually sufficient to stop any leakage and prevent infection of the site. A young child does not need to lay flat for any time after a lumbar puncture. (Besides, laying flat for 8 hours would be difficult, if not impossible, for a 4-year-old.) (I, N, G)

42. 2. The number of drops the client should receive each minute is determined as follows:

500 mL/12 hours
= 41 to 42 mL to be infused each hour

42 mL × 60 (drop factor)/60 minutes = 2520/60
= 42 drops to be infused every minute

(I, T, S)

43. 2. A child in the acute stage of meningitis is irritable and hypersensitive to loud noise and light. The child should be spoken to and bathed gently and calmly; sudden movements should be avoided. (I, T, G)

44. 1. A blood pressure of 122/74 mm Hg is above the 95th percentile for a 4-year-old child. Increased blood pressure is a common sign of increased intracranial pressure. The pulse and respiration rates are within normal limits for this age. Decreased pulse rate and increased or decreased respiratory rate with irregularity may indicate increased intracranial pressure. Temperature of 100.2°F in a child with an infectious process is not related to increased intracranial pressure, but poor temperature control may be a sign of increasing intracranial pressure in older infants and children. (A, N, G)

45. 1. Disseminated intravascular coagulation is characterized by skin petechiae and a purpuric skin rash due to spontaneous bleeding into the tissues. An abnormal coagulation phenomenon causes the condition. Heparin therapy is often used to interrupt the clotting process. (A, N, G)

46. 2. Organisms that cause bacterial meningitis, such as pneumococci or meningococci, are commonly spread in the body by vascular dissemination from a middle ear infection. The meningitis may also be a direct extension from the paranasal and mastoid sinuses. The causative organism is a pneumococcus. A chronically draining ear is frequently also found. (A, N, G)

47. 3. Preschool-aged children worry about having an intact body and become fearful of any threat to body integrity. Allowing the child to participate with required care helps protect her image of an intact body. Finding diversional activities, relieving the anxiety of separation from the home, and enhancing her confidence in the personnel caring for her are invalid reasons for allowing her to place a dressing on the area where an intravenous needle has been positioned. (I, N, L)

48. 3. An emotionally tense child with pent-up hostilities needs a physical activity that will release energy and frustration. Pounding on a peg board offers this opportunity. Activities such as stacking blocks and painting require concentration and fine movements, which could add to frustration. Listening to a story does not allow the child to express emotions and casts her in a passive role. (I, N, L)

49. 3. The nurse identifies a decreased consciousness, bradycardia, hypertension, irregular respirations, and tense fontanel as signs of increased intracranial pressure. The first action should be to attempt to lower the pressure by raising the head of the bed, which should improve venous return and decrease the pressure. The nurse can then notify the physician and administer the antipyretic. Because temperature, pulse, and respirations are fairly objective data, the nurse does not have to verify these findings. (I, N, G)

The Client With Reye's Syndrome

50. 2. The etiology of Reye's syndrome is unknown, but symptoms usually develop a few days to several weeks after the onset of a mild viral illness. Upper respiratory tract infections are usually viral in nature. (A, N, G)

51. 1. Research suggests that giving aspirin (salicylates) to a child with a viral illness can contribute to the development of Reye's syndrome. Acetaminophen is recommended for any child with a viral infection. The disease is not communicable and is not linked to immunizations or bacterial infections. (I, N, H)

The Client With Near Drowning

52. 2. Hypoxia is the primary problem because it results in brain cell damage. Hypothermia occurs rapidly in infants and children because of their large body surface area. Hypothermia is more of a problem when a child is in cold water. (D, N, G)

53. 1. Submerged children struggle initially. Only about 10% of drowning children die without aspirating fluid. There is no difference in survivors in those who nearly drown in salt or fresh water. (I, T, G)

54. 1. There is a combined respiratory acidosis from retained carbon dioxide and metabolic acidosis from the buildup of acid metabolites due to anaerobic metabolism. (P, N, G)

55. 3. The priority nursing diagnosis is Aspiration. The exact condition of the child is not known, so Activity Intolerance would not be appropriate, neither would Impaired Mobility or Altered Parenting. (D, T, G)

56. 2. Guilt is a common parental response; the parents should be allowed to express their feelings. Near drownings occur quickly, usually with lack of supervision. Denying the parents' feelings of guilt is not helpful. (I, N, L)

The Client With Infectious Polyneuritis (Guillain-Barré Syndrome)

57. 2. Muscle paralysis in Guillain-Barré syndrome is usually progressive and ascending in nature. Assessment of progressive muscle weakness helps determine the extent of involvement. (A, T, G)

58. 3. In a child with Guillain-Barré syndrome, decreased volume and clarity of speech and decreased ability to cough voluntarily indicate ascending progression of neural inflammation. These are not signs

of increasing intracranial pressure or regression. A child with laryngeal inflammation retains the ability to cough. (A, T, G)

59. 2. Although Total Incontinence and Impaired Swallowing are both appropriate nursing diagnoses for this child during the acute phase of the illness, addressing Ineffective Breathing Pattern to maintain an adequate oxygen supply takes precedence. Progressive neurologic impairment will likely have an effect on the child's ability to maintain respirations. Potential for Infection relates to an altered immune system, which is not the situation. (D, N, G)

60. 1. Impaired autonomic function in Guillain-Barré syndrome can result in cardiac dysrhythmia, possibly leading to cardiovascular shock and death. The vital centers in the medulla oblongata may be affected, not by edema, but by patchy demyelination. Neither hyperkalemia nor hypoglycemia is associated with this syndrome. (A, T, G)

61. 4. Even in the absence of respiratory problems or distress, the child must be turned frequently to help prevent the cardiopulmonary complications associated with immobility. During the acute disease phase, vigorous physiotherapy is contraindicated because the child may experience muscle pain and be hypersensitive to touch. The child should be handled extremely gently. (I, N, G)

62. 2. Impaired gag and swallowing reflexes associated with cranial nerve involvement require nasogastric tube feedings in a child with Guillain-Barré syndrome. The presence of a gag reflex indicates the return of normal swallowing. (E, T, G)

63. 1. The family should be involved early in developing a rehabilitation plan. The convalescent period for a child with Guillain-Barré syndrome is lengthy, and full recovery may require 1 to 2 years. Most children recover completely; only 10% to 15% have neurologic sequelae. Maintaining peer relationships during convalescence is important for psychosocial development. Children with Guillain-Barré syndrome can attend regular schools. (P, N, G)

64. 3. Developmentally appropriate activities and therapeutic play should be used as rehabilitation modalities. Inappropriate rewards or threats should not be used to coerce a child into compliance. Missing therapy will delay her recovery; it is up to the parents to help set her schedule to ensure she gets adequate rest to be able to follow her treatment plan. (E, N, H)

The Client With a Head Injury

65. 3. The first priority in caring for a child who has sustained a head injury is to establish and maintain ventilation. All other activities are secondary to adequate ventilation. (I, T, G)

66. 1. Lack of response to pain yields the lowest score. From the highest to lowest, the order of eye-opening response to stimuli on the Glasgow coma scale is spontaneous opening, response to speech, response to pain, no response. (A, T, G)

67. 2. A nasogastric tube is initially placed after serious head trauma to decompress the stomach and to prevent vomiting and aspiration. (P, T, S)

68. 1. Because a basilar skull fracture can involve the frontal and ethmoid bones, inserting a nasogastric tube carries the risk of introducing the tube into the cranial cavity through the fracture. An oral gastric tube is preferred for a client with basilar skull fracture. (I, T, G)

69. 3. Using the ratio–proportion method, the equation is:

$$4 \text{ mg}/1 \text{ mL} = 7.6 \text{ mg}/x \text{ mL}$$

$$4x = 7.6$$

$$x = 7.6/4$$

$$x = 1.9 \text{ mL}$$

(I, T, G)

70. 3. As a rule, children demonstrate more rapid and more complete recovery from coma than do adults. However, it is extremely difficult to predict a specific outcome. Assuring the parents that they will be kept informed helps open lines of communication and establish trust. (I, N, L)

71. 2. Mannitol is an osmotic diuretic used to help decrease intracranial pressure by decreasing cerebral edema. It does contribute to the calorie intake of the child but is not used for the purpose of increasing caloric intake because of its diuretic effect. (I, N, G)

72. 2. The unconscious child is positioned to prevent aspiration of saliva and to minimize intracranial pressure. The head of the bed should be elevated, and the child should be either in the semiprone or side-lying position. (I, T, S)

73. 3. The parents' presence may help calm the child. Restraints can frighten and frustrate a child, and straining against them can lead to an increase in intracranial pressure. (I, T, S)

The Client With a Brain Tumor

74. 4. Common signs and symptoms of infratentorial brain tumor in children are headache, visual disturbance, vomiting with or without nausea, and ataxia in the form of gait disturbances. (D, N, G)

75. 4. When a brain tumor is suspected, the child and parents are likely to be very apprehensive and anxious. It is unrealistic to expect to eliminate their fears; rather, the nurse's goal is to decrease them. Preparing both the child and family during hospitalization can help them cope with some of their fears. Children with infratentorial tumors seldom have seizures. Introducing the child to other children is a positive action, but not the most important action at this time. (P, N, L)

76. 2. Both the child and parents should receive preoperative teaching about head shaving, bulky bandages, possible facial edema, and the intensive care unit stay. The prognosis and treatment plan cannot be determined until after surgery, when the type of tumor is diagnosed. (P, N, G)

77. 3. Stage I indicates localized disease without evidence of spread. Such a tumor has a favorable prognosis, if all tumor tissue is removed. Poor prognosis, undifferentiation, rapid growth, and metastasis are characteristics of stage III and IV tumors. (I, K, G)

78. 1. Postoperatively, the child undergoing neurosurgery for brain tumor removal is at risk for cardiopulmonary compromise due to anesthesia, surgical complications, or increased intracranial pressure. The other issues are important but are not the nurse's first priority. (I, N, G)

79. 3. After surgery for an infratentorial tumor, the child is usually positioned flat on either side, with the head and neck in midline and the body slightly extended. Pillows against the back, not the head, help maintain position. Such a position helps avoid pressure on the operative site. Trendelenburg position is usually contraindicated because keeping the head below the level of the heart increases intracranial pressure as well as the risk of hemorrhage. (I, N, G)

80. 1. Hypercapnia, hypoxia, and acidosis are potent cerebral vasodilating mechanisms that can cause increased intracranial pressure. Lowering the CO_2 level and increasing the O_2 level through hyperventilation is the most effective short-term method of reducing intracranial pressure. (I, N, G)

81. 3. Glucose in this clear, colorless fluid indicates the presence of cerebrospinal fluid. Excessive fluid leakage should be reported to the physician. The nurse should not change the dressing of a postoperative craniotomy client unless instructed to do so by the surgeon. The head of the bed would not ordinarily be elevated because this would put pressure on the sutures. (I, T, G)

82. 1. It is not uncommon for a child to be concerned about a change in appearance when the entire head or only part has been shaved. The child should be encouraged to participate in decisions about her care when possible. Assuring her that her hair will grow back does not address the immediate change in appearance; neither does explaining that this type of reaction is normal. (I, N, L)

83. 1. Parents of a child who has undergone neurosurgery can easily become overprotective; yet the parents must foster independence in the convalescing child. It is important for the child to resume age-appropriate activities, and parents play an important role in encouraging this. (D, N, L)

The Client With a Spinal Cord Injury

84. 2. The client's history and symptoms suggest a spinal cord injury. A client with suspected spinal cord injury should not be moved until the spine has been immobilized. Flexing his knees could aggravate a spinal cord injury. (D, N, G)

85. 1. The first priority in emergency care of the client with spinal cord injury is to maintain cardiovascular and respiratory function. Preventing fluid and electrolyte imbalance, providing nutritional support, and providing emotional support are important goals but not priority. (P, N, G)

86. 4. Spinal shock occurs 30 to 60 minutes after a spinal cord injury owing to the sudden disruption of central and autonomic pathways. This disruption causes flaccid paralysis, loss of reflexes, vasodilation, hypotension, and increased pulse and respiratory rates. Autonomic dysreflexia occurs only after the return of spinal reflexes and is characterized by hypertension. Increased intracranial pressure is associated with widened pulse pressure and decreased pulse and respiratory rates. Metabolic alkalosis does not occur with spinal shock. (D, N, G)

87. 1. In spinal cord injury, temperature regulation is lost distal to the injury. Body temperature must be maintained by adjusting room temperature or bed linens. Changing position does not alleviate the temperature regulation problem and could be harmful, considering the client's diagnosis. Reporting this finding to the physician is unnecessary because it is an expected development. (I, T, G)

88. 3. A thoracic spinal cord injury involves the muscles of the lower extremities, bladder, and rectum. Paralytic ileus often occurs; the nurse evaluates this by auscultating the abdomen. (A, T, G)

89. 3. Spinal cord shock causes a loss of reflex activity below the level of the injury, resulting in bladder atony and flaccid paralysis. When the reflex arc returns, it tends to be overactive, resulting in spasticity. The bladder becomes hypertonic during this phase of spinal shock resolution; sensation does not return. (D, N, G)

90. 1. Initially after a catastrophic injury, denial is a common response. With gradual awareness of the situation, anger commonly occurs. The four major stages of grief are denial, anger, depression, and acceptance. (D, N, G)

91. 3. The adolescent is striving for independence and self-definition. A sudden accident with long-term consequences requires many adjustments in terms of self-concept. Autonomy is the task of preschoolers. Industry is a task of children age 6 to 12 years; ego integrity is the task of adult development. (I, N, H)

92. 1. These are signs of autonomic dysreflexia, a generalized sympathetic response usually caused by bladder or bowel distention. Immediate treatment involves eliminating the cause. Because bladder distention is a common cause of this problem, the nurse should immediately determine the patency of the Foley catheter. The nurse should assist the client to a sitting position to help decrease blood pressure. Epinephrine is contraindicated because it elevates blood pressure and thus can exacerbate the problem. (I, N, G)

93. 2. A high priority is placed on leaving the house so that the client can participate in his or her normal activities as much as possible, and a short-term goal toward leaving the house is to maneuver inside first. Although independent performance of activities of daily living is important, complete independence may be a long-term goal. (P, N, H)

NURSING CARE OF CHILDREN

TEST 7: The Child With Neurologic Health Problems

Directions: Use this answer grid to determine areas of strength or need for further study.

NURSING PROCESS

A = Assessment
D = Analysis, nursing diagnosis
P = Planning
I = Implementation
E = Evaluation

COGNITIVE LEVEL

K = Knowledge
C = Comprehension
T = Application
N = Analysis

CLIENT NEEDS

S = Safe, effective care environment
G = Physiologic integrity
L = Psychosocial integrity
H = Health promotion and maintenance

Question #	Answer #	A	D	P	I	E	K	C	T	N	S	G	L	H
1	4	A						C				G		
2	2	A							T			G		
3	1			P						N			L	
4	1				I				T			G		
5	1				I					N		G		
6	1				I				T		S			
7	2					E				N		G		
8	3			P						N	S			
9	3			P					T		S			
10	1		D							N		G		
11	2			P					T		S			
12	3	A							T			G		
13	4			P						N			L	
14	3					E				N		G		
15	2	A								N		G		
16	2				I					N	S			
17	1					E				N		G		
18	4			P					T			G		
19	3				I				T			G		
20	1				I				T		S			
21	3				I				T		S			
22	4					E				N		G		
23	2				I					N	S			
24	3					E				N	S			
25	4				I					N		G		

ANSWER GRID: 1

NURSING PROCESS	COGNITIVE LEVEL	CLIENT NEEDS
A = Assessment	K = Knowledge	S = Safe, effective care environment
D = Analysis, nursing diagnosis	C = Comprehension	G = Physiologic integrity
P = Planning	T = Application	L = Psychosocial integrity
I = Implementation	N = Analysis	H = Health promotion and maintenance
E = Evaluation		

Question #	Answer #	Nursing Process					Cognitive Level				Client Needs			
		A	D	P	I	E	K	C	T	N	S	G	L	H
26	4			P					T					H
27	1				I				T		S			
28	3				I				T		S			
29	2			P						N				H
30	3					E				N				H
31	4					E				N				H
32	3			P						N				H
33	1			P						N				H
34	4	A								N		G		
35	1					E			T			G		
36	2					E				N				H
37	3					E				N				H
38	3				I				T		S			
39	4				I				T			G		
40	1	A								N		G		
41	2				I					N		G		
42	2				I				T		S			
43	2				I				T			G		
44	1	A								N		G		
45	1	A								N		G		
46	2	A								N		G		
47	3				I					N			L	
48	3				I					N			L	
49	3				I					N		G		
50	2	A								N		G		
51	1				I					N				H
52	2		D							N		G		
53	1				I				T			G		
54	1			P						N		G		
55	3		D						T			G		

ANSWER GRID: 2

NURSING PROCESS

A = Assessment
D = Analysis, nursing diagnosis
P = Planning
I = Implementation
E = Evaluation

COGNITIVE LEVEL

K = Knowledge
C = Comprehension
T = Application
N = Analysis

CLIENT NEEDS

S = Safe, effective care environment
G = Physiologic integrity
L = Psychosocial integrity
H = Health promotion and maintenance

Question #	Answer #	Nursing Process					Cognitive Level				Client Needs			
		A	D	P	I	E	K	C	T	N	S	G	L	H
56	2				I					N			L	
57	2	A							T			G		
58	3	A							T			G		
59	2		D							N		G		
60	1	A							T			G		
61	4				I					N		G		
62	2					E			T			G		
63	1			P						N		G		
64	3					E				N				H
65	3				I				T			G		
66	1	A							T			G		
67	2			P					T		S			
68	1				I				T			G		
69	3				I				T			G		
70	3				I					N			L	
71	2				I					N		G		
72	2				I				T		S			
73	3				I				T		S			
74	4		D							N		G		
75	4			P						N			L	
76	2			P						N		G		
77	3				I		K					G		
78	1				I					N		G		
79	3				I					N		G		
80	1				I					N		G		
81	3				I				T			G		
82	1				I					N			L	
83	1		D							N			L	
84	2		D							N		G		
85	1			P						N		G		

NURSING PROCESS

A = Assessment
D = Analysis, nursing diagnosis
P = Planning
I = Implementation
E = Evaluation

COGNITIVE LEVEL

K = Knowledge
C = Comprehension
T = Application
N = Analysis

CLIENT NEEDS

S = Safe, effective care environment
G = Physiologic integrity
L = Psychosocial integrity
H = Health promotion and maintenance

Question #	Answer #	Nursing Process					Cognitive Level				Client Needs			
		A	D	P	I	E	K	C	T	N	S	G	L	H
86	4		D							N		G		
87	1				I				T			G		
88	3	A							T			G		
89	3		D							N		G		
90	1		D							N		G		
91	3				I					N				H
92	1				I					N		G		
93	2			P						N				H
Number Correct														
Number Possible	93	15	10	17	39	12	1	1	34	57	16	56	9	12
Percentage Correct														

Score Calculation: To determine your **Percentage Correct,** divide the **Number Correct** by the **Number Possible.**

ANSWER GRID: 4

The Child With Musculoskeletal Health Problems

- The Client With Musculoskeletal Dysfunction
- The Client With Cerebral Palsy
- The Client With Duchenne's Muscular Dystrophy
- The Client With Developmental Dysplasia of the Hip
- The Client With Congenital Clubfoot
- The Client With Juvenile Rheumatoid Arthritis
- The Client With a Fracture
- The Client With Osteomyelitis
- Correct Answers and Rationale

Select the one best answer, and indicate your choice by filling in the circle in front of the option.

The Client With Musculoskeletal Dysfunction

The nurse works in an orthopedic clinic. The following questions pertain to clients seen in this clinic.

1. A child who limps and complains of pain has been found to have Legg-Calvé-Perthes disease. The right femur is involved. The nurse and family plan for the child's care, which should include
   - ○ 1. controlling pain that is especially acute at night.
   - ○ 2. encouraging the child to walk despite discomfort in the right hip.
   - ○ 3. preventing flexion in the right hip and knee.
   - ○ 4. preventing weight bearing on the head of the right femur.

2. In planning outpatient care for the child with Legg-Calvé-Perthes disease, the nurse should emphasize teaching the family
   - ○ 1. about protein-rich foods.
   - ○ 2. gentle stretching exercises for both legs.
   - ○ 3. management of the corrective appliance.
   - ○ 4. relaxation techniques for pain control.

3. The nurse examines an adolescent who has an abnormally convex angulation in the curvature of the thoracic spine. The nurse would document the findings as

   - ○ 1. equinovarus.
   - ○ 2. kyphosis.
   - ○ 3. lordosis.
   - ○ 4. scoliosis.

4. The nurse would suspect that a child has torticollis (wry neck) after noting a characteristic abnormality of the
   - ○ 1. quadriceps.
   - ○ 2. cervical vertebrae.
   - ○ 3. trapezius muscle.
   - ○ 4. sternocleidomastoid muscle.

5. The mother of a child with flat feet asks the nurse why her child needs to wear corrective shoes. The nurse should reply that the shoes help
   - ○ 1. keep the legs in proper alignment.
   - ○ 2. delay the development of femoral anteversion.
   - ○ 3. prevent the development of internal tibial torsion.
   - ○ 4. strengthen the arches of the feet.

6. The nurse would evaluate the teaching about the etiology of muscular dystrophy as successful when the mother of a child with the disease states, "My son's disease is due to the
   - ○ 1. effects of an automobile accident during my pregnancy."
   - ○ 2. genes he inherited from me."

○ 3. imbalance in his thyroid hormone."

○ 4. viral infection I had when I was pregnant with him."

7. The nurse would assess a female adolescent for lateral deviation of the spine by having her

○ 1. bend forward at the waist and clasp her hands together.

○ 2. lie flat on the floor and extend her legs straight from her trunk.

○ 3. sit in a chair while lifting her feet and legs to a right angle with her trunk.

○ 4. standing against a wall while pressing the length of her back against the wall.

8. The nurse would suspect that the adolescent has scoliosis after observing a skeletal defect that results in a slight limp and

○ 1. a shorter-than-average trunk.

○ 2. a rib hump.

○ 3. a forward body thrust while walking.

○ 4. a waddling gait.

9. A child needs to wear a Milwaukee brace for scoliosis, and the nurse teaches his family about when he can remove it. The nurse would evaluate the teaching as successful when the child and parents indicate that the brace will be removed when he

○ 1. bathes, for about 1 hour per day.

○ 2. eats, for about 3 hours a day.

○ 3. is in school, for about 8 hours a day.

○ 4. sleeps, for about 10 hours a day.

10. The nurse would teach exercises to a child wearing the Milwaukee brace primarily to help

○ 1. decrease back muscle spasms.

○ 2. improve the brace's traction effect.

○ 3. prevent spinal contractures.

○ 4. strengthen the back and abdominal muscles.

11. The nurse would assess an adolescent who complains of pain over the tibial tuberosity for participation in which of the following exercises?

○ 1. Running.

○ 2. Jumping.

○ 3. Biking.

○ 4. Swimming.

The Client With Cerebral Palsy

A mother of a toddler with cerebral palsy brings the child to the clinic for developmental screening.

12. The nurse would explain to the mother that screening tests are done to recognize primary developmental delays early to

○ 1. encourage health maintenance.

○ 2. facilitate communication.

○ 3. prevent secondary developmental delays.

○ 4. maintain current development.

13. The nurse judges that the mother understands the term *cerebral palsy* when she states, "It's a term applied to impaired nerve and muscle control as a result of

○ 1. injury to the cerebrum due to viral infection."

○ 2. malformation of the blood vessels in the ventricles due to inheritance."

○ 3. nonprogressive brain damage due to injury."

○ 4. progressive brain disease due to metabolic imbalances."

14. The nurse would explain to the toddler's mother that spastic cerebral palsy is the most common type. The nurse would describe it to the mother as

○ 1. increased muscle tone and stretch reflexes.

○ 2. slow, wormlike writhing movements.

○ 3. wide-based gait and poor muscle coordination.

○ 4. tremors and lack of active movement.

15. The nurse interviews the mother about the toddler's development. Not attaining which of the following developmental milestones would indicate delay in this 18-month-old?

○ 1. Stoops and recovers.

○ 2. Kicks a ball forward.

○ 3. Builds tower of two cubes.

○ 4. Scribbles.

16. The nurse would expect the toddler with spasticity to do which of the following?

○ 1. Walk on his toes.

○ 2. Use his unaffected arm and leg to propel himself.

○ 3. Exhibit facial grimacing.

○ 4. Have a wide-based gait.

17. The nurse should encourage the mother to position the child upright and to offer toys to his affected side to

○ 1. challenge the use of the affected limb.

○ 2. increase strength in the affected limb.

○ 3. provide diversional activities.

○ 4. test visual acuity.

18. The mother asks the nurse if her child will be able to walk normally because he can pull himself to a standing position. What would be the nurse's best reply?

○ 1. "Ask the doctor what he thinks at your next appointment."

○ 2. "He might but he might not. How old were you when you first walked?"

○ 3. "It's not easy to predict, but the fact that he's able to bear weight is a positive factor."

○ 4. "If he really wants to walk, and works hard, he'll probably be able to do so eventually."

19. The nurse evaluates the family's ability to cope with the child's cerebral palsy. Which of the following

would be indicative of their inability to cope with the disease?

○ 1. Limiting interaction with the extended family and friends.

○ 2. Needing to learn to meet the child's physical needs.

○ 3. Requesting teaching about cerebral palsy in general.

○ 4. Not seeking financial help to pay for medical bills.

The Client With Duchenne's Muscular Dystrophy

A family with a 3-year-old child with Duchenne's muscular dystrophy has been referred to a home health agency.

20. During the initial visit, the nurse would expect the child to demonstrate which of the following early signs of Duchenne's muscular dystrophy?

○ 1. Contractures of the large joints.

○ 2. Enlarged calf muscles.

○ 3. Difficulty riding a tricycle.

○ 4. Small, weak muscles.

21. The nurse explains to the mother that the inheritance pattern of Duchenne's muscular dystrophy is primarily

○ 1. autosomal recessive.

○ 2. autosomal dominant.

○ 3. X-linked.

○ 4. Y-linked.

22. The nurse observes the child attempt to rise from a sitting position on the floor. After attaining a kneeling position, the child "walks" his hands up his legs to stand. The nurse documents this as which of the following?

○ 1. Galeazzi's sign.

○ 2. Goodell's sign.

○ 3. Goodenough's sign.

○ 4. Gowers' sign.

23. The primary nursing diagnosis for the preschool-aged child with early Duchenne's muscular dystrophy would be

○ 1. Altered Family Processes.

○ 2. Self-Care Deficits.

○ 3. Impaired Physical Mobility.

○ 4. Potential for Injury.

24. The primary nursing goal for the child is to

○ 1. encourage early wheelchair use.

○ 2. foster social interactions.

○ 3. maintain function in unaffected muscles.

○ 4. prevent circulatory impairment.

25. When interacting with the child's mother, the nurse observes behavior indicating that she may feel guilty about her child's condition. The nurse would suspect that this guilt stems from the

○ 1. terminal nature of the disease.

○ 2. dependent behavior of the children.

○ 3. genetic mode of transmission.

○ 4. sudden onset of the disease.

26. One of the child's aunts tells the nurse that she understands that the child will not have a normal life-span and asks the nurse to explain what the usual cause of death is in children with muscular dystrophy. The nurse replies,

○ 1. "Most children die of renal failure."

○ 2. "The usual cause of death is respiratory tract infection or cardiac failure."

○ 3. "You should talk to the child's parents about this subject."

○ 4. "Would you like to talk to the child's doctor about this?"

27. The nurse teaches the mother about the course of the disease, therapeutic management, and nursing considerations. Which of the following statements by the mother would indicate that she has understood the teaching?

○ 1. "My son will probably be unable to walk independently by the time he is 9 to 11 years old."

○ 2. "Muscle relaxants are effective for some children."

○ 3. "When my son is a little older, he can have surgery to improve his ability to walk."

○ 4. "I need to help my son be as active as possible to prevent progression of the disease."

The Client With Developmental Dysplasia of the Hip

The nurse performs a newborn assessment.

28. While gently abducting the hips, the nurse feels the femoral head slip into the acetabulum. The nurse documents this finding as a positive

○ 1. Barlow's test.

○ 2. Galeazzi sign.

○ 3. Ortolani's sign.

○ 4. Trendelenburg's sign.

29. In examining an older infant, the nurse would use which of the following as a part of the assessment?

○ 1. Barlow's test.

○ 2. Trendelenburg's sign.

○ 3. Ortolani's test.

○ 4. Symmetric gluteal folds.

A child is fitted with a Pavlik harness to correct developmental dysplasia of the hip.

30. The nurse would teach the parents how to handle the infant in a Pavlik harness. Which of the following interventions would be most appropriate?
○ 1. The diaper is fitted under the straps.
○ 2. The diaper is placed over the straps.
○ 3. Check the skin every other day for red spots under the straps.
○ 4. Put powder on the skin under the straps every day.

31. When teaching the parents about use of orthopedic appliances, the nurse's *initial* step should be to
○ 1. assess their coping strategies.
○ 2. determine their knowledge of the device.
○ 3. provide written instructions.
○ 4. provide the parents with a list of community resources.

An 8-month-old infant with developmental dysplasia of the hip is fitted with a spica cast.

32. The nurse should teach the parents that the abduction stabilizer bar
○ 1. can be adjusted to a position of comfort.
○ 2. can be used to lift the child.
○ 3. is designed to add strength to the cast.
○ 4. is used to turn the child.

33. Three weeks after the application of the spica cast, the mother calls the clinic nurse because the infant's toes are swollen and cool to the touch. The nurse would suspect that these findings are due to the fact that the
○ 1. child has had his feet in a dependent position.
○ 2. child has outgrown the cast.
○ 3. cotton wadding lining of the cast has shrunk.
○ 4. child has an infection in the tissue under the cast.

34. The mother asks the nurse about using a car seat for her infant in a hip spica cast. What would be the nurse's best reply?
○ 1. "You can use a seat belt because of the spica cast."
○ 2. "You will need a specially designed car seat for your infant."
○ 3. "You will still be able to use the one you already have."
○ 4. "There is no car seat you will be able to use."

35. The nurse judges that the mother understands how to feed her 8-month-old in a hip spica cast when she states
○ 1. "I can lay her down flat and feed her that way."
○ 2. "I can raise her head and leave her hips and legs on a pillow at her side."
○ 3. "I can borrow a feeding table to use for her."
○ 4. "I know it will take two of us to feed her—one to hold her, and the other to feed her."

The Client With Congenital Clubfoot

A neonate is diagnosed as having a congenital clubfoot.

36. The infant's parents ask the nurse how his foot will be treated. The nurse would respond that treatment usually includes
○ 1. traction for 6 months.
○ 2. corrective shoes.
○ 3. serial leg casting.
○ 4. waiting until he is 6 months old.

37. The parents convey anxiety about how the problem will be treated and express feelings of helplessness and guilt. *Initially,* the nurse should
○ 1. ask them to share these concerns with the physician.
○ 2. arrange a meeting with other parents whose infants have undergone successful clubfoot treatment.
○ 3. discuss the problem and the feelings that the parents are experiencing.
○ 4. suggest that they make an appointment with a counselor.

38. A plaster cast is applied to correct the deformity. In the immediate postapplication period, the nurse should
○ 1. change the client's position at least every 2 hours.
○ 2. coat the cast with a clear acrylic spray finish.
○ 3. dry the cast rapidly with a hair dryer.
○ 4. handle the cast with the fingertips only.

39. The nurse has taught the parents about caring for the cast. Which of the following statements would indicate that they have understood the teaching? "We'll
○ 1. clean the cast with soap and water if it becomes soiled."
○ 2. elevate the leg with the cast on pillows, so the leg will be above heart level."
○ 3. observe the color and temperature of the toes frequently."
○ 4. remove the petals from the edge of the cast after 24 hours."

40. The parents ask why they have to have so many doctor appointments. The nurse would explain that the cast needs to be changed frequently
    ○ 1. to keep it clean and dry.
    ○ 2. to prevent an infection under the cast.
    ○ 3. because their child's leg grows so rapidly.
    ○ 4. because of the difficulty in caring for an infant with a cast.

41. After clubfoot deformity is overcorrected by serial casting, the client is to wear a Denis Browne splint. The nurse should explain to the parents that the splint is applied to
    ○ 1. assess the strength of calf and thigh muscles.
    ○ 2. help maintain the feet in the desired position.
    ○ 3. prevent kicking.
    ○ 4. prevent possible bone deformities.

42. The nurse teaches the parents how to maintain the function of the Denis Browne splint. Which of the parents' following actions during the return demonstration would indicate that they have understood the teaching?
    ○ 1. Repositioning the angle of the shoes on the bar.
    ○ 2. Putting the child's feet into the shoes without socks.
    ○ 3. Tightening a loose shoe against the splint.
    ○ 4. Using the bar to help lift the child.

43. After the child has been wearing the Denis Browne splint for a while, his mother reports that he is able to wobble across the floor on his hands and knees while wearing the splint. The nurse should tell the mother to
    ○ 1. notify the physician so corrective shoes can be prescribed.
    ○ 2. put the child in a playpen to restrict movements.
    ○ 3. remove the splint for 2 hours daily so the child can be more mobile.
    ○ 4. remove tablecloths from all rooms to which the child has access.

The Client With Juvenile Rheumatoid Arthritis

A preschool-aged girl is admitted with a tentative diagnosis of juvenile rheumatoid arthritis (JRA).

44. The father asks which test can definitely diagnose JRA. The nurse should explain that
    ○ 1. the latex fixation test is diagnostic.
    ○ 2. an elevated erythrocyte sedimentation rate is diagnostic.
    ○ 3. a positive synovial fluid culture is diagnostic.
    ○ 4. no specific laboratory test is diagnostic.

45. The diagnosis of JRA is confirmed. The parents tell the nurse that the diagnosis frightens them because they know nothing about the prognosis. The nurse should explain that
    ○ 1. in most children, the disease will go into permanent remission.
    ○ 2. many children go into long remissions but have severe deformities and loss of function.
    ○ 3. the disease usually progresses to crippling rheumatoid arthritis as the child reaches adulthood.
    ○ 4. most affected children recover completely within a few years.

46. The child's mother is worried that the child will have to stop attending preschool because of the illness. The nurse should explain that the child
    ○ 1. may find it difficult to attend school because of the side effects of the prescribed medication regimen.
    ○ 2. should be encouraged to attend school, but will need time to work out early-morning stiffness.
    ○ 3. should be kept home from school whenever she experiences joint discomfort.
    ○ 4. will need to wear splints and braces to give her more support.

47. The nurse and family develop a care plan to alleviate joint stiffness in the child. Which of these interventions should be included?
    ○ 1. Applying moist heat to affected joints.
    ○ 2. Applying cool compresses to affected joints.
    ○ 3. Performing repetitive weight-bearing exercises using the affected joints.
    ○ 4. Use a soft mattress that is comfortable.

48. The child will be treated with aspirin. The nurse will explain to the parents which of the following?
    ○ 1. It will take 8 weeks before the antiinflammatory effect takes place.
    ○ 2. Within 24 hours, the child will have antiinflammatory relief.
    ○ 3. Call the nurse before giving any over-the-counter medications.
    ○ 4. If you forget to give a dose, do not make it up.

49. Which of the following nursing diagnoses would be appropriate for this preschooler with JRA?
    ○ 1. Total Incontinence.
    ○ 2. Ineffective Airway Clearance.
    ○ 3. Impaired Swallowing.
    ○ 4. Impaired Physical Mobility.

50. The child has become withdrawn, and the mother asks the nurse what she should do. The nurse would suggest that the mother
    ○ 1. introduce the child to other children with JRA.
    ○ 2. spend extra time with the child and less time with her other children.
    ○ 3. send the child to a counselor.
    ○ 4. try to be supportive and understanding of the child.

The Client With a Fracture

A 1-year-old child has a fractured left femur as the result of an automobile accident. He is placed in Bryant traction.

51. The nurse should explain to the parent that this traction's primary purpose is to
- ○ 1. keep the broken bone in proper alignment.
- ○ 2. reduce muscle spasms so common in children.
- ○ 3. minimize demineralization of the femur.
- ○ 4. prevent infection at the insertion site.

52. When the child is in Bryant traction, the nurse should make sure that he is positioned on his back with his legs
- ○ 1. flexed at a 30-degree angle at the hips, with the hips touching the bed.
- ○ 2. flexed at a 90-degree angle, with the hips slightly off the bed.
- ○ 3. separated, with the affected leg at a right angle to the body and the unaffected leg in any comfortable position.
- ○ 4. straight in line, with his body resting flat on the bed.

53. The nurse should assess
- ○ 1. the line of pull of the traction.
- ○ 2. and replace the nonadhesive straps daily.
- ○ 3. the pin sites for signs of infection.
- ○ 4. for nighttime enuresis.

54. When caring for a child in Bryant traction, the nurse should
- ○ 1. allow the weights on the traction to hang freely.
- ○ 2. change the moleskin used on the legs for obtaining traction every other day.
- ○ 3. decrease the amount of weight on the traction to hang freely.
- ○ 4. remove the weights while inspecting the legs for evidence of friction over bony prominences.

A 15-month-old child is admitted with a fractured femur. The parents give different explanations for the injury.

55. Which of the following observations by the nurse would strongly suggest that this child has been abused? The child
- ○ 1. appears happy when personnel work with him.
- ○ 2. plays alongside others contentedly.
- ○ 3. is physically and emotionally underdeveloped for his age.
- ○ 4. sucks his thumb.

56. A nurse suspecting that this child has been abused by his parents should
- ○ 1. continue to collect information until there is no doubt that abuse has occurred.
- ○ 2. ensure that the findings are reported to the proper state authorities.
- ○ 3. keep the findings confidential because they are considered legal privileged communication between the nurse and the client.
- ○ 4. report the findings to the physician because that falls within the province of medical practice.

57. When planning interventions for abusive parents, the nurse should take into account that a common finding regarding abusive parents is that they
- ○ 1. are from a lower socioeconomic group.
- ○ 2. are unemployed.
- ○ 3. have low self-esteem.
- ○ 4. have lost emotional attachments to the family.

A preschool-aged child is brought to the emergency room with a broken right humerus. The child is fearful and cries, "Mommy, I want to go home. Is the doctor going to cut my arm? I hate the nurse."

58. Which of the following would be the most appropriate action for the nurse?
- ○ 1. Tell the parents they will need to wait out in the lobby.
- ○ 2. Ask the charge nurse to assign this client to another nurse.
- ○ 3. Use a doll to show the child what will be done to her arm.
- ○ 4. Ask the parents to discipline her so that the doctor can treat her.

59. Which of the following nursing diagnoses would be the *priority* for this child?
- ○ 1. Altered Self-Esteem.
- ○ 2. Fear.
- ○ 3. Altered Family Processes.
- ○ 4. Pain.

60. A cast is placed on the child's arm in the emergency department, and the nurse gives the parents discharge instructions. The nurse would evaluate the teaching as successful when the parents agree to seek medical advice if the child
- ○ 1. cannot extend the fingers on her right hand.
- ○ 2. vomits after her cast is applied.
- ○ 3. complains that the cast is cool and damp after 5 hours.
- ○ 4. is irritable and complains that the cast is heavy.

61. The nurse should teach the mother that for the first few days at home after casting
- ○ 1. she can use a hair dryer to dry the cast.

○ 2. the child should refrain from strenuous activities.

○ 3. she should check movement and sensation of the fingers once a day.

○ 4. allow the child to do the activities she wants to do.

The nurse examines a 3-year-old with a history of a recent injury to the left leg who refuses to walk and complains of pain when moving the leg.

62. The nurse would suspect the etiology of the problem to be
○ 1. behavioral regression.
○ 2. fracture.
○ 3. hysteria.
○ 4. traumatic paralysis.

63. When assessing the affected leg, the nurse would expect to find muscles that are
○ 1. atrophied
○ 2. contracted.
○ 3. flabby.
○ 4. normal.

64. The nurse notes that the child's left thigh is swollen. What should the nurse do next?
○ 1. Assess the neurologic status of the toes.
○ 2. Determine the circulatory status of the upper thigh.
○ 3. Take the child's vital signs.
○ 4. Notify the physician immediately.

65. The physician diagnoses a complete fracture of the femur and orders that the child be placed in Buck extension. When the mother asks why this treatment is being used, the nurse should explain that it is to
○ 1. immobilize the fracture before surgery.
○ 2. immobilize the fracture until realignment occurs.
○ 3. increase muscle spasms to enhance circulation.
○ 4. hold the bones in place until the cast can be applied tomorrow.

66. The nurse explains to the mother that Buck traction uses the weights that pull forward on the distal bone fragments to produce
○ 1. countertraction.
○ 2. friction.
○ 3. pressure.
○ 4. traction.

67. Anticipating the immobilized child's diversional needs, the nurse would offer him
○ 1. a video game.
○ 2. blocks.
○ 3. hand puppets.
○ 4. marbles.

68. The parents are unable to visit their son for more than 1 hour a day. (They have five other children and both work outside of the home.) The nurse recognizes expressions of guilt in both parents. To help alleviate this guilt, the nurse would make which of the following remarks?
○ 1. "I'm sure you feel guilty about not being able to visit often."
○ 2. "It's important that you visit even if only for 1 hour."
○ 3. "Not all parents can stay all the time."
○ 4. "Perhaps you could take turns visiting."

A spica cast is applied to a school-aged child with a fractured femur.

69. The child seems to adjust to the cast, except that he complains that it is too tight after each meal. The nurse should plan to
○ 1. give an enema that was ordered PRN.
○ 2. give smaller, more frequent meals.
○ 3. offer the child a mechanical soft diet.
○ 4. offer the child more fruits and grains.

70. The nurse would identify the need to do more teaching concerning skin care with the child's mother if she
○ 1. applies powder to the skin under the cast.
○ 2. checks the smoothness of the cast edges.
○ 3. covers the cast around the perineum with plastic film.
○ 4. inspects inside the cast.

71. The child suddenly develops chest pain, dyspnea, diaphoresis, and tachycardia. The nurse would suspect
○ 1. atelectasis.
○ 2. pneumonia.
○ 3. pulmonary edema.
○ 4. pulmonary emboli.

72. The nurse planning care for a child placed in a spica cast would identify the highest-priority nursing goal during the immediate postcasting period as preventing
○ 1. altered skin integrity.
○ 2. neurovascular impairment.
○ 3. respiratory impairment.
○ 4. gastrointestinal discomfort.

73. The nurse is helping a family plan for the discharge of their child, who will be going home in a spica cast. What information would be of *most* concern to the nurse?

○ 1. The bathrooms are all on the second floor.
○ 2. The child's bedroom is on the second floor.
○ 3. The child's 16-year-old sister will be responsible for the child during the day hours.
○ 4. There are three steps up to the front door.

A child goes home after having a cast put on for an open reduction of the radius. Several hours later, the child's mother telephones the hospital and tells the nurse that he is complaining of severe pain, has swollen and pale fingers, and cannot extend his fingers because of discomfort.

74. The nurse should advise the mother to
○ 1. administer an extra dose of pain medication.
○ 2. bring the child to the emergency room immediately.
○ 3. elevate the child's arm over the level of his heart.
○ 4. apply an ice bag over the fractured area.

The Client With Osteomyelitis

An 8-year-old child is hospitalized with osteomyelitis.

75. During initial assessment of a child with osteomyelitis of the left tibia, the nurse would expect the area over the tibia to have
○ 1. diffuse tenderness.
○ 2. decreased pain.
○ 3. increased warmth.
○ 4. localized edema.

76. The nurse assessing a child diagnosed with osteomyelitis would expect to find
○ 1. bradycardia.
○ 2. decreased pain on movement.
○ 3. fever.
○ 4. pulse deficits.

77. After receiving orders for laboratory tests and antibiotics, the nurse would plan to start the antibiotic after blood is drawn for
○ 1. creatinine.
○ 2. culture.
○ 3. hemoglobin.
○ 4. white blood cell count.

78. On reviewing the preliminary laboratory results, the nurse identifies which of the following findings consistent with the diagnosis of osteomyelitis?
○ 1. Hematocrit 30%.
○ 2. Erythrocyte sedimentation rate 17 mm/hour.
○ 3. Serum potassium 5.2 mEq/L.
○ 4. White blood cell count 12,000/mm^3.

79. The nurse explains the medical care plan to the child's mother. The plan would include long-term antibiotic therapy, bed rest, immobilization of the affected leg, and
○ 1. abduction of the affected leg.
○ 2. application of cool, moist packs to the affected leg.
○ 3. elevation of the affected leg.
○ 4. active range-of-motion exercises to the affected leg.

80. The nurse knows that a child being treated for osteomyelitis will be receiving intravenous antibiotic therapy for 3 to 4 weeks. Therefore, the nurse would plan to monitor the child's
○ 1. blood glucose level.
○ 2. thrombin times.
○ 3. urine glucose level.
○ 4. urine specific gravity.

81. To meet the developmental needs of a hospitalized 8-year-old with osteomyelitis, the nurse would include which measure in the plan of care?
○ 1. Encouraging the child to communicate with schoolmates.
○ 2. Encouraging the parents to stay with the child.
○ 3. Allowing siblings to visit freely.
○ 4. Talking to the child about his interests twice daily.

82. The nurse caring for a child on bed rest plans interventions to prevent skin breakdown. The nurse should keep in mind that the most effective way to prevent skin breakdown is
○ 1. attaching a trapeze to the bed.
○ 2. inspecting the skin every 8 hours.
○ 3. giving a back rub at bedtime.
○ 4. repositioning every 2 hours.

83. The nurse would encourage the child with osteomyelitis to choose which of the following meals?
○ 1. Beef and bean burrito with cheese, carrot and celery sticks, and an orange.
○ 2. Buttered wheat bread, cream of broccoli soup, tossed salad with dressing, and an apple.
○ 3. Potato soup; bacon, lettuce, and tomato sandwich; and an orange.
○ 4. Tomato soup, grilled cheese sandwich, and banana.

84. After 2 weeks of treatment for osteomyelitis, the child responds to the nurse's request to begin the bath by throwing the soap across the room. The nurse should recognize that the child is most likely responding to
○ 1. a dislike for the nurse.
○ 2. lack of control over the situation.
○ 3. separation from friends and classmates.
○ 4. pain from the doctor's check of her leg a few minutes before.

CORRECT ANSWERS AND RATIONALE

The letters in parentheses following the rationale identify the step of the nursing process (A, D, P, I, E), cognitive level (K, C, T, N), and client needs (S, G, L, H). See the Answer Grid for the key.

The Client With Musculoskeletal Dysfunction

1. 4. Legg-Calvé-Perthes disease, also known as *coxa plana* or *osteochondrosis,* is characterized by aseptic necrosis at the head of the femur when the blood supply to the area is interrupted. Avoiding weight bearing is especially important to prevent the head of the femur from leaving the acetabulum. Devices such as an abduction brace, a leg cast, or a harness sling are used to protect the affected joint while revascularization and bone healing occur. Surgical procedures are used in some cases. (P, N, G)

2. 3. Because most of the child's care takes place on an outpatient basis, the major emphasis for nursing care is to teach the family the care and management of the corrective device. Pain is usually not a problem once therapy has been initiated. There is no need to perform stretching exercises or increase protein intake if the child is eating a well-balanced diet. (P, N, G)

3. 2. *Kyphosis* is an abnormally increased convex angulation in the curvature of the thoracic spine. The most common cause of kyphosis in children is postural. *Equinovarus* refers to the foot being pointed downward and inward. *Lordosis* is the excessive anterior curvature of the lumbar spine due most often to an underlying neuromuscular disease or spinal deformity. *Scoliosis* is a lateral curvature of the spine. (A, K, G)

4. 4. In torticollis, the sternocleidomastoid muscle appears contracted, or shortened. Range of motion in the neck is limited. This condition causes the neck to turn laterally to one side, with the chin directed to the opposite side. (A, K, G)

5. 1. There is no treatment for flat feet; however, corrective shoes are often prescribed to keep the legs in proper alignment. Femoral anteversion (toeing in) is not associated with flat feet. Corrective shoes will not strengthen the arches or change weight bearing on the feet. (I, N, H)

6. 2. Muscular dystrophy, a genetically determined, sex-linked condition, is a progressive degenerative disease of the skeletal muscles. There are several different forms of muscle involvement. The various deviations that involve progressive weakness of muscle groups form the largest group of muscular diseases of childhood. (E, N, G)

7. 1. Lateral deviation of the spine (scoliosis) is assessed by having the child bend forward at the waist with her hands clasped, then looking for lateral curvature of the spine and a rib hump. (A, N, H)

8. 2. A characteristic sign of scoliosis is rib hump. The hump is best observed from the back and front when the child, undressed to the waist, bends over and lets her arms hang freely. The rib hump and flank asymmetry then become obvious. A slight limp, a crooked hemline, and complaints of back pain are other common findings in a child with scoliosis. (A, N, G)

9. 1. One of the most effective spinal braces for correcting scoliosis, the Milwaukee brace should be worn at all times, except when carrying out personal hygiene measures. (E, T, G)

10. 4. Exercises are prescribed for the child with scoliosis wearing a Milwaukee brace to help strengthen muscles that will help overcome the spinal curvature. Exercise also helps improve the correction of the spine and ribs and improves the child's stamina. (I, T, G)

11. 2. The osteochondroses are a group of diseases affecting various parts of the body; the most common one of this group is Osgood-Schlatter disease. This condition occurs mostly in boys between age 13 and 15 years, when epiphyseal growth is rapid. This growth places stress on muscles and tendons and eventually produces tendinitis, usually at the tibial tuberosity. Osgood-Schlatter disease is ordinarily self-limiting and usually responds to rest. It is seen in children who jump a lot. Ice applied over the painful area can promote comfort. (A, T, G)

The Client With Cerebral Palsy

12. 3. The goal of early recognition of primary developmental delays in children with cerebral palsy is to prevent secondary and tertiary delays. For example, a young infant who is unable to reach or focus on objects would be unable to attain various levels of sensory-perceptual development described by Piaget. Facilitating communication and encouraging health maintenance are all nursing goals for the child with cerebral palsy, but none is as important as the goal of early recognition of primary developmental delays. (I, N, H)

13. 3. *Cerebral palsy* is a collective term applied to nonprogressive cerebellar damage that results in various alterations in neuromuscular tone or function. (E, N, G)

14. 1. Spastic cerebral palsy, the most common clinical type, represents an upper motor neuron muscular impairment that may result in increased muscle tone and stretch reflexes, persistent reflexes, and a lack or delay of postural control. Dyskinetic movements are involuntary and may be manifested in athetoid movements. Ataxia is the least common type of cerebral palsy. Children have a wide-based gait and perform rapid repetitive movements poorly. With the atonic type, which is common, children have tremors and lack active movement. (I, N, G)

15. 1. Delay in reaching developmental milestones is a valuable clue in recognizing cerebral palsy. About 90% of toddlers can stoop and recover by 14 months of age. (A, N, H)

16. 1. Spasticity can cause the toddler to stand or walk on his toes. Use of the unaffected arm and leg to move is characteristic of hemiplegia. Facial grimacing is found with athetoid type, and wide-based gait is found with ataxic type. (A , N, G)

17. 1. Challenging the use of the affected limb facilitates increased function. Positioning the child upright and handing toys to his affected side will keep him occupied and may test his visual acuity, but neither of these is the reason for the activity. Similarly, this activity is not done to increase strength of the affected limb. (I, T, G)

18. 3. Most children with hemiparesis spastic cerebral palsy are able to walk. The motor deficit is usually greater in the upper extremity. The nurse should answer the mother's question honestly. The will to walk is important, but without neurologic stability, the child may be unable to do so. There is no need for the nurse to refer the mother to the physician for an answer to the question. (I, N, G)

19. 1. Lack of interaction with friends and family indicates an inability to cope with others' reactions and responses to the child with cerebral palsy. The need for further teaching and financial problems are of concern but do not indicate the type of response the family is having to the child's problems. (E, N, L)

The Client With Duchenne's Muscular Dystrophy

20. 3. Usually the first clinical manifestations of Duchenne's muscular dystrophy are difficulty running, riding a bicycle, and climbing stairs. Occasionally, enlarged calves may be noted. Muscular atrophy and contractures of the large joints are later signs (A, C, G)

21. 3. Duchenne's muscular dystrophy is an X-linked disorder primarily, and males are affected almost

exclusively because the mother carries the gene that is expressed in males. (I, C, G)

22. 4. In Gowers' sign, the child walks the hands up the legs in an attempt to stand. This is the common manner in which children afflicted with Duchenne's muscular dystrophy arise from sitting to standing. Galeazzi's sign refers to the shortening of the affected limb in congenital hip dislocation. Goodenough's sign refers to a test of mental age. Goodell's sign refers to the softening of the cervix, considered a sign of probable pregnancy. (D, C, G)

23. 3. The primary nursing diagnosis would be impaired physical mobility because of the disease process. All of the diagnoses listed are important, but impaired mobility is the most important. (D, N, G)

24. 3. The primary goal is to maintain function in unaffected muscles for as long as possible. There is no effective treatment for childhood muscular dystrophy. Children who remain active are able to avoid wheelchair confinement longer. Children with muscular dystrophy become socially isolated as their condition deteriorates and they can no longer keep up with friends. Maintaining function helps prevent social isolation. Circulatory impairment is not associated with muscular dystrophy. (P, N, H)

25. 3. The guilt feelings that mothers of children with muscular dystrophy commonly experience stem from the mother-to-son transmission of the defective gene. Disease onset is usually gradual. Congenital forms of muscular dystrophy are rare. (D, N, G)

26. 2. The usual cause of death in children with muscular dystrophy is respiratory tract infection or cardiac failure. The aunt is asking for information about the disease. The answer is not privileged information, so the nurse does not refer her to the parents. Talking to the child's doctor is not necessary at this point because the nurse can answer the question. (I, N, G)

27. 1. Muscular dystrophy is a progressive disease; affected children are usually unable to walk independently by age 9 to 11 years. There is no effective treatment for childhood muscular dystrophy. Children who remain active are able to avoid wheelchair confinement for a longer period, but activity does not prevent disease progression. (E, N, G)

The Client With Developmental Dysplasia of the Hip

28. 3. Ortolani's sign refers to the feeling of the femoral head slipping forward into the acetabulum when forward pressure is exerted from behind the greater trochanter and the knee is held laterally. This sign indicates hip dislocation. A positive Barlow's test indicates that the hip is unstable with increased risk of dislocation. Galeazzi's sign refers to shortening of the affected limb in congenital hip dysplasia. Trendelenburg's sign refers to a downward tilting of the pelvis toward the normal side when a child with a dislocated hip stands on the affected side with the uninvolved leg elevated. (D, C, G)

29. 2. In an older infant, the child may have a limp when weight bearing. With weight bearing, the pelvis tilts downward on the unaffected side instead of upward as it would normally. This is Trendelenburg's sign. Asymmetric thigh and gluteal folds and limited abduction of the affected leg are also seen. (A, C, G)

30. 1. The Pavlik (or Paulik) harness is worn over a diaper. Knee socks are also worn to prevent the straps and foot and leg pieces from rubbing directly on the skin. Lotions and powders can cake and irritate the skin. The skin should be inspected several times a day for red or irritated areas. (I, N, G)

31. 2. Assessing the learner's knowledge is the initial step in teaching. Giving parents written instructions and a list of community resources are appropriate strategies, but neither is the most appropriate initial step. Assessing coping strategies can provide important information to the development of the teaching plan but is not the initial step. (P, N, H)

32. 3. The abduction bar is incorporated into the cast to increase strength and cannot be removed or adjusted, unless the cast is removed and a new cast applied. The bar should never be used to lift or turn the client. (I, T, S)

33. 2. Neonates grow rapidly, and a cast that was adequate for a neonate may be outgrown in less than 1 month. The cast then becomes too tight, and circulation is impaired. If the child had surgery, the chances of infection are minimal after a 4-week period and would be accompanied by other symptoms such as fever. The cotton wadding used to line the cast does not shrink over time. (D, N, G)

34. 2. The child in a hip spica cast needs a specially designed car seat. The one that the mother already has will not be appropriate because of the need for the car seat to accommodate the cast. (I, N, H)

35. 3. Using a feeding table or modified high chair are best for a child who is used to sitting up for feedings. (I, T, H)

The Client With Congenital Clubfoot

36. 3. Management of the infant with a clubfoot deformity starts as soon as possible after birth. Treatment in early infancy is conservative. Depending on the severity of the deformity, it may consist of manipulating the feet into a functional position and applying a series of casts until a marked overcorrection

is achieved. Corrective shoes may be used once the deformity has been corrected. (I, N, G)

37. 3. When an infant is born with an unexpected anomaly, parents are faced with questions, uncertainties, and possible disappointments. They may feel inadequate, helpless, and anxious. The nurse can help the parents initially by assessing their concerns and providing appropriate information to help them clarify or resolve the immediate problems. (I, N, L)

38. 1. Complete drying of a plaster cast takes several hours. Turning the child with a newly applied cast at least every 2 hours helps the cast dry uniformly. The drying cast must be handled with the palms only, to prevent indentations from the fingers, which could cause pressure areas. Dryers are not used to dry the cast because they dry the cast on the surface but not underneath. Furthermore, heat may be conducted to the tissues through the wet cast, causing burns. The cast must not be coated with any substance that would inhibit the evaporation of moisture from the plaster. (I, T, S)

39. 3. A too-tight cast can cause a tourniquet effect and compromise the neurovascular integrity of the extremity. Manifestations of neurovascular impairment include pain, edema, pulselessness, coolness, altered sensation, and inability to move the distal exposed extremity. The cast should be assessed frequently. Wetting a cast with water and soap softens the plaster, which may alter the cast's effectiveness. Adhesive tape petals are applied to cover the rough edges of the cast and are left in place. There is no reason to elevate the casted extremities when a child is being treated for clubfoot with nonsurgical measures. (E, N, G)

40. 3. Casts may have to be changed every 1 to 2 weeks in an infant with a clubfoot deformity because of the infant's rapid growth. The frequent cast changes have nothing to do with infection. Infants with a cast are a little more awkward to care for, but that does not necessitate frequent appointments. (I, N, G)

41. 2. The Denis Browne splint is an adjustable metal bar to which special shoes are attached. This splint provides an appropriate degree of eversion, dorsiflexion, and rotation to keep the feet in a slightly overcorrected position. When the infant kicks, the feet are automatically moved into a corrected position. (I, T, G)

42. 3. If the shoes become loose, they are tightened against the Denis Browne splint. The shoes and foot pieces are set at a particular angle to maintain the correction achieved through casting. The angle of the shoes on the bar should not be repositioned. Parents should put socks on the child's feet before applying the splint to decrease irritation. The splint should not be used as a weight-bearing device when lifting the child. (E, T, S)

43. 4. When an infant begins to become mobile, child-proofing the home is necessary. One important aspect of child-proofing is removing tablecloths, so the child cannot pull on them in an attempt to stand, and thus either fall or pull objects on top of him. The child in the Denis Browne splint needs opportunities to increase mobility to achieve developmental tasks. Increasing mobility is not an indication to remove the splint or to obtain corrective shoes. (I, N, S)

The Client With Juvenile Rheumatoid Arthritis

44. 4. There is no definitive test for JRA. The latex fixation test, which is commonly used to diagnose arthritis in adults, is negative in 90% of children. Synovial fluid cultures are done to rule out septic arthritis. Erythrocyte sedimentation rate may or may not be elevated during active disease. (I, T, G)

45. 1. In most children with JRA, the disease will be in permanent remission by adolescence. Seventy-five percent of the children go into long remissions without severe deformity or functional loss. Only relatively few children recover completely within a few years. (I, T, G)

46. 2. Socialization is important for this preschool-aged child, and activity is important to maintain function. Because children with JRA have the most trouble in the early morning after arising, however, they need more time to "warm up." Splints are worn during periods of rest, not activity, to maintain function. (I, N, G)

47. 1. Applying moist heat to affected joints at any time may facilitate joint movement. Heat increases circulation, decreases pain, and increases mobility. Although exercise is important, weight bearing on affected joints is restricted when joints are affected by the disease, as evidenced by pain and edema. Cool compresses constrict and decrease circulation. The mattress should be firm for better support of the joints. (P, N, G)

48. 3. The first group of drugs prescribed are the nonsteroidal antiinflammatory drugs. Aspirin is included in this group. Aspirin is in some over-the-counter medications, so the family should check with the nurse before buying them. Once aspirin is started, it takes a matter of hours or days for the relief of pain to occur. In 3 to 4 weeks, the antiinflammatory effects occur, including reduction in swelling and less pain with movement. The missed dose will need to be made up to maintain the serum level of aspirin. (P, N, H)

49. 4. A child with juvenile rheumatoid arthritis would have as a nursing diagnosis Impaired Physical Mobility. Impaired Swallowing, Ineffective Airway Clearance, and Total Incontinence are not related to this medical diagnosis. (D, T, G)

50. 4. Parents need to be supportive and understanding of the child while dealing with the grief and loss associated with chronic illness. The child needs to feel valued but may experience secondary gain from the illness if the family interaction patterns are altered. Psychological counseling is not needed at this time because the reaction is normal. Peer support is not effective with a 4-year-old, because a child at this age is developmentally egocentric. (I, N, L)

The Client With a Fracture

51. 1. The primary purpose of traction is to achieve appropriate anatomic alignment. Traction immobilizes bone fragments until sufficient healing has occurred to allow cast application. Muscle spasms are much more common in adults. Traction has no role in preventing infection. (I, C, G)

52. 2. When placed in Bryant traction, the child should be on the back, with the legs flexed at a 90-degree angle at the hips and with the hips raised slightly off the bed. This position provides adequate countertraction to reduce and immobilize the fracture. (I, T, S)

53. 1. The nurse should assess the line of pull of the traction frequently. Nonadhesive straps are used to anchor this type of traction, not pins, and these strips are changed only when ordered by the physician. Nighttime enuresis is bed-wetting at night; a 1-year-old would not be expected to be toilet-trained. (A, N, S)

54. 1. Weights for traction must be allowed to hang freely to maintain consistent traction. Changing the moleskins used for securing an infant's traction and decreasing the amount of weight could result in a return of the bone fragments to a misaligned position, with possible resulting soft tissue damage. The bony prominence can be assessed without releasing weights. Traction should be maintained unless a specific order is given with other directions. (I, N, S)

55. 3. An almost universal finding in descriptions of abused children is underdevelopment for age. This may be reflected in small physical size or in poor psychosocial development. The child should be evaluated further until a plausible diagnosis can be established. A child sucking his thumb contentedly and playing alongside others is exhibiting normal behavior. Abused children tend to be suspicious of others, especially adults. (A, N, L)

56. 2. Evidence of child abuse is legally reportable by anyone who works with children. The nurse should ensure that the findings are reported. Laws ordinarily provide immunity from legal actions for people required to report suspicion of child abuse, if the report is done in good faith. Suspicion, not absolute proof, is necessary for reporting abuse. The nurse's primary responsibility is to the primary client, the child. (I, C, S)

57. 3. Parents who are abusive often suffer from low self-esteem, and the nurse should work to bolster their self-esteem. This can be achieved by praising the parents for appropriate parenting. Employment status and socioeconomic status are not indicators of abusive parents. Abusive parents usually are attached to their children and do not want to give them up to foster care. (P, C, L)

58. 3. Explaining what will happen in language that a child can comprehend through the use of a doll is enough to dispel fears of the unknown. The child needs the parents for support. The child's reaction to the nurse is normal for a child this age and does not usually call for a change in staff assignments. Asking the parents to discipline her for her behavior is inappropriate. (I, N, L)

59. 2. Fear in a preschool-age child normally centers around mutilation and disfigurement. Infants and toddlers most fear separation from parents. School-aged children most fear loss of self-control. The child who has little experience with casting may not be worried about pain specifically. (D, N, L)

60. 1. Inability to extend the fingers of the involved arm may indicate neurologic impairment caused by pressure on soft tissue. The cast will seem heavy until the child adjusts to the extra weight. Cast drying may take 12 or more hours; the dampness causes the sensation of coolness. It is not unusual for a child to vomit after sustaining an injury. (E, N, G)

61. 2. The child should not engage in strenuous activities for a few days. Using a hair dryer to complete the drying of the cast is not encouraged because the hair dryer only dries the outside of the cast. Movement and sensation of the fingers need to be checked several times a day for the first few days. (I, T, S)

62. 2. A fracture should be suspected if an injured child who previously walked without problems refuses to walk after the injury. Pseudoparalysis from pain is found in young children with fractures. Behavioral regression usually does not take the form of refusing to walk. Hysteria usually presents with seizures, abdominal pain, and headaches and is the result of a traumatic situation. (A, T, G)

63. 2. Immediately after a fracture, the muscles contract and physiologically splint the injured area. This phenomenon also accounts for the deformity that results as the muscles pull the bone ends out of alignment. (A, C, G)

64. 1. Assessing the neurologic and circulatory status of the toes, the tissues distal to the fracture, is important. Soft tissue contusions, which frequently accompany femur fractures, can result in severe hemorrhage into the tissue and subsequent circulatory and neurologic impairment. The nurse can document the findings after assessing the leg. There is no need to notify the physician with the finding of edema surrounding the fracture site unless it is causing problems. Vital signs do not help determine why the thigh is swollen. (I, N, G)

65. 2. Buck extension is a type of skin traction used to align and immobilize bone fragments. It is also used to relieve muscle spasms, which enhances circulation and decreases pain. (I, C, G)

66. 4. *Traction* is the forward force produced by attaching weight to a distal bone fragment. *Countertraction* is the backward force of the muscle pull. *Friction* is the force between the client and bed; together with countertraction, it achieves balance. Pressure is not a component of traction. (I, T, G)

67. 3. Hand puppets would enable a 3-year-old child in Buck traction to act out feelings within the constraints imposed by the traction. Marbles are unsafe at this age because they can be swallowed. Blocks are appropriate for a younger child; besides, there is no flat surface available for the child to set blocks. Video games can make him too active in bed and do not meet the child's developmental needs. (P, N, H)

68. 2. Stressing that the parents visit when they can will help to alleviate the guilt they feel. Acknowledging the guilt gives the parents an opportunity to talk about it but does not help alleviate it. Suggesting that the parents take turns visiting implies that they should feel guilty because they may not be doing all they could. Comparing them with other parents does not alleviate guilt feelings. (I, N, L)

69. 2. The spica cast encircles the abdomen, and the addition of a large meal to the stomach may cause the cast to become too snug. If the child's appetite was decreased in conjunction with a feeling of fullness, the nurse might suspect that the child was becoming constipated and plan to use laxatives or a higher-fiber diet. A soft diet is indicated when the child has difficulty chewing food adequately. (P, N, G)

70. 1. Powder should not be applied to skin beneath the cast because it can cause irritation and skin breakdown. Checking the smoothness of the cast edges, covering the cast around the perineum, and inspecting inside the cast can help prevent skin breakdown. (E, T, S)

71. 4. Chest pain and dyspnea in an immobilized adolescent with a large bone fracture suggests a fat embolus, in which fat droplets are transferred from the marrow into the general blood stream by the venous arterial route and may eventually reach the lung or brain. Atelectasis and pneumonia can occur but do not usually develop suddenly. Pulmonary edema should not be a problem in a healthy adolescent who has sustained a fracture. (D, N, G)

72. 2. A cast that is too tight (always a possibility in the immediate postcasting period) can cause neurovascular impairment. Respiratory, skin, and gastrointestinal problems would not develop in the immediate postcasting period, although their prevention would be a long-term nursing goal. (P, N, G)

73. 2. The child will need to have his bed moved to an area that is more central to the family life. The child can be carried up and down the three steps to the house the few times necessary after discharge, but negotiating a flight of steps with a school-aged child in a cast at least twice a day would be difficult, if not dangerous. The child will need to use a bedpan or urinal, so the bathrooms can be on any floor. Because the family is involved in the discharge, the 16-year-old should be taught appropriate care with the rest of the family. (P, N, H)

74. 2. Extreme pain (especially when the part distal to the injury is moved), sudden edema, and pale extremities distal to the injury are symptoms of compartment syndrome. Compartment syndrome must be treated immediately to prevent major neurologic and circulatory impairment. The first step usually is to split the cast to accommodate the edema. Elevating the arm, administering more medication, and applying ice over the fracture would not be effective at this time. (I, N, G)

The Client With Osteomyelitis

75. 3. Findings associated with osteomyelitis commonly include pain over the area, increased warmth, localized tenderness, and diffuse swelling over the involved bone. The area over the affected bone is red. (A, T, G)

76. 3. Elevated temperature, increased pulse and respiratory rates, and increased pain with movement are clinical manifestations of osteomyelitis. Pulse deficit is associated with atrial fibrillation. (A, T, G)

77. 2. Antibiotic therapy starts after blood cultures are drawn. The blood cultures determine the causative organism. The initial antibiotic therapy may be inappropriate for the causative organism and may need to be altered. (I, T, G)

78. 2. In osteomyelitis, the erythrocyte sedimentation rate is elevated (for a child, the normal range is 0 to 13 mm/hour). The erythrocyte sedimentation rate rises in the presence of severe localized or systemic inflammation. The leukocyte count in osteomyelitis is elevated (15,000 to 25,000 mm^3). Hematocrit and potassium levels should be normal. (D, N, G)

79. 3. The affected leg should be elevated and warm moist packs applied to the affected area. This helps decrease the swelling and improves circulation. Good body alignment is maintained; neither leg is abducted. Active range-of-motion exercises are performed on the unaffected leg. (I, T, G)

80. 4. Long-term, high-dose antibiotic therapy can adversely affect renal, hepatic, and hematopoietic function. Therefore, these systems should be assessed carefully. Antibiotics do not usually affect blood glucose level, thrombin time, or urine glucose level. Renal impairment, however, may be reflected in the kidneys' decreased ability to concentrate or dilute urine. (A, N, G)

81. 1. Encouraging contact with schoolmates allows the school-aged child to maintain and develop socialization with peers, an important developmental task of this age group. Although having family visits and interacting with the child are important, they do not meet developmental needs. (I, N, H)

82. 4. The most effective intervention to prevent skin breakdown is to reposition the client frequently. Although a trapeze might encourage the child to change position, it does not guarantee that the child will do so. Inspecting the skin is not an intervention to prevent skin breakdown, but rather an evaluation strategy. A back rub will increase circulation to the back and sacral areas but is not the most effective intervention to prevent skin breakdown. A high-fiber diet will help prevent constipation. (I, N, S)

83. 1. Children with osteomyelitis need a diet high in protein and calories. Milk, eggs, cheese, meat, fish, and vegetables such as beans are the best sources of these nutrients. (I, N, G)

84. 2. School-aged children have an increasing need for independence. Anger and resentment are common responses to dependence and loss of control over the environment, with minimal opportunity to participate in planning and decision making. (D, N, L)

NURSING CARE OF CHILDREN

TEST 8: The Child With Musculoskeletal Health Problems

Directions: Use this answer grid to determine areas of strength or need for further study.

NURSING PROCESS

A = Assessment
D = Analysis, nursing diagnosis
P = Planning
I = Implementation
E = Evaluation

COGNITIVE LEVEL

K = Knowledge
C = Comprehension
T = Application
N = Analysis

CLIENT NEEDS

S = Safe, effective care environment
G = Physiologic integrity
L = Psychosocial integrity
H = Health promotion and maintenance

Question #	Answer #	A	D	P	I	E	K	C	T	N	S	G	L	H
1	4			P						N		G		
2	3			P						N		G		
3	2	A					K					G		
4	4	A					K					G		
5	1				I					N				H
6	2					E				N		G		
7	1	A								N				H
8	2	A								N		G		
9	1					E			T			G		
10	4				I				T			G		
11	2	A							T			G		
12	3				I					N				H
13	3					E				N		G		
14	1				I					N		G		
15	1	A								N				H
16	1	A								N		G		
17	1				I				T			G		
18	3				I					N		G		
19	1					E				N			L	
20	3	A						C				G		
21	3				I			C				G		
22	4		D					C				G		
23	3		D							N		G		
24	3			P						N				H
25	3		D							N		G		

NURSING PROCESS

A = Assessment
D = Analysis, nursing diagnosis
P = Planning
I = Implementation
E = Evaluation

COGNITIVE LEVEL

K = Knowledge
C = Comprehension
T = Application
N = Analysis

CLIENT NEEDS

S = Safe, effective care environment
G = Physiologic integrity
L = Psychosocial integrity
H = Health promotion and maintenance

Question #	Answer #	Nursing Process					Cognitive Level				Client Needs			
		A	D	P	I	E	K	C	T	N	S	G	L	H
26	2				I					N		G		
27	1					E				N		G		
28	3		D					C				G		
29	2	A						C				G		
30	1				I					N		G		
31	2			P						N				H
32	3				I				T		S			
33	2		D							N		G		
34	2				I					N				H
35	3				I				T					H
36	3				I					N		G		
37	3				I					N			L	
38	1				I				T		S			
39	3					E				N		G		
40	3				I					N		G		
41	2				I				T			G		
42	3					E			T		S			
43	4				I					N	S			
44	4				I				T			G		
45	1				I					N		G		
46	2				I					N		G		
47	1			P						N		G		
48	3			P						N				H
49	4		D						T			G		
50	4				I					N			L	
51	1				I			C				G		
52	2				I				T		S			
53	1	A								N	S			
54	1				I					N	S			
55	3	A								N			L	

NURSING PROCESS

A = Assessment
D = Analysis, nursing diagnosis
P = Planning
I = Implementation
E = Evaluation

COGNITIVE LEVEL

K = Knowledge
C = Comprehension
T = Application
N = Analysis

CLIENT NEEDS

S = Safe, effective care environment
G = Physiologic integrity
L = Psychosocial integrity
H = Health promotion and maintenance

Question #	Answer #	Nursing Process					Cognitive Level				Client Needs			
		A	D	P	I	E	K	C	T	N	S	G	L	H
56	2				I			C			S			
57	3			P				C					L	
58	3				I					N			L	
59	2		D							N			L	
60	1					E				N		G		
61	2				I				T		S			
62	2	A							T			G		
63	2	A						C				G		
64	1				I					N		G		
65	2				I			C				G		
66	4				I				T			G		
67	3			P						N				H
68	2				I					N			L	
69	2			P						N		G		
70	1					E			T		S			
71	4		D							N		G		
72	2			P						N		G		
73	2			P						N				H
74	2				I					N		G		
75	3	A							T			G		
76	3	A							T			G		
77	2				I				T			G		
78	2		D							N		G		
79	3				I				T			G		
80	4	A								N		G		
81	1				I					N				H
82	4				I					N	S			
83	1				I					N		G		
84	2		D							N			L	

ANSWER GRID: 3

NURSING PROCESS

A = Assessment
D = Analysis, nursing diagnosis
P = Planning
I = Implementation
E = Evaluation

COGNITIVE LEVEL

K = Knowledge
C = Comprehension
T = Application
N = Analysis

CLIENT NEEDS

S = Safe, effective care environment
G = Physiologic integrity
L = Psychosocial integrity
H = Health promotion and maintenance

Question #	Answer #	Nursing Process					Cognitive Level				Client Needs			
		A	D	P	I	E	K	C	T	N	S	G	L	H
Number Correct														
Number Possible	84	16	10	11	38	9	2	10	21	51	11	52	9	12
Percentage Correct														

Score Calculation: To determine your **Percentage Correct,** divide the **Number Correct** by the **Number Possible.**

ANSWER GRID: 4

The Child With Dermatologic, Endocrine, and Other Health Problems

- **The Client Who Is Preterm**
- **The Client Who Is Septic**
- **The Client With Failure to Thrive**
- **The Client With Atopic Dermatitis**
- **The Client With Burns**
- **The Client With Hypothyroidism**
- **The Client With Insulin-Dependent Diabetes Mellitus**
- **The Client Who Is Abused**
- **Correct Answers and Rationale**

Select the one best answer, and indicate your choice by filling in the circle in front of the option.

The Client Who Is Preterm

A male neonate born prematurely and who is small for gestational age is placed in the intensive care nursery.

1. On assessment, the nurse would expect this neonate to display
   - ○ 1. firm cartilage to the edge of the ear pinna.
   - ○ 2. elbows that can be brought to the midline of the chest with resistance past the midline.
   - ○ 3. fine, downy hair over the upper arms and back.
   - ○ 4. prominent creases on the soles and heels.
2. During the physical assessment, the nurse would also expect to see
   - ○ 1. an abundance of scalp hair.
   - ○ 2. a thin, wasted appearance.
   - ○ 3. descended testicles.
   - ○ 4. numerous rugae on the scrotum.
3. The neonate is suffering from cold stress. The nurse should be especially alert for
   - ○ 1. a yellowish undercast to the skin color.
   - ○ 2. increased abdominal girth.
   - ○ 3. hyperactivity and twitching.
   - ○ 4. slow respirations.
4. Which of the following laboratory values would the nurse associate with cold stress in a 1-day-old preterm neonate?
   - ○ 1. Bilirubin level of 13 mg/dL.
   - ○ 2. Glucose level of 15 mg/dL.
   - ○ 3. Hematocrit of 65%.
   - ○ 4. Hemoglobin level of 23.5 g/dL.
5. The infant is subjected to repeated blood withdrawals for laboratory specimens. The nurse should plan to maintain a careful record of the
   - ○ 1. amount of blood drawn for each specimen.
   - ○ 2. color of each blood specimen.
   - ○ 3. vital signs before each blood draw.
   - ○ 4. last time the neonate was fed before each specimen is collected.
6. The neonate weighs 1870 g and has a respiratory rate of 46 breaths/minute, a pulse rate of 175 beats/minute, and a serum pH of 7.11. He is to receive sodium bicarbonate intravenously. The nurse would know that the sodium bicarbonate is being given to alleviate

○ 1. edema.

○ 2. dehydration.

○ 3. metabolic acidosis.

○ 4. respiratory alkalosis.

7. The neonate is being given oxygen as a treatment for cold stress. The nurse would evaluate the oxygen therapy as achieving the desired effect when the child's

○ 1. heart rate is 200 beats/minute at rest.

○ 2. respiratory rate is 48 breaths/minute at rest.

○ 3. axillary temperature is 98°F.

○ 4. blood pressure is 56/30 mm Hg.

8. The nurse is careful to document the neonate's response to oxygen therapy and to deliver only as much oxygen as is necessary to prevent the development of

○ 1. cataracts.

○ 2. glaucoma.

○ 3. ophthalmia neonatorum.

○ 4. retinopathy of prematurity.

9. The neonate is to be fed by gavage. The nurse should introduce the catheter into the stomach and check placement by

○ 1. aspirating stomach contents through the catheter with a syringe.

○ 2. inserting a small amount of air into the catheter and auscultating for clear breath sounds.

○ 3. introducing water into the catheter and aspirating it back.

○ 4. flushing the catheter with a small amount of water.

10. The neonate is receiving his first feeding by nipple. The nurse would plan to first give the neonate a 5 mL feeding of sterile water to

○ 1. ascertain the patency of the neonate's esophagus.

○ 2. determine whether the neonate can retain the feeding.

○ 3. ensure that the neonate has the energy to take oral feedings.

○ 4. ensure that the mother will be able to feed the neonate.

11. The parents express concern about their neonate's condition. To meet the short-term goals of decreasing the parent's fears and fostering bonding, the nurse should plan to

○ 1. allow the parents to see and touch their neonate.

○ 2. arrange for a visit with another couple who have an ill preterm neonate.

○ 3. encourage the parents to participate in the neonate's care.

○ 4. tell the parents how well their son is doing and not to worry.

12. A nurse working in a neonatal intensive care unit is developing policies to help control infection. Which

policy would dictate the use of the single most effective means of preventing the spread of infection?

○ 1. Having everyone who comes in contact with neonates perform frequent hand and arm washing.

○ 2. Keeping each neonate in an isolation incubator that is opened as infrequently as possible.

○ 3. Maintaining a ventilation system in the unit that provides for continuous clean-air exchange.

○ 4. Requiring everyone who comes in contact with neonates to wear gowns and masks.

The Client Who Is Septic

A 10-day-old neonate is brought to the clinic by the parents. The neonate is lethargic and tachypneic and has a heart rate of 200 beats/minute.

13. The nurse's initial focus should be on the neonate's

○ 1. temperature pattern.

○ 2. number of wet diapers in the past 24 hours.

○ 3. pupillary response.

○ 4. sleep patterns.

14. The mother feels guilty because she did not realize her newborn was sick. What would be the nurse's best response to the mother's statement of her feelings?

○ 1. "You should have realized something was wrong; he is your son."

○ 2. "Did you read the newborn booklet sent home with you from the hospital?"

○ 3. "What you are feeling is normal; next time, you will know what to look for."

○ 4. "Babies can get sick quickly, and parents do not always realize it."

15. In planning care, the nurse would anticipate which of the following?

○ 1. Vital signs will be monitored every 6 hours.

○ 2. The intravenous line will only be used to administer antibiotics.

○ 3. The infant will have formula withheld.

○ 4. The infant will be weighed every other day.

16. The nurse and doctor plan care for the neonate. The pharmacologic plan of care would likely include

○ 1. ampicillin and gentamicin.

○ 2. furosemide and kanamycin.

○ 3. gentamicin and vitamin K.

○ 4. phenytoin sodium and ampicillin.

17. The nurse caring for the neonate would be worried about the onset of septic shock if the neonate's

○ 1. axillary temperature is 99.8°F.

○ 2. blood pressure is 45/25 mm Hg.

○ 3. heart rate during sleep is 205 beats/minute.

○ 4. respiratory rate while awake is 32 breaths/minute.

18. The neonate is to be admitted to the hospital. The mother is crying and is very upset. The nurse's best response to the mother would be
○ 1. "Please don't worry; everything will be all right."
○ 2. "The doctor knows what he's doing, so there is nothing to worry about."
○ 3. "What is it that is making you cry right now?"
○ 4. "You did the right thing to bring your infant here when you did."

19. The nurse notes that the neonate is using the abdominal muscles to breathe and has a respiratory rate of 30 breaths/minute. The nurse should
○ 1. chart the findings.
○ 2. check oxygen saturation with a pulse oximeter.
○ 3. notify the physician of the findings.
○ 4. apply oxygen immediately to the infant.

The Client With Failure to Thrive

A 5-month-old infant is brought to the clinic by his parents because he "cries too much" and "vomits a lot." The infant's birth weight was 6 pounds, 10 ounces, and his current weight is 7 pounds, 4 ounces.

20. Which of the following data would the nurse identify as most important?
○ 1. Regular checkups at the neighborhood clinic.
○ 2. Feeding pattern.
○ 3. Pattern of weight gain.
○ 4. Family dynamics.

21. Which of the following information obtained during a health history is consistent with the diagnosis of failure to thrive? The child
○ 1. fusses during feedings.
○ 2. is fearful of strangers.
○ 3. is quiet only when being held.
○ 4. has to be awakened for feedings.

22. The nurse formulates the nursing diagnosis Altered Nutrition: Less than Body Requirements related to negative feeding patterns. To meet the short-term goals of the infant's care plan, the nurse would plan to
○ 1. have the parents feed the infant whenever possible.
○ 2. give infant formula that has 24 calories per ounce.
○ 3. provide consistent staff to care for the infant.
○ 4. have the infant sit in a high chair during feedings.

23. When observing the infant's mother feed the infant, the nurse would be concerned if the mother

○ 1. tries to maintain eye contact with the infant.
○ 2. talks to the infant during the feeding.
○ 3. places the infant in the crib for the feeding.
○ 4. sits on the floor to feed the infant.

24. The infant is to be discharged, and the health team believes that the family will need follow-up care. The most effective type of follow-up would be
○ 1. daily phone calls from the hospital nurse.
○ 2. enrollment in community parenting classes.
○ 3. twice-weekly clinic appointments.
○ 4. weekly visits by a community health nurse.

25. The mother expresses concern that picking up the infant whenever he cries will spoil him. What would be the nurse's best response?
○ 1. "Allow him to cry for no longer than 45 minutes, then pick him up."
○ 2. "Babies need comforting and cuddling; meeting these needs will not spoil him."
○ 3. "Babies this young cry when they're hungry; try feeding him when he cries."
○ 4. "If it seems as if nothing is wrong, don't pick him up; the crying will stop eventually."

The Client With Atopic Dermatitis

A 4-month-old infant comes to the clinic with persistent pruritic eczema. The lesions have become infected, and the physician has ordered oral antibiotics.

26. The nurse tells the mother that she can best meet the needs of this infant by
○ 1. limiting how many times the grandmother can visit.
○ 2. putting him in a room with a sibling.
○ 3. having the television on in his room so he can hear other voices.
○ 4. picking him up when he fusses.

27. When choosing nightclothes for an infant with atopic dermatitis, which of the following would the nurse suggest to the mother?
○ 1. A diaper and short-sleeved shirt.
○ 2. One-piece cotton pajamas with long sleeves.
○ 3. Two-piece flannel pajamas with short sleeves.
○ 4. A woolen sleeper with feet and mittens.

28. The mother is to apply a lotion containing lanolin and urea to the infant's skin lesions. The goal of this treatment is to
○ 1. decrease the inflammatory response.
○ 2. dry the lesions.
○ 3. hydrate the skin.
○ 4. prevent infection.

29. The nurse would instruct the mother about the care of the skin to

○ 1. soak the child in a tub for 30 minutes to soften the skin.

○ 2. use a mild soap followed by patting the skin to dry it.

○ 3. use an antibacterial soap two times a week.

○ 4. wash clothes in a strong detergent to prevent infections.

The mother and nurse are planning home care for a 3-year-old child with eczema.

30. The nurse should teach the mother to remove which of the following from the child's environment at home?

○ 1. Metal toy trucks.

○ 2. Plastic figures.

○ 3. Stuffed animals.

○ 4. Wooden blocks.

31. The mother tells the community health nurse that her child usually scratches his lesions until they bleed during the night. The nurse would recommend which medication to sedate the child and help relieve the pruritus?

○ 1. Acetaminophen.

○ 2. Chloral hydrate.

○ 3. Diphenhydramine.

○ 4. Auralgan.

The Client With Burns

A 5-year-old boy is admitted to the hospital with severe burns on his legs, head, and lower abdomen and minor burns on other surfaces.

32. The nurse, using the "rule of nines" to estimate the burned area on the body, would allocate a larger percentage of total surface area for this child if the burns were on the child's

○ 1. head and neck.

○ 2. lower extremities.

○ 3. upper extremities.

○ 4. posterior and anterior chest.

33. The nurse would immediately do which of the following?

○ 1. Start an intravenous line.

○ 2. Begin ordered antibiotics orally.

○ 3. Anchor a Foley catheter.

○ 4. Obtain baseline laboratory studies.

34. The nurse would formulate a plan of care for the child that includes the nursing diagnosis Fluid Volume Deficit related to an initial primary shift in plasma from

○ 1. intracellular to intravascular spaces.

○ 2. intravascular to interstitial spaces.

○ 3. intracellular to interstitial spaces.

○ 4. interstitial to intravascular spaces.

35. The nurse anchors a Foley catheter to

○ 1. monitor for a urinary tract infection.

○ 2. measure urine output accurately.

○ 3. prevent urine retention.

○ 4. assess urine specific gravity.

36. The nurse observing which of the following signs would suspect that the child is receiving too much intravenous fluid too rapidly?

○ 1. Marked increase in abdominal girth.

○ 2. Protein in the urine.

○ 3. Dark amber urine.

○ 4. Moist rales in the lung fields.

37. The child becomes angry and combative when it is time to change the dressings and apply mafenide acetate (Sulfamylon). The child will respond best if he

○ 1. has parental support during the dressing changes.

○ 2. is allowed to assist the nurse in removing the dressings and applying the cream.

○ 3. is given permission to cry during the procedure.

○ 4. can schedule the time for his dressing changes.

38. The child has a decreased interest in food. The nurse and mother develop a plan of care to increase the child's intake. Which of the following suggestions made by the mother would indicate that she needs additional teaching?

○ 1. Allowing the mother to feed the child.

○ 2. Withholding dessert and treats unless meals are eaten.

○ 3. Offering the child finger foods that he likes.

○ 4. Serving smaller and more frequent meals.

39. On reviewing the child's laboratory results, the nurse notes a serum potassium level of 3.3 mEq/L. The nurse would decide to encourage the child to drink

○ 1. cranberry juice.

○ 2. apple juice.

○ 3. grape juice.

○ 4. orange juice.

40. When administering the 15th dose of an antibiotic intravenously to the child, the nurse notes that the child is scratching at the intravenous site on the forearm and also notes small, circumscribed, elevated areas on the same arm. The nurse would

○ 1. apply a cold compress to the area and continue to deliver the antibiotic.

2. assess the intravenous site for localized edema or redness.
3. remove the intravenous line, and restart it in another area.
4. stop the infusion of the antibiotic, but continue the intravenous fluids.

41. The nurse is concerned about the child's fluid balance. The nurse would judge that the child is receiving too little fluid when he
1. becomes increasingly irritable.
2. has a urine output of 26 mL for the past hour.
3. has a urine specific gravity of 1.033.
4. has had an increase in blood pressure within the past 3 hours.

42. The nurse teaches the child's mother about the importance of specific nutritional support in burn management. The nurse would judge that the teaching needs to be reinforced if the mother chose which of the following from the diet menu for her child?
1. A bacon, lettuce, and tomato sandwich; milk; and celery and carrot sticks.
2. A cheeseburger, cottage cheese and pineapple salad, chocolate milk, and a brownie.
3. Chicken nuggets, orange and grapefruit sections, and a vanilla milkshake.
4. A beef, bean, and cheese burrito; a banana; fruit-flavored yogurt; and skim milk.

43. The nurse would follow the Centers for Disease Control and Prevention guidelines concerning sterile gloves by wearing them
1. as an optional precautionary measure.
2. when delivering care that would necessitate touching the child.
3. when entering the child's room.
4. when giving direct care to burned areas.

44. The child has infected burns, and the physician orders 250 mg of an antibiotic every 6 hours. The normal dosage for this antibiotic and condition is 20 to 50 mg/kg/24 hours. The child weighs 25 kg. The nurse should
1. carry out the order.
2. give the dose recommended by the pharmacy reference material.
3. question the order because the dose is too low.
4. question the order because the dose is too high.

45. The nurse would be concerned that the child may be hemolyzing red blood cells after noting that the child's
1. abdomen is enlarged.
2. intact skin appears flushed.
3. stools are black.
4. urine is dark brown.

The Client With Hypothyroidism

A 6-week-old infant was normal at birth but has begun to breastfeed poorly. The infant's skin is dry and scaly, and her tongue protrudes. A diagnosis of congenital hypothyroidism is made.

46. The mother asks the nurse why the child was not diagnosed with this condition at birth. The nurse would reply,
1. "We had the results of the newborn screen, but you did not bring the baby in for the 2-week checkup."
2. "Your baby had little need for thyroid hormone until 1 month of age."
3. "Newborns generally receive enough thyroid hormone through breast milk to get by the first few weeks."
4. "We could not reach you at home to give you the test results."

47. The infant is to receive levothyroxine sodium (Synthroid) orally. The nurse would instruct the mother to observe the infant carefully for signs of overdose, which include
1. anorexia.
2. constipation.
3. sweating.
4. sleepiness.

48. After teaching the mother about tests performed to monitor the success of the infant's treatment, the nurse would judge that the teaching was effective when the mother states that the child will need frequent blood tests and regular assessment of
1. blood electrolyte levels.
2. metabolic rate.
3. muscular coordination.
4. bone age.

49. The mother asks the nurse what would happen if her child did not receive treatment. The nurse would explain that one of the outcomes of untreated congenital hypothyroidism is
1. hearing loss.
2. epilepsy.
3. emotional instability.
4. mental retardation.

50. The parents are being taught to administer Synthroid to the infant. The nurse would plan to teach the parents to dissolve the pills and mix the medication in
1. a large amount of water.
2. milk or orange juice.
3. a small amount of formula.
4. the infant's bowl of cereal.

Nursing Care of Children

The Client With Insulin-Dependent Diabetes Mellitus

An 8-year-old boy is admitted to the hospital unconscious owing to severe ketoacidosis.

51. The nurse obtaining a history from the mother would consider which statement by the mother to support a diagnosis of insulin-dependent diabetes mellitus?
○ 1. "He has become almost hyperactive in the past month."
○ 2. "He has begun to wet his bed at night for the first time in 3 years."
○ 3. "He seems to be gaining weight."
○ 4. "He has lost his appetite in the past 2 weeks."

52. The nurse may observe which typical sign of ketoacidosis in the child?
○ 1. Slow, bounding pulse rate.
○ 2. Deep, rapid respirations.
○ 3. Diaphoretic, warm skin.
○ 4. Elevated blood pressure.

53. The mother asks why the child's breath smells. The nurse would explain that the smell is due to the release of
○ 1. amino acids.
○ 2. glycogen.
○ 3. acetone.
○ 4. urea.

54. The nurse has been teaching the parents about insulin. The nurse would judge the teaching about why insulin needs to be injected as successful when the father states that the child cannot take oral insulin because it
○ 1. cannot be digested in the stomach.
○ 2. does not come in a pill form.
○ 3. is destroyed in the stomach before it can work.
○ 4. will cause him to be nauseated.

55. When preparing to give the child his dose of combination regular and NPH humulin insulin, the nurse should
○ 1. take the premixed insulin out of the refrigerator and then withdraw the amount needed in one syringe.
○ 2. use two syringes, one for each type of insulin.
○ 3. withdraw the NPH insulin first, then withdraw the regular insulin into one syringe.
○ 4. withdraw the regular insulin first, then withdraw the NPH insulin into one syringe.

56. A child diagnosed with insulin-dependent diabetes mellitus is attending a camp for diabetic children. He gives himself regular and Lente insulin at 8 AM. The nurse would plan to observe him for pallor, sweating, tachycardia, headache, dizziness, and dif-

ficulty speaking as a result of the effects of the Lente insulin between
○ 1. 8:30 and 10:30 PM.
○ 2. 10 AM and noon.
○ 3. noon and 2 PM.
○ 4. 2 PM and 4 PM.

57. The camp nurse is called to the arts and crafts room because the child is behaving strangely. The nurse's first action should be to
○ 1. make sure the child receives some form of easily digested simple sugar to prevent brain damage and cardiac arrest.
○ 2. ask the child if he took his insulin this morning to determine if he is ketoacidotic.
○ 3. call the child's physician before taking any action.
○ 4. have the child run around the camp track to improve insulin use.

58. The mother of a newly diagnosed diabetic client is being taught the principles of the diabetic diet. The nurse would judge that the mother understands the place of snacks in the diet when the mother states
○ 1. "By spreading the calories throughout the day in small frequent meals, the risk of hyperglycemia is eliminated."
○ 2. "Most children find it difficult to eat all the calories required on their diets in three main meals."
○ 3. "Snacks are used to keep blood glucose at acceptable levels during times when the insulin level peaks."
○ 4. "Snacks are used to offset the desire for sweets and to keep the meals smaller."

59. The nurse and mother are planning interventions that will allow the child to participate in an early morning tennis program at school. The mother has already developed several interventions. Which of the following would the nurse recommend eliminating?
○ 1. Inject the morning insulin dose in an area away from major muscles used in playing tennis.
○ 2. Have the child eat more calories for breakfast on tennis-playing days.
○ 3. Have the child carry a source of quickly absorbed carbohydrate to the program.
○ 4. Teach the other children in the class the signs and symptoms of hyperglycemia.

60. The child attends diet class with her mother. The nurse understands that the diet class has been effective when the child reports to the nurse that she learned,
○ 1. "If I don't eat all my meal, I can make-up the carbohydrates at the next meal."
○ 2. "If I'm not hungry for a meal, I can eat the carbohydrates for a snack later."

382

○ 3. "When I don't finish a meal, I must make up the carbohydrates right then."

○ 4. "When I don't finish a meal, I just need to take more insulin."

61. The client tells the nurse that she does not want her friends to know about the disease. The nurse talks to her about how she could tell her friends. The nurse would judge that the talk had positive results when the child

○ 1. asks the nurse for material on diabetes for a school paper.

○ 2. introduces the nurse to several of her friends as "the nurse who taught me all about my diabetes."

○ 3. says, "I'll try to tell my friends, but they'll probably quit hanging out with me."

○ 4. stays out of the hospital for 6 months.

62. The nurse offers to meet with the mother and the child's teacher before school starts to discuss the teacher's responsibilities in relation to the child's illness. In this meeting, the nurse would plan to discuss

○ 1. how to give an insulin injection.

○ 2. how to perform a glucometer test.

○ 3. signs and symptoms of hypoglycemia.

○ 4. the American Diabetic Association diet.

63. The nurse is teaching the mother and child about sick day management. The nurse judges that the teaching was effective when the mother states that she will

○ 1. keep to the same schedule and type and amount of insulin.

○ 2. immediately call her physician so he can tell her what to do.

○ 3. test the blood glucose more frequently and give regular insulin.

○ 4. take her child to the emergency room for care.

A child is brought to the hospital with ketoacidosis. The child is to receive an insulin drip.

64. The nurse would give *only* which of the following solutions, as ordered?

○ 1. 100 units of regular insulin in 2.5% dextrose.

○ 2. 100 units of regular insulin in 100 mL of 5% dextrose.

○ 3. 100 units of regular insulin in 100 mL of 0.45% saline.

○ 4. 100 units of regular insulin in 100 mL of 0.9% saline.

65. The mother asks the nurse how to manage her child's morning hyperglycemia. The nurse would

○ 1. tell the mother that this is normal and to continue with the ordered doses.

○ 2. ask the mother what her child's blood glucose levels have been for the last few days.

○ 3. tell the mother that this is unusual and she had better take her child to the emergency room now.

○ 4. ask the mother if her child has been avoiding sweets.

66. An adolescent with diabetes is being taught the importance of rotating the sites of his insulin injections. The nurse would judge that the teaching was successful when the adolescent states, "I need to rotate sites because using the same site can cause

○ 1. destruction of the fat tissue and poor absorption."

○ 2. destruction of nerves and painful neuritis."

○ 3. destruction of the tissue and too-rapid insulin uptake."

○ 4. development of resistance to insulin and the need for increased amounts."

67. The nurse tells the diabetic adolescent and mother that, about every 3 months, which of the following tests will be done to assess diabetic management?

○ 1. Hemoglobin electrophoresis.

○ 2. Glycosylated hemoglobin.

○ 3. Glucose tolerance test.

○ 4. Postprandial blood test.

68. The mother of a 10-year-old girl with diabetes asks the nurse's advice about whether her child, who has always been compliant with treatment, should be allowed to go trick-or-treating on Halloween with several of her friends. What would be the nurse's best response?

○ 1. "No, it would be a life-threatening emergency if she eats sweets."

○ 2. "Only if you go with her and watch her so she doesn't eat any sweets."

○ 3. "Yes, just give her a little extra insulin before she goes."

○ 4. "Yes, she needs to be with friends and do the things other children do."

69. The nurse plans to teach a diabetic adolescent about exercise and how it relates to diet and insulin. Which of the following would be part of the teaching plan?

○ 1. Before running, be sure to inject insulin into the leg muscle for quicker absorption.

○ 2. If your blood glucose is 240 ng/dL or above, do not run.

○ 3. You will need extra insulin before running.

○ 4. Do not eat your snack before running because you'll get a stomach ache.

70. A nurse evaluating the knowledge of a 9-year-old who has had diabetes for several years would incor-

porate which of the following developmental considerations in the teaching plan? The client is ready to
- ○ 1. recognize symptoms of hypoglycemia.
- ○ 2. measure insulin accurately in the syringe.
- ○ 3. begin to give own injections with adult supervision.
- ○ 4. assume responsibility for self-care.

The Client Who Is Abused

A 3-year-old child is seen in the emergency room because of a dislocated shoulder. The child has multiple bruises on the thighs and upper arms, and the nurse suspects child abuse.

71. When obtaining a nursing history from parents who are suspected of abusing their injured child, the nurse would typically find that the parents
- ○ 1. are attentive to their child's needs.
- ○ 2. blame themselves for the injury.
- ○ 3. give information about the child's developmental achievements.
- ○ 4. show little concern about the extent of the injury.

72. The nurse would identify which of the following statements made by a mother of a 3-year-old child with unexplained injuries as supporting suspicions of abuse?
- ○ 1. "A good friend and I go shopping at least weekly."
- ○ 2. "I'm disappointed that my child can't tie his shoes."
- ○ 3. "My mother helps me with the children."
- ○ 4. "My child helps dress himself."

73. When the nurse asks the child how his shoulder was hurt, he replies, "It was my fault; I was bad." What would be the nurse's best response?
- ○ 1. "Perhaps it wasn't your fault; can we talk about what happened?"
- ○ 2. "Tell me what you did that made your father hurt you."
- ○ 3. "We'll make you better and won't let your father do this to you again."
- ○ 4. "You'll have to behave better so this won't happen again."

74. The child has blood drawn. The child lies very still and makes no sound during the procedure. What would be the nurse's most appropriate comment?
- ○ 1. "It's okay to cry when something hurts."
- ○ 2. "That really didn't hurt, did it?"
- ○ 3. "We're mean to hurt you that way, aren't we?"
- ○ 4. "You were very good about not crying when the needle went in."

75. The child is admitted to the hospital, and the nurse is aware that a court appearance may be necessary. To plan for this eventuality, the nurse should place priority on
- ○ 1. remembering the parents' and child's behavior when the child was admitted.
- ○ 2. documenting physical findings and behaviors observed during the child's admission.
- ○ 3. formulating subjective opinions about the cause of any injuries.
- ○ 4. preparing answers to questions that may be asked by the attorneys.

76. Which of the following nursing diagnoses would the nurse include in the care plan of a preschooler who has been physically abused?
- ○ 1. High risk for trauma.
- ○ 2. Impaired mobility.
- ○ 3. Self-care deficit.
- ○ 4. Anticipatory grieving.

77. A nurse is approached by an adolescent who has been admitted to the hospital for headaches. She confides that she is being sexually abused by a family friend. What would be the nurse's best initial response?
- ○ 1. "Can you tell me what happened?"
- ○ 2. "I believe you; you were right to tell me."
- ○ 3. "Have you told your mother and father about this?"
- ○ 4. "Who else have you told about this?"

78. A 3-year-old girl has been sexually abused. While interviewing the child, the nurse should ask her to
- ○ 1. describe what happened during the abusive act.
- ○ 2. draw a picture and explain what it means.
- ○ 3. "play out" the event using anatomically correct dolls.
- ○ 4. use puppets to recreate the sexual abuse and observe the child's reactions.

79. A nurse caring for a 15-month-old girl suspects that she has been sexually abused. The nurse's decision regarding reporting the abuse should be based on the fact that
- ○ 1. the parents need to be notified before it can be reported.
- ○ 2. physicians are primarily responsible for reporting suspected abuse.
- ○ 3. a nurse can be sued when reporting abuse on suspicions only.
- ○ 4. a nurse who suspects child abuse is required by law to report these suspicions.

CORRECT ANSWERS AND RATIONALE

The letters in parentheses following the rationale identify the step of the nursing process (A, D, P, I, E), cognitive level (K, C, T, N), and client needs (S, G, L, H). See the Answer Grid for the key.

The Client Who Is Preterm

1. 3. Lanugo (fine, downy hair) covers the entire body until about 20 weeks of gestation, when it begins to disappear from the face, trunk, and extremities, in that order. Lanugo is a consistent finding in preterm neonates. Firm cartilage to the edge of the ear pinna, Scarf sign, and creases on the soles and heels are examples of physical characteristics found in neonates born at term. (A, N, G)

2. 2. Common physical characteristics of preterm neonates include a thin, wasted appearance; scarce scalp hair; thin, pink, smooth skin; and in males, absence of rugae on the scrotum and testicles high in the inguinal canal. (A, T, G)

3. 3. Hyperirritability and twitching are signs of hypoglycemia. Preterm neonates, as well as small-for-gestational-age and large-for-gestational-age neonates, are prone to develop hypoglycemia. A neonate with cold stress must produce heat through increased metabolism, causing oxygen use to increase and glycogen stores to be quickly depleted. Jaundice, abdominal distention, and slow respirations are not associated with neonatal hypoglycemia. (A, N, G)

4. 2. A common finding in neonates with cold stress is low serum glucose level. The normal range for this infant is 20 to 60 mg/dL. Hemoglobin, bilirubin, and hematocrit determinations are not used to confirm hypoglycemia. (D, N, G)

5. 1. When repeated blood specimens are obtained from a preterm neonate, it is a nursing responsibility to keep a record of the amount of blood taken for each specimen. The total blood volume of a preterm neonate is small, and repeated blood collections can deplete blood volume. A record of the amount of blood taken for specimens is a guide to help determine whether the neonate needs a transfusion. Blood color is not a reliable indicator of blood constituents or volume. (P, N, G)

6. 3. Metabolic acidosis results from the metabolic changes associated with cold stress. End products of metabolism increase the acidity of the blood. Therefore, sodium bicarbonate, a buffer base, is often used. Respiratory alkalosis results from excessive carbon dioxide loss, a condition that would be

unusual in this neonate. Sodium bicarbonate is not used to combat edema or dehydration. (P, N, G)

7. 3. Oxygen is given to a cold-stressed neonate to support an increase in the metabolic rate through a complex process of increasing metabolism. In this situation, both the respiratory rate and heart rate are above the normal range for a neonate at rest, which may reflect the need for more oxygen at the cellular level. Normal blood pressure readings would not indicate that the therapy is effective. (E, N, G)

8. 4. High levels of oxygen delivered to a preterm neonate can result in retinopathy of prematurity. The immature blood vessels in the eye constrict and then overgrow, resulting in edema and hemorrhage, which produces scarring, retinal detachment, and eventual blindness. Cataracts and glaucoma are congenital abnormalities in the neonate. Ophthalmia neonatorum is a gonorrheal infection of the eyes that is likely to occur if a mother has the gonorrheal organism in her birth canal. (I, T, S)

9. 1. The method most often recommended to determine whether the gavage catheter is in the stomach is to aspirate stomach contents with a syringe. The presence of stomach contents indicates that the catheter is in the stomach. Any stomach contents obtained should be reintroduced into the stomach to prevent loss of electrolytes. Water introduced into the catheter before placement is confirmed may end up in the lungs. Air introduced into the catheter can be auscultated as a "whoosh" in the stomach area. Any air introduced in this manner should be removed to prevent overdistention of the stomach. (I, T, S)

10. 1. Sterile water is given to a neonate to ascertain whether the esophagus is patent and to prevent the aspiration of formula if it is not. Assessment of the neonate's ability to retain feedings and energy consumption during feedings takes time. Waiting to give formula would be contraindicated in a neonate who is hypoglycemic from cold stress because the condition will worsen if calories are withheld. (P, N, G)

11. 1. Permitting the parents to see and touch the neonate allows for visual searching and information gathering, one of the first steps in the bonding process. Fingertip touching also helps promote the bonding process. Seeing and touching the neonate can often help the parents feel less concerned and more comfortable. The nurse should be present to help the parents understand therapeutic measures

that may be in use for the neonate. Meeting with parents of another ill neonate may only increase the parents' concerns. Although parents are generally encouraged to care for their ill children, a high-risk neonate's care involves special skills that the parents may lack. A long-term nursing goal would be to instruct the parents in such care. Telling the parents not to worry ignores their feelings and tends to cut off communication. (P, N, L)

12. 1. Authorities agree that the single most effective way to control the spread of infection is to have personnel perform frequent arm and hand washing techniques. Measures that are beneficial but not as effective include wearing gowns and masks, using isolation incubators, and providing clean-air exchange. (P, N, S)

The Client Who Is Septic

13. 2. These symptoms in a neonate would lead the nurse to suspect infection. In a neonate who has an immature immunologic response, any infection can rapidly become systemic and result in sepsis. The primary focus of assessment is to determine the neonate's hydration status, especially since sepsis can result in shock. The better hydrated the neonate, the better he can handle the septic state. Because a neonate's kidneys are immature, they cannot conserve water as necessary. This fact makes dehydration a rapid process in the ill neonate. The number of wet diapers in 24 hours would provide data on the neonate's hydration status. Other important assessment data would include skin turgor, mucous membrane status, and status of the fontanel. (A sunken fontanel indicates dehydration.) (A, N, G)

14. 4. The signs and symptoms of sepsis in a neonate are almost imperceptible, such as changes in appearance and behavior. Often, the parents' only complaint is that the neonate does not "look right." Fever or a localized response, which are clues to infections in older children, are often absent in the neonate. (I, N, G)

15. 3. The infant who is septic with lethargy and tachycardia is NPO. Feeding places too much stress on the infant. Vital signs are monitored at least every 4 hours, and an intravenous line is placed for fluid and electrolyte replacement. The infant is weighed every day to determine hydration status. (P, T, G)

16. 1. Sepsis in a neonate is usually treated with a combination of antibiotics that cover a wide spectrum of causative agents. This is done because treatment is begun immediately, before the causative agent is identified. Furosemide is a diuretic and is not indicated for a neonate at risk for septic shock. Phenytoin sodium is an anticonvulsant and is not indicated

for this neonate. Vitamin K is a necessary ingredient for blood clotting and is not necessary for this neonate at this time. (P, N, G)

17. 3. A sleeping heart rate of 205 beats/minute is above normal for this age, which is at most 200 beats/minute. Increased heart rate is an early indication of ensuing shock. The blood pressure is normal. The neonate's respiratory rate is within normal limits for age. The temperature is slightly elevated but is not an indication of shock. A low axillary temperature may indicate shutdown of the peripheral blood supply, which occurs early in shock. (D, N, G)

18. 3. The nurse's best response is an open-ended question that gives the mother an opportunity to share concerns and ask for information. Telling the mother that she did the right thing to bring her infant to the clinic does not address her concerns. In this situation, the mother is right to be worried, and telling her to not do so would be inappropriate. (I, N, L)

19. 1. It is normal for a neonate to breathe using the abdominal muscles. A respiratory rate of 30 breaths/minute is normal for an infant this age. The nurse need not do anything but chart the findings. (I, N, G)

The Client With Failure to Thrive

20. 2. *Failure to thrive* is a term applied to an infant who is not growing at an acceptable rate. One of the parameters for determining whether the growth rate is acceptable is comparison of the infant's weight with the weights of other infants the same age. If the infant's weight falls below the 5th percentile, the infant is considered to have failure to thrive. Pattern of weight gain, whether the infant has received regular checkups, and family dynamics are all important data the nurse would collect, but are not of primary importance. Other characteristics of failure to thrive include eating disorders and developmental retardation. (A, T, H)

21. 1. Infants who have failure to thrive often are fussy during feedings. Although they protest being put down, they are often not content while being held. They are typically unafraid of strangers, which would be abnormal for a 5-month-old. These children also have difficulty sleeping for any length of time. (A, T, G)

22. 3. In the short-term care of this infant, it is important that the same person feed the infant at each meal and that this person be able to assess for negative feeding patterns and replace them with positive patterns. Once the infant is gaining weight and shows progress in the feeding patterns, the parents can be instructed in proper feeding techniques. This is a long-term goal of nursing care. A 5-month-old infant is still too young to be expected to sit in a high chair for feedings and should still be bottle-fed. Because there is no organic reason for the failure to thrive, it should not be necessary to increase the formula calorie content from 20 to 24 calories. (P, N, H)

23. 3. Engagement with an infant during feeding is important. This is achieved through physical contact, eye contact, and voice contact. Most important of these three is physical contact with the person feeding the infant. Holding the infant in a relaxed manner that provides the most physical contact is important. The locale of feeding is unimportant as long as the infant's need for contact is met. (A, T, H)

24. 4. The most effective follow-up care would occur in the home environment. The community health nurse can be supportive of the parents and observe the parent–infant interactions in a natural environment. The community health nurse can evaluate the infant's progress in gaining weight, offer suggestions to the parents, and help the family solve problems as they arise. (P, N, G)

25. 2. It is a common misconception that picking up an infant whenever he or she cries will spoil the child. Infants need to be cuddled and comforted when they are upset. Comforting may be as simple as feeding or changing a wet diaper. Assuming that the infant is hungry each time he cries could lead to overfeeding. (I, T, L)

The Client With Atopic Dermatitis

26. 4. A 4-month-old infant will not be comforted by limiting the number of times the grandmother can visit, sharing a room with a sibling, or listening to the television. (I, N, L)

27. 2. Atopic dermatitis results in pruritus; the infant's skin should be covered as completely as possible to keep him from scratching himself. Cotton is the preferred material. Flannel may be too warm and cause the child to perspire, which will aggravate the condition. Because atopic dermatitis is often associated with allergies, wool garments should be avoided. (I, N, G)

28. 3. The goal of treatment for eczema is to hydrate the skin. The lanolin and urea make an occlusive barrier that keeps moisture in the skin. These preparations will not prevent infection or decrease an inflammatory response. (D, N, G)

29. 2. Care of the skin is basic to the treatment of atopic dermatitis. Use of a mild soap, such as Dove; not allowing the child to soak in the tub, which dries the skin; and patting the skin with a towel after the bath help keep moisture in the skin. (I, N, S)

30. 3. Suitable toys for a 3-year-old include all of the items listed. However, a child with allergies should not be given stuffed animals because they tend to collect dust and are difficult to clean. Eczema is often related to an allergic response. (P, N, H)

31. 3. Diphenhydramine (Benadryl) has both a sedative and antihistamine effect. Chloral hydrate has a sedative effect. Acetaminophen (Tylenol) has an analgesic effect. Auralgan is used to treat painful ears. (I, N, G)

The Client With Burns

32. 4. For a child under age 5 years, 6.5% is allocated to half the head and 1% to the neck when using the rule of nines. For each lower extremity, one half of one thigh is 4%, and one half of one leg is 2.75%. The upper extremities receive 8.5% each, and the posterior and anterior chest receive 13% each. (A, T, G)

33. 1. The child will need fluid replacement therapy as soon as possible, primarily due to the shift of plasma from intravascular to interstitial spaces when the burn occurs. Blisters and edema result from this process and lead to fluid and electrolyte loss. Severe burns are usually sterile; antibiotic treatment, if used at all, would not be a priority at this time. Anchoring a Foley catheter would be done after the intravenous line is started. Laboratory studies would be drawn after the intravenous line is started. (I, N, G)

34. 2. The primary fluid shift in burns is from the intravascular to interstitial spaces. The first effect of a burn is dilation of the capillaries and small vessels in the area, leading to increased capillary permeability. Plasma seeps into the surrounding tissues, producing blisters and edema. There is also an exchange for the electrolyte potassium. (D, N, G)

35. 2. Accurate determination of urine output is a crucial factor in the care of a burn victim. The benefits of using an indwelling catheter to measure urine output to the nearest milliliter outweigh the risk of infection and other problems associated with use. Unless the burns cover the perineal area, making urination painful, urine retention is usually not a problem. Determining urine specific gravity can be done to assess hydration. (I, N, G)

36. 4. Moist rales are an indication that fluid is accumulating in the lung field due to overhydration or too-rapid delivery of fluids. Dark urine would be an indication of underhydration. Abdominal girth would not provide information about fluid status. (D, N, G)

37. 2. Expressions of anger and combativeness are often the result of loss of control and a feeling of powerlessness. Some control over the situation is regained by allowing the child to participate in care. Neither parental support nor permission to cry will give the child a feeling of control over the situation. The treatments are important to the child's physical well-being and should not be delayed. (P, N, L)

38. 2. Allowing the mother to feed the child, serving smaller and more frequent meals, and offering finger foods are all acceptable interventions for a 5-year-old child. This is true whether the child is well or ill. Withholding certain foods until the child complies is punitive and rarely successful. (P, T, H)

39. 4. A serum potassium level of 3.3 mEq/L is low for a child; the normal range is 3.5 to 5.0 mEq/L. Orange juice is the best source of potassium. Grape, apple, and cranberry juices have less potassium. Additional sources of potassium are bananas, cantaloupe, grapefruit juice, tomato juice, honeydew melon, nectarines, and boiled and baked potatoes. (I, N, G)

40. 4. Because it is likely that an allergic reaction is occurring, the nurse should stop the antibiotic. Lesions that are circumscribed, elevated, and pruritic (wheals) are a manifestation of an urticarial reaction. The fact that the child has received multiple doses of the drug is important information because the body needs to be exposed to an antigen to develop an allergic response to it. The intravenous line should be maintained in case the child has an anaphylactic reaction, which could occur if the antibiotic is continued, and needs intravenous access for resuscitation purposes. (I, N, S)

41. 3. The specific gravity of urine increases as the kidneys are forced to conserve water, a sign of dehydration. Normal specific gravity for a child would range from 1.002 to 1.030. Decreased blood pressure would also indicate too little fluid is being infused. Normal minimal urine output for a child between ages 4 and 7 is 24 to 28 mL/hour. Irritability is not a reliable indicator of the need for more fluids. (D, N, G)

42. 1. Hypoproteinemia is common following severe burns. The child's diet should be high in protein to compensate for protein loss and to promote tissue healing. The child will also require a diet high in calories and rich in iron. The menu of bacon, lettuce, and tomato sandwich, apple juice, and celery sticks is lacking in sufficient protein and calories. The other choices include items that are high in protein and in calories. (E, N, G)

43. 4. The Centers for Disease Control and Prevention recommend that sterile gloves be worn when giving any care to a burn area. The gloves should be changed after removing soiled dressings and a new pair put on before applying new dressings. Nonster-

ile gloves should be used for universal precautions, as in caring for any other client. (I, T, S)

44. 1. The ordered dose is 250 mg every 6 hours, which is 1000 mg in 24 hours. The recommended dose is 20 to 50 mg times the weight of 25 kg in 24 hours, which is 500 to 1250 mg in 24 hours. The ordered dose is within the range for the recommended dose. The nurse cannot independently rewrite a medication order. (I, N, S)

45. 4. A sign of hemolysis is hemoglobinuria, which causes the urine to appear dark brown. This condition can result from severe trauma. (D, T, G)

The Client With Hypothyroidism

46. 3. Thyroxine can pass through the placenta to the fetus. This exogenous maternal hormone masks the signs of hypothyroidism at birth in most neonates with congenital hypothyroidism. Failure of normal development occurs during the embryonic period, or an inborn error of metabolism prevents the normal synthesis of thyroxine. These conditions are present at birth. The fetus and neonate require thyroxine, but the exogenous maternal hormone seems to be sufficient. Clinical manifestations may be delayed in breastfed infants, who may not display symptoms until weaned. (I, T, G)

47. 3. Insomnia, rapid pulse, dyspnea, irritability, fever, sweating, and weight loss are all signs indicating Synthroid overdose. Fatigue, sleepiness, decreased or absent appetite (anorexia), and constipation are signs of thyroid insufficiency. (I, T, G)

48. 4. A child with congenital hypothyroidism receiving thyroid replacement therapy should be regularly assessed for blood levels of thyroxine and triiodothyronine. The child also should undergo frequent bone age surveys to ensure optimum growth. Evaluation of metabolic rate, electrolytes, and muscle coordination is not done to determine the success of therapy. (E, T, G)

49. 4. The hallmark signs of untreated congenital hypothyroidism are mental retardation and poor physical development. Congenital hypothyroidism is the most preventable cause of mental retardation. Its effects can be prevented by starting therapy early in the first year of life. Hearing loss, epilepsy, and emotional instability are not associated. (I, T, G)

50. 3. Mixing medications in large amounts of fluid is not recommended because the infant may not take all the liquid. Mixing medication with food is also contraindicated for this infant, who would not be able to digest orange juice, milk, or cereal. Mixing medications with food is also avoided for older children because food aversions can result. Placing the dissolved pill in a small amount of formula would be acceptable for this infant. Cereal is not to be given to an infant younger than 4 months of age. (P, N, S)

The Client With Insulin-Dependent Diabetes Mellitus

51. 2. A sign suggesting hyperglycemia is bed-wetting in a previously continent child. The enuresis is due to polyuria, one of the cardinal signs of insulin-dependent diabetes mellitus. Other cardinal signs are polydipsia (excessive thirst) and polyphagia (excessive hunger). The child also loses weight even though he eats more. The hyperglycemic child is usually slightly lethargic. (A, N, G)

52. 2. Ketones, which are organic acids, readily release free hydrogen ions that cause the blood pH to fall. When ketoacidosis is present, the body attempts to compensate by activating the respiratory buffering process. As a result, the child makes an extra effort to rid himself of excess carbon dioxide, taking deep, rapid breaths and breathing as though he is experiencing air hunger. This characteristic breathing pattern is known as *Kussmaul's respirations.* (A, T, G)

53. 3. In the client with ketoacidosis due to diabetes mellitus, fats break down into fatty acids and glycerol in fat cells and the liver, then convert to ketone bodies. Ketones accumulate in the blood and are expelled by the kidneys into the urine and by the lungs as acetone. (I, T, G)

54. 3. Insulin is rendered inactive by gastric enzymes. (E, T, G)

55. 4. It is recommended that the client taking regular insulin along with an intermediate- or long-acting insulin use only one syringe. Using two syringes is not recommended because the insulin types can be mixed; also, using two syringes is more expensive. NPH does not remain stable for extended periods when mixed with regular insulin, so premixing is rarely recommended. Insulin types such as protamine zinc, globin zinc, and NPH contain an additional modifying protein that slows absorption. A vial of insulin that does not contain the protein (ie, regular insulin) should never be contaminated with insulin that does have the added protein. (I, T, S)

56. 4. The action of an intermediate-acting insulin, such as Lente, begins 2 to 4 hours after injection and peaks 6 to 8 hours after injection. This information is important for timing meals and snacks and recognizing when insulin reactions (hypoglycemia) are likely to occur. Symptoms of hypoglycemia include labile mood, confusion, hunger, headache, shakiness, dizziness, pallor, sweating, and tachycardia. (P, N, G)

57. 1. Assessing a child with hypoglycemia can be difficult. The only sign may be a change in behavior.

Because hypoglycemia is a life-threatening condition, the nurse must assume that the child is hypoglycemic and proceed with interventions for that condition. If the child is hyperglycemic, an increase in blood glucose level at this point would not be lethal. Exercise increases the efficiency of insulin and would only aggravate a hypoglycemic reaction. There is no time to confer with a physician. (I, N, G)

58. 3. Snacks are included in the diabetic diet to offset periods of peak insulin action. Because of the lack of pancreatic functioning, the child does not receive differing amounts of insulin in response to the level of glucose available in the bloodstream. The child with diabetes mellitus is given insulin at specific times, and dietary intake must be matched to the insulin peaks and troughs. The risk of hyperglycemia is not eliminated through regular snacks, although spreading the calories over the day may help the child achieve a more steady blood glucose level. Snacks are not used to offset hunger for sweets or to decrease the amount of food eaten at meals. (E, N, G)

59. 4. It is not necessary that the other children be able to identify hyperglycemia in this child. Hyperglycemia is not life-threatening, but hypoglycemia can be. The other children can be taught signs and symptoms of hypoglycemia and how to treat the condition. Because exercise increases both the efficiency of insulin and the amount of energy required by the body, the child should eat something before participating in a strenuous activity. In this case, increasing caloric intake at breakfast will offset the increased need for energy and increased insulin efficiency. An easily absorbed carbohydrate should be available in case the child experiences hypoglycemia. Insulin uptake from the subcutaneous tissue is increased when the circulation is increased in the area, as occurs around large muscle groups when they are used in strenuous exercise. (P, N, G)

60. 3. The diabetic diet is usually based on an exchange system that takes into account the fact that some foods have similar fat, carbohydrate, and protein components and thus can be exchanged one for another. The meal or snack must be eaten in its entirety because it is calculated with the dose of insulin. If a child does not eat all the meal or snack, then a make-up meal should be given. (E, N, G)

61. 2. The ability to mention her disability indicates that the child feels good enough about herself to share her problem with her peers. Asking for reference material and staying out of the hospital would not indicate that the nurse's interventions targeted toward improving self-esteem have been successful. Saying that her friends will probably desert her if she tells them about the disability indicates that the child still needs to work on her self-esteem and her feelings about the disease. (E, N, L)

62. 3. An insulin reaction can be a life-threatening event. Because the child may have an insulin reaction in the classroom, the nurse and mother should discuss with the child's teachers the seriousness of the condition and how to evaluate the child for hypoglycemia. The teacher also needs to know what measures to take if an insulin reaction occurs. There is no reason why a teacher would need to be able to give an insulin injection, nor does a teacher need to understand the American Diabetic Association diet plan. The child should be responsible for insulin injections, diet, and testing blood glucose levels. (P, N, G)

63. 3. The child who can tolerate oral feedings of simple sugars can be kept at home. The parents should keep careful track of the child's glucose level and confer with the physician and nurse about regular insulin dosages. Using long-acting or intermediate insulin would be risky because the child's ability to take in food and absorb nutrients can change rapidly. (E, N, G)

64. 4. A client in ketoacidosis receives normal saline as a solution until the blood glucose level approaches the normal range. Only regular insulin can be given intravenously. The insulin concentration is the physician's preference. The rate, or units given per hour, is based on the child's weight. (I, N, S)

65. 2. Management of children with early morning hyperglycemia depends on whether the hyperglycemia is insulin-waning or rebound hyperglycemia (Somogyi effect). Insulin waning is a progressive rise in blood glucose throughout the day. The Somogyi effect often shows as an increase in blood sugar glucose at bedtime, a drop at about 2 AM and then a rebound rise early in the morning. (I, T, S)

66. 1. Repeated use of the same infusion site can result in atrophy of the fat in the subcutaneous tissue and lead to poor insulin absorption. The neuritis common in diabetic patients is not related to infusion sites. (E, T, S)

67. 2. Glycosylated hemoglobin is a reflection of the average blood glucose level for the past 2 to 3 months. (P, T, G)

68. 4. The nurse would advise the mother to allow the child to go trick-or-treating. It would not be advisable to give extra insulin because this action could result in severe hypoglycemia, especially if this usually compliant child remains faithful to the treatment regimen. Eating sweets can result in hyperglycemia, which is not desired but is not life-threatening in this context. Children need to be treated like their peers; sheltering them from all

temptation does not allow them the opportunity to develop coping strategies for dealing with the restraints made necessary by their disease. (I, N, G)

69. 2. Exercise decreases blood glucose levels, and to compensate for this, snacks would be given before strenuous exercise. Insulin should not be reduced unless the child cannot tolerate the extra needed food. Vigorous muscle contraction increases local blood flow and absorption of insulin that is injected into that area. The nurse would advise the adolescent to avoid strenuous exercise if the blood glucose is 240 ng/dL or above. (I, N, H)

70. 3. Eight- to 10-year-olds are developmentally ready to begin to give their own injections with adult supervision. Beginning to recognize symptoms of hypoglycemia is appropriate for 4- to 6-year-olds. Measuring insulin accurately in a syringe is appropriate for 10- to 12-year-olds. Assuming responsibility for self-care is appropriate for an older adolescent. (I, N, H)

The Client Who Is Abused

71. 4. Parents of an abused child are typically unconcerned about the child's injury. They may blame the child or others for the injury, may not ask questions about treatment, and may not know developmental information. (A, T, L)

72. 2. Parents who are abusive typically lack knowledge of the child's development and needs. A child at age 3 can help dress himself but would not be expected to tie his shoes. Abusive parents also usually lack social support from family and friends. (D, N, L)

73. 1. Encouraging the abused child to talk about or play out events surrounding the "accident" can help the child and also provide assessment data. An abused child may feel to blame; even if the parent is accused of abuse, the child may still accept responsibility for the act. The nurse should never make promises that cannot be kept. (I, N, L)

74. 1. It is not normal for a preschooler to be totally passive during a painful procedure. An abused child may become "immune" to pain and find that crying may bring on more pain. The child needs to learn that appropriate emotional expression is acceptable. (I, N, L)

75. 2. It is most important for the nurse to document physical findings and observed behaviors on the client's record. Court proceedings usually occur sometime after the nurse's involvement with the child and family, and memories fade. Thus, careful documentation of the facts, not hearsay or subjective opinion, is essential. (P, N, S)

76. 1. An abused child would have as a priority nursing diagnosis High Risk for Trauma. Impaired Mobility and Self-Care Deficit may be pertinent after serious abuse has occurred. (D, N, L)

77. 2. A child who reports abuse must be believed. Often, the child has tried to tell the parents about the abuse but has not been believed or has been rejected. The child may be afraid to tell the parents. The nurse should start with neutral questions and later ask the child for an account of the event. (I, N, L)

78. 3. A 3-year-old child has limited verbal skills and should not be asked to describe an event, explain a picture, or respond verbally or nonverbally to questions. More appropriately, the child can act out an event using dolls. (A, N, L)

79. 4. All states have mandatory reporting laws relating to child abuse and neglect. A nurse or other health care professional who fails to report suspected abuse may be charged with a misdemeanor. Nurses who report suspected child abuse have immunity from being sued. (I, T, H)

NURSING CARE OF CHILDREN

TEST 9: The Child With Dermatologic, Endocrine, and Other Health Problems

Directions: Use this answer grid to determine areas of strength or need for further study.

NURSING PROCESS

A = Assessment
D = Analysis, nursing diagnosis
P = Planning
I = Implementation
E = Evaluation

COGNITIVE LEVEL

K = Knowledge
C = Comprehension
T = Application
N = Analysis

CLIENT NEEDS

S = Safe, effective care environment
G = Physiologic integrity
L = Psychosocial integrity
H = Health promotion and maintenance

Question #	Answer #	Nursing Process					Cognitive Level				Client Needs			
		A	D	P	I	E	K	C	T	N	S	G	L	H
1	3	A								N		G		
2	2	A							T			G		
3	3	A								N		G		
4	2		D							N		G		
5	1			P						N		G		
6	3			P						N		G		
7	3					E				N		G		
8	4				I				T		S			
9	1				I				T		S			
10	1			P						N		G		
11	1			P						N			L	
12	1			P						N	S			
13	2	A								N		G		
14	4				I					N		G		
15	3			P					T			G		
16	1			P						N		G		
17	3		D							N		G		
18	3				I					N			L	
19	1				I					N		G		
20	2	A							T					H
21	1	A							T			G		
22	3			P						N				H
23	3	A							T					H
24	4			P						N		G		
25	2				I				T				L	

ANSWER GRID: 1

NURSING PROCESS

A = Assessment
D = Analysis, nursing diagnosis
P = Planning
I = Implementation
E = Evaluation

COGNITIVE LEVEL

K = Knowledge
C = Comprehension
T = Application
N = Analysis

CLIENT NEEDS

S = Safe, effective care environment
G = Physiologic integrity
L = Psychosocial integrity
H = Health promotion and maintenance

Question #	Answer #	Nursing Process					Cognitive Level				Client Needs			
		A	D	P	I	E	K	C	T	N	S	G	L	H
26	4				I					N			L	
27	2				I					N		G		
28	3		D							N		G		
29	2				I					N	S			
30	3			P						N				H
31	3				I					N		G		
32	4	A							T			G		
33	1				I					N		G		
34	2		D							N		G		
35	2				I					N		G		
36	4		D							N		G		
37	2			P						N			L	
38	2			P					T					H
39	4				I					N		G		
40	4				I					N	S			
41	3		D							N		G		
42	1					E				N		G		
43	4				I				T		S			
44	1				I					N	S			
45	4		D						T			G		
46	3				I				T			G		
47	3				I				T			G		
48	4					E			T			G		
49	4				I				T			G		
50	3			P						N	S			
51	2	A								N		G		
52	2	A							T			G		
53	3				I				T			G		
54	3					E			T			G		
55	4				I				T		S			

NURSING PROCESS

A = Assessment
D = Analysis, nursing diagnosis
P = Planning
I = Implementation
E = Evaluation

COGNITIVE LEVEL

K = Knowledge
C = Comprehension
T = Application
N = Analysis

CLIENT NEEDS

S = Safe, effective care environment
G = Physiologic integrity
L = Psychosocial integrity
H = Health promotion and maintenance

Question #	Answer #	Nursing Process					Cognitive Level				Client Needs			
		A	D	P	I	E	K	C	T	N	S	G	L	H
56	4			P						N		G		
57	1				I					N		G		
58	3					E				N		G		
59	4			P						N		G		
60	3					E				N		G		
61	2					E				N			L	
62	3			P						N		G		
63	3					E				N		G		
64	4				I					N	S			
65	2				I				T		S			
66	1					E			T		S			
67	2			P					T			G		
68	4				I					N		G		
69	2				I					N				H
70	3				I					N				H
71	4	A							T				L	
72	2		D							N			L	
73	1				I					N			L	
74	1				I					N			L	
75	2			P						N	S			
76	1		D							N			L	
77	2				I					N			L	
78	3	A								N			L	
79	4				I				T					H
Number Correct														
Number Possible	79	12	9	18	31	9	0	0	25	54	13	45	13	8
Percentage Correct														

BIBLIOGRAPHY

American Academy of Pediatrics. Committee on Infectious Disease. (1994). *Report of the Committee on Infectious Disease.* Evanston, IL: Author.

Ball, J., & Bindler, R. (1995). *Pediatric nursing: Caring for children.* Norwalk, CT: Appleton & Lange.

Benson, D.S., & Conte, R.S. (1991). *91/92 Nursing meds.* Norwalk, CT: Appleton & Lange.

Bernardo, L.M., & Bove, M. (1993). *Pediatric emergency nursing procedures.* Boston: Jones & Bartlett.

Betz, C., & Sowdon, L. (1996). *Mosby's pediatric nursing reference* (3rd ed.). St. Louis: Mosby-Year Book.

Binder R.M., & Howry, L.B. (1991). *Pediatric drugs and nursing interventions.* San Mateo, CA: Appleton & Lange.

Castiglia, P.Y., & Harbin, R.E. (1992). *Child health care: Process and practice.* Philadelphia: JB Lippincott.

Davis, J., & Sherer, K. (1993). *Applied nutrition and diet therapy for nurses* (2nd ed.). Philadelphia: W.B. Saunders.

Fischbach, F. (1995). *Quick reference to common laboratory and diagnostic tests.* Philadelphia: JB Lippincott.

Foster, R.L., Hunsberger, M.M., & Anderson, J.J. (1989). *Family-centered nursing care of children.* Philadelphia: WB Saunders.

Fuller, J., & Schaller-Ayers, J. (1994). *Health assessment: a nursing approach.* Philadelphia: JB Lippincott.

Gordon, M. (1995). *Manual of nursing diagnosis: 1995–1996.* St. Louis: Mosby-Year Book.

Gordon, M. (1994). *Nursing diagnosis: Process and application.* (3rd ed.). St. Louis: Mosby-Year Book.

Gulanick, M., Puzas, M.K., & Wilson, C.R. (1992). *Nursing care plans for newborns and children: Acute and critical care.* St. Louis: Mosby-Year Book.

Hazinski, M.F. (1992). *Nursing care of the critically ill child* (2nd ed.). St. Louis: Mosby-Year Book.

Hymovich, D.P., and Hagopian, G.A. (1992). *Chronic illness in children and adults: A psychosocial approach.* Philadelphia: WB Saunders.

Jackson, D.B., & Saunders, R. (1993). *Child health nursing: A comprehensive approach to the care of children and their families.* Philadelphia: JB Lippincott.

Jackson, P.L., & Vessey, J.A. (1996). *Primary care of the child with a chronic condition.* St. Louis: Mosby-Year Book.

James, S., & Mott, S. (1988). *Child health nursing: Essential care of children and families.* Menlo Park, CA: Addison-Wesley.

Klaus, M.H., & Fanaroff, A.A. (1993). *Care of the high-risk neonate.* Philadelphia: WB Saunders.

Lewis, S., Grainger, R.D., McDowell, W.A., Gregory, R.J., & Messner, R.L. (1989). *Manual of psychosocial nursing interventions: Promoting mental health in medical-surgical settings.* Philadelphia: WB Saunders.

Marlow, D.R., & Redding, B.A. (1988). *Textbook of pediatric nursing.* (6th ed.). Philadelphia: WB Saunders.

Mott, S., Frazekas, N., & James, S. (1985). *Nursing care of children and families: A holistic approach.* Menlo Park, CA: Addison-Wesley.

Pillitteri, A. (1992). *Maternal and child health nursing care of the childbearing and childbearing family.* Philadelphia: JB Lippincott.

Pipes, P., and Trahms, C.M. (1992). *Nutrition in infancy and childhood* (5th ed.). St. Louis: Mosby-Year Book.

Rose, M., & Thomas, R.B. (1987). *Children with chronic conditions: Nursing in a family and community context.* Philadelphia: WB Saunders.

Schuster, C.S., & Ashburn, S.S. (1992). *The process of human development: A holistic life-span approach* (3rd ed.). Philadelphia: JB Lippincott.

Scipien, G.M., Chard, M.A., Howe, J., & Barnard, M. (1990). *Pediatric nursing care.* St. Louis: Mosby-Year Book.

Smith, P.S., Nix, K.S., Kemper, J.Y., Ligouri, R., Brantly, D.K., Rollins, J.H., Stevens, N.V., & Clutter, L.B. (1991). *Comprehensive child and family nursing skills.* St. Louis: Mosby-Year Book.

Thompson, S.W. (1990). *Emergency care of children.* Boston: Jones & Bartlett.

Waechter, E., Phillips, J., & Holadaz, B. (1985). *Nursing care of children.* Philadelphia: JB Lippincott.

Whaley, L.F., & Wong, D.L. (1995). *Nursing care of infants and children* (5th ed.). St. Louis: Mosby-Year Book.

Part IV

The Nursing Care of Adults With Medical and Surgical Health Problems

The Client With Respiratory Health Problems

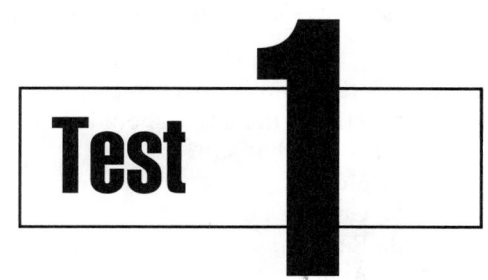

- **The Client With Pneumonia**
- **The Client With Tuberculosis**
- **The Client With Chronic Obstructive Pulmonary Disease**
- **The Client With Lung Cancer**
- **The Client With Chest Trauma**
- **Correct Answers and Rationale**

Select the one best answer, and indicate your choice by filling in the circle in front of the option.

The Client With Pneumonia

A female client, aged 79 years, is admitted to the hospital with a diagnosis of bacterial pneumonia. She has a temperature of 102.6 F, is diaphoretic, has a productive cough, and is experiencing moderate shortness of breath.

1. When obtaining the client's health history, the nurse learns that she has long-standing osteoarthritis, follows a vegetarian diet, has never been seriously ill, and is very concerned with cleanliness. The client says, "I hope I can take a bath each day. I feel so dirty if I don't bathe every day." Which of the following factors would add most to the danger posed by her illness?
   - ○ 1. The client's age.
   - ○ 2. History of osteoarthritis.
   - ○ 3. Following a vegetarian diet.
   - ○ 4. Bathing daily in cold water.
2. A priority nursing diagnosis for this hospitalized client with bacterial pneumonia and shortness of breath would be
   - ○ 1. Altered Cardiopulmonary Tissue Perfusion related to myocardial damage.
   - ○ 2. Potential Self-Care Deficit related to fatigue.
   - ○ 3. Fluid Volume Deficit related to nausea and vomiting.

   - ○ 4. Altered Thought Processes related to inadequate pain relief.
3. The client is to be started on intravenous antibiotics immediately. Which of the following must be completed before antibiotic therapy begins?
   - ○ 1. Urinalysis.
   - ○ 2. Sputum examination.
   - ○ 3. Chest radiograph.
   - ○ 4. Red blood cell count.
4. When administering an aminoglycoside antibiotic to the client, the nurse monitors which of the following?
   - ○ 1. Serum sodium.
   - ○ 2. Serum potassium.
   - ○ 3. Serum creatinine.
   - ○ 4. Red blood cell count.
5. Considering the client's symptoms and condition, the nurse should include which of the following measures in the plan of care?
   - ○ 1. Position changes every 4 hours.
   - ○ 2. Nasotracheal suctioning to clear secretions.
   - ○ 3. Frequent linen changes.
   - ○ 4. Frequent offering of a bedpan.
6. Bed rest is prescribed for the client during the acute phase of her illness. The purpose of bed rest in this situation is to
   - ○ 1. reduce the cellular demand for oxygen.
   - ○ 2. decrease the basal metabolic rate.
   - ○ 3. promote safety.
   - ○ 4. promote clearance of secretions.

7. For the client with a productive cough and difficulty breathing, the nurse should obtain the body temperature at what site?
○ 1. Mouth.
○ 2. Groin fold.
○ 3. Rectum.
○ 4. Axillae.

8. The cyanosis that accompanies bacterial pneumonia is primarily due to
○ 1. decreased cardiac output.
○ 2. iron-deficiency anemia.
○ 3. inadequate peripheral circulation.
○ 4. decreased oxygenation of the blood.

9. A client with pneumonia is experiencing pleuritic chest pain. This type of chest pain is usually described as being
○ 1. a mild but constant aching in the chest.
○ 2. severe mid-sternal pain.
○ 3. moderate pain that worsens on inspiration.
○ 4. muscle spasm pain that accompanies coughing.

10. Which of the following measures would most likely be successful in reducing the client's pleuritic chest pain due to pneumonia?
○ 1. Encourage the client to breathe shallowly.
○ 2. Have the client practice abdominal breathing.
○ 3. Offer the client incentive spirometry.
○ 4. Teach the client to splint the rib cage when coughing.

11. Aspirin is administered to clients with pneumonia because of its antipyretic and
○ 1. analgesic effects.
○ 2. anticoagulant effects.
○ 3. adrenergic effects.
○ 4. antihistamine effects.

12. A client with bacterial pneumonia is coughing up tenacious, purulent sputum. Which of the following measures would most likely help liquefy these viscous secretions?
○ 1. Performing postural drainage.
○ 2. Breathing humidified air.
○ 3. Clapping and percussing over the affected lung.
○ 4. Performing coughing and deep-breathing exercises.

13. Mental status changes that may occur when the client with pneumonia is experiencing hypoxia include which of the following?
○ 1. Coma.
○ 2. Apathy.
○ 3. Irritability.
○ 4. Depression.

14. After 1 day of antibiotic therapy, a client's white blood cell count is 14,000/mm^3. In response to this report, the nurse should
○ 1. notify the physician.
○ 2. increase the next dose of the antibiotic.

○ 3. initiate reverse isolation precautions.
○ 4. administer the next scheduled antibiotic dose early.

15. The client with pneumonia develops mild constipation, and the nurse administers docusate sodium (Colace) as ordered. This drug works by
○ 1. softening the stool.
○ 2. lubricating the stool.
○ 3. increasing stool bulk.
○ 4. stimulating peristalsis.

16. Which of the following would be most important to teach a client older than 65 years to prevent a recurrence of bacterial pneumonia?
○ 1. Change current diet habits.
○ 2. Seek prompt antibiotic therapy for viral infections.
○ 3. Receive prophylactic antibiotic therapy.
○ 4. Obtain annual influenza and pneumococcal vaccines.

The Client With Tuberculosis

A male client has been diagnosed with tuberculosis. He had not been feeling well for the past several weeks and sought medical attention when he began expectorating bloody secretions.

17. Which of the following symptoms are common in clients with active tuberculosis?
○ 1. Marked weight loss.
○ 2. Increased appetite.
○ 3. Dyspnea on exertion.
○ 4. Mental status changes.

18. The nurse obtains a sputum specimen from the client for laboratory study. Which of the following laboratory techniques is most commonly used to identify tubercle bacilli in sputum?
○ 1. Acid-fast staining.
○ 2. Sensitivity testing.
○ 3. Agglutination testing.
○ 4. Dark-field illumination.

19. Which of the following antituberculosis drugs that the client is receiving can damage the eighth cranial nerve?
○ 1. Streptomycin.
○ 2. Isoniazid (INH).
○ 3. Aminosalicylic acid (PAS).
○ 4. Ethambutol hydrochloride (Myambutol).

20. The client who experiences eighth cranial nerve damage will most likely report which of the following symptoms?
○ 1. Vertigo.
○ 2. Facial paralysis.

○ 3. Impaired vision.

○ 4. Difficulty swallowing.

21. In teaching the client about self-care at home, the nurse will include all of the following measures. Which of the measures would have the highest priority?

○ 1. Getting adequate rest.

○ 2. Eating a nourishing diet.

○ 3. Taking medications as prescribed.

○ 4. Living in an area with clean air.

22. The nurse should teach clients that the most common route of transmitting tubercle bacilli from person to person is through contaminated

○ 1. dust particles.

○ 2. droplet nuclei.

○ 3. water.

○ 4. eating utensils.

23. The single most effective way to decrease the spread of microorganisms is

○ 1. frequent handwashing.

○ 2. having separate personal care items for each person.

○ 3. using disposable equipment whenever possible.

○ 4. isolating people known to be harboring disease-causing microorganisms.

24. Many clients with tuberculosis take two antitubercular drugs simultaneously. The primary reason for this is to

○ 1. potentiate the drugs' actions.

○ 2. reduce undesirable drug side effects.

○ 3. allow reduced drug dosages to be given.

○ 4. reduce development of resistant strains of the bacteria.

25. The client with tuberculosis is to be discharged home with community health nursing follow-up. Of the following goals, which would have the highest priority?

○ 1. Offer the client emotional support.

○ 2. Teach the client about the disease.

○ 3. Coordinate various agency services.

○ 4. Assess the client's environment for sanitation.

26. Which of the following techniques for administering the Mantoux test is correct?

○ 1. Hold the needle and syringe almost parallel to the client's skin.

○ 2. Pinch the skin when inserting the needle.

○ 3. Aspirate before injecting the medication.

○ 4. Massage the site after injecting the medication.

27. Which member of a family exposed to tuberculosis would be at highest risk for contracting tuberculosis?

○ 1. The 45-year-old mother.

○ 2. The teenage daughter.

○ 3. The grade-school–aged son.

○ 4. The 76-year-old grandmother.

28. Medical therapy for a client with a positive Mantoux skin test who does not have active tuberculosis would involve

○ 1. reevaluating the client's condition every 6 months.

○ 2. performing a repeat skin test every 6 months.

○ 3. administering isoniazid for about 9 months.

○ 4. administering isoniazid until the skin test reverts to negative.

29. The nurse's best evaluation of a client who exhibits a positive Mantoux test would be that the client has

○ 1. clinical tuberculosis.

○ 2. had contact with the tubercle bacilli.

○ 3. developed a resistance to the tubercle bacilli.

○ 4. developed passive immunity to tuberculosis.

30. To prevent development of peripheral neuropathies associated with isoniazid administration, clients taking this drug are usually advised to

○ 1. follow a low cholesterol diet.

○ 2. supplement the diet with pyridoxine (vitamin B_6).

○ 3. get extra rest.

○ 4. avoid excessive sun exposure.

31. The nurse should caution sexually active female clients taking isoniazid that the drug

○ 1. increases the risk of vaginal infection.

○ 2. has mutagenic effects on ova.

○ 3. decreases the effectiveness of oral contraceptives.

○ 4. inhibits ovulation.

32. Clients who have had active tuberculosis need to be informed that they are at risk for recurrence of tuberculosis during periods of

○ 1. cool and damp weather.

○ 2. active exercise and exertion.

○ 3. physical and emotional stress.

○ 4. rest and inactivity.

33. In which areas of the United States does tuberculosis most commonly occur?

○ 1. Rural farming areas.

○ 2. Inner-city areas.

○ 3. Areas where clean water standards are low.

○ 4. Suburban areas with significant industrial pollution.

The Client With Chronic Obstructive Pulmonary Disease

A client is admitted to the hospital with an acute exacerbation of long-standing chronic obstructive pulmonary disease (COPD) brought on by an upper respiratory infection. He is tachypneic and acutely short of breath. Both he and his wife are extremely anxious.

34. The client is admitted to room 13, but he states that he does not want to remain in the room because the number will bring him bad luck. Personnel in the admitting office say that a change can be made if the nurse feels that it is wise to do so. Which of the following statements offers the best guide for the nurse in this situation?
○ 1. Move the client; the client's fears, even when unfounded, can impede recovery.
○ 2. Move the client; superstitions have a good chance of coming true for those who believe them.
○ 3. Do not move the client; having the client use the room will help him overcome an unwarranted fear.
○ 4. Do not move the client; the client may become unmanageable and demanding when he knows he can have his way.

35. Oxygen at the rate of 2 liters per minute through nasal cannula is prescribed for the client. Which of the following statements best describes why the oxygen therapy is maintained at a relatively low concentration?
○ 1. The oxygen will be lost at the client's nostrils if given at a higher level with a nasal cannula.
○ 2. The client's long history of respiratory problems indicates that he would be unable to absorb oxygen given at a higher rate.
○ 3. The cells in the alveoli are so damaged by the client's long history of respiratory problems that increased oxygen levels and reduced carbon dioxide levels likely will cause the cells to burst.
○ 4. The client's respiratory center is so accustomed to high carbon dioxide and low blood oxygen concentrations that changing these concentrations with oxygen therapy may eliminate his stimulus for breathing.

36. The client reports steady weight loss and that he "is too tired from just breathing to eat." Which of the following nursing diagnoses would be most appropriate when planning nutritional interventions for this client?
○ 1. Altered Nutrition: Less Than Body Requirements related to fatigue.
○ 2. Altered Nutrition: Less Than Body Requirements related to COPD.
○ 3. Weight Loss related to COPD.
○ 4. Ineffective Breathing Patterns related to alveolar hypoventilation.

37. When developing the client's discharge plan, the nurse should be guided by an understanding that the client is most likely to
○ 1. develop infections easily.
○ 2. maintain his current status.
○ 3. require less supplemental oxygen.
○ 4. show permanent improvement.

38. On discharge from the hospital to home, outcome criteria for the client with COPD would include that he
○ 1. promises to do pursed-lip breathing at home.
○ 2. states actions to reduce pain caused by the disease process.
○ 3. exhibits temperature not exceeding 100°F.
○ 4. agrees to call the physician if dyspnea on exertion increases.

39. Which of the following physical assessment findings is typical in a client with advanced COPD?
○ 1. Increased anteroposterior chest diameter.
○ 2. Underdeveloped neck muscles.
○ 3. Collapsed neck veins.
○ 4. Increased chest excursions with respiration.

40. To decrease the risk of COPD, people should be instructed to
○ 1. refrain from drinking more than one alcoholic beverage per day.
○ 2. maintain a high-protein diet.
○ 3. avoid exposure to people with known respiratory infections.
○ 4. abstain from cigarette smoking.

41. The primary reason to teach pursed-lip breathing to clients with emphysema is to help
○ 1. promote oxygen intake.
○ 2. strengthen the diaphragm.
○ 3. strengthen the intercostal muscles.
○ 4. promote carbon dioxide elimination.

42. Theophylline ethylenediamide is administered to a client with COPD to
○ 1. reduce bronchial secretions.
○ 2. relax bronchial smooth muscle.
○ 3. strengthen myocardial contractions.
○ 4. decrease alveolar elasticity.

43. A priority goal for the client with COPD is to
○ 1. maintain functional ability.
○ 2. minimize pain due to the disease process.
○ 3. increase carbon dioxide levels in the blood.
○ 4. treat the infectious agent.

Questions 44 through 47 pertain to the following set of arterial blood gas (ABG) values: pH, 7.52; PaO_2, 50 mm Hg; $PaCO_2$, 28 mm Hg; HCO_3^-, 24 mEq/L.

44. The nurse would interpret these ABG values as indicating
○ 1. metabolic acidosis.
○ 2. metabolic alkalosis.
○ 3. respiratory acidosis.
○ 4. respiratory alkalosis.

45. From the client's $PaCO_2$ level, the nurse determines that the client is
- ○ 1. hypoxemic.
- ○ 2. hypoventilating.
- ○ 3. hyperventilating.
- ○ 4. using oxygen therapy.

46. From the client's PaO_2 level, the nurse concludes that the
- ○ 1. client is hypoxic.
- ○ 2. oxygen level is low but poses no risk for the client.
- ○ 3. client's PaO_2 level is within normal range.
- ○ 4. client requires oxygen therapy with very low oxygen concentrations.

47. The nurse determines that which of the following is a possible etiology for these ABG values?
- ○ 1. COPD.
- ○ 2. Diabetic ketoacidosis with Kussmaul's respirations.
- ○ 3. Myocardial infarction.
- ○ 4. Pulmonary embolus.

48. A client's ABG values are pH, 7.29; PaO_2, 48 mm Hg; $PaCO_2$, 76 mm Hg; HCO_3^-, 36 mEq/L. The plan of care for a client with these values would include close monitoring for which of the following signs and symptoms?
- ○ 1. Cyanosis and restlessness.
- ○ 2. Flushed skin and lethargy.
- ○ 3. Weakness and irritability.
- ○ 4. Anxiety and fever.

49. During postural drainage, movement of secretions from the lower respiratory tract to the upper respiratory tract occurs due to
- ○ 1. friction between the cilia.
- ○ 2. the force of gravity.
- ○ 3. the sweeping motion of cilia.
- ○ 4. involuntary muscle contractions.

50. Clients with COPD may be bedridden at home and get little exercise. Which of the following is a normal physiologic reaction to prolonged periods of bed rest and inactivity?
- ○ 1. Increased sodium retention.
- ○ 2. Increased calcium excretion.
- ○ 3. Increased insulin use.
- ○ 4. Increased red blood cell production.

51. For a client with COPD who has trouble raising respiratory secretions, which of the following nursing measures would help reduce the tenacity of secretions?
- ○ 1. Ensuring that the client's diet is low in salt.
- ○ 2. Ensuring that the client's oxygen therapy is continuous.
- ○ 3. Helping the client maintain a high fluid intake.
- ○ 4. Keeping the client in a semi-sitting position as much as possible.

52. When teaching the client with COPD ways to conserve energy, the nurse should teach the client to lift objects
- ○ 1. while inhaling through pursed lips.
- ○ 2. while exhaling through pursed lips.
- ○ 3. after exhaling but before inhaling.
- ○ 4. after inhaling but before exhaling.

53. The nurse teaches the client with COPD to assess for signs and symptoms of right-sided heart failure, which include
- ○ 1. clubbing of nail beds.
- ○ 2. hypertension.
- ○ 3. ankle edema.
- ○ 4. increased appetite.

The Client With Lung Cancer

A 58-year old client is admitted with a diagnosis of lung cancer. She enjoyed good health until 2 months ago, when she developed a persistent cough that became productive of blood-tinged sputum 1 week ago. She has experienced increasing fatigue during the past month. She reports anorexia and is very thin (5-feet, 7-inches tall, 110 pounds). She has smoked a pack of cigarettes a day for 28 years. A chest radiograph and sputum cytology done a week ago are the basis for the diagnosis.

54. As part of the client's diagnostic work-up, she is to have a bronchoscopy under local anesthesia. Her preoperative medication will be atropine sulfate, 0.4 mg, and meperidine hydrochloride (Demerol), 100 mg intramuscularly. Which of the following interventions should the nurse perform after the test?
- ○ 1. Irrigate the nasogastric tube with 30 mL of normal saline every 2 hours.
- ○ 2. Offer 200 mL of oral fluids every hour to liquefy lung secretions.
- ○ 3. Observe the abdomen for signs of distention and board-like rigidity.
- ○ 4. Position the client on her side and keep her NPO for several hours.

55. The client is to have a left lung lobectomy. Certain data are more important than others in planning her postoperative nursing care. Of the following assessment data obtained in the nurse's admission interview and nursing history, which would increase the client's risk of developing postoperative pulmonary complications? The client
- ○ 1. is 5-feet, 7-inches tall and weighs 110 pounds.
- ○ 2. tends to keep her real feelings to herself.
- ○ 3. ambulates and can climb one flight of stairs without dyspnea.
- ○ 4. is 58 years of age.

56. The night before surgery, the nurse remarks to the client that she looks sad and is quieter than usual. The client says, "I'm scared of having cancer. It's so horrible and I brought it on myself. I should have quit smoking years ago." What would be the nurse's best response to the client?
- ○ 1. "It's okay to be scared. What is it about cancer that you're afraid of?"
- ○ 2. "It's normal to be scared. I would be, too. We'll help you through it."
- ○ 3. "Don't be so hard on yourself. You don't know if your smoking caused the cancer."
- ○ 4. "Do you feel guilty because you smoked?"

57. The client had a left lower lobectomy this morning. She is receiving morphine sulfate by a patient-controlled analgesia (PCA) system. The client complains of moderately severe pain in her left thorax that worsens when she coughs. The nurse should
- ○ 1. let the client rest; no further assessment is needed.
- ○ 2. encourage the client to ignore the pain because some pain is expected after surgery.
- ○ 3. reassure the client that the PCA is working and will relieve her pain.
- ○ 4. assess the pain systematically with the hospital-approved scale.

58. To help control the client's pain during coughing, the nurse should
- ○ 1. place the bed in slight Trendelenburg's position and help the client turn onto her operative side to splint the incision.
- ○ 2. raise the bed to semi-Fowler's position and place one hand on the client's back, on the left side, and one hand under the incision.
- ○ 3. keep the bed flat and tell the client to place her hands over the incision before taking a deep breath.
- ○ 4. raise the bed to complete Fowler's position and help the client turn onto her operative side to splint the incision.

59. Which of the following areas are a priority to evaluate when completing discharge planning for this client?
- ○ 1. The support available to assist the client at home.
- ○ 2. The distance the client lives from the hospital.
- ○ 3. The client's ability to do home blood pressure monitoring.
- ○ 4. The client's knowledge of the causes of lung cancer.

60. A major intervention to help prevent lung cancer would be to
- ○ 1. encourage cigarette smokers to have yearly chest radiographs.
- ○ 2. instruct people about techniques for smoking cessation.

- ○ 3. recommend that people have their houses and apartments checked for asbestos leakage.
- ○ 4. encourage people to install central air cleaners in their homes.

61. When administering atropine sulfate preoperatively to the client scheduled for lung surgery, the nurse should tell the client which of the following? "This medication will
- ○ 1. make you drowsy."
- ○ 2. help you relax."
- ○ 3. make your mouth feel dry."
- ○ 4. reduce the risk of postoperative infection."

62. After lobectomy, clients should be instructed to perform deep-breathing exercises to
- ○ 1. elevate the diaphragm, which enlarges the thorax and increases the lung surface available for gas exchange.
- ○ 2. decrease blood flow to the lungs to allow them to rest and increase the surface available for ventilation.
- ○ 3. control the rate of air flow to the remaining lobe so that it will not become hyperinflated.
- ○ 4. expand the alveoli and increase the lung surface available for ventilation.

63. Which of the following signs and symptoms would alert the nurse to possible internal bleeding in a client who has undergone pulmonary lobectomy?
- ○ 1. Increased blood pressure and decreased pulse and respiratory rates.
- ○ 2. Sanguineous drainage from the chest tube at a rate of 50 mL per hour during the past 3 hours.
- ○ 3. Restlessness and shortness of breath.
- ○ 4. Urine output of 180 mL during the past 3 hours.

64. Which of the following is the most important aspect of pain management for the client after lobectomy?
- ○ 1. Repositioning the client immediately after administering pain medication.
- ○ 2. Reassessing the client 30 minutes after administering pain medication.
- ○ 3. Verbally reassuring the client after administering pain medication.
- ○ 4. Readjusting the pain medication dosage as needed according to the client's condition.

65. While assessing the incisional area from a lobectomy in which a chest tube exits, the nurse feels a crackling sensation under the fingertips along the entire incision. The nurse's first action should be to
- ○ 1. lower the head of the bed and call the physician.
- ○ 2. check the client's blood pressure and ready an aspiration tray.
- ○ 3. mark the area with a skin pencil at the outer periphery of the crackling.
- ○ 4. turn off the suction of the chest drainage system.

66. When caring for a client with a chest tube and water-seal drainage system, the nurse should

○ 1. ensure that the air vent on the water-seal drainage system is capped when the suction is off.

○ 2. strip the chest drainage tubes at least every 4 hours if excessive bleeding occurs.

○ 3. ensure that the chest tube is clamped when moving the client out of the bed.

○ 4. ensure that the collection and suction bottles are below the client's chest level at all times.

67. In a chest tube water-seal drainage system, cessation of fluid fluctuation in the chest tube and the water-seal column generally means that the

○ 1. lung has fully expanded.

○ 2. lung has collapsed.

○ 3. chest tube is in the pleural space.

○ 4. mediastinal space has decreased.

68. The nurse observes a constant gentle bubbling in the water-seal column of a water-seal chest drainage system. This observation should prompt the nurse to

○ 1. continue monitoring as usual; this is a normal observation.

○ 2. check the connectors between the chest and drainage tubes and where the drainage tube enters the collection bottle.

○ 3. decrease the suction to − 15 cm H_2O or less and continue observing the system for changes in bubbling during the next several hours.

○ 4. drain half the water from the underwater-seal chamber.

69. A client who underwent a lobectomy and has a water-seal chest drainage system is breathing with a little more effort and at a faster rate than an hour ago. The client's pulse rate is also increased. The nurse should

○ 1. check the tubing to ensure that the client is not lying on it or kinking it.

○ 2. increase the suction.

○ 3. lower the drainage bottles 2 to 3 feet below the level of the client's chest.

○ 4. ensure that the chest tube has two clamps on it to prevent air leaks.

70. Which of the following items should be readily available at the bedside of a client with a chest tube in place?

○ 1. A tracheostomy tray.

○ 2. Another sterile chest tube.

○ 3. Rubber-capped hemostats.

○ 4. A spirometer.

The Client With Chest Trauma

A 21-year old male client is transported by ambulance to the emergency department after a serious automobile accident. He complains of severe pain in his right chest where he struck the steering wheel. He also has a compound fracture of his right tibia and fibula and multiple lacerations and contusions.

71. The primary patient goal at this point should be to

○ 1. reduce the client's anxiety.

○ 2. maintain adequate oxygenation.

○ 3. decrease chest pain.

○ 4. maintain adequate circulating volume.

72. With a diagnosis of right rib fracture and closed pneumothorax, the client should be placed in

○ 1. modified Trendelenburg's position with his lower extremities elevated.

○ 2. reverse Trendelenburg's position with his head down.

○ 3. left side-lying position with his head elevated 15 to 30 degrees.

○ 4. semi- to high-Fowler's position, tilted toward his right side.

73. On admission, the client's arterial blood gas values were: pH, 7.20; PaO_2, 64 mm Hg; $PaCO_2$, 60 mm Hg; and HCO_3^-, 22 mEq/L. A chest tube is inserted, and oxygen at 4 liters/minute is started. Thirty minutes later, his repeat blood gas values are: pH, 7.30; PaO_2, 76 mm Hg; $PaCO_2$, 50 mm Hg; and HCO_3^-, 22 mEq/L. This change would indicate

○ 1. impending respiratory failure.

○ 2. improving respiratory status.

○ 3. developing respiratory alkalosis.

○ 4. obstruction in the chest tubes.

74. The client's chest tube is connected to a chest tube drainage system with a water seal. The nurse notes that the fluid in the water-seal column is fluctuating with each breath that the client takes. The fluctuation means

○ 1. an obstruction is present in the chest tube.

○ 2. the client is developing subcutaneous emphysema.

○ 3. the chest tube system is functioning properly.

○ 4. there is a leak in the chest tube system.

75. The client's wife arrives on the unit 6 hours after her husband's accident, explaining that she has been out of town. She is distraught because she was not with her husband when he needed her. The most appropriate initial intervention for her would be to

○ 1. allow her to verbalize her feelings and concerns.

○ 2. describe her husband's medical treatment since admission.

○ 3. explain the nature of the injury and reassure her that her husband's condition is stable.

○ 4. reassure her that the important fact is that she is here now.

76. The client is to be discharged to home with the chest tube drainage system intact. The nurse should instruct the client to call the physician for which of the following?

   ○ 1. Respiratory rate greater than 16 breaths/minute.
   ○ 2. Continuous bubbling in the water-seal chamber.
   ○ 3. Fluid in the chest tube.
   ○ 4. Fluctuation of fluid in the water-seal chamber.

77. Which of the following findings would suggest pneumothorax in a trauma victim?

   ○ 1. Pronounced crackles.
   ○ 2. Inspiratory wheezing.
   ○ 3. Dullness on percussion.
   ○ 4. Absent breath sounds.

78. Oxygen toxicity results from oxygen concentrations above

   ○ 1. 21%.
   ○ 2. 28%.
   ○ 3. 40%.
   ○ 4. 60%.

79. For a client with rib fractures and pneumothorax, the physician prescribes morphine sulfate, 1 to 2 mg/hour, given intravenously as needed for pain. The primary objective of this order is to provide adequate pain control so the client can breathe effectively. Which of the following outcomes would indicate successful achievement of this objective?

   ○ 1. Pain rating of "no pain" by the client.
   ○ 2. Decreased client anxiety.
   ○ 3. Respiratory rate of 26 breaths/minute.
   ○ 4. PaO_2 greater than 70 mm Hg.

80. A client undergoes surgery to repair lung injuries. Postoperative orders include the transfusion of one unit of packed red blood cells at a rate of 60 mL/hour. About how long would this transfusion take?

   ○ 1. 2 hours.
   ○ 2. 4 hours.
   ○ 3. 6 hours.
   ○ 4. 8 hours.

81. The primary reason for infusing blood at a rate of 60 mL/hour is to help prevent

   ○ 1. emboli formation.
   ○ 2. fluid volume overload.
   ○ 3. red blood cell hemolysis.
   ○ 4. allergic reaction.

82. When teaching a client to deep breathe effectively after a lobectomy, it would be best for the nurse to instruct the client to

   ○ 1. contract the abdominal muscles, take a slow deep breath through the nose, and hold it for 3 to 5 seconds.
   ○ 2. contract the abdominal muscles, take a deep breath through the mouth, and exhale slowly as if trying to blow out a candle.
   ○ 3. relax the abdominal muscles, take a slow deep breath through the nose, and hold it for 3 to 5 seconds.

   ○ 4. relax the abdominal muscles, take a deep breath through the mouth, and exhale slowly over 10 seconds.

83. On a client's second postoperative day after lung surgery, the nurse auscultates scattered crackles bilaterally. Which of the following interventions would be most appropriate?

   ○ 1. Encourage coughing and check the water-seal system.
   ○ 2. Encourage deep breathing and ambulation as soon as the client is able.
   ○ 3. Perform endotracheal suctioning once per shift and ask the physician to order an expectorant.
   ○ 4. Reduce the frequency of pain medication and increase the suction in the water-seal bottle.

84. Which of the following rehabilitative measures should the nurse teach the client who has undergone chest surgery to perform to prevent shoulder ankylosis?

   ○ 1. Turn from side to side.
   ○ 2. Raise and lower the head.
   ○ 3. Raise the arm on the affected side over the head.
   ○ 4. Flex and extend the elbow on the affected side.

85. A client's chest tube is to be removed by the physician. Which of the following items should the nurse have ready to be placed directly over the wound when the chest tube is removed?

   ○ 1. Butterfly dressing.
   ○ 2. Montgomery strap.
   ○ 3. Fine-mesh gauze dressing.
   ○ 4. Petrolatum gauze dressing.

86. Complications associated with a tracheostomy tube include

   ○ 1. decreased cardiac output.
   ○ 2. damage to the laryngeal nerve.
   ○ 3. pneumothorax.
   ○ 4. adult respiratory distress syndrome (ARDS).

87. A priority goal for the hospitalized client with a new tracheostomy would be to

   ○ 1. decrease secretions.
   ○ 2. instruct the client in caring for the tracheostomy.
   ○ 3. relieve anxiety related to the tracheostomy.
   ○ 4. maintain a patent airway.

88. Measures to prevent ARDS include which of the following?

   ○ 1. Cigarette smoking cessation.
   ○ 2. Maintenance of adequate levels of serum potassium.
   ○ 3. Monitoring clients for signs of hypercapnia.
   ○ 4. Adequate fluid replacement during hypovolemic states.

89. Which of the following would be a priority nursing diagnosis category for a client with ARDS?

   ○ 1. Ineffective Breathing Pattern.
   ○ 2. Pain.

○ 3. Altered Health Maintenance.

○ 4. High Risk for Infection.

90. The nurse interprets which of the following as an early sign of ARDS in a client at risk?

○ 1. elevated carbon dioxide level.

○ 2. hypoxia refractory to oxygen therapy.

○ 3. metabolic acidosis.

○ 4. severe, unexplained electrolyte imbalance.

CORRECT ANSWERS AND RATIONALE

The letters in parentheses following the rationale identify the step of the nursing process (A, D, P, I, E), cognitive level (K, C, T, N), and client needs (S, G, L, H). See the Answer Grid for the key.

The Client With Pneumonia

1. 1. The client described in this item is 79 years old; pneumonia most commonly occurs in the elderly and debilitated. Arthritis, vegetarian diet, and cold-water bathing are unlikely predisposing factors for pneumonia. (A, T, G)

2. 2. Fatigue is a major problem for the client with pneumonia and makes it difficult for clients to perform their self-care activities. Fatigue is due to reduced oxygenation and inability to sleep and rest because of coughing. The hospital environment further contributes to interrupted sleep patterns. Myocardial damage, fluid volume deficit, and pain are not typically related to pneumonia. The client's history does not suggest impaired thought processes. (D, N, G)

3. 2. A sputum specimen is obtained for culture to determine the causative organism. After the organism is identified, an appropriate antibiotic can be prescribed. (I, T, S)

4. 3. It is essential to monitor serum creatinine in the client receiving an aminoglycoside antibiotic because an adverse effect of these antibiotics is acute tubular necrosis, which leads to elevated serum creatinine. (A, T, G)

5. 3. Frequent linen changes take priority for this client because she has shared her concerns for feeling clean. Diaphoresis may produce general discomfort. Position changes need to be done every 2 hours. Nasotracheal suctioning is not indicated with the client's productive cough. Frequent offering of a bed pan is not indicated in this situation. (I, N, L)

6. 1. Pneumonia interferes with ventilation. It is essential to reduce the body's need for oxygen at the cellular level, and bed rest is the most effective method for doing so. (I, C, G)

7. 3. The recommended site for assessing temperature in a client with pneumonia who is coughing and having difficulty breathing is the rectum. The groin and axilla are usually used when the oral and rectal sites are contraindicated. (A, T, S)

8. 4. A client with pneumonia has a ventilation problem due to the infection that causes reduced oxygenation of the blood. This will cause the client to become cyanotic because blood is not adequately oxygenated in the lungs before it enters the peripheral circulation. (A, T, G)

9. 3. Chest pain in pneumonia is generally caused by friction between the pleural layers. It is more severe on inspiration than expiration owing to chest movement. (A, T, G)

10. 4. The pleuritic pain is triggered by chest movement and is particularly severe during coughing. Splinting the chest wall will help reduce the discomfort of coughing. Deep breathing is essential to prevent further atelectasis; an incentive spirometer facilitates effective deep breathing. (I, T, G)

11. 1. Aspirin is administered to clients with pneumonia because it is an analgesic that helps control pain and an antipyretic that helps reduce fever. It is also an antiinflammatory agent that reduces inflammation. Additionally, it reduces blood platelet aggregation and may be used to help prevent clotting in clients prone to heart attacks and strokes. (I, T, G)

12. 2. Humidified air helps liquefy respiratory secretions, making them easier to raise and expectorate. Postural drainage, vibration and percussion of the chest wall, and coughing and deep-breathing exercises may be helpful for respiratory hygiene but will not affect the nature of secretions. (I, T, G)

13. 3. Clients characteristically exhibit irritability or anxiety when hypoxia is present. Coma, apathy, and depression are not typical signs or symptoms of hypoxia. (A, T, L)

14. 1. This client has a white blood cell count of 14,000/mm^3. Normal total white blood cell count is between 5,000 and 10,000/mm^3 in adults. Because this client's white blood cell count remains elevated, the physician should be notified. Altering prescribed medication doses is not a nursing responsibility. Initiating isolation is not indicated. (I, T, S)

15. 1. Docusate sodium is a stool softener that acts similarly to a detergent. It allows fluid and fatty substances to enter the stool and soften it. (I, K, G)

16. 4. Annual influenza and pneumococcal vaccines are effective in reducing the recurrence of pneumonia. Dietary changes are not indicated. Antibiotic therapy for viral infections does not prevent bacterial infection. Prophylactic antibiotic therapy is not typically prescribed because of the increasing prevalence of resistant bacterial strains. (P, N, H)

The Client With Tuberculosis

17. 1. Tuberculosis typically produces anorexia and weight loss. Other signs and symptoms may include

fatigue, afternoon fever, and night sweats. Dyspnea on exertion is not a common symptom of tuberculosis. (A, K, G)

18. 1. The most commonly used technique to identify tubercle bacilli is acid-fast staining. The bacilli have a waxy surface, which makes them difficult to stain in the laboratory. When stained, however, the stain is resistant to removal, even with acids. Therefore, tubercle bacilli are often called acid-fast bacilli. (A, C, S)

19. 1. Streptomycin is an aminoglycoside, and eighth cranial nerve damage is a common side effect of aminoglycosides. Common side effects of isoniazid, aminosalicylic acid, and ethambutol hydrochloride are peripheral neuritis, gastrointestinal intolerance, and optic neuritis, respectively. (A, C, G)

20. 1. The most common side effect of streptomycin is vertigo, resulting from damage to part of the eighth cranial nerve. Other symptoms of eighth cranial nerve toxicity include tinnitus, hearing loss, and ataxia. (E, T, G)

21. 3. It is essential that a client with tuberculosis take medications exactly as prescribed. Sufficient rest, a nourishing diet, and clean air are important but do not rate the same high priority as drug therapy. (I, N, H)

22. 2. Tubercle bacilli may be spread in various ways, most commonly by droplet nuclei carried in air currents. Droplet nuclei are residue of evaporated droplets containing the bacilli, which remain suspended and are circulated in the air. (I, T, S)

23. 1. Unclean hands are thought to spread most organisms. Many techniques can be used to help control the spread of organisms, such as having separate personal care items, using disposable equipment, and isolating people known to be harboring disease-causing organisms—but the most important technique is washing the hands thoroughly and frequently. (I, K, S)

24. 4. Using a combination of antitubercular drugs slows the rate at which organisms develop resistance to the drugs. Combination therapy also appears to be more effective than single-drug therapy. (P, T, G)

25. 2. Ensuring that clients are well educated about the disease is the highest priority. Offering emotional support, teaching about the disease, coordinating agency services, and assessing environment are all part of additional care for clients with tuberculosis. (P, N, G)

26. 1. The appropriate technique for an intradermal injection includes holding the needle and syringe almost parallel to the client's skin, keeping the skin slightly taut when the needle is inserted, and inserting the needle with the bevel side up. The area into

which an intradermal injection is made is not massaged. (I, N, S)

27. 4. Tuberculosis once affected primarily the young; currently, elderly and immunosuppressed people are believed to be at higher risk. (A, T, H)

28. 3. Clients with newly positive skin tests are aggressively treated with isoniazid for about 9 months. Repeat skin testing should not be performed, and skin tests do not convert to negative once a positive response has been obtained. (P, N, H)

29. 2. A positive Mantoux skin test indicates that the client has had contact with tubercle bacilli. It does not mean that the client has active tuberculosis, nor that the client has developed a resistance to tubercle bacilli or a passive immunity to tuberculosis. (E, N, G)

30. 2. Isoniazid competes for the available vitamin B_6 in the body and leaves the client at risk for developing neuropathies related to vitamin deficiency. Supplemental B_6 is routinely prescribed. (P, T, G)

31. 3. Isoniazid interferes with the effectiveness of oral contraceptives, and female clients of childbearing age should be counseled to use an alternate form of birth control while taking the drug. (I, T, H)

32. 3. Tuberculosis can be controlled but never completely eradicated from the body. Periods of intense physical or emotional stress increase the likelihood of recurrence. (I, T, H)

33. 2. Statistics show that of the four geographic areas described in this item, most cases of tuberculosis are found in inner-core residential areas of large cities, where health and sanitation standards tend to be low. These city areas are also generally characterized by substandard housing and poverty. (A, K, S)

The Client With Chronic Obstructive Pulmonary Disease

34. 1. Fear, even when unfounded, can stand in the way of recovery. When this client expresses a fear of being in room 13 because he thinks the number would bring him bad luck, it would be best for the nurse to try to eliminate the reason for the client's fear. Refusing to move the client to another room fails to take the client's fears into account. Moving the client because superstitions have a good chance of coming true relies on an unproven phenomenon. A superstition becomes truth only on the basis of chance. (I, N, L)

35. 4. Relatively low concentrations of oxygen are administered to clients with COPD so as not to eliminate their respiratory drive. Carbon dioxide content in the blood normally regulates respirations. But clients with COPD are often accustomed to high carbon dioxide levels, and the low oxygen blood level is their stimulus to breathe. If they receive excessive oxygen and experience a drop in the blood carbon dioxide, they may stop breathing. (P, T, S)

36. 1. The client's problem is altered nutrition—specifically, less than he requires. The etiology, as stated by the client, is the fatigue associated with his disease process. Therefore, option 1 is the most specific nursing diagnosis, which leads the nurse directly to the nursing actions required. COPD is not an appropriate etiology, because nurses cannot treat the disease process. Altered Breathing Patterns may be a problem, but this diagnosis does not specifically address the problem described by the client. Additionally, Weight Loss as such is not a nursing diagnosis. (D, N, G)

37. 1. A client with COPD is subject to respiratory infections. COPD is slowly progressive; therefore, maintaining current status, requiring less supplemental oxygen, and showing permanent improvement are unrealistic expectations. (P, N, G)

38. 4. Increasing dyspnea on exertion indicates that the client may be experiencing complications of COPD, and therefore the physician should be notified. Extracting promises from clients is not an outcome criterion. Pain is not a common symptom of COPD. Fever is not an acceptable outcome criterion. (E, N, G)

39. 1. Increased anteroposterior chest diameter is characteristic of advanced COPD. Air is trapped in the overextended alveoli, and the ribs are fixed in an inspiratory position. The result is the typical barrel-chested appearance. Other physical changes associated with COPD include overly developed neck muscles, distended neck veins, and diminished chest excursion on respiration. (A, K, G)

40. 4. Cigarette smoking is a major risk factor for COPD. Other risk factors include exposure to environmental pollutants and chronic asthma. Insufficient protein intake and exposure to people with respiratory infection do not increase the risk of COPD. (I, N, H)

41. 4. Pursed-lip breathing increases pressure within the alveoli and makes it easier to empty the air in the alveoli, thereby promoting carbon dioxide elimination. By decreasing the expiratory rate and helping the client relax, pursed-lip breathing helps the client learn to control the rate and depth of respiration. (I, T, G)

42. 2. Theophylline ethylenediamide is a xanthine derivative that acts directly on bronchial smooth muscle to relax and dilate the bronchi and relieve bronchial constriction and spasms. When the drug exerts its primary desired effect, dyspnea and shortness of breath decrease. This drug neither reduces bronchial secretions nor decreases alveolar elasticity. It does increase strength of myocardial contractility,

but this is not the action for which it is used. (P, T, G)

43. 1. A priority goal for the client with COPD is to manage the signs and symptoms of the disease process to maintain the client's ability to function. Pain is not a typical symptom of COPD. Carbon dioxide levels are elevated to an abnormal level with COPD. Clients with COPD do not need treatment for an infectious agent unless such an agent is present. (P, T, G)

44. 4. The client's pH is alkalotic and the $PaCO_2$ is decreased, indicating respiratory alkalosis. The PaO_2 level has little direct bearing on acid-base status but is important in evaluating the client's overall condition. In this client, the low PaO_2 level could be contributing to an increased respiratory rate and the respiratory alkalosis. (D, N, G)

45. 3. This $PaCO_2$ level indicates that the client is hyperventilating. Normal $PaCO_2$ levels are between 35 and 45 mm Hg. In hyperventilation, carbon dioxide is excreted at an increased rate, and the $PaCO_2$ falls below 35 mm Hg. (D, N, G)

46. 1. Normal PaO_2 level ranges between 80 and 100 mm Hg. When the PaO_2 value falls to 50 mm Hg, as described in this item, the nurse should be alert for signs of hypoxia and impending respiratory failure. (D, N, G)

47. 4. $PaCO_2$ of 28 mm Hg and PaO_2 of 50 mm Hg are both abnormal; the PaO_2 of 50 mm Hg signifies acute respiratory failure. In evaluating possible etiologies for this disorder, the nurse should consider conditions that lead to hypoxia and hyperventilation, such as pulmonary embolus. COPD is typically associated with respiratory acidosis and elevated $PaCO_2$. The client with diabetic ketoacidosis most often has metabolic acidosis. A myocardial infarction does not often cause an acid-base imbalance because the primary problem is cardiac in origin. (D, N, G)

48. 2. The high $PaCO_2$ level causes flushing due to vasodilation. The client becomes drowsy and lethargic because carbon dioxide has a depressant effect on the central nervous system. Restlessness, irritability, and anxiety are not common with a $PaCO_2$ level of 80 mm Hg. (A, T, G)

49. 2. In postural drainage, gravity helps move secretions from smaller to larger airways. Postural drainage is best used after percussion has loosened secretions. (I, T, S)

50. 2. Prolonged inactivity causes the body to excrete excessive calcium. This leads to breakdown of bone tissue; as a result, the bones become brittle and fracture easily, a condition known as *osteoporosis*. The excessive calcium excretion that occurs during bed rest also predisposes the client to formation of renal calculi. (A, C, G)

51. 3. A fluid intake of 2 to 3 L/day, in the absence of cardiovascular or renal disease, helps liquefy bronchial secretions. A low-salt diet, continuous oxygen therapy, and a semi-sitting position do not help reduce the viscosity of mucus. (I, T, G)

52. 2. Exhaling normally requires less energy than inhaling. Therefore, lifting while exhaling saves energy and reduces perceived dyspnea. (I, T, H)

53. 3. Right-sided heart failure is a complication of COPD that occurs because of pulmonary hypertension. Signs and symptoms of right-sided heart failure include peripheral edema, jugular venous distention, hepatomegaly, and weight gain due to increased fluid volume. Clubbing of nail beds, hypertension, and increased appetite are not necessarily associated with right-sided heart failure. (I, T, H)

The Client With Lung Cancer

54. 4. Positioning on the side allows any vomitus to roll out by gravity, thereby reducing the risk of aspiration. A nasogastric tube is not placed after a bronchoscopy because the gastrointestinal tract is not entered. Oral fluids are withheld until the gag-and-swallow reflexes return. Preoperative sedation and local anesthesia impair swallowing and the laryngeal reflex, which is protective in nature. The trachea can be perforated inadvertently, not the bowel; abdominal distention and rigidity would indicate bowel perforation. (I, N, G)

55. 1. Risk factors for postoperative pulmonary complications include malnourishment, which is indicated by this client's height and weight. The client's age does not place her at increased risk for complications. Although keeping feelings inside can be problematic, it probably would not be a major contributing factor in postoperative pulmonary complications. (A, T, G)

56. 1. Acknowledging the basic feeling that the client expressed and asking an open-ended question allows the client to explain her fears. The first option addresses the main feeling expressed—fear of cancer—and attempts to explore it further. The second option does not focus on the client's feelings; rather, it merely gives reassurance. The third option does not acknowledge the client's feelings at all. The fourth option assumes guilt, which might be present, but additional information is needed before taking further action. (I, N, L)

57. 4. Systematic pain assessment is necessary for adequate pain management in the postoperative client. Guidelines from the Agency for Health Care Policy Research recommend institutions adopt a pain assessment scale to assist in facilitating pain management. Even though the client is receiving morphine sulfate by PCA, assessment is needed if she is experiencing pain. Reassuring the client or encouraging her to ignore the pain are inappropriate interventions. (A, T, G)

58. 2. Semi-Fowler's position allows for downward displacement of the diaphragm and relaxation of the abdominal muscles, which are needed for good ventilatory excursion. The hand placement supports the operative area and splints it without causing pain from pressure. Trendelenburg's position is contraindicated because abdominal contents pushing against the diaphragm will decrease effective lung volume. Keeping the bed flat does not allow the diaphragm to descend. Positioning the client on the operative side prevents maximum inflation of the left lung, and placing the hands on the operative area before inhalation can restrict thoracic movement. (I, N, G)

59. 1. Because clients are discharged as soon as possible from the hospital, it is essential to evaluate the support they have to assist them with self-care at home. The distance the client lives from the hospital is not a critical factor in discharge planning. There are no data to support that home blood pressure monitoring is needed. Causes of lung cancer, while important, are not the most essential area to evaluate given the client's status. (E, T, S)

60. 2. Epidermoid cancer involving the larger bronchi is almost entirely associated with heavy cigarette smoking. The American Cancer Society reports that smoking is responsible for more than 80% of lung cancers in men and women. The prevalence of lung cancer is related to the duration and intensity of the smoking, so nurses can best prevent lung cancer by persuading clients to stop smoking. Chest radiographs aid in detection of lung cancer; they do not prevent it. Exposure to asbestos has been implicated as a risk factor for lung cancer, but cigarette smoking is the major risk factor. (I, C, H)

61. 3. Atropine sulfate is an anticholinergic drug that decreases mucous secretions in the respiratory tract and dries the mucous membranes of the mouth, nose, pharynx, and bronchi. Atropine does not cause drowsiness; in large doses, it causes excitement and maniacal behavior. It causes the skin to become hot and dry and, in doses less than 0.5 mg, can cause bradycardia. Moderate to large doses cause tachycardia and palpitations. (I, T, G)

62. 4. Deep breathing helps prevent microatelectasis and pneumonitis and also helps force air and fluid out of the pleural space into the chest tubes. The diaphragm is the major muscle of respiration; deep breathing causes it to descend, thereby increasing the ventilating surface. More than half the ventilatory process is accomplished by the rise and fall of the diaphragm. Deep breathing increases blood flow to the lungs. The remaining lobe will naturally hyperinflate to fill the space created by the resected lobe. This is an expected phenomenon. (I, T, G)

63. 3. Restlessness indicates cerebral hypoxia due to decreased circulating volume. Shortness of breath occurs because blood collecting in the pleural space faster than suction can remove it prevents the lung from reexpanding. Increased blood pressure and decreased pulse and respiratory rates are classic late signs of increased intracranial pressure. Decreasing blood pressure and increasing pulse and respiratory rates occur with hypovolemic shock. Sanguineous drainage that changes to serosanguineous drainage at a rate less than 100 mL/hour is normal in the early postoperative period. Urine output of 180 mL over the past 3 hours indicates normal kidney perfusion. (A, N, G)

64. 2. It is essential that the nurse evaluate the effects of pain medication after the medication has had time to act. Although the other interventions are appropriate, reassessment is necessary to determine effectiveness and intervention if needed. (I, N, G)

65. 3. This crackling sensation is most likely subcutaneous emphysema. Subcutaneous emphysema is not an unusual finding and is not dangerous if confined. But progression can be serious, especially if the neck is involved; tracheotomy may be needed. If emphysema progresses noticeably in 1 hour, the physician should be notified. Lowering the head of the bed and assessing blood pressure will not arrest the progress or provide any further information. A tracheotomy tray, not an aspiration tray, would be useful if emphysema progresses to the neck. Emphysema may progress if the chest drainage system does not adequately remove air and fluid; therefore, the system would not be turned off. (I, N, G)

66. 4. The drainage apparatus is always kept *below* the client's chest level to prevent back flow of fluid into the pleural space. The air vent must always be open in the closed chest drainage system to allow air from the client to escape. Stripping a chest tube causes excessive negative intrapleural pressure and is not recommended. Clamping a chest tube when moving a client is not recommended. (I, T, G)

67. 1. Cessation of fluid fluctuation in the tubing can mean one of several things: the lung has fully expanded, and negative intrapleural pressure has been reestablished; the chest tube is occluded; or the chest tube is not in the pleural space. Fluid fluctuation occurs because during inspiration, intrapleural pressure exceeds the negative pressure generated in the water-seal system. Therefore, drainage moves toward the client. During expiration, the pleural pressure exceeds that generated in the

water-seal system, and fluid moves away from the client. (A, C, S)

68. 2. There should never be constant bubbling in the water-seal bottle. Constant bubbling in the water-seal bottle indicates an air leak, which means that less negative pressure is being exerted on the pleural space. Decreasing the suction will not reduce the leak, nor will draining part of the water in the water-seal chamber. (I, T, G)

69. 1. In this case, there may be some obstruction to the flow of air and fluid out of the pleural space, causing air and fluid to collect and build up pressure. This prevents the remaining lung from reexpanding and can cause a mediastinal shift to the opposite side. Increasing the suction is not done without a physician's order. The normal position of the drainage bottles is 2 to 3 feet below chest level. Clamping the tubes obstructs the flow of air and fluid out of the pleural space. (I, T, G)

70. 3. Rubber-capped clamps should be readily available and in view when a client has chest drainage. In some institutions, the protocol to follow after accidental disconnection of a chest tube is to clamp the tube close to the client and notify the physician immediately. (P, C, S)

The Client With Chest Trauma

71. 2. Blunt chest trauma may lead to respiratory failure, and maintenance of adequate oxygenation is the priority for the client. Although pain is distressing to the client and can increase anxiety and decrease respiratory effectiveness, pain control is secondary to maintaining oxygenation. Decreasing the client's anxiety is related to maintaining effective respirations and oxygenation. Maintaining adequate circulatory volume is also secondary to maintaining adequate oxygenation. (P, N, G)

72. 4. Pneumothorax will cause a client to feel extremely short of breath. Semi- or high-Fowler's position will facilitate ventilation by the unaffected lung. A flat or reverse Trendelenburg's position places additional pressure on the chest and inhibits ventilation. Likewise, positioning the client on the unaffected side compromises the remaining functional lung. (I, T, G)

73. 2. The ABG values at admission reveal respiratory acidosis and are consistent with a diagnosis of pneumothorax. The ABG values after chest tube insertion are returning to normal, indicating that treatment is effective. Impending respiratory failure would be indicated by a decreasing PaO_2 or an increasing $PaCO_2$. The client is not alkalotic because the pH values are below 7.35. If the chest tubes were obstructed, the client's respiratory status would deteriorate. (E, N, G)

74. 3. Fluctuation of fluid with respirations in the water-seal column indicate that the system is functioning properly. If an obstruction is present in the chest tube, fluid fluctuation is absent. A leak in the system is indicated when bubbling occurs in the water-seal column. Subcutaneous emphysema occurs when air pockets can be palpated beneath the client's skin around the chest tube insertion site. (E, N, S)

75. 1. Verbalizing feelings and concerns helps decrease anxiety and allows the family member to move on to understanding the current situation. Describing events or explaining equipment is appropriate when the person is not distraught and is ready to learn. Reassuring the family member does not allow verbalization of feelings and discounts the person's feelings. (I, N, L)

76. 2. Continuous bubbling in the water-seal chamber indicates a leak in the system, and the client needs to be instructed to notify the physician if continuous bubbling occurs. Fluid in the chest tube and fluctuation of the fluid in the water-seal chamber are expected. A respiratory rate of greater than 16 breaths/minute may not be unusual and does not always mean that the client should notify the physician. (I, T, S)

77. 4. Pneumothorax indicates that the lung has collapsed and is not functioning. The nurse will hear no sounds of air movement on auscultation. (A, C, G)

78. 3. Oxygen concentration greater than 40% has been found to cause oxygen toxicity in adults. (A, K, S)

79. 1. If the client reports no pain, then the objective of adequate pain relief has been met. Decreased anxiety is not related only to the stated objective; it could also be related to other factors. The respiratory rate of 26 and a PaO_2 of greater than 70 are not related to pain management and are not within normal limits. (E, N, G)

80. 2. One unit of packed red blood cells is about 250 mL. If the blood is delivered at a rate of 60 mL/hour, it will take about 4 hours to infuse the entire unit. (I, T, S)

81. 2. Too-rapid infusion of blood, or of any intravenous fluid, is likely to cause fluid volume overload and related problems such as pulmonary edema. Emboli formation, red blood cell hemolysis, and allergic reaction are not related to rapid infusion. (I, T, G)

82. 1. The recommended procedure for teaching clients postoperatively to deep breathe includes contracting (pulling in) the abdominal muscles and taking a slow, deep breath through the nose. This breath is held 3 to 5 seconds, which facilitates alveolar ventilation by improving the inspiratory phase of ventilation. Ex-

haling slowly as if trying to blow out a candle is a technique used in pursed-lip breathing to facilitate expiration in people with COPD. (I, T, G)

83. 2. Shallow breathing is a common problem after chest surgery owing to the pain associated with deep breathing. Assisting the client to deep breathe and ambulate will help reduce crackles and improve oxygenation. There is no indication in this situation of malfunction in the water-seal system. Reducing pain medication would make effective deep breathing and ambulating more difficult. Endotracheal suctioning is not indicated at this time. (I, T, G)

84. 3. A client who has undergone chest surgery should be taught to raise the arm on the affected side over the head to help prevent shoulder ankylosis. This exercise helps restore normal shoulder movement, prevents stiffening of the shoulder joint, and improves muscle tone and power. (I, T, G)

85. 4. Immediately after chest tube removal, a petrolatum gauze is placed over the wound and covered with a dry sterile dressing. This serves as an airtight seal to prevent air leakage or air movement in either direction. Bandages or straps are not applied directly over wounds. Mesh gauze would allow air movement. (I, T, G)

86. 2. Tracheostomy tubes carry several potential complications, including laryngeal nerve damage, bleeding, and infection. They do not cause decreased cardiac output, pneumothorax, or ARDS. (A, C, G)

87. 4. The main goal for a client with a new tracheostomy is to maintain a patent airway. New tracheostomies frequently cause bleeding and excess secretions, and clients may require frequent suctioning to maintain patency. (P, N, G)

88. 4. One of the major risk factors for development of ARDS is hypovolemic shock. Adequate fluid replacement is essential to minimize the risk of development of ARDS in these clients. Smoking cessation, serum potassium levels, and hypercapnia are not risk factors for development of ARDS. (I, C, H)

89. 1. Ineffective Breathing Pattern is a priority nursing diagnosis category for the client with ARDS. The massive shift of fluid from the capillaries to the alveoli, as well as the reduced surfactant, greatly increases the work of breathing. The lungs become stiff and noncompliant, and the client becomes severely hypoxic. (D, N, G)

90. 2. A hallmark of early ARDS is refractory hypoxemia. The client's PaO_2 level continues to fall, despite higher concentrations of administered oxygen. Elevated carbon dioxide levels and metabolic acidosis occur late in the disorder. Severe electrolyte imbalances are not indicators of ARDS. The client with ARDS usually requires endotracheal intubation and mechanical ventilation. (A, T, G)

NURSING CARE OF ADULTS WITH MEDICAL AND SURGICAL HEALTH PROBLEMS

TEST 1: The Client With Respiratory Health Problems

Directions: Use this answer grid to determine areas of strength or need for further study.

NURSING PROCESS	COGNITIVE LEVEL	CLIENT NEEDS
A = Assessment	K = Knowledge	S = Safe, effective care environment
D = Analysis, nursing diagnosis	C = Comprehension	G = Physiologic integrity
P = Planning	T = Application	L = Psychosocial integrity
I = Implementation	N = Analysis	H = Health promotion and maintenance
E = Evaluation		

Question #	Answer #	Nursing Process A	D	P	I	E	Cognitive Level K	C	T	N	Client Needs S	G	L	H
1	1	A							T			G		
2	2		D							N		G		
3	2				I				T		S			
4	3	A							T			G		
5	3				I					N			L	
6	1				I			C				G		
7	3	A							T		S			
8	4	A							T			G		
9	3	A							T			G		
10	4				I				T			G		
11	1				I				T			G		
12	2				I				T			G		
13	3	A							T				L	
14	1				I				T		S			
15	1				I		K					G		
16	4			P						N				H
17	1	A					K					G		
18	1	A						C			S			
19	1	A						C				G		
20	1					E			T			G		
21	3				I					N				H
22	2				I				T		S			
23	1				I		K				S			
24	4			P					T			G		
25	2			P						N		G		

ANSWER GRID: 1

NURSING PROCESS

A = Assessment
D = Analysis, nursing diagnosis
P = Planning
I = Implementation
E = Evaluation

COGNITIVE LEVEL

K = Knowledge
C = Comprehension
T = Application
N = Analysis

CLIENT NEEDS

S = Safe, effective care environment
G = Physiologic integrity
L = Psychosocial integrity
H = Health promotion and maintenance

Question #	Answer #	Nursing Process					Cognitive Level				Client Needs			
		A	D	P	I	E	K	C	T	N	S	G	L	H
26	1				I					N	S			
27	4	A							T					H
28	3			P						N				H
29	2					E				N		G		
30	2			P					T			G		
31	3				I				T					H
32	3				I				T					H
33	2	A					K				S			
34	1				I					N			L	
35	4			P					T		S			
36	1		D							N		G		
37	1			P						N		G		
38	4					E				N		G		
39	1	A					K					G		
40	4				I					N				H
41	4				I				T			G		
42	2			P					T			G		
43	1			P					T			G		
44	4		D							N		G		
45	3		D							N		G		
46	1		D							N		G		
47	4		D							N		G		
48	2	A							T			G		
49	2				I				T		S			
50	2	A						C				G		
51	3				I				T			G		
52	2				I				T					H
53	3				I				T					H
54	4				I					N		G		
55	1	A							T			G		

NURSING PROCESS

A = Assessment
D = Analysis, nursing diagnosis
P = Planning
I = Implementation
E = Evaluation

COGNITIVE LEVEL

K = Knowledge
C = Comprehension
T = Application
N = Analysis

CLIENT NEEDS

S = Safe, effective care environment
G = Physiologic integrity
L = Psychosocial integrity
H = Health promotion and maintenance

Question #	Answer #	Nursing Process					Cognitive Level				Client Needs			
		A	D	P	I	E	K	C	T	N	S	G	L	H
56	1				I					N			L	
57	4	A							T			G		
58	2				I					N		G		
59	1					E			T		S			
60	2				I			C						H
61	3				I				T			G		
62	4				I				T			G		
63	3	A								N		G		
64	2				I					N		G		
65	3				I					N		G		
66	4				I				T			G		
67	1	A						C			S			
68	2				I				T			G		
69	1				I				T			G		
70	3			P				C			S			
71	2			P						N		G		
72	4				I				T			G		
73	2					E				N		G		
74	3					E				N	S			
75	1				I					N			L	
76	2				I				T		S			
77	4	A						C				G		
78	3	A					K				S			
79	1					E				N		G		
80	2				I				T		S			
81	2				I				T			G		
82	1				I				T			G		
83	2				I				T			G		
84	3				I				T			G		
85	4				I				T			G		

ANSWER GRID: 3

NURSING PROCESS

A = Assessment
D = Analysis, nursing diagnosis
P = Planning
I = Implementation
E = Evaluation

COGNITIVE LEVEL

K = Knowledge
C = Comprehension
T = Application
N = Analysis

CLIENT NEEDS

S = Safe, effective care environment
G = Physiologic integrity
L = Psychosocial integrity
H = Health promotion and maintenance

Question #	Answer #	Nursing Process					Cognitive Level				Client Needs			
		A	D	P	I	E	K	C	T	N	S	G	L	H
86	2	A						C				G		
87	4			P						N		G		
88	4				I			C						H
89	1		D							N		G		
90	2	A							T			G		
Number Correct														
Number Possible	90	22	7	12	42	7	6	10	44	30	17	57	5	11
Percentage Correct														

Score Calculation: To determine your **Percentage Correct,** divide the **Number Correct** by the **Number Possible.**

ANSWER GRID: 4

The Client With Cardiac Health Problems

Test 2

- **The Client With Myocardial Infarction**
- **The Client With Heart Failure**
- **The Client With Valvular Heart Disease**
- **The Client With Hypertension**
- **The Client With Angina**
- **The Client With a Permanent Pacemaker**
- **Correct Answers and Rationale**

Select the one best answer, and indicate your choice by filling in the circle in front of the option.

The Client With Myocardial Infarction

A 60-year-old male client is admitted through the emergency department with crushing substernal chest pain that radiates to the shoulder, jaw, and left arm. The admitting diagnosis is acute myocardial infarction (MI).

1. Immediate admission orders include oxygen by nasal cannula at 4 L/minute, blood work, a chest radiograph, a 12-lead electrocardiogram (ECG), and 2 mg of morphine sulfate given intravenously. The nurse should *first*
- ○ 1. Administer the morphine.
- ○ 2. Obtain a 12-lead ECG.
- ○ 3. Obtain the blood work.
- ○ 4. Order the chest radiograph.

2. When administering a thrombolytic drug to the client experiencing an MI, the nurse explains to him that the purpose of the drug is to
- ○ 1. help keep him well hydrated.
- ○ 2. dissolve clots that he may have.
- ○ 3. prevent kidney failure.
- ○ 4. treat potential cardiac dysrhythmias.

3. If the client develops cardiogenic shock, which characteristic sign should the nurse expect to observe?
- ○ 1. Oliguria.
- ○ 2. Bradycardia.
- ○ 3. Elevated blood pressure.
- ○ 4. Fever.

4. The physician orders continuous intravenous nitro-

glycerin infusion for the client. Essential nursing actions include
- ○ 1. obtaining an infusion pump for the medication.
- ○ 2. monitoring blood pressure every shift.
- ○ 3. monitoring urine output hourly.
- ○ 4. obtaining serum potassium levels daily.

5. The client says to the nurse, "My father died of a heart attack when he was 60, and I suppose I will too." Which of the following responses by the nurse would be the most appropriate?
- ○ 1. "Tell me more about what you are feeling."
- ○ 2. "Are you thinking that you won't recover from this illness?"
- ○ 3. "You have a fine doctor. Everything will be all right soon, I'm sure."
- ○ 4. "Would you agree that this would be very unlikely?"

6. A priority nursing diagnosis during the first 24 hours following an MI is
- ○ 1. Impaired Gas Exchange.
- ○ 2. High Risk for Infection.
- ○ 3. Fluid Volume Deficit.
- ○ 4. Constipation.

7. The pain associated with MI is due to
- ○ 1. left ventricular overload.
- ○ 2. impending circulatory collapse.
- ○ 3. extracellular electrolyte imbalances.
- ○ 4. insufficient oxygen reaching the heart muscle.

8. Aspirin is administered to the client experiencing an MI because of its
- ○ 1. antipyretic action.

○ 2. antithrombotic action.
○ 3. antiplatelet action.
○ 4. analgesic action.

9. While caring for a client who has sustained an MI, the nurse notes eight premature ventricular contractions (PVCs) in 1 minute on the cardiac monitor. The client is receiving an intravenous infusion of 5% dextrose in water and 2 liters/minute of oxygen. The nurse's first course of action should be to
○ 1. increase the intravenous infusion rate.
○ 2. notify the physician promptly.
○ 3. increase the oxygen concentration.
○ 4. administer a prescribed analgesic.

10. Which of the following findings is indicative of MI?
○ 1. Elevated serum cholesterol value.
○ 2. Elevated creatinine phosphokinase (CPK) value.
○ 3. Below-normal erythrocyte sedimentation rate.
○ 4. Elevated white blood cell count.

11. Which of the following is expected for a client on the second day of hospitalization after an MI? The client
○ 1. has minimal chest pain.
○ 2. can identify risk factors for MI.
○ 3. agrees to participating in cardiac rehabilitation program.
○ 4. can perform personal self-care activities without pain.

12. Nursing measures for the client who has had an MI include helping the client to avoid activity that results in Valsalva's maneuver. Which of the following actions would help prevent Valsalva's maneuver? Have the client
○ 1. take fewer but deeper breaths.
○ 2. clench her teeth while moving in bed.
○ 3. drink fluids through a straw.
○ 4. avoid holding her breath during activity.

13. Expected outcomes following intravenous administration of furosemide include
○ 1. increased blood pressure.
○ 2. increased urine output.
○ 3. decreased pain.
○ 4. decreased premature ventricular contractions.

14. After an MI, the hospitalized client is taught to move his or her legs about while resting in bed. This type of exercise is recommended primarily to help
○ 1. prepare the client for ambulation.
○ 2. promote urinary and intestinal elimination.
○ 3. prevent thrombophlebitis and blood clot formation.
○ 4. decrease the likelihood of decubitus ulcer formation.

15. Which of the following accurately reflects the principles on which a client's diet will most likely be based during the acute phase of MI?
○ 1. Liquids as desired.
○ 2. Small, easily digested meals.
○ 3. Three regular meals per day.
○ 4. Nothing by mouth.

16. A client whose condition remains stable after an MI is gradually allowed increased activity. Of the following criteria, the best one on which to judge whether the activity is appropriate is to note the degree of
○ 1. edema.
○ 2. cyanosis.
○ 3. dyspnea.
○ 4. weight loss.

17. Which of the following activities would be least appropriate to prevent sensory deprivation during a client's stay in the cardiac care unit?
○ 1. Watching television.
○ 2. Visiting with the client's daughter.
○ 3. Reading the newspaper.
○ 4. Keeping the client's door closed to provide privacy.

18. Of the following factors, which appears most closely linked to the development of coronary artery disease?
○ 1. Diet.
○ 2. Climate.
○ 3. Heredity.
○ 4. Excessive exercise.

19. A client loses 3.2 kg while hospitalized. About how many pounds has the client lost?
○ 1. 1 pound.
○ 2. 3 pounds.
○ 3. 5 pounds.
○ 4. 7 pounds.

20. A basic principle of any rehabilitation program, including cardiac rehabilitation, is that rehabilitation begins
○ 1. on discharge from the hospital.
○ 2. on discharge from the cardiac care unit.
○ 3. on admission to the hospital.
○ 4. four weeks after the onset of illness.

21. A client is discharged from the hospital after an MI. The client is walking and is taught to continue walking, gradually progressing the distance walked. Which vital sign should the nurse teach the client to monitor to determine whether to increase or decrease progression?
○ 1. Pulse rate.
○ 2. Blood pressure.
○ 3. Body temperature.
○ 4. Respiratory rate.

22. If a client displays behavior detrimental to health, such as smoking cigarettes, eating a diet high in saturated fat, or leading a sedentary lifestyle, techniques of behavior modification may be used to help the client change behavior. The nurse can best reinforce new adaptive behaviors by

○ 1. explaining how the old behavior leads to poor health.
○ 2. withholding praise until the new behavior is well established.
○ 3. rewarding the client whenever the acceptable behavior is performed.
○ 4. instilling mild fear into the client to extinguish the behavior.

23. Alteplase recombinant, or tissue plasminogen activator (tPA), a thrombolytic enzyme, is administered during the first 6 hours after onset of MI to
○ 1. control chest pain.
○ 2. reduce coronary artery vasospasm.
○ 3. control the dysrhythmias associated with MI.
○ 4. revascularize the blocked coronary artery.

24. A priority nursing assessment measure related to tPA administration is to
○ 1. observe for chest pain.
○ 2. monitor for increased atrial dysrhythmias.
○ 3. monitor the 12-lead ECG every 4 hours.
○ 4. observe for signs of crackles.

25. Contraindications to the administration of tPA include which of the following?
○ 1. Age greater than 60 years.
○ 2. History of cerebral hemorrhage.
○ 3. History of heart failure.
○ 4. Cigarette smoking.

26. Crackles heard on lung auscultation indicate
○ 1. pulmonary edema.
○ 2. bronchospasm.
○ 3. airway narrowing.
○ 4. fluid-filled alveoli.

27. The client with angina has been taking nifedipine. The client should be taught to
○ 1. monitor blood pressure weekly.
○ 2. perform daily weights.
○ 3. inspect gums daily.
○ 4. limit intake of green leafy vegetables.

The Client With Heart Failure

A 69-year-old woman has a history of heart failure. She is admitted to the emergency department with heart failure complicated by pulmonary edema.

28. A priority assessment for this client at admission is
○ 1. blood pressure.
○ 2. skin breakdown.
○ 3. serum potassium.
○ 4. urine output.

29. In which of the following positions should the nurse place the client?
○ 1. Semi-sitting (low-Fowler's position).
○ 2. Lying on her right side (Sims' position).
○ 3. Sitting nearly upright (high-Fowler's position).
○ 4. Lying on her back with her head lowered (Trendelenburg's position).

30. Which of the following would be a priority nursing diagnosis for the client with heart failure and pulmonary edema?
○ 1. High Risk for Infection related to stasis of secretions in alveoli.
○ 2. Impaired Skin Integrity related to pressure.
○ 3. Activity Intolerance related to imbalance between oxygen supply and demand.
○ 4. Constipation related to immobility.

31. The major goal of therapy for this client would be to
○ 1. increase cardiac output.
○ 2. improve respiratory status.
○ 3. decrease peripheral edema.
○ 4. enhance comfort.

32. Digoxin is administered intravenously to this client, primarily because the drug acts to
○ 1. dilate coronary arteries.
○ 2. increase myocardial contractility.
○ 3. decrease cardiac dysrhythmias.
○ 4. decrease electrical conductivity in the heart.

33. The nurse is preparing the client to go home. The nurse should instruct the client to
○ 1. monitor urine output daily.
○ 2. maintain bed rest for at least 1 week.
○ 3. monitor daily potassium intake.
○ 4. weigh daily.

34. The client asks the nurse about the reason for taking enalapril maleate. The nurse bases her response on the fact that enalapril is prescribed for people with heart failure to
○ 1. lower the blood pressure by increasing peripheral vasoconstriction.
○ 2. lower the heart rate by slowing the conduction system.
○ 3. block the conversion of angiotensin I to angiotensin II.
○ 4. increase myocardial contractility and thereby improve cardiac output.

35. Metoprolol tartrate, a β-adrenergic antagonist, may be administered to a client with heart failure because it acts to
○ 1. reduce peripheral vascular resistance.
○ 2. increase peripheral vascular resistance.
○ 3. reduce fluid volume.
○ 4. improve myocardial contractility

36. Furosemide is administered intravenously to a client with heart failure. How soon after administration should the nurse begin to see evidence of the drug's desired effect?
○ 1. 5 to 10 minutes.

○ 2. 30 minutes to 1 hour.

○ 3. 2 to 4 hours.

○ 4. 6 to 8 hours.

37. A client with heart failure will take oral furosemide at home. To help the client evaluate the effectiveness of furosemide therapy, the nurse should teach the client to

○ 1. weigh daily.

○ 2. take blood pressure daily.

○ 3. keep a daily record of urinary output.

○ 4. have a serum potassium level drawn weekly.

38. The nurse teaches a client with heart failure to take oral furosemide in the morning. The primary reason for this is to help

○ 1. decrease gastrointestinal irritation.

○ 2. retard rapid drug absorption.

○ 3. excrete fluids accumulated during the night.

○ 4. prevent sleep disturbances during the night.

39. Clients with heart failure are prone to atrial fibrillation. During physical assessment, the nurse would suspect atrial fibrillation when palpation of the radial pulse reveals

○ 1. two regular beats followed by one irregular beat.

○ 2. an irregular pulse rhythm.

○ 3. pulse rate below 60 beats/minute.

○ 4. a weak, thready pulse.

40. Complications of atrial fibrillation can be caused by

○ 1. stasis of blood in the atria.

○ 2. increased cardiac output.

○ 3. decreased pulse rate.

○ 4. elevated blood pressure.

41. The nurse should teach the client that signs of digitalis toxicity include

○ 1. skin rash over the chest and back.

○ 2. increased appetite.

○ 3. colored vision.

○ 4. elevated blood pressure.

42. The nurse should be especially alert for signs and symptoms of digoxin toxicity if serum levels indicate that the client has a

○ 1. low sodium level.

○ 2. high glucose level.

○ 3. high calcium level.

○ 4. low potassium level.

43. Which of the following foods should the nurse teach the client with heart failure to avoid or limit when following a 2-g sodium diet?

○ 1. Apples.

○ 2. Tomato juice.

○ 3. Alcoholic beer.

○ 4. Beef tenderloin.

44. To help maintain a normal blood level of potassium, the client receiving a loop diuretic should be encouraged to eat such foods as bananas, orange juice, and

○ 1. spinach.

○ 2. skimmed milk.

○ 3. baked chicken.

○ 4. brown rice.

The Client With Valvular Heart Disease

A 70-year old woman is scheduled to undergo mitral valve replacement for severely calcific mitral stenosis and mitral regurgitation. Although the diagnosis was made during childhood, she did not have symptoms until 4 years ago. Recently, she noticed increased symptoms despite daily doses of digoxin and furosemide.

45. During the initial interview with the client, the nurse would most likely learn that the client's childhood health history that contributed to mitral valve disease included

○ 1. chicken pox.

○ 2. poliomyelitis.

○ 3. rheumatic fever.

○ 4. meningitis.

46. The client undergoes a mitral valve replacement. Postoperatively, she develops multiple PVCs. The physician orders lidocaine hydrochloride given intravenously with a 50-mg initial bolus followed by continuous infusion at 2 mg/minute. The intravenous bag contains 2 g of lidocaine in 500 mL of dextrose 5% in water. If the infusion pump delivers 60 microdrops/mL, how many microdrops would provide 4 mg of lidocaine each minute?

○ 1. 15 microdrops.

○ 2. 30 microdrops.

○ 3. 45 microdrops.

○ 4. 60 microdrops.

47. After the client experiences some initial excitation, the nurse would judge that she is demonstrating a typical adverse reaction to lidocaine hydrochloride when she complains of

○ 1. palpitations.

○ 2. tinnitus.

○ 3. urinary frequency.

○ 4. lethargy.

48. The physician orders pulmonary artery pressure monitoring, including pulmonary capillary wedge pressure, with a pulmonary artery catheter. The purpose of this is to help assess the

○ 1. degree of coronary artery stenosis.

○ 2. blood pressure within the right ventricle.

○ 3. pressure from fluid within the left ventricle.

○ 4. oxygen and carbon dioxide pressure in the blood.

49. The client's chest tube accidentally disconnects from the drainage tube when she turns onto her

side. Which of the following actions should the nurse take first?
- ○ 1. Notify the physician.
- ○ 2. Clamp the chest tube.
- ○ 3. Raise the level of the drainage bottle.
- ○ 4. Reconnect the tube.

50. Which of the following signs and symptoms would most likely be found in a client with mitral regurgitation?
- ○ 1. Exertional dyspnea.
- ○ 2. Confusion.
- ○ 3. Elevated CPK value.
- ○ 4. Chest pain.

51. The nurse expects that a client with mitral stenosis would likely demonstrate symptoms associated with congestion in the
- ○ 1. aorta.
- ○ 2. right atrium.
- ○ 3. superior vena cava.
- ○ 4. pulmonary circulation.

52. Because a client has mitral stenosis and is a prospective valve recipient, the nurse preoperatively assesses the client's past compliance with medical regimens. Lack of compliance with which of the following regimens would pose the greatest health hazard to this client?
- ○ 1. Medication therapy.
- ○ 2. Diet modification.
- ○ 3. Activity restrictions.
- ○ 4. Lifestyle modifications.

53. In preparing a client and the client's family for a postoperative intensive care unit stay, the nurse should explain that
- ○ 1. the client will remain in the intensive care unit for 5 days.
- ○ 2. the client will sleep most of the time while in the intensive care unit.
- ○ 3. noise and activity within the intensive care unit are minimal.
- ○ 4. the client will receive medication to relieve pain.

54. A client who has undergone a mitral valve replacement experiences persistent bleeding from the surgical incision during the early postoperative period. Which of the following pharmaceutical agents should the nurse be prepared to administer to this client?
- ○ 1. Vitamin C.
- ○ 2. Protamine sulfate.
- ○ 3. Quinidine sulfate.
- ○ 4. Warfarin sodium (Coumadin).

55. The most effective measure the nurse can use to prevent wound infection when changing a client's dressing after coronary artery bypass surgery is to
- ○ 1. observe careful handwashing procedures.
- ○ 2. cleanse the incisional area with an antiseptic.
- ○ 3. use prepackaged sterile dressings to cover the incision.
- ○ 4. place soiled dressings in a waterproof bag before disposing of them.

56. For a client who excretes excessive amounts of calcium during the postoperative period after open heart surgery, which of the following measures should the nurse institute to help prevent complications associated with excessive calcium excretion?
- ○ 1. Ensure a liberal fluid intake.
- ○ 2. Provide an alkaline-ash diet.
- ○ 3. Prevent constipation.
- ○ 4. Enrich the client's diet with dairy products.

57. The nurse teaches the client who is receiving warfarin sodium that
- ○ 1. partial thromboplastin time values determine the dosage of warfarin sodium.
- ○ 2. protamine sulfate is used to reverse the effects of warfarin sodium.
- ○ 3. the international normalized ratio (INR) is used to assess effectiveness.
- ○ 4. warfarin sodium will facilitate clotting of the blood.

58. Good dental care is an important measure in reducing the risk of endocarditis. A teaching plan to promote good dental care in a client with mitral stenosis should include demonstrating the proper use of
- ○ 1. a manual toothbrush.
- ○ 2. an electric toothbrush.
- ○ 3. an irrigation device.
- ○ 4. dental floss.

59. Before a client's discharge after mitral valve replacement surgery, the nurse should evaluate the client's understanding of postcardiac surgery activity restrictions. Which of the following should the client not engage in until after the 1-month postdischarge appointment with the surgeon?
- ○ 1. Showering.
- ○ 2. Lifting anything heavier than 10 pounds.
- ○ 3. A program of gradually progressive walking.
- ○ 4. Light housework.

The Client With Hypertension

An industrial health nurse at a large printing plant finds a male employee's blood pressure to be elevated on two occasions 1 month apart and refers him to his private physician. The employee is about 25 pounds overweight and has smoked a pack of cigarettes daily for more than 20 years.

60. During a nursing assessment, the client says, "I don't really know why I'm here. I feel fine and

haven't had any symptoms." The nurse would recognize the importance of explaining to the client that symptoms of hypertension
- ○ 1. are often not present.
- ○ 2. signify a high risk of stroke.
- ○ 3. occur only with malignant hypertension.
- ○ 4. appear after irreversible kidney damage has occurred.

61. The client's physician prescribes atenolol for the hypertension. The nurse should instruct the client to
- ○ 1. avoid sudden discontinuation of the drug.
- ○ 2. monitor the blood pressure annually.
- ○ 3. follow a 2-g sodium diet.
- ○ 4. discontinue the medication if severe headaches develop.

62. The nurse teaches the client about his dietary restrictions: a low-calorie, low-fat, low-sodium diet. Which of the following menu selections would best meet his needs?
- ○ 1. Mixed green salad with blue cheese dressing, crackers, and cold cuts.
- ○ 2. Ham sandwich on rye bread and an orange.
- ○ 3. Baked chicken, an apple, and a slice of white bread.
- ○ 4. Hot dogs, baked beans, and celery and carrot sticks.

63. The client's job involves working in a warm dry room, frequently bending and crouching to check the underside of a high-speed press, and wearing eye guards. Given this information, the nurse should assess the client for
- ○ 1. Muscle aches.
- ○ 2. Thirst.
- ○ 3. Lethargy.
- ○ 4. Postural hypotension.

64. An exercise program is prescribed for the client. Which intervention would be most likely to assist the client in maintaining an exercise program?
- ○ 1. Giving him a written exercise program.
- ○ 2. Explaining the exercise program to the client's wife.
- ○ 3. Reassuring the client that he can do the exercise program.
- ○ 4. Tailoring a program to the client's needs and abilities.

65. The client realizes the importance of quitting smoking, and the nurse develops a plan to help him achieve his goal. Which of the following nursing interventions should be the initial step in this plan?
- ○ 1. Review the negative effects of smoking on the body.
- ○ 2. Discuss the effects of passive smoking on environmental pollution.
- ○ 3. Establish the client's daily smoking pattern.

- ○ 4. Explain how smoking worsens high blood pressure.

66. Essential hypertension would be diagnosed in a 40-year-old man whose blood pressure readings were consistently at or above
- ○ 1. 120/90 mm Hg.
- ○ 2. 130/85 mm Hg.
- ○ 3. 140/90 mm Hg.
- ○ 4. 160/80 mm Hg.

67. The plan of care for a client with hypertension taking propranolol hydrochloride would include
- ○ 1. instructing the client to discontinue the drug if nausea occurs and to monitor blood pressure.
- ○ 2. monitoring blood pressure every week and adjusting the medication dose accordingly.
- ○ 3. measuring partial thromboplastin time weekly to evaluate blood clotting status.
- ○ 4. instructing the client to notify the physician of irregular or slowed pulse rate.

68. When teaching a client about propranolol hydrochloride, the nurse should base the information on the knowledge that propranolol hydrochloride
- ○ 1. blocks β-adrenergic stimulation and thus causes decreased heart rate, myocardial contractility, and conduction.
- ○ 2. increases norepinephrine secretion and thus decreases blood pressure and heart rate.
- ○ 3. is a potent arterial and venous vasodilator that reduces peripheral vascular resistance and lowers blood pressure.
- ○ 4. is an angiotensin-converting enzyme inhibitor that reduces blood pressure by blocking the conversion of angiotensin I to angiotensin II.

69. A priority nursing diagnostic category for the client with hypertension would be
- ○ 1. Pain.
- ○ 2. Fluid Volume Deficit.
- ○ 3. Impaired Skin Integrity.
- ○ 4. Altered Health Maintenance.

70. Nonpharmacologic approaches to hypertension control that the nurse may be involved in teaching the client with hypertension include
- ○ 1. proper administration of antihypertensive agents.
- ○ 2. activity restrictions.
- ○ 3. low potassium diet therapy.
- ○ 4. a regular exercise program.

71. The most important long-term goal for a client with hypertension would be to
- ○ 1. learn how to avoid stress.
- ○ 2. explore a job change or early retirement.
- ○ 3. make a commitment to long-term therapy.
- ○ 4. control high blood pressure.

72. Long-term complications of hypertension include
- ○ 1. renal insufficiency and failure.

○ 2. valvular heart disease.

○ 3. endocarditis.

○ 4. peptic ulcer disease.

The Client With Angina

During the past few months, a 56-old woman has felt brief twinges of chest pain while working in her garden and has had frequent episodes of indigestion. She comes to the hospital after experiencing severe anterior chest pain while raking leaves. Her evaluation confirms a diagnosis of stable angina pectoris.

73. The woman says, "I really thought I was having a heart attack. How can you tell the difference?" Which response by the nurse would provide the client with the most accurate information about the difference between the pain of angina and that of MI?

○ 1. "The pain associated with a heart attack is much more severe."

○ 2. "The pain associated with a heart attack radiates into the jaw and down the left arm."

○ 3. "It is impossible to differentiate anginal pain from that of a heart attack without an ECG."

○ 4. "The pain of angina is usually relieved by resting or lying down."

74. After stabilization and treatment, the client is discharged from the hospital. At her follow-up appointment, she is discouraged because she is experiencing pain with increasing frequency. She states that she visits an invalid friend twice a week and now cannot walk up the second flight of steps to the friend's apartment without pain. Which measure that the nurse could suggest would most likely help the client deal with this problem?

○ 1. Visit her friend early in the day.

○ 2. Rest for at least an hour before climbing the stairs.

○ 3. Take a nitroglycerin tablet before climbing the stairs.

○ 4. Lie down once she reaches the friend's apartment.

75. The nurse teaches the client that which of the following meals would be best on her low-cholesterol diet?

○ 1. Hamburger, salad, and milkshake.

○ 2. Baked liver, green beans, and coffee.

○ 3. Spaghetti with tomato sauce, salad, and coffee.

○ 4. Fried chicken, green beans, and skim milk.

76. The nurse should teach the client to report immediately which of the following symptoms to her physician?

○ 1. A change in the pattern of her pain.

○ 2. Pain during sexual activity.

○ 3. Pain during an argument with her husband.

○ 4. Absence of pain during or after an activity such as lawn-mowing.

77. The physician refers the client for a cardiac catheterization. The nurse explains to the client that this procedure is used to

○ 1. open and dilate blocked coronary arteries.

○ 2. assess the extent of arterial blockage.

○ 3. bypass obstructed vessels.

○ 4. assess the functional adequacy of the valves and heart muscle.

78. The client is scheduled for a percutaneous transluminal coronary angioplasty (PTCA) to treat her angina. Priority goals for the client immediately after PTCA would include

○ 1. minimizing dyspnea.

○ 2. maintaining adequate urine output.

○ 3. decreasing myocardial contractility.

○ 4. preventing fluid volume deficit.

79. Which of the following are generally considered to be risk factors for the development of atherosclerosis?

○ 1. Family history of early MI, hypertension, and anemia.

○ 2. Diabetes mellitus, smoking, and late onset of puberty.

○ 3. Male gender, total blood cholesterol level above 150 mg/dL, and low protein intake.

○ 4. Heredity, physical inactivity, and hypertension.

80. Under age 50 years, many more men than women suffer from coronary artery disease due to atherosclerosis. The leading cause of death in women is

○ 1. acquired immunodeficiency syndrome.

○ 2. breast cancer.

○ 3. coronary artery disease.

○ 4. chronic obstructive pulmonary disease.

81. A client with angina asks the nurse, "What information does an ECG provide?" The nurse would respond that an ECG primarily gives information about the

○ 1. electrical conduction of the myocardium.

○ 2. oxygenation and perfusion of the heart.

○ 3. contractile status of the ventricles.

○ 4. physical integrity of the heart muscle.

82. As an initial step in treating a client with angina, the physician prescribes nitroglycerin tablets, 0.3 mg given sublingually. This drug's principal effects are produced by

○ 1. antispasmodic effects on the pericardium.

○ 2. stimulation of α- and β-receptor sites.

○ 3. vasodilation of peripheral vasculature.

○ 4. improved conductivity in the myocardium.

83. The nurse teaches the client with angina about the

common expected side effects of nitroglycerin, including

○ 1. headache, hypotension, and dizziness.

○ 2. hypertension, flushing, and dizziness.

○ 3. hypotension, shock, and shortness of breath.

○ 4. stomach cramps, flushing, and dizziness.

84. Sublingual nitroglycerin tablets begin to work within 1 to 2 minutes. How should the nurse instruct the client to use the drug when chest pain occurs?

○ 1. "Take one tablet every 2 to 5 minutes until the pain stops."

○ 2. "Take one tablet and rest for 10 minutes. Call the physician if pain persists after 10 minutes."

○ 3. "Take one tablet, then an additional tablet every 5 minutes for a total of three tablets. Call the physician if pain persists after 3 tablets."

○ 4. "Take one tablet. If pain persists after 5 minutes, take two tablets. If pain still persists 5 minutes later, call the physician."

85. Which of the following points should the nurse include when instructing the client with angina about sublingual nitroglycerin?

○ 1. The drug will cause increased urine output.

○ 2. Store the tablets in a tight, light-resistant container.

○ 3. Use the tablets only when the pain is severe.

○ 4. The shelf life of nitroglycerin is long; it keeps for up to 2 years.

86. Nitroglycerin is also available in ointment or paste form. Before applying nitroglycerin ointment, the nurse should

○ 1. cleanse the skin where the ointment will be placed with alcohol.

○ 2. obtain the client's pulse rate and cardiac rhythm.

○ 3. remove the ointment previously applied.

○ 4. instruct the client to expect pain relief in the next 15 minutes.

87. In explaining the procedure of PTCA to a client, the nurse should describe that the procedure involves

○ 1. opening a stenosed artery with an inflatable balloon-tipped catheter.

○ 2. increased blood clotting after the procedure.

○ 3. passing a catheter through the coronary arteries to find blocked arteries.

○ 4. inserting grafts to divert blood from blocked coronary arteries.

88. The nurse interprets the rhythm strip in Figure 1 from a client's bedside monitor as

○ 1. normal sinus rhythm.

○ 2. sinus tachycardia.

○ 3. atrial fibrillation.

○ 4. ventricular fibrillation.

89. The nurse interprets the rhythm strip in Figure 2 from a client's bedside monitor as

○ 1. normal sinus rhythm.

○ 2. sinus tachycardia.

○ 3. atrial fibrillation.

○ 4. pacemaker rhythm.

90. The nurse interprets the rhythm strip in Figure 3 from a client's bedside monitor as

○ 1. normal sinus rhythm.

○ 2. sinus tachycardia.

○ 3. atrial fibrillation.

○ 4. ventricular tachycardia.

The Client With a Permanent Pacemaker

A 74-year-old woman is admitted to the telemetry unit for placement of a permanent pacemaker for sinus bradycardia.

91. A priority goal for the client within 24 hours of insertion of a permanent pacemaker would be to

○ 1. maintain skin integrity.

○ 2. maintain cardiac conduction stability.

○ 3. decrease cardiac output.

○ 4. increase activity level.

92. Outcome criteria for the client being discharged from the hospital who had a permanent pacemaker implanted 2 days ago include that the client

○ 1. selects a low-cholesterol diet to control coronary artery disease.

○ 2. states need for bed rest for 1 week after discharge.

○ 3. verbalizes safety precautions needed to prevent pacemaker malfunction.

○ 4. explains signs and symptoms of MI.

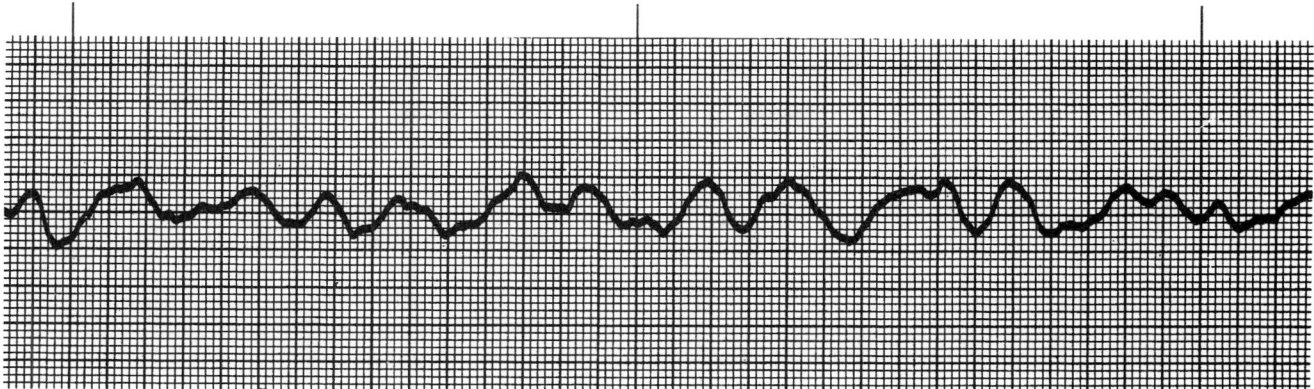

Figure 1.

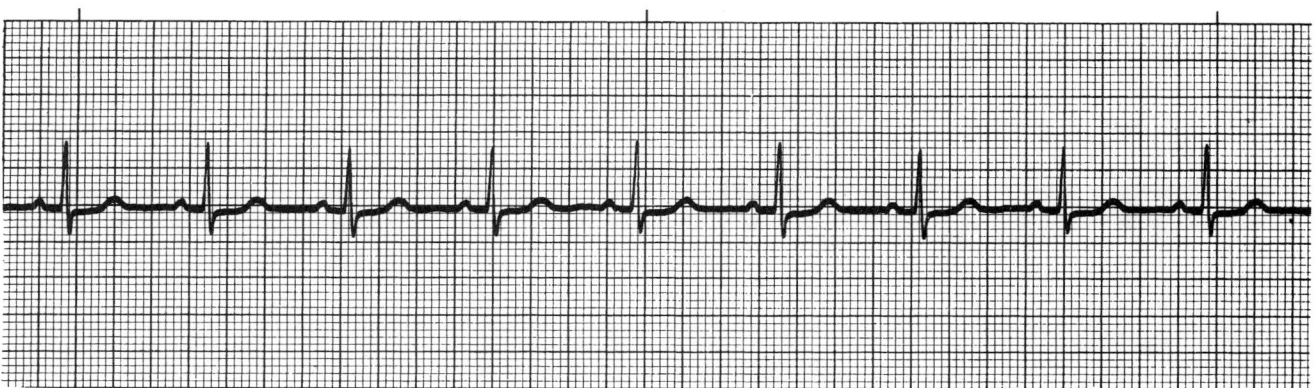

Figure 2.

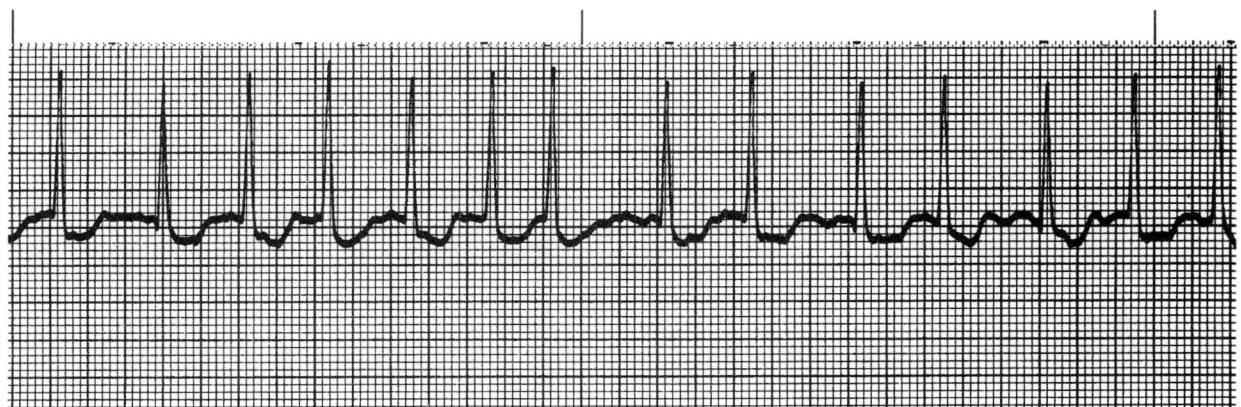

Figure 3.

CORRECT ANSWERS AND RATIONALE

The letters in parentheses following the rationale identify the step of the nursing process (A, D, P, I, E), cognitive level (K, C, T, N), and client needs (S, G, L, H). See the Answer Grid for the key.

The Client With Myocardial Infarction

1. 1. Although obtaining the ECG, chest radiograph, and blood work are all important, the nurse's priority action should be to relieve the crushing chest pain. Thus, administering morphine sulfate is the priority action. (I, T, G)

2. 2. Thrombolytic drugs are administered within the first 6 hours of onset of an MI to lyse clots and reduce the extent of myocardial damage. (I, T, G)

3. 1. Oliguria occurs during cardiogenic shock because there is reduced blood flow to the kidneys. Typical signs of cardiogenic shock include low blood pressure, rapid and weak pulse, decreased urine output, and signs of diminished blood flow to the brain, such as confusion and restlessness. Cardiogenic shock is a serious complication of an MI, with a mortality rate approaching 90%. (A, T, G)

4. 1. Intravenous nitroglycerin infusion requires an infusion pump for precise control of the medication. Blood pressure monitoring would be done with a continuous system, and more frequently than every shift. Hourly urine outputs are not always required for this client. Obtaining serum potassium levels is not associated with nitroglycerin infusion. (I, N, G)

5. 1. When a client makes a comment about death, it is best for the nurse to help the client express his or her feelings. Asking a question that requires no more than a yes or no answer is unlikely to elicit how the client really feels and offers the client no support. Cliches such as "everything will be all right soon" are not helpful because they ignore the client's feelings. Trying to explain away the client's feelings will also be of no help to the client and ignores the way the client feels. (I, T, L)

6. 1. Impaired Gas Exchange related to poor oxygenation and dysrhythmias is a major problem immediately after MI. Therapy is directed toward improving cardiac output and decreasing myocardial workload. High Risk for Infection, Fluid Volume Deficit, and Constipation are not priority problems during the first 24 hours. (D, N, G)

7. 4. An MI interferes with or blocks blood circulation to the heart muscle. This causes ischemia, or poor myocardial oxygenation, producing the characteristic ischemic pain. (A, C, G)

8. 2. The primary reason aspirin is administered to the client experiencing an MI is because of its antithrombotic action. In clinical trials, the antithrombotic action of aspirin has been thought to account for improved outcomes in clients with MI. Aspirin does have antipyretic, antiplatelet, and analgesic actions, but these are not the primary reasons it is used in clients experiencing MI. (P, C, G)

9. 2. PVCs are often a precursor of life-threatening dysrhythmias, including ventricular tachycardia and ventricular fibrillation. An occasional PVC is not considered dangerous, but if PVCs occur at a rate greater than five or six a minute in the post-MI client, the physician should be notified promptly. More than six PVCs per minute is considered serious and usually calls for decreasing ventricular irritability by administering medications such as lidocaine hydrochloride. (I, T, G)

10. 2. Common laboratory findings in the client who has suffered a MI include elevated CPK level. CPK is the first of three enzymes to rise in response to myocardial damage; levels peak within the first 24 hours after myocardial damage. CPK is also released during muscle injury and brain injury. The CPK isoenzyme CPK-MB elevates only in response to myocardial damage. The other two enzymes that elevate in response to myocardial injury, but after CPK, are lactic dehydrogenase (LDH) and serum glutamic oxaloacetic transaminase (SGOT). White blood cell count and erythrocyte sedimentation rate are typically elevated but not diagnostic for MI. Serum cholesterol level can predict possible risk for MI but is not a diagnostic tool for MI. (A, T, G)

11. 4. By day two of hospitalization after an MI, clients are expected to be able to perform personal care without chest pain. Experiencing chest pain, even at a minimal level, is not an acceptable outcome for day two. Day two of hospitalization may be too soon for clients to be able to identify risk factors or definitely agree to participate in cardiac rehabilitation. (E, N, S)

12. 4. Bearing down against a closed glottis can best be prevented by instructing the client to avoid holding her breath during activity. For example, the client should avoid bearing down when having a bowel movement, vomiting, coughing, or moving around in bed by exhaling during activity. Valsalva's maneuver may cause a change in the heartbeat, with cardiac dysrhythmias, increased venous pressure, increased intrathoracic pressure, and thrombi dislodgement. Valsalva's maneuver is not prevented by such activities as taking deep breaths (unless they are taken through the mouth), clenching the teeth, or taking fluids through a drinking tube. (I, T, G)

13. 2. Furosemide is a loop diuretic that acts to increase urine output. It does not increase blood pressure, decrease pain, or decrease dysrhythmias. (E, T, G)

14. 3. Exercise helps prevent stasis of blood, which predisposes to thrombophlebitis and blood clot formation. (I, T, H)

15. 2. Recommended dietary principles in the acute phase of MI include avoiding large meals because small, easily digested foods are better tolerated. Clients are not prescribed diets of liquids only or nothing by mouth unless their condition is very unstable. Fluids are given according to the client's needs, and sodium restrictions may be prescribed, especially for clients with manifestations of heart failure. Cholesterol restrictions may be ordered as well. (P, T, G)

16. 3. Physical activity is gradually increased after an MI while the client is still hospitalized and through a period of rehabilitation. Activity progression requires adjustments if the client has suffered complications, however. One of the recommended ways to evaluate progression of activity is to determine how activity affects the client's degree of fatigue. The client is becoming fatigued and progressing too rapidly if activity causes dyspnea, chest pain, a rapid heartbeat, or fatigue. When any of these symptoms appear, the client should reduce activity and progress more slowly. (E, T, G)

17. 4. Keeping the client's door closed is likely to contribute to feelings of isolation and sensory deprivation. Such activities as watching television, visiting with a relative, and reading a newspaper help prevent sensory deprivation and do not require physical effort. (I, T, L)

18. 3. Heredity appears most closely linked to coronary heart disease. (A, T, G)

19. 4. 1 kg = 2.2 pounds; 3.2 × 2.2 = 7.04 pounds. (A, T, G)

20. 3. A basic principle of rehabilitation, including cardiac rehabilitation, is that rehabilitation begins on hospital admission. Early rehabilitation is essential to promote maximum functional ability as the client recovers from an illness. (P, K, S)

21. 1. Clients who continue on a progressive exercise program at home after suffering an MI should be taught to monitor pulse rate. The pulse rate can be expected to increase with exercise, but exercise should not be increased if pulse rate increases more than about 25 beats/minute from baseline or exceeds 100 to 125 beats/minute. Clients should also

be taught to decrease exercise if chest pain or dyspnea occurs. (I, T, H)

22. 3. A basic principle of behavior modification is that behavior that is learned and continued is behavior that has been rewarded. Other reinforcement techniques have not been found to be as effective as reward. (I, T, H)

23. 4. Alteplase recombinant (tPA), a thrombolytic agent administered intravenously, lyses the clot blocking the coronary artery. The drug is most effective when administered within the first 6 hours after onset of MI. (I, T, G)

24. 1. Observing for chest pain is a priority assessment because closure of the previously obstructed coronary artery may recur. Clients who receive tPA frequently receive heparin to prevent closure of the artery after tPA. Spontaneous bleeding, such as gastrointestinal bleeding, cerebral hemorrhage, or bruising, is another adverse effect of thrombolytic therapy. Careful assessment for signs of bleeding and monitoring of partial thromboplastin time are essential to detect complications. (A, T, G)

25. 2. A past history of cerebral hemorrhage is a contraindication to administration of tPA because the risk of hemorrhage may be further increased. (P, C, G)

26. 4. Crackles are auscultated over fluid-filled alveoli. Wheezes are heard when airway narrowing occurs, as with bronchospasm. Pulmonary edema is a medical emergency. Crackles may occur without pulmonary edema. (A, N, G)

27. 3. The client taking nifedipine should inspect his or her gums daily to monitor for gingival hyperplasia. This is an uncommon side effect but requires monitoring and intervention if it occurs. (I, T, H)

The Client With Heart Failure

28. 1. Blood pressure is the priority assessment at admission because people with pulmonary edema typically experience severe hypertension that requires early intervention. (A, T, G)

29. 3. Sitting nearly upright in bed with the feet and legs resting on the mattress decreases venous return to the heart, thus reducing myocardial workload. Also, the sitting position allows maximum space for lung expansion. (I, T, G)

30. 3. Activity intolerance is a primary problem for clients with heart failure and pulmonary edema. The decreased cardiac output associated with heart failure leads to reduced oxygen and fatigue. Clients frequently complain of dyspnea and fatigue. (D, N, G)

31. 1. Increasing cardiac output is the main goal of therapy for the client with heart failure or pulmonary edema. Pulmonary edema is an acute medical emergency requiring immediate intervention. In the client with heart failure or pulmonary edema, improved respiratory status will occur when cardiac output is improved. Peripheral edema is not typically associated with pulmonary edema. Comfort will be improved when cardiac output increases to an acceptable level. (P, N, G)

32. 2. Digoxin is a cardiac glycoside with positive inotropic activity. This inotropic activity causes increased strength of myocardial contractions and thereby increases output of blood from the left ventricle. As a result, there is less blood shifting from the capillaries into the alveoli. Although digoxin does decrease the electrical conductivity of the myocardium, this is not the primary reason for its use in clients with heart failure and pulmonary edema. Digoxin does not dilate coronary arteries. (P, T, G)

33. 4. People with heart failure are taught to weigh themselves daily to maintain a target weight and monitor increasing fluid retention. Increasing fluid retention in these clients may lead to decompensation and hospitalization. Monitoring daily urine output and weekly serum potassium levels are not required of these clients. A week of bed rest is not indicated for most people with heart failure. (I, T, H)

34. 3. Enalapril maleate is an angiotensin-converting enzyme (ACE) inhibitor that prevents conversion of angiotensin I to angiotensin II. Angiotensin II is a potent vasoconstrictor and also contributes to aldosterone secretion. Thus, enalapril acts as an antihypertensive. In clinical trials of people with heart failure, enalapril has been associated with reduced mortality rates. Enalapril decreases peripheral vasoconstriction but does not lower the heart rate or increase myocardial contractility. (I, N, G)

35. 1. β-Adrenergic antagonists such as metoprolol tartrate act on β_1-adrenoreceptors in the cardiac muscle and thereby reduce heart rate and lower blood pressure. These drugs may also compete with catecholamines at neuron sites, which would further their ability to lower blood pressure. (P, C, G)

36. 1. After intravenous injection of furosemide, diuresis normally begins in about 5 minutes and reaches its peak within about 30 minutes. Medication effects last 2 to 4 hours. When furosemide is given intramuscularly or orally, drug action begins more slowly and lasts longer than when it is given intravenously. (E, T, G)

37. 1. Monitoring daily weights will help determine the effectiveness of diuretic therapy. A client who gains weight without diet changes most probably is retaining fluids, and the diuretic therapy should be adjusted. Blood pressure monitoring, urinalysis, and serum potassium levels are not used to determine the effectiveness of diuretic therapy. (I, T, G)

38. 4. When diuretics are given early in the day, the client's need to void more frequently will not disturb nighttime sleep. (I, T, G)

39. 2. Characteristics of atrial fibrillation include pulse rate greater than 100 beats/minute, totally irregular rhythm, and no definite P waves on the ECG. During assessment, the nurse is likely to note the irregular rate and should report it to the physician. (A, T, G)

40. 1. Atrial fibrillation occurs when the SA node no longer functions as the heart's pacemaker and impulses are initiated at sites within the atria. Because conduction through the atria is disturbed, atrial contractions are reduced, and stasis of blood in the atria occurs, predisposing to emboli. Some estimates predict that 30% of clients with atrial fibrillation develop emboli. (E, T, G)

41. 3. Colored vision and seeing yellow spots are symptoms of digitalis toxicity. Anorexia, nausea, and vomiting are other common symptoms of digitalis toxicity. Additional signs of toxicity include dysrhythmias, such as atrial fibrillation or bradycardia, and diarrhea. (E, T, G)

42. 4. A low serum potassium level predisposes the client to digoxin toxicity. Thus, the nurse should be especially alert for signs and symptoms of toxicity if the client's serum levels reveal hypokalemia. Because potassium inhibits cardiac excitability, a low serum potassium level increases cardiac excitability. (I, T, G)

43. 2. Canned foods and juices, such as tomato juice, are typically high in sodium and should be avoided in a sodium-restricted diet. Canned foods and juices in which sodium has been removed are available. Apples, beer, and beef tenderloin are not as high in sodium as many canned items, and the client should read the labels. (I, T, G)

44. 1. Foods rich in potassium include bananas, orange juice, honeydew melon, cantaloupe, and watermelons. Other good sources of potassium are grapefruit juice, nectarines, potatoes, canned tomato juice, dried prunes, raisins, figs, and green, leafy vegetables, such as spinach. (I, T, G)

The Client With Valvular Heart Disease

45. 3. Most clients with mitral stenosis have a history of rheumatic fever or bacterial endocarditis. Such infectious diseases as scarlet fever, poliomyelitis, and meningococcal meningitis are not associated with mitral stenosis. (A, T, G)

46. 4. The solution to this problem is as follows:

$$2 \text{ g} = 2000 \text{ mg}$$

$2000 \text{ mg}/500 \text{ mL} = 4 \text{ mg}/x \text{ mL}$

$2000x = 2000$

$x = 2000/2000 = 1 \text{ mL of solution/minute}$

mL $\times$ 60 microdrops $= 60$ microdrops/minute.

(I, T, S)

47. 2. The desired effect of lidocaine hydrochloride is to depress automaticity in the His-Purkinje fibers and elevate the stimulation threshold in the ventricles, thereby decreasing ectopic ventricular beats. Common adverse effects of lidocaine hydrochloride include dizziness, tinnitus, blurred vision, tremors, numbness and tingling of extremities, excessive perspiration, hypotension, convulsions, and finally coma. Cardiac effects include slowed conduction and cardiac arrest. (E, T, G)

48. 3. The pulmonary artery pressures are used to assess the heart's ability to receive and pump blood. Pulmonary capillary wedge pressure reflects the left ventricular end-diastolic pressure and guides the physician in determining fluid management for clients. The degree of coronary artery stenosis is assessed during a cardiac catheterization. (P, T, G)

49. 2. When a chest tube becomes disconnected, the nurse should take immediate steps to prevent air from entering the chest cavity, which may cause the lung to collapse. Therefore, when a chest tube is accidentally disconnected from the drainage tube, the nurse should either double-clamp the chest tube as close to the client as possible or place the open end of the tube in a container of sterile water or saline solution. Then the physician should be notified. The specific course of action depends on institutional policy, and each nurse should be aware of the policy within the institution. (I, T, G)

50. 1. Weight gain due to fluid retention and worsening heart failure cause exertional dyspnea in clients with mitral regurgitation. The rise in left atrial pressure that accompanies mitral valve disease is transmitted backward to the pulmonary veins, capillaries, and arterioles and eventually to the right ventricle. Signs and symptoms of pulmonary and systemic venous congestion follow. (A, T, G)

51. 4. When mitral stenosis is present, the left atrium has difficulty emptying its contents into the left ventricle. Hence, because there is no valve to prevent backward flow into the pulmonary vein, the pulmonary circulation is under pressure. Functioning of the aorta, the right atrium, and the superior vena cava are not immediately influenced by mitral stenosis. (A, T, G)

52. 1. Preoperatively, anticoagulants may be prescribed for the client with advanced valvular heart disease to prevent emboli. Postoperatively, all clients with mechanical valves, and some clients with bioprostheses, are maintained indefinitely on anticoagulant therapy. Adhering strictly to a dosage schedule and observing specific precautions are necessary to prevent hemorrhage or thromboembolism. Some clients are maintained on lifelong antibiotic prophylaxis to prevent recurrence of rheumatic fever. Episodic prophylaxis is required to prevent infective endocarditis after dental procedures or instrumentation or upper respiratory, gastrointestinal, or genitourinary tract surgery. (A, T, G)

53. 4. Management of postoperative pain is a priority for the client after surgery, including valve replacement surgery, according to the Agency for Health Care Policy Research. The client and family should be informed that pain will be assessed by the nurse and medications will be given to relieve the pain. The client will stay in the intensive care unit as long as monitoring and intensive care are needed. Sensory deprivation and overload, high noise levels, and disrupted sleep and rest patterns are some environmental factors that impact recovery from valve replacement surgery. (I, T, S)

54. 2. Protamine sulfate is used to help combat persistent bleeding in a client who has had open heart surgery. Warfarin sodium is an anticoagulant, as is heparin, and these two agents would tend to cause the client to bleed even more. Vitamin C and quinidine sulfate do not influence blood clotting. (I, T, G)

55. 1. Many factors help prevent wound infections, including washing hands carefully, using sterile prepackaged supplies and equipment, cleansing the incisional area well, and disposing of soiled dressings properly. However, most authorities say that the single most effective measure in preventing wound infections is to wash the hands carefully before and after changing dressings. Careful handwashing is also important in helping reduce other infections often acquired in hospitals, such as urinary tract and respiratory system infections. (I, T, S)

56. 1. In an immobilized client, calcium leaves the bone and concentrates in the extracellular fluid. When a large amount of calcium passes through the kidneys, calcium can precipitate and form calculi. Nursing interventions that help prevent calculi include ensuring a liberal fluid intake, unless contraindicated; providing a diet rich in acid to keep the urine acidic, which increases the solubility of calcium; and limiting foods rich in calcium, such as dairy products. (I, T, S)

57. 3. The INR is the value used to assess effectiveness of the warfarin sodium therapy. INR is the prothrombin time ratio that would be obtained if the thromboplastin reagent from the World Organization was used for the plasma test. It is now the recommended method to monitor effectiveness of warfarin sodium. Generally, the INR for clients administered warfarin sodium should range from 2 to 3. In the past, prothrombin time was used to assess effectiveness of warfarin sodium and was maintained at 1.5 to 2.5 times the control value. Fresh frozen plasma or vitamin K is used to reverse warfarin sodium's anticoagulant effect. Partial thromboplastin time is used to assess the effectiveness of heparin therapy, whereas protamine sulfate reverses the effects of heparin. (I, T, S)

58. 1. Daily dental care and frequent checkups by a dentist who is informed about the client's condition are required to maintain good oral health. Using an irrigation device, an electric toothbrush, or dental floss may cause gums to bleed and allow bacteria to enter mucous membranes and the bloodstream, increasing the risk of endocarditis. (I, T, H)

59. 2. Most cardiac surgical clients have median sternotomy incisions, which take about 3 months to heal. Measures that promote healing include avoiding heavy lifting, performing muscle reconditioning exercises, and using caution when driving. Showering or bathing is allowed as long as the incision is well approximated with no open areas or drainage. Activities should gradually be resumed on discharge. (I, T, G)

The Client With Hypertension

60. 1. Most people with hypertension have no symptoms, even with dangerous elevations in blood pressure. Therefore, the presence or absence of symptoms is not an accurate reflection of a person's status. Symptoms are not directly related to the status of the kidney. The severity of the hypertension, rather than the presence of absence of symptoms, determines the risk of some complications such as stroke. (I, T, G)

61. 1. Atenolol is a β-adrenergic antagonist indicated for management of hypertension. Sudden discontinuation of this drug is dangerous because it may exacerbate symptoms. Blood pressure needs to be monitored more frequently than annually in a client newly diagnosed and treated for hypertension. Clients are not usually placed on a 2-g sodium diet for hypertension. (I, T, H)

62. 3. Processed and cured meat products, such as cold cuts, ham, and hot dogs, are all high in both fat and sodium and should be avoided on a low-calorie, low-fat, low-salt diet. Dietary restrictions of all types are complex and difficult to implement with clients who are basically asymptomatic. (I, T, H)

63. 4. Possible dizziness from postural hypotension when rising from a crouched or bent position increases the client's risk of being injured by the equipment. The nurse should assess the client's blood pressure in all three positions (lying, sitting, and standing) at all routine visits. The other adverse effects listed could also cause complications in the work environment but are not as potentially dangerous as postural hypotension. (A, T, G)

64. 4. Tailoring, or individualizing, a program to the client's lifestyle has been shown to be an effective strategy for changing health behaviors. Providing a written program, explaining the program to the spouse, and reassuring the client about the program may be helpful but are not as likely to promote adherence as tailoring the program. (P, T, H)

65. 3. A plan to reduce or stop smoking begins with establishing the client's personal daily smoking pattern and activities associated with smoking. It is important that the client understand the associated health risks, but this knowledge has not been shown to help clients change their smoking behavior. (I, T, H)

66. 3. American Heart Association standards define hypertension as a consistent systolic blood pressure level above 140 mm Hg and a consistent diastolic blood pressure level above 90 mm Hg. (A, T, G)

67. 4. Propranolol hydrochloride is a β-adrenergic blocking agent used to treat hypertension. In addition to lowering blood pressure by blocking sympathetic nervous system stimulation, the drug lowers the heart rate. Therefore, the client should be assessed for bradycardia and other dysrhythmias. The client needs to be instructed *not* to discontinue medication because sudden withdrawal of propranolol hydrochloride may cause rebound hypertension. Propranolol dosage is not typically adjusted based on weekly blood pressure readings or partial thromboplastin time values. (I, T, G)

68. 1. Actions of propranolol hydrochloride include reducing heart rate, decreasing myocardial contractility, and slowing conduction. (I, T, G)

69. 4. Managing hypertension is a priority for the client with hypertension. Clients with hypertension frequently do not experience other signs and symptoms, such as pain, fluid volume deficit, or altered skin integrity. It is this asymptomatic nature that makes hypertension so difficult to treat because clients may not recognize they are hypertensive or may not perceive the need for aggressive management of the hypertension. (D, N, H)

70. 4. A regular exercise program is a nonpharmacologic approach that aids weight management, an essential component of hypertension control. Activity restrictions are not commonly part of therapy for clients with hypertension. A low-sodium rather than low-potassium diet may be adjunct therapy. Proper administration of antihypertensive agents is a pharmacologic approach. (I, N, H)

71. 3. Compliance is the most critical element of hypertension therapy. Most hypertensive clients require lifelong treatment and cannot be managed successfully without drug therapy. Stress and weight management are important components of hypertension therapy, but the priority goal is related to compliance. (P, N, H)

72. 1. Renal disease, including renal insufficiency and failure, is a complication of hypertension. Effective treatment of hypertension assists in preventing this complication. (D, C, G)

The Client With Angina

73. 4. The characteristic of anginal pain that helps differentiate it from the pain of a heart attack is that anginal pain is transient and usually alleviated by resting or lying down. In unstable angina, however, there is increasing frequency, intensity, or duration of pain. Anginal pain is not always less severe than that of an MI, and it may radiate down the arm or into the jaw. (I, T, G)

74. 3. Nitroglycerin may be used prophylactically before stressful physical activities such as stair-climbing to help the client remain pain free. Resting before or after an activity is not as likely to help prevent an activity-related pain episode. (I, N, G)

75. 3. Pasta, tomato sauce, salad, and coffee would be the best selection for the client following a low-cholesterol diet. Hamburgers, milkshakes, liver, and fried foods tend to be high in cholesterol. (I, T, H)

76. 1. The client should report a change in the pattern of chest pain. It may indicate increasing severity of coronary artery disease. Pain occurring during stress or sexual activity would not be unexpected, and the client can be instructed to take nitroglycerin to prevent this pain. (I, T, G)

77. 2. Cardiac catheterization is done in clients with angina primarily to assess the extent and severity of the coronary artery blockage. A decision about medical management, angioplasty, or coronary artery bypass surgery will be based on the catheterization results. (I, T, G)

78. 4. Because the contrast medium used in PTCA acts as an osmotic diuretic, the client may experience diuresis with resultant fluid volume deficit after the procedure. Additionally, potassium levels must be closely monitored for decreases. Increased myocardial contractility would be a goal, not decreased contractility. Dyspnea would not be anticipated after this procedure. (P, T, G)

79. 4. Risk factors for atherosclerosis include cigarette smoking, hypertension, high blood cholesterol level, male gender, family history of atherosclerosis, diabetes mellitus, obesity, and physical inactivity. (A, K, G)

80. 3. Coronary artery disease is the leading cause of death in women as well as men. Although it is generally agreed that estrogen helps protect women from atherosclerotic changes before menopause, women are still at risk for coronary artery disease. Much attention has focused on the lack of research studies dealing with cardiac disease in women and minorities, and work is under way to gain a better understanding of cardiac disease in these populations. (A, K, G)

81. 1. An ECG directly reflects the transmission of electrical cardiac impulses through the heart. This information makes it possible to evaluate indirectly the functional status of the heart muscle and the contractile response of the ventricles. However, these elements are not measured directly. (I, T, S)

82. 3. Nitroglycerin produces peripheral vasodilation, which reduces myocardial oxygen consumption and demand. Vasodilation in coronary arteries and collateral vessels may also increase blood flow to the ischemic areas of the heart. Nitroglycerin affects neither α- nor β-receptors. It does not affect pericardial spasticity or myocardial conductivity. (I, T, G)

83. 1. Because of its widespread vasodilating effects, nitroglycerin often produces such side effects as headache, hypotension, and dizziness. The client should sit or lie down to avoid fainting. Nitroglycerin does not cause shortness of breath or stomach cramps. (I, T, G)

84. 3. The correct protocol for nitroglycerin use involves immediate administration with subsequent doses taken at 5-minute intervals as needed, for a total dose of three tablets. Sublingual nitroglycerin appears in the bloodstream within 2 to 3 minutes and is metabolized within about 10 minutes. (I, T, G)

85. 2. Clients should be instructed to keep nitroglycerin in a tightly closed, dark container and to replenish it frequently because it deteriorates rather rapidly. Clients should be instructed to use nitroglycerin at the first indication of chest pain and not to wait before using the drug. (I, T, G)

86. 3. When applying nitroglycerin ointment to a client's skin, the nurse should first remove the ointment applied during previous administration, otherwise the client will be receiving too much medication. The blood pressure should be assessed before administration because the ointment may decrease blood pressure. Nitroglycerin ointment is not used for relief of acute cardiac pain. (I, T, G)

87. 1. PTCA is best described as insertion of a balloon-tipped catheter into the coronary artery to compress a plaque and thereby open a stenosed artery. PTCA does not directly affect blood clotting mechanisms, even though the client may receive heparin after the procedure to reduce the incidence of recurring obstruction. Inserting grafts to divert blood from blocked arteries describes coronary artery bypass graft surgery. (P, T, G)

88. 4. This rhythm is ventricular fibrillation, which is characterized by absence of any definite pattern. Ventricular fibrillation causes pulselessness and complete cardiac arrest in the victim, and treatment is defibrillation. Lidocaine hydrochloride may be administered after defibrillation to suppress additional ventricular ectopi. (D, N, G)

89. 1. This rhythm is normal sinus rhythm. It is characterized by a regular ventricular rate of 60 to 100 beats/minute, and each QRS complex is preceded by a P wave. The PR and QRS intervals are within normal limits. (D, N, G)

90. 3. This rhythm is atrial fibrillation. It is characterized by an irregular QRS interval, no definite P waves before the QRS waves, and a ventricular rate greater than 100 beats/minute. (D, N, G)

The Client With a Permanent Pacemaker

91. 2. Maintaining cardiac conduction stability to prevent dysrhythmias is a priority immediately following artificial pacemaker implantation. The client should have continuous ECG monitoring until proper pacemaker function is verified. (P, N, G)

92. 3. Education is a major component of the discharge plan for a client with an artificial pacemaker. The client with a permanent pacemaker needs to be able to state specific information about safety precautions necessary to maintain proper pacemaker function. (E, N, G)

NURSING CARE OF ADULTS WITH MEDICAL AND SURGICAL HEALTH PROBLEMS

TEST 2: The Client With Cardiac Health Problems

Directions: Use this answer grid to determine areas of strength or need for further study.

NURSING PROCESS

A = Assessment
D = Analysis, nursing diagnosis
P = Planning
I = Implementation
E = Evaluation

COGNITIVE LEVEL

K = Knowledge
C = Comprehension
T = Application
N = Analysis

CLIENT NEEDS

S = Safe, effective care environment
G = Physiologic integrity
L = Psychosocial integrity
H = Health promotion and maintenance

Question #	Answer #	A	D	P	I	E	K	C	T	N	S	G	L	H
1	1				I				T			G		
2	2				I				T			G		
3	1	A							T			G		
4	1				I					N		G		
5	1				I				T				L	
6	1		D							N		G		
7	4	A						C				G		
8	2			P				C				G		
9	2				I				T			G		
10	2	A							T			G		
11	4					E				N	S			
12	4				I				T			G		
13	2					E			T			G		
14	3				I				T					H
15	2			P					T			G		
16	3					E			T			G		
17	4				I				T				L	
18	3	A							T			G		
19	4	A							T			G		
20	3			P			K				S			
21	1				I				T					H
22	3				I				T					H
23	4				I				T			G		
24	1	A							T			G		
25	2			P				C				G		

NURSING PROCESS

A = Assessment
D = Analysis, nursing diagnosis
P = Planning
I = Implementation
E = Evaluation

COGNITIVE LEVEL

K = Knowledge
C = Comprehension
T = Application
N = Analysis

CLIENT NEEDS

S = Safe, effective care environment
G = Physiologic integrity
L = Psychosocial integrity
H = Health promotion and maintenance

Question #	Answer #	Nursing Process					Cognitive Level				Client Needs			
		A	D	P	I	E	K	C	T	N	S	G	L	H
26	4	A								N		G		
27	3				I				T					H
28	1	A							T			G		
29	3				I				T			G		
30	3		D							N		G		
31	1			P						N		G		
32	2			P					T			G		
33	4				I				T					H
34	3				I					N		G		
35	1			P				C				G		
36	1					E			T			G		
37	1				I				T			G		
38	4				I				T			G		
39	2	A							T			G		
40	1					E			T			G		
41	3					E			T			G		
42	4				I				T			G		
43	2				I				T			G		
44	1				I				T			G		
45	3	A							T			G		
46	4				I				T		S			
47	2					E			T			G		
48	3			P					T			G		
49	2				I				T			G		
50	1	A							T			G		
51	4	A							T			G		
52	1	A							T			G		
53	4				I				T		S			
54	2				I				T			G		
55	1				I				T		S			

ANSWER GRID: 2

436

NURSING PROCESS

A = Assessment
D = Analysis, nursing diagnosis
P = Planning
I = Implementation
E = Evaluation

COGNITIVE LEVEL

K = Knowledge
C = Comprehension
T = Application
N = Analysis

CLIENT NEEDS

S = Safe, effective care environment
G = Physiologic integrity
L = Psychosocial integrity
H = Health promotion and maintenance

Question #	Answer #	Nursing Process					Cognitive Level				Client Needs			
		A	D	P	I	E	K	C	T	N	S	G	L	H
56	1				I				T		S			
57	3				I				T		S			
58	1				I				T					H
59	2				I				T			G		
60	1				I				T			G		
61	1				I				T					H
62	3				I				T					H
63	4	A							T			G		
64	4			P					T					H
65	3				I				T					H
66	3	A							T			G		
67	4				I				T			G		
68	1				I				T			G		
69	4		D							N				H
70	4				I					N				H
71	3			P						N				H
72	1		D					C				G		
73	4				I				T			G		
74	3				I					N		G		
75	3				I				T					H
76	1				I				T			G		
77	2				I				T			G		
78	4			P					T			G		
79	4	A					K					G		
80	3	A					K					G		
81	1				I				T		S			
82	3				I				T			G		
83	1				I				T			G		
84	3				I				T			G		
85	2				I				T			G		

ANSWER GRID: 3

NURSING PROCESS

A = Assessment
D = Analysis, nursing diagnosis
P = Planning
I = Implementation
E = Evaluation

COGNITIVE LEVEL

K = Knowledge
C = Comprehension
T = Application
N = Analysis

CLIENT NEEDS

S = Safe, effective care environment
G = Physiologic integrity
L = Psychosocial integrity
H = Health promotion and maintenance

Question #	Answer #	Nursing Process					Cognitive Level				Client Needs			
		A	D	P	I	E	K	C	T	N	S	G	L	H
86	3				I				T			G		
87	1			P					T			G		
88	4		D							N		G		
89	1		D							N		G		
90	3		D							N		G		
91	2			P						N		G		
92	3					E				N		G		
Number Correct														
Number Possible	92	17	7	13	47	8	3	5	68	16	8	68	2	14
Percentage Correct														

Score Calculation: To determine your **Percentage Correct,** divide the **Number Correct** by the **Number Possible.**

ANSWER GRID: 4

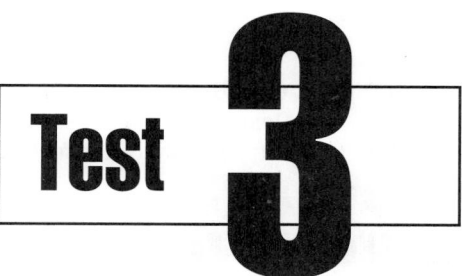

The Client With Cardiovascular and Hematologic Health Problems; the Client Who Is Dying

- The Client With Pernicious Anemia
- The Client With Hodgkin's Disease
- The Client Requiring Cardiopulmonary Resuscitation
- The Client in Shock
- The Client With Anemia
- The Client Who Is Dying
- Correct Answers and Rationale

Select the one best answer, and indicate your choice by filling in the circle in front of the option.

The Client With Pernicious Anemia

A 75-year-old female client is evaluated for pernicious anemia.

1. The nurse prepares the client for a gastric analysis as part of the initial assessment. A typical laboratory finding of gastric analysis in a client with pernicious anemia is
   ○ 1. high bile concentration.
   ○ 2. absence of intrinsic factor.
   ○ 3. low bicarbonate concentration.
   ○ 4. immature red blood cells.
2. The client is given radioactive B_{12} in water for a Shilling test. The primary purpose of this test is to measure the client's ability to
   ○ 1. store vitamin B_{12}.
   ○ 2. digest vitamin B_{12}.
   ○ 3. absorb vitamin B_{12}.
   ○ 4. produce vitamin B_{12}.
3. The client likely will suffer from the symptoms of vitamin B_{12} deficiency, even though she consumes normal amounts of food containing this vitamin. What is the reason for her vitamin deficiency?
   ○ 1. Inability to absorb the vitamin because the stomach is not producing sufficient acid.
   ○ 2. Inability to absorb the vitamin because the stomach is not producing sufficient intrinsic factor.
   ○ 3. Excessive excretion of the vitamin because of kidney dysfunction.
   ○ 4. Increased requirement for the vitamin because of rapid red blood cell production.
4. A priority nursing diagnostic category for the client with pernicious anemia is
   ○ 1. Alteration in Comfort: Pain.
   ○ 2. Fluid Volume Deficit.
   ○ 3. Activity Intolerance.
   ○ 4. Ineffective Breathing Pattern.
5. The client's husband is taught to administer vitamin B_{12} injections to his wife, using the ventrogluteal site. Which of the following positions would most help to decrease the client's discomfort when her husband injects the vitamin B_{12}? Having the client
   ○ 1. lie on her side with her legs extended.
   ○ 2. lie on her abdomen with her toes pointed inward.

○ 3. lean over the edge of a low table with her hips well flexed.

○ 4. stand upright with her feet comfortably apart.

The Client With Hodgkin's Disease

A 47-year-old male client diagnosed with Hodgkin's disease is admitted to the hospital for staging. He is to undergo bone marrow biopsy.

6. The nurse assesses the client's nutritional status to be adequate. Which of the following blood examinations would be most helpful in determining whether the client's diet contains inadequate protein?

○ 1. Red blood cell count.

○ 2. Bilirubin level.

○ 3. Reticulocyte count.

○ 4. Albumin level.

7. Three different chemotherapeutic agents are administered to the client. The nurse explains to the client that three drugs are given over an extended period because

○ 1. the second and third drugs increase the effectiveness of the first drug.

○ 2. the first two drugs destroy the cancer cells, and the third drug minimizes side effects.

○ 3. the three drugs can then be given in lower doses.

○ 4. the three drugs have a synergistic effect and different actions.

8. A priority nursing diagnostic category for a client receiving chemotherapy would be

○ 1. Fluid Volume Excess.

○ 2. Impaired Physical Mobility.

○ 3. Potential for Infection.

○ 4. Altered Health Maintenance.

9. The client experiences episodes of severe nausea and vomiting, with more than 1000 mL of emesis in 4 hours. The nurse's most appropriate action would be to

○ 1. notify the physician.

○ 2. maintain the client on a liquid diet.

○ 3. continue to monitor the client for another 4 hours.

○ 4. administer pain medication as ordered.

10. The chemotherapy is extremely toxic to bone marrow, and the client develops thrombocytopenia. The nurse would recognize that a priority goal of care would be to take precautions to control

○ 1. bleeding.

○ 2. diarrhea.

○ 3. infection.

○ 4. hypotension.

11. The client is placed in protective (reverse) isolation.

The nurse explains to the client and family that protective isolation helps prevent the spread of organisms

○ 1. to the client from sources outside the client's environment.

○ 2. from the client to health care personnel, visitors, and other clients.

○ 3. by using special techniques to destroy discharges from the client's body.

○ 4. by using special techniques to handle the client's linen and personal items.

12. An early sign of Hodgkin's disease is

○ 1. difficulty swallowing.

○ 2. swollen cervical lymph nodes.

○ 3. difficulty breathing.

○ 4. a feeling of fullness over the liver.

13. Hodgkin's disease typically affects people in which of the following age groups?

○ 1. Children (ages 6 to 12 years).

○ 2. Teenagers (ages 13 to 20 years).

○ 3. Young adults (ages 21 to 40 years).

○ 4. Older adults (ages 41 to 50 years).

14. The process of staging Hodgkin's disease provides health care personnel with information useful for all of the following purposes except

○ 1. prescribing therapy.

○ 2. determining the extent of the disease.

○ 3. estimating the activity of the disease.

○ 4. identifying the cell causing the disease.

15. The nurse explains to the client with Hodgkin's disease that a bone marrow specimen will be obtained from the sternum or iliac crest because

○ 1. these sites contain the most bone marrow of any bones.

○ 2. the marrow from these sites is the most pure form.

○ 3. bone marrow is only available from these sites.

○ 4. these sites are accessible and away from major organs.

16. A client with Hodgkin's disease is readmitted to the hospital frequently with exacerbations that prove to be resistant to the aggressive treatment protocol. The client is finally readmitted as death appears imminent. The nurse should be aware that one of the greatest emotional problems that hospitalized terminally ill clients face is

○ 1. fear of pain.

○ 2. fear of further therapy.

○ 3. feelings of isolation.

○ 4. feelings of social inadequacy.

The Client Requiring Cardiopulmonary Resuscitation

A rescuer is called to a neighbor's home after a 56-year-old man collapses. After quickly assessing the victim, the rescuer determines that cardiopulmonary resuscitation (CPR) is necessary.

17. To determine that chest compressions are necessary, the rescuer
- ○ 1. calls the victim's name.
- ○ 2. performs the chin-tilt to open the victim's airway.
- ○ 3. palpates the carotid pulse for 1 minute.
- ○ 4. watches the victim's chest for respirations.

18. Proper hand placement for chest compressions is essential to reduce the risk of which of the following complications?
- ○ 1. gastrointestinal bleeding.
- ○ 2. myocardial infarction.
- ○ 3. emesis.
- ○ 4. rib fracture.

19. The victim's teenage son tells the rescuer that he knows CPR and can help. The first rescuer continues external cardiac compressions while the son administers artificial ventilations. The cardiac compressions should be administered at which rate?
- ○ 1. 40 to 60 per minute.
- ○ 2. 60 to 80 per minute.
- ○ 3. 80 to 100 per minute.
- ○ 4. 100 to 120 per minute.

20. The victim is transported by ambulance to the hospital's emergency room, where the admitting nurse quickly assesses his condition. Of the following observations, the one most often recommended for determining the effectiveness of CPR is noting whether
- ○ 1. pulse rate is normal.
- ○ 2. pupils are reacting to light.
- ○ 3. mucous membranes are pink.
- ○ 4. systolic blood pressure is at least 80 mm Hg.

21. The client receives epinephrine in the emergency room. This drug is administered primarily because of its ability to
- ○ 1. dilate bronchioles.
- ○ 2. constrict arterioles.
- ○ 3. free glycogen from the liver.
- ○ 4. enhance myocardial contractility.

22. Criteria for a rescuer to discontinue CPR include which of the following?
- ○ 1. When it is obvious that the victim will not survive.
- ○ 2. When the rescuer is exhausted.
- ○ 3. After 30 minutes of CPR without a pulse rate.
- ○ 4. When the family requests discontinuation.

23. What is the compression-to-ventilation ratio for one-rescuer CPR?
- ○ 1. 5:1.
- ○ 2. 15:1.
- ○ 3. 5:2.
- ○ 4. 15:2.

24. During CPR, the xiphoid process at the lower end of the sternum should not be deeply compressed when performing external cardiac compression because of the danger of lacerating the victim's
- ○ 1. lung.
- ○ 2. liver.
- ○ 3. stomach.
- ○ 4. diaphragm.

25. When performing external chest compressions on an adult during CPR, the rescuer should depress the sternum
- ○ 1. 0.5 to 1 inch.
- ○ 2. 1 to 1.5 inches.
- ○ 3. 1.5 to 2 inches.
- ○ 4. 2 to 2.5 inches.

26. During two-rescuer CPR, the adult victim's pulse should be checked by the rescuer
- ○ 1. who is delivering chest compressions.
- ○ 2. who is delivering breaths.
- ○ 3. every 2 minutes.
- ○ 4. using the brachial artery.

27. If the victim's chest wall fails to rise with each inflation when rescue breathing is administered during CPR, the most likely reason is that the
- ○ 1. airway is not clear.
- ○ 2. victim is beyond resuscitation.
- ○ 3. inflations are being given at too rapid a rate.
- ○ 4. rescuer is using inadequate force for cardiac massage.

28. During rescue breathing in CPR, the victim will exhale by
- ○ 1. normal relaxation of the chest.
- ○ 2. gentle pressure of the rescuer's hand on the upper chest.
- ○ 3. the pressure of cardiac compressions.
- ○ 4. turning the head to the side.

29. What is the estimated maximum time a person can be without cardiopulmonary function and still not experience permanent brain damage?
- ○ 1. 1 to 2 minutes.
- ○ 2. 4 to 6 minutes.
- ○ 3. 8 to 10 minutes.
- ○ 4. 12 to 15 minutes.

30. The nurse would know to administer the Heimlich maneuver on a suspected choking victim when the victim
- ○ 1. becomes cyanotic.
- ○ 2. cannot speak owing to airway obstruction.
- ○ 3. can make only minimal vocal noises.
- ○ 4. is coughing vigorously.

31. When performing the Heimlich maneuver on a conscious adult victim, the rescuer delivers inward and upward thrusts
- ○ 1. above the umbilicus.
- ○ 2. at the level of the xiphoid process.

○ 3. over the victim's mid-abdominal area.
○ 4. below the xiphoid process and above the umbilicus.

The Client in Shock

A 47-year-old woman has had a gastric ulcer for years. After she started vomiting blood today, her neighbor drove her to the emergency room.

32. In the early stage of shock, the nurse would expect the results of arterial blood gas (ABG) analysis to indicate
○ 1. respiratory alkalosis.
○ 2. respiratory acidosis.
○ 3. metabolic alkalosis.
○ 4. metabolic acidosis.

33. The client receives an intravenous infusion of packed red blood cells and normal saline solution. A priority for this client includes assessing her for
○ 1. hypovolemia.
○ 2. anaphylactic reaction.
○ 3. pain.
○ 4. altered level of consciousness.

34. The client does not respond adequately to fluid replacement, and an intravenous infusion of dopamine hydrochloride is started. Dopamine hydrochloride in moderate dosages is frequently the drug of choice for treating shock primarily because it
○ 1. acts as a potent vasoconstrictor.
○ 2. increases myocardial contractility.
○ 3. supports renal perfusion.
○ 4. has no serious side effects.

35. Which of the following would be an essential nursing action for the client receiving dopamine hydrochloride to treat shock?
○ 1. Administer pain medication concurrently.
○ 2. Monitor blood pressure continuously.
○ 3. Evaluate arterial blood gases at least every 2 hours.
○ 4. Monitor for signs of infection.

36. The client's condition stabilizes, but medical intervention fails to stop gastric bleeding. She is scheduled for surgery within the next 6 hours. The nurse ensures that the client is warm but not overheated and that the light in the room is lowered. The nurse gives the client and her family calm, simple answers to their questions about the surgery. What is the primary rationale behind these interventions?
○ 1. To stabilize fluid and electrolyte balance.
○ 2. To minimize oxygen consumption.
○ 3. To increase client and family comfort.
○ 4. To prevent infection.

37. The underlying pathophysiologic alteration in all types of shock is
○ 1. hemorrhage of blood or body fluids.
○ 2. decreased cardiac output.
○ 3. inadequate tissue perfusion.
○ 4. vasodilation of vascular beds.

38. Which of the following assessment findings indicates hypovolemic shock?
○ 1. Pulse less than 60 beats/minute.
○ 2. Respiratory rate more than 30 breaths/minute.
○ 3. Pupils unequally dilated.
○ 4. Systolic blood pressure less than 90 mm Hg.

39. If none of the following bed positions is contraindicated, which position would be preferred for the client with hypovolemic shock?
○ 1. Supine.
○ 2. Semi-Fowler's.
○ 3. Supine with the legs elevated 15 degrees.
○ 4. Trendelenburg's.

40. Which of the following would be the best indication that fluid replacement for the client in hypovolemic shock is adequate?
○ 1. Urine output greater than 30 mL/hour.
○ 2. Systolic blood pressure above 110 mm Hg.
○ 3. Diastolic blood pressure above 90 mm Hg.
○ 4. Urine output of 20 to 30 mL/hour.

41. When assessing a client for early septic shock, the nurse should observe for
○ 1. cool, clammy skin.
○ 2. warm, flushed skin.
○ 3. decreased systolic blood pressure.
○ 4. hemorrhage.

42. The nurse can contribute to preventing septic shock by
○ 1. administering intravenous fluid therapy replacement as ordered.
○ 2. obtaining vital signs every 4 hours for all clients.
○ 3. monitoring red blood cell counts for elevation.
○ 4. maintaining asepsis of indwelling urinary catheters.

43. The underlying pathophysiologic alterations in septic shock include which of the following?
○ 1. Production of antibodies in response to an antigen introduced by therapy.
○ 2. Release of histamine and other vasoactive substances that increase capillary permeability.
○ 3. Shifting of fluids from the interstitial space to the vascular space.
○ 4. Release of a myocardial factor that increases contractility.

44. Complications of septic shock include
○ 1. anaphylaxis.
○ 2. adult respiratory distress syndrome.
○ 3. chronic obstructive pulmonary disease.
○ 4. mitral valve prolapse.

45. Which of the following best describes cardiogenic shock? The client experiences
○ 1. decreased cardiac output due to hypovolemia.
○ 2. shock due to decreased circulating blood volume.
○ 3. shock due to decreased myocardial contractility.
○ 4. decreased cardiac output due to infarction.

The Client With Anemia

46. In relation to the toxic effects of vitamin B_{12}, the nurse should teach the client with pernicious anemia that
○ 1. this vitamin is remarkably free of toxicity.
○ 2. ringing in the ears is a common symptom of toxicity.
○ 3. nausea and vomiting are common symptoms of toxicity.
○ 4. skin rashes and itching are common symptoms of toxicity.

47. A priority nursing diagnosis for a client with iron deficiency anemia would be
○ 1. Fluid Volume Excess related to anemia.
○ 2. Alteration in Nutrition related to nausea.
○ 3. Self-Care Deficit related to fatigue.
○ 4. Inadequate Home Maintenance related to immobility.

48. The client with iron deficiency anemia should be instructed to eat which of the following foods high in iron, if it is not contraindicated for other medical reasons?
○ 1. Eggs.
○ 2. Lettuce.
○ 3. Citrus fruits.
○ 4. Cheese.

49. The nurse should instruct the client to eat which of the following foods to obtain the best supply of vitamin B_{12}?
○ 1. Fresh fruits.
○ 2. Green leafy vegetables.
○ 3. Meats and dairy products.
○ 4. Whole-wheat breads and cereals.

The Client Who Is Dying

50. Which of the following statements best explains the common observation that health care personnel avoid terminally ill people?
○ 1. The family members who are present can provide essential care.
○ 2. Health care personnel do not understand their own feelings about death and dying.
○ 3. The dying person requires minimal physical care to be comfortable.
○ 4. It is best to avoid interrupting the person, to protect his right to die with dignity.

51. Which statement by a dying person would indicate that the client has accepted death?
○ 1. "I've lived a good life all in all."
○ 2. "I really don't think you're trying to help me anymore."
○ 3. "I'm too young to die, but I know I have no choice."
○ 4. "I wish I could spend one more night with my friends."

52. A terminally ill client slips into a coma. In offering sound advice to the client's family, the nurse explains that the last of the senses to lapse into unconsciousness is thought to be
○ 1. smell.
○ 2. sight.
○ 3. touch.
○ 4. hearing.

53. When the wife of a terminally ill client cries and expresses her grief, one thing that the nurse should do is
○ 1. call the physician to speak with the client and his wife.
○ 2. find a place where the nurse and the client's wife can talk privately.
○ 3. leave her alone to work through her emotions in private.
○ 4. explain that everything possible was done for her husband.

CORRECT ANSWERS AND RATIONALE

The letters in parentheses following the rationale identify the step of the nursing process (A, D, P, I, E), cognitive level (K, C, T, N), and client needs (S, G, L, H). See the Answer Grid for the key.

The Client With Pernicious Anemia

1. 2. Clients with pernicious anemia demonstrate a lack of intrinsic factor in gastric secretions. (A, T, S)

2. 3. Pernicious anemia is caused by the body's inability to absorb vitamin B_{12}. This results from a lack of intrinsic factor in the gastric juices. The Shilling test helps diagnose pernicious anemia by determining the client's ability to absorb vitamin B_{12}. (A, C, G)

3. 2. Most clients with pernicious anemia have deficient production of intrinsic factor in the stomach. Intrinsic factor attaches to the vitamin in the stomach and forms of complex that allows the vitamin to be absorbed in the small intestine. (A, N, G)

4. 3. Clients with anemia experience activity intolerance and fatigue, which is a priority problem for them that requires intervention. (D, T, G)

5. 2. To promote comfort when injecting at the ventrogluteal site, the position of choice is the client lying on the abdomen with the toes pointing inward. This positioning promotes muscle relaxation, which in turn decreases the discomfort of making an injection into a tense muscle. (I, T, G)

The Client With Hodgkin's Disease

6. 4. Serum albumin levels help determine whether protein intake is sufficient. Proteins are broken down into amino acids during digestion. Amino acids are absorbed in the small intestine, and albumin is built from amino acids. (A, T, G)

7. 4. Three chemotherapeutic drugs are given over a period of time. Multiple drug regimens are used because when given in combination, the drugs have a synergistic effect. Additionally, drugs that have different cycles, different actions, and different toxic side effects are given in combination to enhance therapy. (I, T, G)

8. 3. A common priority problem of chemotherapy is potential for infection because chemotherapeutic agents may suppress formation of white blood cells and their components, leading to increased risk of infection. Careful monitoring of white blood cell levels is warranted in clients receiving immunosuppressive drugs. Fluid volume deficit is more typical than fluid volume excess. Impaired physical mobility and altered health maintenance are not necessarily priority problems encountered during chemotherapy. (D, N, G)

9. 1. The nurse should notify the physician of extreme amounts of emesis because further treatment may be warranted. Administering pain medication is important but will not relieve the nausea and vomiting. Placing the client on a liquid diet is the physician's decision. (I, N, G)

10. 1. Thrombocytopenia (low platelet count) leaves the client at risk for potentially life-threatening spontaneous hemorrhage. (I, T, G)

11. 1. The primary purpose of protective (reverse) isolation is to reduce transmission of organisms to the client from sources outside the client's environment. (I, T, G)

12. 2. A characteristic early sign of Hodgkin's disease is swollen cervical lymph nodes. The disease originates in the lymphatic system. (A, T, G)

13. 3. Hodgkin's disease most often strikes young adults, usually between ages 21 and 40 years. A resurgence in incidence then occurs after age 50 years. The disease occurs somewhat more often in men than in women. (A, K, G)

14. 4. Staging of Hodgkin's disease determines the extent and activity of the disease to guide appropriate therapy. The nature of the cell causing the disease is studied microscopically, not by staging. (A, K, G)

15. 4. The iliac crest and the sternum are the most common sites for obtaining bone marrow specimens in adults. These sites are usually selected because they are easily accessible and are away from major organs. (P, K, G)

16. 3. Terminally ill clients most often describe feelings of isolation because they tend to be ignored, are often left out of conversations (especially those dealing with the future), and sense the attitudes of discomfort that many people feel in their presence. Helpful nursing measures include taking the time to be with these clients, offering them opportunities to talk about their feelings, and answering their questions honestly. (P, T, L)

The Client Requiring Cardiopulmonary Resuscitation

17. 3. Before performing chest compressions, it is essential to establish pulselessness of the victim. Chest

compressions performed on a victim with a pulse can lead to further injury. Based on recommendations from the American Heart Association, pulselessness is established by palpating the carotid pulse for 1 minute. (I, T, S)

18. 4. Proper hand placement during chest compressions is essential to reduce the risk of rib fractures, which may lead to pneumothorax and other internal injuries. (I, T, S)

19. 3. The external cardiac compression rate for two-rescuer CPR is 80 to 100 compressions per minute to ensure adequate oxygenation. (I, T, G)

20. 2. Pupillary reaction is the best indication of whether oxygenated blood is reaching the client's brain. Pupils that remain widely dilated and do not react to light likely indicate that serious brain damage has occurred. (E, T, G)

21. 4. Epinephrine is administered during CPR primarily for its ability to improve cardiac activity. Epinephrine has great affinity for adrenergic receptors in cardiac tissue and acts to strengthen and speed the heart rate as well as to increase impulse conduction from atria to ventricles. Epinephrine constricts arterioles, but this is not the primary reason for administering it during CPR. (I, T, G)

22. 2. According to the American Heart Association, once initiated, CPR may only be discontinued when the rescuer is exhausted or when a physician is present to determine client status. Other reasons, such as the rescuer thinking the victim will not survive or the family requesting discontinuation, are not acceptable reasons. (E, N, G)

23. 4. With one-rescuer CPR, the compression-to-ventilation ratio is 15:2, with a 1- to 1.5-second pause for ventilation. (I, K, G)

24. 2. Because of its location near the xiphoid process, the liver is the organ most easily damaged from pressure exerted over the xiphoid process during CPR. The pressure on the victim's chest wall should be sufficient to compress the heart but not so great as to damage internal organs. Injury may result, however, even when CPR is performed properly. (I, K, G)

25. 3. An adult's sternum must be depressed 1.5 to 2 inches with each compression to ensure adequate heart compression. (I, K, G)

26. 2. The carotid artery pulse is most easily assessed by the rescuer performing ventilations because that person is closest to the victim's carotid area, and assessment will not disturb the hand placement of the rescuer delivering chest compressions. Pulse assessment is done about every 5 to 10 minutes. (I, K, G)

27. 1. If the airway is not clear, it is impossible to inflate the lungs during CPR. A common sign of airway

obstruction is failure of the victim's chest wall to rise with each inflation. (E, C, G)

28. 1. The exhalation phase of ventilation is a passive activity and will occur during CPR as part of the normal relaxation of the victim's chest. No action by the rescuer is necessary. (E, T, G)

29. 2. After a person is without cardiopulmonary function for 4 to 6 minutes, permanent brain damage is almost certain. To prevent permanent brain damage, it is important to begin CPR promptly after a victim suffers cardiopulmonary failure. (E, T, G)

30. 2. The Heimlich maneuver should be administered only to a victim who cannot make *any* sounds due to airway obstruction. If the victim can whisper words, some air exchange is occurring, and the emergency medical system should be called instead of attempting the Heimlich maneuver. (A, T, G)

31. 4. The thrusts should be delivered below the xiphoid process but above the umbilicus to minimize the risk of internal injuries. (I, C, S)

The Client in Shock

32. 1. As a compensatory measure in the early stage of shock, the client hyperventilates in response to hypoxemia. Hyperventilation is an attempt to provide more oxygen to the tissues in the face of a decreased circulating volume. It increases minute volume and results in decreased $PaCO_2$, while PaO_2 remains normal. This is the classic picture of respiratory alkalosis. Metabolic acidosis and respiratory acidosis occur in the advanced stage of shock. (A, N, G)

33. 2. The client receiving a blood product requires astute assessment for signs and symptoms of allergic reaction and anaphylaxis, including pruritus (itching), urticaria (hives), facial or glottal edema, and shortness of breath. If such a reaction occurs, the nurse should stop the transfusion immediately and notify the physician. Usually, an antihistamine, such as diphenhydramine hydrochloride (Benadryl), is administered. Epinephrine and corticosteroids may be administered in severe reactions. (A, T, G)

34. 2. Dopamine hydrochloride is a potent inotropic agent that increases myocardial contractility. Increased myocardial contractility leads to improved cardiac output and improved tissue perfusion. When given in moderate doses, dopamine can maintain systolic blood pressure above 90 mm Hg in clients with shock. An added benefit of dopamine is that it dilates the renal and mesenteric arteries, supporting renal perfusion. In high doses, dopamine is a vasoconstrictor and may cause serious side effects; thus, it is not administered in high doses. (I, T, G)

35. 2. The client receiving dopamine hydrochloride requires continuous blood pressure monitoring with an invasive or noninvasive device. The nurse may titrate the intravenous infusion to maintain a systolic blood pressure of 90 mm Hg. (I, T, G)

36. 2. The interventions of providing warmth and bed rest and minimizing anxiety are aimed at decreasing the body's need for oxygen and nutrients, substances already deficient in the client in shock. These interventions are not directly related to fluid and electrolyte balance or to infection prevention. These interventions may increase the client and family's comfort, but this is not the primary goal. (I, N, G)

37. 3. The primary pathophysiologic alteration in shock is inadequate tissue perfusion. This alteration may be caused by hemorrhage, as in hypovolemic shock; decreased cardiac output, as in cardiogenic shock; or massive vasodilation of the vascular bed, as in neurogenic, anaphylactic, and septic shock. (A, N, G)

38. 4. Typical signs and symptoms of hypovolemic shock include systolic blood pressure less than 90 mm Hg, narrowing pulse pressure, tachycardia, tachypnea, cool and clammy skin, decreased urine output, and mental status changes such as irritability or anxiety. (A, T, G)

39. 3. A client in hypovolemic shock is best positioned supine in bed with the feet elevated 15 degrees to bring peripheral blood into the central circulation. Trendelenburg's position was formerly recommended but has been found to inhibit respiratory expansion and possibly to cause increased intracranial pressure. Semi-Fowler's position would not facilitate venous return. (I, T, G)

40. 1. Urine output provides the most sensitive indication of the client's response to therapy for hypovolemic shock. Urine output should be consistently greater than 30 to 35 mL/hour. Blood pressure is a more accurate reflection of the adequacy of vasoconstriction than of tissue perfusion. (E, N, G)

41. 2. Warm, flushed skin occurs in the hyperdynamic, "warm shock" phase of septic shock. Other signs and symptoms of early septic shock include restlessness, confusion, tachypnea, and tachycardia. As the shock stage progresses, the signs and symptoms resemble those of hypovolemic shock, with cool, clammy skin and oliguria. (A, T, G)

42. 4. Interventions such as maintaining asepsis of indwelling urinary catheters are essential to prevent infection. Preventing septic shock is a major focus of nursing care because the mortality rate for septic shock is as high as 90% in some populations. Very young and elderly clients (those younger than 2 years and older than 65 years) are at increased risk for septic shock. (I, N, H)

43. 2. In septic shock, the major pathophysiologic alterations are due to the release of vasoactive substances that increase capillary permeability. These vasoactive substances lead to massive vasodilation and fluid shifts from the vascular to the interstitial spaces. Myocardial depressant factor is also released, which causes decreased myocardial contractility. (D, C, G)

44. 2. Adult respiratory distress syndrome (ARDS) is a complication associated with septic shock. ARDS causes respiratory failure and may lead to death, even after the client has recovered from shock. (A, C, G)

45. 3. Cardiogenic shock occurs when myocardial contractility diminishes and cardiac output greatly decreases. Cardiogenic shock does not result from hypovolemia; in fact, the circulating blood volume is within normal limits or increased in cardiogenic shock. Infarction is not always the cause of cardiogenic shock. (A, C, G)

The Client With Anemia

46. 1. Vitamin B_{12} is remarkably free of toxicity. Allergic reactions that have occurred are believed to be caused by impurities or the preservative in B_{12} preparations. (I, T, H)

47. 3. Fatigue is commonly experienced by clients with iron deficiency anemia due to reduced oxygen-carrying capacity from low hemoglobin. The fatigue may lead to the client's inability to perform his or her own care. Fluid volume deficit is another possible problem. Nausea and immobility are not necessarily related to iron deficiency anemia. (D, N, G)

48. 1. Eggs are high in iron. Other foods high in iron include organ meats (liver, kidney, heart), muscle meats (dark meat from poultry), shellfish, whole-grain cereals and breads, dark green vegetables, legumes, nuts, and dried fruits (apricots, raisins, dates). (I, N, H)

49. 3. Good sources of vitamin B_{12} include meats and dairy products. Many fresh fruits are good sources of vitamin A, vitamin B_2, and vitamin B_9 (folic acid). Whole-wheat breads and cereals are good sources of vitamin B_1, vitamin B_2, vitamin B_3, vitamin B_6, and vitamin E. (I, T, G)

The Client Who Is Dying

50. 2. Health care personnel may avoid the terminally ill client because they are uncomfortable about death and do not understand their own feelings about dying. Family members should not be expected to assume responsibility for the client's care, but they should be involved in the client's care to the extent they desire. Skilled and knowledgeable nursing care is required to make a dying person comfortable. Interrupting the client does not necessarily interfere with the right to die with dignity. (A, N, S)

51. 1. A terminally ill person has generally accepted finiteness when he or she expresses satisfaction with the way he or she has lived life. The terminally ill person still needs attention, and the nurse should be alert to comments that may reflect defeat rather than acceptance during this time. Criticism of caretakers typically occurs when a person is angry and is asking, "Why me?" Depression and sadness may occur and may be associated with crying. The per-

son may not have not accepted death even though it is imminent. Trying to bargain for time to do one more thing before dying may occur before acceptance. (E, N, L)

52. 4. Hearing is thought to be the last sense to leave the body. Although unconscious, the client may still be able to hear. (P, K, G)

53. 2. When a family member expresses grief, it is best if the nurse can find a private place where the person will be comfortable in expressing grief and crying. Offering to call the physician, leaving the family member alone, or reassuring her that everything possible was done for her husband are not as likely to facilitate expression of grief and promote healing. (I, T, L)

NURSING CARE OF ADULTS WITH MEDICAL AND SURGICAL HEALTH PROBLEMS

TEST 3: The Client With Cardiovascular and Hematologic Health Problems; the Client Who Is Dying

Directions: Use this answer grid to determine areas of strength or need for further study.

NURSING PROCESS

A = Assessment
D = Analysis, nursing diagnosis
P = Planning
I = Implementation
E = Evaluation

COGNITIVE LEVEL

K = Knowledge
C = Comprehension
T = Application
N = Analysis

CLIENT NEEDS

S = Safe, effective care environment
G = Physiologic integrity
L = Psychosocial integrity
H = Health promotion and maintenance

Question #	Answer #	A	D	P	I	E	K	C	T	N	S	G	L	H
1	2	A							T		S			
2	3	A						C				G		
3	2	A								N		G		
4	3		D						T			G		
5	2				I				T			G		
6	4	A							T			G		
7	4				I				T			G		
8	3		D							N		G		
9	1				I					N		G		
10	1				I				T			G		
11	1				I				T			G		
12	2	A							T			G		
13	3	A					K					G		
14	4	A					K					G		
15	4			P			K					G		
16	3			P					T				L	
17	3				I				T		S			
18	4				I				T		S			
19	3				I				T			G		
20	2					E			T			G		
21	4				I				T			G		
22	2					E				N		G		
23	4				I		K					G		
24	2				I		K					G		
25	3				I		K					G		

NURSING PROCESS

A = Assessment
D = Analysis, nursing diagnosis
P = Planning
I = Implementation
E = Evaluation

COGNITIVE LEVEL

K = Knowledge
C = Comprehension
T = Application
N = Analysis

CLIENT NEEDS

S = Safe, effective care environment
G = Physiologic integrity
L = Psychosocial integrity
H = Health promotion and maintenance

Question #	Answer #	A	D	P	I	E	K	C	T	N	S	G	L	H
26	2				I		K					G		
27	1					E		C				G		
28	1					E			T			G		
29	2					E			T			G		
30	2	A							T			G		
31	4				I			C			S			
32	1	A								N		G		
33	2	A							T			G		
34	2				I				T			G		
35	2				I				T			G		
36	2				I					N		G		
37	3	A								N		G		
38	4	A							T			G		
39	3				I				T			G		
40	1					E				N		G		
41	2	A							T			G		
42	4				I					N				H
43	2		D					C				G		
44	2	A						C				G		
45	3	A						C				G		
46	1				I				T					H
47	3		D							N		G		
48	1				I					N				H
49	3				I				T			G		
50	2	A								N	S			
51	1					E				N			L	
52	4			P			K					G		
53	2				I				T				L	

ANSWER GRID: 2

449

NURSING PROCESS

A = Assessment
D = Analysis, nursing diagnosis
P = Planning
I = Implementation
E = Evaluation

COGNITIVE LEVEL

K = Knowledge
C = Comprehension
T = Application
N = Analysis

CLIENT NEEDS

S = Safe, effective care environment
G = Physiologic integrity
L = Psychosocial integrity
H = Health promotion and maintenance

Question #	Answer #	Nursing Process					Cognitive Level				Client Needs			
		A	D	P	I	E	K	C	T	N	S	G	L	H
Number Correct														
Number Possible	53	16	4	3	23	7	8	6	26	13	5	42	3	3
Percentage Correct														

Score Calculation: To determine your **Percentage Correct,** divide the **Number Correct** by the **Number Possible.**

ANSWER GRID: 3

The Client With Upper Gastrointestinal Tract Health Problems

- **The Client With Peptic Ulcer Disease**
- **The Client With Cholecystitis**
- **The Client With Cancer of the Stomach**
- **The Client With Pancreatitis**
- **The Client With Hiatal Hernia**
- **Correct Answers and Rationale**

Select the one best answer, and indicate your choice by filling in the circle in front of the option.

The Client With Peptic Ulcer Disease

A client is brought to the hospital after vomiting bright red blood and is admitted through the emergency department with a bleeding duodenal ulcer.

1. While the client is bleeding, it will be essential for the nurse to assess frequently for signs of early shock. Which one of the following is an important indicator of early shock?
   - ○ 1. Tachycardia.
   - ○ 2. Dry, flushed skin.
   - ○ 3. Increased urine output.
   - ○ 4. Loss of consciousness.
2. If the client develops a sudden sharp pain in the mid-epigastric region along with a rigid, board-like abdomen, the nurse should understand that these clinical manifestations most likely indicate that
   - ○ 1. an intestinal obstruction has developed.
   - ○ 2. additional ulcers have developed.
   - ○ 3. the esophagus has become inflamed.
   - ○ 4. the ulcer has perforated.
3. The client tells the nurse that he had black stools before admission to the hospital but had not reported this to his physician. Based on this information, which nursing diagnosis would be appropriate for this client?
   - ○ 1. Ineffective Individual Coping related to fear of diagnosis of chronic illness.

   - ○ 2. Knowledge Deficit related to unfamiliarity with significant signs and symptoms.
   - ○ 3. Constipation related to decreased gastric motility.
   - ○ 4. Altered Nutrition: Less Than Body Requirements related to gastric bleeding.
4. The client asks the nurse what causes an ulcer to develop. The nurse responds that recent research indicates that many peptic ulcers are the result of
   - ○ 1. work-related stress.
   - ○ 2. *Helicobacter pylori* infection.
   - ○ 3. diets high in fat and spicy foods.
   - ○ 4. a genetic defect in the gastric mucosa.
5. The client has been taking propantheline bromide (Pro-Banthine) at home. The nurse should prepare a teaching plan for the client that indicates the medication acts primarily to
   - ○ 1. suppress gastric secretions.
   - ○ 2. neutralize acid in the stomach.
   - ○ 3. shorten the time required for digestion in the stomach.
   - ○ 4. improve the mixing of foods and gastric secretions.
6. The client reports frequent episodes of epigastric pain that awaken him during the night, a feeling of fullness in the abdomen, and anxiety about his health. Based on these data, which nursing diagnosis would be most appropriate?
   - ○ 1. Altered Nutrition: Less than Body Requirements related to anorexia.

2. Sleep Pattern Disturbance related to epigastric pain.
3. Ineffective Individual Coping related to exacerbation of duodenal ulcer.
4. Activity Intolerance related to abdominal pain.

7. Which of the following expected outcomes would be most appropriate for this client? The client will
1. verbalize absence of epigastric pain.
2. accept the need to inject himself with vitamin B_{12} for the rest of his life.
3. understand the need to increase his exercise activity.
4. eliminate all stress from his life.

8. The nurse is preparing to teach the client about the diet he should follow at home after discharge. The nurse should explain that his diet will most likely consist of
1. full liquids and pureed food.
2. high-fat, high-protein foods.
3. any foods that he can tolerate.
4. six small meals a day.

9. Which one of the following statements indicates that the client understands the dietary modifications he will need to follow at home?
1. "I should eat a bland, soft diet."
2. "It is important to eat six small meals a day."
3. "I should drink several glasses of milk a day."
4. "I should avoid alcohol and caffeine."

10. The client undergoes an upper gastrointestinal endoscopy to help the physician visualize the ulcer's location and severity. Immediately after the endoscopy, what should the nurse evaluate besides his vital signs?
1. Return of the gag reflex.
2. Bowel sounds.
3. Breath sounds.
4. Intake and output.

11. The nurse finds the client surrounded by papers from his briefcase and arguing on the telephone with a coworker. The nurse's interaction with him should be based on knowledge that
1. involvement with his job will keep him from becoming bored in the hospital.
2. rest is an essential component of ulcer healing.
3. not keeping up with his job will increase his stress level.
4. setting limits on a client's behavior is an essential aspect of the nursing role.

12. The client has been instructed to avoid intense physical activity and stress. Which activity should the client incorporate into his home care plan?
1. Conduct all physical activity early in the morning so he can rest all afternoon.
2. Have his wife agree to perform the necessary yard work at home.

3. Give up his weekly golf game.
4. Develop a plan that provides for periods of physical and mental rest.

13. Which of the following statements would indicate that the client understands how to adjust his response to work-related stress effectively?
1. "My job is too stressful. I will have to find a different career."
2. "I don't have any control over my stressors at work. My coworkers are difficult to work with."
3. "Well, I guess this ulcer means I won't be able to work toward a promotion."
4. "I will have to improve my ability to cope with stress."

14. Which of the following activities should the nurse encourage the client with a peptic ulcer to avoid?
1. Chewing gum.
2. Smoking cigarettes.
3. Eating chocolate.
4. Taking acetaminophen (Tylenol).

15. The client will take a daily dose of ranitidine (Zantac) at home. The nurse would know that the client understands about proper drug administration when he says that he will take the drug
1. before meals.
2. with meals.
3. at bedtime.
4. when pain occurs.

16. The client has been taking aluminum hydroxide (Amphojel), 30 mL six times per day, at home. He tells the nurse at the clinic that he has not been able to have a bowel movement for 3 days. Based on this information, the nurse would determine that the client most likely
1. has not been including enough fiber in his diet.
2. needs to increase his daily exercise.
3. is experiencing a side effect of the aluminum hydroxide.
4. has developed a gastrointestinal obstruction.

The Client With Cholecystitis

A client is admitted to the hospital with a diagnosis of cholecystitis from cholelithiasis.

17. Which of the following symptoms would the nurse most likely observe in a client with cholecystitis from cholelithiasis?
1. Black stools.
2. Nausea after ingestion of high-fat foods.
3. Elevated temperature of 103°F.
4. Decreased white blood cell count.

18. The client is complaining of severe abdominal pain

and extreme nausea and has vomited several times. Based on these data, which nursing diagnosis would have the highest priority for intervention at this time?
- ○ 1. Anxiety related to severe abdominal discomfort.
- ○ 2. Fluid Volume Deficit related to vomiting.
- ○ 3. Pain related to gallbladder inflammation.
- ○ 4. Altered Nutrition: Less Than Body Requirements related to vomiting.

19. Which of the following nursing interventions should have the highest priority during the first hour after this client's admission?
- ○ 1. Administering pain medication.
- ○ 2. Completing the admission history.
- ○ 3. Maintaining hydration.
- ○ 4. Teaching about planned diagnostic tests.

20. Propantheline bromide (Pro-Banthine) is ordered for the client. This drug is used to
- ○ 1. relieve pain.
- ○ 2. decrease biliary contraction.
- ○ 3. treat infection.
- ○ 4. relieve nausea.

21. The client is receiving propantheline bromide (Pro-Banthine). The nurse would evaluate the client's response to the medication by observing for which one the following side effects?
- ○ 1. Urinary retention.
- ○ 2. Diarrhea.
- ○ 3. Hypertension.
- ○ 4. Diaphoresis.

22. If a gallstone becomes lodged in the common bile duct, the nurse should anticipate that the client's stools would most likely be
- ○ 1. green.
- ○ 2. gray.
- ○ 3. black.
- ○ 4. yellow.

23. When the common bile duct is obstructed, the nurse should evaluate the client for signs of
- ○ 1. respiratory distress.
- ○ 2. circulatory overload.
- ○ 3. urinary tract infection.
- ○ 4. prolonged bleeding time.

24. The client is scheduled for cholecystography. Which one of the following actions would the nurse plan to implement before the test?
- ○ 1. Have the client drink 1000 mL of water.
- ○ 2. Ask the client about possible allergies to iodine or shellfish.
- ○ 3. Administer an intravenous contrast agent the evening before the test.
- ○ 4. Administer tap-water enemas until clear.

25. Preoperatively, the client expresses anxiety about having surgery. Which of the following nursing interventions would help achieve the goal of reducing the client's anxiety?
- ○ 1. Provide the client with information, but only if he requests it.
- ○ 2. Tell the client what to expect in the postoperative period.
- ○ 3. Reassure the client by telling him about the high percentage of clients who are not afraid of surgery.
- ○ 4. Stress to the client the importance of following his physician's instructions after surgery.

26. The nurse is preparing to start an intravenous infusion. Before inserting the needle into a vein, the nurse would apply a tourniquet to the client's arm to
- ○ 1. distend the veins.
- ○ 2. stabilize the veins.
- ○ 3. immobilize the arm.
- ○ 4. occlude arterial circulation.

27. Preoperatively, the nurse instructs the client in the correct use of an incentive spirometer. This treatment is essential after surgery in the upper abdominal area because
- ○ 1. the client is maintained on bed rest for several days.
- ○ 2. ambulation is restricted by the presence of drainage tubes.
- ○ 3. the operative incision is near the diaphragm.
- ○ 4. the presence of a nasogastric tube makes it difficult for the client to cough effectively.

28. To evaluate the effectiveness of the incentive spirometer, the nurse should understand that this device is used primarily to
- ○ 1. stimulate circulation.
- ○ 2. prepare for ambulation.
- ○ 3. strengthen abdominal muscles.
- ○ 4. increase respiratory effectiveness.

29. The nurse should understand that the primary reason for withholding food and fluids from a client who will receive general anesthesia is to help prevent
- ○ 1. constipation during the immediate postoperative period.
- ○ 2. vomiting and possible aspiration of vomitus during surgery.
- ○ 3. pressure on the diaphragm with poor lung expansion during surgery.
- ○ 4. gas pains and distention during the immediate postoperative period.

30. The nurse administers a preoperative intramuscular medication at the ventrogluteal site. The nurse will inject the medication into which muscle?
- ○ 1. Rectus femoris.
- ○ 2. Gluteus minimus.
- ○ 3. Vastus lateralis.

○ 4. Gluteus maximus.

31. The client undergoes a traditional cholecystectomy and choledochotomy and returns from surgery with a T tube in place. To evaluate the effectiveness of the T tube, the nurse should understand that the primary reason for the T tube is to
○ 1. promote wound drainage.
○ 2. provide a way to irrigate the biliary tract.
○ 3. minimize the passage of bile into the duodenum.
○ 4. prevent bile from entering the peritoneal cavity.

32. How much bile would the nurse expect the T tube to drain during the first 24 hours after a cholecystectomy?
○ 1. 50 to 100 mL.
○ 2. 150 to 250 mL.
○ 3. 300 to 500 mL.
○ 4. 550 to 700 mL.

33. The nurse should measure the amount of drainage from the T tube and record it by
○ 1. adding it to the client's urine output.
○ 2. charting it separately on the output record.
○ 3. adding it to the amount of wound drainage.
○ 4. subtracting it from the total intake for each day.

34. The nurse develops a plan of care for a client with a T tube. Which one of the following nursing interventions should be included?
○ 1. Inspect skin around the T tube daily for irritation.
○ 2. Irrigate the T tube every 4 hours to maintain patency.
○ 3. Maintain client in a supine position while T tube is in place.
○ 4. Keep T tube clamped except for during mealtimes.

35. Prochlorperazine (Compazine) is prescribed for postoperative administration. The nurse would evaluate that the drug has had a therapeutic effect when the client no longer complains of
○ 1. nausea.
○ 2. dizziness.
○ 3. abdominal spasms.
○ 4. abdominal distention.

36. Which nursing measure would be most effective in helping the client cough and deep breathe after a cholecystectomy?
○ 1. Having the client take rapid, shallow breaths to decrease pain.
○ 2. Having the client lay on the right side while coughing and deep breathing.
○ 3. Teaching the client to use a folded blanket or pillow to splint the incision.
○ 4. Withholding pain medication so the client can be alert enough to follow the nurse's instructions.

37. Which of the following nursing interventions would best accomplish the goal of preventing atelectasis and pneumonia in a postoperative client?
○ 1. Administer oxygen therapy p.r.n. to maintain adequate oxygenation.
○ 2. Offer meperidine hydrochloride (Demerol) 30 minutes before having the client cough and deep breathe.
○ 3. Encourage the client to cough, deep breathe, and turn in bed once every 4 hours.
○ 4. Maintain the client on bed rest for at least 48 hours to minimize incisional pain.

38. Which of the following signs and symptoms would be an early indication that the client's serum potassium level is below normal?
○ 1. Diarrhea.
○ 2. Sticky mucous membranes.
○ 3. Muscle weakness in the legs.
○ 4. Tingling in the fingers.

39. The correct procedure for auscultating the client's abdomen for bowel sounds would include
○ 1. palpating the abdomen first to determine correct stethoscope placement.
○ 2. encouraging the client to cough to stimulate movement of fluid and air through the abdomen.
○ 3. placing the client on the left side to aid auscultation.
○ 4. listening for 5 minutes in all four quadrants to confirm absence of bowel sounds.

40. During the first few weeks after a cholecystectomy, the client should plan to follow a diet that includes
○ 1. a decreased intake of fruits, vegetables, whole grains, and nuts, to minimize pressure within the small intestine.
○ 2. at least four servings of meat, cheese, and peanut butter daily to increase protein intake to aid incisional healing.
○ 3. a limited intake of fat distributed throughout the day so there is not an excessive amount in the intestine at any one time.
○ 4. ingestion of pancreatic enzymes with meals to replace the normal enzyme secretion that has been surgically altered.

41. After a cholecystectomy, it is recommended that the client follow a low-fat diet at home. Which of the following foods would be most appropriate to include in a low-fat diet?
○ 1. Cheese omelet and vanilla pudding.
○ 2. Egg salad sandwich and fresh fruit cup.
○ 3. Ham salad sandwich and baked custard.
○ 4. Roast beef and green beans.

42. A client has had a laparoscopic cholecystectomy. Which of the following statements indicates that the client understands the nurse's discharge instructions about activity restrictions?

○ 1. "I will need to stay in bed the first 2 days I am home."

○ 2. "I will not be able to lift objects until 6 weeks after my surgery."

○ 3. "I can return to my normal activities within 7 days."

○ 4. "I should avoid sitting upright for 1 week after my surgery."

The Client With Cancer of the Stomach

A client has been diagnosed with adenocarcinoma of the stomach. A subtotal gastric resection is planned.

43. The nurse determines that the client's nutritional status has been severely compromised through prolonged episodes of nausea and vomiting. Which of the following therapies would the nurse anticipate to be the most effective in correcting his nutritional deficits before surgery?

○ 1. High-protein between-meal nourishment four times a day.

○ 2. Continuous enteral feedings at 200 mL/hour.

○ 3. Total parenteral nutrition (TPN) for several days.

○ 4. Intravenous infusion of normal saline solution at 125 mL/hour.

44. The client is scheduled to undergo a subtotal gastrectomy (Billroth II procedure). When providing preoperative client teaching, the nurse should explain that the surgical procedure will allow stomach contents to bypass the

○ 1. ileum.

○ 2. duodenum.

○ 3. cardiac sphincter.

○ 4. fundus of the stomach.

45. The client tells the nurse that since his diagnosis of cancer, he has been having trouble sleeping and is frequently preoccupied with thoughts about how his life will change. He says, "I wish my life could stay the same." Based on these data, which one of the following nursing diagnoses would be appropriate at this time?

○ 1. Ineffective Individual Coping related to the diagnosis of cancer.

○ 2. Sleep Pattern Disturbance related to fear of the unknown.

○ 3. Anticipatory Grieving related to diagnosis of cancer.

○ 4. Anxiety related to the need for gastric surgery.

46. After surgery, the client will have a nasogastric tube in place for several days postoperatively to

○ 1. prevent excessive pressure on suture lines.

○ 2. prevent the development of ascites.

○ 3. provide enteral feedings in the immediate postoperative period.

○ 4. enable administration of antacids to promote healing of the anastomosis.

47. The nurse should anticipate that drainage from the nasogastric tube would be what color about 12 to 24 hours after a subtotal gastrectomy?

○ 1. Brown.

○ 2. Green.

○ 3. Red.

○ 4. White.

48. After a subtotal gastrectomy, care of the client's nasogastric tube and drainage system should include which of the following nursing interventions?

○ 1. Irrigate the tube with 30 mL of sterile water every hour, if needed.

○ 2. If the tube is not draining well, reposition it.

○ 3. Monitor the client for nausea, vomiting, and abdominal distention.

○ 4. If the drainage is sluggish on low suction, turn the machine to high suction.

49. From an analysis of the data collected about the client and his surgery, the nurse formulates the nursing diagnosis High Risk for Altered Respiratory Function. Which of the following postoperative factors would this diagnosis be related to?

○ 1. A high abdominal incision.

○ 2. Ambulating three times a day.

○ 3. Possibility of reoccurring nausea.

○ 4. Maintenance of a semi-Fowler's position.

50. After gastric resection surgery, which of the following signs and symptoms would alert the nurse to the development of a leaking anastomosis?

○ 1. Pain, fever, and abdominal rigidity.

○ 2. Diarrhea with fat in the stool.

○ 3. Palpitations, pallor, and diaphoresis after eating.

○ 4. Feelings of fullness and nausea after eating.

51. As part of the client's discharge planning, the nurse has identified Altered Nutrition: Less Than Body Requirements as a major nursing diagnosis. To help the client meet nutritional goals at home, the nurse should develop a plan of care that includes

○ 1. instructing him to increase the amount eaten at each meal by doubling that eaten at the previous meal.

○ 2. encouraging him to eat smaller amounts more frequently and to stop when he feels full.

○ 3. explaining that if he vomits after a meal, he should eat nothing more that day.

○ 4. informing him that bland foods are less nutritional, and instructing him to use them minimally in his diet.

52. Which of the following outcomes would indicate that the client's nutritional goal is being achieved?

○ 1. Gradual increase in food intake and tolerance.

○ 2. Occasional episodes of nausea and vomiting.
○ 3. Ingestion of 2000 mL/day of water.
○ 4. Rapid weight gain within 1 week.

53. As a result of his gastric resection, the client is at risk for developing dumping syndrome. The nurse would develop a plan of care for this client based on knowledge that this problem primarily stems from
○ 1. excess secretion of digestive enzymes in the intestines.
○ 2. rapid emptying of stomach contents into the small intestine.
○ 3. excess glycogen production by the liver.
○ 4. the loss of gastric juices.

54. To reduce the risk of dumping syndrome, the nurse should teach the client which of the following strategies?
○ 1. Sit upright after meals.
○ 2. Drink fluids with meals.
○ 3. Decrease the protein content of meals.
○ 4. Decrease the carbohydrate content of meals.

55. Which one of the following expected outcomes about nutrition would be appropriate for a client who has had a subtotal gastrectomy for gastric cancer? The client will
○ 1. regain any weight lost within 4 weeks of the surgical procedure.
○ 2. eat three full meals a day without experiencing gastric complications.
○ 3. learn to self-administer enteral feedings every 4 hours.
○ 4. maintain adequate nutrition through oral or parenteral feedings.

The Client With Pancreatitis

A client is admitted with a possible diagnosis of pancreatitis.

56. Which of the following symptoms would the nurse anticipate observing in a client with pancreatitis?
○ 1. Hypertension, elevated white blood cell count, and peripheral edema.
○ 2. Left upper quadrant abdominal pain, nausea, and vomiting.
○ 3. Hypoglycemia, tachycardia, and cyanosis.
○ 4. Decreased white blood cell count, clubbing of fingernails, and mid-epigastric discomfort.

57. The initial diagnosis of pancreatitis would be confirmed if the client's bloodwork showed a significant elevation in serum
○ 1. amylase.
○ 2. glucose.
○ 3. potassium.

○ 4. trypsin.

58. The client rarely drinks alcohol because of her religious convictions. She becomes upset when the physician persists in asking her about alcohol intake. The nurse should explain that the reason for these questions is that
○ 1. there is a strong link between alcohol use and acute pancreatitis.
○ 2. alcohol intake can interfere with the tests used to diagnose pancreatitis.
○ 3. alcoholism is a major health problem, and all hospitalized clients are questioned about alcohol intake.
○ 4. the physician must obtain the pertinent facts, and religious beliefs cannot be considered.

59. Pain control is an important nursing goal for the client with pancreatitis. Which of the following medications would the nurse plan to administer in this situation?
○ 1. Meperidine hydrochloride (Demerol).
○ 2. Cimetidine (Tagamet).
○ 3. Morphine sulfate.
○ 4. Codeine sulfate.

60. The nurse monitors the client for early signs of shock. Shock is extremely difficult to manage in pancreatitis primarily because of the
○ 1. severity of gastrointestinal hemorrhage.
○ 2. vasodilating effects of kinin peptides.
○ 3. tendency toward congestive heart failure.
○ 4. frequent incidence of acute tubular necrosis.

61. The nurse evaluates the client's most recent laboratory data. Which laboratory finding would be consistent with a diagnosis of acute pancreatitis?
○ 1. Hyperglycemia.
○ 2. Leukopenia.
○ 3. Thrombocytopenia.
○ 4. Hyperkalemia.

62. The nurse notices muscle twitching in the client's hands and forearms. The nurse would report these symptoms immediately because clients with pancreatitis are at serious risk for
○ 1. hypermagnesemia.
○ 2. hypoglycemia.
○ 3. hyperkalemia.
○ 4. hypocalcemia.

63. The initial treatment plan for this client most likely would focus on
○ 1. resting the gastrointestinal tract.
○ 2. ensuring adequate nutrition.
○ 3. maintaining fluid and electrolyte balance.
○ 4. treating infection.

64. When providing care for a client with pancreatitis, the nurse would anticipate which of the following orders?
○ 1. Force fluids to 3000 mL/24 hours.

○ 2. Insert a nasogastric tube and connect it to low suction.
○ 3. Place the client in reverse Trendelenburg's position.
○ 4. Place the client in enteric isolation.

65. The client is to have an nasogastric tube inserted. Appropriate technique for insertion of the tube should include
○ 1. lubricating the tube with petroleum-based lubricant.
○ 2. asking the client to not breathe while the tube is advanced to the stomach.
○ 3. placing the client in a supine position.
○ 4. having the client tilt the head toward the ceiling while inserting the tube into the nose.

66. Which of the following techniques is considered the best way to determine whether a nasogastric tube is positioned in the stomach?
○ 1. Aspirating with a syringe and observing for the return of gastric contents.
○ 2. Irrigating with normal saline and observing for the return of solution.
○ 3. Placing the tube's free end in water and observing for air bubbles.
○ 4. Instilling air and auscultating over the epigastric area for the presence of the tube.

67. The nurse uses 30 mL of solution to irrigate a nasogastric tube and notes that 20 mL returns promptly into the drainage container. When the nurse records the results of the irrigation, how much solution should be recorded as intake?
○ 1. 10 mL.
○ 2. 20 mL.
○ 3. 30 mL.
○ 4. 50 mL.

68. The client complains of sore nares while the nasogastric tube is in place. Which of the following nursing measures would be most appropriate to help alleviate the client's discomfort?
○ 1. Repositioning the tube in the nares.
○ 2. Irrigating the tube with a cool solution.
○ 3. Applying a water-soluble lubricant to the nares.
○ 4. Having the client change position more frequently.

69. For a client with a nasogastric tube attached to low suction postoperatively, intravenous replacement therapy will be needed primarily to
○ 1. maintain bladder function.
○ 2. facilitate osmotic diuresis.
○ 3. equalize intake and output.
○ 4. maintain fluid and electrolyte balance.

70. The client begins to complain of abdominal distention. The nasogastric tube is still inserted. Which of the following measures should the nurse implement first?

○ 1. Call the physician.
○ 2. Irrigate the nasogastric tube.
○ 3. Check the function of the suction equipment.
○ 4. Reposition the nasogastric tube.

71. Which of the following medications would most likely be given to the client to augment pain control?
○ 1. Ibuprofen (Motrin).
○ 2. Magnesium hydroxide (Maalox).
○ 3. Propantheline bromide (Pro-Banthine).
○ 4. Propranolol (Inderal).

72. Which of the following would most likely be a major nursing diagnosis for a client with acute pancreatitis?
○ 1. Ineffective Airway Clearance.
○ 2. Fluid Volume Excess.
○ 3. Impaired Swallowing.
○ 4. Altered Nutrition: Less Than Body Requirements.

73. The client develops chronic pancreatitis. What would be the appropriate home diet for a client with chronic pancreatitis?
○ 1. A low-protein, high-fiber diet distributed over four to five moderate-sized meals daily.
○ 2. A low-fat, bland diet distributed over five to six small meals daily.
○ 3. A high-calcium, soft diet distributed over three meals and an evening snack daily.
○ 4. A diabetic exchange diet distributed over three meals and two snacks daily.

74. Pancreatic enzyme replacements are ordered for the client to take at home. The nurse should instruct the client to take them
○ 1. three times daily between meals.
○ 2. with each meal and snack.
○ 3. in the morning and at bedtime.
○ 4. every 4 hours, at specified times.

75. The nurse should teach the client to monitor the effectiveness of pancreatic enzyme replacement therapy by
○ 1. monitoring her fluid intake.
○ 2. performing regular finger stick tests for glucose.
○ 3. observing her stools for steatorrhea.
○ 4. testing her urine for ketones.

The Client With Hiatal Hernia

A client is being evaluated for a possible hiatal hernia.

76. The client is scheduled to have an upper gastrointestinal tract series. Which of the following treatments should the nurse anticipate after the examination?
○ 1. A laxative.
○ 2. A clear liquid diet.

457

○ 3. An enema.

○ 4. An intravenous infusion.

77. The nurse would expect a client with a hiatal hernia to report that the symptoms worsen when the client is

○ 1. lying down.

○ 2. physically active.

○ 3. upset or angry.

○ 4. sitting.

78. Based on awareness that the primary symptoms of a sliding hiatal hernia are associated with reflux, the nurse should particularly assess the client for

○ 1. heartburn, regurgitation, and dysphagia.

○ 2. jaundice, ascites, and edema.

○ 3. a visible abdominal bulge, diarrhea, and anorexia.

○ 4. vomiting, stomatitis, and board-like abdominal rigidity.

79. Which of the following factors most likely would have contributed to the development of the client's hiatal hernia?

○ 1. Her desk job as a secretary.

○ 2. Her height (5 feet, 3 inches) and weight (190 pounds).

○ 3. Frequent laxative use.

○ 4. Her age.

80. Which of the following nursing interventions would most likely promote self-care behaviors in the client with a hiatal hernia?

○ 1. Introduce the client to other people who are successfully managing their care.

○ 2. Include the client's daughter in the teaching so she can help implement the plan.

○ 3. Ask the client to identify other situations in which she demonstrated responsibility for herself.

○ 4. Assure the client that she will be able to implement all aspects of the plan successfully.

81. The client has been taking magnesium hydroxide (Milk of Magnesia) at home in an attempt to control her symptoms. The nurse should be aware that the most common complaint associated with the ongoing use of magnesium-based antacids is

○ 1. anorexia.

○ 2. weight gain.

○ 3. diarrhea.

○ 4. constipation.

82. Which of the following lifestyle modifications should the nurse encourage the client with a hiatal hernia to include in activities of daily living?

○ 1. Daily aerobic exercise.

○ 2. Eliminating smoking and alcohol use.

○ 3. Carefully balancing activity and rest.

○ 4. Avoiding high-stress situations.

83. The nurse assesses the client's understanding of the relationship between body position and gastroesophageal reflux. Which response would indicate that the client understands measures to avoid problems with reflux while sleeping?

○ 1. "I can elevate the foot of the bed 4 to 6 inches."

○ 2. "I can sleep on my stomach with my head turned to the left."

○ 3. "I can sleep on my back without a pillow under my head."

○ 4. "I can elevate the head of the bed 4 to 6 inches."

84. In developing a teaching plan for the client, the nurse's assessment of which work-related factors would be most useful?

○ 1. Number and length of breaks.

○ 2. Body mechanics used in lifting.

○ 3. Temperature in the work area.

○ 4. Cleaning solvents used.

85. The client attends two sessions with the dietitian to learn about diet modifications to minimize gastroesophageal reflux. The teaching would be judged successful if the client says that she will decrease her intake of

○ 1. fats.

○ 2. high-sodium foods.

○ 3. carbohydrates.

○ 4. high-calcium foods.

86. Which of the following dietary measures would be useful in preventing esophageal reflux?

○ 1. Eating small, frequent meals; avoiding overeating.

○ 2. Belching frequently to reduce abdominal distention.

○ 3. Avoiding air swallowing with meals.

○ 4. Reducing the size of the evening meal and adding a bedtime snack.

87. The nurse instructs the client on health maintenance activities to help control her symptoms from hiatal hernia. Which of the following statements would indicate the client has understood the instructions?

○ 1. "I'll avoid lying down after a meal."

○ 2. "I can still enjoy my potato chips and cola at bedtime."

○ 3. "I wish I didn't have to give up swimming."

○ 4. "If I wear a girdle, I'll have more support for my stomach."

88. The physician prescribes metoclopramide hydrochloride (Reglan) for the client. The nurse plans to instruct the client that this drug is used in hiatal hernia therapy to

○ 1. increase the resting tone of the esophageal sphincter.

○ 2. neutralize gastric secretions.

○ 3. delay gastric emptying.

○ 4. reduce secretion of digestive juices.

89. The nurse should instruct the client to avoid which of the following drugs while taking metoclopramide hydrochloride (Reglan)?
- ○ 1. Antacids.
- ○ 2. Antihypertensives.
- ○ 3. Anticoagulants.
- ○ 4. Alcohol.

90. Cimetidine (Tagamet) may also be used to treat hiatal hernia. The nurse should understand that this drug is used to prevent
- ○ 1. esophageal reflux.
- ○ 2. the feeling of fullness after meals.
- ○ 3. esophagitis.
- ○ 4. ulcer formation.

91. The client asks the nurse whether she will need surgery to correct her hiatal hernia. Which reply by the nurse would be most accurate?
- ○ 1. Surgery is usually required, although medical treatment is attempted first.
- ○ 2. The symptoms of hiatal hernia can usually be successfully managed with diet modifications, medications, and lifestyle changes.
- ○ 3. Surgery is not performed for this type of hernia.
- ○ 4. A minor surgical procedure to reduce the size of the diaphragmatic opening will probably be planned.

CORRECT ANSWERS AND RATIONALE

The letters in parentheses following the rationale identify the step of the nursing process (A, D, P, I, E), cognitive level (K, C, T, N), and client needs (S, G, L, H). See the Answer Grid for the key.

The Client With Peptic Ulcer Disease

1. 1. In early shock, the body attempts to meet its perfusion needs through tachycardia, vasoconstriction, and fluid conservation. The skin becomes cool and clammy. The client may experience increased restlessness and anxiety from hypoxia, but loss of consciousness is a late sign of shock. Urine output in early shock may be normal or slightly decreased. (A, C, G)

2. 4. The body reacts to perforation of an ulcer by immobilizing the area as much as possible. This results in board-like abdominal rigidity, usually with extreme pain. This may occur over several hours or days. It is a medical emergency requiring immediate intervention. (D, N, G)

3. 2. Black tarry stools are an important warning sign of bleeding in peptic ulcer disease. Digested blood in the stool causes it to be black. The odor of the stool is very offensive. Clients with peptic ulcer disease should be instructed to report the incidence of black stools promptly to their primary health care provider. (D, N, G)

4. 2. Recent research has indicated that most peptic ulcers may be caused by *Helicobacter pylori*, which is a gram-negative organism. This is especially true in developing countries, where housing and sanitation are poor. If this organism is detected through diagnostic tests, then treatment of the ulcer will include the use of antibiotics and bismuth compounds (eg, Pepto-Bismol). (I, C, G)

5. 1. Propantheline bromide is an anticholinergic drug that reduces secretion by the gastric, salivary, bronchial, and sweat glands. Anticholinergic drugs act by blocking ganglionic action in the autonomic nervous system. (P, K, G)

6. 2. Based on the data provided, the most appropriate nursing diagnosis would be Sleep Pattern Disturbance. A client with a duodenal ulcer commonly awakens during the night with pain. There are not enough data to support the other nursing diagnoses. (D, N, G)

7. 1. A realistic goal for this client would be to gain relief from epigastric pain. There is no need for vitamin B_{12} injections because this client has not had

any gastric surgery that would lead to vitamin B_{12} deficiency. Exercise should be modified, not increased, because it can stimulate further production of gastric acid. It is not possible to eliminate all stress from a client's life. Instead, the client should be assisted to develop effective coping and problem-solving strategies as necessary. (E, N, H)

8. 3. Diet therapy for ulcer disease is a controversial issue. There is no scientific evidence that diet therapy promotes healing. Most clients are instructed to follow a diet that they can tolerate. There is no need for the client to ingest only liquid and pureed food. A high-fat diet would not be healthy or necessary. Bedtime snacks should be avoided because they may increase gastric acid secretion. (P, T, H)

9. 4. The client should avoid foods that cause discomfort; however, there is no need to follow a soft, bland diet. Eating six small meals daily is no longer a common treatment for peptic ulcer disease. Milk in large quantities in not recommended because it actually stimulates further production of gastric acid. Caffeinated beverages and alcohol should be avoided because they appear to stimulate gastric acid production. (E, T, H)

10. 1. The client who has had an upper gastrointestinal endoscopy should be monitored for return of the gag reflex. An upper gastrointestinal endoscopy does not affect bowel sounds or breath sounds. (E, T, S)

11. 2. Rest is an essential component of ulcer healing. Nurses can help clients understand the importance of rest and find ways to balance work and family demands to promote permanent healing. Nurses cannot demand these changes; clients must choose them. (P, C, L)

12. 4. It would be most effective for the client to develop a health maintenance plan that incorporates regular periods of physical and mental rest. Strategies should be identified that are appropriate to the types of physical and mental stressors that the client needs to cope with in his home and work environments. There is no need for the client to avoid yard work or golf if these activities are not stressful to him. Scheduling all physical activity to occur only in the morning would not be restful. (P, N, H)

13. 4. Although clients cannot eliminate stress, they can improve their ability to cope with it. Identifying stressors at work, setting professional goals a little lower, and considering a job change may help a client deal with stress, but improving the ability to cope with stress is most effective. (E, N, L)

14. 2. Cigarette smoking should be avoided because of its stimulatory effect on gastric secretions. Nicotine also increases the release of epinephrine, which leads to vasoconstriction. A client with a peptic ulcer should check with the physician before taking any over-the-counter drug, but acetaminophen does not typically cause gastric irritation. The client may chew gum and eat chocolate if desired. (I, T, H)

15. 3. Ranitidine blocks secretion of hydrochloric acid. Clients who take only one daily dose of ranitidine are usually recommended to take it at bedtime. Clients who take the drug twice a day are recommended to take it in the morning and at bedtime. (E, C, H)

16. 3. Aluminum products, such as aluminum hydroxide, form insoluble salts in the body. These precipitate and accumulate in the intestines, possibly causing constipation. (D, N, G)

The Client With Cholecystitis

17. 2. A client with cholecystitis from cholelithiasis may experience nausea, vomiting, abdominal discomfort, and other gastrointestinal symptoms after eating high-fat foods. This is due to decreased fat absorption related to lack of normal bile flow from the gallbladder. Clients are more likely to have a low-grade fever and an elevated white blood cell count due to inflammation. Black stools would be unexpected. (A, T, G)

18. 3. The primary goal of nursing care at this time is to decrease the client's severe abdominal pain. The pain, which is frequently accompanied by nausea and vomiting, is caused by biliary spasm. Opioid analgesics, such as meperidine, are given to relieve the severe pain and spasm of cholecystitis. Relief of pain may decrease nausea and vomiting and thus decrease the client's likelihood of developing further complications, such as fluid volume deficit (D, N, G)

19. 1. Administering pain medication would have the highest priority during the first hour after the client's admission. Completing the admission history, maintaining hydration, and teaching about planned diagnostic tests are aspects of this client's care but are not the highest priority. (I, N, G)

20. 2. Propantheline bromide is an anticholinergic used to decrease biliary contractions and aid in the reduction of pain. (P, C, G)

21. 1. Propantheline bromide is an anticholinergic drug. Common side effects include constipation; flushed, dry skin; and dry mouth, nose, and throat. Urinary retention may also occur, as may orthostatic hypotension. (E, C, S)

22. 2. When bile is not reaching the intestine, the feces do not contain bile pigments. The stool then be-comes gray, clay-like, or putty-like in color. Black stool can be caused by upper gastrointestinal bleeding and by certain medications, such as iron supplements. (A, K, G)

23. 4. A client with an obstructed common bile duct should be monitored for prolonged bleeding time. Such an obstruction prevents bile from entering the intestinal tract, thus decreasing the absorption of fat-soluble vitamins A, D, E, and K. Vitamin K is necessary for prothrombin formation. Prothrombin deficiency causes delayed blood clotting, which results in prolonged bleeding time. (E, T, G)

24. 2. Iodine compounds used as radiographic contrast agents, such as iopanoic acid (Telepaque), should not be administered to the client with iodine and seafood allergies because anaphylaxis may occur. The contrast agent is administered orally 1 to 12 hours before the test. The client is NPO after administration of the contrast agent. Enemas are not required for cholecystography. (P, C, S)

25. 2. If the client understands the reasons for prescribed treatments, he is more likely to cooperate with the plan. Fear of the unknown can increase anxiety. Telling the client to follow his physician's orders or comparing him with others will not decrease anxiety. (I, N, L)

26. 1. Applying a tourniquet obstructs venous blood flow and distends the veins. (I, K, G)

27. 3. The incisions made for upper abdominal surgery are near the diaphragm and make deep breathing painful. Incentive spirometry is essential to prevent the development of atelectasis after surgery. (I, T, G)

28. 4. Incentive spirometry promotes lung expansion and increases respiratory function. When used properly, an incentive spirometer causes sustained maximal inspiration and increased cardiac output. (E, K, G)

29. 2. Oral food and fluids are withheld before surgery when a client receives general anesthesia primarily to help prevent vomiting and possible aspiration of stomach contents. Withholding food and fluids before surgery does not prevent constipation, gas pains, or abdominal distention in the postoperative period, nor does it relieve pressure on the diaphragm. (I, C, G)

30. 2. When using the ventrogluteal site, the nurse injects the medication into the gluteus minimus muscle. (I, C, S)

31. 4. A T tube is used after exploration of the common duct to help prevent bile from spilling into the peritoneal cavity. The tube also helps maintain patency of the common duct and helps ensure bile drainage out of the body until the edema in the common duct subsides sufficiently for bile to drain into the duodenum. A T tube is not used to irrigate the biliary tract, promote wound drainage, or minimize passage of bile into the duodenum. (E, C, S)

32. 3. The T tube usually drains 300 to 500 mL in the first 24 hours after a cholecystectomy and choledochotomy. After 3 to 4 days, the amount decreases to less than 200 mL per 24 hours. (A, K, S)

33. 2. T tube drainage is recorded separately on the output record. Adding it to other output makes it difficult to determine the amount of bile drainage. The client's total intake will be incorrect if drainage is subtracted from it. (I, C, S)

34. 1. Bile is erosive and extremely irritating to the skin. Therefore, it is essential that skin around the T tube be kept clean and dry. T tubes are not routinely irrigated; they are irrigated only on order of the physician. There is no need to maintain the client in a supine position; assist the client into a position of comfort. T tubes are never clamped without a physician's order. If ordered to be clamped, however, this typically is done 1 to 2 hours before and after meals. (P, T, S)

35. 1. Prochlorperazine is administered to control nausea, vomiting, and retching. In doses larger than those needed to control nausea and vomiting, prochlorperazine is used in psychotherapy because of its effects on mood and behavior. (E, C, S)

36. 3. A folded bath blanket or pillow placed over the incision will be most effective in helping the client cough and deep breathe after a cholecystectomy. Taking rapid, shallow breaths would not be effective. Lying on the right side would cause increased incisional pain and decreased lung expansion. The client should be positioned in Fowler's position when possible to promote maximum lung expansion. Withholding pain medication will make the client less likely to cough and deep breathe owing to the discomfort. (I, T, S)

37. 2. Coughing and deep breathing are more effective when pain is minimal. A client in severe pain tends to limit movement and to breathe shallowly to decrease the pain. Enough pain medication should be given to decrease pain without depressing respirations; this allows the client to cough effectively. Deep-breathing exercises should be performed at least every 2 hours. Ambulation to increase ventilation and gas exchange should be encouraged as soon as possible postoperatively (usually on the first postoperative day). Administration of oxygen will not prevent atelectasis or pneumonia. (I, N, G)

38. 3. An early indication of hypokalemia is muscle weakness in the legs. Potassium is essential for proper neuromuscular impulse transmission. When neuromuscular impulse transmission is impaired, as in hypokalemia, leg muscles become weak and flabby. If hypokalemia progresses, respiratory muscles become involved, and the client becomes apneic. Hypokalemia also causes electrocardiogram changes. Diarrhea is common in hyperkalemia. Tingling in the fingers and around the mouth occurs in hypocalcemia. Sticky mucous membranes are common in hypernatremia. (D, K, G)

39. 4. Because of the irregularity of bowel sounds, the nurse should listen for 5 minutes in each quadrant to confirm the absence of bowel sounds. Auscultation is performed before palpation because palpation may affect peristaltic activity. The client should be positioned supine to provide adequate access to the abdomen. (A, C, G)

40. 3. Bile flows almost continuously into the intestine for the first few weeks after gallbladder removal. Limiting the amount of fat in the intestine at any one time ensures that adequate bile will be available to facilitate digestion. There is no need to eliminate high-fiber foods, and doing so would tend to increase (rather than decrease) pressure within the large intestine (not the small intestine). Eating large amounts of meat, cheese, and peanut butter would be undesirable because these foods are often high in fat. Removing the gallbladder does not decrease pancreatic secretions. (P, N, H)

41. 4. Lean meats, such as beef, lamb, veal, and well-trimmed lean ham and pork, are low in fat. Ham salad and egg salad are high in fat from the fat in salad dressing. Rice, pasta, and vegetables are low in fat when not served with butter, cream, or sauces. Fruits are low in fat. The amount of fat allowed in a client's diet after a cholecystectomy will depend on the client's ability to tolerate fat. Typically, the client does not require a special diet. (P, C, H)

42. 3. Laparoscopic cholecystectomy is performed through a small incision at the umbilicus. Hospital stays postoperatively are minimal, and clients are encouraged to ambulate early. Clients typically resume all normal activities within 7 days of surgery. (E, T, H)

The Client With Cancer of the Stomach

43. 3. TPN bypasses the enteral route and provides total nutrition: protein, carbohydrates, fats, vitamins, minerals, and trace elements. Oral and enteral feedings would enter the stomach and could increase any feelings of fullness, nausea, and vomiting that the client has had. Intravenous isotonic saline, which contains only water, sodium, and chloride, provides incomplete nutrition. (P, N, G)

44. 2. A Billroth II procedure bypasses the duodenum and connects the stump of the stomach directly to the jejunum. The pyloric sphincter is sacrificed, along with some of the stomach fundus. The cardiac sphincter remains intact. (I, K, G)

45. 3. The data presented most clearly support a nursing diagnosis of Anticipatory Grieving. The client is grieving about the changes occurring in his life due to the diagnosis of gastric cancer. (D, N, L)

46. 1. Nasogastric suctioning is ordered to remove accumulated gas or fluid (secretions). Excessive fluid can cause pressure on suture lines, resulting in injury, rupture, or dislodgement. Ascitic fluid collects in the peritoneal space, not the stomach. The gastrointestinal tract should remain empty (no food or fluids) until peristalsis returns and suture lines have healed adequately, at which time the nasogastric tube is removed. Enteral feedings in the immediate postoperative period would be inappropriate. Antacids are not used to promote healing of suture lines. (I, C, S)

47. 1. About 12 to 24 hours after subtotal gastrectomy, gastric drainage is normally brown, which indicates digested blood. Drainage during the first 6 to 12 hours contains some bright red blood, but large amounts of blood or excessive bloody drainage should be reported to the physician promptly. Green or cloudy white drainage is not expected during the first 12 to 24 hours after a subtotal gastrectomy. (E, C, G)

48. 3. These symptoms would indicate that gas and secretions are accumulating within the remaining gastric pouch due to impaired peristalsis or edema at the operative site, and may indicate that the drainage system is not working properly. Saline solution is used to irrigate nasogastric tubes. Hypotonic solutions (eg, water) would increase electrolyte loss. After gastric surgery, only the surgeon repositions the nasogastric tube because of the danger of rupturing or dislodging the suture line. In addition, a physician's order is needed to irrigate the nasogastric tube because this may also disrupt the suture line. The amount of suction varies with the type of tube used and is ordered by the physician. (I, N, S)

49. 1. Breathing and coughing cause pain in clients with high abdominal incisions. Splinting of the chest occurs, which decreases coughing and deep-breathing efforts. Shallow breathing leads to hypoventilation and atelectasis. Semi-Fowler's position facilitates drainage of the remaining stomach contents, thus decreasing the risk of regurgitation, which could result in aspiration of gastric contents. The position also allows for greater chest wall expansion and diaphragm contraction. Frequent ambulation helps decrease the likelihood of respiratory complications. The possibility of recurring nausea is not related to respiratory complications. (D, N, G)

50. 1. Pain, fever, and abdominal rigidity are symptoms of inflammation or peritonitis. Diarrhea with fat in the stool is steatorrhea and is not present in peritonitis. Palpitations, pallor, and diaphoresis after eating are vasomotor symptoms of gastric retention. (A, N, G)

51. 2. Because of the client's reduced stomach capacity, frequent small feedings are recommended. Early satiety can result, and large quantities of food are not well tolerated. Each client should progress at his or her own pace, gradually increasing the amount of food eaten at each meal. The goal is three meals daily if possible, but this can take 6 months or longer to achieve. Nausea can be episodic and can result from eating too fast or eating too much at one time. Eating less and more slowly, rather than not eating at all, can be a solution. Bland foods are recommended as starting foods because they are easily digested and less irritating to the healing mucosa. (P, T, H)

52. 1. Weight gain will be slow and gradual because less food can be eaten at one time due to the decreased stomach size. More food and fluid will be tolerated as edema at the suture line decreases and healing progresses. The remaining stomach may stretch over time to accommodate more food. Rapid weight gain may be due to fluid retention (1 pint of fluid equals 1 pound of weight). Food intake will be greater if nausea and vomiting are absent. Water provides hydration but not nutrients. (E, T, G)

53. 2. After gastric resection, ingested food moves rapidly from the remaining stomach into the duodenum or jejunum. The food has not undergone adequate preliminary digestion in the stomach. It is concentrated, distends the intestine, and stimulates significant secretion of insulin by the pancreas. The dumping syndrome results from these factors, which are initiated by the rapid movement of food out of the stomach. (P, K, G)

54. 4. Carbohydrates are restricted, but protein is recommended because it is digested more slowly. Fluids are restricted to reduce the bulk of food, and lying on the left side is encouraged to decrease movement of the food bolus. (I, T, G)

55. 4. An appropriate expected outcome is for the client to maintain nutrition either through oral or total parenteral feedings. Oral and total parenteral nutrition may also be used concurrently. It is not realistic to expect the client to regain weight loss within 4 weeks of surgery. After surgery, it is recommended that the client eat six small meals a day rather than three full meals to decrease symptoms of dumping syndrome. Enteral feedings are not part of the expected outcome for gastric surgery. (E, T, G)

The Client With Pancreatitis

56. 2. The most common symptom of pancreatitis is intense abdominal pain in the mid-epigastric area or the left upper quadrant. The pain may radiate to the back. Nausea and vomiting, hyperglycemia, and elevated white blood count are also common. Hypotension and tachycardia may occur as a result of pancreatic hemorrhage, excessive fluid volume shifting, or enzyme damage. Peripheral edema, cyanosis, and fingernail clubbing are not typical symptoms of pancreatitis. (A, C, G)

57. 1. The primary diagnostic tests for pancreatitis are serum amylase and lipase and urine amylase. Serum amylase is the most common test; the result may be above 200 Somogyi units/dL. (A, K, G)

58. 1. Alcoholism is the major cause of acute pancreatitis in the United States. Because some clients are reluctant to discuss their alcohol use, staff may inquire about it in several ways. Alcohol intake does not interfere with the pertinent tests used to diagnose pancreatitis. Recent ingestion of large amounts of alcohol, however, may cause an increased serum amylase level, and large amounts of ethyl and methyl alcohol may produce elevated urinary amylase levels. All hospitalized clients are asked about alcohol and drug use on admission but are not repeatedly asked about it during hospitalization. Physicians do seek all the facts, but this can be done while considering the client's religious beliefs. Religious beliefs are pertinent to total client care. (I, T, L)

59. 1. Meperidine hydrochloride, a strong narcotic analgesic, effectively reduces the pain of acute pancreatitis. Morphine sulfate and codeine sulfate are contraindicated in pancreatitis because they may cause spasm and exacerbate pain. Cimetidine, a histamine receptor antagonist, decreases gastric acidity. (P, T, G)

60. 2. Life-threatening shock is a potential complication of pancreatitis. Kinin peptides activated by the trapped trypsin cause vasodilation and increased capillary permeability. These effects exacerbate shock and are not easily reversed with pharmacologic agents such as vasopressors. (A, K, G)

61. 1. Pancreatitis interferes with β-cell functioning, and clients must be monitored carefully for hyperglycemia. (E, C, G)

62. 4. Hypocalcemia is a major potential complication of pancreatitis. Muscle twitching and irritability are primary symptoms of hypocalcemia. Calcium replacement must begin as soon as hypocalcemia is validated. Hypomagnesemia may result from vomiting in clients with pancreatitis, especially if they are malnourished. Serum glucose is elevated. Hypokalemia may occur with loss of gastric juice through vomiting or nasogastric suction. (A, C, G)

63. 1. There is little definitive treatment for pancreatitis. It is important to suppress enzymes to reduce

pancreatic stimulation. This is done by keeping the client NPO to rest the gastrointestinal tract. Preventing infection and ensuring adequate nutrition and fluid and electrolyte balance are related issues but are not the primary focus of treatment. (P, N, G)

64. 2. Nasogastric suction is frequently used in the treatment of pancreatitis to decrease pancreatic secretion and gastric distention. Food and fluids are withheld during the acute phase of pancreatitis to rest the pancreas. Intravenous fluids are administered to provide hydration. Placing the client in reverse Trendelenburg's position and maintaining enteric isolation are not appropriate for treating pancreatitis. (P, T, S)

65. 4. Having the client look toward the ceiling as the nurse inserts a nasogastric tube facilitates tube insertion. When the tube reaches the nasopharynx, the client should be instructed to bring the head forward a bit by flexing the neck. This technique closes the trachea and opens the esophagus to receive the tube. Correct techniques include having the client assume an upright position, lubricating the tube with a water-soluble lubricant, and having the client swallow as the tube is passed into the stomach. (I, T, S)

66. 1. The best way to determine whether a nasogastric tube is in the stomach is to apply suction to the tube with a syringe and observe for the return of stomach contents. Another satisfactory method is to instill air into the tube with a syringe while auscultating over the epigastric area. Hearing the air enter the stomach helps ensure proper placement, but the method is not foolproof. If the tube is not in the stomach and solution is introduced, the solution could enter respiratory passages and harm the client. Observing for air bubbles when the free end of the tube is placed under water is an unacceptable, unsafe method of determining tube placement. (I, N, S)

67. 3. The nurse records the total amount of solution used to irrigate a gastric tube as intake and the total amount of return in the drainage bottle as output. (I, T, S)

68. 3. Applying a water-soluble lubricant to the nares helps alleviate sore nares when a nasogastric tube is in place. Measures such as irrigating and repositioning the tube and changing the client's position will not relieve irritation from the tube. (I, T, S)

69. 4. The primary purpose of fluid replacement therapy for a client receiving gastric suction is to maintain fluid and electrolyte balance. Gastric suctioning interrupts the normal intake of fluids; thus, intravenous replacement therapy is indicated. (I, T, G)

70. 3. When a client with a nasogastric tube exhibits abdominal distention, the nurse should first check the suction machine. If the equipment is functioning properly, then the nurse should take other steps, such as checking tube patency. (I, N, S)

71. 3. Antispasmodic drugs such as proprantheline bromide may be administered along with narcotics to deal with the intense pain associated with pancreatitis. (I, C, G)

72. 4. Altered Nutrition: Less Than Body Requirements is likely to be a priority nursing diagnosis because the abdominal pain, nausea, and vomiting typical of pancreatitis can affect the client's food and fluid intake. Treatment of pancreatitis also frequently involves stopping all oral intake until the inflammation is resolved. Clients with pancreatitis are at risk for developing malnutrition. Intravenous therapy is used for fluid replacement, and total parenteral nutrition may be ordered to prevent malnourishment. (D, N, G)

73. 2. A low-fat, bland diet prevents stimulation of the pancreas while providing adequate nutrition. Although calcium is important, the low fat content is more significant. Dietary protein and fiber are not directly related to pancreatitis. The hyperglycemia of acute pancreatitis is usually transient and does not require long-term dietary modification. (I, C, H)

74. 2. Pancreatic enzymes are prescribed to facilitate the digestion of protein and fats and should be taken in conjunction with every meal and snack. Specified hours for administration are ineffective because the enzymes must be taken in conjunction with food ingestion. (I, C, H)

75. 3. If the dosage and administration of pancreatic enzymes are adequate, the client's stool will be relatively normal. Any increase in odor or fat content would indicate the need for dosage adjustment. Stable body weight would be another indirect indicator. (E, C, H)

The Client With Hiatal Hernia

76. 1. A laxative is administered after an upper gastrointestinal series. This examination involves the administration of barium, which must be eliminated from the body because it may harden and cause an obstruction. (P, C, S)

77. 1. Hiatal hernia produces symptoms of esophageal reflux as the sphincter slides up into the negative-pressure environment of the thorax. The symptoms typically occur when the client is in a recumbent position. Neither emotions nor normal activity influence the incidence of reflux. (A, C, G)

78. 1. Heartburn, the most common symptom of a sliding hiatal hernia, results from reflux of gastric secretions into the esophagus. Regurgitation of gastric contents and dysphagia are other common symptoms. (A, C, G)

79. 2. Any factor that increases intraabdominal pressure can contribute to the development of hiatal hernia. Such factors include obesity, abdominal straining, and pregnancy. Hiatal hernia is also associated with aging and occurs in both males and females. (A, T, H)

80. 3. Self-responsibility is the key to individual health maintenance. Using examples of situations in which the client has demonstrated self-responsibility can be reinforcing and supporting. Meeting other people who are managing their care and involving family members can be helpful, but individual motivation is more important. Reassurance can be helpful but is less important than individualization of care. The client has ultimate responsibility for her personal health habits. (I, T, H)

81. 3. The magnesium salts in magnesium hydroxide are related to those found in laxatives and may cause diarrhea. Aluminum salt products can cause constipation. Many clients find that a combination product is required to maintain normal bowel elimination. (P, K, G)

82. 2. Smoking and alcohol use both reduce esophageal sphincter tone and can result in reflux and thus should be avoided or minimized by clients with hiatal hernia. The other factors may increase the client's general health and well-being but are not directly associated with hiatal hernia. (P, T, H)

83. 4. Sleeping with the head of the bed elevated encourages movement of food through the esophagus by gravity. By fostering esophageal acid clearance, gravity helps keep the acidic pepsin and alkaline biliary secretions from contacting the esophagus. Neither elevating the foot of the bed nor sleeping flat without a pillow under the head enhances this clearance. Sleeping on the right side minimizes the problem for some clients. (E, T, G)

84. 2. Bending, especially after eating, can cause gastroesophageal reflux; lifting heavy objects increases intraabdominal pressure. Knowing the client's lifting techniques enables the nurse to assess the client's knowledge of factors contributing to hiatal hernia and of methods that prevent complications. The other factors are not directly related to hiatal hernia. (A, N, H)

85. 1. Fats are associated with decreased esophageal sphincter tone, which increases reflux. Obesity contributes to the development of hiatal hernia, and a low-fat diet might also aid in weight loss. Fat is the most concentrated source of calories. The other options do not affect reflux. (E, T, H)

86. 1. Esophageal reflux worsens when the stomach is overdistended with food. Thus, an important measure is to eat small, frequent meals. Food intake in the evening should be strictly limited to reduce the incidence of nighttime reflux. (I, T, H)

87. 1. A client with a hiatal hernia should avoid the recumbent position immediately after meals to minimize gastric reflux. Wearing tight, constrictive clothing, such as a girdle, can increase intraabdominal pressure and thus lead to reflux of gastric juices. Bedtime snacks, as well as high-fat foods and carbonated beverages, should be avoided. Excessive vigorous exercise also should be avoided, especially after meals, but there is no reason why the client must give up swimming. (E, N, H)

88. 1. Metoclopramide hydrochloride increases sphincter tone and facilitates gastric emptying; both actions reduce the incidence of reflux. Antacids or histamine receptor antagonists may also be prescribed to help control reflux and esophagitis. (P, K, G)

89. 4. Metoclopramide hydrochloride can cause sedation. Alcohol and other central nervous system depressants add to this sedation. A client taking this drug should be cautioned to avoid driving or other hazardous activities for a few hours after taking the drug. (I, C, G)

90. 3. Cimetidine is a histamine receptor antagonist that decreases the quantity of gastric secretions. It may be used in hiatal hernia therapy to prevent or treat the esophagitis and heartburn associated with reflux. (P, K, G)

91. 2. Most clients can be treated successfully with a combination of diet restrictions, medications, weight control, and lifestyle modifications. Surgery to correct hiatal hernia is extensive and commonly produces complications. It is performed only when medical therapy fails to control the symptoms. (I, C, G)

NURSING CARE OF ADULTS WITH MEDICAL AND SURGICAL HEALTH PROBLEMS

TEST 4: The Client With Upper Gastrointestinal Tract Health Problems

Directions: Use this answer grid to determine areas of strength or need for further study.

NURSING PROCESS	COGNITIVE LEVEL	CLIENT NEEDS
A = Assessment	K = Knowledge	S = Safe, effective care environment
D = Analysis, nursing diagnosis	C = Comprehension	G = Physiologic integrity
P = Planning	T = Application	L = Psychosocial integrity
I = Implementation	N = Analysis	H = Health promotion and maintenance
E = Evaluation		

Question #	Answer #	Nursing Process A	D	P	I	E	Cognitive Level K	C	T	N	Client Needs S	G	L	H
1	1	A						C				G		
2	4		D							N		G		
3	2		D							N		G		
4	2				I			C				G		
5	1			P			K					G		
6	2		D							N		G		
7	1					E				N				H
8	3			P					T					H
9	4					E			T					H
10	1					E			T		S			
11	2			P				C					L	
12	4			P						N				H
13	4					E				N			L	
14	2				I				T					H
15	3					E		C						H
16	3		D							N		G		
17	2	A							T			G		
18	3		D							N		G		
19	1				I					N		G		
20	2			P				C				G		
21	1					E		C			S			
22	2	A					K					G		
23	4					E			T			G		
24	2			P				C			S			
25	2				I					N			L	

NURSING PROCESS

A = Assessment
D = Analysis, nursing diagnosis
P = Planning
I = Implementation
E = Evaluation

COGNITIVE LEVEL

K = Knowledge
C = Comprehension
T = Application
N = Analysis

CLIENT NEEDS

S = Safe, effective care environment
G = Physiologic integrity
L = Psychosocial integrity
H = Health promotion and maintenance

Question #	Answer #	Nursing Process					Cognitive Level				Client Needs			
		A	D	P	I	E	K	C	T	N	S	G	L	H
26	1				I		K					G		
27	3				I				T			G		
28	4					E	K					G		
29	2				I			C				G		
30	2				I			C			S			
31	4					E		C			S			
32	3	A					K				S			
33	2				I			C			S			
34	1			P					T		S			
35	1					E		C			S			
36	3				I				T		S			
37	2				I					N		G		
38	3		D				K					G		
39	4	A						C				G		
40	3			P						N				H
41	4			P				C						H
42	3					E			T					H
43	3			P						N		G		
44	2				I		K					G		
45	3		D							N			L	
46	1				I			C			S			
47	1					E		C				G		
48	3				I					N	S			
49	1		D							N		G		
50	1	A								N		G		
51	2			P					T					H
52	1					E			T			G		
53	2			P			K					G		
54	4				I				T			G		
55	4					E			T			G		

ANSWER GRID: 2

NURSING PROCESS

A = Assessment
D = Analysis, nursing diagnosis
P = Planning
I = Implementation
E = Evaluation

COGNITIVE LEVEL

K = Knowledge
C = Comprehension
T = Application
N = Analysis

CLIENT NEEDS

S = Safe, effective care environment
G = Physiologic integrity
L = Psychosocial integrity
H = Health promotion and maintenance

Question #	Answer #	A	D	P	I	E	K	C	T	N	S	G	L	H
56	2	A						C				G		
57	1	A					K					G		
58	1				I				T				L	
59	1			P					T			G		
60	2	A					K					G		
61	1					E		C				G		
62	4	A						C				G		
63	1			P						N		G		
64	2			P					T		S			
65	4				I				T		S			
66	1				I					N	S			
67	3				I				T		S			
68	3				I				T		S			
69	4				I				T			G		
70	3				I					N	S			
71	3				I			C				G		
72	4		D							N		G		
73	2				I			C						H
74	2				I			C						H
75	3					E		C						H
76	1			P				C			S			
77	1	A						C				G		
78	1	A						C				G		
79	2	A							T					H
80	3				I				T					H
81	3			P			K					G		
82	2			P					T					H
83	4					E			T			G		
84	2	A								N				H
85	1					E			T					H

NURSING PROCESS

A = Assessment
D = Analysis, nursing diagnosis
P = Planning
I = Implementation
E = Evaluation

COGNITIVE LEVEL

K = Knowledge
C = Comprehension
T = Application
N = Analysis

CLIENT NEEDS

S = Safe, effective care environment
G = Physiologic integrity
L = Psychosocial integrity
H = Health promotion and maintenance

Question #	Answer #	Nursing Process					Cognitive Level				Client Needs			
		A	D	P	I	E	K	C	T	N	S	G	L	H
86	1				I				T					H
87	1					E				N				H
88	1			P			K					G		
89	4				I			C				G		
90	3			P			K					G		
91	2				I			C				G		
Number Correct														
Number Possible	91	14	9	20	29	19	13	28	27	23	19	47	5	20
Percentage Correct														

Score Calculation: To determine your **Percentage Correct,** divide the **Number Correct** by the **Number Possible.**

ANSWER GRID: 4

The Client With Lower Gastrointestinal Tract Health Problems

- The Client With Cancer of the Colon
- The Client With Hepatitis A
- The Client With Hepatitis B
- The Client With Hemorrhoids
- The Client With Inflammatory Bowel Disease
- The Client With an Intestinal Obstruction
- The Client With Cirrhosis
- The Client With an Ileostomy
- The Client on Total Parenteral Nutrition
- The Client With Diverticular Disease
- Correct Answers and Rationale

Select the one best answer, and indicate your choice by filling in the circle in front of the option.

The Client With Cancer of the Colon

A client has been experiencing cramping lower abdominal pain and has noticed a gradual change in his bowel elimination pattern.

1. As part of the preparation for a barium enema, the client is instructed to take 60 mL of castor oil orally. Castor oil facilitates cleansing of the bowel primarily by
   - ○ 1. softening the feces.
   - ○ 2. lubricating the feces.
   - ○ 3. increasing the volume of intestinal contents.
   - ○ 4. irritating the nerve endings in the intestinal mucosa.
2. As part of the client's outpatient teaching plan, the nurse would instruct him to take which of the medications below after the barium enema?
   - ○ 1. A laxative.
   - ○ 2. An emetic.
   - ○ 3. An antacid.
   - ○ 4. A digestant.

3. The client is scheduled for an abdominoperineal resection with permanent colostomy. Which of the following measures would most likely be included in the plan for the client's preoperative preparation?
   - ○ 1. Keep the client NPO for 2 days before surgery.
   - ○ 2. Administer kanamycin (Kantrex) the night before surgery.
   - ○ 3. Inform the client that chest tubes will be in place after surgery.
   - ○ 4. Advise the client to limit activity.
4. The client asks, "Where will my colostomy be placed?" What would be the nurse's best response?
   - ○ 1. "The surgeon will decide that during surgery."
   - ○ 2. "It doesn't matter; you'll have to wear an ostomy pouch anyway."
   - ○ 3. "In the midline of the abdomen, near your umbilicus."
   - ○ 4. "A permanent colostomy is usually located on the left side of the abdomen."
5. The client had a nasogastric tube inserted at the time of surgery. This tube will most likely be removed when the client demonstrates
   - ○ 1. absence of nausea and vomiting.

○ 2. passage of mucus from the rectum.

○ 3. passage of flatus and feces from the colostomy.

○ 4. absence of stomach drainage for about 24 hours.

6. Which of the following nursing actions would be most appropriate immediately after nasogastric tube removal?

○ 1. Provide the client with mouth care.

○ 2. Auscultate for bowel sounds.

○ 3. Palpate for abdominal distention.

○ 4. Give the client some orange sherbet.

7. Which of the following would be an appropriate expected outcome for the client who has had an abdominoperineal resection with a colostomy? The client will

○ 1. demonstrate an understanding of the need to maintain a high-fiber diet.

○ 2. verbalize that he feels free to discuss concerns about his sexual functioning.

○ 3. indicate that he understands the need to avoid physical exertion.

○ 4. limit fluid intake to 1000 mL/day.

8. The client indicates that he is ready to learn about his colostomy. Which of the following nursing interventions would most likely be effective in preparing the client to look at the colostomy?

○ 1. Telling the client how normal body functions will continue.

○ 2. Encouraging the client to ask questions about the colostomy.

○ 3. Asking a member of the local ostomy club to visit the client.

○ 4. Using illustrative material during teaching sessions with the client.

9. The nurse irrigates the client's colostomy. If the client complains of abdominal cramping after receiving about 150 mL of solution during the colostomy irrigation, the nurse should temporarily

○ 1. stop the flow of solution.

○ 2. have the client sit up in bed.

○ 3. remove the irrigating cone or tube.

○ 4. insert the cone or tube further into the colon.

10. The nurse evaluates the client's stoma during the initial postoperative period. Which of the following signs should be reported immediately to the physician? The stoma

○ 1. is slightly edematous.

○ 2. is dark red to purple.

○ 3. oozes a small amount of blood.

○ 4. does not expel stool.

11. The nurse changes the client's colostomy bag and dressing. Which of the following would be an indication that the client is ready to participate in his care? The client

○ 1. asks what time the doctor will visit that day.

○ 2. asks about the supplies used during the dressing change.

○ 3. talks about something he read in the morning newspaper.

○ 4. complains about the way the night nurse changed the dressing.

12. Which of the following skin preparations would be best to apply around the client's colostomy?

○ 1. Karaya.

○ 2. Petrolatum.

○ 3. Cornstarch.

○ 4. Antiseptic cream.

13. Which of the following measures would most effectively promote wound healing after the client's perineal drains have been removed?

○ 1. Taking sitz baths.

○ 2. Taking daily showers.

○ 3. Applying warm, moist dressings to the area.

○ 4. Applying a protected heating pad to the area.

14. When planning diet teaching for the client with a colostomy, the nurse would develop a plan that emphasizes that

○ 1. foods containing roughage should be eliminated from the diet.

○ 2. liquids are best limited to prevent diarrhea.

○ 3. clients with colostomies must experiment to determine the balance of food that is best for them.

○ 4. a high-fiber diet will produce a formed stool that can be passed with more regularity through a colostomy.

15. Which of the following statements indicates that the client understands the home care of his colostomy?

○ 1. "I can attach my colostomy pouch directly to my skin as long as it is not irritated."

○ 2. "I can anticipate some pain around my stoma when I clean it."

○ 3. "I can expect to see some blood in my stool on occasion."

○ 4. "I should be able to establish a regular pattern of elimination with my colostomy."

The Client With Hepatitis A

A 22-year-old college student is admitted to the hospital acutely ill with hepatitis A (formerly infectious hepatitis).

16. The nurse would expect the client to exhibit which of the following symptoms during the acute phase of hepatitis A?

○ 1. Diarrhea.

○ 2. Yellowed sclera.

○ 3. Shortness of breath.

○ 4. Light, frothy urine.

17. The nurse plans care for the client with hepatitis A with the understanding that the causative virus will be excreted from the client's body primarily through the
    ○ 1. skin.
    ○ 2. feces.
    ○ 3. urine.
    ○ 4. mucus.

18. The nurse is planning a staff development in-service for health care staff on how to care for clients with hepatitis A. Which of the following precautions would the nurse indicate as *not* essential to the care of clients with hepatitis A?
    ○ 1. Gowning if contact with infective material is likely.
    ○ 2. Tagging soiled linens.
    ○ 3. Assigning the client to a private room.
    ○ 4. Wearing gloves when giving direct care.

19. When developing a plan of care for the client, the nurse should incorporate nursing orders that reflect that the primary treatment for the client will be concerned with ensuring that the client receives
    ○ 1. adequate bed rest.
    ○ 2. a generous fluid intake.
    ○ 3. regular antibiotic therapy.
    ○ 4. daily intravenous electrolyte therapy.

20. Which of the following test results would the nurse use to assess the client's liver function?
    ○ 1. Glucose tolerance.
    ○ 2. Creatinine clearance.
    ○ 3. Serum transaminase.
    ○ 4. Serum electrolytes.

21. Which of the following diets would most likely be prescribed for a client with hepatitis A?
    ○ 1. High-fat, low-protein diet.
    ○ 2. High-protein, low-fat diet.
    ○ 3. High-carbohydrate, high-calorie diet.
    ○ 4. Low-sodium, low-fat diet.

22. The nurse develops a teaching plan for the client about how to prevent the transmission of hepatitis A. The nurse should instruct the client that when he goes home he should
    ○ 1. spray the yard to eliminate infected insects.
    ○ 2. set traps to catch infected rodents.
    ○ 3. tell family members to wash their hands frequently.
    ○ 4. disinfect all clothing and eating utensils with bleach.

23. The nurse assesses that the client is experiencing fatigue, weakness, and a general feeling of malaise. He tires rapidly during his morning care. Based on this data, which of the following would be an appropriate nursing diagnosis?
    ○ 1. Impaired Physical Mobility related to malaise.
    ○ 2. Self-Care Deficit related to fatigue.

○ 3. Ineffective Individual Coping related to long-term illness.
○ 4. Activity Intolerance related to fatigue.

24. The client expresses concern because he fears that his friends may also acquire hepatitis. Which of the following is most commonly used for prophylactic treatment of people exposed to hepatitis A?
    ○ 1. Penicillin.
    ○ 2. Sulfadiazine (Microsulfon).
    ○ 3. Immune serum globulin.
    ○ 4. Interferon.

25. When preparing the client for extended convalescence, the nurse teaches him about problems that may occur. The nurse knows that the client has understood the teaching when he says that he is most likely to have difficulty
    ○ 1. controlling pain.
    ○ 2. maintaining a regular bowel elimination pattern.
    ○ 3. preventing respiratory complications.
    ○ 4. maintaining a positive, optimistic outlook.

26. The client who has had hepatitis A should be instructed never to
    ○ 1. drink alcohol.
    ○ 2. donate blood.
    ○ 3. smoke.
    ○ 4. eat fatty foods.

The Client With Hepatitis B

The client has been admitted to the hospital with a diagnosis of hepatitis B.

27. Which of the following situations would most likely expose the nurse to the hepatitis B virus?
    ○ 1. Coming in contact with client's feces.
    ○ 2. Spraying the client's blood into the nurse's eyes.
    ○ 3. Touching the client's arm with ungloved hands while taking a blood pressure.
    ○ 4. Disposing of syringes and needles without recapping.

28. The community health nurse develops a health education program about preventing the transmission of hepatitis B. The nurse evaluates that the teaching has been effective when the community residents identify which of the following activities to be high risk for acquiring hepatitis B?
    ○ 1. Frequent use of marijuana.
    ○ 2. Ingestion of large amounts of acetaminophen (Tylenol).
    ○ 3. Intravenous drug use.
    ○ 4. Ingestion of contaminated seafood.

29. Which of the following goals would be appropriate for the client with hepatitis B? The client will

○ 1. adhere to measures to prevent the spread of infection to others.

○ 2. adhere to a low sodium, low protein diet.

○ 3. verbalize the importance of using sedatives to provide adequate rest.

○ 4. avoid social activities with friends after discharge from the hospital.

30. The client tells the nurse, "I feel so isolated from my friends and family. Nobody wants to be around me." What would be the most appropriate nursing diagnosis for this client?

○ 1. Anxiety related to feelings of isolation.

○ 2. Social Isolation related to significant other's fear of contracting disease.

○ 3. Powerlessness related to lack of social support.

○ 4. Self-Esteem Disturbance related to feelings of rejection.

31. What would be the nurse's best response to the client's expressed feelings of isolation?

○ 1. "Don't worry. It's normal to feel this way."

○ 2. "Your friends are probably afraid of contracting hepatitis from you."

○ 3. "I'm sure you're imagining that!"

○ 4. "Tell me more about your feelings of isolation."

The Client With Hemorrhoids

A 36-year-old client has been diagnosed with hemorrhoids.

32. Which of the following factors in the client's nursing history most likely would be a primary cause of her hemorrhoids?

○ 1. Her age.

○ 2. Three pregnancies with vaginal deliveries.

○ 3. Her job as a schoolteacher.

○ 4. Varicosities in her legs.

33. Which of the following interventions would be most appropriate for the nurse to recommend to the client to decrease her hemorrhoid discomfort?

○ 1. Decrease fiber in the diet.

○ 2. Take laxatives to promote bowel movements.

○ 3. Use warm sitz baths.

○ 4. Decrease physical activity.

34. The client has an elective hemorrhoidectomy. Immediately after a hemorrhoidectomy, the priority goal of nursing care for the client should be to

○ 1. prevent venous stasis.

○ 2. promote ambulation.

○ 3. control pain.

○ 4. prevent infection.

35. Which position would be ideal for the client in the early postoperative period?

○ 1. High-Fowler's.

○ 2. Supine.

○ 3. Side-lying.

○ 4. Trendelenburg's.

36. The nurse instructs the client not to use sitz baths until at least 12 hours postoperatively to avoid inducing

○ 1. hemorrhage.

○ 2. rectal spasm.

○ 3. urine retention.

○ 4. constipation.

37. The nurse teaches the client the proper procedure for using sitz baths. The nurse would know that the client has understood the teaching when she says that it is most important to take a sitz bath

○ 1. first thing each morning.

○ 2. as needed for discomfort.

○ 3. after a bowel movement.

○ 4. at bedtime.

38. The nurse has been teaching the client ways to avoid recurrence of hemorrhoids, including the importance of a high-fiber diet. The client's selection of which of the following breakfast menus would indicate that she understands the instructions?

○ 1. Danish pastry, prune juice, coffee, and milk.

○ 2. Oatmeal, milk, grapefruit wedges, and bran muffin.

○ 3. Corn flakes, milk, white toast, and orange juice.

○ 4. Scrambled eggs, bacon, English muffin, and apple juice.

The Client With Inflammatory Bowel Disease

A client who has suffered from ulcerative colitis for the past 5 years is admitted to the hospital with an exacerbation of her disease.

39. The nurse assesses the client's bowel elimination pattern. Which of the following signs are most typical of ulcerative colitis?

○ 1. Constipation.

○ 2. Bloody, diarrheal stools.

○ 3. Steatorrhea.

○ 4. Alternating periods of constipation and diarrhea.

40. Which of the following factors was most likely of greatest significance in causing an exacerbation of the client's ulcerative colitis?

○ 1. She reports that her work is very demanding and she's worried about "measuring up."

○ 2. She has recently begun following a modified vegetarian diet.

○ 3. She has been working out with weights for the past 3 months.

○ 4. She has begun attending a holistic health group.

41. Which goal for the client's care should take priority during the first days of her hospitalization?
○ 1. Promoting self-care and independence.
○ 2. Stopping the diarrhea.
○ 3. Maintaining adequate nutrition.
○ 4. Promoting rest and comfort.

42. The client is following orders for bed rest with bathroom privileges. What would be the primary rationale for her activity restriction?
○ 1. To conserve energy.
○ 2. To reduce intestinal peristalsis.
○ 3. To promote rest and comfort.
○ 4. To prevent injury.

43. The client's symptoms have been present for more than a week. The nurse recognizes that she should be assessed carefully for signs of
○ 1. congestive heart failure.
○ 2. deep vein thrombosis.
○ 3. hypokalemia.
○ 4. hypocalcemia.

44. The client says to the nurse, "I can't take this anymore! I'm constantly in pain, and I can't leave my room because I need to stay by the toilet. I don't know how to deal with this." Based on these comments, an appropriate nursing diagnosis for this client would be
○ 1. Impaired Physical Mobility related to fatigue.
○ 2. Altered Thought Processes related to pain.
○ 3. Social Isolation related to chronic fatigue.
○ 4. Ineffective Individual Coping related to chronic abdominal pain.

45. The nurse should include which of the following measures in this client's care?
○ 1. Encouraging the use of stool softeners.
○ 2. Suggesting sitz baths p.r.n.
○ 3. Keeping the client's bathroom available for use.
○ 4. Wearing a gown to provide direct care.

46. The client's diarrhea persists. She is thin and has lost 12 pounds since the exacerbation of her ulcerative colitis. The nurse should anticipate that the physician will order which of the following treatment approaches to help the client meet her nutritional needs?
○ 1. Initiating continuous enteral feedings.
○ 2. Encouraging a high-calorie, high-protein diet.
○ 3. Implementing total parenteral nutrition (TPN).
○ 4. Providing six small meals a day.

47. The physician prescribes sulfasalazine for the client to continue taking at home. What instructions should the nurse give the client about taking this medication?
○ 1. Avoid taking it with food.
○ 2. Take the total dose at bedtime.
○ 3. Take it with a full glass (240 mL) of water.
○ 4. Stop taking it if urine turns orange-yellow.

48. The client expresses serious concerns about his career as an attorney because of the effects of stress on ulcerative colitis. Which course of action would it be best for the nurse to suggest?
○ 1. Review his current coping mechanisms and develop alternatives, if needed.
○ 2. Consider a less stressful career in which he would still use his education and experience.
○ 3. Ask his colleagues to help decrease his stress by giving him the easier cases.
○ 4. Prepare family members for the fact that he will have to work part-time.

49. Which of the following diets would be most appropriate for the client with ulcerative colitis to follow?
○ 1. High-calorie, low-protein diet.
○ 2. High-protein, low-residue diet.
○ 3. Low-fat, high-fiber diet.
○ 4. Low-sodium, high-carbohydrate diet.

50. Which of the following statements indicates the client understands the lifestyle modifications he needs to make because of his ulcerative colitis?
○ 1. "I may have coffee with my meals."
○ 2. "I am allowed to have alcohol as long as I only drink wine."
○ 3. "I will have to stop smoking."
○ 4. "I can eat popcorn for an evening snack."

51. Which of the following would be an appropriate expected outcome of nursing care for the client with ulcerative colitis? The client
○ 1. maintains an ideal body weight.
○ 2. verbalizes the importance of restricting fluids.
○ 3. experiences decreased frequency of constipation.
○ 4. accepts that an ileostomy will be necessary.

The Client With an Intestinal Obstruction

A client is admitted to the hospital complaining of nausea, vomiting, and abdominal pain. Bowel obstruction is suspected.

52. During the initial assessment, the nurse hears high-pitched tinkling bowel sounds on auscultation and dull sounds on percussion. The dull sounds are caused by
○ 1. hyperactive peristalsis.
○ 2. excessive gas trapped in the intestine.
○ 3. the presence of a mass or tumor in the bowel.
○ 4. fluid trapped in the intestine.

53. Of the following symptoms of bowel obstruction, which is related primarily to small bowel obstruction rather than to large bowel obstruction?
○ 1. Profuse vomiting.

○ 2. Cramping abdominal pain.

○ 3. Abdominal distention.

○ 4. High-pitched bowel sounds above the obstruction.

54. The physician orders intestinal decompression for the client using a Cantor tube. The primary purpose of a nasoenteric tube such as a Cantor tube is to

○ 1. remove fluid and gas from the intestine.

○ 2. prevent fluid accumulation in the stomach.

○ 3. break up the obstruction.

○ 4. provide an alternative route for drug administration.

55. As soon as the Cantor tube has been inserted, the nurse should instruct the client to

○ 1. lie still on her back.

○ 2. lie on her right side.

○ 3. lie on her left side.

○ 4. get up and sit in a chair.

56. Which of the following statements about nasoenteric tubes, such as the Cantor tube, are correct? The tube

○ 1. cannot be attached to suction.

○ 2. contains a soft rubber bag filled with mercury.

○ 3. is taped securely to the client's cheek after insertion.

○ 4. can have its placement determined only by auscultation.

57. Which of the following measures would most likely be included in the client's care as soon as the Cantor tube has passed into the duodenum?

○ 1. Maintain bed rest with bathroom privileges.

○ 2. Advance the tube 2 to 4 inches at specified times.

○ 3. Provide frequent mouth care.

○ 4. Provide ice chips for the client to suck.

58. Which of the following nursing measures would be inappropriate when caring for a client with a Cantor tube?

○ 1. Injecting 10 mL of air into the tube to facilitate drainage.

○ 2. Applying a water-soluble lubricant to the client's nares.

○ 3. Coiling extra tubing on the client's bed.

○ 4. Irrigating the tube with 50 mL of normal saline solution.

59. Which of the following nursing diagnoses most likely would be appropriate for a client with an intestinal obstruction?

○ 1. Impaired Swallowing related to NPO status.

○ 2. Urinary Retention related to fluid volume depletion.

○ 3. Fluid Volume Deficit related to nausea and vomiting.

○ 4. Chronic Pain related to abdominal distention.

60. The client continues to have pain even though the Cantor tube is patent and draining. The physician wants to delay administering pain medication. When the client asks why, what would be the nurse's best response?

○ 1. "Narcotics trigger the vomiting center and would cause more fluid loss."

○ 2. "Narcotics may mask symptoms of increased obstruction or complications."

○ 3. "There is some risk of becoming addicted to narcotics, so it is best to take them only when necessary."

○ 4. "Narcotics will interfere with the anesthetic if surgery is needed."

61. Intestinal decompression has been successful, but the client needs surgery to relieve the obstruction. The day before surgery, the nurse receives the following set of orders for the client. Which order should the nurse question before performing?

○ 1. Tap-water enemas until clear.

○ 2. Out of bed as tolerated.

○ 3. Neomycin sulfate 1 g every 4 hours.

○ 4. Betadine scrub to abdomen b.i.d.

62. Before surgery, the nurse monitors the client's urine output and finds that the total output for the past 2 hours is 35 mL. This would indicate

○ 1. successful intestinal intubation.

○ 2. inadequate pain relief.

○ 3. extension of the obstruction.

○ 4. inadequate fluid replacement.

63. The client underwent a bowel resection and was in the postanesthesia recovery unit for 1 hour. She returns from the recovery room with an intravenous line, a nasogastric tube, and a Foley catheter in place. She complains of pain and asks for medication. What action should the nurse take first?

○ 1. Administer the ordered narcotic.

○ 2. Establish the location and severity of the pain.

○ 3. Determine if she was medicated for pain in the postanesthesia recovery unit.

○ 4. Reposition her and give her a back rub.

64. During the evening shift on the day of the client's surgery, the nasogastric tube drains 500 mL of green-brown fluid. The nurse should

○ 1. call the physician immediately.

○ 2. increase the intravenous infusion rate.

○ 3. record the amount of drainage on the client's chart.

○ 4. irrigate the tube with normal saline solution.

The Client With Cirrhosis

A male client with a history of cirrhosis related to chronic alcoholism has been experiencing a slow but steady decline in his general health. Recent bloodwork reveals hypokalemia, anemia, elevated liver function studies, prolonged prothrombin time, and elevated circulating estrogen level.

65. Because of the elevated circulating estrogen level, the nurse would expect the client to exhibit which of the following symptoms?
○ 1. Gynecomastia.
○ 2. Increased chest and body hair.
○ 3. Testicular hypertrophy.
○ 4. Increased libido.

66. The client complains that his skin always feels itchy and he "scratches himself raw" while he sleeps. The nurse should recognize that the itching is the result of which abnormality associated with cirrhosis?
○ 1. Folic acid deficiency.
○ 2. Prolonged prothrombin time.
○ 3. Increased bilirubin levels.
○ 4. Hypokalemia.

67. During this stage of his illness, the client should be encouraged to follow which diet?
○ 1. High-calorie, restricted protein, low-sodium diet.
○ 2. Bland, low-protein, low-sodium diet.
○ 3. Well-balanced normal nutrients, low-sodium diet.
○ 4. High-protein, high-calorie, high-potassium diet.

68. The client's wife asks the nurse about health-promoting activities that she could help her husband include in his daily routine at home. Which one of the following measures would be appropriate for the nurse to suggest?
○ 1. Supplement the diet with daily multivitamins.
○ 2. Limit daily alcohol intake.
○ 3. Take a sleeping pill at bedtime.
○ 4. Avoid contact with other people whenever possible.

69. The client's weight has not changed during the last 6 months, but his abdominal girth has increased. The nurse should recognize that the pathologic basis for the development of ascites is portal hypertension and
○ 1. excess serum sodium level and increased aldosterone excretion.
○ 2. increased aldosterone excretion and decreased serum albumin level.
○ 3. decreased colloid osmotic pressure and lymphatic obstruction.
○ 4. decreased serum albumin level and decreased colloid osmotic pressure.

70. The position of choice for a client with severe ascites would be
○ 1. high-Fowler's.
○ 2. side-lying.
○ 3. modified Trendelenburg's.
○ 4. any position, as long as frequent position changes are ensured.

71. The physician decreases the client's dietary sodium restriction to 1 g/day and orders a diuretic. The nurse would plan to administer a diuretic that facilitates sodium excretion while conserving body potassium such as
○ 1. furosemide (Lasix).
○ 2. spironolactone (Aldactone).
○ 3. hydrochlorothiazide (HydroDIURIL).
○ 4. ethacrynic acid (Edecrin).

72. The client receives 100 mL of 25% serum albumin intravenously. Which assessment finding would best indicate that the albumin was having its desired effect?
○ 1. Increased urine output.
○ 2. Increased serum albumin level.
○ 3. Decreased anorexia and itching.
○ 4. Increased ease of breathing.

73. Four months later, the same client is admitted through the emergency department. He is vomiting bright red blood, and the physician suspects bleeding esophageal varices. The physician decides to insert a Sengstaken-Blakemore tube. The nurse should explain to the client that the tube acts by
○ 1. providing a large diameter for effective gastric lavage.
○ 2. applying direct pressure to gastric bleeding sites.
○ 3. blocking blood flow to the stomach and esophagus.
○ 4. applying direct pressure to the esophagus.

74. Once the Sengstaken-Blakemore tube is successfully inserted, which of the following nursing interventions would be appropriate?
○ 1. Provide him with an emesis basin to expectorate secretions.
○ 2. Obtain an order for lozenges to counteract dry mouth.
○ 3. Moisten the internal nares with a petroleum-based lubricant.
○ 4. Obtain an order for lidocaine hydrochloride (Xylocaine Viscous) to decrease the discomfort of swallowing.

75. About 30 minutes after the tube is inserted, the nurse observes that the client appears to be having difficulty breathing. The nurse's first action should be to
○ 1. remove the tube.
○ 2. deflate the esophageal portion of the tube.
○ 3. determine whether the tube is obstructing the airway.
○ 4. raise the head of the bed and increase the oxygen flow rate.

76. The client's condition stabilizes, and the Sengstaken-Blakemore tube is removed. The physician orders oral neomycin as well as a neomycin enema. The purpose of this therapy is to

○ 1. reduce abdominal pressure and prevent further bleeding.

○ 2. prevent the client from straining during defecation and stimulating rebleeding.

○ 3. remove intestinal contents and block ammonia formation.

○ 4. reduce the irritating effect of blood on the intestinal mucosa.

77. The nurse monitors the client for the development of portal systemic encephalopathy, being alert for changes in the client's

○ 1. level of consciousness.

○ 2. vital signs.

○ 3. urine output.

○ 4. respiratory status.

78. The client's serum ammonia level begins to rise, and the physician orders 30 mL of lactulose (Cephulac). Which of the following effects of this drug would the nurse expect to see?

○ 1. Increased urine output.

○ 2. Improved level of consciousness.

○ 3. Diarrhea.

○ 4. Nausea and vomiting.

79. The client recovers slowly. He is to be discharged home with a prescription for lactulose (Cephulac). The nurse teaches the client and his wife how to administer this medication. Which of the following statements would indicate that the client has understood the teaching?

○ 1. "I'll take it with Maalox."

○ 2. "I'll mix it with apple juice."

○ 3. "I'll take it with a laxative."

○ 4. "I'll mix the crushed tablets in some gelatin."

The Client With an Ileostomy

A client has been admitted to the hospital for an ileostomy.

80. The client asks the nurse, "Is it really possible to lead a normal life with an ileostomy?" Which action by the nurse would likely be the most effective response to this question?

○ 1. Have the client talk to her clergyman about her concerns.

○ 2. Tell the client to worry about those concerns after surgery.

○ 3. Arrange for a person with an ostomy to visit the client preoperatively.

○ 4. Notify the surgeon of the client's question.

81. The client is learning about caring for her ileostomy. Which of the following statements would indicate that she understands how to care for her ileostomy pouch?

○ 1. "I'll empty my pouch when it's about one-third full."

○ 2. "I can take my pouch off at night."

○ 3. "I should change my pouch immediately after lunch."

○ 4. "I must apply a new pouch system every day."

82. The nurse explains to the client that some form of skin barrier must be used around the stoma at all times. A skin barrier

○ 1. helps prevent the formation of odor.

○ 2. helps maintain an accurate output record.

○ 3. protects against irritation from effluent from the ileostomy.

○ 4. will allow the client to keep the ostomy pouch on for a longer time.

83. The client is receiving diet instructions from the nurse. Which of the following instructions would be appropriate?

○ 1. "Limit your fluids to 1000 mL/day."

○ 2. "Chew your food thoroughly."

○ 3. "There's no need to monitor your diet."

○ 4. "Six small meals a day will prevent abdominal distention."

84. The nurse should instruct the client to report immediately which of the following symptoms to the physician?

○ 1. Passage of liquid stool from the stoma.

○ 2. Occasional presence of undigested food in the effluent.

○ 3. Absence of drainage from the ileostomy for 6 or more hours.

○ 4. Temperature of 99.8°F.

85. The nurse finds the client crying. The client explains to the nurse, "I'm upset because I know I won't be able to have children now that I have an ileostomy." Which of the following would be the best response for the nurse?

○ 1. "Many individuals in your position decide to adopt. Why don't you consider that option?"

○ 2. "Having an ileostomy does not necessarily mean that you can't bear children. Let's talk to your doctor about your concerns."

○ 3. "I can understand your reasons for being upset. Having children must be important to you."

○ 4. "I'm sure you will adjust to this situation with time. Try not to be too upset."

The Client on Total Parenteral Nutrition

A client with inflammatory bowel disease is receiving TPN.

86. The basic component of the client's TPN solution is most likely to be

○ 1. an isotonic glucose solution.

○ 2. a hypertonic glucose solution.

○ 3. a hypotonic dextrose solution.

○ 4. a low-molecular-weight dextrose solution.

87. The nurse would regularly assess the client's ability to metabolize the TPN solution adequately by monitoring him for

○ 1. tachycardia.

○ 2. hypertension.

○ 3. elevated blood urea nitrogen.

○ 4. hyperglycemia.

88. Which of the following interventions should the nurse include in the client's care plan to prevent complications associated with TPN administered through a central line?

○ 1. Use a strict clean technique for all dressing changes.

○ 2. Tape all connections of the system.

○ 3. Encourage bed rest.

○ 4. Cover the insertion site with a moisture-proof dressing.

89. Which of the following would be the best indication that the goals for TPN are being achieved for the client?

○ 1. Urine negative for glucose.

○ 2. Serum potassium level of 4 mEq/L.

○ 3. Serum glucose level of 96.

○ 4. Weight gain of 0.5 pounds/day.

90. The nurse notices that the client's TPN solution is infusing too slowly. The nurse calculates that the client has received 300 mL less than was ordered for the day. The nurse should

○ 1. quickly increase the flow rate to infuse an additional 300 mL over the next hour.

○ 2. maintain the flow rate at the current rate and document any discrepancy in the chart.

○ 3. assess the infusion system, note the client's condition, and notify the physician.

○ 4. discontinue the solution and administer dextrose in 5% water until the infusion problem is resolved.

91. When developing a care plan for a client who is receiving TPN, which one of the following potential nursing diagnoses would be most appropriate?

○ 1. Impaired Swallowing.

○ 2. Impaired Gas Exchange.

○ 3. Fluid Volume Excess.

○ 4. Altered Tissue Perfusion.

92. The nurse is changing the subclavian dressing over the catheter insertion site. Which one of the following actions would be appropriate for the nurse to incorporate into the dressing change?

○ 1. Place the client in high-Fowler's position.

○ 2. Check for tubing kinks and leakage.

○ 3. Cleanse the area, starting 2 inches from the insertion site and moving inward.

○ 4. Remove old ointment from the insertion site with soap and warm water.

The Client With Diverticular Disease

93. Which of the following laboratory findings would the nurse expect to find in a client with diverticulitis?

○ 1. Elevated red blood count.

○ 2. Decreased platelet count.

○ 3. Elevated white blood count.

○ 4. Elevated serum blood urea nitrogen.

94. The nurse is aware that the diagnostic tests typically ordered for acute diverticulitis do not include a barium enema. The reason for this is that a barium enema

○ 1. can perforate an intestinal abscess.

○ 2. would greatly increase the client's pain.

○ 3. is of minimal diagnostic value in diverticulitis.

○ 4. is too lengthy a procedure for the client to tolerate.

95. The client is treated as an outpatient with drug therapy. The nurse would anticipate drug therapy for diverticulitis to include

○ 1. tranquilizers.

○ 2. laxatives.

○ 3. broad-spectrum antibiotics.

○ 4. opioid analgesics.

96. Which of the following measures should the client be taught to integrate into his daily routine at home?

○ 1. Using enemas to relieve periods of constipation.

○ 2. Decreasing fluid intake to increase formed consistency of stool.

○ 3. Eating a high-fiber diet when symptomatic with diverticulitis.

○ 4. Refraining from straining and lifting activities that increase intraabdominal pressure.

CORRECT ANSWERS AND RATIONALE

The letters in parentheses following the rationale identify the step of the nursing process (A, D, P, I, E), cognitive level (K, C, T, N), and client needs (S, G, L, H). See the Answer Grid for the key.

The Client With Cancer of the Colon

1. 4. Castor oil breaks down in the intestines to form ricinoleic acid. This acid irritates nerve endings in the intestinal mucosa, producing evacuation. Mineral oil is a laxative that softens and lubricates the stool. Saline cathartics, such as magnesium sulfate and citrate, increase the volume of intestinal content, thus stimulating evacuation. (I, K, G)

2. 1. After a barium enema, a laxative is ordinarily prescribed. This is done to promote elimination of the barium. Retained barium predisposes the client to constipation and fecal impaction. (P, K, H)

3. 2. Antibiotics are administered preoperatively to reduce the bacterial count in the colon. The client will be placed on a low residue diet to help cleanse the bowel before surgery but typically is not placed on NPO status until 8 to 12 hours before surgery. Laxatives and enemas may also be administered. Chest tubes would not be expected postoperatively. There is no need to limit the client's activity before surgery. (P, N, S)

4. 4. The preferred site for a permanent colostomy is in the lower portion of the descending colon, when possible; hence, placement is on the left side of the body. Because the colon normally absorbs large quantities of water, placing the colostomy near the end of the colon will result in near-normal stool consistency. Optimal placement of an ostomy is usually determined before surgery by an enterostomal therapist. (I, T, G)

5. 3. A sign indicating that a client's colostomy is open and ready to function is passage of feces and flatus. When this occurs, gastric suction is ordinarily discontinued, and the client is allowed to start taking fluids and food orally. Absence of bowel sounds would indicate that the tube should remain in place because peristalsis has not yet returned. Passage of mucus from the rectum will not occur in this client because of the nature of the surgery. Absence of stomach drainage or absence of nausea and vomiting is not a criterion for judging whether or not gastric suction should be continued. (A, C, G)

6. 1. Mouth care should be provided after nasogastric tube removal. Auscultating and palpating the abdomen should have been done before tube removal. After tube removal, the nurse will continue to assess the client's abdomen, but there is no need to do this immediately after removal. Giving the client something to eat or drink would not be appropriate until after mouth care has been provided. (I, T, S)

7. 2. The client should be encouraged to discuss any concerns about sexual functioning. The client will not need to maintain a high-fiber diet, but instead will be encouraged to avoid any foods that cause odor and flatulence. While the client with a colostomy will be instructed to avoid high contact sports, further changes in physical activity are unnecessary. Fluid intake will be encouraged, not restricted. (E, T, H)

8. 4. When a client demonstrates readiness to learn about colostomy, it is usually best to start with simple techniques such as using illustrative material during teaching sessions. This will help the client visualize how the colostomy will appear. Telling the client how normal body functions will continue and encouraging him to ask questions are recommended, but these measures will do less to prepare the client for the sight of a colostomy than will using illustrative material. Visits from members of an ostomy club are also recommended, but these visits usually are more beneficial when the client has knowledge of the colostomy and how it looks and functions. (I, N, L)

9. 1. Abdominal cramping that may occur during a colostomy irrigation results from stimulation of the colon by the irrigating solution. The best course of action is to stop the flow of solution temporarily until cramping subsides. Having the client sit up in bed or advancing the cone or tube further will not help stop cramping. There is no need to remove the cone or tube because it will need to be reinserted when irrigation is continued. (I, T, S)

10. 2. A dark red to purple stoma indicates inadequate blood supply. Mild edema is normal in the early postoperative period, as is slight oozing of blood. The colostomy would typically not begin functioning for 2 to 4 days after surgery. (E, T, S)

11. 2. A client who asks about supplies used for dressings may be ready to participate in self-care. Inquiring about the physician's visit, discussing news events, and complaining about a dressing change are behaviors that avoid the subject of the colostomy. (E, N, L)

12. 1. Karaya and Stomahesive are both effective agents for protecting the skin around a colostomy. They keep the skin healthy and prevent skin irritation from stoma drainage. Petrolatum, cornstarch,

and antiseptic creams do not protect the skin adequately. (I, T, S)

13. 1. Sitz baths are an effective way to cleanse the operative area following an abdominoperineal resection. Sitz baths bring warmth to the area, improve circulation, and promote healing and cleanliness. Most clients find them comfortable and relaxing. (I, N, G)

14. 3. Experience has shown that it is best to adjust the diet of a client with a colostomy in a manner that best suits the client rather than trying special diets. Promoting a high-fiber diet and limiting roughage and liquids are not recommended. (P, C, H)

15. 4. Many colostomies, especially those located in the descending colon, can be regulated to evacuate on a regular schedule. All ostomy appliances should be applied using a peristomal skin barrier. There should be no pain associated with touching the stoma. After the immediate postoperative period, it is not normal for blood to be present in the stool. Bleeding should be reported to the client's health care provider. (E, T, H)

The Client With Hepatitis A

16. 2. Liver inflammation and obstruction block the normal flow of bile. Excess bilirubin turns the skin and sclera yellow and the urine dark and frothy. Profound anorexia is also common. Shortness of breath would be unexpected. (A, C, G)

17. 2. The organism causing hepatitis A leaves the body primarily through feces. The respiratory route has not been ruled out entirely as a possible portal but is not considered the most common route of exit. (P, T, S)

18. 3. Enteric precautions are recommended for clients with hepatitis A, but a private room for an adult client is unnecessary. These recommendations are made by the Centers for Disease Control and Prevention. (P, N, S)

19. 1. Treatment during the acute phase of hepatitis consists primarily of bed rest with bathroom privileges. Bed rest is maintained during the acute phase to reduce metabolic demands on the liver, thus increasing its blood supply and supporting cell regeneration. When activity is gradually resumed, the client should be taught to rest before he feels overly tired. (I, T, G)

20. 3. Bilirubin levels and liver enzymes, such as serum glutamic pyruvic transaminase (SGPT) and serum glutamic oxaloacetic transaminase (SGOT), are carefully monitored during hepatitis. Their levels provide important data about liver function. Blood glucose, creatinine clearance, and serum electrolytes provide no information about liver function. (A, K, G)

21. 3. Unlike the hepatitis of alcoholism, viral forms of hepatitis are not usually associated with nutritional depletion. Therefore, a well-balanced diet is advocated to ensure nutritional status. It is a challenge to ensure that clients with hepatitis A ingest a balanced diet with sufficient carbohydrates and calories because these clients are generally anorexic and have little interest in eating. (P, T, G)

22. 3. The hepatitis A virus is transmitted through the fecal–oral route. Common vehicles spreading the virus include contaminated hands, water, and food, especially shellfish growing in contaminated water. Certain animal handlers are at risk for hepatitis A, particularly those handling primates. (I, T, H)

23. 4. The most appropriate diagnosis for this client is Activity Intolerance related to fatigue. The major goal of care is to increase activity gradually as the client can tolerate. Periods of alternating rest and activity should be included in the plan of care. There is no evidence that the client is physically immobile, coping ineffectively, or unable to provide self-care. (D, N, G)

24. 3. Immune serum globulin is administered prophylactically to people exposed to hepatitis A. Recently, a vaccine for hepatitis A, VAQTA, has been developed and may be used in conjunction with immune globulin for immediate and long-term protection. Interferons are a family of naturally occurring proteins that can be used to treat several forms of cancer, and antibiotics are not used to prevent or treat viral hepatitis. (I, C, H)

25. 4. Convalescence after hepatitis may take weeks or even months. Boredom and depression are common problems that the client should anticipate. Problems with pain, maintaining a regular bowel elimination pattern, and preventing respiratory complications are unlikely. Bed rest is not prescribed, but activity is strictly limited to support healing. (E, T, G)

26. 2. Uncomplicated hepatitis A does not require any particular lifestyle modifications once healing has occurred. Moderation in alcohol consumption is recommended. Clients should never donate blood, however. (I, T, H)

The Client With Hepatitis B

27. 2. Hepatitis B virus is spread through contact with blood, body fluids contaminated with blood, and such body fluids as cerebrospinal, pleural, peritoneal, and synovial fluids; semen; and vaginal secretions. The risk of transmission of hepatitis B through feces is low. Touching the client without gloves when there is no danger of contact with blood or body fluids is acceptable. Preventive measures for the nurse include using barrier protection (gloves, goggles, and gown) when appropriate and not recapping needles. A hepatitis B vaccine exists and is recommended for high-risk people. (E, N, S)

28. 3. People at high risk for hepatitis B include users of illicit intravenous drugs, people with multiple sex partners, homosexual males, and health care personnel who have frequent contact with blood. Hepatitis B is not spread through marijuana use or ingestion of contaminated seafood. Acetaminophen taken in large amounts can cause severe hepatic necrosis but does not cause hepatitis B. (E, T, H)

29. 1. The client should be taught how to prevent the spread of hepatitis B to others. It is not necessary for the client to isolate himself from family and friends. Sedatives should be avoided because these are usually detoxified by the liver. The client should eat a well-balanced, nutritional diet. There is no need to restrict sodium or protein. (P, N, H)

30. 2. The most appropriate nursing diagnosis for this client is Social Isolation. Clients with hepatitis frequently feel guilty about possibly exposing others to the disease. Family and friends may experience fear of contracting the disease. (D, T, L)

31. 4. The nurse should encourage the client to further verbalize feelings of isolation. Instead of belittling or dismissing these feelings, the nurse should allow clients to verbalize their fears and provide education on how to prevent infection transmission. (I, T, L)

The Client With Hemorrhoids

32. 2. Hemorrhoids are associated with prolonged sitting or standing, portal hypertension, chronic constipation, and prolonged increased intraabdominal pressure, as associated with pregnancy and the strain of vaginal delivery. (A, C, G)

33. 3. Use of warm sitz baths can help relieve the rectal discomfort of hemorrhoids. Fiber in the diet should be increased to promote regular bowel movements. Laxatives are irritating and should be avoided. Decreasing physical activity will not decrease discomfort. (P, T, H)

34. 3. Rectal surgery is accompanied by severe pain resulting from spasms of sphincters and muscles. Therefore, controlling pain is a priority goal of posthemorrhoidectomy nursing care. Preventing venous stasis, promoting ambulation, and preventing infection are important goals but not priority goals given the nature of the surgery. (P, T, G)

35. 3. Positioning in the early posthemorrhoidectomy phase should avoid stress and pressure on the operative site. The prone and side-lying positions are ideal from a comfort perspective. Any sitting position is less than ideal, and there is no need for Trendelenburg's position. (I, T, S)

36. 1. Applying heat during the immediate postoperative period may cause hemorrhage at the surgical site. Moist heat may relieve rectal spasms after bowel movements. Urine retention caused by reflex spasm may also be relieved by moist heat. Increasing fiber and fluid in the diet can help prevent constipation. (I, C, S)

37. 3. Adequate cleansing of the anal area is difficult but essential. After rectal surgery, sitz baths assist in this process, so the posthemorrhoidectomy client should take a sitz bath after defecating. Other times are dictated by client comfort. (E, T, H)

38. 2. Oatmeal, grapefruit wedges, and bran muffins are all high-fiber foods. Processed foods such as pastries, processed cereals, and white bread are low in fiber. Protein foods contain little if any fiber. Prune juice is not high in fiber but has a laxative effect caused by dihydroxyphenyl isatin. (E, K, H)

The Client With Inflammatory Bowel Disease

39. 2. Diarrhea is the primary symptom of ulcerative colitis. It is profuse and severe; the client may pass as many as 15 to 20 watery stools per day. Stools may contain blood, mucus, and pus. The frequent diarrhea is often accompanied by anorexia and nausea. Steatorrhea (fatty stools) is more typical of pancreatitis and cholecystitis. Alternating diarrhea and constipation is associated with irritable bowel syndrome. (A, T, G)

40. 1. Stressful and emotional events have been clearly linked to exacerbations of ulcerative colitis, although their role in the etiology of the disease has been disproved. Diet and exercise are unlikely causes of acute exacerbation. (A, N, G)

41. 2. Diarrhea is the primary symptom, and stopping it is the first goal of treatment. The other goals are ongoing and will be best achieved by halting the exacerbation. The client may receive antidiarrheal agents, antispasmodic agents, bulk hydrophilic agents, or antiinflammatory drugs. (P, N, G)

42. 2. Modified bed rest helps conserve energy and promote comfort, but its primary purpose is to help reduce the hypermotility of the colon. (P, C, G)

43. 3. Massive diarrhea causes significant depletion of the body's stores of sodium and potassium as well as fluid. The client should be closely monitored for hypokalemia and hyponatremia. (A, C, G)

44. 4. It is not uncommon for clients with ulcerative colitis to become apprehensive and upset about the frequency of stools and presence of abdominal cramping. During these acute exacerbations, clients need emotional support and encouragement to verbalize their feelings about their chronic health concerns and assistance in developing effective coping methods. (D, N, L)

45. 2. Anal excoriation is inevitable with profuse diarrhea, and meticulous perianal hygiene is essential. Sitz baths are comforting and cleansing. Diarrhea necessitates the ready availability of a bedpan or bedside commode. It is not appropriate to administer stool softeners to a client with diarrhea. A gown is not indicated because no infectious agent is involved. (I, T, G)

46. 3. A client with severe symptoms of ulcerative colitis will be kept NPO to rest the bowel. To maintain the client's nutritional status, the client usually is started on TPN. (P, T, G)

47. 3. Adequate fluid intake prevents crystalluria and stone formation during sulfasalazine therapy. This drug can cause gastrointestinal distress and is best taken after meals and in equally divided doses. It gives alkaline urine an orange-yellow color, but it is not necessary to stop the drug. (I, K, G)

48. 1. A client with a chronic disease need not curtail career goals. Self-care is the cornerstone of long-term management, and learning to cope with and modify stressors will enable the client to live with the disease. Giving up a desired career could discourage and even depress the client. Placing the responsibility for minimizing stressors at work in the hands of others leads to a feeling of loss of control and stunts the sense of responsibility needed for sound self-care. Working part-time rather than full-time is unnecessary. (I, N, L)

49. 2. Clients with ulcerative colitis should follow a well-balanced high-protein, high-calorie, low-residue diet, avoiding such foods as whole wheat grains, nuts, and raw fruits and vegetables. (I, T, H)

50. 3. Caffeine, tobacco, and alcohol are gastrointestinal stimulants and should be avoided by clients with ulcerative colitis. High-fiber foods such as popcorn and nuts are not allowed. (E, T, H)

51. 1. An appropriate expected outcome for a client with ulcerative colitis is maintaining an ideal body weight. It would not be appropriate to restrict fluid intake; the client should strive to remain well hydrated. Ulcerative colitis produces episodic diarrhea, not constipation. It is not inevitable that the client with ulcerative colitis will need an ileostomy. The decision to perform surgery depends on the extent of the disease and the severity of the symptoms. (E, N, G)

The Client With an Intestinal Obstruction

52. 4. On percussion, air produces a resonant sound, and fluid produces a dull sound. An intestinal obstruction traps large amounts of fluid in the intes-

tine. Hyperperistalsis would be apparent on auscultation. (A, C, G)

53. 1. Profuse vomiting is the classic sign of small bowel obstruction. Abdominal distention and discomfort tend to be more pronounced with large bowel obstruction. High-pitched bowel sounds indicate hyperperistalsis, which occurs early in obstruction. (A, C, G)

54. 1. Intestinal decompression is accomplished with a Cantor, Harris, or Miller-Abbott tube. These 6- to 10-foot tubes are passed through the gastrointestinal tract to the obstruction. They remove accumulated fluid and gas, relieving the pressure. (I, C, S)

55. 2. The client is placed on her right side to facilitate movement of the mercury-weighted tube through the pyloric sphincter. After the tube is in the intestine, the client will be turned from side to side or encouraged to ambulate to facilitate tube movement through the intestinal loops. (I, C, S)

56. 2. An intestinal tube is not taped in position until it has reached the obstruction. A Cantor tube is attached to suction, and the small balloon at its tip is injected with mercury. Because the tube has a radiopaque strip, its progress through the intestinal tract can be followed by fluoroscopy. (I, C, S)

57. 2. Once the intestinal tube has passed into the duodenum, it is usually advanced, as ordered, 2 to 4 inches every 30 to 60 minutes. This enables peristalsis to carry the tube forward. The client is encouraged to walk, which also facilitates tube progression. A client with an intestinal tube needs frequent mouth care to stimulate saliva secretion, to maintain a healthy oral cavity, and to promote comfort. Ice chips are contraindicated because hypotonic fluid will draw extra fluid into an already distended bowel. (I, T, S)

58. 4. Intestinal tubes are not irrigated. The other nursing measures are appropriate. (I, N, S)

59. 3. A client with an intestinal obstruction is particularly susceptible to fluid volume deficit and electrolyte imbalances. The client's pain is acute in nature, not chronic. The other nursing diagnoses are not appropriate. (D, N, G)

60. 2. Medications that mask symptoms may delay accurate diagnosis and appropriate treatment. Narcotics are thought to stimulate a chemoreceptor emetic trigger zone in the medulla, causing nausea and vomiting. Potential fluid loss is not the reason that such medications are not administered to clients with suspected intestinal obstruction; a patent intestinal tube minimizes vomiting. Addiction is unlikely when pain medication is administered to control pain. Narcotics are often used to facilitate anesthesia induction. (I, C, G)

61. 1. High colonic irrigation can increase the risk of

perforation in a distended and inflamed colon. Tap water is hypotonic in the bowel and would draw increased fluid into the area. The other measures are part of standard preparation for intestinal surgery. (I, N, S)

62. 4. The kidney is sensitive to circulating fluid volume. Urine output below 30 mL/hour indicates that the kidney is concentrating urine and that fluid replacement needs to be increased. The intestinal tube removes sequestered fluid in the bowel, not fluid in the general circulation. The effect of pain on renal function is not so dramatic as described here. (E, N, G)

63. 2. Assessing pain, including location and severity, is essential before administering pain medication. Because the client spent an hour in the postanesthesia recovery unit, the nurse would next determine whether she had been medicated for pain in that unit. The pain is most likely incisional but could result from positioning, a too-tight dressing, or anxiety. (I, N, S)

64. 3. Because peristalsis has not been reestablished, this amount of gastric drainage would be expected. The green-brown color would also be expected. The appropriate nursing action is to chart the amount and color of output and continue monitoring the client. (I, N, G)

The Client With Cirrhosis

65. 1. The normal liver acts to metabolize and inactivate hormones. Loss of this function increases the levels of circulating hormones. Excess estrogen in a male may cause gynecomastia; loss of axillary, chest, and pubic hair; testicular atrophy; and impotence. It will not increase libido. Palmar erythema and spider angiomas are also common results of hormone excess. (A, K, G)

66. 3. Excess retained bilirubin produces an irritating effect on the peripheral nerves, causing intense itching. Folic acid, prothrombin, and potassium imbalances cause varied symptoms, but itching is not directly related to these imbalances. (E, C, G)

67. 3. Cirrhosis is a slowly progressive disease. Inadequate nutrition is the primary ongoing problem. Clients are encouraged to eat normal, well-balanced diets, restricting sodium to prevent fluid retention. Protein is not restricted until the liver actually fails, which is usually late in the disease. (I, T, G)

68. 1. General health promotion measures include maintaining good nutrition, avoiding infection, and abstaining from alcohol. Rest and sleep are essential, but an impaired liver may not be able to detoxify sedatives and barbiturates. Such drugs must be used cautiously, if at all, by clients with cirrhosis. The client does not need to avoid contact with others but should exercise caution to stay away from ill people. (I, N, H)

69. 4. Ascites results from increased pressure in the venous system, low levels of serum albumin (which contributes to decreased colloid osmotic pressure), and sodium retention, resulting in part from decreased aldosterone clearance. (A, C, G)

70. 1. Ascites can compromise the action of the diaphragm and increase the client's risk of respiratory problems. Frequent position changes are important, but the preferred position is high-Fowler's. Ascites also greatly increases the risk of skin breakdown. (I, T, S)

71. 2. Hypokalemia is an ongoing problem for a client with cirrhosis. When a diuretic is needed, the ideal choice is a potassium-sparing agent. Spironolactone is the diuretic of choice for clients with cirrhosis because it facilitates sodium excretion while conserving potassium. Furosemide, hydrochlorothiazide, and ethacrynic acid are thiazide diuretics, which cause potassium loss. (P, K, G)

72. 1. Normal serum albumin is administered to reduce ascites. Hypoalbuminemia, a mechanism underlying ascites formation, results in decreased colloid osmotic pressure. Administering serum albumin increases plasma colloid osmotic pressure, which causes fluid to flow from the tissue space into the plasma. Increased urine output is the best indication that the albumin is having the desired effect. A client receiving albumin should be monitored for such complications as fluid overload and pulmonary edema. (E, N, G)

73. 4. The Sengstaken-Blakemore tube has a small gastric balloon that anchors the tube and applies pressure to the area of the cardiac sphincter. The large esophageal balloon applies direct pressure on the bleeding sites in the esophagus. A tube passing through the balloons allows for aspiration and irrigation. (P, C, S)

74. 1. An inflated esophageal balloon prevents swallowing. Therefore, the nurse should provide the client with tissues and encourage him to spit into the tissues or an emesis basin. If the client cannot manage his secretions, gentle oral suctioning is needed. Oral and nasal care is provided every 1 to 2 hours. A water-soluble lubricant is applied to the external nares. (I, T, S)

75. 3. If the gastric balloon should rupture or deflate, the esophageal balloon can move and partially or totally obstruct the airway. The client must be observed closely. No direct action should be taken, however, until the condition is accurately diagnosed. (I, N, S)

76. 3. Neomycin is administered to decrease the bacterial effect on digested blood in the intestines, which results in ammonia production. This ammonia, if not detoxified by the liver, can result in hepatic coma. (P, C, G)

77. 1. Ammonia has a toxic effect on central nervous system tissue and produces altered level of consciousness, marked by drowsiness and irritability. If this process is unchecked, the client may lapse into coma. (A, C, G)

78. 3. Lactulose increases intestinal motility, thereby decreasing ammonia formation in the intestine. An expected effect, therefore, would be diarrhea. (P, K, G)

79. 2. The taste of lactulose is a problem for some clients; mixing it with fruit juice can make it more palatable. For clients without dietary sodium restrictions, lactulose can also be mixed with milk. Lactulose should not be given with antacids, which may inhibit its action. Lactulose is a laxative that expels trapped ammonia from the colon. It comes as a syrup for oral or rectal administration. (E, T, S)

The Client With an Ileostomy

80. 3. If the client agrees, having a person who has successfully adjusted to living with an ileostomy visit her would be the most helpful measure. This would let the client actually see that she will be able to pursue typical activities of daily life postoperatively. Her questions can be answered by someone who has felt some of the same concerns. Disregarding the client's concerns is not helpful. Although the physician should know about the client's concerns, this in itself will not reassure the client about life after an ileostomy. A visit from a clergyman may be helpful to some clients but may not provide this client with the information she is seeking. (I, N, L)

81. 1. The pouch should be emptied when it is about one-third full to prevent the weight of the pouch from breaking the seal. The client with an ileostomy must wear a pouch at all times to collect stool. A pouch can be worn for 3 to 7 days before being changed. The client should change the pouch at a time when the stoma is least likely to function; 2 to 4 hours after a meal is generally the most appropriate time. (E, N, H)

82. 3. Due to high concentrations of digestive enzymes, ileostomy effluent is irritating to skin and can cause excoriation and ulceration. Some form of protection must be used to keep the effluent from contacting the skin. (I, N, S)

83. 2. The client is instructed to chew food well to aid digestion and prevent obstruction. The client is usually placed on a regular diet but is encouraged to eat high-fiber and high-cellulose foods (eg, nuts, pop-

corn, corn, peas, tomatoes) with caution; these foods may swell in the intestine and cause an obstruction. The client should maintain an adequate fluid intake. Eating six small meals a day is not necessary. (I, T, H)

84. 3. The ileostomy drains liquid stool at frequent intervals throughout the day. Any sudden decrease in drainage or onset of severe abdominal pain should be reported to the physician immediately. (A, T, H)

85. 2. The fact that the client has an ileostomy does not necessarily mean that she cannot get pregnant and bear children. Women of childbearing age should be encouraged to discuss their concerns with their physician. (I, N, L)

The Client on Total Parenteral Nutrition

86. 2. The TPN solution is usually a hypertonic glucose solution. If a commercial preparation is unavailable, the solution is best prepared in a pharmacy under strict aseptic conditions. Electrolytes may be added to meet a client's particular needs. (I, K, S)

87. 4. During TPN administration, the client should be monitored regularly for hyperglycemia. The client may require small amounts of insulin to improve glucose metabolism. The client should also be observed for signs of hypoglycemia, which may occur if the body overproduces insulin in response to a high-glucose intake or if too much insulin is administered to help improve glucose metabolism. (A, T, G)

88. 2. Complications associated with administering TPN through a central line include infection and air embolism. To prevent these complications, strict aseptic technique is used for all dressing changes, the insertion site is covered with an air-occlusive dressing, and all connections of the system are taped. Ambulation and activities of daily living are encouraged. (I, T, S)

89. 4. A steady and progressive weight gain is the best indication that the client's nutritional goals are being met by TPN. These laboratory values are within normal limits but do not indicate attainment of nutritional goals. (E, N, G)

90. 3. The nurse's most appropriate action is to assess the infusion system to determine the cause of the inaccurate flow rate and to note the client's response to the decreased infusion. The physician should be notified of the infusion discrepancy. When adjusted, the flow rate of TPN solution should be gradually increased or decreased to prevent fluid and electrolyte imbalances. It should never be discontinued abruptly. (I, N, S)

91. 3. The most appropriate anticipated nursing diagnosis is Fluid Volume Excess. Clients receiving TPN are at high risk for developing fluid imbalances, either deficit or excess. The rate of the infusion and the client's response to the infusion must be carefully monitored by the nurse to prevent fluid disturbances. (D, T, G)

The Client With Diverticular Disease

92. 2. The client should be placed in a low-Fowler's position for the dressing change. When cleansing the insertion site, the nurse must always start at the site and work outward to maintain asepsis of the area. It is inappropriate to remove old ointments with warm water and soap. The area may be cleansed with acetone or alcohol swabs, as institution policy dictates. It is important to inspect the site carefully for fluid leakages or kinks in the tubing lying under the dressing. (I, T, S)

93. 3. Because of the inflammatory nature of diverticulitis, the nurse would anticipate an elevated white blood count. The remaining laboratory findings are not associated with diverticulitis. (A, C, G)

94. 1. Barium enemas are contraindicated in clients with acute diverticulitis because they can lead to perforation of the colon. A barium enema may be ordered after the client has been treated with antibiotic therapy and the inflammation has subsided. (A, T, S)

95. 3. Clients with diverticulitis are usually treated with broad-spectrum antibiotics. Mild analgesics and anticholinergics may also be administered. Clients with severe diverticulitis may be hospitalized for intravenous antibiotic therapy and may receive opioid analgesics such as meperidine (Demerol) and morphine. Laxatives are not used because they increase intestinal motility. Tranquilizers are not used for treatment of diverticulitis. (P, T, G)

96. 4. Clients with diverticular disease should refrain from any activities, such as lifting, straining, or coughing, that increase intraabdominal pressure. Enemas are contraindicated because they increase intestinal pressure. Fluid intake should be increased, rather than decreased, to promote soft, formed stools. A low-fiber diet is used when inflammation is present. (I, T, H)

NURSING CARE OF ADULTS WITH MEDICAL AND SURGICAL HEALTH PROBLEMS

TEST 5: The Client With Lower Gastrointestinal Tract Health Problems

Directions: Use this answer grid to determine areas of strength or need for further study.

NURSING PROCESS

A = Assessment
D = Analysis, nursing diagnosis
P = Planning
I = Implementation
E = Evaluation

COGNITIVE LEVEL

K = Knowledge
C = Comprehension
T = Application
N = Analysis

CLIENT NEEDS

S = Safe, effective care environment
G = Physiologic integrity
L = Psychosocial integrity
H = Health promotion and maintenance

Question #	Answer #	Nursing Process					Cognitive Level				Client Needs			
		A	D	P	I	E	K	C	T	N	S	G	L	H
1	4				I		K					G		
2	1			P			K							H
3	2			P						N	S			
4	4				I				T			G		
5	3	A						C				G		
6	1				I				T		S			
7	2					E			T					H
8	4				I					N			L	
9	1				I				T		S			
10	2					E			T		S			
11	2					E				N			L	
12	1				I				T		S			
13	1				I					N		G		
14	3			P				C						H
15	4					E			T					H
16	2	A						C				G		
17	2			P					T		S			
18	3			P						N	S			
19	1				I				T			G		
20	3	A					K					G		
21	3			P					T			G		
22	3				I				T					H
23	4		D							N		G		
24	3				I			C						H
25	4					E			T			G		

NURSING PROCESS

A = Assessment
D = Analysis, nursing diagnosis
P = Planning
I = Implementation
E = Evaluation

COGNITIVE LEVEL

K = Knowledge
C = Comprehension
T = Application
N = Analysis

CLIENT NEEDS

S = Safe, effective care environment
G = Physiologic integrity
L = Psychosocial integrity
H = Health promotion and maintenance

Question #	Answer #	A	D	P	I	E	K	C	T	N	S	G	L	H
26	2				I				T					H
27	2					E				N	S			
28	3					E			T					H
29	1			P						N				H
30	2		D						T				L	
31	4				I				T				L	
32	2	A						C				G		
33	3			P					T					H
34	3			P					T			G		
35	3				I				T		S			
36	1				I			C			S			
37	3					E			T					H
38	2					E	K							H
39	2	A							T			G		
40	1	A								N		G		
41	2			P						N		G		
42	2			P				C				G		
43	3	A						C				G		
44	4		D							N			L	
45	2				I				T			G		
46	3			P					T			G		
47	3				I		K					G		
48	1				I					N			L	
49	2				I				T					H
50	3					E			T					H
51	1					E				N		G		
52	4	A						C				G		
53	1	A						C				G		
54	1				I			C			S			
55	2				I			C			S			

ANSWER GRID: 2

NURSING PROCESS

A = Assessment
D = Analysis, nursing diagnosis
P = Planning
I = Implementation
E = Evaluation

COGNITIVE LEVEL

K = Knowledge
C = Comprehension
T = Application
N = Analysis

CLIENT NEEDS

S = Safe, effective care environment
G = Physiologic integrity
L = Psychosocial integrity
H = Health promotion and maintenance

Question #	Answer #	Nursing Process					Cognitive Level				Client Needs			
		A	D	P	I	E	K	C	T	N	S	G	L	H
56	2				I			C			S			
57	2				I				T		S			
58	4				I					N	S			
59	3		D							N		G		
60	2				I			C				G		
61	1				I					N	S			
62	4					E				N		G		
63	2				I					N	S			
64	3				I					N		G		
65	1	A					K					G		
66	3					E		C				G		
67	3				I				T			G		
68	1				I					N				H
69	4	A						C				G		
70	1				I				T		S			
71	2			P			K					G		
72	1					E				N		G		
73	4			P				C			S			
74	1				I				T		S			
75	3				I					N	S			
76	3			P				C				G		
77	1	A						C				G		
78	3			P			K					G		
79	2					E			T		S			
80	3				I					N			L	
81	1					E				N				H
82	3				I					N	S			
83	2				I				T					H
84	3	A							T					H
85	2				I					N			L	

ANSWER GRID: 3

489

NURSING PROCESS

A = Assessment
D = Analysis, nursing diagnosis
P = Planning
I = Implementation
E = Evaluation

COGNITIVE LEVEL

K = Knowledge
C = Comprehension
T = Application
N = Analysis

CLIENT NEEDS

S = Safe, effective care environment
G = Physiologic integrity
L = Psychosocial integrity
H = Health promotion and maintenance

Question #	Answer #	Nursing Process					Cognitive Level				Client Needs			
		A	D	P	I	E	K	C	T	N	S	G	L	H
86	2				I		K				S			
87	4	A							T			G		
88	2				I				T		S			
89	4					E				N		G		
90	3				I					N	S			
91	3		D						T			G		
92	2				I				T		S			
93	3	A						C				G		
94	1	A							T		S			
95	3			P					T			G		
96	4				I				T					H
Number Correct														
Number Possible	96	16	5	17	41	17	9	20	39	28	28	41	8	19
Percentage Correct														

Score Calculation: To determine your **Percentage Correct,** divide the **Number Correct** by the **Number Possible.**

ANSWER GRID: 4

The Client With Endocrine Health Problems

- **The Client With Hyperthyroidism**
- **The Client With Diabetes Mellitus**
- **The Client With Pituitary Adenoma**
- **The Client With Addison's Disease**
- **The Client With Cushing's Disease**
- **Correct Answers and Rationale**

Select the one best answer, and indicate your choice by filling in the circle in front of the option.

The Client With Hyperthyroidism

A 42-year-old business woman visits her physician complaining of nervousness, irritability, and difficulty sleeping. A tentative diagnosis of Graves' disease is made.

1. Another typical symptom of Graves' disease is
- ○ 1. anorexia.
- ○ 2. tachycardia.
- ○ 3. weight gain.
- ○ 4. goiter.

2. Which symptom related to the client's menstrual cycle would she likely report during initial assessment?
- ○ 1. Dysmenorrhea.
- ○ 2. Metrorrhagia.
- ○ 3. Oligomenorrhea.
- ○ 4. Menorrhagia.

3. Propylthiouracil (PTU) is prescribed for the client. The nurse should teach the client to report immediately which of the following signs and symptoms?
- ○ 1. Sore throat and fever.
- ○ 2. Painful and excessive menstruation.
- ○ 3. Constipation and abdominal distention.
- ○ 4. Increased urine output and itchy skin.

4. The client says to the nurse, "I am so irritable, I feel like yelling a lot of the time." Which of the following responses by the nurse would give the client the most accurate explanation of her behavior?

- ○ 1. "This type of behavior may be caused by temporary confusion brought on by your illness."
- ○ 2. "This type of behavior may be caused by the excess thyroid hormone in your system."
- ○ 3. "This type of behavior is caused by your worrying about the seriousness of her illness."
- ○ 4. "This type of behavior is caused by the stress of trying to manage a career and cope with illness."

5. A radioactive iodine uptake (RAIU) test and a protein-bound iodine (PBI) test are planned for the client with hyperthyroidism. These two tests would have falsely elevated results if the client has recently taken medications containing
- ○ 1. iodine.
- ○ 2. digitalis.
- ○ 3. ferrous salts.
- ○ 4. antihistamines.

6. Measures to prevent eye damage from exophthalmos include
- ○ 1. massaging the eyes at regular intervals.
- ○ 2. instilling an ophthalmic anesthetic as ordered.
- ○ 3. taping the eyelids closed with nonirritating tape.
- ○ 4. covering both eyes with moistened gauze pads.

7. This client is treated with sodium iodide I 131. The nurse explains to the client that this drug will
- ○ 1. stabilize the thyroid hormone levels before a thyroidectomy.
- ○ 2. reduce uptake of thyroxine and thereby improve the client's condition.

491

○ 3. lower the level of thyroid hormones by slowing the body's production of them.

○ 4. destroy thyroid tissue so that thyroid hormones are no longer produced.

8. Which of the following nursing diagnoses would most likely be appropriate for the client after treatment with sodium iodide I 131?

○ 1. High Risk for Injury related to altered level of consciousness.

○ 2. Ineffective Breathing Patterns related to effects of radioactive iodine.

○ 3. Self-Care Deficit related to the need for immobilization after radioactive iodine therapy.

○ 4. Altered Health Maintenance related to lack of knowledge about disease management.

9. After treatment with sodium iodide I 131, the nurse teaches the client

○ 1. how to monitor for signs and symptoms of hyperthyroidism.

○ 2. that immobility is necessary for 1 week to prevent complications of the medication.

○ 3. that thyroxine replacement will be necessary for the remainder of the client's life.

○ 4. to assess for hypertension and tachycardia resulting from altered thyroid activity.

A client is scheduled for a subtotal thyroidectomy to treat hyperthyroidism.

10. Saturated solution of potassium iodide (SSKI) is prescribed preoperatively for the client. The primary reason for using this drug is that it helps

○ 1. slow progression of exophthalmos.

○ 2. reduce the vascularity of the thyroid gland.

○ 3. decrease the body's ability to store thyroxine.

○ 4. increase the body's ability to excrete thyroxine.

11. Which of the following measures is most often recommended when preparing SSKI for administration?

○ 1. Pour the solution over ice chips.

○ 2. Mix the solution with an antacid.

○ 3. Dilute the solution with water, milk, or fruit juice.

○ 4. Disguise the solution in a pureed fruit or vegetable.

12. The nurse asks the client to state her name as soon as she regains consciousness postoperatively after a subtotal thyroidectomy, then repeats this request from time to time. The nurse does this primarily to monitor for signs of

○ 1. internal hemorrhage.

○ 2. decreasing level of consciousness.

○ 3. laryngeal nerve damage.

○ 4. upper airway obstruction.

13. After the subtotal thyroidectomy, which of the following items should be kept in the client's room to treat postoperative complications that may develop?

○ 1. Equipment to begin total parenteral nutrition.

○ 2. A cutdown tray.

○ 3. Equipment for tube feedings.

○ 4. Equipment to perform a tracheostomy.

14. Which of the following symptoms might indicate that a client was developing tetany after a subtotal thyroidectomy?

○ 1. Backache and joint pains.

○ 2. Tingling in the fingers.

○ 3. Hoarseness.

○ 4. Retraction of neck muscles with inspiration.

15. Which of the following medications should be available to provide emergency treatment if the client develops tetany after a subtotal thyroidectomy?

○ 1. Sodium phosphate.

○ 2. Calcium gluconate.

○ 3. Echothiophate iodide.

○ 4. Sodium bicarbonate.

A 60-year-old woman is diagnosed with hypothyroidism.

16. Signs and symptoms of hypothyroidism include

○ 1. tachycardia.

○ 2. weight gain.

○ 3. diarrhea.

○ 4. anorexia.

17. Appropriate nursing diagnoses for the client would likely include which of the following?

○ 1. High Risk for Injury: Corneal Abrasion related to incomplete closure of eyelid.

○ 2. Altered Nutrition: Less Than Body Requirements related to hypermetabolism.

○ 3. Fluid Volume Deficit related to diarrhea.

○ 4. Activity Intolerance related to fatigue associated with the disorder.

18. When discussing the client's complaint of feelings of sadness and depression that have just begun, the nurse should inform the client that these feelings are

○ 1. the effects of thyroid hormone replacement therapy and will diminish over time.

○ 2. related to the thyroid hormone replacement therapy and will not diminish over time.

○ 3. a normal part of aging and having a chronic illness.

○ 4. most likely related to low thyroid hormone levels and will improve with treatment.

The Client With Diabetes Mellitus

A 55-year-old male client has recently been diagnosed with non-insulin–dependent diabetes mellitus (NIDDM) and is being started on the sulfonylurea compound tolbutamide. He is concerned about the diagnosis and says he knows nothing about diabetes. The nurse determines that he needs much teaching and support.

19. Tolbutamide is believed to lower blood glucose level by
  ○ 1. potentiating the action of insulin.
  ○ 2. lowering the renal threshold of glucose.
  ○ 3. stimulating pancreatic cells to release insulin.
  ○ 4. combining with glucose to render it inert.
20. When teaching the client about foot care, the nurse should instruct him to
  ○ 1. avoid going barefoot.
  ○ 2. wear hard-soled shoes.
  ○ 3. apply toenail polish.
  ○ 4. use bar soap to wash the feet.
21. The client asks the nurse to recommend something to remove corns from his toes. The nurse should advise him to
  ○ 1. apply a high-quality corn plaster to the area.
  ○ 2. consult his physician about removing the corns.
  ○ 3. apply iodine to the corns before peeling them off.
  ○ 4. soak his feet in borax solution to peel off the corns.
22. The nurse notes several small bandages covering cuts on the client's hands. The client says, "I'm so clumsy. I'm always cutting or burning myself." Which of the following responses by the nurse would be most appropriate?
  ○ 1. "Don't worry about it, but keep all your cuts clean and covered."
  ○ 2. "Even small cuts can be serious for people with diabetes and need special care."
  ○ 3. "Why do you think you injure yourself so frequently?"
  ○ 4. "You really should have your doctor check all injuries, even small ones."
23. The client says, "If I could just avoid what you call carbohydrates in my diet, I guess I would be okay." The nurse should base the response to this comment on the knowledge that diabetes affects metabolism of
  ○ 1. carbohydrates only.
  ○ 2. fats and carbohydrates only.
  ○ 3. protein and carbohydrates only.
  ○ 4. proteins, fats, and carbohydrates.
24. The client says he eats a lot of pasta products, such as macaroni and spaghetti. He asks if he can still eat them. Which of the following would be the nurse's best response?
  ○ 1. "Because you're overweight, it's better to eliminate pasta from your diet."
  ○ 2. "Pasta can be a part of your diet. It's included in the bread and cereal exchange."
  ○ 3. "Pasta can be included in your diet, but it shouldn't be served with sauces."
  ○ 4. "Eating pasta can predispose to various complications, so it's better to eliminate it."
25. The nurse should caution this client with diabetes mellitus who is taking tolbutamide (Orinase) that alcoholic beverages must be included when calculating total caloric intake and, if used in excess, tend to cause symptoms of
  ○ 1. hypokalemia.
  ○ 2. hyperkalemia.
  ○ 3. hyperglycemia.
  ○ 4. hypoglycemia.

A 48-year-old female client has adult-onset diabetes mellitus that will now require insulin for management. The plan is to change her from an oral agent to insulin, which will be done on an outpatient basis. Education will be completed by the home care nurse.

26. Of the following factors, which one is most important in predisposing a person to adult-onset diabetes mellitus?
  ○ 1. Cigarette smoking.
  ○ 2. High-cholesterol diet.
  ○ 3. Obesity.
  ○ 4. Hypertension.
27. The nurse should assess the client for which of the following disorders, to which clients with diabetes mellitus are predisposed?
  ○ 1. Arthritis.
  ○ 2. Hypertension.
  ○ 3. Osteoporosis.
  ○ 4. Leukemia.
28. When educating the client about activity level, the nurse bases the information on the knowledge that exercise affects the body's physiologic functioning relative to glucose usage in which of the following ways?
  ○ 1. Exercise helps avoid hypoglycemia.
  ○ 2. Exercise stimulates insulin overproduction.
  ○ 3. Exercise decreases the renal threshold for glucose.
  ○ 4. Exercise increases the use of glucose by muscles.
29. When teaching the client about diet, the nurse informs the client that which of the following dietary

constituents has been observed to minimize a rise in blood glucose level after meals in clients with diabetes mellitus?

○ 1. Dietary fiber.
○ 2. Dairy products.
○ 3. Vitamin-fortified foods.
○ 4. Organ meats.

30. The client is taught to take isophane (NPH) insulin at 5 PM each day. The client should be instructed that she will be at greatest risk for hypoglycemia at about

○ 1. 11 AM, shortly before lunch.
○ 2. 1 PM, shortly after lunch.
○ 3. 6 PM, shortly after dinner.
○ 4. 1 AM, during bedtime.

31. The client is being taught to self-administer insulin. Learning goals most likely will be attained when they are established by the

○ 1. nurse and client, because both need to be responsible for teaching.
○ 2. physician and client, because the physician is the manager of care and the client is the main participant.
○ 3. client, because the client is best able to identify his or her own needs and how to meet those needs.
○ 4. client, nurse, and physician, so the client can participate in planning care with the nurse and physician.

32. The most accurate indication that the client has learned how to give an insulin self-injection correctly is the client's ability to

○ 1. perform the procedure safely.
○ 2. critique the nurse's performance of the procedure.
○ 3. explain all steps of the procedure correctly.
○ 4. correctly answer a post-test about the procedure.

33. Angiotensin-converting enzyme inhibitors may be prescribed for the client to reduce vascular changes associated with diabetes mellitus and possibly prevent or delay development of

○ 1. chronic obstructive pulmonary disease.
○ 2. pancreatic cancer.
○ 3. renal failure.
○ 4. cerebral vascular accident.

34. The nurse should assess the client for which of the following problems, most likely to be related to diabetes mellitus?

○ 1. Cataracts.
○ 2. Retinopathy.
○ 3. Astigmatism.
○ 4. Blurred vision.

35. The nurse should teach the client that the most common symptoms of hypoglycemia are

○ 1. nervousness and diaphoresis.

○ 2. anorexia and incoherent speech.
○ 3. Kussmaul's respirations and confusion.
○ 4. bradycardia and blurred vision.

36. What is the most important reason why it is vital to recognize and treat hypoglycemia promptly in the client with diabetes mellitus?

○ 1. The client may become dehydrated quickly.
○ 2. Hypoglycemia can lead to brain damage.
○ 3. Hypoglycemia necessitates increased insulin dosage.
○ 4. The client may become confused, increasing the risk of injury.

37. When teaching the client how to manage her diabetes mellitus during episodes of minor illness such as colds or flu, the nurse should include which of the following measures in the teaching plan?

○ 1. Increase the frequency of blood or urine glucose testing.
○ 2. Try to reduce food intake to reduce nausea.
○ 3. Call the physician if glucose appears in the blood or urine.
○ 4. Stop taking long-acting insulin temporarily.

38. A priority nursing diagnosis category for this client would be

○ 1. Altered Nutrition.
○ 2. Ineffective Breathing Pattern.
○ 3. Pain.
○ 4. Activity Intolerance.

39. During a home visit, the client begins to cry and says, "I just cannot stand the thought of having to give myself a shot everyday." Which of the following would be the best response by the nurse?

○ 1. "If you do not give yourself your insulin shots, you will die."
○ 2. "We can teach your daughter to give the shots so you will not have to do it."
○ 3. "I can arrange to have a home care nurse give you the shots every day."
○ 4. "What is it about giving yourself the insulin shots that bothers you?"

40. The client comes to the emergency room with diabetic ketoacidosis. The nurse would identify which of the following nursing diagnosis categories as a priority problem?

○ 1. Sleep Pattern Disturbance.
○ 2. Altered Health Maintenance.
○ 3. Altered Nutrition.
○ 4. Fluid Volume Deficit.

The Client With Pituitary Adenoma

A 42-year-old male client is admitted for surgery to treat a pituitary tumor. On admission, he says that he is "happy the doctor finally discovered what's wrong." He had been experiencing symptoms for the last 5 months.

41. The client reports, with some embarrassment, that he has been experiencing mild galactorrhea. The nurse explains that this problem is caused by overproduction of which hormone?
- ○ 1. Prolactin.
- ○ 2. Adrenocorticotropic hormone (ACTH).
- ○ 3. Growth hormone (GH).
- ○ 4. Thyroid-stimulating hormone (TSH).

42. The nurse would anticipate that the client's primary symptoms were probably
- ○ 1. severe lethargy and fatigue.
- ○ 2. decreased libido and impotence.
- ○ 3. bony proliferation of the hands, jaw, and feet.
- ○ 4. deepening or coarsening of the voice.

43. The client is scheduled for a transsphenoidal hypophysectomy. The nurse would explain that the surgery will be performed through an incision in the
- ○ 1. back of the mouth.
- ○ 2. nose.
- ○ 3. sinus channel below the right eye.
- ○ 4. space between the upper gums and lip.

44. To help minimize the risk of postoperative respiratory complications, the nurse would focus the client's preoperative teaching on the importance of
- ○ 1. using blow bottles.
- ○ 2. making frequent position changes.
- ○ 3. deep breathing.
- ○ 4. coughing.

45. Which of the following would be a major focus of planning nursing care for the client after transsphenoidal hypophysectomy? Monitoring for
- ○ 1. cerebrospinal fluid leak.
- ○ 2. fluctuating blood glucose level.
- ○ 3. Cushing's syndrome.
- ○ 4. respiratory complications.

46. The client expresses concern about how surgery will affect his sexual ability. Which of the following statements provides the most accurate information about the physiologic effects of hypophysectomy?
- ○ 1. Removing the source of excess hormone will restore the client's natural potency and fertility.
- ○ 2. Potency will be restored, but the client will remain infertile.
- ○ 3. Fertility will be restored, but decreased libido and potency will persist.
- ○ 4. Exogenous hormones will be needed to restore potency after the adenoma is removed.

47. Before undergoing a transsphenoidal hypophysectomy for pituitary adenoma, the client asks the nurse how the surgeon closes the incision made in the dura. The nurse would respond based on the knowledge that
- ○ 1. dissolvable sutures are used to close the dura.

- ○ 2. the nasal packing provides pressure until normal wound healing occurs.
- ○ 3. a patch is made with a piece of fascia.
- ○ 4. a synthetic mesh is placed to facilitate healing.

48. Initial treatment for a cerebrospinal fluid leak after a transsphenoidal hypophysectomy for pituitary tumor would most likely involve
- ○ 1. repacking the nose.
- ○ 2. returning the client to surgery.
- ○ 3. enforcing bed rest with the head of the bed elevated.
- ○ 4. administering high-dose corticosteroid therapy.

49. Diabetes insipidus is a possible complication after pituitary surgery. For which symptom should the nurse observe to aid detection of diabetes insipidus?
- ○ 1. Urine specific gravity less than 1.010.
- ○ 2. Urine output between 1 and 2 liters per day.
- ○ 3. Blood glucose level above 300 mg/100 mL.
- ○ 4. Urine negative for glucose and ketones.

50. Vasopressin is administered to the client with diabetes insipidus because it acts to
- ○ 1. decrease tubular reabsorption of water.
- ○ 2. increase tubular reabsorption of water.
- ○ 3. increase release of insulin from the pancreas.
- ○ 4. decrease glucose production within the liver.

51. A priority outcome criterion for the client with diabetes insipidus would include which of the following?
- ○ 1. Maintains normal fluid balance.
- ○ 2. Selects American Diabetes Association diet correctly.
- ○ 3. States dietary restrictions.
- ○ 4. Exhibits serum glucose level within normal range.

52. Nursing care planning for a client recovering from transsphenoidal hypophysectomy would include which of the following?
- ○ 1. rinsing the mouth with saline solution.
- ○ 2. performing frequent toothbrushing.
- ○ 3. cleaning the teeth with an electric toothbrush.
- ○ 4. rinsing the mouth with peroxide.

53. The nurse teaches the client to monitor for signs and symptoms of which potential complication after hypophysectomy?
- ○ 1. Acromegaly.
- ○ 2. Cushing's disease.
- ○ 3. Diabetes mellitus.
- ○ 4. Hypopituitarism.

The Client With Addison's Disease

A 48-year-old salesman came down with what initially appeared to be a routine case of the flu. He awakened during the night extremely ill, anxious, and very weak. Afraid that he was dying, the man's wife drove him to the emergency room, where he is tentatively diagnosed as having Addison's disease and being in crisis.

54. Which of the following would be the priority goal for this client in the emergency room?
○ 1. Controlling hypertension.
○ 2. Preventing irreversible shock.
○ 3. Preventing infection.
○ 4. Relieving anxiety.

55. Which of the following would be an expected finding in this client?
○ 1. Fluid retention.
○ 2. Pain.
○ 3. Peripheral edema.
○ 4. Hunger.

56. The client is receiving an intravenous infusion of 5% dextrose in normal saline running at 125 mL/hour. When hanging a new bottle of fluid, the nurse notes swelling and hardness at the infusion site. Which immediate action would be indicated?
○ 1. Discontinue the infusion.
○ 2. Apply a warm dressing to the site.
○ 3. Stop the flow of solution temporarily.
○ 4. Irrigate the needle with normal saline.

57. The client's wife asks the nurse if the intravenous infusion is meeting her husband's nutritional needs because he has vomited several times. The nurse's response should be based on the knowledge that 1 liter of 5% dextrose in normal saline delivers
○ 1. 170 calories.
○ 2. 250 calories.
○ 3. 340 calories.
○ 4. 500 calories.

58. The client is admitted to the medical unit. The nurse formulates the nursing diagnosis Fluid Volume Deficit related to inadequate fluid intake and to fluid loss secondary to inadequate adrenal hormone secretion. As his oral intake increases, which of the following fluids would be most appropriate for the client?
○ 1. Milk and diet soda.
○ 2. Water and eggnog.
○ 3. Bouillon and juice.
○ 4. Coffee and milkshakes.

59. After stabilization of his condition, the client attends a stress management class because stress can precipitate addisonian crisis. Which of the following actions taught by the nurse in the class is based on principles of stress management?
○ 1. Remove all sources of stress from your life.
○ 2. Find alternative relaxation techniques such as music.
○ 3. Take antianxiety drugs daily.

○ 4. Avoid discussing stressful experiences.

60. When teaching the client newly diagnosed with primary Addison's disease, the nurse should explain that the disease results from
○ 1. insufficient secretion of adrenocorticotropic hormone (ACTH).
○ 2. dysfunction of the hypothalamic pituitary.
○ 3. idiopathic atrophy of the adrenal gland.
○ 4. oversecretion of the adrenal medulla.

61. The nurse would expect the client with Addison's disease to exhibit which of the following signs and symptoms?
○ 1. Weight gain and irritability.
○ 2. Hunger and double vision.
○ 3. Lethargy and depression.
○ 4. Muscle spasms and tetany.

62. All of the following results from routine blood tests would be typical of Addison's disease *except*
○ 1. hyperkalemia.
○ 2. hyponatremia.
○ 3. hyperglycemia.
○ 4. elevated blood urea nitrogen (BUN) level.

63. The client with Addison's disease who is taking glucocorticoids at home should base medication administration on the principle that
○ 1. various circumstances increase the need for glucocorticoids, so dosage adjustments will be needed.
○ 2. the need for glucocorticoids stabilizes, and a predetermined dose is taken every third day.
○ 3. glucocorticoids are cumulative, so a dose is taken every third day.
○ 4. a dose is taken every 6 hours because of the pattern of glucocorticoid secretion.

64. Cortisone acetate (Cortone Acetate) and fludrocortisone acetate (Florinef Acetate) are prescribed as replacement therapy for a client with Addison's disease. What administration schedule should be followed for this therapy?
○ 1. Take both drugs three times a day.
○ 2. Take the entire dose of both drugs first thing in the morning.
○ 3. Take all the fludrocortisone acetate and two-thirds of the cortisone acetate in the morning, and take the remaining cortisone acetate in the afternoon.
○ 4. Take half of each drug in the morning and the remaining half of each drug at bedtime.

65. The nurse should instruct the client taking oral glucocorticoids to take them
○ 1. with a full glass of water.
○ 2. on an empty stomach.
○ 3. between meals.
○ 4. with meals or an antacid.

66. Which of the following is the best indicator for determining whether a client with Addison's disease is receiving the correct amount of glucocorticoid replacement?

○ 1. Skin turgor.
○ 2. Temperature.
○ 3. Thirst.
○ 4. Daily weight.

67. Which of the following signs and symptoms would likely indicate that the client with Addison's disease is receiving too much glucocorticoid replacement?

○ 1. Anorexia.
○ 2. Dizziness.
○ 3. Rapid weight gain.
○ 4. Poor skin turgor.

68. A priority goal for the client with Addison's disease is

○ 1. Maintain medication compliance.
○ 2. Reduce daily activities to avoid overstressing the body.
○ 3. Follow a 2-g sodium diet.
○ 4. Prevent hypertensive episodes.

69. The client with Addison's disease should anticipate the need for increased glucocorticoid supplementation in which of the following situations?

○ 1. Returning to work after a weekend.
○ 2. Going on vacation.
○ 3. Having dental work performed.
○ 4. Having a routine medical checkup.

70. The nurse should teach the client with Addison's disease that the side effect of bronze-colored skin is thought to be due to

○ 1. hypersensitivity to sun exposure.
○ 2. increased serum bilirubin level.
○ 3. side effects of the glucocorticoid therapy.
○ 4. increased secretion of adrenocorticotropic hormone (ACTH).

71. A priority nursing diagnosis for the client during addisonian crisis would most likely be

○ 1. Self-Care Deficit related to weakness and fatigue.
○ 2. Altered Nutrition: More Than Body Requirements related to increased appetite.
○ 3. Altered Nutrition: More Than Body Requirements related to decreased exercise.
○ 4. Fluid Volume Excess related to reduced urinary excretion of fluid.

The Client With Cushing's Disease

A 42-year-old female client reports that she has gained weight and that her face and body are "rounder," while her legs and arms have become thinner. A tentative diagnosis of Cushing's disease is made.

72. When examining this client, the nurse would expect to find

○ 1. orthostatic hypotension.
○ 2. muscle hypertrophy in the extremities.
○ 3. bruised areas on the skin.
○ 4. decreased body hair.

73. Other signs and symptoms of Cushing's disease include

○ 1. weight loss.
○ 2. thin, fragile skin.
○ 3. hypotension.
○ 4. abdominal pain.

74. Cushing's disease can result from several different causes. Possible etiologies of Cushing's disease include all of the following *except*

○ 1. adrenal cortex atrophy.
○ 2. pituitary oversecretion of ACTH.
○ 3. adrenal gland tumor.
○ 4. high-dose steroid therapy.

75. Which of the following test results would be consistent with a diagnosis of Cushing's disease?

○ 1. Postprandial hypoglycemia.
○ 2. Hypokalemia.
○ 3. Hyponatremia.
○ 4. Decreased urinary calcium level.

76. The client tells the nurse that the physician said her morning serum cortisol level was within normal limits. She asks, "How can that be? I'm not imagining all these symptoms!" The nurse's response should be based on the knowledge that

○ 1. some clients are very sensitive to the effects of cortisol and develop symptoms even with normal levels.
○ 2. a single random blood test cannot provide reliable information about endocrine levels.
○ 3. the excessive cortisol in Cushing's disease commonly results from loss of the normal diurnal secretion pattern.
○ 4. tumors tend to secrete hormones irregularly, and the hormones are often not present in the blood.

77. The woman's diet needs to be modified to control her symptoms. Which diet would be most appropriate?

○ 1. High protein, high calorie, and restricted sodium.
○ 2. High protein, low calorie, and restricted sodium.
○ 3. High protein, high calorie, and high potassium.
○ 4. Low protein, restricted sodium, and high potassium.

78. Bone resorption is a possible complication of Cushing's disease. To counter the damage done by the disease, the nurse should encourage the client to

○ 1. increase the amount of calcium in the diet.
○ 2. maintain a regular program of weight-bearing exercise.

○ 3. limit her dietary phosphate intake.

○ 4. include isometric exercise in her daily routine.

The client has been found to have an adrenal tumor and is scheduled for a bilateral adrenalectomy.

79. The nurse begins extensive preoperative teaching, which includes the importance of deep breathing. Which of the following would be the most accurate instructions?

○ 1. "Sit in an upright position and take a deep breath."

○ 2. "Hold your abdomen firmly and take several deep breaths."

○ 3. "Tighten your stomach muscles as you inhale and breathe normally."

○ 4. "Raise your shoulders to expand your chest."

80. A priority goal in the first 24 hours after the client undergoes a bilateral adrenalectomy is to

○ 1. begin oral nutrition.

○ 2. promote self-care activities.

○ 3. prevent adrenal crisis.

○ 4. ambulate in the hallway.

81. The client's postoperative orders include an order for hydromorphone hydrochloride (Dilaudid), 2 mg given subcutaneously every 4 hours p.r.n. for pain. This drug is administered in relatively small doses primarily because it is

○ 1. less likely to cause dependency in small doses.

○ 2. less irritating to subcutaneous tissues in small doses.

○ 3. as potent as most other analgesics in larger doses.

○ 4. excreted before accumulating in toxic amounts in the body.

82. Which of the following factors would be most important in selecting the needle length to use for a subcutaneous injection of hydromorphone hydrochloride?

○ 1. The diameter of the needle.

○ 2. The amount of adipose tissue at the administration site.

○ 3. The viscosity of the solution to be injected.

○ 4. The amount of medication to be administered.

83. The nurse should recognize that the most probable cause of temperature elevation in the early postoperative period is

○ 1. dehydration.

○ 2. poor lung expansion.

○ 3. wound infection.

○ 4. urinary tract infection.

84. The client recovering from a bilateral adrenalectomy now has a patient-controlled analgesia system with morphine sulfate. Priority nursing actions for the client would include

○ 1. observing the client at regular intervals for narcotic addiction.

○ 2. encouraging the client to reduce analgesic use and tolerate the pain.

○ 3. evaluating pain control at least every 2 hours.

○ 4. increasing the amount of morphine if the client does not administer the medication.

85. After surgery for bilateral adrenalectomy, the client is kept on bed rest for several days to stabilize the body's need for steroids postoperatively. Which of the following exercises has been found to be especially helpful in preparing a client for ambulation after a period of bed rest? Alternately

○ 1. flexing and extending the knees.

○ 2. abducting and adducting the legs.

○ 3. tensing and relaxing the Achilles tendons.

○ 4. flexing and relaxing the quadriceps femoris muscles.

86. As the nurse helps the postoperative client out of bed, the client complains of gas pains in her abdomen. The most effective nursing intervention to relieve this discomfort would be to

○ 1. encourage the client to ambulate.

○ 2. insert a rectal tube.

○ 3. insert a nasogastric tube.

○ 4. encourage the client to drink carbonated liquids.

87. Because of steroid excess, the client who has undergone a bilateral adrenalectomy is at an increased risk for

○ 1. postoperative confusion.

○ 2. delayed wound healing.

○ 3. emboli.

○ 4. malnutrition.

88. The client who has undergone a bilateral adrenalectomy is nearing discharge. She tells the nurse that she is concerned about persistent body changes and the fact that her moods are still so unpredictable. She says, "I thought surgery was supposed to fix all that." The most appropriate nursing goal for this client would be to help her accept that

○ 1. her body changes are permanent.

○ 2. her body and mood will gradually return to near normal.

○ 3. the physical changes are permanent, but the mood swings will disappear.

○ 4. the physical changes are temporary, but the mood swings are permanent.

89. After bilateral adrenalectomy for Cushing's disease, the client is told by her physician that she needs periodic testosterone injections. She asks the nurse, "What is that for? Did he forget I'm a woman?" What would be the nurse's best response? "Androgens are

○ 1. needed to balance the reproductive cycle."

○ 2. needed to restore the body's sodium and potassium balance."

○ 3. given to stimulate protein anabolism."

○ 4. given to stabilize mood swings."

90. Which of the following should the nurse include in the client's teaching plan?

○ 1. Emphasizing that the client will need steroid replacement for the rest of her life.

○ 2. Instructing the client about the importance of tapering steroid medication carefully to prevent crisis.

○ 3. Informing the client that steroids will be required only until her body can manufacture sufficient quantities.

○ 4. Emphasizing that the client will need to take steroids whenever her life involves physical or emotional stress.

CORRECT ANSWERS AND RATIONALE

The letters in parentheses following the rationale identify the step of the nursing process (A, D, P, I, E), cognitive level (K, C, T, N), and client needs (S, G, L, H). See the Answer Grid for the key.

The Client With Hyperthyroidism

1. 2. Hyperthyroidism is a state of hypermetabolism. Graves' disease is the most common type of hyperthyroidism. The increased metabolic rate generates heat and produces tachycardia and fine muscle tremors. It also causes weight loss and increased appetite. Anorexia and goiter are associated with hypothyroidism. (A, T, G)

2. 3. A change in the menstrual interval, diminished menstrual flow (oligomenorrhea), or even the absence of menstruation (amenorrhea) may result from the hormonal imbalances of hyperthyroidism. Dysmenorrhea is painful menstruation. Metrorrhagia is blood loss between menstrual periods, and menorrhagia is excessive bleeding during menstrual periods. (A, T, G)

3. 1. Two serious side effects of propylthiouracil are leukopenia and agranulocytosis. The client should be taught to promptly report any signs and symptoms of infection, such as a sore throat and fever, because the drug must be discontinued if adverse reactions occur. Other side effects include skin rash, edema, and enlarged salivary and lymph nodes. Painful menstruation, constipation, abdominal distention, increased urine output, and itching are not associated with propylthiouracil therapy. (I, T, S)

4. 2. A typical sign of hyperthyroidism is irritability due to the high level of thyroid hormone in the body. Such behavior decreases as the client responds to therapy. The other explanations for this client's behavior are not satisfactory. (I, N, L)

5. 1. A client is likely to have falsely elevated RAIU and PBI tests if he or she has taken a medication containing iodine within the past month or so. Many medications can falsely elevate or depress test results, but medications containing iodine are most commonly used by clients with hyperthyroidism. Digitalis, antihistamines, and ferrous sulfate do not influence these tests. The RAIU and PBI tests are used to evaluate thyroid function. (A, T, S)

6. 3. Because the eyelids tend to not close completely during sleep in exophthalmos, they should be taped shut to prevent drying. Sleeping masks have also proved helpful for some people. Massaging the eyes,

instilling ointment into the eyes, and covering the eyes with moist gauze pads are not satisfactory nursing measures to protect the eyes of a client with exophthalmos during sleep. (I, T, G)

7. 4. Sodium iodide I 131 destroys the thyroid tissue, and thyroid hormones are no longer produced. (I, T, G)

8. 4. Management of the disease process is a priority for the client after therapy with sodium iodide I 131. Signs of hyperthyroidism persist until thyroid hormone production stops. At that time, the client will need to be able to recognize symptoms of hypothyroidism and will need thyroid replacement hormones for life. Significant changes in level of consciousness and breathing pattern are not expected. The client does not need to be immobilized following radioactive treatment. (D, N, H)

9. 3. The client needs to be informed that she will need thyroid replacement hormone for the remainder of her life. (I, T, G)

10. 2. SSKI is frequently administered before a thyroidectomy because it helps decrease the vascularity of the thyroid gland. A highly vascular thyroid gland is very friable, a condition that presents a hazard during surgery. SSKI does not decrease the progression of exophthalmos, decrease the body's ability to store thyroxine, or increase the body's ability to excrete thyroxine. (P, T, G)

11. 3. SSKI should be well diluted in milk, water, juice, or a carbonated beverage before administration to help disguise the strong, bitter taste. Also, this drug is irritating to mucosa if taken undiluted. The client should sip the diluted preparation through a drinking straw to help prevent staining of the teeth. (I, T, G)

12. 3. Laryngeal nerve damage is a potential complication of thyroid surgery because of the proximity of the thyroid gland and the recurrent laryngeal nerve. Asking the client to speak helps assess for signs of laryngeal nerve damage. The client's level of consciousness can be partially assessed by asking her to speak, but in this situation, this is not the primary reason for doing so. (I, T, G)

13. 4. Equipment for an emergency tracheostomy should be kept in the room, in the event that tracheal edema and airway occlusion occur. The other equipment is not used in the anticipated emergency care. (P, T, S)

14. 2. Tetany may occur after thyroidectomy if the parathyroid glands are accidentally injured or re-

moved during surgery. This would cause a disturbance in calcium metabolism. An early sign of tetany is numbness with tingling of the fingers and in the circumoral region. (A, T, G)

15. 2. The client with tetany is suffering from hypocalcemia, which is treated by administering a preparation of calcium, such as calcium gluconate. (I, T, G)

16. 2. Typical symptoms of hypothyroidism include weight gain, fatigue, apathy, brittle nails, dry skin, and numbness and tingling in the fingers. (A, K, G)

17. 4. A major problem for the person with hypothyroidism is fatigue. Other signs and symptoms include lethargy, personality changes, generalized edema, impaired memory, slowed speech, cold intolerance, dry skin, muscle weakness, constipation, weight gain, and hair loss. Incomplete closure of the eyelids, hypermetabolism, and diarrhea are associated with hyperthyroidism. (D, N, G)

18. 4. Hypothyroidism may contribute to sadness and depression. This client needs to know that these feelings may be related to her low thyroid hormone levels and may improve with treatment. (I, T, L)

The Client With Diabetes Mellitus

19. 3. Oral hypoglycemic agents of the sulfonylurea group, such as tolbutamide (Orinase), lower blood glucose level by stimulating pancreatic cells to release insulin. These agents also increase insulin's ability to bind to the body's cells, thereby increasing the number of insulin receptors in the body. (P, K, G)

20. 1. The client with diabetes is prone to serious foot problems when circulation is impaired because the foot becomes insensitive to temperature and pressure. The client should be taught to avoid going barefoot to prevent injury. Other interventions for proper foot care include wearing properly fitting shoes, using mild soap with warm water to wash the feet, and inspecting the feet daily. (I, T, H)

21. 2. A client with diabetes should be advised to consult the physician for corn removal because of the danger of traumatizing foot tissue. (I, T, G)

22. 2. Proper and careful first-aid treatment is important when a client with diabetes has a skin break; the client should be taught to consult a physician promptly if any signs of infection, such as redness, swelling, pain, or blistering, occur. The client with diabetes should understand that any skin break, no matter how small, warrants concern. (I, N, G)

23. 4. A disease of glucose intolerance, diabetes mellitus affects the metabolism of carbohydrates, fats, and proteins. The client's diet should contain appropriate amounts of all three nutrients, plus adequate minerals and vitamins. The nurse evaluates that the client does not understand his diet and needs further instructions. (I, C, G)

24. 2. Special foods are not required for a client with diabetes, nor should certain foods (except refined sugars) be eliminated entirely from the diet. More important is that mealtimes, meal size, and meal composition be consistent. Pasta may be included in the diet as part of the bread and cereal exchange. For example, one-half cup of pasta is equivalent to one slice of bread. Pasta sauces may be used if they are taken into account in the total diet. A client's ethnic, religious, and cultural food preferences should be taken into account in meal planning. If these preferences are not considered, a client may eat foods without making proper adjustments or may reject the diet entirely. (I, N, G)

25. 4. A client with diabetes who takes tolbutamide should be advised to limit alcohol intake. Tolbutamide in combination with alcohol can cause hypoglycemia. (I, T, G)

26. 3. Factors predisposing to the development of adult-onset diabetes mellitus include obesity. Cigarette smoking and hypertension are not predisposing factors. Factors such as a high-cholesterol diet and sedentary lifestyle do not predispose to diabetes mellitus but may contribute to obesity. (A, C, H)

27. 2. The client with diabetes mellitus is especially prone to hypertension due to atherosclerotic changes. Atherosclerotic complications such as hypertension, myocardial infarction, cerebrovascular accident, uremia, and gangrene, are reported to cause 70% of deaths in people with diabetes mellitus. Mortality from cardiovascular and renal complications is rising in people with diabetes mellitus. (A, K, G)

28. 4. Exercise increases the use of blood glucose by the muscles and therefore reduces the body's insulin requirements. Exercise also tends to lower blood cholesterol and triglyceride levels, which is especially important for clients with diabetes mellitus because they are prone to cardiovascular disease. In addition, exercise is a healthful diversional activity, helps control weight, and promotes circulation. The client should be taught the effects of exercise on blood glucose levels and the importance of snacking before exercise, unless the amount and time of exercise is the same every day and has already been taken into account when determining the dosage of hypoglycemic agents. (I, C, G)

29. 1. Foods high in dietary fiber are recommended by the American Diabetes Association because they tend to blunt the rise in blood glucose levels after meals. Dietary fiber is the part of food not broken down and absorbed during digestion. Most fibers come from plants; good sources include whole grains, legumes, vegetables, fruits, and nuts. Poor sources of fiber include dairy products and meats. Foods fortified with vitamins are satisfactory if they also contain fiber. However, many foods fortified with vitamins contain either no dietary fiber (such as fortified milk) or little fiber (such as products fortified with vitamins but made with refined grains). (I, C, G)

30. 4. The client with diabetes mellitus taking NPH insulin in the evening is most likely to become hypoglycemic shortly after midnight because this insulin peaks in 8 to 12 hours. (I, T, G)

31. 4. Learning goals are most likely to be attained when they are established mutually by the client and members of the health care team, including the nurse and the physician. Learning is motivated by perceived problems or goals arising out of unmet needs. The perception of the unmet needs must be the client's; the nurse and physician help the client arrive at his own perception of the need or reason to learn. (P, N, H)

32. 1. The nurse would judge that learning has occurred from evidence of a change in the client's behavior. A client who performs a procedure safely demonstrates that he or she has acquired a skill. Evaluating skill acquisition requires performance of that skill. (E, T, H)

33. 3. Renal failure frequently results from the vascular changes associated with diabetes mellitus. Mortality in people with diabetes mellitus due to renal and cardiovascular diseases is increasing. Heart disease and stroke are twice as common among people with diabetes mellitus than among people without the disease. Damage to organs such as the liver, lungs, and pancreas is less life-threatening. (I, C, G)

34. 2. The leading cause of blindness in the United States is diabetes mellitus, and the major cause of blindness in people with diabetes mellitus is diabetic retinopathy. Corneal problems, cataracts, refractive changes, and extraocular muscle changes are also noted. Astigmatism has not been associated with diabetes mellitus. (A, C, G)

35. 1. The four most commonly reported signs and symptoms of hypoglycemia are nervousness, weakness, perspiration, and confusion. Other signs and symptoms include hunger, incoherent speech, tachycardia, and blurred vision. Anorexia and Kussmaul's respirations are clinical manifestations of hyperglycemia or ketoacidosis. (I, T, G)

36. 2. Hypoglycemia is dangerous because it can lead to permanent brain damage. Changes in cerebral function occur because the brain uses glucose for metabolism and is unable to use alternative sources of energy as well as glucose. Prompt treatment of hypoglycemia is essential to prevent cellular dam-

age. Although injury due to confusion is a concern, it is not the most important reason for prompt treatment of hypoglycemia. Dehydration is more frequently associated with hyperglycemia. Hypoglycemia is treated with glucose or glucagon, not insulin. (I, N, G)

37. 1. Colds and influenza present special challenges to the client with diabetes mellitus because the body's need for insulin increases during illness. Therefore, the client must take the prescribed insulin dose, increase the frequency of blood or urine testing, maintain an adequate fluid intake to counteract the dehydrating effect of hyperglycemia, and contact the physician if urine ketone levels rise significantly. (I, N, H)

38. 1. Altered Nutrition is a priority diagnosis for this client with adult-onset diabetes mellitus. (D, T, G)

39. 4. The best response would be to allow the client to verbalize her fears about giving herself a shot each day. If possible, the client needs to be responsible for her own care, including giving her own injections. Using tactics that will increase fear are not effective in changing behavior. (I, T, L)

40. 4. Fluid Volume Deficit, or dehydration, is the main problem in diabetic ketoacidosis because increased osmolarity from the glucose leads to a fluid shift from the intracellular to the extracellular space. The fluid shift leads to increased renal excretion of glucose and fluid. Severe dehydration is a medical emergency requiring immediate insulin and fluid administration. (D, N, G)

The Client With Pituitary Adenoma

41. 1. Galactorrhea, or abnormal flow of breast milk, results from overproduction of prolactin. Pituitary tumors can cause oversecretion of adrenocorticotropic hormone (ACTH), growth hormone (GH), and thyroid-stimulating hormone (TSH). Prolactin-secreting tumors account for 30% to 50% of pituitary adenomas. (I, T, G)

42. 2. Excessive prolactin secretion in males results in decreased libido and impotence; these are often the only significant symptoms until the tumor becomes large. Bony alterations and voice changes are associated with excessive growth hormone. (A, T, G)

43. 4. With transsphenoidal hypophysectomy, the sella turcica is entered from below, through the sphenoid sinus. There is no external incision; the incision is made between the upper lip and gums. (P, C, G)

44. 3. Deep breathing helps prevent atelectasis, but coughing is contraindicated because it increases intracranial pressure. Increased intracranial pressure should be avoided because it increases pressure on the graft site. The opening made in the dura mater

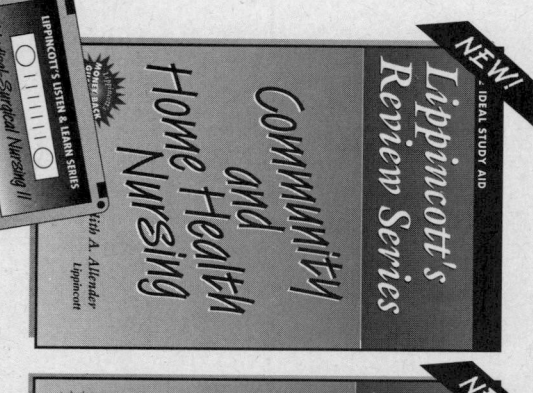
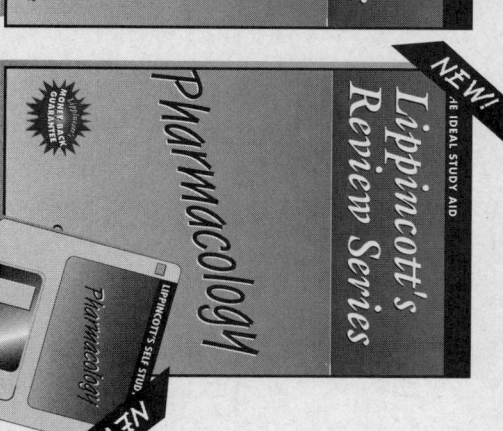
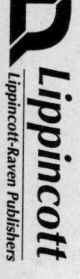

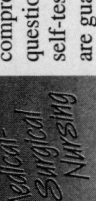
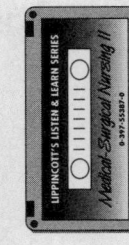
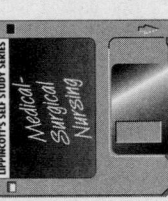

on entering the sella turcica is frequently patched with a piece of fascia from the leg. Blow bottles are not effective in preventing atelectasis because they do not promote sustained alveolar inflation to maximal lung capacity. Frequent position changes help loosen lung secretions, but deep breathing is most important in preventing atelectasis. (I, T, S)

45. 1. A major focus of nursing care after transsphenoidal hypophysectomy is preventing and monitoring for a cerebrospinal fluid leak. Hypoglycemia and adrenocortical insufficiency may occur. Monitoring for postoperative respiratory complications is always important but is not related specifically to transsphenoidal hypophysectomy. (P, N, G)

46. 1. The client's sexual problems are directly related to the excessive prolactin level. Removing the source of excessive hormone secretion should allow the client to return gradually to a normal physiologic pattern, but psychological effects may persist. (I, T, L)

47. 3. The dural opening is typically repaired with a patch of muscle or fascia taken from the leg. The client should be prepared preoperatively for the presence of a leg incision. (I, T, S)

48. 3. Significant or persistent cerebrospinal fluid leaks are treated initially with bed rest, with the head of the bed elevated to decrease pressure on the graft site. Most leaks heal spontaneously, but occasionally surgical repair is needed. (I, T, G)

49. 1. Major manifestations of diabetes insipidus are polyuria and polydipsia. The polyuria leads to a decreased urine specific gravity (between 1.001 and 1.010). The client may drink and excrete 5 to 40 liters of fluid daily. Diabetes insipidus does not affect metabolism. Blood glucose level above 250 mg/100 mL is associated with ketoacidosis. Urine negative for sugar and acetone is normal. (A, T, G)

50. 2. Vasopressin is administered to the client with diabetes insipidus because it acts to increase tubular reabsorption of water. (P, T, G)

51. 1. Because diabetes insipidus involves excretion of large amounts of fluid, maintaining normal fluid balance is a priority for this client. Dietary restrictions and serum glucose levels are priorities in diabetes mellitus but not in diabetes insipidus. (E, T, G)

52. 1. After transsphenoidal surgery, the client must be careful not to disturb the suture line while healing occurs. Frequent oral care will be provided with rinses of saline, and the teeth may be gently cleaned with Toothettes, but frequent and vigorous toothbrushing is contraindicated. (P, T, G)

53. 4. Most clients who undergo adenoma removal experience a gradual return of normal pituitary secretion, but the development of hypopituitarism is a possibility that should be monitored. There would

be no reason for the excessive secretion of other hormones. (I, T, H)

The Client With Addison's Disease

54. 2. Addison's disease is caused by a deficiency of adrenocortical hormone. Causes of this deficiency include surgical removal of the adrenal cortex or its destruction from infection, such as histoplasmosis. Immediate treatment for the client in addisonian crisis is directed toward combating shock by restoring circulating volume and administering hydrocortisone. Hypotension occurs due to shock. Relieving anxiety is appropriate when the client's condition is stabilized, but the calm, competent demeanor of the emergency department staff will be initially reassuring. Preventing infection is not an appropriate goal in this situation. (P, N, G)

55. 2. Adrenal hormone deficiency can cause profound changes. The client may experience severe pain (headache, abdominal pain, back pain, or pain in the extremities). Inhibited gluconeogenesis commonly produces hypoglycemia, and impaired sodium retention causes decreased fluid volume and hypotension. Edema would not be expected. Gastrointestinal disturbances are expected findings in Addison's disease. (A, C, G)

56. 1. Signs of infiltration include slowing of the infusion and swelling, pain, hardness, pallor, and coolness of the skin at the site. If these signs occur, the intravenous line should be discontinued and restarted at another infusion site. (I, T, S)

57. 1. Each liter of 5% dextrose in normal saline solution contains 170 calories. (I, K, G)

58. 3. Electrolyte imbalances associated with Addison's disease include hypoglycemia, hyponatremia, and hyperkalemia. Salted bouillon and fruit juices provide glucose and sodium to replenish these deficits. Water could cause further sodium dilution. Coffee's diuretic effect would aggravate the fluid deficit. Milk contains potassium and sodium, and diet soda does not contain sugar. (I, N, G)

59. 2. Finding alternative methods of dealing with stress, such as relaxation techniques, is a cornerstone of stress management. Removing all sources of stress from one's life is not possible. Avoiding discussion of stressful situations will not necessarily reduce stress. Antianxiety drugs are prescribed by physicians, not as a part of stress management classes. (I, N, L)

60. 3. Primary disease refers to a problem in the gland itself. Primary Addison's disease occurs from idiopathic atrophy of the glands. The process is believed to be autoimmune in nature. Pituitary dysfunction can cause Addison's disease, but this is not a primary disease process. (I, K, G)

61. 3. The onset of Addison's disease is usually insidious, and this disease is relatively asymptomatic until a major stressor such as illness triggers a crisis. Although many of the disease symptoms are vague and nonspecific, most clients experience lethargy and depression as early symptoms. Other early symptoms include irritability, weight loss, nausea, and vomiting. (A, K, G)

62. 3. Hyperkalemia and hyponatremia are characteristic of Addison's disease. There is decreased renal perfusion and excretion of waste products, which causes the BUN to elevate. Decreased hepatic gluconeogenesis and increased tissue glucose uptake cause hypoglycemia, not hyperglycemia, which is associated with cortisol excess. (A, C, G)

63. 1. The need for glucocorticoids changes with circumstances. The basal dose is established when the client is discharged, but this dose covers only normal daily needs and does not provide for additional stressors. As the manager of the medication schedule, the client needs to know signs of excessive and insufficient dosages. Glucocorticoids are not cumulative and must be taken daily. They must never be discontinued suddenly; in the absence of endogenous production, addisonian crisis could result. Glucocorticoids are taken daily, with two thirds of the daily dose taken at about 8 AM and the remainder at about 4 PM. This schedule stimulates the diurnal pattern of normal secretion, with highest levels between 4 AM and 6 AM and lowest levels in the evening. (I, N, H)

64. 3. Fludrocortisone acetate can be administered once a day, but cortisone acetate administration should follow the body's natural diurnal pattern of secretion, with greater amounts secreted during the day to meet increased demand. Typically, baseline administration of cortisone acetate is 25 mg in the morning and 12.5 mg in the afternoon. (I, C, G)

65. 4. Oral steroids have pronounced ulcerogenic properties and should be administered with meals, if possible, or otherwise with an antacid. They should never be taken on an empty stomach. (I, T, H)

66. 4. Measuring daily weight is a reliable, objective way to monitor fluid balance. Rapid variations in weight reflect changes in fluid volume. Tongue turgor is a more reliable indicator of fluid volume changes than skin turgor in older people, whose skin is less elastic. Temperature is not a direct measurement of fluid balance. (E, T, H)

67. 3. A client taking glucocorticoids walks a fine line between underdosage and overdosage. Fluid balance is an important indicator of the adequacy of hormone replacement. Rapid weight gain is a warn-

ing sign that the client is receiving too much hormone replacement. (E, T, G)

68. 1. Medication compliance is an essential part of the self-care required to manage Addison's disease. The client must learn to adjust the glucocorticoid dose in response to the normal and unexpected stresses of daily living. Regularity in daily habits will make adjustment easier, but the client should not be encouraged to withdraw from normal activities to avoid stress. (P, T, H)

69. 3. Illness or surgery places tremendous stress on the body, necessitating increased glucocorticoid dosage. Dental work is a good example. Extreme emotional or psychological stress will also necessitate dosage adjustment. (P, T, S)

70. 4. Bronzing, or general deepening of skin pigmentation, is a classic sign of Addison's disease and is due to melanocyte-stimulating hormone produced in response to increased ACTH secretion. The hyperpigmentation is typically found in the distal portion of extremities and areas exposed to sun. Additionally, areas that may not be exposed to sun, such as the nipples, genitalia, tongue, and knuckles, become bronze-colored. Treatment of Addison's disease usually reverses the hyperpigmentation. (I, T, G)

71. 1. Weakness and fatigue are major problems for the client experiencing addisonian crisis. A client in crisis requires bed rest until the crisis has been resolved. Fluid volume deficit and nausea and vomiting are other problems during crisis. (D, N, G)

The Client With Cushing's Disease

72. 3. Skin bruising from increased skin and blood vessel fragility is a classic sign of Cushing's disease. Muscle wasting occurs in the extremities, and fluid retention causes hypertension. Hair on the head typically thins, while body hair increases. (A, T, G)

73. 2. In Cushing's disease, excessive cortisol secretion causes rapid protein catabolism, depleting the collagen support of the skin. The skin becomes thin and fragile and susceptible to easy bruising. Weight gain, mood swings, and slow wound healing are other symptoms of Cushing's disease. (A, K, G)

74. 1. Cushing's disease is caused by hormone oversecretion, which can be caused by a tumor, overstimulation from the pituitary, or the use of prescription steroid drugs. It does not result from glandular atrophy. (A, T, G)

75. 2. Sodium retention is typically accompanied by potassium depletion. The client with Cushing's disease exhibits postprandial or persistent hyperglycemia, and bone resorption of calcium increases the urine calcium load. Kidney stones also may form. (A, T, S)

76. 3. The most prominent feature of Cushing's disease is often the loss of the diurnal cortisol secretion pattern. The client's random morning cortisol level may be within normal limits, but secretion continues at that level throughout the entire day. Twenty-four–hour urine collections are often useful in identifying the cumulative excess. (I, T, G)

77. 2. Primary dietary interventions include reducing weight by restricting total calories and reducing water weight by restricting sodium. Increased protein catabolism necessitates supplemental protein intake. In addition, the client should be encouraged to eat potassium-rich foods because serum levels are typically depleted. (P, T, G)

78. 2. Osteoporosis is a serious outcome of prolonged cortisol excess because calcium is resorbed out of the bone. Regular daily weight-bearing exercise is the most effective way to drive calcium back into the bones. (I, T, H)

79. 2. Effective splinting for a high incision reduces stress on the incision line, reduces pain, and increases the client's ability to deep breathe effectively. Deep breathing should be done hourly by the client after surgery. (I, T, G)

80. 3. The primary goal in the first 24 hours after adrenalectomy is to identify and prevent adrenal crisis. Monitoring vital signs is the most important evaluation measure; the other interventions are either not a priority or inappropriate during the first postoperative day. (P, N, G)

81. 3. Hydromorphone hydrochloride is about five times more potent than morphine sulfate, from which it is prepared. Thus, it is administered only in small doses. It has the same, but generally less severe, side effects as morphine. (I, C, G)

82. 2. Needle length depends on the amount of adipose tissue at the site and the angle at which the injection is given. The viscosity of the medication determines the needle diameter. The amount of medication could influence the injection site, which, in turn, could affect the needle length; however, this is not the most important factor in this situation. (I, C, S)

83. 2. Pulmonary problems become evident in the early postoperative period. Poor lung expansion from bed rest, pain, and retained anesthesia is a common cause of slight postoperative temperature elevation. Wound infections typically appear 4 to 7 days after surgery. (A, C, G)

84. 3. Pain control should be evaluated at least every 2 hours for the client with a patient-controlled analgesia system. Addiction is not a common problem for the postoperative client. A client should not be encouraged to tolerate pain; in fact, other nursing actions besides patient-controlled analgesia should be implemented to enhance the action of narcotics. Such nursing actions include providing back rubs, position changes, and a calm, restful environment. One of the purposes of patient-controlled analgesia is for the patient to determine frequency of administering the medication; the nurse should not interfere unless the patient is not obtaining pain relief. (I, T, G)

85. 4. Alternately flexing and relaxing the quadriceps muscles helps prepare the client for ambulation. The other exercises listed do nothing to increase a client's readiness for walking. (I, T, S)

86. 1. Decreased mobility is one of the most common causes of abdominal distention. Ambulation increases peristaltic activity and helps move gas. (I, T, G)

87. 2. Persistent cortisol excess undermines the collagen matrix of the skin, impairing wound healing. It also carries an increased risk of infection and of bleeding. (I, T, G)

88. 2. As the body readjusts to normal cortisol levels, mood and many physical changes will gradually return to a near-normal state. (P, N, L)

89. 3. The testosterone is needed not to support sexual functioning but to support protein anabolism. Thus, it is needed by both males and females. (I, T, H)

90. 1. Bilateral adrenalectomy requires lifelong adrenal hormone replacement therapy. If unilateral surgery is performed, most clients gradually reestablish a normal secretion pattern. (P, N, G)

NURSING CARE OF ADULTS WITH MEDICAL AND SURGICAL HEALTH PROBLEMS

TEST 6: The Client With Endocrine Health Problems

Directions: Use this answer grid to determine areas of strength or need for further study.

NURSING PROCESS

A = Assessment
D = Analysis, nursing diagnosis
P = Planning
I = Implementation
E = Evaluation

COGNITIVE LEVEL

K = Knowledge
C = Comprehension
T = Application
N = Analysis

CLIENT NEEDS

S = Safe, effective care environment
G = Physiologic integrity
L = Psychosocial integrity
H = Health promotion and maintenance

Question #	Answer #	Nursing Process					Cognitive Level				Client Needs			
		A	**D**	**P**	**I**	**E**	**K**	**C**	**T**	**N**	**S**	**G**	**L**	**H**
1	2	A							T			G		
2	3	A							T			G		
3	1				I				T		S			
4	2				I					N			L	
5	1	A							T		S			
6	3				I				T			G		
7	4				I				T			G		
8	4		D							N				H
9	3				I				T			G		
10	2			P					T			G		
11	3				I				T			G		
12	3				I				T			G		
13	4			P					T		S			
14	2	A							T			G		
15	2				I				T			G		
16	2	A					K					G		
17	4		D							N		G		
18	4				I				T				L	
19	3			P			K					G		
20	1				I				T					H
21	2				I				T			G		
22	2				I					N		G		
23	4				I			C				G		
24	2				I					N		G		
25	4				I				T			G		

ANSWER GRID: 1

NURSING PROCESS

A = Assessment
D = Analysis, nursing diagnosis
P = Planning
I = Implementation
E = Evaluation

COGNITIVE LEVEL

K = Knowledge
C = Comprehension
T = Application
N = Analysis

CLIENT NEEDS

S = Safe, effective care environment
G = Physiologic integrity
L = Psychosocial integrity
H = Health promotion and maintenance

Question #	Answer #	Nursing Process					Cognitive Level				Client Needs			
		A	D	P	I	E	K	C	T	N	S	G	L	H
26	3	A						C						H
27	2	A					K					G		
28	4				I			C				G		
29	1				I			C				G		
30	4				I				T			G		
31	4			P						N				H
32	1					E			T					H
33	3				I			C				G		
34	2	A						C				G		
35	1				I				T			G		
36	2				I					N		G		
37	1				I					N				H
38	1		D						T			G		
39	4				I				T				L	
40	4		D							N		G		
41	1				I				T			G		
42	2	A							T			G		
43	4			P				C				G		
44	3				I				T		S			
45	1			P						N		G		
46	1				I				T				L	
47	3				I				T		S			
48	3				I				T			G		
49	1	A							T			G		
50	2			P					T			G		
51	1					E			T			G		
52	1			P					T			G		
53	4				I				T					H
54	2			P						N		G		
55	2	A						C				G		

ANSWER GRID: 2

NURSING PROCESS

A = Assessment
D = Analysis, nursing diagnosis
P = Planning
I = Implementation
E = Evaluation

COGNITIVE LEVEL

K = Knowledge
C = Comprehension
T = Application
N = Analysis

CLIENT NEEDS

S = Safe, effective care environment
G = Physiologic integrity
L = Psychosocial integrity
H = Health promotion and maintenance

Question #	Answer #	Nursing Process					Cognitive Level				Client Needs			
		A	D	P	I	E	K	C	T	N	S	G	L	H
56	1				I				T		S			
57	1				I		K					G		
58	3				I					N		G		
59	2				I					N			L	
60	3				I		K					G		
61	3	A					K					G		
62	3	A						C				G		
63	1				I					N				H
64	3				I			C				G		
65	4				I				T					H
66	4					E			T					H
67	3					E			T			G		
68	1			P					T					H
69	3			P					T		S			
70	4				I				T			G		
71	1		D							N		G		
72	3	A							T			G		
73	2	A					K					G		
74	1	A							T			G		
75	2	A							T		S			
76	3				I				T			G		
77	2			P					T			G		
78	2				I				T					H
79	2				I				T			G		
80	3			P						N		G		
81	3				I			C				G		
82	2				I			C			S			
83	2	A						C				G		
84	3				I				T			G		
85	4				I				T		S			

ANSWER GRID: 3

NURSING PROCESS

A = Assessment
D = Analysis, nursing diagnosis
P = Planning
I = Implementation
E = Evaluation

COGNITIVE LEVEL

K = Knowledge
C = Comprehension
T = Application
N = Analysis

CLIENT NEEDS

S = Safe, effective care environment
G = Physiologic integrity
L = Psychosocial integrity
H = Health promotion and maintenance

Question #	Answer #	Nursing Process					Cognitive Level				Client Needs			
		A	D	P	I	E	K	C	T	N	S	G	L	H
86	1				I				T			G		
87	2				I				T			G		
88	2			P						N			L	
89	3				I				T					H
90	1			P						N		G		
Number Correct														
Number Possible	90	18	5	15	48	4	7	13	52	18	10	61	6	13
Percentage Correct														

Score Calculation: To determine your **Percentage Correct,** divide the **Number Correct** by the **Number Possible.**

ANSWER GRID: 4

The Client With Urinary Tract Health Problems

- The Client With Cancer of the Bladder
- The Client With Renal Calculi
- The Client With Acute Renal Failure
- The Client With Urinary Tract Infection
- The Client With Pyelonephritis
- The Client With Chronic Renal Failure
- The Client With Urinary Incontinence
- Correct Answers and Rationale

Select the one best answer, and indicate your choice by filling in the circle in front of the option.

The Client With Cancer of the Bladder

A client is admitted to the outpatient surgery unit for a cystoscopy to rule out cancer of the bladder.

1. The most common symptom associated with bladder cancer is
   - ○ 1. painless hematuria.
   - ○ 2. decreasing urine output.
   - ○ 3. burning on urination.
   - ○ 4. frequent infections.
2. Which of the following symptoms would indicate that the client has developed a complication after the cystoscopy?
   - ○ 1. Dizziness.
   - ○ 2. Chills.
   - ○ 3. Pink-tinged urine.
   - ○ 4. Bladder spasms.
3. If the client develops lower abdominal pain, the nurse should instruct him to
   - ○ 1. apply an ice pack to his pubic area.
   - ○ 2. massage his abdomen gently.
   - ○ 3. ambulate as much as possible.
   - ○ 4. sit in a tub of warm water.
4. The diagnosis of bladder cancer is made, and the client is scheduled for an ileal conduit. Preoperatively, the nurse reinforces the client's understanding of the surgical procedure by explaining that an ileal conduit

   - ○ 1. is a temporary procedure that can be reversed later.
   - ○ 2. diverts urine into the sigmoid colon, where it is expelled through the rectum.
   - ○ 3. conveys urine from the ureters to a stoma opening on the abdomen.
   - ○ 4. creates an opening in the bladder that allows urine to drain into an external pouch.
5. Which of the following postoperative complications would the nurse particularly anticipate in a client undergoing a pelvic surgical procedure such as an ileal conduit?
   - ○ 1. Bleeding.
   - ○ 2. Infection.
   - ○ 3. Thrombophlebitis.
   - ○ 4. Atelectasis.
6. The nurse notes that the client's urinary appliance contains pale yellow urine with large amounts of mucus. How would the nurse best interpret these data?
   - ○ 1. The client is developing an infection of the urinary tract.
   - ○ 2. The mucus is caused by elevated levels of glucose in the urine.
   - ○ 3. These findings are normal for a client with an ileal conduit.
   - ○ 4. There is irritation of the stoma.
7. The nurse assesses the client's stoma regularly for edema. Which of the following signs and symptoms would indicate excessive stomal edema?

511

○ 1. Elevated temperature.
○ 2. Urine dribbling from the stoma.
○ 3. Complaints of discomfort around the stoma.
○ 4. Urine output below 30 mL/hour.

8. When teaching the client to care for his ileal conduit, the nurse instructs him to empty the appliance frequently to help prevent
   ○ 1. tearing of the ileal conduit.
   ○ 2. interruption of urine production.
   ○ 3. forcing urine into the kidneys.
   ○ 4. separation of the appliance from the skin.

9. The nurse should teach the client to prevent urine leakage when changing the appliance by
   ○ 1. inserting a gauze wick into the stoma.
   ○ 2. closing the opening temporarily with a cellophane seal.
   ○ 3. suctioning the stoma for a few minutes before changing the appliance.
   ○ 4. avoiding oral fluids for several hours before changing the appliance.

10. The client will be using a reusable appliance at home. The nurse should teach him to clean it routinely with
    ○ 1. baking soda.
    ○ 2. soap.
    ○ 3. hydrogen peroxide.
    ○ 4. alcohol.

11. Which of the following solutions will be useful in helping control odor in the collecting bag after it has been cleaned?
    ○ 1. Salt.
    ○ 2. Vinegar.
    ○ 3. Ammonia.
    ○ 4. Bleach.

12. The client tells the nurse, "This urinary pouch is embarrassing. Everyone will know that I'm not normal. I don't see how I can go out in public anymore." The most appropriate nursing diagnosis for this client is
    ○ 1. Anxiety related to presence of urinary diversion.
    ○ 2. Knowledge Deficit about how to care for the urinary diversion.
    ○ 3. Self-Esteem Disturbance related to feelings of worthlessness.
    ○ 4. Body Image Disturbance related to creation of a urinary diversion.

13. The nurse teaches the client to attach his appliance to a standard urine collection bag at night. The most important reason for doing this is to
    ○ 1. prevent urine reflux into the stoma.
    ○ 2. prevent appliance separation.
    ○ 3. prevent urine leakage.
    ○ 4. eliminate the need to restrict fluids.

14. The nurse teaches the client measures to prevent urinary tract infection. Which of the following measures would likely be most effective?
    ○ 1. Avoiding people with respiratory tract infections.
    ○ 2. Maintaining a daily fluid intake of 2000 to 3000 mL.
    ○ 3. Using sterile technique to change the appliance.
    ○ 4. Irrigating the stoma daily.

15. The nurse evaluates the effectiveness of the client's postoperative plan of care. Which of the following would be an expected outcome for a client with an ileal conduit? The client
    ○ 1. verbalizes the understanding that his physical activity must be significantly curtailed.
    ○ 2. states that he will place an aspirin in the drainage pouch to help control odor.
    ○ 3. demonstrates how to catheterize the stoma.
    ○ 4. states that he will empty the drainage pouch frequently throughout the day.

The Client With Renal Calculi

A client is admitted to the hospital with a diagnosis of renal calculi. She is experiencing severe flank pain and complains of nausea. Her temperature is 100.6°F.

16. The immediate nursing goal should be to
    ○ 1. prevent urinary tract complications.
    ○ 2. alleviate nausea.
    ○ 3. alleviate pain.
    ○ 4. maintain fluid and electrolyte balance.

17. The client is to have a kidney, ureter, and bladder (KUB) radiograph. Which of the following would be ordered to prepare her for this radiograph?
    ○ 1. Fluid and food will be withheld the morning of the examination.
    ○ 2. A tranquilizer will be given before the examination.
    ○ 3. An enema will be given before the examination.
    ○ 4. No special preparation is required for the examination.

18. Besides nausea and severe flank pain, the client complains of pain in her groin and bladder. The nurse would determine that these symptoms most likely result from
    ○ 1. nephritis.
    ○ 2. referred pain.
    ○ 3. urine retention.
    ○ 4. additional stone formation.

19. The client is scheduled for an intravenous pyelogram (IVP) to determine the location of the stone. Which of the following measures would be most important for the nurse to include in pretest preparation?

○ 1. Ensuring adequate fluid intake the day of the test.

○ 2. Preparing her for the possibility of bladder spasms during the test.

○ 3. Checking her history for allergy to iodine.

○ 4. Determining when she had her last bowel movement.

20. When starting the client's intravenous line, the nurse applies a tourniquet and selects the site for inserting the needle. When should the nurse remove the tourniquet?

○ 1. When the skin has been cleansed.

○ 2. As soon as the needle is in the vein.

○ 3. As soon as the needle is positioned under the skin.

○ 4. When the needle has been secured with tape.

21. In preparation for starting intravenous therapy, the nurse selects a site to insert the needle. Which of the following areas should the nurse try first?

○ 1. Back of the hand.

○ 2. Inner aspect of the elbow.

○ 3. Inner aspect of the forearm.

○ 4. Outer aspect of the forearm.

22. After the IVP, the nurse should anticipate incorporating which of the following measures into the client's plan of care?

○ 1. Maintaining bed rest.

○ 2. Encouraging adequate fluid intake.

○ 3. Assessing for hematuria.

○ 4. Administering a laxative.

23. The the correct procedure for collecting a urine specimen from an indwelling catheter is to

○ 1. open the spigot on the collecting bag and allow urine to empty into the specimen container.

○ 2. disconnect the drainage tube from the collecting bag and allow urine to flow from the tubing into the specimen container.

○ 3. disconnect the drainage tube from the indwelling catheter and allow urine to flow from the tubing into the specimen container.

○ 4. remove urine from the drainage tube with a sterile needle and syringe and place urine from the syringe into the specimen container.

24. The nurse finds a container with the client's urine specimen sitting on a counter in the bathroom. The client states that the specimen has been sitting in the bathroom at least 2 hours. What would be the nurse's most appropriate action?

○ 1. Discard the urine and obtain a new specimen.

○ 2. Send the urine to the laboratory as quickly as possible.

○ 3. Add fresh urine to the collected specimen and send the specimen to the laboratory.

○ 4. Place the specimen in the refrigerator until it can be transported to the laboratory.

25. A client has a ureteral catheter in place after renal surgery. A priority nursing action for care of the ureteral catheter would be to

○ 1. irrigate the catheter with 30 mL of normal saline every 8 hours.

○ 2. ensure that the catheter is draining freely.

○ 3. clamp the catheter every 2 hours for 30 minutes.

○ 4. ensure that the catheter drains at least 30 mL/hour.

26. To reduce urethral irritation, the nurse should tape the client's Foley catheter to her

○ 1. inner thigh.

○ 2. gown.

○ 3. lower abdomen.

○ 4. lower thigh.

27. Which of the following interventions would be the most appropriate for preventing the development of a paralytic ileus in the client after renal surgery?

○ 1. Encourage her to ambulate every 2 to 4 hours.

○ 2. Offer her 3 to 4 ounces of a carbonated beverage every hour.

○ 3. Encourage her to use the incentive spirometer every 2 hours while awake.

○ 4. Continue intravenous fluid therapy with 1000 mL of 5% dextrose in water every 8 hours.

28. Which of the following best indicates that the client's peristaltic activity is returning to normal?

○ 1. The client passes flatus.

○ 2. The client says that she is hungry.

○ 3. Bowel sounds are absent on auscultation.

○ 4. Peristalsis can be felt on abdominal palpation.

29. The day after surgery, the nurse is conducting a postoperative assessment of the client. Which of the following findings would be most important for the nurse to report to the physician?

○ 1. Temperature of 99.8°F.

○ 2. Urine output of 20 mL/hour.

○ 3. Absence of bowel sounds.

○ 4. A 2-inch by 2-inch area of serous sanguineous drainage on the flank dressing.

30. Of the following findings in the client's nursing history, which would be the least likely to have predisposed her to renal calculi?

○ 1. Having had several urinary tract infections in the past 2 years.

○ 2. Having taken large doses of vitamin C over the past several years.

○ 3. Drinking less than the recommended amount of milk.

○ 4. Having been on prolonged bed rest after an accident the previous year.

31. What instructions should the nurse plan to include in the client's home care plan because of her history of stone formation?

○ 1. Increase her daily fluid intake to at least 2 to 3 liters.

○ 2. Strain her urine at home regularly.

○ 3. Eliminate dairy products from her diet.

○ 4. Follow measures to alkalinize her urine.

32. Because the client's stone was found to be composed of uric acid, a low purine, alkaline-ash diet was ordered. The client's incorporation of which of the following food items into her home diet would indicate that she understands the necessary diet modifications?

○ 1. Milk, apples, tomatoes, and corn.

○ 2. Eggs, spinach, dried peas, and gravy.

○ 3. Salmon, chicken, caviar, and asparagus.

○ 4. Grapes, corn, cereals, and liver.

33. Allopurinol (Zyloprim), 200 mg/day, is prescribed for the client to take at home. The nurse should teach the client about which of the following side effects of this medication?

○ 1. Abdominal pain, retinopathy, and anorexia.

○ 2. Drowsiness, maculopapular rash, and anemia.

○ 3. Nausea, vomiting, and nasal congestion.

○ 4. Dizziness, erythema, and palpitations.

34. The client has a clinic appointment scheduled for 10 days after discharge. Which laboratory finding at that time would indicate that allopurinol (Zyloprim) has had a therapeutic effect?

○ 1. Decreased urinary alkaline phosphatase level.

○ 2. Increased urinary calcium excretion.

○ 3. Increased serum calcium level.

○ 4. Decreased serum uric acid level.

35. A client undergoes extracorporeal shock wave lithotripsy (ESWL) to break up and remove renal calculi. Which of the following nursing measures is appropriate for the postoperative care of this client?

○ 1. Maintain client on strict bed rest for 48 hours after the procedure.

○ 2. Instruct client to anticipate a decrease in urinary output.

○ 3. Instruct client to anticipate hematuria for about 24 hours after the procedure.

○ 4. Limit fluid intake to 1000 mL/day until all stone fragments have been passed.

36. When caring for a client after a closed renal biopsy, the nurse would anticipate implementing which of the following nursing measures?

○ 1. Maintaining the client on strict bed rest in a supine position for 6 hours.

○ 2. Inserting an indwelling catheter to monitor urine output.

○ 3. Applying a sandbag to the biopsy site to prevent bleeding.

○ 4. Administering intravenous narcotic medications to promote comfort.

The Client With Acute Renal Failure

A client developed shock after a severe myocardial infarction and has now developed acute renal failure.

37. The client's family asks the nurse why the client has developed acute renal failure. The nurse should base the response on the knowledge that there was

○ 1. a decrease in the blood flow through the kidneys.

○ 2. an obstruction of urine flow from the kidneys.

○ 3. a blood clot formed in the kidneys.

○ 4. structural damage to the kidney resulting in acute tubular necrosis.

38. The most significant sign of acute renal failure is

○ 1. increased blood pressure.

○ 2. elevated body temperature.

○ 3. decreased urine output.

○ 4. increased urine specific gravity.

39. The client's blood urea nitrogen (BUN) level is elevated. This most likely resulted from

○ 1. destruction of kidney cells.

○ 2. hemolysis of red blood cells.

○ 3. below-normal metabolic rate.

○ 4. reduced renal blood flow.

40. The client's potassium blood level is elevated, and the nurse administers sodium polystyrene sulfonate (Kayexalate). This drug is administered because of its ability to

○ 1. increase potassium excretion from the colon.

○ 2. release hydrogen ions for sodium ions.

○ 3. increase calcium absorption in the colon.

○ 4. exchange sodium for potassium ions in the colon.

41. If the client's potassium level continues to rise, the nurse should be prepared for which of the following emergency situations?

○ 1. Cardiac arrest.

○ 2. Pulmonary edema.

○ 3. Circulatory collapse.

○ 4. Hemorrhage.

42. A high-carbohydrate, low-protein diet is prescribed for the client. The rationale for the high-carbohydrate diet is that carbohydrates will

○ 1. act as a diuretic.

○ 2. reduce demands on the liver.

○ 3. help maintain urine acidity.

○ 4. prevent the development of ketosis.

43. The client asks the nurse for a snack. Because the client's potassium level is elevated, which of the following snacks would be most appropriate for the nurse to serve?

○ 1. A gelatin dessert.

○ 2. Yogurt.

○ 3. An orange.

○ 4. Dried peanuts.

44. The client is on a fluid restriction of 500 mL/day, plus replacement for urine output. Because the client's 24-hour urine output yesterday was 150 mL, the total fluid allotment for the next 24 hours is 650 mL. What change-of-shift information given by the nurse who worked 7:30 AM to 3:30 PM would indicate an understanding of how to distribute this fluid? The fluid allotment for this shift was
- ○ 1. supplemented with gelatin and ice cream.
- ○ 2. divided equally between breakfast and lunch.
- ○ 3. given in small amounts throughout the shift.
- ○ 4. given in its entirety in the morning to minimize the client's thirst.

45. The client has an external cannula inserted in the forearm for hemodialysis. Which of the following nursing measures is appropriate for the care of this client?
- ○ 1. Using the unaffected arm for blood pressure measurements.
- ○ 2. Drawing blood from the cannula for routine lab work.
- ○ 3. Percussing the cannula for bruits each shift.
- ○ 4. Injecting heparin into the cannula each shift.

46. The nurse initiates the client's first hemodialysis treatment. The client develops a headache, confusion, and nausea. The nurse recognizes these symptoms as being indicative of
- ○ 1. disequilibrium syndrome.
- ○ 2. myocardial infarction.
- ○ 3. air embolism.
- ○ 4. peritonitis.

47. If disequilibrium syndrome occurs during dialysis, the priority nursing action would be to
- ○ 1. start nasal oxygen administration.
- ○ 2. slow the rate of dialysis.
- ○ 3. reassure the client.
- ○ 4. place the client in Trendelenburg's position.

48. The client receives heparin while on dialysis. Which of the following statements about the anticoagulation that occurs with dialysis is correct?
- ○ 1. Regional anticoagulation can be achieved by infusion of heparin in the machine and protamine sulfate in the client.
- ○ 2. Warfarin sodium (Coumadin) is given to maintain anticoagulation between treatments.
- ○ 3. Heparin does not enter the body, so there is no risk of bleeding.
- ○ 4. Clotting time is seriously prolonged for several hours after each treatment.

49. Which of the following abnormal blood values would not be improved by dialysis treatment?
- ○ 1. Elevated serum creatinine.
- ○ 2. Hyperkalemia.
- ○ 3. Low hemoglobin.
- ○ 4. Hypernatremia.

50. The nurse teaches the client how to recognize signs of infection in the shunt. The client should be taught to observe for
- ○ 1. absence of a bruit.
- ○ 2. sluggish capillary refill time.
- ○ 3. coolness of the involved extremity.
- ○ 4. swelling at the shunt site.

51. The client asks the nurse, "Will my kidneys ever function normally again?" The nurse's response should be based on knowledge that the client's renal status will most likely
- ○ 1. continue to improve over a period of weeks.
- ○ 2. result in the need for permanent hemodialysis.
- ○ 3. improve only if the client receives a renal transplant.
- ○ 4. result in end-stage renal failure.

The Client With Urinary Tract Infection

A 24-year-old female client, who is on her honeymoon, comes to an ambulatory care clinic in moderate distress with a probable diagnosis of acute cystitis.

52. Which of the following symptoms would the nurse expect the client to report during the assessment?
- ○ 1. Fever and chills.
- ○ 2. Frequency and burning on urination.
- ○ 3. Suprapubic pain and nausea.
- ○ 4. Dark, concentrated urine.

53. A midstream urine specimen is ordered, and the nurse teaches the client how to collect the specimen correctly. Which of the following should the nurse include in the instructions?
- ○ 1. Void directly into the sterile specimen container.
- ○ 2. Save the first voided urine.
- ○ 3. Stop collecting urine after the bladder is empty.
- ○ 4. Cleanse the urethral meatus after obtaining the specimen.

54. The client asks the nurse, "How did I get this infection?" The nurse should explain that in most instances, cystitis is caused by
- ○ 1. congenital strictures in the urethra.
- ○ 2. an infection elsewhere in the body.
- ○ 3. urine stasis in the urinary bladder.
- ○ 4. an ascending infection from the urethra.

55. The physician tells the client that the infection has likely been precipitated by sexual intercourse and that an antibiotic will be ordered. The client becomes upset, and tearfully asks if this means she should abstain from intercourse for the rest of her honeymoon. What advice should the nurse offer her?
- ○ 1. "Avoid intercourse until you've completed the

antibiotic therapy and then limit intercourse to once a week."

○ 2. "Limit intercourse to once a day in the early morning after your bladder has rested."

○ 3. "As long as you're comfortable, you can have intercourse as often as you wish; but be sure to urinate within 15 minutes after intercourse."

○ 4. "You and your husband can enjoy intercourse as often as you wish. Just make sure he wears a condom and uses a spermicide."

56. The client is afraid to discuss this sexual issue with her husband. Which would be the nurse's best approach?

○ 1. Have a group meeting with the client, her husband, the doctor, the nurse, and the pharmacist.

○ 2. Insist that the client talk with her husband alone because good communication is the basis for a successful marriage.

○ 3. Talk first with the husband alone and then with both of them together to share the husband's reactions.

○ 4. Spend time with the client to increase her comfort and then stay with her while she talks with her husband.

57. The client is given a prescription for co-trimoxazole (Bactrim-DS) for her infection. Which of the following statements would indicate that she understands the principles of antibiotic therapy?

○ 1. "I'll take the pills until I feel better and keep the rest for recurrences."

○ 2. "I'll take all the pills and then return to my doctor."

○ 3. "I'll take the pills until the symptoms go away, and then reduce the dose to one pill a day."

○ 4. "I'll take all the pills and then have the prescription renewed once."

58. The nurse teaches the client methods to relieve her discomfort until the antibiotic takes effect. Which of the following responses by the client would indicate that she understands the nurse's instructions? "I will

○ 1. place ice packs on my perineum."

○ 2. take hot tub baths."

○ 3. drink a cup of warm tea every hour."

○ 4. void every 5 to 6 hours."

59. The client is also given a prescription for phenazopyridine hydrochloride (Pyridium). The nurse should teach the client that this drug is used to treat urinary tract infections by

○ 1. releasing formaldehyde and providing bacteriostatic action.

○ 2. potentiating the action of the antibiotic.

○ 3. providing an analgesic effect on the bladder mucosa.

○ 4. preventing the crystallization that can occur with sulfa drugs.

60. Before the client starts taking phenazopyridine hydrochloride (Pyridium), she should be taught about which of the drug's side effects?

○ 1. Bright orange-red urine.

○ 2. Incontinence.

○ 3. Gastric distress.

○ 4. Slight drowsiness.

61. Which of the following statements by the client would indicate that she is at high risk for a recurrence of cystitis?

○ 1. "I can usually go 8 to 10 hours without needing to empty my bladder."

○ 2. "I shower every morning."

○ 3. "I wipe from front to back after voiding."

○ 4. "I drink a lot of water during the day."

62. To prevent recurrence of cystitis, the nurse should plan to encourage the client to include which of the following measures in her daily routine?

○ 1. Wearing cotton underpants.

○ 2. Wearing tight pants.

○ 3. Douching regularly with 0.25% acetic acid.

○ 4. Using bubble baths and vaginal sprays.

63. The nurse explains to the client the importance of drinking large quantities of fluid. To help her understand, the nurse should tell her to drink

○ 1. twice as much fluid as she usually drinks.

○ 2. at least 1 quart more than she usually drinks.

○ 3. a lot of water, juice, and other fluids throughout the day.

○ 4. at least 3 quarts each day.

The Client With Pyelonephritis

A client is admitted to the hospital with a diagnosis of acute pyelonephritis.

64. Which of the following symptoms would most likely indicate pyelonephritis?

○ 1. Ascites.

○ 2. Costovertebral angle (CVA) tenderness.

○ 3. Polyuria.

○ 4. Nausea and vomiting.

65. Which of the following factors would put the client at increased risk for pyelonephritis?

○ 1. A 2-year history of hypertension.

○ 2. Ingestion of large quantities of cranberry juice.

○ 3. Average fluid intake of 2000 mL/day.

○ 4. A 12-year history of diabetes mellitus.

66. The client asks the nurse, "How will I know whether the antibiotics are effectively treating my infection?'' The nurse's most appropriate response would be

○ 1. "After you take the antibiotics for 2 weeks, you'll be cured."

○ 2. "The doctor can tell by the color and odor of your urine."

○ 3. "The doctor can determine your progress through urine cultures."

○ 4. "When your symptoms disappear, you'll know that your infection is gone."

The Client With Chronic Renal Failure

A client who has been treated for long-term hypertension develops chronic renal failure. He had a permanent peritoneal catheter inserted and thus far has been successfully managed with peritoneal dialysis.

67. The nurse assesses the client and notes the following: crackles in the lung bases, elevated blood pressure, and weight gain of 2 pounds in 1 day. Based on these data, which of the following nursing diagnoses is appropriate?

○ 1. Fluid Volume Excess related to the kidney's inability to maintain fluid balance.

○ 2. Increased Cardiac Output related to fluid overload.

○ 3. Altered Tissue Perfusion related to interrupted arterial blood flow.

○ 4. Ineffective Management of Therapeutic Regimen related to lack of knowledge about therapy.

68. Which of the following laboratory results would be *unexpected* in a client with chronic renal failure?

○ 1. Serum potassium 6.0 mEq/L.

○ 2. Serum creatinine 4.9 mg/dL.

○ 3. BUN 15 mg/dL.

○ 4. Serum phosphate 5.2 mg/dL.

69. Which of the following laboratory tests is considered the most reliable indicator of renal function?

○ 1. BUN.

○ 2. Urinalysis.

○ 3. Serum potassium.

○ 4. Serum creatinine.

70. What is the primary disadvantage of using standard peritoneal dialysis for long-term management of chronic renal failure?

○ 1. The danger of hemorrhage is high.

○ 2. It cannot correct severe imbalances.

○ 3. It is a time-consuming method of treatment.

○ 4. The risk of contracting hepatitis is high.

71. The client complains that he feels nauseated at least part of every day. The nurse should explain that the nausea is the result of

○ 1. acidosis caused by his medications.

○ 2. accumulation of waste products in his blood.

○ 3. chronic anemia and fatigue.

○ 4. excess fluid load.

72. The dialysis solution is warmed before use in peritoneal dialysis primarily to

○ 1. encourage the removal of serum urea.

○ 2. force potassium back into the cells.

○ 3. add extra warmth to the body.

○ 4. promote abdominal muscle relaxation.

73. Which of the following assessments would be most appropriate for the nurse to make while the dialysis solution is dwelling within the client's abdomen?

○ 1. Assessing for urticaria.

○ 2. Observing respiratory status.

○ 3. Checking capillary refill time.

○ 4. Monitoring electrolyte status.

74. During the client's dialysis, the nurse observes that the solution draining from his abdomen is consistently blood-tinged. Which interpretation of this observation would be correct? Bleeding

○ 1. is common when the client has a permanent peritoneal catheter.

○ 2. indicates abdominal blood vessel damage.

○ 3. can indicate kidney damage.

○ 4. is caused by too-rapid infusion of the dialysate.

75. During dialysis, the nurse observes that the flow of dialysate stops before all the solution has drained out. The nurse should

○ 1. have the client get out of bed and sit in a chair.

○ 2. turn the client from side to side.

○ 3. reposition the peritoneal catheter.

○ 4. have the client get up and walk.

76. Which of the following nursing interventions should be included in the client's care plan during dialysis therapy?

○ 1. Keep him in isolation.

○ 2. Monitor his blood pressure.

○ 3. Pad the side rails of his bed.

○ 4. Keep him NPO.

77. The most potentially dangerous complication of peritoneal dialysis is

○ 1. abdominal pain.

○ 2. gastrointestinal bleeding.

○ 3. peritonitis.

○ 4. muscle cramps.

78. After completion of dialysis, the nurse would expect the client to exhibit

○ 1. hematuria.

○ 2. weight loss.

○ 3. hypertension.

○ 4. increased urine output.

79. Aluminum hydroxide gel (Amphojel) is prescribed for the client to take at home. The purpose of giving this drug to a client with chronic renal failure is to

○ 1. relieve the pain of gastric hyperacidity.
○ 2. prevent Curling's stress ulcers.
○ 3. bind phosphate in the intestine.
○ 4. reverse metabolic acidosis.

80. The nurse teaches the client when to take the aluminum hydroxide gel. Which of the following statements would indicate that he understands the teaching? "I'll take it
○ 1. every 4 hours around the clock."
○ 2. between meals and at bedtime."
○ 3. when I have a sour stomach."
○ 4. with meals and bedtime snacks."

81. The client tells the nurse he takes magnesium hydroxide (Milk of Magnesia) at home for constipation. The nurse suggests that he switch to psyllium hydrophilic mucilloid (Metamucil) because
○ 1. Milk of Magnesia can cause magnesium intoxication.
○ 2. Milk of Magnesia is too harsh on the bowel.
○ 3. Metamucil is more palatable.
○ 4. Milk of Magnesia is high in sodium.

82. In planning teaching strategies for the client, the nurse must keep in mind the neurologic impact of uremia. Which teaching strategy would be most appropriate?
○ 1. Providing all needed teaching in one extended session.
○ 2. Validating frequently the client's understanding of the material.
○ 3. Conducting a one-on-one session with the client.
○ 4. Using videotapes to reinforce the material as needed.

83. The nurse helps the client develop a home diet plan with the goal of helping him maintain adequate nutritional status. Which of the following diets would be most appropriate for a client with chronic renal failure?
○ 1. High carbohydrate, high protein.
○ 2. High calcium, high potassium, high protein.
○ 3. Low protein, low sodium, low potassium.
○ 4. Low protein, high potassium.

84. Sexual problems can be troublesome to clients with chronic renal failure. Which one of the following strategies would be most useful in helping a client cope with such a problem?
○ 1. Accepting the fact that sexual activity must be decreased owing to the fatigue associated with chronic renal failure.
○ 2. Using alternate forms of sexual expression and intimacy during periods of altered sexual functioning.
○ 3. Planning rest periods after sexual activity.
○ 4. Avoiding sexual activity to prevent the embarrassment of altered sexual functioning.

85. The client has asked to be evaluated for a home continuous ambulatory peritoneal dialysis (CAPD) program. The nurse should explain that the major advantage of this approach in people with chronic renal failure is that it
○ 1. is relatively low in cost.
○ 2. allows the client to be more independent.
○ 3. is faster and more efficient than standard peritoneal dialysis.
○ 4. has fewer potential side effects and complications.

86. The client asks if his diet would change on CAPD. Which of the following would be the nurse's best response? "Diet restrictions
○ 1. are more rigid with CAPD because standard peritoneal dialysis is a more effective technique."
○ 2. are the same for both CAPD and standard peritoneal dialysis."
○ 3. with CAPD are fewer than with standard peritoneal dialysis because dialysis is constant."
○ 4. with CAPD are fewer than with standard peritoneal dialysis because CAPD works more quickly."

87. Peritoneal infection is the most serious potential complication of CAPD. Which of the following is the most significant sign of peritoneal infection?
○ 1. Cloudy dialysate fluid.
○ 2. Swelling in the legs.
○ 3. Poor drainage of the dialysate fluid.
○ 4. Redness at the catheter insertion site.

The Client With Urinary Incontinence

A client has been diagnosed with stress incontinence.

88. When developing a plan of care for the client, the nurse should take into consideration that stress incontinence is best defined as the involuntary loss of urine associated with
○ 1. a strong urge to urinate.
○ 2. overdistention of the bladder.
○ 3. activities that increase abdominal pressure.
○ 4. obstruction of the urethra.

89. The nurse at the ambulatory care clinic completes a nursing history on the client. Which of the following assessment data would most likely be related to the client's current complaint of stress incontinence? The client's
○ 1. intake of 2 to 3 liters of fluid a day.
○ 2. history of three full-term pregnancies.
○ 3. age of 45 years.
○ 4. history of competitive swimming.

90. The primary goal of nursing care for this client is to

○ 1. help the client adjust to the frequent episodes of incontinence.

○ 2. eliminate all episodes of incontinence.

○ 3. prevent the development of urinary tract infections.

○ 4. decrease the number of incontinence episodes.

91. The client asks the nurse what kind of diet she should follow at home. The nurse should recommend that the client

○ 1. avoid alcohol and caffeine.

○ 2. decrease her fluid intake.

○ 3. increase her intake of fruit juice.

○ 4. avoid milk products.

92. The client has been given a pamphlet that describes Kegel exercises. Which of the following statements indicates to the nurse that the client has understood the instructions contained in the pamphlet?

○ 1. "I should perform these exercises every evening."

○ 2. "It will probably take a year before the exercises are effective."

○ 3. "I can do these exercises sitting up, lying down, or standing."

○ 4. "I need to tighten my abdominal muscles to do these exercises correctly."

CORRECT ANSWERS AND RATIONALE

The letters in parentheses following the rationale identify the step of the nursing process (A, D, P, I, E), cognitive level (K, C, T, N), and client needs (S, G, L, H). See the Answer Grid for the key.

The Client With Cancer of the Bladder

1. 1. Painless hematuria is the most common symptom associated with bladder cancer. Bleeding from the lesions occurs fairly early in the disease process, but bladder cancer is basically asymptomatic in early stages. Bladder cancer is not related to infection or renal function. (A, K, G)

2. 2. Pink-tinged urine and bladder spasms are common after cystoscopy, but chills could indicate the onset of acute infection that can progress to septic shock. (E, K, G)

3. 4. Lower abdominal pain after a cystoscopy is frequently caused by bladder spasms. Warm water can help relax muscles. Ice is not effective in relieving spasms. Ambulation may increase bladder irritability. (I, T, G)

4. 3. An ileal conduit is a permanent urinary diversion in which a portion of the ileum is surgically resected and one end of the segment is closed. The ureters are surgically attached to this segment of the ileum, and the open end of the ileum is brought to the skin surface on the abdomen to form the stoma. The client must wear a pouch to collect the urine that continually flows through the conduit. (I, C, G)

5. 3. Clients undergoing pelvic surgery are at increased risk for thrombophlebitis postoperatively. Extensive pelvic surgery, such as that involved in an ileal conduit, removes lymph nodes from the pelvis and results in circulatory congestion from edema and stasis. Bleeding, infection, and atelectasis are not unique to this type of surgery. (P, C, G)

6. 3. A segment of the terminal ileus is used to form the conduit that collects urine from the ureters, and hence the client with an ileal conduit can be expected to excrete urine that contains mucus from this intestinal mucous membrane. Mucus production is not a result of infection, stomal irritation, or glycosuria. There is no reason to expect to find glucose in the client's urine. The nurse would recommend that the client maintain a large fluid intake (if not contraindicated) of 2 to 3 liters per day to maintain adequate urinary output. (D, N, G)

7. 4. Urine output below 30 mL/hour could indicate stomal edema, which obstructs urine output. An ele-

vated temperature should be noted, but it is not related to stomal edema. Discomfort around the stoma is common postoperatively after construction of an ileal conduit. Dribbling of urine from the stoma is normal. (A, N, G)

8. 4. If the appliance becomes too full, it is likely to pull away from the skin completely or leak urine onto the skin. A full appliance will not tear the ileal conduit, interrupt urine production, or force urine into the kidneys. (I, T, H)

9. 1. Inserting a gauze wick into the stoma helps prevent urine leakage when changing the appliance. The stoma should not be sealed or suctioned, and oral fluids should not be avoided. (I, T, H)

10. 2. A reusable appliance should be routinely cleaned with soap and water. (I, T, H)

11. 2. A distilled vinegar solution acts as a good deodorizing agent after an appliance has been cleansed well with soap and water. If the client prefers, a commercial deodorizer may be used. Salt solution does not deodorize. Ammonia and bleaching agents may damage the appliance. (I, T, H)

12. 4. It is normal for clients to express fears and concerns about the body changes associated with a urinary diversion. Allowing the client time to verbalize these concerns in a supportive environment can help the client begin coping with these changes in a positive manner. Encouraging the client to discuss his or her concerns with people who have successfully adjusted to ostomy surgery may be beneficial. Most communities have local support groups that the client can contact for assistance. (D, N, L)

13. 1. The most important reason for attaching the appliance to a standard urine collection bag at night is to prevent urine reflux into the stoma and ureters. Using a standard collection bag also keeps the appliance from separating from the skin and resultant urine leakage. A client with an ileal conduit should drink 2000 to 3000 mL of fluid each day, unless contraindicated. (I, N, H)

14. 2. Maintaining a fluid intake of 2000 to 3000 mL/day is likely to be most effective in preventing urinary tract infection. A high fluid intake results in high urine output, which prevents urinary stasis and bacterial growth. Clean, not sterile, technique is used to change the appliance. An ileal conduit stoma is not irrigated. (I, N, H)

15. 4. It is important that the client empty the drainage pouch throughout the day to decrease the risk of leakage. An ileal conduit stoma is not catheterized

by the client. The client does not normally need to curtail physical activity. Aspirin should never be placed in a pouch because the aspirin can irritate the stoma. (E, T, H)

The Client With Renal Calculi

16. 3. The immediate nursing goal for this client is to alleviate pain, which can be excruciating. The other goals are appropriate throughout the client's hospitalization but are not immediate. (P, N, G)

17. 4. A KUB radiographic examination ordinarily requires no preparation. It is usually done while the client lies supine. It does not involve the use of radiopaque substances. (P, K, S)

18. 2. The pain associated with renal colic due to calculi is often referred to the groin and bladder in female clients and to the testicles in male clients. Nausea, vomiting, abdominal cramping, and diarrhea may also be present. Unlikely causes of pain from renal colic in the groin and bladder or testicles include urine retention or nephritis. The type of pain described in this situation is unlikely to be due to additional stone formation. (D, C, G)

19. 3. A client scheduled for an IVP should be assessed for allergies to iodine and shellfish. Clients with such allergies may be allergic to the IVP dye and be at risk for an anaphylactic reaction. Bowel preparation is important before an IVP to allow visualization of the ureters and bladder, but checking for allergies is most important. (I, N, S)

20. 2. When starting an intravenous infusion, the nurse should remove the tourniquet as soon as the needle is in the vein. Until then, the tourniquet keeps the vein distended so that it is more visible and easier to enter. After the needle is in the vein, the tourniquet should be removed before applying tape so that fluid can enter the vein promptly. (I, T, S)

21. 1. When starting an intravenous infusion, the nurse initially uses veins low on the hand or arm. Should the vein be damaged, veins higher on the arm are still available for use. After a vein higher up on the arm has been damaged, veins below it on the arm cannot be used. (I, T, S)

22. 2. After an IVP, the nurse should encourage fluids to decrease the risk of renal complications caused by the contrast agent. There is no need to place the client on bed rest or to administer a laxative. An IVP would not cause hematuria. (I, T, S)

23. 4. To obtain a urine specimen from a client with an indwelling Foley catheter attached to a closed urine drainage system, the nurse removes the specimen from the drainage tube using a sterile needle and syringe. This technique is not likely to predispose to a urinary tract infection because the drainage sys-

tem is not opened to the air. Furthermore, this urine specimen would be fresh, unlike the urine collected in the drainage bag. (I, T, S)

24. 1. The appropriate action would be to discard the specimen and obtain a new one. Urine allowed to stand at room temperature will become alkaline. (I, T, S)

25. 2. The ureteral catheter should drain freely without bleeding at the site. The catheter is rarely irrigated and is never clamped. The client's total urine output (ureteral catheter plus voiding or Foley catheter output) should be 30 mL/hour. (I, N, S)

26. 1. To reduce urethral irritation, the nurse should tape the Foley catheter to a female client's inner thigh or a male client's thigh or abdomen. Taping the catheter to the client's gown does not prevent urethral irritation and may lead to accidental removal of the catheter as the client moves. (I, T, S)

27. 1. Ambulation stimulates the return of peristalsis. A client with paralytic ileus is kept NPO until peristalsis returns. Intravenous fluid infusion and incentive spirometry are routine postoperative orders. (I, N, G)

28. 1. Passing flatus indicates the return of peristalsis, as do active bowel sounds. Peristalsis is difficult to palpate, and palpation is not an appropriate method of assessing bowel activity. Hunger is not the best indicator of peristaltic return. (E, N, G)

29. 2. The decrease in urine output may reflect inadequate renal perfusion and should be reported immediately. Urine output of 30 mL/hour or greater is considered acceptable. The other assessment findings are not unusual during the early postoperative period. (E, N, S)

30. 3. A high, rather than low, milk intake predisposes to renal calculi formation. Such conditions as urinary tract infections, low fluid intake, prolonged immobility, and high daily doses of vitamins C and D tend to predispose to stone formation. Men between 30 and 50 years of age develop calculi more often than women. Clients who have had renal calculi experience recurrence twice as often. People living in hot climates can develop calculi due to an increased insensible fluid loss combined with inadequate fluid intake. This results in concentration of urine and precipitation of urinary salts. (A, C, G)

31. 1. A high daily fluid intake is essential in clients at risk for calculi formation because it prevents urinary stasis, which can cause crystallization. Depending on the composition of the stone, the client also may be instructed to limit calcium by instituting specific dietary measures aimed at preventing calcium phosphate stone formation. (P, T, H)

32. 1. Because a high purine diet contributes to the formation of uric acid, a low-purine diet is advocated.

An alkaline-ash diet is also advocated because uric acid crystals are more likely to develop in acid urine. Foods that may be eaten as desired in a low-purine diet include milk, all fruits, tomatoes, cereals, and corn. Foods high in purines include liver, caviar, and gravy. Foods containing moderate to large amounts of purine include spinach, dried peas, salmon, chicken, and asparagus. Foods allowed on an alkaline-ash diet include milk, fruits (except cranberries, plums, and prunes), vegetables (especially legumes and green vegetables), and small amounts of ham, beef, trout, and salmon. (E, K, H)

33. 2. Side effects of allopurinol include drowsiness, maculopapular rash, anemia, abdominal pain, retinopathy, nausea, vomiting, and bone marrow depression. (I, C, G)

34. 4. By inhibiting uric acid synthesis, allopurinol decreases its excretion. The drug's effectiveness is assessed by evaluating for decreased serum uric acid level. (E, K, G)

35. 3. It is normal for hematuria to occur for up to 24 hours after ESWL. Hematuria that occurs for longer than 24 hours should be reported to the physician. ESWL is usually performed on an outpatient basis, and strict bed rest is not necessary after the procedure. Urinary output should not be decreased, and any difficulty urinating should be reported. Fluid intake should be increased to 2 to 3 liters per day, not decreased. (I, T, S)

36. 1. After a renal biopsy, the client is maintained on strict bed rest in a supine position for at least 6 hours to prevent bleeding. If no bleeding occurs, the client typically resumes general activity after 24 hours. Narcotics to control pain would not be anticipated; local discomfort at the biopsy site can be controlled with analgesics. Urine output is monitored, but an indwelling catheter is not typically inserted. (I, T, S)

The Client With Acute Renal Failure

37. 1. There are three categories of acute renal failure: prerenal, intrarenal, and postrenal. Causes of prerenal failure occur outside the kidney and include poor perfusion and a decrease in circulating volume due to such factors as trauma, septic shock, impaired cardiac function, and dehydration. Causes of intrarenal failure, such as hypersensitivity (allergic disorders), renal vessel obstruction, and nephrotoxic agents, result in structural damage to the kidney due to acute tubular necrosis. Postrenal failure, or obstruction within the urinary tract, results from kidney stones, tumors, or benign prostatic hypertrophy. (P, C, G)

38. 3. A sudden change in urine output is typical of acute renal failure. Most commonly, the initial change is greatly decreased urine output. Later in the course of acute renal failure, the client may have marked diuresis (nonoliguric failure). Other common signs and symptoms of acute renal failure include lethargy, nausea and vomiting, diarrhea, headaches, muscle twitching, and convulsions. Serum creatinine and BUN levels are elevated. Urine-specific gravity usually is within a low-normal range because the kidneys have difficulty concentrating urine. High body temperatures and sudden blood pressure elevation are not typically associated with acute renal failure. (A, C, G)

39. 4. Reduced renal blood flow causes an elevated BUN level. Urea, an end product of protein metabolism, is normally excreted by the kidneys. Any impairment in renal function causes an increase in plasma urea level. (A, C, G)

40. 4. Polystyrene sulfonate, a cation-exchange resin, causes the body to excrete potassium through the gastrointestinal tract. In the intestines, particularly the colon, the sodium of the resin is partially replaced by potassium. The potassium is then eliminated when the resin is eliminated with feces. Polystyrene sulfonate may be administered orally or rectally and is used specifically to treat hyperkalemia. (I, K, G)

41. 1. Hyperkalemia predisposes to serious cardiac dysrhythmias and cardiac arrest. Therefore, the nurse should be prepared to treat cardiac arrest when caring for a client with hyperkalemia. (P, C, G)

42. 4. High-carbohydrate foods meet the body's caloric needs during acute renal failure. Protein is limited because its breakdown may result in accumulation of toxic waste products. (I, T, G)

43. 1. Gelatin desserts contain little or no potassium and can be served to a client on a potassium-restricted diet. Foods high in potassium include bran and whole grains; most dried, raw, and frozen fruits and vegetables; most milk and milk products; chocolate, nuts, raisins, coconut, and strong brewed coffee. Highly refined foods, fruits and vegetables cooked in large amounts of water, butter, cream, and hard candies are generally low in potassium. (I, N, G)

44. 3. Thirst is a strong motivator to drink. Giving small amounts of fluid during an 8-hour shift helps minimize thirst. Gelatin and ice cream are inappropriate supplements because they become liquid at room temperature. Some fluids should be given with meals, but not the entire 8-hour allotment. (I, N, S)

45. 1. Heparin is not injected into the cannula to maintain patency. Because it is part of the general circulation, the cannula cannot be heparinized. The external cannula must be handled carefully and protected from damage and disruption. The arm with the cannula is not used for blood pressure measurement, intravenous therapy, or venipuncture. Patency is assessed by auscultating for bruits every shift. In addition, a tourniquet or clamps should be kept at the bedside because dislodgement of the cannula would cause arterial hemorrhage. (I, T, S)

46. 1. Typical symptoms of disequilibrium syndrome include headache, nausea and vomiting, confusion, and even seizures. Disequilibrium syndrome typically occurs near the end or after the completion of hemodialysis treatment. (D, N, G)

47. 2. If disequilibrium syndrome occurs during dialysis, the most appropriate intervention is to slow the rate of dialysis. The syndrome is believed to result from too-rapid removal of urea and excess electrolytes from the blood; this causes transient cerebral edema, which produces the symptoms. (I, N, G)

48. 1. Regional anticoagulation can be achieved by infusing heparin in the dialyzer and protamine sulfate, its antagonist, in the client. The client's clotting time will not be seriously affected, although some rebound effect may occur. The clotting time is monitored carefully. Warfarin sodium is not used in dialysis treatment. (I, T, S)

49. 3. Dialysis will correct electrolyte imbalances and clear metabolic waste products from the body, but it has no effect on anemia. Because some red cells are injured during the procedure, dialysis aggravates a low hemoglobin concentration. (E, N, G)

50. 4. Signs of an external access shunt infection include redness, tenderness, swelling, and drainage from around the shunt site. (A, T, S)

51. 1. The kidneys have a remarkable ability to recover from serious insult. In view of this client's prompt and effective treatment, her prognosis should be good. Effective treatment for acute renal failure consists primarily of restoring normal fluid and electrolyte balance so the body can restore renal functioning and repair renal tissue. The client should be taught how to recognize the symptoms of decreasing renal function and to notify the physician if such problems occur. (P, C, G)

The Client With Urinary Tract Infection

52. 2. The classic symptoms of cystitis are severe burning, urgency, and frequent urination. Some clients also develop fever, hematuria, and suprapubic pain. Systemic symptoms are more likely to accompany pyelonephritis than cystitis. (A, K, G)

53. 1. To collect a midstream urine specimen, the client voids directly into a sterile specimen container. Other correct techniques include discarding the first 30 mL, stopping the collection before the blad-

der is empty, and cleansing the urethral meatus before obtaining the specimen. (I, T, S)

54. 4. Although various conditions may result in cystitis, the most common cause is an ascending infection from the urethra. (I, K, G)

55. 3. Intercourse is not contraindicated in cystitis. Voiding immediately after intercourse flushes bacteria from the urethra, which should help prevent recurrence. There is no reason to wait until the antibiotic therapy is completed or to limit the frequency of intercourse. A condom and spermicide do not prevent cystitis because cystitis results from the introduction of the client's own organisms (usually *Escherichia coli*) into the urethra. (I, N, H)

56. 4. As newlyweds, the client and her husband need to develop a strong communication base. The nurse can facilitate the development of this base by preparing the client and being there for support. Being present also allows the nurse to intervene, if necessary, to facilitate the discussion of a difficult topic. Given this situation, an interdisciplinary conference is inappropriate and would not promote intimacy for the client and her husband. Insisting that the client talk with her husband alone is not complying with her request. Having the nurse speak first with the husband alone shifts responsibility away from the couple. (I, N, L)

57. 2. Antibiotics are prescribed for a definite treatment period, and all the pills should be taken. A urine culture should be done after the course of antibiotic therapy to ensure that the urine is bacteria free. Stopping the medication early may cause the infection to recur. Tapering the dosage is inappropriate with antibiotics because it lowers the therapeutic blood level. Refilling the prescription would be indicated only after urine culture indicates that the urine is not bacteria free and the physician prescribes another course of antibiotics. (E, T, H)

58. 2. Hot tub baths promote relaxation and help relieve urgency, discomfort, and spasm. Applying heat to the perineum is more helpful than cold because heat reduces inflammation. Although liberal fluid intake should be encouraged, tea, coffee, and cola can be irritating to the bladder and should be avoided. Voiding at least every 2 to 3 hours should be encouraged because it reduces urinary stasis. (E, N, H)

59. 3. Phenazopyridine hydrochloride is a urinary analgesic that works directly on the bladder mucosa to relieve the distressing symptoms of dysuria. (I, C, G)

60. 1. The client should be told that phenazopyridine hydrochloride turns the urine a bright orange-red, which may stain underwear. It can be frightening for a client to see orange-red urine without having been forewarned. (I, C, G)

61. 1. Stasis of urine in the bladder is one of the chief causes of bladder infection, and a client who voids infrequently is at greater risk of reinfection. Liberal fluid intake (unless contraindicated) and scrupulous hygiene are excellent preventive measures, but the client also should be taught to void every 2 to 3 hours during the day. (E, T, H)

62. 1. A woman can adopt several health-promotion measures to prevent the recurrence of cystitis, including avoiding too-tight pants, noncotton underpants, and irritating substances such as bubble baths and vaginal soaps and sprays. Regular douching is not recommended; it can alter the pH of the vagina, increasing the risk of infection. (P, T, H)

63. 4. Instructions should be as specific as possible, and the nurse should avoid general statements such as "a lot." A specific goal is most useful. A mix of fluids will increase the likelihood of client compliance. (I, T, H)

The Client With Pyelonephritis

64. 2. Common symptoms of pyelonephritis include CVA tenderness, burning, urinary urgency or frequency, chills, and fever and fatigue. Polyuria, ascites, and nausea and vomiting are not indicative of pyelonephritis. (A, C, G)

65. 4. A client with a history of diabetes mellitus, urinary tract infections, or renal calculi is at increased risk for pyelonephritis. Others at high risk include pregnant women and people with structural alterations of the urinary tract. (A, T, G)

66. 3. Antibiotics are usually prescribed for a 2- to 4-week period. A urine culture is needed to evaluate the effectiveness of antibiotic therapy. (I, T, H)

The Client With Chronic Renal Failure

67. 1. Crackles in the lungs, weight gain, and elevated blood pressure are all indicators of fluid volume excess, a common complication in chronic renal failure. The client's fluid status should be monitored carefully for imbalances on an ongoing basis. (D, N, G)

68. 3. The stated BUN level is within the normal range of 10 to 15 mg/dL and thus would be unexpected in renal failure. BUN level is usually significantly elevated in chronic renal failure, which causes retention of waste products and electrolytes. Elevated serum potassium (normal, 3.5 to 5 mEq/L), elevated serum creatinine (normal, 0.8 to 1.7 mg/dL for males, 0.6 to 1 mg/dL for females), and hyperphos-

phatemia (normal, 2.5 to 4.8 mg/dL) commonly occur in chronic renal failure. (A, K, G)

69. 4. Of the tests listed, serum creatinine is the most reliable indicator of renal function. BUN may be influenced by other factors unrelated to renal disease. A urinalysis may indicate the presence of a renal or urologic disorder. Potassium levels are affected by numerous factors. (E, C, G)

70. 3. A disadvantage of standard peritoneal dialysis in long-term management of chronic renal failure is that it requires large blocks of time. Peritoneal dialysis is effective in maintaining a client's fluid and electrolyte balance. Neither the danger of hemorrhage nor of hepatitis is high with peritoneal dialysis. (E, K, G)

71. 2. Nausea typically results from the chronic presence of retained waste products in the body. The client can control nausea most effectively by following his diet regimen strictly and avoiding wide swings in blood values between treatments. (I, C, G)

72. 1. The main reason for warming the peritoneal dialysis solution is that the warm solution helps dilate peritoneal vessels, which increases urea clearance. Warmed dialyzing solution also contributes to client comfort by preventing chilly sensations, but this is a secondary reason for warming the solution. (I, C, S)

73. 2. During dwell time, the dialysis solution is allowed to remain in the peritoneal cavity for the time ordered by the physician (usually 20 to 45 minutes). During this time, the nurse should monitor the client's respiratory status because the pressure of the dialysis solution on the diaphragm can create respiratory distress. The client's laboratory values are obtained before beginning treatment and are monitored every 4 to 8 hours during the treatment, not just during the dwell time. (A, N, S)

74. 2. Because the client has a permanent catheter in place, blood-tinged drainage should not occur. Persistent blood-tinged drainage could indicate damage to the abdominal vessels, and the physician should be notified. Blood-tinged drainage is common, however, with the initial dialysis runs immediately after peritoneal catheter insertion. (A, N, S)

75. 2. Fluid return with peritoneal dialysis is accomplished by gravity flow. Actions that enhance gravity flow include turning the client from side to side, raising the head of the bed, and gently massaging the abdomen. The nurse should not attempt to reposition the catheter. The client is usually confined to a recumbent position during the dialysis. (I, T, S)

76. 2. Because hypotension is a complication associated with peritoneal dialysis, the nurse records intake and output, monitors vital signs, and observes the client's behavior. The nurse also encourages visiting and other diversional activities. A client on peritoneal dialysis need not be kept NPO, placed in isolation, or placed in a bed with padded side rails. (I, T, S)

77. 3. Peritonitis is a serious risk associated with peritoneal dialysis. Aseptic technique should be maintained during the procedure. Minor abdominal cramping may occur with dialysis; gastrointestinal bleeding is an extremely rare complication. (E, N, G)

78. 2. Weight loss is expected, and blood pressure usually decreases as well. The client's weight before and after dialysis is one measure of the effectiveness of treatment. Dialysis only minimally affects the damaged kidneys' ability to manufacture urine. Hematuria would not occur after completion of peritoneal dialysis. (A, C, G)

79. 3. A client in renal failure develops hyperphosphatemia that causes a corresponding excretion of the body's calcium stores. To decrease this loss, aluminum hydroxide gel is prescribed to bind phosphates in the intestine and facilitate their excretion. (P, T, G)

80. 4. Aluminum hydroxide gel is administered to bind the phosphates in ingested foods and must be given with or immediately after meals and snacks. It is not administered to treat hyperacidity in clients with chronic renal failure and thus is not prescribed between meals or p.r.n. (E, T, G)

81. 1. Magnesium is normally excreted by the kidneys. When the kidneys fail, magnesium can accumulate and cause severe neurologic problems. Milk of Magnesia is harsher than Metamucil, but magnesium toxicity is a more serious problem. A client may find both Milk of Magnesia and Metamucil unpalatable. Milk of Magnesia is not high in sodium. (I, T, G)

82. 2. Uremia can cause decreased alertness, so the nurse needs to validate the client's comprehension frequently. The client's ability to concentrate is limited, so short lessons are most effective. If family members are present at the sessions, they can reinforce material. Written materials that the client can review are superior to videotapes. (P, N, G)

83. 3. Dietary management for clients with chronic renal failure is usually designed to restrict protein, sodium, and potassium intake. The degree of dietary restriction depends on the degree of renal impairment. The client should also receive an adequate caloric intake along with appropriate vitamin and mineral supplements. (P, T, G)

84. 2. Altered sexual functioning commonly occurs in chronic renal failure and can stress marriages and relationships. The client should not avoid sexual activity but instead should modify it. Effective coping strategies also include measures for removing uremic fetor and resting before sexual activity. (I, N, L)

85. 2. The major benefit of CAPD is that it frees the client from daily dependence on dialysis centers, health care personnel, and machines for life-sustaining treatment. This independence is a valuable outcome for some people. (I, C, G)

86. 3. Dietary restrictions with CAPD are fewer than those with standard peritoneal dialysis because dialysis is constant, not intermittent. The constant slow diffusion of CAPD helps prevent accumulation of toxins and allows for a more liberal diet. (I, N, G)

87. 1. Cloudy drainage indicates bacterial activity in the peritoneum. Other signs and symptoms of infection are fever, hyperactive bowel sounds, and abdominal pain. Swollen legs and inadequate dialysate drainage are unrelated to infection. Redness at the insertion site indicates local infection, not peritonitis. If untreated, however, a local infection can progress to the peritoneum. (A, N, G)

The Client With Urinary Incontinence

88. 3. Stress incontinence is the involuntary loss of urine during such activities as coughing, sneezing, laughing, or physical exertion. These activities increase abdominal and detrusor pressure. (P, C, G)

89. 2. The history of three pregnancies is most likely the cause of the client's current episodes of stress incontinence. The client's fluid intake, age, and history of swimming are not causes of her incontinence. (A, T, G)

90. 4. The primary goal of nursing care is to decrease the number on incontinence episodes and the amount of urine expressed in an episode. Behavioral interventions, such as diet and exercise, as well as medications are the nonsurgical management of choice used to treat stress incontinence. (P, T, G)

91. 1. Clients with incontinence should be encouraged to avoid alcohol and caffeine products because both are bladder stimulants. The client should not decrease fluid intake. There is no need to avoid milk products, and increasing the intake of fruit juice may be desirable but will not affect the episodes of incontinence. (I, T, H)

92. 3. The client can perform the Kegel exercises at anytime, in any of the positions listed. To be most effective, the exercises should be performed at least twice a day for a total of 10 minutes a day. Pelvic muscles, not the abdominal muscles, should be contracted during these exercises. The client can learn to identify these muscles by urinating and stopping the flow. If performed regularly, the client should begin to note changes after about 6 weeks. (E, T, H)

NURSING CARE OF ADULTS WITH MEDICAL AND SURGICAL HEALTH PROBLEMS

TEST 7: The Client With Urinary Tract Health Problems

Directions: Use this answer grid to determine areas of strength or need for further study.

NURSING PROCESS

A = Assessment
D = Analysis, nursing diagnosis
P = Planning
I = Implementation
E = Evaluation

COGNITIVE LEVEL

K = Knowledge
C = Comprehension
T = Application
N = Analysis

CLIENT NEEDS

S = Safe, effective care environment
G = Physiologic integrity
L = Psychosocial integrity
H = Health promotion and maintenance

Question #	Answer #	A	D	P	I	E	K	C	T	N	S	G	L	H
1	1	A					K					G		
2	2					E	K					G		
3	4				I				T			G		
4	3				I			C				G		
5	3			P				C				G		
6	3		D							N		G		
7	4	A								N		G		
8	4				I				T					H
9	1				I				T					H
10	2				I				T					H
11	2				I				T					H
12	4		D							N			L	
13	1				I					N				H
14	2				I					N				H
15	4					E			T					H
16	3			P						N		G		
17	4			P			K				S			
18	2		D					C				G		
19	3				I					N	S			
20	2				I				T		S			
21	1				I				T		S			
22	2				I				T		S			
23	4				I				T		S			
24	1				I				T		S			
25	2				I					N	S			

ANSWER GRID: 1

NURSING PROCESS

A = Assessment
D = Analysis, nursing diagnosis
P = Planning
I = Implementation
E = Evaluation

COGNITIVE LEVEL

K = Knowledge
C = Comprehension
T = Application
N = Analysis

CLIENT NEEDS

S = Safe, effective care environment
G = Physiologic integrity
L = Psychosocial integrity
H = Health promotion and maintenance

Question #	Answer #	Nursing Process					Cognitive Level				Client Needs			
		A	D	P	I	E	K	C	T	N	S	G	L	H
26	1				I				T		S			
27	1				I					N		G		
28	1					E				N		G		
29	2					E				N	S			
30	3	A						C				G		
31	1			P					T					H
32	1					E	K							H
33	2				I			C				G		
34	4					E	K					G		
35	3				I				T		S			
36	1				I				T		S			
37	1			P				C				G		
38	3	A						C				G		
39	4	A						C				G		
40	4				I		K					G		
41	1			P				C				G		
42	4				I				T			G		
43	1				I					N		G		
44	3				I					N	S			
45	1				I				T		S			
46	1		D							N		G		
47	2				I					N		G		
48	1				I				T		S			
49	3					E				N		G		
50	4	A							T		S			
51	1			P				C				G		
52	2	A					K					G		
53	1				I				T		S			
54	4				I		K					G		
55	3				I					N				H

ANSWER GRID: 2

NURSING PROCESS

A = Assessment
D = Analysis, nursing diagnosis
P = Planning
I = Implementation
E = Evaluation

COGNITIVE LEVEL

K = Knowledge
C = Comprehension
T = Application
N = Analysis

CLIENT NEEDS

S = Safe, effective care environment
G = Physiologic integrity
L = Psychosocial integrity
H = Health promotion and maintenance

Question #	Answer #	A	D	P	I	E	K	C	T	N	S	G	L	H
56	4				I					N			L	
57	2					E			T					H
58	2					E				N				H
59	3				I			C				G		
60	1				I			C				G		
61	1					E			T					H
62	1			P					T					H
63	4				I				T					H
64	2	A						C				G		
65	4	A							T			G		
66	3				I				T					H
67	1		D							N		G		
68	3	A					K					G		
69	4				E			C				G		
70	3				E		K					G		
71	2				I			C				G		
72	1				I			C			S			
73	2	A								N	S			
74	2	A								N	S			
75	2				I				T		S			
76	2				I				T		S			
77	3					E				N		G		
78	2	A						C				G		
79	3			P					T			G		
80	4					E			T			G		
81	1				I				T			G		
82	2			P						N		G		
83	3			P					T			G		
84	2				I					N			L	
85	2				I			C				G		

ANSWER GRID: 3

NURSING PROCESS

A = Assessment
D = Analysis, nursing diagnosis
P = Planning
I = Implementation
E = Evaluation

COGNITIVE LEVEL

K = Knowledge
C = Comprehension
T = Application
N = Analysis

CLIENT NEEDS

S = Safe, effective care environment
G = Physiologic integrity
L = Psychosocial integrity
H = Health promotion and maintenance

Question #	Answer #	Nursing Process					Cognitive Level				Client Needs			
		A	D	P	I	E	K	C	T	N	S	G	L	H
86	3				I					N		G		
87	1	A								N		G		
88	3			P				C				G		
89	2	A							T			G		
90	4			P					T			G		
91	1				I				T					H
92	3					E			T					H
Number Correct														
Number Possible	92	15	5	13	44	15	10	19	36	27	22	49	3	18
Percentage Correct														

Score Calculation: To determine your **Percentage Correct,** divide the **Number Correct** by the **Number Possible.**

ANSWER GRID: 4

The Client With Reproductive Health Problems

Select the one best answer, and indicate your choice by filling in the circle in front of the option.

The Client With Uterine Fibroids

A 39-year-old female client has been experiencing intermittent vaginal bleeding for the past several months. Her physician tells her that she has uterine fibroids and recommends an abdominal hysterectomy.

1. The nurse is completing the routine admission assessment when the client expresses fear about the surgery. Which of the following statements offers the best guide for the nurse's response? The nurse should
- ○ 1. reassure the client of her physician's competence.
- ○ 2. give the client opportunities to express her fears.
- ○ 3. teach the client that fear impedes recovery.
- ○ 4. change the subject of conversation to pleasantries when the client appears fearful.

2. The client is to be admitted the morning of the surgery. Essential information that the client needs before admission includes
- ○ 1. what to wear to the hospital.
- ○ 2. what she can eat and drink before admission.
- ○ 3. the type of pain medication that will be prescribed postoperatively.
- ○ 4. preoperative teaching about coughing during the postoperative period.

3. The physician prescribes 0.4 mg of atropine sulfate and 75 mg of meperidine hydrochloride to be given intramuscularly 1 hour before surgery. The stock ampule of atropine contains 0.8 mg/mL, and the stock ampule of meperidine hydrochloride contains 100 mg/mL. The two drugs are compatible and can be drawn up in one syringe. How much of the drugs will be in the syringe to give the ordered doses?
- ○ 1. 0.75 mL.
- ○ 2. 1.25 mL.
- ○ 3. 1.50 mL.
- ○ 4. 1.75 mL.

4. The client requires catheterization when she is unable to void. When preparing to insert the catheter into the urinary meatus, the nurse locates the anatomic structures between the labia minora. Starting from the area nearer the pubic bone and moving downward toward the anus, in which of the following order do the clitoris, vaginal opening, and urinary meatus lie?
- ○ 1. Clitoris, vaginal opening, urinary meatus.
- ○ 2. Urinary meatus, vaginal opening, clitoris.
- ○ 3. Vaginal opening, clitoris, urinary meatus.
- ○ 4. Clitoris, urinary meatus, vaginal opening.

5. During the recovery period, the nurse notes that the client is an Orthodox Jew and refuses to eat hospital food. Hospital policy discourages food from outside the hospital. What step should the nurse take first in this situation?

○ 1. Teach the client that it is important for her to eat what she is served.

○ 2. Discuss the situation and possible courses of action with the dietitian.

○ 3. Encourage the client's family to bring food for the client because of the special circumstances.

○ 4. Explain to the client that if she does not eat, the physician will have to order intravenous therapy.

6. Which of the following early signs or symptoms will the client most likely experience if she hyperventilates while performing deep breathing exercises postoperatively?

○ 1. Dyspnea.
○ 2. Dizziness.
○ 3. Blurred vision.
○ 4. Mental confusion.

7. Eight hours after catheterization, the postoperative abdominal hysterectomy client has not voided and says to the nurse, "I don't think I can urinate." The appropriate nursing action is to

○ 1. call and inform the surgeon of the client's status.
○ 2. administer additional pain medication.
○ 3. increase the client's fluid intake.
○ 4. place the client on the bedpan and give her privacy.

8. Which nursing measure would most likely relieve postoperative gas pains after abdominal hysterectomy?

○ 1. Offering the client a hot beverage.
○ 2. Providing extra warmth.
○ 3. Applying a snugly fitting abdominal binder.
○ 4. Helping the client walk.

9. On the second postoperative day after the abdominal hysterectomy, the client develops a fever of 100.4°F. One of the appropriate actions by the nurse is to

○ 1. increase the number of wound changes to minimize infection.
○ 2. obtain a culture and sensitivity of the urine to determine the source of infection.
○ 3. ensure that the client takes at least 10 deep breaths every hour.
○ 4. change the site of her intravenous fluid catheter to reduce the risk of infection.

10. The nursing care plan for a client after gynecologic surgery includes nursing orders intended to help reduce the risk of thrombophlebitis. An order that would be *contraindicated* would be to

○ 1. ambulate the client.
○ 2. massage the client's legs.
○ 3. have the client wear elasticized stockings.
○ 4. have the client perform range-of-motion exercises in bed.

11. The nurse is changing the dressing of the client after an abdominal hysterectomy. Which of the following

nursing measures would be most appropriate if the dressing sticks to the client's incisional area?

○ 1. Pull off the dressing quickly and then apply slight pressure over the area.
○ 2. Lift an easily moved portion of the dressing and then remove it slowly.
○ 3. Moisten the dressing with sterile normal saline solution and then remove it.
○ 4. Remove part of the dressing and then remove the remainder gradually over a period of several minutes.

12. A priority nursing diagnosis category for the client who experiences wound dehiscence postoperatively after an abdominal hysterectomy would be

○ 1. High Risk for Infection.
○ 2. Fluid Volume Excess.
○ 3. Ineffective Airway Clearance.
○ 4. Altered Nutrition: Less Than Body Requirements.

13. The client experiences a wound evisceration on day 2 after the abdominal hysterectomy. The immediate action by the nurse should be to

○ 1. replace the abdominal contents into the wound carefully while wearing gloves.
○ 2. apply a loose-fitting sterile abdominal binder over the wound.
○ 3. approximate the wound edges by applying strips of adhesive over the wound.
○ 4. cover the exposed tissues with sterile dressings moistened with normal saline solution.

14. Which of the following hormones are likely to be prescribed for the client after an abdominal hysterectomy and removal of the ovaries and fallopian tubes?

○ 1. Estrogen.
○ 2. Thyroxine.
○ 3. Prolactin.
○ 4. Testosterone.

15. Which of the following nursing diagnoses would be most appropriate for the client being discharged from the hospital 3 days after an abdominal hysterectomy?

○ 1. Altered Nutrition: Less Than Body Requirements related to nausea and vomiting.
○ 2. Fluid Volume Excess related to surgery.
○ 3. Altered Breathing Pattern related to postoperative pneumonia.
○ 4. Ineffective Individual Coping related to body image disturbance.

16. In preparing discharge instructions for the client after an abdominal hysterectomy, the nurse should *first*

○ 1. have the client read the discharge instructions.
○ 2. assess the client's available social supports.
○ 3. call the social worker to evaluate the client.
○ 4. read the instructions to the client.

The Client With Breast Disease

A lump is discovered by a 46-year-old woman during breast self-examination. She calls the physician's office and informs the nurse of the lump.

17. Risk factors for the development of breast cancer include
○ 1. early menopause before age 40 years.
○ 2. early onset of menstruation.
○ 3. having had more than two children.
○ 4. breast-feeding.

18. The nurse teaches the woman that the best time in the menstrual cycle to examine the breasts is during the
○ 1. week that ovulation occurs.
○ 2. week that menstruation occurs.
⊗ 3. first week after menstruation.
○ 4. week before menstruation occurs.

19. Which of the following positions is the one of choice for palpating tissues during breast self-examination?
○ 1. Sitting in a chair with a pillow under both shoulders to elevate the chest.
○ 2. Standing flat to best expose and palpate the chest area.
○ 3. Flat on the back with a pillow under the head and arms raised over the head.
○ 4. Flat on the back with a pillow under the shoulder on the side being examined.

20. The client states that she has always noticed that her brassiere fits more snugly at certain times of the month. She asks the nurse if this is a sign of breast disease. The nurse should base the reply to this client on the knowledge that
○ 1. benign cysts tend to cause the breasts to vary in size.
○ 2. it is normal for the breasts to increase in size before menstruation begins.
○ 3. a change in breast size warrants further investigation.
○ 4. differences in sizes of the breasts are related to normal growth and development.

21. The client is diagnosed with benign fibrocystic breast disease. Interventions to reduce discomfort from this disease include teaching the client to
○ 1. increase her activity level.
○ 2. wear tight supporting garments.
○ 3. avoid caffeine.
○ 4. obtain estrogen therapy from her physician.

22. The client is advised by the physician to have mammography screening annually. Measures to improve adherence with mammography screening include
○ 1. making sure that the individual barriers to screening are minimized.
○ 2. emphasizing that mammography screening can prevent breast cancer.
○ 3. emphasizing that mammography screening is a low-cost approach to cancer prevention.
○ 4. informing the client that she is at high risk for breast cancer and needs to follow the physician's recommendation.

A 50-year old client is diagnosed with breast cancer and is scheduled for a modified radical mastectomy.

23. During the admission workup, the client is extremely anxious and asks many questions. Which of the following statements would offer the best guide for the nurse to answer questions raised by this apprehensive preoperative client? It is usually best to
○ 1. tell the client as much as she wants to know and is able to understand.
○ 2. delay discussing the client's questions with her until she is convalescing.
○ 3. delay discussing the client's questions with her until her apprehension subsides.
○ 4. explain to the client that she should discuss her questions first with the physician.

24. The client asks the nurse, "Where is cancer usually found in the breast?" On a diagram of a left breast, the nurse would indicate that most malignant tumors occur in which quadrant of the breast?
○ 1. Upper, outer quadrant
○ 2. Upper, inner quadrant
○ 3. Lower, outer quadrant
○ 4. Lower, inner quadrant

25. Atropine sulfate is included in her preoperative orders. The primary reason for giving this drug preoperatively is that it helps
○ 1. promote general muscular relaxation.
○ 2. decrease pulse and respiratory rates.
○ 3. decrease nausea.
○ 4. inhibit oral and respiratory secretions.

26. Which of the following observations should the recovery room nurse plan to make *first* when the client returns from the operating room?
○ 1. Obtaining and recording vital signs.
○ 2. Observing that drainage tubes are patent and functioning.
○ 3. Ensuring that the client's airway is free of obstruction.
○ 4. Checking the client's dressings for drainage.

27. Postoperatively, the client has an incisional drainage tube attached to suction. The primary purpose of this tube is to help

○ 1. decrease intrathoracic pressure and facilitate breathing.

○ 2. increase collateral lymphatic flow toward the operative area.

○ 3. remove accumulated serum and blood in the operative area.

○ 4. prevent formation of adhesions between the skin and chest wall in the operative area.

28. Which of the following positions would be best for the client's right arm when she returns to her room after a right mastectomy?

○ 1. Across her chest wall.

○ 2. At her side at the same level as her body.

○ 3. In the position that affords her the greatest comfort without placing pressure on the incision.

○ 4. On pillows, with her hand higher than her elbow and her elbow higher than her shoulder.

29. On the third postoperative day, the drainage tube is removed, and the dressings are changed. The client appears shocked when she sees the operative area and exclaims, "I look horrible! Will it ever look better?" Which of the following responses by the nurse would be most appropriate?

○ 1. "After it heals and you're dressed, you won't even know you had surgery."

○ 2. "Don't worry. You know the tumor is gone, and the area will heal very soon."

○ 3. "Would you like to meet Ms. Paul? She looks just great and she had a mastectomy, too."

○ 4. "You're shocked by the sudden change in your appearance as a result of this surgery, aren't you?"

30. In providing discharge teaching for the client after a modified radical mastectomy, the nurse should instruct the client that she may need to modify or avoid which of the following activities?

○ 1. Shampooing her dog.

○ 2. Caring for her tropical fish.

○ 3. Working in her rose garden.

○ 4. Taking a late-evening swim.

31. A client is to have radiation therapy after a modified radical mastectomy and discharge from the hospital. When caring for the skin at the site of therapy, the client should be taught to avoid all of the following practices except

○ 1. washing the area with water.

○ 2. exposing the area to sunlight.

○ 3. applying an ointment to the area.

○ 4. using talcum powder on the area.

32. The nurse would teach a client that a normal local tissue response to radiation is

○ 1. atrophy of the skin.

○ 2. scattered pustule formation.

○ 3. redness of the surface tissue.

○ 4. sloughing of two layers of skin.

33. The nurse refers a client to Reach to Recovery. The primary purpose of the American Cancer Society's Reach to Recovery program is to

○ 1. help rehabilitate women who have had mastectomies.

○ 2. raise funds to support early breast cancer detection programs.

○ 3. provide free dressings for women who have had radical mastectomies.

○ 4. collect statistics for research from women who have had mastectomies.

The Client With Benign Prostatic Hypertrophy

A 72-year-old male client is brought to the emergency room by his son. The client is extremely uncomfortable and has been unable to void for the past 12 hours. He has known for some time that he has an enlarged prostate but has wanted to avoid surgery.

34. The best method for the nurse to use when assessing for bladder distention in a male client is to check for

○ 1. a rounded swelling above the pubis.

○ 2. dullness in the lower left quadrant.

○ 3. rebound tenderness below the symphysis.

○ 4. urine discharge from the urethral meatus.

35. During the client's urinary bladder catheterization, the bladder is emptied gradually. The best rationale for the nurse's action is that emptying an overdistended bladder completely at one time tends to cause

○ 1. renal collapse and failure.

○ 2. abdominal cramping and pain.

○ 3. hypotension and possible shock.

○ 4. weakening and atrophy of bladder musculature.

36. The primary reason for lubricating the urinary catheter generously before inserting it into a male client is that this technique helps reduce

○ 1. spasms at the orifice of the bladder.

○ 2. friction along the urethra when the catheter is being inserted.

○ 3. the number of organisms gaining entrance to the bladder.

○ 4. the formation of encrustations that may occur at the end of the catheter.

37. The primary reason for taping an indwelling catheter laterally to the thigh is to help

○ 1. eliminate pressure at the penoscrotal angle.

○ 2. prevent the catheter from kinking in the urethra.

○ 3. prevent accidental catheter removal.

○ 4. allow the client to turn without kinking the catheter.

38. The function of the prostate gland is primarily to
○ 1. store underdeveloped sperm before ejaculation.
○ 2. regulate the acidity and alkalinity environment for proper sperm development.
○ 3. produce a secretion that aids the nourishment and passage of sperm.
○ 4. secrete a hormone that stimulates the production and maturation of sperm.

39. Many older men with prostatic hypertrophy do not seek medical attention until urinary obstruction is almost complete. Investigations have found that the primary reason for this delay in seeking attention is that these men
○ 1. tend to feel too self-conscious to seek help when reproductive organs are involved.
○ 2. expect that it is normal to have to live with some urinary problems as they grow older.
○ 3. are fearful that sexual indiscretions in earlier life may be the cause of their problem.
○ 4. have little discomfort in relation to the amount of pathology because responses to pain stimuli fade with age.

40. The nurse anticipates that the client will most likely report having experienced which of the following symptoms?
○ 1. voiding at less frequent intervals.
○ 2. difficulty starting the flow of urine.
○ 3. painful urination.
○ 4. increased force of the urine stream.

41. The client is prepared for admission to the hospital. Which of the following reports by the emergency room nurse would be most helpful to the nurse responsible for admitting the client?
○ 1. "A urine specimen was obtained from the client and sent to the laboratory for analysis."
○ 2. "The client was catheterized, and 1100 mL of urine was obtained. The urine appeared cloudy, and a specimen was sent to the laboratory."
○ 3. "The client is very cooperative. He is comfortable now that his bladder has been emptied. He had no ill effects from catheterization."
○ 4. "The client was in the emergency room for 3 hours because of bladder distention. He is fine now but is being admitted as a possible candidate for surgery."

42. The client is scheduled to undergo a transurethral resection of the prostate gland. The procedure is to be done under spinal anesthesia. Postoperatively, the nurse should be particularly alert for early signs of
○ 1. convulsions.
○ 2. cardiac arrest.
○ 3. renal shutdown.
○ 4. respiratory paralysis.

43. A common nursing diagnosis for the client in the immediate postoperative phase after transurethral resection is
○ 1. Altered Peripheral Tissue Perfusion related to deep vein thrombosis.
○ 2. Self-Care Deficit related to pain of bladder spasms.
○ 3. Body Image Disturbance related to disfiguring surgery.
○ 4. Altered Peripheral Tissue Perfusion related to bleeding at the incision site.

44. The client has a continuous bladder irrigation after a transurethral resection. A major goal related to the irrigation is to
○ 1. maintain catheter patency.
○ 2. reduce incisional bleeding.
○ 3. recognize signs of prostate cancer.
○ 4. perform activities of daily living.

45. In which of the following circumstances would the nurse increase the flow rate of his continuous bladder irrigation?
○ 1. When the drainage is continuous but slow.
○ 2. When the drainage appears cloudy and dark yellow.
○ 3. When the drainage has become brighter red.
○ 4. When there is no drainage of urine and irrigating solution.

46. The client is to receive belladonna and opium suppositories, as needed, postoperatively after a transurethral resection. The nurse should give the client this drug when he demonstrates signs of
○ 1. urinary tract infection.
○ 2. urine retention.
○ 3. frequent urination.
○ 4. pain from bladder spasms.

47. A nursing assistant tells the nurse, "I think the client is confused. He keeps telling me he has to void, but that isn't possible because he has a catheter in place." Which of the following possible responses would be most appropriate for the nurse to make?
○ 1. "His catheter is probably plugged. I'll irrigate it in a few minutes."
○ 2. "That's a common complaint after prostate surgery. The client only imagines the urge to void."
○ 3. "The urge to void is usually created by the large catheter, and he may be having some bladder spasms."
○ 4. "I think he may be somewhat confused and possibly may be having some internal bleeding."

48. The report on a urine culture indicates numerous white and red blood cells and a moderate amount of bacterial growth. The nurse evaluating these findings accurately would deduce that the client most likely has a
○ 1. urethral stricture.
○ 2. decreased renal filtration rate.

○ 3. urinary tract infection.

○ 4. prostate gland malignancy.

49. In discussing home care with the client after a transurethral resection, the nurse should teach the male client that dribbling of urine

○ 1. may be an chronic problem.

○ 2. may persist for several months.

○ 3. is an abnormal sign that requires intervention.

○ 4. is a sign of healing within the prostate.

50. A priority nursing diagnosis category for the client being discharged to home 3 days after transurethral resection would be

○ 1. Fluid Volume Deficit.

○ 2. Alteration in Nutrition.

○ 3. Self-Care Deficit.

○ 4. Ineffective Airway Clearance.

51. If the client's prostate enlargement had been due to a malignancy, which of the following blood examinations should the nurse have anticipated to assess whether metastasis has occurred?

○ 1. Serum creatinine level.

○ 2. Serum acid phosphatase level.

○ 3. Total nonprotein nitrogen level.

○ 4. Endogenous creatinine clearance time.

The Client With a Sexually Transmitted Disease

A home care nurse begins caring for a 25-year-old female client who has just been diagnosed with human immunodeficiency virus (HIV).

52. The client asks the nurse, "How could this have happened?" The nurse responds to the question based on the most frequent mode of HIV transmission, which is

○ 1. hugging an HIV-positive sexual partner without using barrier precautions.

○ 2. inhaling cocaine.

○ 3. sharing food utensils with an HIV-positive person without proper cleansing of the utensils.

○ 4. having sexual intercourse with an HIV-positive person without using a condom.

53. The physician prescribes zidovudine (AZT), a drug that acts to help

○ 1. destroy the virus.

○ 2. enhance the body's antibody production.

○ 3. slow replication of the virus.

○ 4. neutralize toxins produced by the causative organism.

54. The client develops herpes genitalis and is counseled by the nurse concerning follow-up care.

Women who have this disease are at risk for developing

○ 1. sterility.

○ 2. cervical cancer.

○ 3. uterine fibroid tumors.

○ 4. irregular menses.

55. Which of the following nursing diagnosis categories would most likely be a priority for the client with herpes genitalis?

○ 1. Alteration in Sleep: Sleep Pattern Disturbance.

○ 2. Nutritional Deficit.

○ 3. Alteration in Comfort: Pain.

○ 4. Alteration in Breathing Patterns.

56. The primary reason that a herpes simplex infection is a serious concern to the client with HIV infection is that herpes simplex

○ 1. is an acquired immunodeficiency virus (AIDS)–defining illness.

○ 2. is curable only after 1 year of antiviral therapy.

○ 3. leads to cervical cancer.

○ 4. causes severe electrolyte imbalances.

57. In providing education to the client, the nurse should take into account the fact that the most effective method known to control the spread of HIV infection is

○ 1. premarital serologic screening.

○ 2. prophylactic treatment of exposed people.

○ 3. laboratory screening of pregnant women.

○ 4. ongoing sex education about preventive behaviors.

58. The client becomes depressed about her diagnosis and tells the nurse "I have nothing worth living for now." Which of the following statements would be the best response by the nurse?

○ 1. "There is much to live for; you may not develop AIDS for years."

○ 2. "You should not be too depressed; we are close to finding a cure for AIDS."

○ 3. "You are right; it is very depressing to have HIV."

○ 4. "Tell me more about how you are feeling about being HIV positive."

A 34-year old man is diagnosed with syphilis. The home health care nurse is scheduled to follow the client for 1 month.

59. The organism responsible for causing syphilis is classified as a

○ 1. virus.

○ 2. fungus.

○ 3. rickettsia.

○ 4. spirochete.

60. The typical chancre of syphilis appears as
○ 1. a grouping of small, tender pimples.
○ 2. an elevated wart.
○ 3. a painless, moist ulcer.
○ 4. an itching, crusted area.

61. When interviewing a client with newly diagnosed syphilis, the nurse should anticipate that the most difficult problem likely will be
○ 1. motivating the client to undergo treatment.
○ 2. obtaining a list of the client's sexual contacts.
○ 3. increasing the client's knowledge of the disease.
○ 4. assuring the client that records are confidential.

62. Probenecid is prescribed in conjunction with penicillin as treatment for syphilis because probenecid helps
○ 1. delay detoxification of penicillin.
○ 2. inhibit excretion of penicillin.
○ 3. maintain sensitivity of organisms to penicillin.
○ 4. decrease the likelihood of an allergic reaction to penicillin.

63. A priority nursing diagnosis for a client with primary syphilis would likely be
○ 1. High Risk for Infection Transmission related to lack of knowledge about mode of transmission.
○ 2. Pain related to cutaneous skin lesions on palms and soles.
○ 3. Altered Skin Tissue Perfusion related to a bleeding chancre.
○ 4. Body Image Disturbance related to alopecia.

An 18-year old female college student is seen at the university health center. She undergoes a pelvic examination and is diagnosed with gonorrhea.

64. Which of the following responses by the nurse would be best when the client says that she is nervous about the upcoming pelvic examination?
○ 1. "Can you tell me more about how you're feeling?"
○ 2. "You're not alone. Most women feel uncomfortable about this examination."
○ 3. "Do not worry about Dr. Smith. He's a specialist in female problems."
○ 4. "We'll do everything we can to avoid embarrassing you."

65. In educating this client, the nurse should emphasize that in women, gonorrhea
○ 1. is often marked by symptoms of dysuria or vaginal bleeding.
○ 2. does not lead to serious complications.
○ 3. can be treated but not cured.

○ 4. may not cause symptoms until serious complications occur.

66. Which of the following groups has experienced the greatest rise in the incidence of sexually transmitted diseases over the past two decades?
○ 1. Teenagers.
○ 2. Divorced people.
○ 3. Young married couples.
○ 4. Infants.

67. The client informs the nurse that she has had sexual intercourse with her boyfriend, and asks the nurse "Would he have any symptoms?" The nurse responds that in males, symptoms of gonorrhea include
○ 1. impotence.
○ 2. scrotal swelling.
○ 3. urine retention.
○ 4. dysuria.

The Client With Cancer of the Cervix

A 45-year old female client makes a clinic appointment for a routine gynecologic examination. She reports that she had not had an examination for 10 years.

68. Correct preparation of the client for a Papanicolaou's (Pap) smear would include which of the following measures?
○ 1. The test should be scheduled while the client is menstruating.
○ 2. The client should not bathe on the morning before the examination.
○ 3. The woman should not douche on the morning before the examination.
○ 4. The woman should take a laxative the night before the examination.

69. The position of choice for a client undergoing a vaginal examination is the
○ 1. Sims' position.
○ 2. lithotomy position.
○ 3. genupectoral position.
○ 4. dorsal recumbent position.

70. A client asks the nurse to explain the meaning of the Pap smear results. Which of the following concepts should the nurse include in the response?
○ 1. A typical Pap smear means that abnormal—but not necessarily neoplastic—cells were found in the smear.
○ 2. An atypical Pap smear means that cancer cells were found in the smear.
○ 3. A positive Pap smear alone is not very important diagnostically because there are many false-positive results.

○ 4. Abnormal cells in a Pap smear may be caused by conditions other than cancer.

71. Which of the following is a risk factor for cervical cancer?

○ 1. Sexual experiences with one partner.

○ 2. Multiple pregnancies.

○ 3. Positive family history for cervical cancer.

○ 4. Adolescent pregnancy.

72. The American Cancer Society recommends that the average adult woman follow which schedule for Pap smear screening?

○ 1. Annually after 18 years of age.

○ 2. Annually if sexually active; every 5 years if sexually abstinent.

○ 3. Every 3 years after three initial negative tests taken annually.

○ 4. Every 3 years until age 40 and annually thereafter.

A 27-year-old female client makes an appointment with a gynecologist for a routine examination and Pap smear. The woman has always been in good health.

73. The woman tells the nurse that she is always nervous about these examinations because "there's been a lot of cancer in my family." The nurse should be aware that an early sign of cervical cancer is

○ 1. a thick, foul-smelling vaginal discharge.

○ 2. bleeding after intercourse.

○ 3. a change in the menstrual cycle.

○ 4. watery vaginal discharge.

74. After examination and diagnostic testing, the client is diagnosed with cancer of the cervix in situ. A conization is scheduled. Which of the following nursing interventions would take priority during the first 24 postoperative hours?

○ 1. Monitoring vital signs hourly.

○ 2. Maintaining strict bed rest.

○ 3. Monitoring vaginal bleeding.

○ 4. Maintaining electrolyte balance.

75. The client's husband says to the nurse, "The doctor told my wife that her cancer is curable. Is he just trying to make us feel better?" Which would be the nurse's most accurate response?

○ 1. "When cervical cancer is detected early and treated aggressively, the cure rate is almost 100%."

○ 2. "The 5-year survival rate is about 75%, which makes the odds pretty good."

○ 3. "Saying a cancer is curable means that 50% of all women with the cancer survive at least 5 years."

○ 4. "Cancers of the female reproductive tract tend to be slow growing and respond well to treatment."

76. The client's cancer recurs, and internal radiation treatment with a radium implant is planned. On hospital admission, the client says that she is concerned about being radioactive and has been having nightmares about the treatment. What would be a reasonable explanation for the nurse to give to the client?

○ 1. "The radioactive material is controlled and stays with the source; once the material is removed, no radioactivity will remain."

○ 2. "The radioactivity will gradually decrease, and you will be discharged when the radioactive material reaches its half-life."

○ 3. "These nightmares indicate that you're in the denial phase of accepting the diagnosis."

○ 4. "Careful shielding prevents the area above your waist from radioactivity."

77. A lead-lined container and a pair of long forceps are kept in the client's hospital room for

○ 1. disposal of emesis or other bodily secretions.

○ 2. handling of the dislodged radiation source.

○ 3. disposal of the client's eating utensils.

○ 4. storage of the radiation booster dose.

78. The client's mother asks why so many nurses are involved in her daughter's care and says, "The doctor said I can be in the room for up to 2 hours each day, but the nurses say they're restricted to 30 minutes." The nurse explains that this variation is based on the fact that nurses

○ 1. touch the client, which increases their exposure to radiation.

○ 2. work with many clients and could carry infection to a client receiving radiation therapy, if exposure is prolonged.

○ 3. work with radiation on an ongoing basis, while visitors have infrequent exposure to radiation.

○ 4. are at greater risk from the radiation because they are younger than the mother.

79. A priority nursing diagnosis for a client with cervical cancer and an internal radium implant would be

○ 1. Pain related to cervical tumor.

○ 2. Anxiety related to self-care deficit from imposed immobility during radiation.

○ 3. Altered Health Maintenance related to surgery.

○ 4. Sleep Pattern Disturbance related to interruptions of sleep by health care personnel.

80. What activity orders would be appropriate for a client with an internal radium implant for cervical cancer?

○ 1. Out of bed as tolerated within the room.

○ 2. Bed rest with bathroom privileges.

○ 3. Bed rest in position of comfort.

○ 4. Bed rest with the head of the bed flat.

81. Which of the following would be standard nursing

care for a client with cervical cancer and an internal radium implant in place?

○ 1. Offer the bedpan every 2 hours.

○ 2. Provide perineal care twice daily.

○ 3. Check the position of the applicator hourly.

○ 4. Offer a low residue diet.

82. The nurse should carefully observe a client with internal radium implants for typical side effects associated with radiation therapy to the cervix. These effects include

○ 1. cramping pain and severe vaginal itching.

○ 2. confusion and sleep disturbances.

○ 3. high fever in the afternoon or evening.

○ 4. nausea, vomiting, and a foul discharge.

The Client With Testicular Disease

A 28-year-old male client is diagnosed with acute epididymitis.

83. The nurse would expect to find that the classic symptoms of epididymitis that caused the client to seek medical care were

○ 1. burning and pain on urination.

○ 2. severe tenderness and swelling in the scrotum.

○ 3. foul-smelling ejaculate and severe scrotal swelling.

○ 4. foul-smelling urine and pain on urination.

84. All of the following would be appropriate interventions for this client *except*

○ 1. maintaining bed rest.

○ 2. elevating the testes.

○ 3. increasing fluid intake.

○ 4. applying hot packs to the scrotum.

85. When teaching a client to perform testicular self-examination, the nurse should explain that the examination should be performed

○ 1. after intercourse.

○ 2. at the end of the day.

○ 3. after a warm bath or shower.

○ 4. after exercise.

86. The normal testis can be described as

○ 1. soft.

○ 2. egg shaped.

○ 3. spongy.

○ 4. lumpy.

87. A year later, the client returns to the physician, saying that he thinks the epididymitis has returned.

The physician examines him and makes a preliminary diagnosis of testicular cancer. Which clinical manifestation helps differentiate testicular cancer from epididymitis?

○ 1. The inability to achieve or sustain an erection.

○ 2. Scrotal pain.

○ 3. A dragging sensation in the scrotum.

○ 4. Scrotal swelling.

88. Although the cause of testicular cancer is unknown, it is associated with a history of

○ 1. undescended testis.

○ 2. sexual relations at an early age.

○ 3. seminal vesiculitis.

○ 4. epididymitis.

89. The diagnosis of testicular cancer is confirmed, and the client is scheduled for a right orchiectomy. The day before surgery, the client tells the nurse that he is concerned about the effect that losing a testicle will have on his manhood. Which of the following facts about orchiectomy should form the basis for the nurse's response?

○ 1. Testosterone levels are decreased.

○ 2. Sexual drive and libido are unchanged.

○ 3. Sperm count increases in the remaining testicle.

○ 4. Secondary sexual characteristics change.

90. Because the client will have a high inguinal incision, a priority problem for the immediate postoperative period would be

○ 1. bladder spasms.

○ 2. urinary elimination.

○ 3. pain.

○ 4. nausea.

91. The orchiectomy is performed, and the pathology report reveals a diagnosis of malignant seminoma. Chemotherapy is ordered. The nurse teaches the client about the potential side effects of chemotherapy, which include

○ 1. fluid volume retention.

○ 2. dyspnea.

○ 3. sterility.

○ 4. anemia.

92. A client diagnosed with testicular cancer expresses fear and questions the nurse about his prognosis. The nurse should base the response on the knowledge that

○ 1. testicular cancer is almost always fatal.

○ 2. testicular cancer has a cure rate of 90% when diagnosed early.

○ 3. surgery is the treatment of choice for testicular cancer.

○ 4. testicular cancer has a 50% cure rate when diagnosed early.

CORRECT ANSWERS AND RATIONALE

The letters in parentheses following the rationale identify the step of the nursing process (A, D, P, I, E), cognitive level (K, C, T, N), and client needs (S, G, L, H). See the Answer Grid for the key.

The Client With Uterine Fibroids

1. 2. The best approach for a client who is fearful about having surgery is to allow the client opportunities to express her fears. Such courses of action as assuring a client of the physician's competence, saying that fear impedes recovery, and changing the subject are nonsupportive and deny her an opportunity to express her feelings. (I, N, L)

2. 2. It is a priority that the client knows that she will not be able to eat or drink for 8 hours before admission. The clothing she should wear to the hospital and the type of medication she will receive are important, but not the priority. Coughing is not routinely recommended for postoperative clients unless they experience pulmonary congestion. (I, T, S)

3. 2. The correct amount to administer is determined by using ratios, as follows:

0.8 mg$/1$ mL $= 0.4$ mg$/x$ mL.

$0.8x = 0.4$

$x = 0.5$ mL of atropine sulfate

100 mg$/1$ mL $= 75$ mg$/x$ mL.

$100x = 75$

$x = 0.75$ mL of meperidine hydrochloride

0.5 mL of atropine $+ 0.75$ mL of meperidine hydrochloride $= 1.25$ mL total

(I, C, S)

4. 4. Starting from the area nearer the pubic bone and moving toward the anus, the anatomic order is clitoris, urinary meatus, and vaginal opening. (I, K, G)

5. 2. The best course of action when a client refuses to eat food that is contrary to her religious beliefs is to discuss the situation with the client and the dietitian. Health team members may need to confer about this client's needs. Telling the client that it is important for her to eat what is served is unlikely to help because she has already refused the food. Encouraging her family to bring suitable food to the hospital for her is ordinarily against agency policy and should not be considered until the situation has been discussed with an agency dietitian. Threatening a client by saying that if she does not eat, intravenous therapy will be necessary is nonsupportive and is unlikely to gain her cooperation. (I, N, G)

6. 2. Hyperventilation occurs when the client breathes so rapidly and deeply that she exhales excessive amounts of carbon dioxide. A characteristic symptom of hyperventilation is dizziness. Dyspnea, blurred vision, and mental confusion are not associated with hyperventilation. (A, T, G)

7. 4. The nurse should suspect that a client has urinary retention when she is unable to void in an 8-hour period. Before calling the physician for an order to catheterize the client, the nurse should assist the client in trying to void by placing her on the bedpan and allowing her privacy. Increasing fluid intake is not indicated at this time in this situation. (I, T, G)

8. 4. Usually, the discomfort associated with gas pains is likely to be relieved when the client ambulates. The gas will be more easily expelled with exercise. Such techniques as applying an abdominal binder, offering the client a hot beverage, and providing extra warmth are not recommended and may even aggravate the discomfort of postoperative gas pains. (I, T, G)

9. 3. Elevated temperature on the second postoperative day is most suggestive of a respiratory tract infection. Respiratory infections most often occur during the first 48 hours after surgery. Signs of infection, if present in the wound or urinary tract, are likely to occur later in the postoperative period. There is no indication that the intravenous catheter is the source of infection. (I, T, G)

10. 2. Massaging the legs postoperatively is contraindicated because it may dislodge small clots of blood, if present, and cause even more serious problems. Such measures as ambulating the client, having her wear elasticized stockings, and having her move her legs about in bed have been found to help reduce the incidence of postoperative thrombophlebitis. (I, T, G)

11. 3. When a dressing sticks to a wound, it is best to moisten the dressing with sterile normal saline solution and then remove it carefully. Trying to remove a dry dressing is likely to irritate the skin and wound. (I, T, S)

12. 1. Dehiscence, the opening of a wound, places the client at an immediate increased risk for infection. (D, N, G)

13. 4. The nurse should cover the exposed tissues with

sterile dressings moistened with sterile normal saline solutions if the wound opens and tissues are exposed (wound evisceration). The nurse should also cover an eviscerated wound with sterile dressings moistened with sterile normal saline solution. The physician should be notified immediately when a wound dehisces or eviscerates. Such measures as trying to replace the exposed tissues or organs, applying an abdominal binder, or trying to approximate the wound edges with adhesive strips are contraindicated and are likely to aggravate the problem. (I, T, G)

14. 1. The primary ovarian hormone is estrogen. It is likely to be prescribed for a woman whose ovaries, fallopian tubes, and uterus have been surgically removed. Many physicians now use both estrogen and progesterone, cyclically or combined, in postoperative hormone replacement therapy. (I, C, G)

15. 4. Body image disturbance related to loss of female reproductive organs may lead to ineffective coping in some women. Therefore, interventions to address this problem should be incorporated into discharge planning. Nausea, vomiting, and fluid volume overload are not problems expected 3 days after an abdominal hysterectomy. (D, N, L)

16. 2. Assessment is the first step in planning client education. Assessing social support resources is a key aspect of discharge planning that begins when the client is admitted to the hospital. Calling the social worker is not the first action the nurse should take. Having the client read the instructions or reading instructions to the client is not the first step of discharge planning. (I, N, S)

The Client With Breast Disease

17. 2. A family history of breast cancer, early onset of menstruation, delayed onset of menopause, and childlessness all appear to increase a woman's risk of breast cancer. Breast-feeding does not increase the risk. (A, K, G)

18. 3. It is generally recommended that the breasts be examined during the first week after menstruation. During this period, the breasts are least likely to be tender or swollen because the secretion of estrogen, which prepares the uterus for implantation, is at its lowest level. (I, T, H)

19. 4. For a self-breast examination, placing a pillow or towel under the shoulder on the side being examined elevates the chest wall while the woman lies flat on her back. This positioning allows for better distribution of breast tissue over the chest wall and allows for the most thorough examination of tissues by palpation. A standing position, facing a mirror, is used to examine the breasts for changes in size and shape, for skin dimpling, and for nipple changes. The standing or sitting positions are not appropriate for palpating breast tissues. (I, C, H)

20. 2. The breasts normally are about the same size. They may vary in size somewhat before menstruation, owing to breast engorgement caused by hormonal changes. A woman may then note that her brassiere fits more tightly than usual. (I, T, H)

21. 3. Avoiding caffeine is thought to alleviate discomfort associated with fibrocystic breast disease. Wearing tighter garments could increase discomfort. Activity level is not associated with fibrocystic breast disease. A nurse should not recommend estrogen therapy as an intervention for discomfort from fibrocystic breast disease. (I, T, G)

22. 1. Reducing barriers to mammography scan is the best way to improve adherence with screening. Mammography can detect breast cancer in the early stages but cannot prevent it. Mammography is not a low-cost approach for all clients, and in fact, it may cost the client a significant amount of money. The client is not at high risk for developing breast cancer at this point. (I, N, H)

23. 1. An important nursing responsibility is preoperative teaching, and the most frequently recommended guide for teaching is to tell the client as much as she wants to know and is able to understand. Delaying discussion of issues about which the client has concerns is likely to aggravate the situation and cause the client to feel distrust. (I, T, L)

24. 1. About half of malignant breast tumors occur in the upper, outer quadrant of the breast. Interestingly, but for no known reason, cancer appears in the left breast more often than in the right breast. (A, K, G)

25. 4. Atropine sulfate, a cholinergic blocking agent, is given preoperatively primarily to reduce secretions in the mouth and respiratory tract. It is not used to promote muscle relaxation, decrease pulse and respiratory rates, or decrease nausea and vomiting. (I, C, G)

26. 3. The highest priority when a nurse receives a client from the operating room is to assess airway patency. If the airway is not clear, immediate steps should be taken so that the client is able to breathe. After ensuring that the airway is clear and the client is breathing well, the nurse should proceed with such measures as obtaining the vital signs, assessing that drainage tubes are functioning properly, and checking the client's dressing. (A, T, G)

27. 3. A drainage tube is placed in the wound after a modified radical mastectomy to help remove accumulated blood and fluid in the area. Drainage tubes placed in a wound do not decrease intrathoracic pressure, increase collateral lymphatic flow, or prevent the adhesion formation. (I, T, G)

28. 4. Lymph nodes are ordinarily removed from the axillary area when a modified radical mastectomy is done. Therefore, to facilitate drainage from the arm on the affected side, the client's arm should be elevated on pillows with her hand higher than her elbow and her elbow higher than her shoulder. The other techniques for positioning the arm on the affected side do not facilitate drainage from the arm. (I, T, G)

29. 4. When a client appears shocked by her appearance after surgery, such as after having a mastectomy, the nurse should help her express her feelings and offer supportive care, which she needs at this time. Telling the client not to worry or that her disfigurement will not show when she is dressed are nonsupportive and are likely to cause more concerns. Having the client meet someone who has had breast surgery is often helpful but is better done later, when the client is convalescing and accustomed to the appearance of the operative site. The client needs the nurse's support when the dressings are removed, not sometime later. (I, N, L)

30. 3. After a mastectomy, every effort should be made to avoid cuts, bruises, and burns on the affected arm because normal circulation has been impaired. Working in a rose or cactus garden is a risk because of the danger of skin pricks. The client should be advised to wear protective clothing to prevent cuts, bruises, and burns. Such activities as caring for pets and swimming are not contraindicated for the postmastectomy client. (I, N, H)

31. 1. A client receiving radiation therapy should avoid lotions, ointments, and anything that may cause irritation to the skin, such as exposure to sunlight and talcum powder. The area may safely be washed with water if it is done gently and if care is taken not to injure the skin. (I, T, S)

32. 3. The most common reaction of the skin to radiation therapy is redness of the surface tissues. Dryness, desquamation, tanning, and capillary dilation are also common. (I, T, H)

33. 1. The American Cancer Society's Reach to Recovery is a rehabilitation program for women who have had breast surgery. It is designed to meet their physical, psychological, and cosmetic needs but does not provide funds or dressings. Research is not part of the program. (I, T, L)

The Client With Benign Prostatic Hypertrophy

34. 1. The best way to assess for a distended bladder is to check for a rounded swelling above the pubis. This swelling represents the distended bladder ris-

ing above the pubis into the abdominal cavity. (A, C, G)

35. 3. Rapidly emptying an overdistended bladder may cause hypotension and shock due to the sudden change of pressure within the abdominal viscera. Renal collapse is not likely, nor are abdominal cramping and bladder weakening and atrophy. (I, T, G)

36. 2. Lubricating the catheter liberally before catheterizing a male decreases friction along the urethra and reduces irritation and trauma to urethral tissues. Because the male urethra is tortuous, a liberal amount of lubrication is advised to ease catheter passage. The female urethra is not tortuous, and although the catheter should be lubricated before insertion, not as much lubricant is necessary as for a male. (I, C, S)

37. 1. The primary reason for taping an indwelling catheter to a male client so that the penis is held in a lateral position is to prevent pressure at the penoscrotal angle. Prolonged pressure at the penoscrotal angle can cause a ureterocutaneous fistula. (I, T, S)

38. 3. The prostate gland serves one primary purpose: it produces a secretion that aids the nourishment and passage of sperm. (A, K, G)

39. 2. It has been found that older men tend to believe that it is normal to live with some urinary problems. As a result, these men often overlook symptoms and simply attribute them to aging. (E, K, H)

40. 2. Signs and symptoms of prostatic hypertrophy include difficulty starting the flow of urine, urinary frequency and hesitancy, decreased force of the urine stream, interruptions in the urine stream when voiding, and nocturia. (A, T, G)

41. 2. A report about the client's condition should be as clear, pertinent, and concise as possible, and it should be free of subjective information that could be interpreted differently by different caregivers. In this situation, the nurse should indicate how much urine had been drained from the client's bladder and how the urine appeared. The nurse should also report that a urine specimen has been sent to the laboratory for analysis. The fact that the specimen is cloudy should cause others to evaluate the client further. (E, T, S)

42. 4. If paralysis of vasomotor nerves in the upper spinal cord occurs when spinal anesthesia is used, the client is likely to develop respiratory paralysis. Artificial ventilation is required until the effects of anesthesia subside. Other possible complications of spinal anesthesia include hypotension, nausea and vomiting, postanesthesia headache, and neurologic complications, such as muscle weakness in the legs. (A, T, G)

43. 2. The pain of bladder spasms frequently necessitates intervention. Deep vein thrombosis and bleeding at the incisional site are not common after a transurethral resection. The surgery is not disfiguring. (D, N, G)

44. 1. Maintaining catheter patency during the immediate postoperative period after a transurethral resection is a priority. Incisional bleeding is not expected unless a complication occurs. Performing activities of daily living, such as bathing, is not a priority immediately after surgery. The client in the immediate postoperative period is not ready for teaching. (P, T, S)

45. 3. During continuous bladder irrigation after a prostatectomy, the rate at which the solution enters the bladder should be increased when the drainage becomes brighter red. The color indicates the presence of blood. Increasing the flow of irrigating solution helps flush the catheter well so that clots do not plug it. There would be no reason to increase the flow rate when the return is continuous or appears cloudy and dark yellow. Increasing the flow would be contraindicated if there is no return of urine and irrigating solution. (I, T, G)

46. 4. Belladonna and opium suppositories are prescribed and administered to reduce bladder spasms that cause pain after a transurethral resection. (I, T, G)

47. 3. The Foley catheter creates the urge to void and may also cause bladder spasms. Less likely reasons for the client's urge to void include a plugged catheter, imagining the urge, confusion, and internal bleeding. (I, N, G)

48. 3. The presence of red and white blood cells in the urine is most typical of a urinary tract infection. (E, T, G)

49. 2. Dribbling of urine may occur for several months after transurethral resection, and the client needs to be informed that this is expected. (I, T, H)

50. 3. Self-Care Deficit is a priority diagnosis because the client may need assistance with activities that involve bending or lifting. Fluid volume deficit, alteration in nutrition, and ineffective airway clearance are not anticipated priority problems after transurethral resection. (D, N, H)

51. 2. The most specific examination to determine whether a malignancy extends outside of the prostatic capsule is a study of the serum acid phosphatase level. The level increases when a malignancy has been metastasized. (A, K, S)

The Client With a Sexually Transmitted Disease

52. 4. HIV infection is transmitted through blood and body fluids, particularly vaginal and seminal fluids.

A blood transfusion is one way the disease can be contracted. Other modes of transmission are sexual intercourse with an infected partner and sharing needles for intravenous drug injections with an infected person. (A, C, S)

53. 3. Zidovudine interferes with replication of HIV and thereby slows progression of HIV to AIDS. There is no known cure for HIV infection. (I, C, G)

54. 2. Women who have herpes genitalis are more likely to develop cervical cancer than women who have never had the disease. Regular examinations, including Pap tests, are recommended. (I, T, H)

55. 3. Pain is a common problem in women with herpes genitalis. Analgesia may be prescribed for the pain. Sleep disturbances, nutritional deficits, and altered breathing patterns are not problems frequently associated with herpes genitalis. (D, T, G)

56. 1. Herpes simplex is one of a group of disorders that, when diagnosed in the presence of HIV infection, are considered to be diagnostic for AIDS. Other AIDS-defining illnesses include Kaposi's sarcoma; cytomegalovirus of the liver, spleen, or lymph nodes; and *Pneumocystis carinii* pneumonia. (A, N, G)

57. 4. Education to prevent behaviors that cause HIV transmission is the primary method of controlling HIV infection. Behaviors that place people at risk for HIV infection include unprotected sexual intercourse and sharing of intravenous drug needles. Educating clients about using condoms during sexual relations is a priority in controlling HIV transmission. (E, N, H)

58. 4. The nurse should respond with a statement that allows the client to express her thoughts and feelings. Encouraging statements do not provide an opportunity for the client to express herself, nor does a statement agreeing that she is right. (I, N, L)

59. 4. *Treponema pallidum,* the organism that causes syphilis, is classified as a spirochete because of its corkscrew appearance. (A, K, G)

60. 3. The chancre of syphilis is characteristically a painless, moist ulcer. The serous discharge is very infectious. The chancre most often occurs on the penis but may also occur on the anus, rectum, lips, and mouth. It also occasionally occurs on the skin where the causative organism entered the body. (A, K, G)

61. 2. An important aspect of controlling the spread of sexually transmitted diseases is obtaining a list of the sexual contacts of an infected client. These contacts, in turn, should be encouraged to obtain immediate care. Many people with sexually transmitted diseases are reluctant to reveal their sexual contacts, which makes controlling sexually transmitted diseases difficult. There are fewer reported difficulties in motivating people with sexually transmitted diseases to seek treatment, increasing their knowledge of the disease, and assuring them that their records are confidential. (P, N, S)

62. 2. Normally, the kidneys effectively clear penicillin from the blood. Probenecid inhibits excretion of penicillin and thereby helps maintain high blood levels of penicillin. (I, C, G)

63. 1. A client with primary syphilis is at risk of transmitting the disease to sexual partners if he or she is not knowledgeable about how the disease is spread. Cutaneous lesions on the palms and soles and alopecia are signs of secondary syphilis. Chancres do not bleed sufficiently to alter tissue perfusion. (D, N, H)

64. 1. Asking the client to describe her nervousness gives her the opportunity to express her concerns and allows the nurse to understand her better. Responses that make assumptions about the source of the concern or offer reinforcement are nonsupportive and block successful communication. (I, N, L)

65. 4. Many women are unaware that they have gonorrhea because they are symptom-free or experience only very mild symptoms until the disease progresses to pelvic inflammatory disease. (I, T, H)

66. 1. Statistics reveal that the incidence of sexually transmitted diseases is rising more rapidly among teenagers than among any other age group. Many reasons have been given for this trend, including a change in societal mores and increasing sexual activity among teenagers. (E, N, H)

67. 4. Gonorrhea in men is characterized by dysuria and a mucopurulent urethral discharge. (I, T, G)

The Client With Cancer of the Cervix

68. 3. Douching within 24 to 48 hours before a Pap smear may wash away cells and secretions needed for accurate test results. The test should be scheduled for a time when the client is not menstruating. No bowel preparation is needed, and the client may bathe as desired. (I, C, S)

69. 2. Although other positions may be used, the preferred position for a vaginal examination is the lithotomy position because it is convenient for the examiner and offers the best visualization. (I, T, S)

70. 4. The Pap smear identifies atypical cervical cells that may be present for various reasons. Cancer is the most common possible cause, but not the only one. An adequate smear provides accurate diagnostic data; the false-positive rate is only about 5%. (I, T, G)

71. 3. A positive family history is a risk factor for cervical cancer. The incidence of cervical cancer is closely linked to sexual experience with multiple partners and a history of sexually transmitted dis-

ease (ie, syphilis, gonorrhea, herpes genitalis). Multiple pregnancies and pregnancy at an early age do not increase the risk. (A, T, G)

72. 3. Current American Cancer Society guidelines advocate Pap smears every 3 years after an initial negative pattern is established and the woman is deemed to be at low risk for development of cervical cancer. Annual screening is recommended for any woman in the high-risk category. (P, C, H)

73. 4. In its early stages, cancer of the cervix is usually asymptomatic, which underscores the importance of regular Pap smears. A watery vaginal discharge is often the first noticeable symptom. Discomfort, foul-smelling discharge, and weight loss are late signs. (A, T, G)

74. 3. Uncontrolled vaginal bleeding is the priority concern during the first 24 hours after conization of the cervix. This is best monitored by keeping an accurate pad count, which assesses the extent of bleeding. Hourly vital signs and strict bed rest are unnecessary unless complications develop. Electrolyte imbalance is not anticipated with this procedure. (I, T, G)

75. 1. When cervical cancer is detected early and treated aggressively, the cure rate approaches 100%. (I, T, G)

76. 1. The radioactivity comes from a radioactive material such as radium or cesium. Radioactivity affects tissues but does not make them radioactive. Once the radioactive source is removed, no radioactivity remains. Accurate information can help alleviate ungrounded fears. The time required for a radioactive substance to be half-dissipated is called its half-life, but this does not determine discharge time. The client receiving sealed internal radiotherapy is not discharged until the radioactive source is removed. Nightmares probably indicate the client's concern about the therapy. There is no way to shield the area above the waist from radiation with cervical implants. (I, N, L)

77. 2. Dislodged radioactive materials should not be touched with bare or gloved hands. Forceps are used to place the material in the lead-lined container, which shields the radiation. Exposure to radiation can occur only by direct exposure to the encased radioactive substance; it cannot result from contact with emesis or urine or from touching the client. Radioactive materials are kept only in the radiation department. It is not usual to boost an applicator. (I, T, S)

78. 3. The three factors related to radiation safety are time, distance, and shielding. Nurses on radiation oncology units work with radiation frequently and so must limit their contact. Nurses are physically closer to clients than are visitors, who are often asked to sit 6 feet away. Touching the client does not increase the amount of radiation exposure. Aseptic technique and isolation prevent the spread of infection. Age is a risk factor for people in their reproductive years. (I, N, S)

79. 2. A client may experience anxiety because she is immobilized on strict bed rest and is unable to care for herself while the implant is in place. The other diagnoses are not priorities; typically, the tumor is surgically removed before the implant is placed. (D, N, L)

80. 4. The client with a cervical implant is kept on strict bed rest, flat in bed. Limitation of movement is designed to prevent accidental displacement or even dislodgment of the implant. Client knowledge and understanding are critical to compliance with these restrictions. (I, T, S)

81. 4. Bowel movements can be difficult with the radium applicator in place. The purpose of the low residue diet is to decrease the need for a bowel movement. To prevent dislodging the applicator, the client is maintained on strict bed rest and allowed only to turn from side to side. Perineal care is omitted during radium implant therapy, although any vaginal discharge should be reported to the doctor. It is rare for the applicator to extrude, so this need not be checked every hour. (I, T, G)

82. 4. Nausea, vomiting, and foul vaginal discharge are common side effects of internal radiation therapy for cervical cancer. (A, T, G)

The Client With Testicular Disease

83. 2. Epididymitis causes acute tenderness and pronounced swelling of the scrotum. It is occasionally, but not routinely, associated with urinary tract infection. (A, T, G)

84. 4. Rest is the foundation of treatment. Elevating the scrotum may increase the client's comfort. Intermittent ice application will enhance comfort and reduce swelling. Hot packs are not used because the temperature in the scrotum should remain below body temperature; excessive exposure to heat can cause destruction of sperm cells. (I, T, G)

85. 3. After a warm bath or shower, the testes hang low and relaxed and are in ideal position for manual evaluation and palpation. (I, T, H)

86. 2. Normal testes feel smooth, egg-shaped, and firm to the touch, without lumps. They should not be soft or spongy to the touch. (A, K, G)

87. 3. A dragging sensation in the scrotum is associated with testicular cancer, not epididymitis. The manifestations of testicular cancer are less dramatic than those of epididymitis. Other clinical manifestations of testicular cancer include a lump in or swelling of the testis, a dull ache in the lower abdomen or inguinal area, and occasional pain. Sexual performance is unaffected. (A, C, G)

88. 1. Cryptorchidism (undescended testis) carries a greatly increased risk for testicular cancer. Other possible causes include chemical carcinogens, trauma, orchitis, and environmental factors. Testicular cancer is not associated with early sexual relations in men, although cervical cancer is associated with early sexual relations in women. (A, C, H)

89. 2. The remaining testicle undergoes hyperplasia and produces enough testosterone to maintain sexual drive, libido, and secondary sexual characteristics. Sperm count can decrease after a unilateral orchiectomy; this is attributed to the stress of the surgery. (I, N, G)

90. 3. Due to the location of the incision, pain is a major problem during the immediate postoperative period. Bladder spasms and elimination problems are more commonly associated with prostate surgery. (D, N, G)

91. 3. Sterility is a potential side effect of the chemotherapeutic agents used to treat testicular cancer. (I, T, S)

92. 2. When diagnosed early and treated aggressively, testicular cancer has a cure rate of about 90%. Surgery is only one mode of treatment and is combined with chemotherapy and radiation therapy. The chemotherapeutic regimen used currently is responsible for the successful treatment of testicular cancer. (P, T, G)

NURSING CARE OF ADULTS WITH MEDICAL AND SURGICAL HEALTH PROBLEMS

TEST 8: The Client With Reproductive Health Problems

Directions: Use this answer grid to determine areas of strength or need for further study.

NURSING PROCESS

A = Assessment
D = Analysis, nursing diagnosis
P = Planning
I = Implementation
E = Evaluation

COGNITIVE LEVEL

K = Knowledge
C = Comprehension
T = Application
N = Analysis

CLIENT NEEDS

S = Safe, effective care environment
G = Physiologic integrity
L = Psychosocial integrity
H = Health promotion and maintenance

Question #	Answer #	Nursing Process					Cognitive Level				Client Needs			
		A	D	P	I	E	K	C	T	N	S	G	L	H
1	2				I					N			L	
2	2				I				T		S			
3	2				I			C			S			
4	4				I		K					G		
5	2				I					N		G		
6	2	A							T			G		
7	4				I				T			G		
8	4				I				T			G		
9	3				I				T			G		
10	2				I				T			G		
11	3				I				T		S			
12	1		D							N		G		
13	4				I				T			G		
14	1				I			C				G		
15	4		D							N			L	
16	2				I					N	S			
17	2	A					K					G		
18	3				I				T					H
19	4				I			C						H
20	2				I				T					H
21	3				I				T			G		
22	1				I					N				H
23	1				I				T				L	
24	1	A					K					G		
25	4				I			C				G		

ANSWER GRID: 1

NURSING PROCESS

A = Assessment
D = Analysis, nursing diagnosis
P = Planning
I = Implementation
E = Evaluation

COGNITIVE LEVEL

K = Knowledge
C = Comprehension
T = Application
N = Analysis

CLIENT NEEDS

S = Safe, effective care environment
G = Physiologic integrity
L = Psychosocial integrity
H = Health promotion and maintenance

Question #	Answer #	Nursing Process					Cognitive Level				Client Needs			
		A	D	P	I	E	K	C	T	N	S	G	L	H
26	3	A							T			G		
27	3				I				T			G		
28	4				I				T			G		
29	4				I					N			L	
30	3				I					N				H
31	1				I				T		S			
32	3				I				T					H
33	1				I				T				L	
34	1	A						C				G		
35	3				I				T			G		
36	2				I			C			S			
37	1				I				T		S			
38	3	A					K					G		
39	2					E	K							H
40	2	A							T			G		
41	2					E			T		S			
42	4	A							T			G		
43	2		D							N		G		
44	1			P					T		S			
45	3				I				T			G		
46	4				I				T			G		
47	3				I					N		G		
48	3					E			T			G		
49	2				I				T					H
50	3		D							N				H
51	2	A					K				S			
52	4	A						C			S			
53	3				I			C				G		
54	2				I				T					H
55	3		D						T			G		

ANSWER GRID: 2

NURSING PROCESS

A = Assessment
D = Analysis, nursing diagnosis
P = Planning
I = Implementation
E = Evaluation

COGNITIVE LEVEL

K = Knowledge
C = Comprehension
T = Application
N = Analysis

CLIENT NEEDS

S = Safe, effective care environment
G = Physiologic integrity
L = Psychosocial integrity
H = Health promotion and maintenance

Question #	Answer #	Nursing Process					Cognitive Level				Client Needs			
		A	D	P	I	E	K	C	T	N	S	G	L	H
56	1	A								N		G		
57	4					E				N				H
58	4				I					N			L	
59	4	A					K					G		
60	3	A					K					G		
61	2			P						N	S			
62	2				I			C				G		
63	1		D							N				H
64	1				I					N			L	
65	4				I				T					H
66	1					E				N				H
67	4				I				T			G		
68	3				I			C			S			
69	2				I				T		S			
70	4				I				T			G		
71	3	A							T			G		
72	3			P				C						H
73	4	A							T			G		
74	3				I				T			G		
75	1				I				T			G		
76	1				I					N			L	
77	2				I				T		S			
78	3				I					N	S			
79	2		D							N			L	
80	4				I				T		S			
81	4				I				T			G		
82	4	A							T			G		
83	2	A							T			G		
84	4				I				T			G		
85	3				I				T					H

ANSWER GRID: 3

NURSING PROCESS

A = Assessment
D = Analysis, nursing diagnosis
P = Planning
I = Implementation
E = Evaluation

COGNITIVE LEVEL

K = Knowledge
C = Comprehension
T = Application
N = Analysis

CLIENT NEEDS

S = Safe, effective care environment
G = Physiologic integrity
L = Psychosocial integrity
H = Health promotion and maintenance

Question #	Answer #	Nursing Process					Cognitive Level				Client Needs			
		A	D	P	I	E	K	C	T	N	S	G	L	H
86	2	A					K					G		
87	3	A						C				G		
88	1	A						C						H
89	2				I					N		G		
90	3		D							N		G		
91	3				I				T		S			
92	2			P					T			G		
Number Correct														
Number Possible	92	20	8	4	55	5	9	13	47	23	18	48	9	17
Percentage Correct														

Score Calculation: To determine your **Percentage Correct,** divide the **Number Correct** by the **Number Possible.**

ANSWER GRID: 4

The Client With Neurologic Health Problems

- **The Client With a Head Injury**
- **The Client With Seizures**
- **The Client With a Cerebrovascular Accident**
- **The Client With Parkinson's Disease**
- **The Client With Multiple Sclerosis**
- **The Unconscious Client**
- **The Client in Pain**
- **Correct Answers and Rationale**

Select the one best answer, and indicate your choice by filling in the circle in front of the option.

The Client With a Head Injury

A 22-year-old man is brought to the emergency room with an apparent head injury after being involved in a serious motor vehicle accident. He is unconscious on arrival and exhibits signs of increasing intracranial pressure. He is accompanied by his fiancee and an adult friend.

1. Which of the following methods would be best, from a legal standpoint, for obtaining permission to treat the unconscious client?
   - ○ 1. Having his fiancee sign the consent form.
   - ○ 2. Having three physicians agree on the treatment he needs.
   - ○ 3. Obtaining a verbal consent by telephone from a responsible relative.
   - ○ 4. Obtaining written consent from the adult friend who accompanied the client to the emergency room.

2. When the client arrives in the emergency room, which of the following considerations should receive the highest priority?
   - ○ 1. Establishing an airway.
   - ○ 2. Replacing blood losses.
   - ○ 3. Stopping bleeding from open wounds.
   - ○ 4. Determining whether he has a neck fracture.

3. The client's initial blood pressure is 124/80 mm Hg. As his condition worsens, pulse pressure increases. Which of the following blood pressure readings indicates a pulse pressure greater than the initial pulse pressure?
   - ○ 1. 102/60 mm Hg.
   - ○ 2. 110/90 mm Hg.
   - ○ 3. 140/100 mm Hg.
   - ○ 4. 160/100 mm Hg.

4. The nurse assesses the client frequently for signs of increasing intracranial pressure, including
   - ○ 1. unequal pupil size.
   - ○ 2. decreasing systolic blood pressure.
   - ○ 3. tachycardia.
   - ○ 4. decreasing body temperature.

5. Which of the following respiratory signs would indicate increasing intracranial pressure in the brain stem?
   - ○ 1. Slow, irregular respirations.
   - ○ 2. Rapid, shallow respirations.
   - ○ 3. Asymmetric chest excursion.
   - ○ 4. Nasal flaring.

6. The nurse checks the client's gag reflex. The recommended technique for testing the gag reflex is to
   - ○ 1. touch the back of the client's throat with a tongue depressor.
   - ○ 2. observe the client for evidence of spontaneous swallowing when the neck is stroked.

○ 3. place a few milliliters of water on the client's tongue and note whether he swallows.

○ 4. observe the client's response to the introduction of a catheter for endotracheal suctioning.

7. Which of the following clinical manifestations would be an early indicator of a deterioration in the client's neurologic status?

○ 1. Widening pulse pressure.

○ 2. Decrease in the pulse rate.

○ 3. Dilated, fixed pupil.

○ 4. Decrease in level of consciousness.

8. The nurse obtains a specimen from clear fluid that is draining from the client's nose. To determine whether this fluid is mucus or cerebrospinal fluid (CSF), it should be tested for

○ 1. pH level.

○ 2. specific gravity.

○ 3. glucose.

○ 4. microorganisms.

9. Which of the following positions would be most appropriate for a client with a head injury?

○ 1. Head of the bed elevated 30 to 45 degrees.

○ 2. Trendelenburg's position.

○ 3. Left Sims' position.

○ 4. Head elevated on two pillows.

10. The client receives mannitol (Osmitrol) during surgery to help decrease intracranial pressure. Which of the following nursing observations would most likely indicate that the drug is having the desired effect?

○ 1. Urine output increases.

○ 2. Pulse rate decreases.

○ 3. Blood pressure decreases.

○ 4. Muscular relaxation increases.

11. Which of the following comments by the nurse would most help the client become oriented when he regains consciousness?

○ 1. "I'm your nurse, and I'll take care of you."

○ 2. "Can you tell me your name and where you live?"

○ 3. "I'll bet you're a little confused right now. Don't worry, everything is going to be all right."

○ 4. "You are in the hospital. You were in an accident and needed to have surgery."

12. As the client gradually regains consciousness, he becomes restless and attempts to pull out his intravenous line. Which action should the nurse take to protect the client without increasing his intracranial pressure?

○ 1. Place him in a jacket restraint.

○ 2. Wrap his hands in soft "mitten" restraints.

○ 3. Hold his hands firmly in place at his sides.

○ 4. Apply a wrist restraint to each arm.

13. When the client is fully conscious, the nurse would best assess his motor strength by

○ 1. comparing equality of hand grasps.

○ 2. observing spontaneous movements.

○ 3. observing the client feed himself.

○ 4. asking him to signal if he feels pressure applied to his feet.

14. Which of the following postoperative care measures would be contraindicated for a client at risk for increased intracranial pressure?

○ 1. Deep breathing.

○ 2. Turning.

○ 3. Coughing.

○ 4. Passive range-of-motion exercises.

15. Of the following nursing orders on the client's care plan, which would be most helpful in determining whether he may be developing diabetes insipidus?

○ 1. Obtain vital signs every 2 hours.

○ 2. Measure urine specific gravity hourly.

○ 3. Determine arterial blood gas values every other day.

○ 4. Test a urine specimen for glucose every morning.

16. The client is suffering from short-term memory loss. Which of the following nursing actions would be appropriate to help him cope with his memory loss?

○ 1. Instruct family members to ignore his behavior.

○ 2. Place a single-date calendar where he can view it.

○ 3. Tell him every morning what activities he will be expected to perform that day.

○ 4. Explain that he will have to try harder to remember things.

17. After 4 weeks of hospitalization, the client is to be discharged to a rehabilitation facility to continue his recovery. Which one of the following expected outcomes would be appropriate for the client at this stage of his rehabilitation? The client will

○ 1. exhibit no further episodes of short-term memory loss.

○ 2. be able to return to his construction job in 3 months.

○ 3. actively participate in the rehabilitation process as appropriate.

○ 4. be emotionally stable and display personality traits present before injury.

The Client With Seizures

A young adult has had several episodes of seizures. He is admitted to the hospital for diagnostic studies.

18. The client is placed on seizure precautions. Which of the following measures would be contraindicated?

○ 1. Encourage him to perform his own personal hygiene.

○ 2. Allow him to wear his own clothing.

○ 3. Assess oral temperature with a glass thermometer.

○ 4. Encourage him to be out of bed.

19. Which of the following statements would best describe the seizure activity of a tonic-clonic (grand mal) seizure?
    ○ 1. Seizure activity begins in one extremity and spreads gradually to adjacent areas.
    ○ 2. The client's eyes become vacant with an abrupt cessation of all activity.
    ○ 3. The client exhibits facial grimaces, patting motions, and lip smacking.
    ○ 4. The seizure activity is marked by sudden loss of consciousness and stiffening of the body, followed by violent muscle contractions.

20. The nurse plans to teach the client about the computed tomography (CT) scan that will be done at noon the next day. Which of the following statements by the nurse would be most accurate?
    ○ 1. "You must shampoo your hair tonight to remove all oil and dirt."
    ○ 2. "You may drink fluids until about 8 AM. Then we will give you a cleansing enema."
    ○ 3. "We will partially shave your head tonight so that electrodes can be securely attached to your scalp."
    ○ 4. "There is no special preparation necessary. You will need to hold your head very still during the examination."

21. An electroencephalogram (EEG) is ordered for the client. What action should the nurse take when the client is served a breakfast consisting of a soft-boiled egg, toast with butter and marmalade, orange juice, and coffee on the morning of the EEG?
    ○ 1. Remove all the food.
    ○ 2. Remove the coffee.
    ○ 3. Remove the toast, butter, and marmalade only.
    ○ 4. Substitute vegetable juice for the orange juice.

22. The client asks the nurse, "What caused me to have a seizure? I've never had one before." The nurse's reply should be based on the knowledge that a primary cause of tonic-clonic seizures in adults older than 20 years is
    ○ 1. head trauma.
    ○ 2. electrolyte imbalance.
    ○ 3. a congenital defect.
    ○ 4. an episode of high fever.

23. The nurse enters the client's room as the client, who is sitting in a chair, begins to have a seizure. Which of the following actions should the nurse take first?
    ○ 1. Lift the client onto his bed.
    ○ 2. Ease the client to the floor.
    ○ 3. Restrain the client's body movements.
    ○ 4. Insert an airway into the client's mouth.

24. A priority goal for the client after the seizure has subsided is to
    ○ 1. monitor for an aura.
    ○ 2. determine what the client was doing when the seizure began.
    ○ 3. maintain a patent airway.
    ○ 4. place the client in a position of comfort.

25. Which of the following interventions would be effective in minimizing the risk of seizure activity in this client?
    ○ 1. Maintain the client on bed rest.
    ○ 2. Administer sedatives as ordered.
    ○ 3. Close the door to the room to minimize stimulation.
    ○ 4. Administer anticonvulsant medications on schedule.

26. During the seizure, which of the following would be appropriate for the nurse to note?
    ○ 1. Heart rate and blood pressure.
    ○ 2. When the last dose of anticonvulsant medication was administered.
    ○ 3. What type of aura the client had.
    ○ 4. Movement of the extremities.

27. Which of the following observations would the nurse expect in the client after a tonic-clonic (grand mal) seizure? The client
    ○ 1. may be drowsy after the seizure.
    ○ 2. may be unable to move after the seizure.
    ○ 3. will remember what triggered the seizure.
    ○ 4. will be hypotensive.

28. Phenytoin sodium (Dilantin) is prescribed for the client. He asks the nurse how the medication will help him. The nurse's best response should be based on knowledge that the drug is thought to act by
    ○ 1. correcting the abnormal synthesis of norepinephrine in the body.
    ○ 2. depressing transmission of abnormal impulses in the spinal cord.
    ○ 3. reducing the responsiveness of neurons in the brain to abnormal impulses.
    ○ 4. interrupting the flow of abnormal impulses from the viscera to the brain.

29. The nurse plans to teach the client about prescribed phenytoin sodium therapy. It is important that the client understand that the medication must not be stopped suddenly because
    ○ 1. a physical dependency on the drug develops over time.
    ○ 2. this can precipitate the development of status epilepticus.
    ○ 3. this would lead to a hypoglycemic reaction.
    ○ 4. phenytoin is the only effective drug for tonic-clonic seizures.

30. The client states that he is afraid he will not be able to drive again because of his seizures. The nurse

should respond by telling him that driving will depend on local laws but that most laws require

○ 1. that a person with a history of seizures drive only during daytime hours.

○ 2. evidence that the seizures are under medical control.

○ 3. evidence that seizures occur no more often than every 6 months.

○ 4. that the person with a history of seizures carry a medical identification card at all times when driving.

31. The client tells the nurse that he is unclear about what an aura is. The nurse would correctly define an *aura* as

○ 1. a postseizure state of amnesia.

○ 2. hallucinations occurring during a seizure.

○ 3. a symptom that occurs just before a seizure.

○ 4. a feeling of relaxation as the seizure begins to subside.

32. Which of the following interventions will assist the client in taking phenytoin as prescribed?

○ 1. Calling him daily for the first week after hospital discharge.

○ 2. Having a family member monitor him to ensure compliance.

○ 3. Providing him with written and verbal instructions about the medicine.

○ 4. Emphasizing that embarrassing seizures may occur again is he does not take the medicine.

33. Which of the following findings should suggest to the nurse that a client is having a typical reaction to long-term phenytoin sodium therapy? The client

○ 1. has gained considerable weight.

○ 2. reports insomnia.

○ 3. exhibits an excessive growth of his gum tissue.

○ 4. says that he now needs to wear eyeglasses.

The Client With a Cerebrovascular Accident

A 72-year-old retired man experiences a thrombotic cerebrovascular accident (CVA) and is admitted to the hospital. The diagnosis is a left CVA with flaccid hemiplegia of his right side.

34. When planning the client's care, the nurse should keep in mind that rehabilitation begins

○ 1. as soon as anticoagulant therapy is started.

○ 2. when the client is admitted to the hospital.

○ 3. when the client is first able to work cooperatively with health care personnel.

○ 4. as soon as a physical therapist can be brought into the client's health care team.

35. Regular oral hygiene is an essential intervention for the client. Which of the following nursing measures would be inappropriate when providing oral hygiene?

○ 1. Placing the client on his back with a small pillow under his head.

○ 2. Keeping portable suctioning equipment at the bedside.

○ 3. Opening the client's mouth with a padded tongue blade.

○ 4. Cleansing the client's mouth and teeth with a toothbrush.

36. Nursing assessment data include: inability to move the right arm and leg; absence of muscle tone in the right arm and leg; and lack of knowledge about how to turn in bed. Based on these data, which of the following would be the most appropriate nursing diagnosis for this client?

○ 1. Activity Intolerance.

○ 2. Sleep Pattern Disturbance.

○ 3. Impaired Physical Mobility.

○ 4. Unilateral Neglect.

37. A priority assessment in the first 24 hours of admission for this client is assessment of

○ 1. risk factors for vascular disease.

○ 2. pupil size and pupillary response.

○ 3. urinary elimination patterns.

○ 4. health behaviors before the CVA.

38. Assessment of the client's functional status before and after the CVA is essential because

○ 1. the rehabilitation plan will be guided by it.

○ 2. functional status before the CVA will help predict outcomes.

○ 3. it will help the client recognize his physical limitations.

○ 4. the client can be expected to regain much of his functioning.

39. The nurse changes the client's position in bed regularly. Which of the following techniques would most likely cause friction and predispose to pressure ulcer formation?

○ 1. Rolling the client onto his side.

○ 2. Sliding the client to move him up in bed.

○ 3. Lifting the client on a drawsheet when moving him up in bed.

○ 4. Having the client help lift himself off the bed using a trapeze.

40. The nurse is concerned about the possible development of plantar flexion. Which of the following measures has been found to be the most effective means of preventing plantar flexion in a stroke client?

○ 1. Placing the client's feet against a firm footboard.

○ 2. Repositioning the client every 2 hours.

○ 3. Having the client wear ankle-high tennis shoes at intervals throughout the day.

○ 4. Massaging the client's feet and ankles regularly.

41. Because the CVA affected the left side of the client's brain, the nurse should anticipate that the client will most likely experience
○ 1. expressive aphasia.
○ 2. dyslexia.
○ 3. apraxia.
○ 4. agnosia.

42. For the client experiencing expressive aphasia, which of the following nursing actions would be most helpful in promoting communication?
○ 1. Speaking loudly.
○ 2. Using short sentences.
○ 3. Writing all directions so the client can read them.
○ 4. Correcting all of the client's speech errors.

43. For the client with dysphagia, which of the following measures would be ineffective in decreasing the risk of aspiration while eating?
○ 1. Maintaining an upright position.
○ 2. Restricting the diet to liquids until swallowing improves.
○ 3. Introducing foods on the unaffected side of the mouth.
○ 4. Keeping distractions to a minimum.

44. When helping the client learn self-care skills, the nurse should use which of the following interventions to help him learn to dress himself?
○ 1. Encourage the client to wear clothing designed especially for people who have had a stroke.
○ 2. Dress the client, explaining each step of the process as it is completed.
○ 3. Teach the client to put on clothing on the affected side first.
○ 4. Encourage the client to ask his wife for help when dressing.

45. The CVA has caused homonymous hemianopia (blindness in half of the visual field). Homonymous hemianopia would probably manifest itself in which of the following food-related behaviors?
○ 1. Increased preference for foods high in salt.
○ 2. Eating food on only half of the plate.
○ 3. Forgetting the names of foods.
○ 4. Inability to swallow liquids.

46. Although all of the following measures might be useful in reducing the client's visual disability, which measure should the nurse teach him primarily as a safety precaution?
○ 1. Wear a patch over one eye.
○ 2. Place personal items on his sighted side.
○ 3. Lie in bed with the unaffected side toward the door.
○ 4. Turn his head from side to side when walking.

47. The client is experiencing mood swings and often has "crying jags" that are distressing to his family. It would be best for the nurse to instruct family members to do which of the following when these crying jags occur?
○ 1. Sit quietly with the client until the episode is over.
○ 2. Ignore the behavior and continue what they were doing.
○ 3. Attempt to divert the client's attention.
○ 4. Tell the client that this behavior is unacceptable.

48. The client is aware of and discouraged by his physical handicaps. The nurse can best help him overcome a negative self-concept by conveying
○ 1. helpfulness and sympathy.
○ 2. concern and charity.
○ 3. direction and firmness.
○ 4. encouragement and patience.

49. The nurse is preparing the client for discharge to home. Which of the following factors would most likely influence the client's continuing progress in rehabilitation at home?
○ 1. The family's ability to provide support to the client.
○ 2. The client's ability to ambulate.
○ 3. The availability of a home health aide to care for the client.
○ 4. The frequency of follow-up visits with the physician.

50. The client is receiving a thrombolytic agent. The expected outcome of this drug therapy is
○ 1. increased vascular permeability and improved cerebral perfusion.
○ 2. decreased vascular permeability and improved cerebral perfusion.
○ 3. dissolved emboli and thus minimization of the damage of the CVA.
○ 4. prevention of further hemorrhage within the cerebral vasculature.

The Client With Parkinson's Disease

A 67-year-old man is admitted to the hospital for a diagnostic workup for probable Parkinson's disease.

51. When assessing the client, the nurse would anticipate which of the following signs and symptoms?
○ 1. Dry mouth.
○ 2. Aphasia.
○ 3. An exaggerated sense of euphoria.
○ 4. A stiff, mask-like facial expression.

52. A priority nursing diagnosis category for this client is
○ 1. Alteration in Nutrition.
○ 2. Lack of Knowledge.
○ 3. Ineffective Breathing Pattern.

○ 4. Potential for Injury.

53. The nurse observes that the client's upper arm tremors disappear as he unbuttons his shirt. Which of the following statements would best guide the nurse when analyzing these observations about the client's tremors?
    ○ 1. The tremors are probably psychological and can be controlled at will.
    ○ 2. The tremors sometimes disappear with purposeful and voluntary movements.
    ○ 3. The tremors often increase in severity when the client's attention is diverted by some activity.
    ○ 4. There is no explanation for the observation, which is probably a chance occurrence.

54. To minimize the effects of hypokinesia, the client should be taught to schedule his most demanding physical activities
    ○ 1. early in the morning, when his energy level is high.
    ○ 2. to coincide with the peak action of drug therapy.
    ○ 3. immediately after a rest period.
    ○ 4. when family members will be available.

55. Which of the following goals would be most realistic and appropriate when planning the client's nursing care?
    ○ 1. To cure the disease.
    ○ 2. To stop progression of the disease.
    ○ 3. To begin preparations for terminal care.
    ○ 4. To maintain optimal body function.

56. The physical therapy regimen developed for a client with Parkinson's disease is aimed primarily at
    ○ 1. maintaining joint flexibility and relaxing muscles.
    ○ 2. building muscle strength.
    ○ 3. improving muscle endurance.
    ○ 4. reducing ataxia.

57. The client is started on levodopa (L-dopa) therapy. The nurse would evaluate that the drug is exerting its desired effect when the client experiences an improvement in
    ○ 1. mood.
    ○ 2. muscle rigidity.
    ○ 3. appetite.
    ○ 4. alertness.

58. To maintain the therapeutic effects of levodopa, most clients require gradually increasing dosages. The nurse should teach the client's family that important symptoms of levodopa toxicity are
    ○ 1. lethargy and sleepiness.
    ○ 2. anorexia and nausea.
    ○ 3. diarrhea and cramping.
    ○ 4. delusions and hallucinations.

59. When administering the prescribed medications to the client, the nurse knows it is essential that

○ 1. the client can explain each medication before taking it.
○ 2. the client take all of the medications at one time.
○ 3. the medications are taken at mealtime.
○ 4. the medications are taken at the time scheduled.

60. The client needs a long time to complete his morning hygiene, but he becomes annoyed when the nurse offers assistance and refuses all help. Which would be the nurse's best initial response in this situation?
    ○ 1. Tell him firmly that he needs assistance and help him with his care.
    ○ 2. Praise him for his desire to be independent and give him extra time and encouragement.
    ○ 3. Tell him that he is being unrealistic about his abilities and must accept the fact that he needs help.
    ○ 4. Suggest that if he insists on self-care, he should at least modify his routine.

61. Pallidotomy is a surgery developed to reduce the detrimental effects of Parkinson's disease. The main goal for the client after pallidotomy would be
    ○ 1. improved functional ability.
    ○ 2. decreased episodes of depression.
    ○ 3. improved neurologic functioning.
    ○ 4. increased oxygenation.

The Client With Multiple Sclerosis

A 48-year-old woman is admitted to the hospital with a bladder infection and incontinence. She has had multiple sclerosis for 15 years.

62. Clients with multiple sclerosis experience many different symptoms. Which of the following symptoms is atypical of multiple sclerosis?
    ○ 1. Double vision.
    ○ 2. Sudden bursts of energy.
    ○ 3. Weakness in the extremities.
    ○ 4. Muscle tremors.

63. When developing a plan of home care for the client, the nurse should teach the client about which of the following complications that would be most likely to occur?
    ○ 1. Ascites.
    ○ 2. Contractures.
    ○ 3. Fluid volume overload.
    ○ 4. Myocardial infarction.

64. Baclofen is prescribed for the client. The nurse would evaluate that the drug is accomplishing its intended purpose when it
    ○ 1. induces sleep.
    ○ 2. stimulates the client's appetite.

○ 3. relieves muscular spasticity.

○ 4. reduces the urine bacterial count.

65. The client has received various drug therapies for multiple sclerosis over the years. It is difficult to evaluate the effectiveness of any particular drug because clients with multiple sclerosis tend to

○ 1. exhibit intolerance to many drugs.

○ 2. experience spontaneous remissions from time to time.

○ 3. require multiple drugs that are used simultaneously.

○ 4. endure long periods of exacerbation before the illness responds to a particular drug.

66. The client has slurred speech. When the nurse talks with her, which of the following techniques would be contraindicated?

○ 1. Encouraging her to speak slowly.

○ 2. Encouraging her to speak distinctly.

○ 3. Asking her to repeat indistinguishable words.

○ 4. Asking her to speak louder when tired.

67. The client's right hand trembles severely whenever she attempts a voluntary action. She spills her coffee twice at lunch and cannot get her dress fastened securely. Which of the following nurse's notes offers the best account of these observations?

○ 1. "Has an intention tremor of the right hand."

○ 2. "Right-hand tremor worsens with purposeful acts."

○ 3. "Needs assistance with dressing and eating due to severe trembling and clumsiness."

○ 4. "Slight shaking of right hand increases to severe tremor when client tries to button her clothes or drink from a cup."

68. The client may eventually lose control of her bowels and require bowel retraining. If this occurs, which of the following measures would likely be least helpful?

○ 1. Eating a diet high in roughage.

○ 2. Setting a regular time for elimination.

○ 3. Raising the toilet seat for easy access by wheelchair.

○ 4. Limiting fluid intake to 1000 mL/day.

69. The client sometimes exhibits signs or symptoms of emotional distress. The nurse should be aware that clients with multiple sclerosis are most likely to exhibit

○ 1. mood disorders.

○ 2. thought disorders.

○ 3. psychosomatic illnesses.

○ 4. drug dependency problems.

70. As part of the rehabilitation program planned for the client, therapy and hobbies would be used to help develop her

○ 1. diligence and persistence.

○ 2. muscles and motivation.

○ 3. intellect and imagination.

○ 4. productivity and personality.

71. As the client prepares for discharge, the nurse should encourage her to

○ 1. accept the necessity for a quiet and inactive lifestyle.

○ 2. keep active while avoiding emotional upset and fatigue.

○ 3. follow good health habits to change the course of the disease.

○ 4. practice using the mechanical aids that she will need when future disabilities arise.

72. The client has various sensory impairments associated with her disease. Which of the following would be an appropriate safety precaution for this client?

○ 1. Carefully testing the temperature of bath water.

○ 2. Avoiding kitchen activities owing to the high risk of injury.

○ 3. Avoiding hot-water bottles or heating pads.

○ 4. Inspecting the skin daily for injury or pressure points.

73. Which of the following nursing interventions would most likely be used to help the client avoid episodes of urinary incontinence?

○ 1. Maintain a fluid intake of 1500 mL/day.

○ 2. Insert an indwelling urinary catheter.

○ 3. Establish a regular voiding schedule.

○ 4. Administer prophylactic antibiotics, as ordered.

74. The client's daughter and 3-year-old granddaughter live with her. The daughter asks the nurse what she can do to most help her mother at home. From which of the following measures would the client probably benefit most at home?

○ 1. A course of psychotherapy.

○ 2. A regular program of daily activities.

○ 3. A day-care center for the granddaughter.

○ 4. A weekly visit by another person with multiple sclerosis.

The Unconscious Client

A 38-year-old man is admitted to the emergency room after being found unconscious at the wheel of his car in the hospital parking lot. The client is comatose and does not respond to stimuli. A drug overdose is suspected.

75. Which of the following assessment findings would lead the nurse to suspect that the coma is a result of a toxic drug overdose?

○ 1. Hypertension.

○ 2. Fever.

○ 3. Dilated pupils.

○ 4. Facial asymmetry.

76. Blood and urine analysis confirm a diagnosis of salicylate overdose. The client is treated with gastric lavage. Which of the following positions would be most appropriate for the client during this procedure?
- ○ 1. Lateral.
- ○ 2. Supine.
- ○ 3. Trendelenburg's.
- ○ 4. Lithotomy.

77. In anticipation of further emergency treatment for the client, which of the following medications should the nurse have available?
- ○ 1. Vitamin K.
- ○ 2. Dextrose 50%.
- ○ 3. Activated charcoal powder.
- ○ 4. Sodium thiosulfate.

78. The client's wife and sister arrive at the hospital, distraught about his comatose condition as well as the possibility that this appears to be an intentional overdose. Which of the following would be an appropriate initial nursing intervention with this family?
- ○ 1. Explain that since the client was found on hospital property, he was probably asking for help and did not intentionally overdose.
- ○ 2. Give the wife and sister a big hug and assure them that he is in good hands.
- ○ 3. Encourage the wife and sister to ventilate their feelings and concerns, and listen carefully.
- ○ 4. Allow the wife and sister to help care for the client by rubbing his back when he is turned.

79. A priority goal for this client during the first 24 hours of admission is to
- ○ 1. educate regarding drug abuse.
- ○ 2. minimize pain.
- ○ 3. maintain intact skin.
- ○ 4. monitor for myocardial infarction.

80. The client is at risk for developing a decubitus ulcer. The first warning of an impending decubitus ulcer is when pressure applied to skin turns it
- ○ 1. bluish.
- ○ 2. reddish.
- ○ 3. whitish.
- ○ 4. yellowish.

81. The nurse finds an aide massaging the client's bony prominences. The correct action by the nurse is to
- ○ 1. reinforce the aide's use of this intervention over the bony prominences.
- ○ 2. explain that massage is effective because it improves blood flow to the area.
- ○ 3. inform the aide that massage is even more effective when combined with lotion during the massage.
- ○ 4. instruct the aide that massage is contraindicated because it decreases blood flow to the area.

82. The client has been positioned on his side. The nurse would anticipate that which of the following areas would be a pressure point in this position?
- ○ 1. Sacrum.
- ○ 2. Occiput.
- ○ 3. Ankles.
- ○ 4. Heels.

83. The client is placed in a right side-lying position. Which of the following techniques to position the client is incorrect? The client's
- ○ 1. head is placed on a small pillow.
- ○ 2. right leg is extended without pillow support.
- ○ 3. left arm is rested on the mattress with the elbow flexed.
- ○ 4. left leg is supported on a pillow with the knee flexed.

84. To prevent external rotation of the client's hips while he is lying on his back, it would be best for the nurse to place
- ○ 1. firm pillows under the length of his legs.
- ○ 2. sandbags alongside his legs from knees to ankles.
- ○ 3. trochanter rolls alongside his legs from ilium to mid-thigh.
- ○ 4. a footboard that supports his feet in the normal anatomic position.

85. The nurse's goal for performing passive range-of-motion exercises on an unconscious client would be to
- ○ 1. preserve muscle mass.
- ○ 2. prevent bone demineralization.
- ○ 3. increase muscle tone.
- ○ 4. maintain joint mobility.

86. When the nurse performs oral hygiene for the unconscious client, which of the following actions would be most appropriate?
- ○ 1. Keep a suction machine available.
- ○ 2. Place the client in a prone position.
- ○ 3. Wear sterile gloves while brushing the client's teeth.
- ○ 4. Use gauze wrapped around the fingers to cleanse the client's gums.

87. The nurse observes that the client's right eye does not close totally. Based on this finding, which of the following nursing interventions would be most appropriate?
- ○ 1. Making sure the client wears his eyeglasses at all times.
- ○ 2. Placing an eye patch over his right eye.
- ○ 3. Instilling artificial tears once every shift.
- ○ 4. Cleansing the eye with a clean washcloth every shift.

88. The nurse is assessing the client's respiratory status. Which of the following symptoms may be an early indicator of hypoxia in the unconscious client?
- ○ 1. Cyanosis.
- ○ 2. Decreased respirations.
- ○ 3. Restlessness.

○ 4. Hypotension.

89. Intermittent enteral tube feedings are ordered for the client. When administering the feeding, the nurse should implement which of the following actions?
○ 1. Heat the formula in a microwave.
○ 2. Place the client in semi-Fowler's position.
○ 3. Obtain a sterile gavage bag and tubing for use.
○ 4. Weigh the client before administering the feeding.

90. The client is to receive 200 mL of tube feeding every 4 hours. The nurse checks the client's gastric residual before administering the feeding and obtains 40 mL of gastric residual. What should the nurse do next?
○ 1. Withhold the tube feeding and notify the physician.
○ 2. Dispose of the residual and continue with the feeding.
○ 3. Delay feeding the client for 1 hour and then recheck the residual.
○ 4. Readminister the residual to the client and continue with the feeding.

91. Of the following actions the nurse could take when providing catheter care, which should have the highest priority?
○ 1. Cleansing the area around the urethral meatus.
○ 2. Clamping the catheter periodically to maintain muscle tone.
○ 3. Irrigating the catheter with several ounces of normal saline solution.
○ 4. Changing the location where the catheter is taped to the client's leg.

The Client in Pain

A 34-year-old man of Chinese descent is admitted to the hospital after experiencing multiple trauma as a result of an automobile accident. He has three fractured ribs, a hairline fracture of the pelvis, a compound fracture of his right tibia and fibula, and soft tissue injuries. He is in severe pain when he arrives on the unit after emergency surgery.

92. The client reports severe pain and requests frequent medication. A nursing assistant expresses her surprise, saying, "I thought Asian people were very stoic about pain." Which of the following statements about pain is correct? The level of pain
○ 1. perception varies widely from person to person.
○ 2. tolerance is about the same in all people.
○ 3. tolerance is determined by a person's genetic makeup.
○ 4. perception is about the same in all people.

93. The nurse finds it difficult to relieve the client's pain satisfactorily. Which of the following measures should the nurse take into consideration when continuing efforts to promote comfort?
○ 1. Improving the nurse–client relationship.
○ 2. Enlisting the help of the client's family.
○ 3. Allowing the client additional time for privacy to work through his responses to pain.
○ 4. Arranging to have the client share a room with a client who has little pain.

94. After 5 days of hospitalization, the client asks for pain medication with increasing frequency and exhibits increased anxiety and restlessness. What is the probable cause of his behavior?
○ 1. His physical condition is deteriorating.
○ 2. He is becoming addicted to the narcotic.
○ 3. His coping mechanisms are exhausted.
○ 4. He has developed tolerance to his narcotic dosage.

95. The client tells the nurse, "If I could be among my people, I could receive acupuncture for this pain." The nurse should understand that acupuncture in the Asian culture is based on the theory that it
○ 1. eliminates evil spirits.
○ 2. promotes tranquility with God.
○ 3. restores the balance of energy.
○ 4. blocks nerve pathways to the brain.

96. The client's physician decides to change the medication to oral meperidine hydrochloride (Demerol). His current dose is ordered as 75 mg given intramuscularly every 4 hours p.r.n. What dosage of oral meperidine hydrochloride will be required to provide an equivalent analgesic dose?
○ 1. 25 to 50 mg.
○ 2. 75 to 100 mg.
○ 3. 125 to 150 mg.
○ 4. 250 to 300 mg.

97. Meperidine hydrochloride is an effective pain reliever because of its ability to
○ 1. reduce the perception of pain.
○ 2. decrease the sensitivity of pain receptors.
○ 3. interfere with pain impulses traveling along sensory nerve fibers.
○ 4. block the conduction of pain impulses along the central nervous system.

98. The nurse bases interventions to reduce pain on the gate-control theory of pain. This theory holds that a regulatory process controls impulses reaching the brain. This regulatory process is believed to be located in the
○ 1. brain stem.
○ 2. cerebellum.
○ 3. spinal cord.
○ 4. hypothalamus.

99. The body typically and automatically responds to pain first with attempts to improve its ability to

○ 1. tolerate the pain.
○ 2. decrease the perception of pain.
○ 3. escape the source of pain.
○ 4. divert attention from the source of pain.

100. Ergotamine tartrate (Gynergen) is prescribed for the client's migraine headaches. The nurse would judge correctly that the desired effect of the drug is being accomplished when the client reports that it
○ 1. aborts the migraine attacks.
○ 2. reduces the severity of migraine attacks.
○ 3. relieves the sleeplessness experienced in the past after a migraine attack.
○ 4. decreases the visual problems experienced in the past after a migraine attack.

101. The pain associated with migraine headaches is believed to be due to
○ 1. dilation of the cranial arteries.
○ 2. a temporary decrease in intracranial pressure.
○ 3. irritation and inflammation of the openings of the sinuses.
○ 4. sustained contraction of muscles around the scalp and face.

102. The client is evaluated at the pain center, and biofeedback therapy is suggested. The purpose of biofeedback is to enable the client to exert control over physiologic processes by
○ 1. regulating the body processes through electrical control.
○ 2. shocking himself when an undesirable response is elicited.
○ 3. monitoring his body processes for the therapist to interpret.
○ 4. translating signals of his body processes into observable forms.

103. An expected outcome of a back rub to relieve pain is
○ 1. stimulation of large-diameter cutaneous fibers to block the pain impulses from the spinal cord to the brain.
○ 2. stimulation of small-diameter cutaneous fibers to block the pain impulses from the brain to the spinal cord.
○ 3. stimulation of the release of endorphins.
○ 4. distraction of the client from focusing on the source of the pain.

104. Research studies have demonstrated that patient-controlled analgesia is more effective than intermittent narcotic administration. Which response by the nurse to a client asking about patient-controlled analgesia reflects knowledge of these research findings? "Patient-controlled analgesia is more effective because
○ 1. a different narcotic is used."
○ 2. two narcotics are administered simultaneously."

○ 3. the client controls the amount of pain medication administered."
○ 4. the nurse interrupts the client less frequently, and the client can get more sleep."

105. Nursing responsibilities for the client with a patient-controlled analgesia system would include
○ 1. reassuring the client that pain will be relieved.
○ 2. documenting the client's response to pain medication on a routine basis.
○ 3. instructing the client to continue pressing the system's button whenever pain occurs.
○ 4. titrating pain medication as necessary until the client is free of pain.

106. Which of the following statements represents a major principle of chronic pain management?
○ 1. A physiologic approach is most effective.
○ 2. A psychological approach is most effective.
○ 3. Medication is the mainstay of therapy.
○ 4. A multidisciplinary approach is most effective.

107. When locating the ventrogluteal site before giving an intramuscular injection, the nurse should place her or his hand on the client's
○ 1. iliac crest.
○ 2. greater trochanter.
○ 3. anterior superior iliac spine.
○ 4. posterior superior iliac spine.

108. The nurse holds the gauze pledget against an intramuscular injection site while removing the needle from the muscle. This technique helps
○ 1. seal off the track left by the needle in the tissue.
○ 2. speed the spread of the medication in the tissue.
○ 3. avoid the discomfort of the needle pulling on the skin.
○ 4. prevent organisms from entering the body through the skin puncture.

109. A client asks why the nurse does not give the intramuscular injection into the upper arm. The nurse should explain that the deltoid muscle is rarely used because the muscle
○ 1. is small.
○ 2. is difficult to locate.
○ 3. has many pain receptors.
○ 4. has a poor blood supply.

110. After administering an intramuscular injection with a disposable needle and syringe, the nurse should dispose of the needle and syringe by
○ 1. cutting the needle at the hilt in a needle cutter before disposing of it in the universal precaution container.
○ 2. leaving the needle uncapped and disposing of the needle and syringe in the universal precaution container.
○ 3. recapping the needle and placing the needle and syringe in the universal precaution container.
○ 4. separating the needle and syringe and placing both in the universal precaution container.

CORRECT ANSWERS AND RATIONALE

The letters in parentheses following the rationale identify the step of the nursing process (A, D, P, I, E), cognitive level (K, C, T, N), and client needs (S, G, L, H). See the Answer Grid for the key.

The Client With a Head Injury

1. 3. An operative permit must be signed before any surgical procedure is performed. If the client is unable to sign a permit because of his condition, a responsible relative should be obtained to sign the permit. When a relative is not readily available and when time is of the essence, a letter, telephone call, or telegram may be used to obtain permission. (I, N, S)

2. 1. The highest priority for a client with multiple injuries is to establish an open airway to enable effective ventilation and brain oxygenation. Unless the client has a patent airway, other care measures will be futile. (I, N, S)

3. 4. The pulse pressure is determined by subtracting the diastolic pressure from the systolic pressure. For example, a client with a blood pressure of 102/60 mm Hg has a pulse pressure of 42 mm Hg. Widening pulse pressure is a sign of increased intracranial pressure. (A, T, G)

4. 1. Increasing intracranial pressure causes unequal pupils from pressure on the third cranial nerve, rising body temperature from hypothalmic damage, and rising systolic pressure, which reflects the additional pressure needed to perfuse the brain. Pressure on the vagus nerve produces bradycardia, not tachycardia. (A, T, G)

5. 1. Neural control of respiration takes place in the brain stem. Deterioration and pressure produce irregular respiratory patterns. Rapid, shallow respirations, asymmetric chest movements, and nasal flaring are more characteristic of respiratory distress or hypoxia. (A, T, G)

6. 1. The best technique for assessing the gag reflex is to touch the back of the client's throat in the pharyngeal area with a tongue depressor or cotton swab. The reflex is absent if the client does not gag. Reflexes are typically absent or sluggish in the presence of increased intracranial pressure. It is dangerous to place liquids in the mouth of an unconscious client because of the risk of aspiration. (A, N, S)

7. 4. A decrease in the client's level of consciousness is an early indicator of deterioration of the client's neurologic status. Such a change precedes all other changes that occur. Changes in level of consciousness, such as restlessness and irritability, may be subtle. The nurse needs to monitor the client closely to detect changes as quickly as possible. (A, C, G)

8. 3. The constituents of CSF are similar to those of blood plasma. An examination for glucose content is done to determine whether body fluid is mucus or CSF. Mucus does not contain glucose; CSF does. (A, T, G)

9. 1. The client should be positioned to avoid extreme neck flexion or extension. The head of the bed is usually elevated 30 to 45 degrees to help prevent increased intracranial pressure. (I, T, S)

10. 1. Mannitol is an osmotic diuretic that helps decrease intracranial pressure through its dehydrating effects. The drug is acting in the desired manner when urine output increases. It may be desirable to decrease pulse rate, decrease blood pressure, and relax the muscles in certain situations, but mannitol is not used to accomplish these goals. (A, N, G)

11. 4. Explaining where a client is and why he is there helps him become oriented after a period of unconsciousness. Asking the client his name helps determine his level of orientation. (I, T, G)

12. 2. It would be best to wrap the client's hands in washcloths or to have him wear mitts when he becomes restless while regaining consciousness after brain surgery. Restraining him tends to increase activity and restlessness and thus increase intracranial pressure. (I, T, S)

13. 1. Comparing equality of hand grasps is a technique used to assess motor strength. Noting that the client can feed himself verifies coordination and motor ability but does not help determine muscle strength. The ability to move spontaneously demonstrates motor ability but not strength. Having the client signal when pressure is applied to his feet tests sensory function. (A, T, G)

14. 3. Coughing is contraindicated for a client at risk for increased intracranial pressure because coughing increases intracranial pressure. Deep breathing, turning, and passive range-of-motion exercises can be continued. (I, T, S)

15. 2. Diabetes insipidus results from deficiency of antidiuretic hormone (ADH). The condition may occur in conjunction with head injuries as well as with other disorders. In ADH deficiency, the client is extremely thirsty and excretes large amounts of highly diluted urine. The degree of urine concentration is best assessed by measuring the specific gravity of urine samples. (A, C, G)

16. 2. It is not unusual for a client to be disoriented and suffer short-term memory loss after a head injury. Explanations of activities should be simple and given immediately before the procedure. Family members should be encouraged to bring familiar objects from home for the client to see. Clocks, single-date calendars, and other items to help orient the client should be provided. Frequent reassurance and orientation by the nurse and family members will help the client understand the reason for his hospitalization and recognize that he is in a safe environment. Ignoring the client's behavior would not provide the client with the reassurance and assistance that he needs. (I, N, G)

17. 3. Recovery from a serious head injury is a long-term process that may continue for months or years after the injury. Depending on the extent of the injury, clients who are transferred to rehabilitation facilities most likely will continue to exhibit cognitive and mobility impairments as well as behavior and personality changes. The client would be expected to participate in the rehabilitation efforts to the extent he is capable. Family members and significant others will need long-term support to help them cope with the changes that have occurred in the client. (E, T, L)

The Client With Seizures

18. 3. In a client subject to seizure activity, temperature should be assessed by a route other than oral when using a mercury thermometer. A glass thermometer could break in the client's mouth if a seizure occurred. (I, T, S)

19. 4. Tonic-clonic (grand mal) seizures characteristically begin with a sudden loss of consciousness and generalized tonic muscle contractions. During this phase, which usually lasts less than 1 minute, the client is apneic. The clonic phase of the seizure then begins, characterized by violent, rhythmic muscle contractions. Respirations resume at this time. Most tonic-clonic seizures last a total of 2 to 5 minutes. (A, C, G)

20. 4. In general, there is no special preparation for a CT scan. The client will be asked to hold the head very still during the examination, which lasts about 30 to 60 minutes. In some instances, food and fluids may be withheld for 4 to 6 hours before the procedure if a contrast medium is used because the radiopaque substance sometimes causes nausea. (I, C, S)

21. 2. Beverages containing caffeine, such as coffee, tea, and cola drinks, are withheld before an EEG because of the stimulating effects of the caffeine. A meal should not be omitted before an EEG because low blood sugar could alter brain wave patterns. (I, C, S)

22. 1. Trauma is one of the primary causes of brain damage and seizure activity in adults. This condition is referred to as *posttraumatic epilepsy*. Other common causes of seizure activity in adults include neoplasms, withdrawal from drugs and alcohol, and vascular disease. (P, C, G)

23. 2. If a client has a seizure while sitting in a chair, it would be best to ease him to the floor and place a pillow under his head. No effort should be made to restrain him. The strong muscle contractions may cause the client to injure himself if he is restrained. The nurse is likely to be hurt, as well as the client, if the nurse tries to lift him to a bed. Placing an airway in the client's mouth during a seizure is not necessary or recommended. (I, N, S)

24. 3. A priority goal for the client after a seizure is to maintain the patency of the airway because the tongue may occlude the airway during the seizure. (P, T, S)

25. 4. Anticonvulsant medications administered as scheduled will help prevent further seizures. Bed rest, sedation, and privacy are not interventions that will minimize risk of seizures. (I, T, G)

26. 4. During a seizure, the nurse should note movement of the client's head, eyes, and extremities, especially when the seizure first begins. Other important assessments would include noting the progression and duration of the seizure, respiratory status, loss of consciousness, pupil size, and incontinence of urine and stool. It is typically not necessary to assess the client's pulse and blood pressure during a tonic-clonic seizure. The nurse should focus on maintaining an open airway and preventing injury to the client. (A, N, G)

27. 1. A client is often drowsy after a seizure. Despite drowsiness, however, the client is usually able to move and speak afterward. The client may not remember what, if anything, triggered the seizure. Hypotension is not a frequent problem after a seizure. (A, N, G)

28. 3. Exactly how phenytoin sodium helps control seizures is unclear. The most common theory posits that it reduces the responsiveness of neurons in the brain to abnormal impulses—that is, it depresses neural activity. (P, C, G)

29. 2. Anticonvulsant drug therapy should never be stopped suddenly; doing so can lead to the life-threatening status epilepticus. Phenytoin sodium does not carry a risk of physical dependency. It is one of many drugs used effectively to treat tonic-clonic seizure disorders. (P, C, G)

30. 2. Specific motor vehicle regulations and restrictions for people who experience seizures vary lo-

cally. Most commonly, evidence that the seizures are under medical control is required before the person is given permission to drive. It is recommended that a person subject to seizures carry a card or wear an identification bracelet describing the illness so that in an emergency the condition can be quickly identified. (I, C, H)

31. 3. An aura is a premonition of an impending seizure. Auras usually are of a sensory nature (ie, an olfactory, visual, gustatory, or auditory sensation); some may be of a psychic nature. Evaluating an aura may help identify the area of the brain from which the seizure originates. (I, K, G)

32. 3. Providing the client with written and verbal instructions will increase understanding of the medication regimen. Calling the client daily should not be necessary to ensure compliance. The client should be responsible for taking his own medication rather than relying on a family member. Reinforcing that seizures may be embarrassing is not an appropriate approach to improve medication compliance. (I, N, H)

33. 3. A common side effect of long-term phenytoin therapy is an overgrowth of gingival tissues. Problems may be minimized with good oral hygiene, but in some cases, overgrown tissues must be removed surgically. (E, C, G)

The Client With a Cerebrovascular Accident

34. 2. Rehabilitation for a client who has sustained a cerebrovascular accident should begin at the time the client is admitted to the hospital. The first goal of rehabilitation should be to help prevent the client from developing deformities. This goal is achieved through such techniques as positioning the client properly in bed, changing his position frequently, and supporting all parts of his body in proper alignment. Passive range-of-motion exercises may also be started, unless contraindicated. (P, C, G)

35. 1. A helpless client should be positioned on the side, not on the back, with the head on a small pillow. This positioning helps secretions escape from the throat and mouth and minimizes the risk of aspiration. Suctioning equipment should be available, the client's mouth should be opened with a padded tongue blade, and the mouth and teeth can be cleaned with a toothbrush. (I, N, S)

36. 3. Based on the data provided, the most appropriate nursing diagnosis is Impaired Physical Mobility. There are no data to indicate that this client is suffering from a disturbance in sleep patterns or an inability to tolerate activity. There also is no indication that the client is neglecting the right side of his body. (D, N, G)

37. 2. Monitoring pupil size and pupillary response is part of the neurologic assessment of cranial nerve function and is critical for this client. Risk factors, elimination patterns, and previous health behaviors are important to assess but are not the priority during the acute post-CVA period. (A, T, G)

38. 1. Knowledge of the clients functional status before and after the CVA will guide the plan for rehabilitation and is therefore essential for the nurse to assist. (A, T, G)

39. 2. Sliding a client on a sheet causes friction and should be avoided. Friction tends to injure skin tissues and predispose to pressure ulcer formation. Rolling the client, lifting him on a drawsheet, and having him help lift himself off the bed with a trapeze all help prevent friction from being moved in bed. (I, T, G)

40. 3. Regular repositioning and range-of-motion exercises are important interventions, but the use of ankle-high tennis shoes has been found to be most effective in preventing plantar flexion (footdrop). Foot boards stimulate spasms and are not routinely recommended. (I, N, S)

41. 1. Broca's area, which controls expressive speech, is located on the left side of the brain. Therefore, a client with a cerebrovascular accident in this area is likely to exhibit expressive or motor *aphasia. Dyslexia,* the inability of a person with normal vision to interpret written language, is thought to be due to a central nervous system defect in the ability to organize graphic symbols. *Apraxia* is the inability to perform purposeful movements in the absence or loss of motor power, sensation, or coordination. *Agnosia* is the loss of comprehension of auditory, visual, or other sensations despite an intact sensory sphere. (P, C, G)

42. 2. Although the client with expressive aphasia is unable to communicate verbally, he can understand what is being said to him. The client's communication with others may be helped by a communication or picture board on which he can point to objects or activities he desires. (I, T, S)

43. 2. A client with dysphagia (difficulty swallowing) frequently has the most difficulty ingesting liquids, which are easily aspirated. Measures that minimize the risk of aspiration in a client with dysphagia include maintaining an upright position while eating (unless contraindicated), introducing foods on the unaffected side of the mouth, and keeping distractions to a minimum. (I, N, S)

44. 3. When dressing, the client should put clothing on the affected side first. He should wear normal clothing, if possible. Other people may help the client dress, but the emphasis should be on self-care. (I, T, H)

45. 2. Although many eating behaviors may be disturbed after a CVA, eating food on only half the plate would result from an inability to coordinate visual images and spatial relationships. (E, C, G)

46. 4. To expand the visual field, the partially sighted client should be taught to turn his head from side to side when walking. Neglecting to do so may result in accidents. This technique helps maximize the use of remaining sight. A patch does not address the problem of hemianopia. Appropriate positioning of the client and personal items will increase his ability to cope with the problem but will not affect his safety. (I, T, S)

47. 3. A client who has brain damage may be emotionally labile and may cry or laugh for no explainable reason. Crying jags are best dealt with by attempting to divert the client's attention. Ignoring the behavior or attempting to deal with it behaviorally will not affect it. (I, N, L)

48. 4. When offering emotional support to a client who is discouraged and has a negative self-concept because of physical handicaps, the nurse should display encouragement and patience. The client should be praised when he shows progress in his efforts to overcome handicaps. Sympathy, charity, and firm discipline have little supportive value. (I, N, L)

49. 1. The strong support of family members is frequently identified as an important factor that influences a stroke client's continuing progress in rehabilitation after discharge. Discharge planning should prepare the client and family for the many changes that will be necessary when the client returns home. Family support groups can be beneficial in guiding and supporting families in the care of the client. An effective discharge plan will coordinate the resources of the client, family, and community. (P, N, H)

50. 3. Thrombolytic agents are used for clients with CVA. They act by dissolving emboli, thereby reducing the damage of the event. (E, K, G)

The Client With Parkinson's Disease

51. 4. Typical signs of Parkinson's disease include drooling; a low-pitched, monotonous voice; and a stiff, mask-like facial expression. Aphasia is not a symptom of Parkinson's disease. An exaggerated sense of euphoria would not be typical; more likely, the client would exhibit depression, probably related to the progressive nature of the disease and the client's difficulties in dealing with it. Many clients also begin to show a decline in cognitive, memory, and perceptual abilities. (A, C, G)

52. 4. A priority diagnosis for this client is Potential for Injury because the client with Parkinson's disease often has a propulsive gait, characterized by a tendency to take increasingly quicker steps while walking. This type of gait often causes the client to fall or to have trouble stopping. (D, T, S)

53. 2. Voluntary and purposeful movements often temporarily decrease or stop the tremors associated with Parkinson's disease. In some clients, however, tremors may increase with voluntary effort. Tremors are not psychological in nature and cannot be willfully controlled. (E, C, G)

54. 2. Demanding physical activity should be performed during the peak action of drug therapy. Clients should be encouraged to maintain independence in self-care activities to the greatest extent possible. Adequate time should be allowed to perform these self-care activities. (I, N, G)

55. 4. Parkinson's disease progresses in severity, and there is no known cure or way to stop its progression. Many clients live for years with the disease, however, and it would not be appropriate to start planning terminal care at this time for this client. The most appropriate and realistic goal is to help the client function at his best. (P, N, G)

56. 1. Muscle rigidity, which can lead to contracture, is a major symptom of Parkinson's disease. Physical therapy is aimed at maintaining joint flexibility and relaxing muscles. (P, C, G)

57. 2. Levodopa is prescribed to decrease severe muscle rigidity. Its effectiveness is primarily measured by the client's response in this area. (E, C, G)

58. 4. Increasing doses of levodopa put a client at serious risk for toxicity. Severe mental deterioration, as evidenced by delusions or hallucinations, frequently occurs in the toxic state, and family members must be instructed about this possibility. (I, K, G)

59. 4. While the client is hospitalized for adjustment of medication, it is essential that the medications be administered exactly at the scheduled time, for accurate evaluation of effectiveness. (I, T, G)

60. 2. Ongoing self-care is a major goal for clients with Parkinson's disease. The client should be given additional time as needed and praised for his efforts to remain independent. (I, N, L)

61. 1. Pallidotomy is done to improve the functional ability of the client with Parkinson's disease. Improving functional ability is a priority for these clients. (P, C, G)

The Client With Multiple Sclerosis

62. 2. Visual disturbances, speech impairment, problems with walking associated with loss of muscle tone and tremors, spastic weakness in the extremities, and dizziness with nausea and vomiting are some common symptoms of multiple sclerosis. Hyperexcitability and euphoria may occur, but because of muscle weakness, sudden bursts of energy are unlikely. (A, C, G)

63. 2. Typical complications of multiple sclerosis include contractures, decubitus ulcers, and respiratory infections. Nursing care should be directed toward the goal of preventing these complications. Ascites, fluid volume overload, and myocardial infarction are not associated with multiple sclerosis. (P, C, G)

64. 3. Baclofen is a centrally acting skeletal muscle relaxant that helps relieve the muscle spasms common in multiple sclerosis. Methocarbamol is another skeletal muscle relaxant used to treat multiple sclerosis; the nurse may encounter others in practice. (E, C, G)

65. 2. Evaluating drug effectiveness is difficult because a high percentage of clients with multiple sclerosis exhibit unpredictable episodes of remission, exacerbation, and steady progress without apparent cause. (E, C, G)

66. 4. Such practices as asking a client with slurred speech to speak slowly and distinctly and to repeat indistinguishable words tend to improve her ability to communicate effectively. Asking a client to speak louder even when tired may aggravate the problem. (I, N, G)

67. 4. Nurse's notes should be concise, objective, clearly stated, and relevant. This client trembles when she attempts voluntary action such as drinking a beverage or fastening clothing. This activity should be described exactly as it occurs so that others reading the note will have no doubt about the nurse's observation of the client's behavior. (I, N, S)

68. 4. Limiting fluid intake is likely to aggravate rather than relieve symptoms when a bowel-training program is being implemented. Furthermore, water imbalance, as well as electrolyte imbalance, tends to aggravate symptoms of multiple sclerosis. (I, T, H)

69. 1. Clients with multiple sclerosis often experience psychological disturbances that are best described as mood disorders. Emotional instability is typical. Thought disorders, psychosomatic illnesses, and drug dependency are not typical of clients with multiple sclerosis unless these disorders are present independently. (P, T, L)

70. 2. Care for the client with multiple sclerosis is directed toward muscle rehabilitation and client motivation. The disease is chronic; thus, goals should be those with the most benefit over a prolonged period. (P, T, H)

71. 2. The nurse's most positive approach is to encourage a client with multiple sclerosis to keep active while avoiding emotional upset and fatigue. A quiet, inactive lifestyle is not necessarily indicated. Good health habits will not likely alter the course of the disease, although they may help minimize complications. Practicing using aids that will be needed for future disabilities may be helpful but also can be discouraging. (I, N, L)

72. 1. Safety concerns are essential for a client with sensory impairment. Water temperature should be tested carefully, hot-water bottles should be avoided, and the skin should be inspected regularly. Independence and self-care are also important; the client should not be instructed to avoid kitchen activities out of fear of injury. (I, N, H)

73. 3. Establishing a regular fluid intake of 2000 to 3000 mL/day and maintaining a regular voiding pattern would be the most appropriate measure to help the client avoid urinary incontinence. Inserting an indwelling catheter would be a treatment of last resort because of the increased risk for infection. If catheterization is required, intermittent self-catheterization is preferred because of its lower risk of infection. (P, T, G)

74. 2. A client with multiple sclerosis usually does best and is least frustrated at home when a regular program of daily activities is planned. There is no information given in this item suggesting that psychological counseling is necessary or that it would be helpful to have the granddaughter attend a day-care center. A weekly visit by another person with multiple sclerosis may not be contraindicated, but it is less likely to benefit the client as much as a regular program of planned activities. (I, N, L)

The Unconscious Client

75. 3. Equal, normally reactive pupils indicate adequate neurologic functioning. Progressive pupil dilation indicates increased intracranial pressure, and fixed dilated pupils indicate injury at the midbrain. Overdose of amphetamines, alcohol, or cocaine also causes dilated pupils; overdose of morphine and barbiturates results in constricted pupils. Blood pressure is regulated by various factors, and a finding of hypertension would not pinpoint a toxic disorder. Fever is related either to infection or dehydration. Facial asymmetry indicates paralysis. (A, T, G)

76. 1. An unconscious client is best positioned in a lateral or semiprone position because these positions allow the jaw and tongue to fall forward, facilitate drainage of secretions, and prevent aspiration. Positioning the client supine carries a major risk of airway obstruction from the tongue, vomitus, or nasopharyngeal secretions. Trendelenburg's position, with the head lower than the heart, decreases effective lung volume and increases the risk of cerebral edema. The lithotomy position has no purpose in this situation. (I, N, S)

77. 3. Activated charcoal powder is administered to absorb remaining particles of salicylate. Vitamin K is an antidote for warfarin sodium. Dextrose 50% is an antidote for insulin. Sodium thiosulfate is an antidote for cyanide. (P, K, G)

78. 3. The initial response to crisis is high anxiety. Anxiety must dissipate before a person can deal with the actual situation. Allowing family members to ventilate their feelings can help this dissipation. The reasons for the client's actions are unknown; assumptions must be validated before they become facts. Touch can be appropriate, but not when used as false reassurance. Helping with the client's care is appropriate at a later time. (I, N, L)

79. 3. Maintaining intact skin is a priority goal for the unconscious client. Unconscious clients need to be turned every hour to prevent complications of immobility, which include pressure ulcers and stasis pneumonia. (P, T, S)

80. 3. Staging of pressure ulcers can be found in the Guidelines for Pressure Ulcers published by the Agency for Health Care Policy Research (AHCPR), a division of the Health and Human Services. When pressure is applied to the skin, the area first becomes blanched, or whitish. When pressure is relieved, the circulation tends to carry excess blood to the area to make up for the temporary decrease in blood supply. This effect, called *reactive hyperemia,* causes the skin to redden. Such a reddened area is a precursor of a pressure sore. (A, C, G)

81. 4. Massaging reddened areas that are due to pressure is contraindicated because it further reduces blood flow to the area. In the past, massaging reddened areas was thought to improve blood flow to the area, and some nursing personnel may still believe that massaging the area is effective in preventing pressure ulcer formation. (I, T, S)

82. 3. Common pressure points in the side-lying position include the ears, shoulders, ribs, greater trochanter, medial and lateral condyles, and ankles. (P, T, G)

83. 3. The client will not be in proper body alignment if, when in the right side-lying position, his left arm rests on the mattress with the elbow flexed. This positioning of the arm pulls the left shoulder out of good alignment, restricting respiratory movements. The arm should be supported on a pillow. (I, T, G)

84. 3. Trochanter rolls placed alongside the client's legs from the ilium to midthigh are recommended to prevent external rotation of the hips. Placing sandbags from the knees to the ankle will not effectively support the hips in proper alignment. Pillows can be used only as a temporary measure because they can

not hold the legs and hips in proper alignment over a prolonged period. A footboard does not help keep the legs and hips in proper alignment. (I, T, G)

85. 4. Passive range-of-motion exercises are performed to maintain joint mobility. They will not have a positive effect on the client's muscle tone or bone structure. Active exercise is needed to preserve bone and muscle mass. (P, C, S)

86. 1. The nurse should keep suction equipment available to remove secretions and should place the client in a side-lying position. Performing oral hygiene is a clean procedure; therefore, the nurse wears clean gloves, not sterile gloves. The nurse should never place any fingers in an unconscious client's mouth; the client may bite down. Padded tongue blades, swabs, or a toothbrush should be used instead. (I, T, S)

87. 2. When the blink reflex is absent or the eyes do not close completely, the cornea may become dry and irritated. Placing a patch over the eye is the most appropriate intervention to prevent eye injury. (I, N, S)

88. 3. Restlessness is an early indicator of hypoxia. The nurse should suspect hypoxia in the unconscious client who becomes restless. The most accurate method for determining the presence of hypoxia is to evaluate arterial blood gas values. Cyanosis and decreased respirations are late indicators of hypoxia. Hypertension, not hypotension, is a sign of hypoxia. (A, T, G)

89. 2. The client should be placed in semi-Fowler's position to reduce the risk of aspiration. The formula should be at room temperature, not heated. Administering enteral tube feedings is a clean procedure, not a sterile one; thus, sterile supplies are not required. Clients receiving enteral feedings should be weighed regularly, but not necessarily before each feeding. (I, T, S)

90. 4. Gastric residuals are checked before administration of enteral feedings to determine whether gastric emptying is delayed. A gastric residual of less than 50% of the previous feeding volume is usually considered acceptable. If the amount of gastric residual is excessive, the nurse notifies the physician and holds the feeding. If only a small amount of gastric residual is obtained, the nurse reinstills it through the tube and then administers the feeding. Reinstilling the residual helps prevent electrolyte and fluid losses. (I, N, S)

91. 1. It is generally agreed that bladder infections in a client with an indwelling catheter result from infections that ascend from the urethra into the bladder. Good catheter care, including meticulous cleansing of the area around the urethral meatus, is of the highest priority for the client with an indwelling catheter. Clamping an indwelling catheter is not recommended. (I, N, S)

The Client in Pain

92. 1. Pain perception is an individual experience. Research indicates that pain tolerance and perception vary widely among people due to individual differences. (P, C, G)

93. 1. Experience has demonstrated that clients who feel confidence in the personnel caring for them do not require as much therapy for pain relief as those who have less confidence. Without the client's confidence, developed in an effective nurse–client relationship, other interventions may be less effective. (P, N, L)

94. 4. Physical tolerance to a regular narcotic dose develops rapidly with frequent use. The client experiences increased discomfort, asks for medication more frequently, and exhibits anxious and restless behavior, which is often misinterpreted as indicative of developing dependence or addiction. (A, N, G)

95. 3. Acupuncture, like acumassage and acupressure, is performed in certain Asian cultures to help restore the energy balance within the body. Pressure, massage, and fine needles are applied to "energy pathways" to help restore the body's balance. In the Western world, many researchers think that the gate-control theory of pain may be applicable to acupuncture, acumassage, and acupressure. (P, K, L)

96. 4. The equianalgesic dose of oral meperidine hydrochloride is up to four times the intramuscular dose. Although meperidine hydrochloride can be given orally, it is more effective when given intramuscularly. (I, K, G)

97. 1. Narcotic analgesics relieve pain by reducing or altering the perception of pain. They do not decrease the sensitivity of pain receptors, interfere with pain impulses traveling along sensory nerve fibers, or block the conduction of pain impulses in the central nervous system. (P, C, G)

98. 3. According to the gate-control theory, the regulatory process that controls pain impulses reaching the brain most probably occurs in the spinal cord. (P, C, G)

99. 3. Responses to pain are directed initially toward the body's ability to escape or flee the source of pain. The response is typical of the fight-or-flight phenomenon, first described by Walter B. Cannon when he was working on theories of homeostasis and fear. (A, C, G)

100. 1. Ergotamine tartrate is used to help abort a migraine attack. The drug acts as a vasoconstrictor. It should be taken as soon as prodromal symptoms of migraine appear. The drug is not used to reduce severity of headaches, relieve sleeplessness after an attack, or decrease visual problems after an attack. (A, T, G)

101. 1. A vascular disturbance involving branches of the carotid artery is believed to cause migraine attacks. Vasoconstriction of blood vessels apparently occurs first. The extracranial and intracranial arteries then dilate, causing the headache. Family history of migraine headaches is present in more than half of all people who experience migraines. (A, K, G)

102. 4. Biofeedback aims to translate body processes into observable signs, which the client can use to exercise some control over certain body processes. For example, a biofeedback machine measures a client's pulse rate and displays the information. The client is then instructed to try to lower the pulse rate, using such techniques as listening to relaxing music or thinking of a pleasant scene. If any action lowers the pulse rate, the client learns to continue to do whatever it was that decreased the pulse rate. The reinforcement of learning is immediate because the client can see the results of his actions. (P, T, G)

103. 1. Massage stimulates the large-diameter cutaneous fibers, which block transmission of pain impulses from the spinal cord to the brain. Although massage may have other positive effects, such as distracting the client, the physiologic process of fiber stimulation supports using massage as therapy for pain relief. (A, C, G)

104. 3. Studies have supported that one reason patient-controlled analgesia is effective is because the client has control over the narcotic administration. Morphine is the most commonly used narcotic in patient-controlled analgesia. Only one narcotic is administered at a time. Nursing assessments and actions remain basically the same for the client using patient-controlled analgesia. (I, T, G)

105. 2. It is essential that the nurse documents the client's response to pain medication on a routine, systematic basis. Through careful assessment and documentation, the effectiveness of pain relief interventions can be evaluated and modified, if necessary. Reassuring the client that pain will be relieved is often not realistic. A client who continually presses the patient-controlled analgesia button may not be getting adequate pain relief. Pain medication is not titrated. (I, T, S)

106. 4. A multidisciplinary approach to pain relief is needed for greatest effectiveness. In addition to the client, the nurse, and the physician, others that may be needed on the team include a social worker, an occupational therapist, a dietician, and a psychologist or a psychiatrist. Pain relief interventions based on physiologic and psychological principles can be used simultaneously to obtain greater pain relief. Medication administration is only one option for reducing pain. (E, N, S)

107. 2. To locate the ventrogluteal site, the nurse places the palm on the client's greater trochanter with the index finger on the anterosuperior iliac spine. The posterior iliac spine is a landmark for locating the dorsogluteal site. The site should be carefully and correctly identified to avoid tissue or nerve damage. (I, K, S)

108. 3. Holding a pledget against an injection site while removing the needle helps prevent the needle from pulling on the skin. The technique makes any injection more comfortable. (I, K, S)

109. 1. Because the deltoid muscle is small, any injection into it is relatively uncomfortable. The muscle is easy to locate. It has pain receptors and a good blood supply, just as do the other muscles in the body. (I, K, S)

110. 2. Universal precautions for care of needles and syringes involve *never* recapping used needles. Immediately after giving an injection, the nurse should place the entire needle and syringe set in the universal precautions container in the client's room. (I, K, S)

NURSING CARE OF ADULTS WITH MEDICAL AND SURGICAL HEALTH PROBLEMS

TEST 9: The Client With Neurologic Health Problems

Directions: Use this answer grid to determine areas of strength or need for further study.

NURSING PROCESS

A = Assessment
D = Analysis, nursing diagnosis
P = Planning
I = Implementation
E = Evaluation

COGNITIVE LEVEL

K = Knowledge
C = Comprehension
T = Application
N = Analysis

CLIENT NEEDS

S = Safe, effective care environment
G = Physiologic integrity
L = Psychosocial integrity
H = Health promotion and maintenance

Question #	Answer #	Nursing Process					Cognitive Level				Client Needs			
		A	D	P	I	E	K	C	T	N	S	G	L	H
1	3				I					N	S			
2	1				I					N	S			
3	4	A							T			G		
4	1	A							T			G		
5	1	A							T			G		
6	1	A								N	S			
7	4	A						C				G		
8	3	A							T			G		
9	1				I				T		S			
10	1	A								N		G		
11	4				I				T			G		
12	2				I				T		S			
13	1	A							T			G		
14	3				I				T		S			
15	2	A						C				G		
16	2				I					N		G		
17	3					E			T				L	
18	3				I				T		S			
19	4	A						C				G		
20	4				I			C			S			
21	2				I			C			S			
22	1			P				C				G		
23	2				I					N	S			
24	3			P					T		S			
25	4				I				T			G		

NURSING PROCESS

A = Assessment
D = Analysis, nursing diagnosis
P = Planning
I = Implementation
E = Evaluation

COGNITIVE LEVEL

K = Knowledge
C = Comprehension
T = Application
N = Analysis

CLIENT NEEDS

S = Safe, effective care environment
G = Physiologic integrity
L = Psychosocial integrity
H = Health promotion and maintenance

Question #	Answer #	Nursing Process					Cognitive Level				Client Needs			
		A	D	P	I	E	K	C	T	N	S	G	L	H
26	4	A								N		G		
27	1	A								N		G		
28	3				I			C				G		
29	2				I			C				G		
30	2				I			C						H
31	3				I		K					G		
32	3				I					N				H
33	3					E		C				G		
34	2			P				C				G		
35	1				I					N	S			
36	3		D							N		G		
37	2	A							T			G		
38	1	A							T			G		
39	2				I				T			G		
40	3				I					N	S			
41	1		D					C				G		
42	2				I				T		S			
43	2				I					N	S			
44	3				I				T					H
45	2					E		C				G		
46	4				I				T		S			
47	3				I					N			L	
48	4				I					N			L	
49	1			P						N				H
50	3					E	K					G		
51	4	A						C				G		
52	4		D						T		S			
53	2	A						C				G		
54	2				I					N		G		
55	4			P						N		G		

ANSWER GRID: 2

NURSING PROCESS

A = Assessment
D = Analysis, nursing diagnosis
P = Planning
I = Implementation
E = Evaluation

COGNITIVE LEVEL

K = Knowledge
C = Comprehension
T = Application
N = Analysis

CLIENT NEEDS

S = Safe, effective care environment
G = Physiologic integrity
L = Psychosocial integrity
H = Health promotion and maintenance

Question #	Answer #	A	D	P	I	E	K	C	T	N	S	G	L	H
56	1			P				C				G		
57	2					E		C				G		
58	4				I		K					G		
59	4				I				T			G		
60	2				I					N			L	
61	1			P				C				G		
62	2	A						C				G		
63	2			P				C				G		
64	3					E		C				G		
65	2					E		C				G		
66	4				I					N		G		
67	4	A								N	S			
68	4				I				T					H
69	1	A							T				L	
70	2			P					T					H
71	2				I					N			L	
72	1				I					N				H
73	3				I				T			G		
74	2				I					N			L	
75	3	A							T			G		
76	1				I					N	S			
77	3			P			K					G		
78	3				I					N			L	
79	3			P					T		S			
80	3	A						C				G		
81	4				I				T		S			
82	3			P					T			G		
83	3				I				T			G		
84	3				I				T			G		
85	4			P				C			S			

ANSWER GRID: 3

NURSING PROCESS

A = Assessment
D = Analysis, nursing diagnosis
P = Planning
I = Implementation
E = Evaluation

COGNITIVE LEVEL

K = Knowledge
C = Comprehension
T = Application
N = Analysis

CLIENT NEEDS

S = Safe, effective care environment
G = Physiologic integrity
L = Psychosocial integrity
H = Health promotion and maintenance

Question #	Answer #	Nursing Process					Cognitive Level				Client Needs			
		A	D	P	I	E	K	C	T	N	S	G	L	H
86	1				I				T		S			
87	2				I					N	S			
88	3	A							T			G		
89	2				I				T		S			
90	4				I					N	S			
91	1				I					N	S			
92	1			P				C				G		
93	1			P						N			L	
94	4	A								N		G		
95	3			P			K						L	
96	4				I		K					G		
97	1			P				C				G		
98	3			P				C				G		
99	3	A						C				G		
100	1	A							T			G		
101	1	A					K					G		
102	4			P					T			G		
103	1					E		C				G		
104	3				I				T			G		
105	2				I				T		S			
106	4			P						N	S			
107	2				I		K				S			
108	3				I		K				S			
109	1				I		K				S			
110	2				I		K				S			

ANSWER GRID: 4

NURSING PROCESS

A = Assessment
D = Analysis, nursing diagnosis
P = Planning
I = Implementation
E = Evaluation

COGNITIVE LEVEL

K = Knowledge
C = Comprehension
T = Application
N = Analysis

CLIENT NEEDS

S = Safe, effective care environment
G = Physiologic integrity
L = Psychosocial integrity
H = Health promotion and maintenance

Question #	Answer #	Nursing Process					Cognitive Level				Client Needs			
		A	D	P	I	E	K	C	T	N	S	G	L	H
Number Correct														
Number Possible	110	26	3	20	53	8	11	29	38	32	33	60	10	7
Percentage Correct														

Score Calculation: To determine your **Percentage Correct,** divide the **Number Correct** by the **Number Possible.**

ANSWER GRID: 5

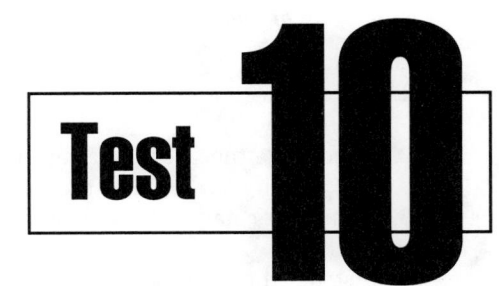

The Client With Musculoskeletal Health Problems

- **The Client With Rheumatoid Arthritis**
- **The Client With Osteoarthritis**
- **The Client With a Hip Fracture**
- **The Client With a Herniated Disk**
- **The Client With Peripheral Vascular Disease Having an Amputation**
- **The Client With a Femoral Fracture**
- **The Client With a Spinal Cord Injury**
- **Correct Answers and Rationale**

Select the one best answer, and indicate your choice by filling in the circle in front of the option.

The Client With Rheumatoid Arthritis

A 60-year-old woman with the diagnosis of rheumatoid arthritis has been hospitalized for an evaluation of her increasingly impaired physical mobility.

1. The client asks the nurse to explain why her joints are becoming increasingly painful. The nurse's response should be based on knowledge that rheumatoid arthritis
   ○ 1. results from degenerative joint damage.
   ○ 2. affects only the weight-bearing joints of the body.
   ○ 3. begins with inflammation of joint synovial tissue.
   ○ 4. is usually caused by aging.

2. The client has been taking large doses of aspirin to relieve her joint pain. The nurse should assess the client for which important symptom of aspirin toxicity?
   ○ 1. Dysuria.
   ○ 2. Tinnitus.
   ○ 3. Chest pain.
   ○ 4. Drowsiness.

3. Which statement by the client would indicate that she needs additional teaching to safely receive the maximum benefit of her aspirin therapy?

   ○ 1. "I always take aspirin with food to protect my stomach."
   ○ 2. "Once I learned to take my aspirin with meals, I was able to start using the inexpensive generic brand."
   ○ 3. "I always watch for bleeding gums or blood in my stool."
   ○ 4. "I try to take aspirin only on days when the pain seems particularly bad."

4. The client tells the nurse, "I can't seem to do my household chores anymore without becoming tired. My knees hurt whenever I walk; it's difficult for me to get around my house and yard." Based on these data, which nursing diagnosis would be most appropriate for this client?
   ○ 1. Activity Intolerance related to fatigue and pain.
   ○ 2. Self-Care Deficit related to increasing joint pain.
   ○ 3. Ineffective Individual Coping related to chronic pain.
   ○ 4. Body Image Disturbance related to fatigue and joint pain.

5. Which of the following activities would the nurse likely choose to implement in response to a nursing diagnosis of Activity Intolerance related to lack of energy conservation?

○ 1. Encourage the client to perform all tasks early in the day.

○ 2. Encourage the client to alternate periods of rest and activity throughout the day.

○ 3. Administer narcotics to promote pain relief and rest.

○ 4. Instruct the client to not perform daily hygienic care until activity tolerance improves.

6. The client tells the nurse, "I have a friend who took gold shots and had a wonderful response. Why didn't my doctor let me try that?" Which of the following replies by the nurse would be best?

○ 1. "It's the doctor's prerogative to decide how to treat you."

○ 2. "Tell me more about your friend's arthritic condition. Maybe I can answer that question for you."

○ 3. "That drug is used for cases that are worse than yours. It wouldn't help you, so don't worry about it."

○ 4. "Every patient is different. What works for one patient may not always be effective for another."

7. In developing a plan of care for the client, the nurse should consider that clients with rheumatoid arthritis should be positioned so as to

○ 1. decrease edema around the joints.

○ 2. promote maximum comfort.

○ 3. prevent venous stasis.

○ 4. prevent flexion deformities of the joints.

8. The client undergoes a right total knee replacement. The nurse would anticipate which of the following activity orders for this client on the first postoperative day?

○ 1. Bed rest for 24 to 48 hours after surgery.

○ 2. Ambulate with walker twice a day.

○ 3. Up to chair with leg elevated.

○ 4. Dangle at bedside for 20 minutes.

9. Postoperatively, the client's right leg is placed in a continuous passive motion (CPM) machine. Nursing responsibilities when caring for a client with this apparatus would include which of the following?

○ 1. Adjusting the settings as needed to prevent client discomfort.

○ 2. Increasing the range-of-motion settings at least every 8 hours.

○ 3. Maintaining proper positioning of the joint on the CPM machine.

○ 4. Discontinuing the CPM therapy when the client's range-of-motion increases.

10. The nurse teaches the client to perform isometric exercises to strengthen her leg muscles after surgery. Isometric exercises are particularly effective for clients with rheumatoid arthritis because they

○ 1. cost little in terms of time and money.

○ 2. strengthen the muscles while keeping the joints stationary.

○ 3. involve clients in their own care and thus improve morale.

○ 4. prevent joint stiffness.

11. The nurse evaluates the client's ability to perform quadriceps-setting exercises. The client would correctly perform these exercises by

○ 1. bending the knee to form a right angle.

○ 2. rotating the leg slowly around in circles.

○ 3. pressing the back of the knee into the mattress.

○ 4. turning the leg inward toward the opposite thigh.

12. The client tells the nurse, "I know it is important to exercise my joints, so I won't lose mobility. But my joints are so stiff and painful that exercising is difficult." Which of the following responses by the nurse would be most appropriate?

○ 1. "You are probably exercising too much. Decrease your exercise to every other day."

○ 2. "Tell the doctor about your symptoms. Maybe he can increase your pain medication."

○ 3. "Stiffness and pain are part of your disease. You can learn to cope by focusing on activities you enjoy."

○ 4. "Take a warm tub bath or shower before exercising. This may relieve some of your discomfort."

13. Which of the following expected outcomes would be appropriate for a client with rheumatoid arthritis? The client will

○ 1. minimize the frequency with which anti-inflammatory drugs are used to control joint discomfort.

○ 2. demonstrate use of adaptive equipment in the home environment as appropriate.

○ 3. learn to limit activity so as to avoid joint pain.

○ 4. verbalize that recovery from rheumatoid arthritis will require several years of treatment.

The Client With Osteoarthritis

A client has been diagnosed with degenerative joint disease (osteoarthritis) of the left hip.

14. Which of the following factors would most likely increase the joint symptoms of osteoarthritis?

○ 1. A long history of smoking.

○ 2. Excessive alcohol use.

○ 3. Obesity.

○ 4. Emotional stress.

15. The nurse would anticipate conservative treatment of osteoarthritis to include

○ 1. isotonic exercises to strengthen muscles.

○ 2. opioid analgesics for pain control.

○ 3. routine injections of intraarticular corticosteroids.

○ 4. orthotic devices to support involved joints.

16. The client's physician orders ibuprofen (Motrin) to treat the left hip pain. To minimize gastric mucosal irritation, the nurse should teach the client to take this medication

○ 1. at bedtime.

○ 2. on arising.

○ 3. immediately after a meal.

○ 4. when her stomach is empty.

17. The client reports increasingly severe pain in the left hip; the physician recommends a total hip replacement. Preoperative nursing care for this client should begin with

○ 1. teaching how to prevent hip flexion.

○ 2. demonstrating coughing and deep breathing techniques.

○ 3. displaying an actual hip prosthesis.

○ 4. assessing the client's understanding of the procedure.

18. The nurse would plan to use an abduction pillow (or splint) after a total hip replacement to

○ 1. prevent hip flexion.

○ 2. decrease formation of sacral decubitus ulcers.

○ 3. prevent dislocation of the prosthesis.

○ 4. increase peripheral circulation.

19. The client tells the nurse that the pain in his operative hip has increased. On assessing the hip and leg, the nurse notes that the leg is internally rotated and shorter than the other leg, and that the client has difficulty moving the leg. Based on this information, the nurse determines that the client

○ 1. has experienced increased pain due to a muscle spasm.

○ 2. requires repositioning to achieve better alignment of the leg.

○ 3. would benefit from additional muscle strengthening exercises.

○ 4. has experienced a dislocation of the hip prosthesis.

20. The nurse has instructed the client on the correct positioning of his leg and hip after hip replacement surgery. Which of the following statements indicate the client has understood these instructions?

○ 1. "I may cross my legs as long as I keep my knees extended."

○ 2. "I should avoid bending over to tie my shoes."

○ 3. "I can sit in any chair that I find comfortable."

○ 4. "I should avoid any unnecessary walking for about 3 months after my surgery."

The Client With a Hip Fracture

A client is admitted to the hospital with a diagnosis of a right hip fracture. She complains of right hip pain and cannot move her right leg.

21. Which of the following assessments made by the nurse indicates that the client has a typical sign of a hip fracture? The client's right leg is

○ 1. rotated internally.

○ 2. held in a flexed position.

○ 3. adducted.

○ 4. shorter than the leg on the unaffected side.

22. The client's fracture is corrected by surgical internal fixation with the insertion of a pin. The nurse's plan of care reflects the understanding that internal fixation with a pin is the treatment of choice for most older people because it

○ 1. is a simpler procedure.

○ 2. promotes rapid healing.

○ 3. carries less danger of infection.

○ 4. makes earlier mobilization possible.

23. The nurse anticipates that the client will return from surgery with a drainage tube at the incision site that is attached to suction. The purpose of this apparatus is to help

○ 1. detect a wound infection.

○ 2. eliminate the need for wound irrigation.

○ 3. prevent fluid accumulation in the wound.

○ 4. provide a way to instill antibiotics into the wound.

24. Which of the following signs or symptoms would be of least importance when the nurse evaluates the client for postoperative peripheral nerve damage?

○ 1. Pain.

○ 2. Sensation.

○ 3. Bleeding.

○ 4. Pulselessness.

25. Which of the following pieces of equipment should the nurse plan to use to help prevent external rotation of the client's right leg postoperatively?

○ 1. Sandbags.

○ 2. A high footboard.

○ 3. A rubber air ring.

○ 4. A metal bed cradle.

26. Which of the following nursing measures would be most important to implement to decrease the risk of a surgical wound infection in this client?

○ 1. Inserting an indwelling urinary catheter to prevent possible soiling of the dressing.

○ 2. Accurately measuring drainage from the surgical drainage tube.

○ 3. Changing the surgical dressings using sterile technique.

○ 4. Monitoring the incision for signs of redness, swelling, and warmth.

27. When the client is lying on her side, the nurse should place pillows or a splint between her legs to prevent

○ 1. flexion of the knees.

○ 2. abduction of the thighs.

○ 3. adduction of the hip joint.

○ 4. hyperextension of the knees.

28. In which of the following chairs would it be best for the client to sit postoperatively?

○ 1. A desk-type swivel chair.

○ 2. A padded upholstered chair.

○ 3. A high-backed chair with armrests.

○ 4. A recliner with an attached footrest.

29. The nurse should teach the client that which of the following leg positions is contraindicated for her while sitting in a chair?

○ 1. Crossing her legs.

○ 2. Elevating her legs.

○ 3. Flexing her ankles.

○ 4. Extending her knees.

30. When assessing the client as a candidate for crutch walking, the nurse should take into account that for some elderly people, crutch walking is an impractical goal primarily because of decreased

○ 1. visual acuity.

○ 2. reaction time.

○ 3. motor coordination.

○ 4. level of comprehension.

31. Which of the following activities should the nurse plan to teach the client to strengthen her hand muscles in preparation for using crutches?

○ 1. Brushing her hair.

○ 2. Squeezing a rubber ball.

○ 3. Flexing and extending her wrists.

○ 4. Pushing her hands into the mattress while raising herself in bed.

32. The nurse assesses the client's home environment for the safe use of crutches. Which one of the following would pose the greatest hazard to the client's safe use of crutches at home?

○ 1. A 4-year-old cocker spaniel.

○ 2. Scatter rugs.

○ 3. Snack tables.

○ 4. Rocking chairs.

The Client With a Herniated Disk

A client is diagnosed with a herniated lumbar disk at the L4-5 interspace.

33. During the initial client interview, the nurse would most likely learn that the symptom that first caused the client to seek health care was

○ 1. loss of bladder control.

○ 2. loss of voluntary muscle control.

○ 3. back pain that is relieved with resting.

○ 4. back pain that radiates to the shoulders.

34. Which of the following positions would be most comfortable for this client?

○ 1. Prone.

○ 2. Supine.

○ 3. Semi-Fowler's.

○ 4. Right or left Sims'.

35. The client is scheduled for a myelogram and asks the nurse about the procedure. The nurse would explain that radiographs will be taken of the client's spine after an injection of

○ 1. sterile water.

○ 2. normal saline solution.

○ 3. liquid nitrogen.

○ 4. radiopaque dye.

36. The client returns from the myelogram, for which an iodized oil (Pantopaque) was used. Which one of the following nursing measures would be included in his care?

○ 1. Bed rest with bathroom privileges.

○ 2. Restricted fluid intake.

○ 3. Head of the bed elevated 45 degrees.

○ 4. Assessment of lower extremity movement and sensation.

37. Which of the following categories of medications would the nurse anticipate being included in the conservative management of a client of with a herniated lumbar disk?

○ 1. Muscle relaxants.

○ 2. Sedatives.

○ 3. Tranquilizers.

○ 4. Parenteral analgesics.

38. The client undergoes a lumbar laminectomy. Which of the following would most likely be a priority nursing diagnosis for this client in the postoperative phase?

○ 1. Impaired Physical Mobility related to fear of back pain.

○ 2. Altered Nutrition: Less Than Body Requirements related to inability to eat in supine position.

○ 3. Bowel Incontinence related to decreased physical activity.

○ 4. Body Image Disturbance related to fear of disfiguring surgical scar.

39. Postoperatively, the nurse administers trimethobenzamide hydrochloride (Tigan) to the client. The nurse would evaluate that the drug was effective if it controlled the client's

○ 1. muscle spasms.

○ 2. nausea.

○ 3. shivering.

○ 4. dry mouth.

40. The client asks to be turned onto his side. It would be appropriate for the nurse to

○ 1. ask the client to help by using an overhead trapeze to turn himself.

○ 2. turn the client's shoulders first, followed by his hips and legs.

○ 3. inform the client that because of his laminectomy, he may only lie supine.

○ 4. get another nurse to help logroll the client into position.

41. The nurse helps the client apply the back brace he is to wear. Which of the following positions should the client assume before the brace is applied?

○ 1. Standing.

○ 2. Lying on his side in bed.

○ 3. Lying on his abdomen in bed.

○ 4. Sitting in a straight chair.

42. To protect the client's skin under the brace, the nurse should

○ 1. place padding as necessary for a snug fit.

○ 2. have the client wear a thin cotton shirt under the brace.

○ 3. lubricate the areas where the client's brace will contact skin surfaces.

○ 4. apply powder to the areas where the client's brace will contact skin surfaces.

43. When the client ambulates for the first time after surgery, he begins to feel faint. Which nursing action would be best until help arrives?

○ 1. Have the client close his eyes for a few minutes.

○ 2. Maneuver the client to a sitting position on the floor.

○ 3. Separate her or his feet to form a wide base of support and have the client rest against the nurse's hip.

○ 4. Have the client separate his feet to form a wide base of support and then bend at the waist to place his head near his knees.

44. The nurse would know that the client understands his postoperative instructions when he places his feet in which of the following positions when sitting in a chair?

○ 1. Flat on the floor.

○ 2. On a low footstool.

○ 3. In any position of comfort while keeping his legs uncrossed.

○ 4. On a high footstool so that his feet are about at the same level as the chair seat.

45. Which of the following activities would be contraindicated for the client in the first postoperative days?

○ 1. Assisting with his daily hygiene.

○ 2. Lying flat on his back in bed.

○ 3. Walking in the hall.

○ 4. Sitting in his room to read or watch television.

46. Which of the following instructions regarding body mechanics would be most appropriate for helping the client avoid further back injury?

○ 1. Pull objects rather than pushing them.

○ 2. Sleep on a soft mattress.

○ 3. Avoid prolonged sitting and standing.

○ 4. Sit in chairs with soft cushions.

The Client With Peripheral Vascular Disease Having an Amputation

A client is admitted to the hospital with peripheral vascular disease of the lower extremities. He is scheduled for an amputation of the left leg.

47. Which of the following symptoms is not typically associated with peripheral arterial disease?

○ 1. Ankle edema.

○ 2. Intermittent claudication.

○ 3. Decreased or absent pulses.

○ 4. Cool skin.

48. To assess the client's dorsalis pedis pulse, the nurse should palpate the

○ 1. medial surface of the ankle.

○ 2. area behind the ankle.

○ 3. ventral aspect of the top of the foot.

○ 4. medial aspect of the dorsum of the foot.

49. The nurse notes the following assessment findings regarding the client's peripheral vascular status: cramping leg pain relieved by rest; cool, pale feet; and delayed capillary refilling. Based on these data, the nurse would make a nursing diagnosis of

○ 1. Impaired Skin Integrity.

○ 2. Impaired Gas Exchange.

○ 3. Altered Peripheral Tissue Perfusion.

○ 4. Impaired Physical Mobility.

50. The client says, "I've really tried to manage my condition well." Which of the following routines would the nurse evaluate as having been appropriate for him?

○ 1. Resting with his legs elevated above the level of his heart.

○ 2. Walking slowly but steadily for 30 minutes twice a day.

○ 3. Minimizing activity.

○ 4. Wearing antiembolism stockings at all times when out of bed.

51. Which of the following clinical manifestations would be most indicative of complete arterial obstruction in the lower extremities?

○ 1. Aching pain.

○ 2. Burning sensations.

○ 3. Numbness and tingling.

○ 4. Coldness.

52. While the nurse is providing preoperative teaching, the client says, "I hate the idea of being an invalid after they cut off my leg." The nurse's most therapeutic response would be

○ 1. "You'll still have one good leg to use."
○ 2. "Tell me more about how you're feeling."
○ 3. "Let's finish the preoperative teaching."
○ 4. "You're fortunate to have a wife who can take care of you."

53. The client asks the nurse, "Why can't the doctor tell me exactly how much of my leg he's going to take off? Don't you think I should know that?" The nurse responds knowing that the final decision on the level of the amputation will depend primarily on
○ 1. the need to remove as much of the leg as possible.
○ 2. the adequacy of the blood supply to the tissues.
○ 3. the ease with which a prosthesis can be fitted.
○ 4. the client's ability to walk with a prosthesis.

54. The client returns from surgery for a below-the-knee amputation with the residual limb covered with dressings and a woven elastic bandage. At first, the bandage was dry, but now, 30 minutes later, the nurse notices a small amount of bloody drainage. What should be the priority action?
○ 1. Notify the physician.
○ 2. Mark the area of drainage.
○ 3. Change the dressing.
○ 4. Reinforce the dressing.

55. The client's room should contain which emergency equipment when he returns from surgery?
○ 1. Suction equipment.
○ 2. Emergency cart.
○ 3. Airway.
○ 4. Tourniquet.

56. What would be the most important nursing intervention in caring for the client's residual limb during the first 24 hours after surgery?
○ 1. Keeping the residual limb flat on the bed.
○ 2. Abducting the residual limb on a scheduled basis.
○ 3. Applying traction to the residual limb.
○ 4. Elevating the residual limb on a pillow.

57. Which of the following nursing goals would take priority when planning for the client's physical mobility after amputation?
○ 1. Preventing contractures.
○ 2. Promoting comfort.
○ 3. Preventing edema.
○ 4. Preventing phantom-limb pain.

58. The second morning after surgery, the client says, "This sounds crazy, but I feel my left toes tingling." This statement would indicate to the nurse that he is experiencing a
○ 1. denial reaction.
○ 2. phantom-limb sensation.
○ 3. hallucination.
○ 4. body image disturbance.

59. The client is to be fitted with a functioning prosthesis. The nurse has been teaching him how to care for his residual limb. Which behavior would demonstrate that the client has an understanding of proper residual limb care? The client
○ 1. applies powder to the residual limb.
○ 2. inspects the residual limb weekly with a mirror.
○ 3. removes the prosthesis whenever he sits down.
○ 4. washes and dries the residual limb daily.

60. The client will use crutches while his prosthesis is being adjusted. Which of the following exercises would best prepare him for using crutches?
○ 1. Range-of-motion exercises of the shoulders.
○ 2. Isometric exercises of the shoulders.
○ 3. Quadriceps and gluteal setting exercises.
○ 4. Triceps exercises.

61. When using crutches, the client should be taught to support his weight primarily on his
○ 1. axillae.
○ 2. elbows.
○ 3. upper arms.
○ 4. hands.

62. The client is to be discharged on a low-fat, low-cholesterol, low-sodium diet. What would be the nurse's first step in planning the dietary instructions?
○ 1. Determine the client's knowledge level about cholesterol.
○ 2. Ask the client to name foods high in fat, cholesterol, and salt.
○ 3. Explain the importance of complying with the diet.
○ 4. Assess the family's food preferences.

63. The nurse has been instructing the client on how to prepare meals that are low in fat, cholesterol, and sodium. Which of these comments would indicate that he needs additional teaching?
○ 1. "I'll eat only water-packed tuna."
○ 2. "I'll use a Teflon-coated pan when cooking."
○ 3. "I'll eat more liver with onions."
○ 4. "I'll avoid using steak sauce and catsup."

The Client With a Femoral Fracture

A 28-year-old male construction worker is brought to the hospital emergency room after a fall from a beam. He has a fractured right femur and multiple cuts and bruises on his upper body and right arm and hand.

64. A booster injection for tetanus is administered in the emergency room after it is determined that the client has not had any immunizations since childhood. Which of the following biologic products would be used to provide the client with passive immunity for tetanus?

○ 1. Tetanus toxoid.
○ 2. Tetanus antigen.
○ 3. Tetanus vaccine.
○ 4. Tetanus antitoxin.

65. The client is admitted to the orthopedic unit in balanced skeletal traction using a Thomas splint and Pearson attachment. The primary purpose of traction in this case is to
○ 1. prevent neurologic damage.
○ 2. realign fracture fragments.
○ 3. control internal bleeding.
○ 4. maintain skin integrity.

66. The nurse is responsible for maintaining effective traction. Which of the following conditions is necessary for effective traction?
○ 1. The weights rest securely on the bed frame.
○ 2. The ropes are in the wheel grooves of the pulleys.
○ 3. The client is positioned low in the bed.
○ 4. The weights are increased by one-half pound each shift.

67. When a client is placed in balanced skeletal traction, which of the following nursing actions would be appropriate?
○ 1. Ensuring that the traction weights hang freely from the bed at all times.
○ 2. Gradually increasing the traction weight as the client's tolerance increases.
○ 3. Applying and removing the traction weights at regular intervals throughout the day.
○ 4. Removing the weights briefly as necessary to reposition the client in bed.

68. The purpose of the Pearson attachment on the traction setup is to
○ 1. support the lower portion of the leg.
○ 2. support the thigh and upper leg.
○ 3. attach the skeletal pin.
○ 4. prevent flexion deformities in the ankle and foot.

69. Because of the nature of his fracture, the client is at risk for fat emboli. Which of the following manifestations would the nurse most likely note if the client developed a fat embolus?
○ 1. Mental confusion.
○ 2. Migraine-like headaches.
○ 3. Numbness in the right leg.
○ 4. Muscle spasms in the right thigh.

70. Which of the following treatments would most likely be used to treat the client if fat emboli developed?
○ 1. Hypothermia.
○ 2. Supplemental oxygen.
○ 3. Intravenous heparin.
○ 4. Anticholesterol drugs.

71. The client is upset and agitated about his injury and its treatment. He says, "How can I stay like this for weeks? I can't even move!" Based on these data, the most likely nursing diagnosis would be

○ 1. Impaired Physical Mobility related to traction.
○ 2. Ineffective Individual Coping related to prolonged immobility.
○ 3. Diversional Activity Deficit related to prolonged hospitalization.
○ 4. Activity Intolerance related to impaired mobility.

72. The client asks the nurse what his activity limitations are while he is in traction. The nurse explains that while he is in traction, he
○ 1. can turn from side to side in bed and sit up.
○ 2. must lie flat in bed and cannot turn at all.
○ 3. can sit up straight in bed but cannot turn.
○ 4. can turn slightly from side to side and sit up at a 30- to 40-degree angle.

73. Because of the Thomas splint, the nurse would need to assess the client regularly for
○ 1. signs of skin pressure in the groin area.
○ 2. decreased breath sounds.
○ 3. skin breakdown behind the heel.
○ 4. urine retention.

74. The client has the nursing diagnosis Self-Care Deficit related to the confinement of traction. Which of the following would indicate a successful outcome for this diagnosis? The client
○ 1. assists as much as possible in his care, and his participation increases over time.
○ 2. allows the nurse to complete his care in an efficient manner and does not interfere.
○ 3. allows his wife to assume total responsibility for his care.
○ 4. allows his wife to complete his care because he knows she needs to feel useful.

75. To prevent infection and osteomyelitis, the nurse provides pin site care and inspects the site daily for evidence of infection. Which of the following clinical manifestations at the pin site would alert the nurse to infection?
○ 1. Slight serous oozing.
○ 2. Lack of scab formation.
○ 3. Itching.
○ 4. Pain.

76. The client has a nursing diagnosis of Constipation related to the decreased mobility imposed by traction. A care plan that incorporates which of the following breakfasts would be most helpful in reestablishing a normal bowel routine?
○ 1. Eggs and bacon, buttered toast, orange juice, and coffee.
○ 2. Corn flakes with sliced banana, milk, and English muffin and jelly.
○ 3. Orange juice, breakfast pastries (doughnut and danish), and coffee.
○ 4. An orange, raisin bran and milk, and wheat toast with butter.

The Client With a Spinal Cord Injury

The client, a 25-year-old woman, fell during a rock-climbing trip. She is alert and conscious but cannot move her arms or legs on command.

77. The priority concern when planning to move a person with a possible spinal cord injury is to
    ○ 1. wrap and support the extremities, which can be easily injured.
    ○ 2. move the person gently to help reduce pain.
    ○ 3. immobilize the head and neck to prevent further injury.
    ○ 4. cushion the back with pillows to ensure comfort.

78. It is determined that the client suffered a C7 spinal cord injury. Which of the following would be the most important nursing intervention during the acute stage of her care?
    ○ 1. Turning and repositioning every 2 hours.
    ○ 2. Maintaining proper alignment.
    ○ 3. Maintaining a patent airway.
    ○ 4. Monitoring vital signs.

79. The nurse recognizes that spinal shock is likely to persist for the first several weeks after the injury. Which of the following symptoms would be unexpected during the period of spinal shock?
    ○ 1. Tachycardia.
    ○ 2. Rapid respirations.
    ○ 3. Hypertension.
    ○ 4. Dry, warm skin.

80. During the period of spinal shock, the nurse should expect the client's bladder function to be
    ○ 1. spastic.
    ○ 2. normal.
    ○ 3. atonic.
    ○ 4. uncontrolled.

81. Passive range-of-motion exercises for the legs and assisted range-of-motion exercises for the arms are part of the client's care regimen. Which observation by the nurse would indicate a successful outcome of this treatment?
    ○ 1. Free, easy movement of the joints.
    ○ 2. Absence of paralytic footdrop.
    ○ 3. External rotation of the hips at rest.
    ○ 4. Absence of tissue ischemia over bony prominences.

82. The client's fracture is surgically repaired. Once healing has begun, daily physical therapy sessions are scheduled that include using a tilt table. After the therapist places the client at a 45-degree angle, the nurse should monitor her for which of the following?
    ○ 1. Hypertension.
    ○ 2. Pedal edema.

○ 3. Facial flushing.
○ 4. Dizziness.

83. After a month of therapy, the client begins to experience muscle spasms in her legs. She calls the nurse in excitement to report the leg movement. Which response by the nurse would be the most accurate?
    ○ 1. "These movements indicate that the damaged nerves are healing."
    ○ 2. "This is a good sign. Keep trying to move all the affected muscles."
    ○ 3. "The return of movement means that eventually you should be able to walk again. The damage is not permanent."
    ○ 4. "The movements occur from muscle reflexes. They can't be initiated or controlled by the brain."

84. The nurse realizes that the client is at risk for autonomic dysreflexia. Which of the following symptoms would indicate this condition?
    ○ 1. Sudden, severe hypertension.
    ○ 2. Bradycardia.
    ○ 3. Paralytic ileus.
    ○ 4. Hot, dry skin.

85. If autonomic dysreflexia occurs, what would be the priority nursing intervention?
    ○ 1. Administer nitroprusside sodium (Nipride) intravenously.
    ○ 2. Call the physician.
    ○ 3. Place the client in Fowler's position.
    ○ 4. Send a urine sample for culture.

86. The nurse assesses the client to determine the cause of the autonomic dysreflexia. The nurse would prioritize assessment based on the knowledge that the most common stimulus for an autonomic dysreflexia episode is
    ○ 1. bowel distention.
    ○ 2. bladder distention.
    ○ 3. anxiety.
    ○ 4. rising intracranial pressure.

87. The orthotics department makes a custom trunk brace for the client. The nurse would plan to apply this brace at which time?
    ○ 1. While the client is sitting in a chair.
    ○ 2. Before the client gets out of bed.
    ○ 3. As soon as the client becomes fatigued.
    ○ 4. When the client is standing on the tilt table.

88. Urinary tract infection is a serious problem after spinal cord injury. Which of the following would be the most important measure to prevent this?
    ○ 1. Drink a glass of citrus fruit juice at every meal.
    ○ 2. Drink at least 2000 mL of fluid daily.
    ○ 3. Add extra protein to the daily diet.
    ○ 4. Ensure that the urine remains alkaline.

89. The client asks the nurse why the dietitian has recommended that she decrease her total daily intake

of calcium. Which of the following responses by the nurse would provide the most accurate information?
- ○ 1. "Excessive intake of dairy products makes constipation more common."
- ○ 2. "Immobility increases calcium absorption from the intestine."
- ○ 3. "Lack of weight-bearing causes demineralization of the long bones and increases the kidneys' calcium load."
- ○ 4. "Dairy products likely will contribute to weight gain."

90. As a first step in teaching the client about her sexual health, the nurse assesses her understanding of the sexual functioning of a quadriplegic. Which of the following statements by the client would indicate good understanding?
- ○ 1. "I won't be able to have sexual intercourse until the Foley catheter is removed."
- ○ 2. "I can participate in sexual activity but might not experience orgasm."
- ○ 3. "I won't be able to have sexual intercourse because it causes hypertension, but other sexual activity is allowed."
- ○ 4. "I'll be able to participate in sexual activity but will be infertile."

91. The client had been active in sports and outdoor activities, and she talks almost obsessively about her past activities. In tears, one day she asks the nurse, "Why can't I stop talking about these things? I know those days are gone forever." Which response by the nurse would convey the best understanding of the client's behavior?
- ○ 1. "Be patient. It takes time to adjust to such a massive loss."
- ○ 2. "Talking about the past is a form of denial. We have to help you focus on today."
- ○ 3. "Reviewing your losses is a way of working through your grief. Someday soon you'll be able to let go."
- ○ 4. "It's a simple escape mechanism to go back and live again in happier times."

CORRECT ANSWERS AND RATIONALE

The letters in parentheses following the rationale identify the step of the nursing process (A, D, P, I, E), cognitive level (K, C, T, N), and client needs (S, G, L, H). See the Answer Grid for the key.

The Client With Rheumatoid Arthritis

1. 3. Synovial joints are characteristically affected by rheumatoid arthritis. Rheumatoid arthritis is an inflammatory disorder that most commonly affects middle-aged women. Osteoarthritis is a degenerative joint disease that affects weight-bearing joints and is associated with aging. (I, K, G)

2. 2. Tinnitus (ringing in the ears) is a common symptom of aspirin toxicity. Dysuria, drowsiness, and chest pain are not associated with aspirin toxicity. (A, K, G)

3. 4. Aspirin therapy in rheumatoid arthritis involves continuous ongoing administration to establish and maintain therapeutic blood levels. Aspirin should not be used on a p.r.n. basis. It should always be buffered with food, and clients should be instructed to observe for symptoms of bleeding. (E, T, H)

4. 1. Activity Intolerance related to fatigue and pain is a common problem of clients with rheumatoid arthritis. The goal of nursing care is to help clients conserve their energy and to decrease episodes of fatigue. (D, N, H)

5. 2. The client with rheumatoid arthritis should be encouraged to alternate periods of activity and rest throughout the day. Neither encouraging the client to perform all activities of daily living at once nor encouraging her to cease all participation in daily activities will increase activity tolerance; instead, these actions may further decrease activity tolerance. Narcotics are not typically administered to control arthritic pain. (I, N, G)

6. 4. When a client compares her therapy with someone else's, it is best for the nurse to explain truthfully that there are various forms of arthritis and arthritis treatment. What helps one person may not help another. Avoiding the question or suggesting that the client should not ask a particular question is nontherapeutic. (I, N, L)

7. 4. Proper positioning to prevent flexion deformities of the joints is an ongoing need for clients with rheumatoid arthritis and should be included in the postoperative care plan. Positioning to promote comfort and avoid venous stasis is important but not unique to clients with rheumatoid arthritis. (P, T, S)

8. 3. Usual postoperative activity orders for a client with a total knee replacement include transferring the client out of bed to a chair on the first postoperative day. The affected leg is protected with a knee immobilizer and elevated while the client is up in the chair. Activity progresses to partial weight-bearing with the use of assistive devices. (P, T, G)

9. 3. The nurse must frequently evaluate the positioning of the client's leg, the range-of-motion setting, and the client's response to the therapy. Using a CPM machine will likely produce initial discomfort for the client. If the client cannot tolerate the discomfort, the physician should be notified for an order to adjust the settings. The settings for the machine are determined by the physician and cannot be changed without an order. Therapy will continue until the client regains 90-degree flexion in the knee. (I, T, S)

10. 2. An exercise program is recommended to strengthen muscles after arthroplasty. Isometric (or muscle-setting) exercises strengthen muscles but keep the joint stationary during the healing process. Isometric exercise costs little in terms of time and money, and may help improve a client's morale by promoting self-care, but these are not necessarily primary reasons for using it. Isometric exercise will not help prevent joint stiffness; the joint is kept stationary. (I, N, G)

11. 3. The quadriceps-setting exercises strengthen the quadriceps femoris, leg muscles important for proper walking. These muscles can be exercised in bed by pushing the back of the knee into the mattress. (E, T, S)

12. 4. Superficial heat applications such as tub baths, showers, and warm compresses can be helpful in relieving pain and stiffness. Exercises can be performed more comfortably and more effectively after heat applications. (I, T, S)

13. 2. Depending on the degree of joint involvement, clients with rheumatoid arthritis may need to learn to function with adaptive equipment. Such equipment can help the client maintain independence with the activities of daily living. The client needs to understand that rheumatoid arthritis cannot be cured and that the consistent use of antiinflammatory drugs is considered important to minimize joint inflammation and damage. Periods of activity should be alternated with rest periods, but limiting activity to avoid joint pain is not a realistic or desirable outcome. (E, T, H)

The Client With Osteoarthritis

14. 3. Osteoarthritis most commonly results from "wear and tear"—excessive and prolonged mechanical stress on the joints. Increased weight increases stress on weight-bearing joints. Therefore, an obese client with osteoarthritis should be encouraged to lose weight. (A, C, G)

15. 4. Orthotic devices such as braces or splints may be used to provide support to affected joints. Isometric exercises are used to strengthen muscles. Opioid analgesics are not used for osteoarthritic pain control. Acetaminophen and selected nonsteroidal anti-inflammatory drugs may be used to achieve pain relief. Intraarticular corticosteroid injections are not used routinely, but instead are cautiously used during periods of acute joint pain. (P, T, H)

16. 3. Drugs that cause gastric irritation are best taken after or with a meal, when stomach contents help minimize the local irritation. (I, T, H)

17. 4. All of the information provided is important. Before implementing a teaching plan, however, the nurse should determine the client's level of understanding about the procedure. Only then can the nurse develop an individualized teaching plan designed to meet the needs of this client. (A, N, L)

18. 3. After a total hip replacement, it is important to maintain the hip in a state of abduction to prevent dislocation of the prosthesis. Use of an abduction pillow or splint will not prevent hip flexion or the formation of sacral decubitus ulcers, and it will not increase peripheral circulation. (P, T, S)

19. 4. Classic signs of dislocation of the hip prosthesis include increasing pain, abnormal rotation, shortened leg, difficulty or inability moving the leg, and misalignment of the leg. The nurse should notify the surgeon so that the prosthesis can be repositioned. (D, N, G)

20. 2. Acute flexion and adduction of the hip should be avoided after hip replacement surgery. The client may need assistance with putting on socks and shoes and should avoid sitting in low chairs and crossing his legs. Stair climbing is typically avoided for about 3 months after surgery. Frequent walks are encouraged to increase muscle strength and provide hip exercises. (E, T, H)

The Client With a Hip Fracture

21. 4. After a hip fracture, the leg on the affected side is characteristically shorter than the unaffected leg. Typically, it is also abducted and rotated externally. Pain is usually present. (A, T, G)

22. 4. Using a pin for the internal fixation of a fractured hip has various advantages. This procedure is especially favored for older clients because it enables earlier postoperative ambulation and provides good fixation at the fracture site. (P, N, G)

23. 3. The primary reason for applying suction to a wound drainage tube is to prevent fluid from accumulating in the wound. This greatly enhances wound healing and helps prevent abscess formation. (P, C, S)

24. 3. Nerve damage may be indicated by the presence of any of the "five Ps": pain, pallor, pulselessness, paresthesia, and paralysis. Bleeding does not indicate peripheral nerve damage. Peripheral nerve damage can occur after almost any orthopedic surgery. (E, N, G)

25. 1. It is best to support the client's leg in its proper anatomic position and to prevent external rotation by supporting the leg with sandbags. A trochanter roll can also be used. Sandbags should be placed along the length of the thigh and lower leg. Neither a footboard, a rubber air ring, nor a metal-frame bed cradle will help prevent external rotation of the leg. (P, T, S)

26. 3. Wound infection can best be prevented by using strict sterile technique during dressing changes. Accurately measuring drainage and monitoring the incision for signs of infection are important nursing actions but will not prevent a wound infection. Inserting a Foley catheter is an unnecessary action in this case and would predispose the client to a urinary tract infection. (I, N, G)

27. 3. After hip surgery for a fractured femur, the client should be positioned on the nonoperative side with pillows or an abductor splint between the legs to help prevent adduction of the operative leg. This positioning places the hip in proper alignment. Dislocation of the hip can occur if the leg on the affected side is allowed to adduct. (I, C, S)

28. 3. A high-backed straight chair with armrests is recommended to help keep the client in the best possible alignment after surgery for a hip fracture. Soft, low, and swivel chairs do not promote good body alignment or good security. (I, N, H)

29. 1. Leg crossing causes adduction of the hips; after hip surgery, this may result in a dislocation of the operated hip. This client should not cross her legs. Elevating the legs, flexing the ankles, and extending the knees are not necessarily contraindicated. (I, T, H)

30. 3. Some elderly people are not good candidates for crutch walking because they are not strong enough to use crutches or are not coordinated enough to walk safely with crutches. Such factors as visual acuity, reaction time, and level of comprehension may influence the ability to learn crutch walking but are not as important as motor coordination. (A, T, S)

31. 2. A client being prepared for crutch walking should be taught to support her weight with her hands when crutch walking. Supporting weight in the axillae is contraindicated owing to the risk of possible nerve damage and circulatory obstruction. The client should be taught to squeeze a ball vigorously to help strengthen her hands in preparation for weight-bearing with the hands. Such activities as brushing the hair, flexing and extending the wrists, and doing pushups may be indicated, but they are not likely to strengthen the hands. (P, C, S)

32. 2. Scatter rugs are the single greatest hazard in the home, especially for elderly people who are unsure of walking. Falls have been found to account for nearly half the accidental deaths that occur in the home. (A, N, S)

The Client With a Herniated Disk

33. 3. A typical symptom of a herniated lumbar disk is low back pain that is usually relieved by rest and aggravated by activity that causes an increase in fluid pressure in the spine, such as sneezing, coughing, lifting, and bending. Muscle weakness and sensory losses may occur, and there is generally a change in tendon reflexes. Pain radiating to the shoulders, which often mimics some symptoms of a heart attack, is a typical symptom of cervical disk herniation. Loss of voluntary muscle control, which may cause chorea-like movements, and loss of urinary control are not typically early symptoms of lumbar disk problems. (A, C, G)

34. 3. This client will be most comfortable in the semi-Fowler's position. Hyperextension of the spine causes discomfort for a client with a herniated disk; thus, the prone position is contraindicated for this client. (I, T, G)

35. 4. A radiopaque dye (usually an iodized oil, but in some instances a water-soluble compound) is used for a myelogram. Air may be used for an air-contrast study. Myelography is used to determine the exact location of a herniated disk. (I, K, G)

36. 4. Nursing care of the client after a myelogram depends in part on the type of dye used. For example, if an oil contrast such as Pantopaque was used, the client will usually lie flat for 8 to 12 hours. If a water-soluble contrast was used, the head of the bed is elevated 45 degrees for 8 to 24 hours. This position reduces the rate of upward dispersion of the contrast medium. Regardless of the type of dye used for the test, bed rest is required for several hours after a myelogram. Fluid intake is encouraged to replace cerebrospinal fluid, to reduce headache, and to facilitate absorption of retained contrast media. Neuro-

logic status in the lower extremities is assessed frequently, as is the client's ability to void. (I, N, G)

37. 1. Muscle relaxants and nonsteroidal anti-inflammatory drugs are frequently prescribed for the conservative management of herniated lumbar disks. In addition, the client may receive oral analgesics. Sedatives, tranquilizers, and parenteral analgesics are not typically used in the conservative treatment of herniated lumbar disks. (P, C, G)

38. 1. Postoperative back pain related to the surgical incision and muscle spasms is common after laminectomy. The client may avoid movement to prevent pain if nursing measures are not implemented to control pain. Depending on the activity order, the client may be turned to his side or have the head of the bed elevated for meals. Constipation is more likely to be a problem postoperatively owing to inactivity. Surgical laminectomy scars are small and typically do not cause fear of disfigurement. (D, N, G)

39. 2. Trimethobenzamide hydrochloride is a centrally acting antiemetic that helps control nausea and vomiting. It does not control muscle spasms, shivering, or dry mouth. (E, C, G)

40. 4. After a laminectomy, the client's spine must be maintained in proper alignment. The client who had a laminectomy may be turned to his side by logrolling him in one unit while keeping his back straight. It takes at least two people to perform this procedure correctly. Having the client turn himself, or moving his shoulders and hips separately, does not allow the back to remain in straight alignment. (I, N, S)

41. 2. A back brace should be applied before the client who has had back surgery is out of bed and placing weight on the legs and back. The brace is placed on the bed while the client assumes a side-lying position. The client is then rolled onto the brace. Hyperextension of the back after back surgery is contraindicated. (I, T, S)

42. 2. Having the client wear a thin cotton shirt under a brace helps to protect the skin and to keep the brace free of skin oils and perspiration. Using padding may increase pressure points. Lubricating and powdering the skin under the brace do not provide the best protection from irritation by the brace. (I, N, S)

43. 3. A client who feels faint while walking with the nurse should rest on the nurse's hip. This maneuver is relatively easy and can be maintained until help is available. Having the client close his eyes is unlikely to relieve symptoms of fainting. Maneuvering the client to the floor requires considerable strength and may injure the client, especially when done quickly. This client should not bend at the waist because of his recent back surgery. (I, N, S)

44. 1. A client who has had back surgery should place the feet flat on the floor. This ordinarily provides the greatest comfort because it places no strain on the operative area. (E, N, G)

45. 4. After a laminectomy, a client should either lie flat in bed in good alignment or should walk. Sitting for long periods is contraindicated because pressure is increased to the operative area and alignment is compromised. (I, T, G)

46. 3. Prolonged sitting and standing should be avoided. When sitting, the client should choose a chair with good support and a straight back. The client should sit with feet flat on the floor. Pushing objects rather than pulling them will help decrease back strain. Clients should select a semi-firm to firm mattress to provide back support. (I, T, H)

The Client With Peripheral Vascular Disease Having an Amputation

47. 1. Inadequate arterial circulation produces symptoms of hypoxia. The skin is cool to the touch, pulses are difficult or impossible to palpate, and exercise causes moderate to severe cramping pain. Ankle edema is associated with venous insufficiency and stasis. (A, C, G)

48. 4. The dorsalis pedis pulse is found on the medial aspect of the dorsal surface of the foot in line with the big toe. The posterior tibial pulse is on the medial surface of the ankle just behind the medial malleolus. The popliteal pulse is behind the knee. (A, K, S)

49. 3. The data obtained by the nurse are major defining characteristics for the nursing diagnosis Altered Peripheral Tissue Perfusion. The data do not indicate that the client's skin integrity or physical mobility has been impaired at this time. The diagnosis Impaired Gas Exchange is used to describe clients with respiratory insufficiency. (D, N, G)

50. 2. Slow, steady walking is a recommended activity for clients with peripheral arterial disease because it stimulates the development of collateral circulation. The client with peripheral arterial disease should not remain inactive. Elevating the legs above the heart and wearing antiembolism stockings are strategies for venous congestion and may worsen peripheral arterial disease. (E, T, G)

51. 4. Coldness is the assessment finding most consistent with complete arterial obstruction. Other expected findings would include paralysis and pallor. Aching pain, burning sensations, and numbness and tingling are earlier signs of tissue hypoxia and ischemia and are associated with incomplete obstruction. (A, C, G)

52. 2. Encouraging the client undergoing amputation to verbalize feelings is the most therapeutic nursing intervention. By eliciting information, the nurse may be able to provide information to help the client cope. The nurse should avoid value-laden responses that may make the client feel guilty or hostile and block further communication. The nurse should not ignore the client's expressed concerns. The nurse should not reinforce the client's concern about invalidism and dependency or assume that his wife is willing to care for him. (I, T, L)

53. 2. The level of amputation often cannot be accurately determined until surgery, when the surgeon can directly assess the adequacy of the circulation of the residual limb. A longer residual limb facilitates prosthesis-fitting, and this aspect will be considered in the final decision, but it is not the primary factor. (P, C, G)

54. 2. The nurse should mark the blood stain and observe it again in 10 minutes. There is no need to notify the physician immediately because some oozing and bloody drainage are expected. Given the slight amount of drainage, there is no need either to replace the dressing or reinforce it. (I, N, S)

55. 4. Hemorrhage is an unexpected, but possible, complication of radical surgery such as amputation. A tourniquet should be available at the bedside during the early postoperative period to deal with such a complication. (P, K, S)

56. 4. Elevating the residual limb on a pillow for the first 24 hours after surgery helps prevent edema and promotes comfort by increasing venous return. Elevating the residual limb for longer than the first 24 hours is contraindicated because of the potential for developing contractures. Adducting the residual limb on a scheduled basis prevents abduction contracture. (I, N, G)

57. 1. Preventing joint contractures is essential to physical mobility. Promoting comfort and preventing edema are appropriate immediate postoperative nursing goals, but attaining them does not affect physical mobility in the immediate and extended postoperative periods. Phantom-limb pain begins 2 weeks to 2 months after amputation. It occurs briefly in about 30% of clients, but only about 2% experience persistent pain. (P, T, G)

58. 2. Descriptions of sensations, painful and otherwise, in the amputated part are common and are known as *phantom-limb sensations*. The client should be reassured that these sensations are normal and are not a sign of a mental problem. Denial may be present after amputation; signs include refusal to look at or talk about the amputation. Hallucinations indicate a serious, possibly psychotic condition and should be thoroughly assessed. Referral to an appropriate health care provider is in order. Body image disturbances can develop after amputation due to fear, grief, loss of locomotion, and decreased self-esteem related to the loss of the body part. (D, K, G)

59. 4. Washing and thoroughly drying the residual limb daily are important hygiene measures to prevent infection. Nothing should be applied to the residual limb after it is cleansed. Powder may cause excessive drying and cracking of the skin, and cream may soften the skin excessively. The residual limb should be inspected daily with a mirror for early signs of skin breakdown. To reduce residual limb swelling, the prosthesis should be removed only at night. (E, T, G)

60. 4. Using crutches requires significant strength from the triceps muscles, and efforts should be focused on strengthening these muscles in anticipation of crutch walking. Bed and wheelchair pushups are excellent exercises targeted at the triceps muscles. (I, N, G)

61. 4. Using crutches properly requires supporting body weight primarily on the hands. Using crutches improperly can cause nerve damage from excess pressure. Careful instruction and evaluation of crutch use is essential. (I, K, S)

62. 4. Before beginning dietary interventions, the nurse must assess the client's pattern of food intake, life cycle, food preferences, and ethnic, cultural, and financial influences. (P, N, H)

63. 3. Liver and organ meats are high in cholesterol and saturated fat and should be limited. Water-packed tuna is one of the leanest fish available. Using a Teflon-coated pan when cooking reduces the need for shortening. Steak sauce and catsup are high in sodium. (E, N, G)

The Client With a Femoral Fracture

64. 4. Passive immunity for tetanus is provided in the form of tetanus antitoxin or tetanus immune globulin. An antitoxin is an antibody to the toxin of an organism. Toxoids, antigens, and vaccines all provide active immunity by stimulating the body to produce its own antibodies. (I, K, G)

65. 2. Traction promotes realignment of the bone fragments. This will facilitate subsequent internal fixation. Traction immobilizes the fracture site and may increase the client's comfort. Mobilization could result in further damage. Traction increases circulation to the affected part but does not control internal bleeding. Traction may create, rather than prevent, a problem with skin integrity. (P, K, G)

66. 2. For the weights to maintain the therapeutic effect of the traction, they must be properly positioned and free hanging and should be removed only in

life-threatening situations. Effective traction depends on the client being positioned at the head of the bed. Sufficient weight is applied initially to overcome spasm in affected muscles. As the muscles relax, the weight may be reduced. (I, T, S)

67. 1. In balanced skeletal traction, the appropriate pressures and counterpressures are applied to the fracture site, with the traction weights hanging freely at all times. These weights are in place continuously and should never be lifted, reduced, or eliminated. Skin traction may be applied intermittently, but balanced skeletal traction is continuous. (I, T, S)

68. 1. The Pearson attachment supports the lower leg and provides increased stability in the overall traction setup. It also makes it easier to maintain correct alignment. (P, C, G)

69. 1. Fat emboli usually result in cerebral disturbances that cause mental confusion or agitation from hypoxia. If severe, hypoxia can produce delirium and coma. (A, C, G)

70. 2. Respiratory failure is a common cause of death after fat emboli. Respiratory support is provided by administering high concentrations of oxygen. Oxygen therapy appears to reduce the surface tension of the fat globules and supports respiratory function by reducing hypoxia. The rest of the treatments are not appropriate for fat emboli. (P, C, G)

71. 2. Although all the nursing diagnoses listed may be appropriate for this client, the diagnosis of Ineffective Individual Coping is the most appropriate given the data provided. The nurse should seek ways to help the client adjust to and cope with his present state of immobility. Emphasis should be placed on what the client can do to care for himself. Encouraging the client to participate in his daily care and to continue exercises to maintain muscle strength are important activities that will help him maintain some control over his situation. (D, N, L)

72. 1. Although normal movement is not possible in skeletal traction, the balanced weights ensure that changes in position do not alter or interfere with the traction pull. Therefore, a client can turn and sit up in bed while the traction is in place. (I, T, L)

73. 1. The Thomas splint is secured by rings that slip over the thigh. They are placed tight up into the groin and may cause discomfort, pressure, or skin irritation. (A, T, S)

74. 1. Self-care minimizes sensory deprivation and allows the client to gain a sense of control. Passivity can indicate denial or depression. Family members can assist, but giving them primary responsibility undermines the client's self-esteem. (E, N, H)

75. 4. Inflammation, evidenced by pain, swelling, and redness, is one of the early signs of infection and needs prompt intervention. Slight oozing at the pin site is expected and decreases bacteria in the pin tract. Crusting or scab formation should be prevented because it may trap bacteria in the pin tract. Itching at the pin site may be due to dryness or irritation. (A, C, G)

76. 4. High-fiber foods provide bulk and decrease water absorption in the bowel. Whole grains and fruits (not juices, which often are strained) are recommended. Processed foods and breads contain little fiber. (P, T, G)

The Client With a Spinal Cord Injury

77. 3. The immediate concern is to immobilize the head and neck to prevent further trauma when the fractured vertebra may be unstable and easily displaced. Pain is usually not a significant consideration with this type of injury. (P, N, S)

78. 3. Initial care is focused on establishing and maintaining a patent airway and supporting ventilation. Innervation to the intercostal muscles is affected; if spinal edema extends to the C4 level, paralysis of the diaphragm usually occurs. The effects and extent of edema are unpredictable in the first hours, and respiratory status must be closely monitored. Suction equipment should be readily available. (I, N, G)

79. 3. Spinal shock produces massive vasodilation and subsequent pooling of blood in the peripheral circulation. The client is relatively hypovolemic and exhibits tachycardia, tachypnea, anxiety, and flushed but dry skin. Hypertension would not be expected. (A, C, G)

80. 3. During the period of spinal shock, the bladder is completely atonic and will continue to fill passively unless the client is catheterized. No reflex activity occurs during this period, so reflex emptying does not occur. (P, C, G)

81. 1. Range-of-motion exercises help preserve joint motion and stimulate circulation. Contractures develop rapidly in clients with spinal cord injuries, and the absence of this complication indicates treatment success. External rotation of the hips is prevented by using trochanter rolls. Local ischemia over bony prominences is prevented by following a regular turning schedule. (E, T, G)

82. 4. Lack of vasomotor tone in the lower extremities causes venous pooling, and the client may become hypotensive and dizzy when positioned upright. The tilt table is used to help the client overcome vasomotor instability and tolerate an upright position. Some pedal edema could occur, but it would develop gradually and would be less problematic than the hypotension. Elastic stockings are sometimes used to facilitate venous return from the legs. Signs and symptoms of insufficient cerebral circulation are pallor, diaphoresis, tachycardia, and nausea. (A, T, G)

83. 4. After the period of spinal shock, the muscles gradually become spastic owing to an increased sensitivity of the lower motor neurons. The movement is not voluntary and cannot be brought under voluntary control. It is expected, but does not indicate that healing is taking place. (I, C, G)

84. 1. With a cervical injury, the client has sympathetic fibers that can be stimulated to fire reflexively. The firing is cut off from brain control and is both reflexive and massive. It classically produces pounding headache and dangerously elevated blood pressure, "goose bumps," and profuse sweating. Hot and dry skin, bradycardia, and paralytic ileus typically occur during spinal shock, not during autonomic dysreflexia. (A, C, G)

85. 3. Autonomic dysreflexia is a medical emergency. Although notifying the physician is important, it is more essential that the nurse intervene immediately in the situation. The rising blood pressure can cause cerebrovascular accident, blindness, or even death. Placing the client in Fowler's position lowers blood pressure. Administering nitroprusside sodium intravenously is appropriate if the conservative measures are ineffective. A urine sample for culture should be obtained if the client has an elevated temperature and no other cause for the dysreflexia is found. A urinary tract infection may be causing symptoms. (I, N, G)

86. 2. The dysreflexia occurs from a sympathetic response to autonomic nervous system stimulation. A distended bladder is the most common cause; bowel fullness may also trigger the syndrome. After placing the client in Fowler's position, the nurse should check the Foley catheter for patency and the rectum for fecal impaction. (A, T, G)

87. 2. Braces are designed to be applied while the client is lying down. They are custom-designed to fit contours of the chest and buttocks and may not fit properly if applied with the client in other positions. A poor fit could result in pressure areas or inadequate support. (P, C, S)

88. 2. As soon as the client's vasomotor status stabilizes, it is essential that she drink at least 2000 mL of fluid daily, unless contraindicated. Increased fluid intake helps flush out bacteria and prevents urinary stasis. Ingesting an acid-ash diet forms acid urine, which helps prevent urinary tract infection. Most citrus fruits are not metabolized as acids in the body. (I, N, H)

89. 3. Long-bone demineralization is a serious consequence of the loss of weight-bearing. An excessive calcium load is brought to the kidneys, and precipitation may occur, predisposing to stone formation. Absorption is not altered. (I, K, G)

90. 2. There are no contraindications to sexual activity in a woman with spinal cord injury, although she may not be able to experience orgasm. A Foley catheter may be left in place during intercourse in both male and female clients. Because a spinal cord injury does not affect fertility, the client should have access to family planning information so that an unplanned pregnancy can be avoided. (E, T, G)

91. 3. Spinal cord injury represents a physical loss; grief is the normal response to this loss. Working through grief entails reviewing memories and eventually letting go of them. The process may take as long as 2 years. (I, N, L)

NURSING CARE OF ADULTS WITH MEDICAL AND SURGICAL HEALTH PROBLEMS

TEST 10: The Client With Musculoskeletal Health Problems

Directions: Use this answer grid to determine areas of strength or need for further study.

NURSING PROCESS

A = Assessment
D = Analysis, nursing diagnosis
P = Planning
I = Implementation
E = Evaluation

COGNITIVE LEVEL

K = Knowledge
C = Comprehension
T = Application
N = Analysis

CLIENT NEEDS

S = Safe, effective care environment
G = Physiologic integrity
L = Psychosocial integrity
H = Health promotion and maintenance

Question #	Answer #	Nursing Process					Cognitive Level				Client Needs			
		A	D	P	I	E	K	C	T	N	S	G	L	H
1	3				I		K					G		
2	2	A					K					G		
3	4					E			T					H
4	1		D							N				H
5	2				I					N		G		
6	4				I					N			L	
7	4			P					T		S			
8	3			P					T			G		
9	3				I				T		S			
10	2				I					N		G		
11	3					E			T		S			
12	4				I				T		S			
13	2					E			T					H
14	3	A						C				G		
15	4			P					T					H
16	3				I				T					H
17	4	A								N			L	
18	3			P					T		S			
19	4		D							N		G		
20	2					E			T					H
21	4	A							T			G		
22	4			P						N		G		
23	3			P				C			S			
24	3					E				N		G		
25	1			P					T		S			

NURSING PROCESS

A = Assessment
D = Analysis, nursing diagnosis
P = Planning
I = Implementation
E = Evaluation

COGNITIVE LEVEL

K = Knowledge
C = Comprehension
T = Application
N = Analysis

CLIENT NEEDS

S = Safe, effective care environment
G = Physiologic integrity
L = Psychosocial integrity
H = Health promotion and maintenance

Question #	Answer #	A	D	P	I	E	K	C	T	N	S	G	L	H
26	3				I					N		G		
27	3				I			C			S			
28	3				I					N				H
29	1				I				T					H
30	3	A							T		S			
31	2			P				C			S			
32	2	A								N	S			
33	3	A						C				G		
34	3				I				T			G		
35	4				I		K					G		
36	4				I					N		G		
37	1			P				C				G		
38	1		D							N		G		
39	2					E		C				G		
40	4				I					N	S			
41	2				I				T		S			
42	2				I					N	S			
43	3				I					N	S			
44	1					E				N		G		
45	4				I				T			G		
46	3				I				T					H
47	1	A						C				G		
48	4	A					K				S			
49	3		D							N		G		
50	2					E			T			G		
51	4	A						C				G		
52	2				I				T				L	
53	2			P				C				G		
54	2				I					N	S			
55	4			P			K				S			

ANSWER GRID: 2

NURSING PROCESS

A = Assessment
D = Analysis, nursing diagnosis
P = Planning
I = Implementation
E = Evaluation

COGNITIVE LEVEL

K = Knowledge
C = Comprehension
T = Application
N = Analysis

CLIENT NEEDS

S = Safe, effective care environment
G = Physiologic integrity
L = Psychosocial integrity
H = Health promotion and maintenance

Question #	Answer #	Nursing Process					Cognitive Level				Client Needs			
		A	D	P	I	E	K	C	T	N	S	G	L	H
56	4				I					N		G		
57	1			P					T			G		
58	2		D				K					G		
59	4					E			T			G		
60	4				I					N		G		
61	4				I		K				S			
62	4			P						N				H
63	3					E				N		G		
64	4				I		K					G		
65	2			P			K					G		
66	2				I				T		S			
67	1				I				T		S			
68	1			P				C				G		
69	1	A						C				G		
70	2			P				C				G		
71	2		D							N			L	
72	1				I				T				L	
73	1	A							T		S			
74	1					E				N				H
75	4	A						C				G		
76	4			P					T			G		
77	3			P						N	S			
78	3				I					N		G		
79	3	A						C				G		
80	3			P				C				G		
81	1					E			T			G		
82	4	A							T			G		
83	4				I			C				G		
84	1	A						C				G		
85	3				I					N		G		

NURSING PROCESS

A = Assessment
D = Analysis, nursing diagnosis
P = Planning
I = Implementation
E = Evaluation

COGNITIVE LEVEL

K = Knowledge
C = Comprehension
T = Application
N = Analysis

CLIENT NEEDS

S = Safe, effective care environment
G = Physiologic integrity
L = Psychosocial integrity
H = Health promotion and maintenance

Question #	Answer #	Nursing Process					Cognitive Level				Client Needs			
		A	**D**	**P**	**I**	**E**	**K**	**C**	**T**	**N**	**S**	**G**	**L**	**H**
86	2	A							T			G		
87	2			P				C			S			
88	2				I					N				H
89	3				I		K					G		
90	2					E			T			G		
91	3				I					N			L	
Number Correct														
Number Possible	91	17	6	20	35	13	10	19	32	30	24	49	6	12
Percentage Correct														

Score Calculation: To determine your **Percentage Correct,** divide the **Number Correct** by the **Number Possible.**

ANSWER GRID: 4

The Client With Sensory Health Problems

- **The Client With Cataracts**
- **The Client With a Retinal Detachment**
- **The Client With Glaucoma**
- **The Client Undergoing Nasal Surgery**
- **The Client With a Hearing Disorder**
- **The Client With Meniere's Disease**
- **The Client With Cancer of the Larynx**
- **The Client With Burns**
- **Correct Answers and Rationale**

Select the one best answer, and indicate your choice by filling in the circle in front of the option.

The Client With Cataracts

A client is admitted to outpatient surgery for a cataract extraction on the right eye. The procedure is to be done under a local anesthetic.

1. The client asks the nurse, "What causes cataracts in old people?" Which of the following statements should form the basis for the nurse's response? Cataracts most commonly
   - ○ 1. result from chronic systemic disease.
   - ○ 2. are a result of aging.
   - ○ 3. result from eye injuries sustained early in life.
   - ○ 4. result from the prolonged use of toxic substances.

2. The client asks, "What does the lens of my eye do?" The nurse should explain that the lens of the eye
   - ○ 1. produces aqueous humor.
   - ○ 2. holds the rods and cones.
   - ○ 3. focuses light rays onto the retina.
   - ○ 4. regulates the amount of light entering the eye.

3. The client tells the nurse that she is afraid of being awake during eye surgery. Which of the following responses by the nurse would be the most appropriate?
   - ○ 1. "Have you ever had any reactions to local anesthetics in the past?"

   - ○ 2. "What is it that disturbs you about the idea of being awake?"
   - ○ 3. "By using a local anesthetic, you won't have nausea and vomiting after the surgery."
   - ○ 4. "There's really nothing to fear about being awake. You'll be given a medication that will help you relax."

4. A client with a cataract would most likely complain of which symptoms?
   - ○ 1. Halos and rainbows around lights.
   - ○ 2. Eye pain and irritation that worsens at night.
   - ○ 3. Blurred and hazy vision.
   - ○ 4. Eye strain and headache when doing close work.

5. Before cataract surgery, the nurse is to instill several types of eye drops into a client's right eye. The accepted abbreviation for the right eye is
   - ○ 1. OD.
   - ○ 2. OS.
   - ○ 3. OU.
   - ○ 4. RE.

6. The nurse is to instill drops of phenylephrine hydrochloride (Neo-Synephrine) into a client's right eye before cataract removal surgery. This preparation acts in the eye to produce
   - ○ 1. dilation of the pupil and blood vessels.
   - ○ 2. dilation of the pupil and constriction of blood vessels.
   - ○ 3. constriction of the pupil and constriction of blood vessels.

    4. constriction of the pupil and dilation of blood vessels.

7. A short time after surgery, the client complains of nausea. The nurse's best course of action would be to

    1. instruct the client to take a few deep breaths until the nausea subsides.
    2. explain that this is a common feeling that will pass quickly.
    3. tell the client to call the nurse promptly if vomiting occurs.
    4. medicate the client with an antiemetic, as ordered.

8. Which of the following statements indicates the client has understood the instructions to follow at home after cataract surgery?

    1. "I may not watch television for 3 weeks."
    2. "I should keep my protective eye shield in place at all times."
    3. "I should not bend over to pick up objects from the floor."
    4. "I can lift what I want."

9. An essential aspect of the plan of care for the client after cataract removal surgery would be to

    1. increase cardiac output.
    2. prevent fluid volume excess.
    3. maintain a darkened environment.
    4. promote safety at home.

10. The client is discharged home on the day of surgery. Which of the following potential nursing diagnoses would be most appropriate for the client at this time?

    1. Diversional Activity Deficit related to activity limitations after surgery.
    2. Chronic Pain related to postoperative incisional discomfort.
    3. High Risk for Injury related to limited vision after surgery.
    4. Self-Feeding Deficit related to inability to visualize food.

11. What information about vision would be most important for the nurse to include in the client's discharge plan?

    1. The client will need to wear corrective glasses or contact lenses.
    2. The client will need to wear glasses only until the eye heals.
    3. Cataract glasses correct vision by magnifying objects.
    4. The client will need to relearn to judge distances accurately.

12. After returning home, the client will need to continue to instill eye drops in the affected eye. The client is instructed to apply slight pressure against the nose at the inner canthus of the eye after instilling the eye drops. Applying the pressure

    1. prevents the medication from entering the tear duct.
    2. prevents the drug from running down the client's face.
    3. allows the sensitive cornea to adjust to the medication.
    4. facilitates distribution of the medication over the eye surface.

13. Which of the following activities would be appropriate for achieving the goal of decreasing intraocular pressure after eye surgery? The client will avoid

    1. lying supine.
    2. coughing.
    3. deep breathing.
    4. ambulation.

14. After cataract removal surgery, the nurse teaches the client about activities that she can do at home. Which of the following activities would be contraindicated?

    1. Walking down the hall unassisted.
    2. Lying in bed on the nonoperative side.
    3. Performing isometric exercises.
    4. Bending over the sink to wash her hair.

15. After cataract removal surgery, the client is instructed to report any complaints of a sharp pain in the operative eye because this could indicate which of the following postoperative complications?

    1. Detached retina.
    2. Prolapse of the iris.
    3. Extracapsular erosion.
    4. Intraocular hemorrhage.

16. Outcome criteria for the client after cataract removal surgery would include which of the following? The client states

    1. her vision is clear.
    2. her infection is under control.
    3. methods to decrease intraocular pressure.
    4. she is able to administer parenteral pain medication.

The Client With a Retinal Detachment

A client is admitted through the emergency department with a diagnosis of detached retina in the right eye. His eyes are bilaterally patched on admission.

17. As the nurse completes the admission history, the client reports that before the physician patched his eye, he saw many spots, or "floaters." The nurse should explain to the client that these spots were caused by

○ 1. pieces of the retina floating in the eye.
○ 2. blood cells released into the eye by the detachment.
○ 3. contamination of the aqueous humor.
○ 4. spasms of the retinal blood vessels traumatized by the detachment.

18. The client does not understand what happened to his eye. Which of the following explanations by the nurse would most accurately describe the pathology of retinal detachment?
○ 1. "A tear in the retina permits the escape of vitreous humor from the eye."
○ 2. "The optic nerve is damaged when it is exposed to vitreous humor."
○ 3. "The two layers of the retina separate, allowing fluid to enter between them."
○ 4. "Retinal injury produces inflammation and edema, which increase intraocular pressure."

19. The client asks the nurse why his eyes have to be patched. The nurse's reply should be based on the knowledge that eye patches serve to
○ 1. reduce rapid eye movements.
○ 2. decrease the irritation of light entering the damaged eye.
○ 3. protect the injured eye from infection.
○ 4. rest the eyes to promote healing.

20. The client is extremely apprehensive. He states, "I'm afraid of going blind. It would be so hard to live that way." What factor should the nurse consider before responding to his statement?
○ 1. Repeat surgery is impossible, so if this procedure fails, vision loss is inevitable.
○ 2. The surgery will only delay blindness in the right eye, but vision is preserved in the left eye.
○ 3. More and more services are available to help newly blind people adapt to daily living.
○ 4. Optimism is justified because surgical treatment has a 90% to 95% success rate.

21. In the immediate postoperative period after scleral buckling, the client's nursing care should include which of the following?
○ 1. Encouraging deep breathing and coughing every 2 hours.
○ 2. Assessing for eye drainage.
○ 3. Applying pressure dressings to both eyes.
○ 4. Enforcing strict bed rest.

22. Which of the following statements would provide the best guide for activity for the client during his rehabilitation period?
○ 1. Activity is resumed gradually, and he can resume his usual activities in 5 to 6 weeks.
○ 2. Activity level is determined by the client's tolerance, and he can be as active as he wishes.
○ 3. Activity levels will be restricted for several months, so he should plan on being sedentary.

○ 4. Activity resumption is controlled by a graduated series of "buckle" exercises.

23. Which of the following clinical manifestations commonly occur in retinal detachment?
○ 1. Sudden, severe eye pain and colored halos around lights.
○ 2. Inability to move the eye and loss of light accommodation.
○ 3. A tearing sensation and increased lacrimation.
○ 4. Flashing lights and visual field loss.

24. Which of the following would be a priority goal for a client who has undergone surgery for retinal detachment?
○ 1. Control pain.
○ 2. Increase intraocular pressure.
○ 3. Promote a low sodium diet.
○ 4. Maintain a darkened environment.

25. Before the surgical repair of a detached retina, the client is placed on flat bed rest. The nurse understands that the rationale for this position is that it
○ 1. helps reduce intraocular pressure.
○ 2. facilitates drainage from the eye.
○ 3. keeps the client safe while confined to bed.
○ 4. helps prevent further retinal detachment or tearing.

26. Scleral buckling, a procedure used to treat retinal detachment, involves
○ 1. removing the torn segment of the retina and stitching down the remaining segment.
○ 2. replacing the torn segment of the retina with a strip of retina from a donor.
○ 3. stitching the retina firmly to the optic nerve to give it support.
○ 4. creating a splint to hold the retina together until a scar can form and seal off the tear.

27. In discharge planning after scleral buckling, the nurse should ensure that the client understands the need for initial activity restriction at home. Which of the following activities would be contraindicated during the early recovery period?
○ 1. Watching television.
○ 2. Reading.
○ 3. Talking on the telephone.
○ 4. Walking in the yard.

28. The nurse would evaluate that the client understands his home care instructions after scleral buckling for a detached retina if he says his activity should include
○ 1. avoiding abrupt movements of the head.
○ 2. exercising the eye muscles each day.
○ 3. turning the entire head rather than just the eyes for sight.
○ 4. avoiding activities requiring good depth perception.

The Client With Glaucoma

A client has been treated for chronic open-angle glaucoma for 5 years.

29. The client asks the clinic nurse, "How does glaucoma damage my eyesight?" The nurse's reply should be based on the knowledge that chronic open-angle glaucoma
    - ○ 1. results from chronic eye inflammation.
    - ○ 2. causes increased intraocular pressure.
    - ○ 3. leads to detachment of the retina.
    - ○ 4. is caused by decreased blood flow to the retina.

30. If the client experienced any symptom of glaucoma, it would most likely be
    - ○ 1. eye pain.
    - ○ 2. excessive lacrimation.
    - ○ 3. colored light flashes.
    - ○ 4. decreasing peripheral vision.

31. The nurse reevaluates the client's ability to instill eye drops correctly. The client correctly demonstrates the procedure when he
    - ○ 1. blows his nose immediately after administering the eye drops.
    - ○ 2. positions himself on his right side to instill the eye drops.
    - ○ 3. instills the eye drops into the conjunctival sac.
    - ○ 4. wipes the tip of the eye drop applicator with a disposable tissue.

32. Miotics are frequently used in the basic treatment of glaucoma. The nurse should understand that miotics work by
    - ○ 1. paralyzing ciliary muscles.
    - ○ 2. constricting intraocular vessels.
    - ○ 3. constricting the pupil.
    - ○ 4. relaxing ciliary muscles.

33. The nurse would plan to teach the client to administer which of the following drugs for open-angle glaucoma?
    - ○ 1. Pilocarpine hydrochloride.
    - ○ 2. Atropine sulfate.
    - ○ 3. Scopolamine hydrobromide.
    - ○ 4. Acetazolamide (Diamox).

34. The most effective health-promotion measure related to glaucoma that the nurse can teach clients is
    - ○ 1. prompt treatment of all eye infections.
    - ○ 2. avoidance of extended-wear contact lenses by older people.
    - ○ 3. annual intraocular pressure measurements for people older than 40 years.
    - ○ 4. appropriate blood pressure control.

35. Which of the following information should the nurse give the client when preparing him for tonometry?

36. The nurse learns that the client uses timolol maleate (Timoptic) eye drops. The nurse would understand that this β-adrenergic blocker helps control glaucoma by
    - ○ 1. constricting the pupils.
    - ○ 2. dilating the canals of Schlemm.
    - ○ 3. reducing aqueous humor formation.
    - ○ 4. improving the ability of the ciliary muscle to contract.

37. The nurse observes the client instill his eye drops. The client says, "I just try to hit the middle of my eyeball so the drops don't run out of my eye." The nurse explains to the client that the method he is now using may cause
    - ○ 1. scleral staining.
    - ○ 2. corneal injury.
    - ○ 3. excessive lacrimation.
    - ○ 4. systemic drug absorption.

38. When reviewing the client's home care plan, the nurse should encourage him to implement which of the following measures?
    - ○ 1. Reducing daily fluid intake.
    - ○ 2. Wearing dark glasses in the bright sun.
    - ○ 3. Minimizing active exercise.
    - ○ 4. Adding extra lighting to his home.

39. The client with glaucoma is scheduled for a minor surgical procedure. Which of the following orders would require clarification or correction before the nurse would carry it out?
    - ○ 1. Administer morphine sulfate.
    - ○ 2. Administer atropine sulfate.
    - ○ 3. Teach deep breathing exercises.
    - ○ 4. Teach leg exercises.

40. The client asks when he can stop taking the eye medication for his chronic open-angle glaucoma. The nurse should tell the client that he
    - ○ 1. can stop using the eye drops when his vision improves.
    - ○ 2. needs to use the eye drops only when he has symptoms.
    - ○ 3. can discontinue the eye drops after 2 months of normal eye examinations.
    - ○ 4. must use the eye medication for the rest of his life.

41. Which of the following clinical manifestations would the nurse associate with acute narrow-angle glaucoma?
    - ○ 1. Sudden loss of vision in one eye and headache.

- ○ 1. Oral pain medication will be given before the procedure.
- ○ 2. It is a painless procedure with no side effects.
- ○ 3. Blurred or double vision may occur after the procedure.
- ○ 4. Medication will be given to dilate the pupils before the procedure.

○ 2. Acute light sensitivity and blurred vision.

○ 3. Double vision and headache.

○ 4. Sudden eye pain and colored halos around lights.

42. A client has been diagnosed with an acute episode of narrow-angle glaucoma. The nurse plans the client's nursing care with the understanding that acute narrow-angle glaucoma

○ 1. frequently resolves without treatment.

○ 2. is typically treated with sustained bed rest.

○ 3. is a medical emergency that can rapidly lead to blindness.

○ 4. is most commonly treated with steroid therapy.

The Client Undergoing Nasal Surgery

A 27-year-old woman is admitted for elective nasal surgery for a deviated septum.

43. The client returns from surgery after a submucosal resection with nasal packing in place. Which of the following assessments would be a priority?

○ 1. Determining the degree of pain the client is experiencing.

○ 2. Assessing for airway obstruction.

○ 3. Observing for ecchymosis in the periorbital region.

○ 4. Assessing the client's appetite.

44. Which of the following techniques is the most appropriate way to assess for posterior nasal bleeding?

○ 1. Change the nasal drip pad frequently and note the amount of drainage.

○ 2. Monitor the client's hemoglobin and hematocrit values every 8 hours.

○ 3. Frequently assess if the client is nauseated.

○ 4. Use a penlight to inspect the back of the pharynx for bleeding.

45. After the client returns from surgery, the nurse would anticipate placing her in what position?

○ 1. Supine.

○ 2. Left side-lying.

○ 3. Semi-Fowler's.

○ 4. Reverse Trendelenburg's.

46. Which of the following interventions would likely be most effective for the client to use at home when managing the discomfort of rhinoplasty the initial 2 days after surgery?

○ 1. Applying warm, moist compresses.

○ 2. Lying in a prone position.

○ 3. Blowing the nose gently.

○ 4. Applying ice compresses.

47. Which of the following would be an important initial clue to the client that bleeding was occurring even if the nasal drip pad remained dry and intact?

○ 1. Complaints of nausea.

○ 2. Repeated swallowing.

○ 3. Rapid respiratory rate.

○ 4. Feelings of anxiety.

48. The client complains that the nasal packing is uncomfortable and asks when it will be removed. What information should the nurse give the client about the removal of the packing? The nasal packing is usually removed

○ 1. the day of surgery.

○ 2. 24 to 48 hours after surgery.

○ 3. after nasal edema subsides.

○ 4. after pain has diminished.

49. Because the packing blocks the client's nose, the client should be instructed to include which of the following measures in her postoperative home care?

○ 1. Frequent mouth care.

○ 2. Examine the nares for ulcerations.

○ 3. Monitor temperature every 4 hours.

○ 4. Normal saline nose drops.

50. Which of the following measures related to food and fluid intake would be appropriate for the client to implement in the early postoperative period after nasal surgery?

○ 1. Increase fluid intake.

○ 2. Drink through a straw.

○ 3. Take an antiemetic before eating.

○ 4. Limit intake of high-fiber foods.

51. The nurse would teach the client to implement which of the following nasal care measures after the nasal packing is removed?

○ 1. Irrigate the nares with normal saline solution daily.

○ 2. Remove old blood from inside the nares with cotton-tipped applicators.

○ 3. Lubricate the membranes for comfort with a water-soluble lubricant.

○ 4. Avoid cleaning the nares for at least 2 days.

52. The nurse should include which of the following information in the client's discharge teaching?

○ 1. The client should expect tarry stools for several days at home.

○ 2. Nausea is an expected outcome of surgery and may persist for several days.

○ 3. Brief episodes of epistaxis are expected after the surgery.

○ 4. The pain from surgery should be resolved within 24 hours of the surgery.

53. The client is ready for discharge. Which of the following discharge instructions would be appropriate for the client?

○ 1. Avoid activities that elicit the Valsalva maneuver.

○ 2. Take aspirin to control nasal discomfort.

○ 3. Avoid brushing teeth until the nasal packing is removed.

○ 4. Apply heat to the nasal area to control swelling.

54. Which one of the following statements would indicate to the nurse that the client has understood the discharge instructions?
○ 1. "I should not shower until my packing is removed."
○ 2. "I will take stool softeners and modify my diet to prevent constipation."
○ 3. "Coughing every 2 hours is important to prevent respiratory complications."
○ 4. "It is important to blow my nose each day to remove the dried secretions."

55. A woman tells the nurse at the ambulatory care clinic that her 6-year-old daughter has severe nosebleeds. Which of the following instructions should the nurse give this woman about managing nosebleeds?
○ 1. Help the child assume a comfortable position with her head tilted backward.
○ 2. Tilt the child's head backward and place firm pressure on the nose.
○ 3. Help the child lie on her stomach and collect the blood on a clean towel.
○ 4. Place the child in a sitting position with her neck bent forward and apply firm pressure on the nasal septum.

The Client With a Hearing Disorder

These questions are representative of a variety of situations with clients who experience a hearing disorder.

56. Which of the following nursing interventions would be most appropriate for facilitating communication with a client who has a hearing impairment?
○ 1. Stand to one side of the client when speaking, to direct the voice directly into the client's ear.
○ 2. Stand close to the client and speak as loudly as possible.
○ 3. Stand in front of the client and speak slowly and clearly.
○ 4. Ask only questions that the client can answer with a "yes" or "no" response.

57. A 75-year-old client who has been taking furosemide (Lasix) regularly for 4 months tells the nurse that he is having trouble hearing. What would be the nurse's best response to this statement?
○ 1. Tell the client that because he is 75 years old, it is inevitable that his hearing should begin to deteriorate.
○ 2. Have the client immediately report the hearing loss to his physician.

○ 3. Schedule the client for audiometric testing and a hearing aid.
○ 4. Tell the client that the hearing loss is only temporary; when his system adjusts to the furosemide, his hearing will improve.

58. Which of the following techniques is appropriate for irrigating an adult client's ear to move cerumen?
○ 1. Allow the irrigating solution to run down the wall of the ear canal.
○ 2. Use sterile solution and equipment.
○ 3. The irrigating solution should be cool.
○ 4. After instilling the solution, pack the ear canal tightly with cotton pledgets.

59. Which of the following best describes the effects of a hearing aid for a client with sensorineural hearing loss?
○ 1. It will make sounds louder and clearer.
○ 2. It will have no effect on hearing.
○ 3. It will make sounds louder but not clearer.
○ 4. It improves the client's ability to separate words from background noises.

60. A client reports progressively worsening hearing problems during the past 5 years. Which one of the following symptoms is a characteristic of sensorineural hearing loss?
○ 1. Has decreased ability to hear high-pitched tones.
○ 2. Maintains ability to distinguish and understand speech.
○ 3. Maintains ability to discriminate between sounds.
○ 4. Has difficulty with clear articulation of speech.

The Client With Meniere's Disease

A client is diagnosed with Meniere's disease.

61. The classic triad of symptoms associated with Meniere's disease is vertigo,
○ 1. nausea, and headache.
○ 2. tinnitus, and hearing loss.
○ 3. headache, and double vision.
○ 4. hearing loss, and vomiting.

62. The symptom of vertigo is a subjective experience. Which of the following is the most accurate description of vertigo?
○ 1. A feeling that the environment is in motion.
○ 2. An episode of blackout.
○ 3. Lightheadedness.
○ 4. Narrowed vision preceding fainting.

63. The client would be experiencing a typical symptom of Meniere's disease if, before an attack, he experienced
○ 1. a severe headache.

○ 2. nausea.

○ 3. blurred vision.

○ 4. a feeling of intra-ear fullness.

64. The client is instructed to modify his diet. The nurse would explain that the most frequently recommended diet modification for Meniere's disease is

○ 1. low sodium.

○ 2. high protein.

○ 3. low carbohydrate.

○ 4. low fat.

65. Which of the following statements by the client would indicate that he understands the expected course of Meniere's disease?

○ 1. The disease process will gradually extend to the eyes.

○ 2. Control of the episodes is usually possible, but a cure is not yet available.

○ 3. Continued medication therapy will cure the disease.

○ 4. Bilateral deafness is an inevitable outcome of the disease.

66. The potential for injury during an attack of Meniere's disease is great. The nurse should instruct the client to take which immediate action when experiencing vertigo?

○ 1. Place his head between his knees.

○ 2. Concentrate on rhythmic deep breathing.

○ 3. Close his eyes tightly.

○ 4. Assume a reclining or flat position.

67. The client's wife expresses concern because during the past year, her husband has curtailed family activities and evenings out. Based on this information, which of the following would be the most appropriate nursing diagnosis?

○ 1. Social Isolation related to attacks of vertigo and hearing loss.

○ 2. Anxiety related to concern about progressive hearing loss.

○ 3. Self-Care Deficit related to labyrinth dysfunction.

○ 4. Altered Sensory Perception related to labyrinth dysfunction.

68. The nurse would anticipate that all of the following drugs may be used in the attempt to control the client's symptoms except

○ 1. antihistamines.

○ 2. antiemetics.

○ 3. diuretics.

○ 4. glucocorticoids.

69. The client finds the chronic tinnitus of Meniere's disease extremely irritating. Which of the following strategies would be best for the nurse to suggest?

○ 1. Maintain a quiet, restful environment.

○ 2. Mask the tinnitus with background music.

○ 3. Ensure adequate dietary levels of vitamin B_6.

○ 4. Explore the use of a hearing aid.

70. An expected outcome of the client's care would be to

○ 1. save his hearing.

○ 2. prevent environmental injury.

○ 3. control his symptoms.

○ 4. help him cope with the disease.

The Client With Cancer of the Larynx

A client with laryngeal cancer is admitted to the hospital for a total laryngectomy.

71. Because the laryngeal cancer was identified early, the nurse would anticipate that the client's primary symptom was most likely

○ 1. difficulty in swallowing.

○ 2. persistent mild hoarseness.

○ 3. chronic foul breath.

○ 4. nagging unproductive cough.

72. The client is scheduled for radical neck surgery and a total laryngectomy. During the preoperative teaching, the nurse should prepare the client for which of the following postoperative possibilities?

○ 1. Endotracheal intubation.

○ 2. Insertion of a laryngectomy tube.

○ 3. Immediate speech therapy.

○ 4. Normal oral and nasal breathing.

73. A priority nursing diagnosis for the client with a laryngectomy would be

○ 1. Fluid Volume Deficit related to difficulty swallowing.

○ 2. Impaired Communication related to removal of the larynx.

○ 3. Self-Care Deficit (Feeding) related to inability to swallow.

○ 4. Powerlessness related to diagnosis of cancer.

74. The priority nursing goal for the client during the immediate postoperative period should be to

○ 1. maintain a patent airway.

○ 2. provide nutrition.

○ 3. prevent strain on suture lines.

○ 4. prevent hemorrhage.

75. The client receives tube feedings to meet his fluid and nutrition needs. The primary rationale for tube feedings in this situation would be to

○ 1. prevent pain from swallowing.

○ 2. ensure adequate intake.

○ 3. prevent fistula development.

○ 4. allow for adequate suture line healing.

76. The client appears withdrawn and depressed. He keeps the curtain drawn, refuses visitors, and says he wants to be left alone. Which nursing intervention would most likely be therapeutic for the client?

○ 1. Discussing his behavior with his wife to determine the cause.

○ 2. Exploring his future plans.

○ 3. Respecting his need for privacy.

○ 4. Encouraging him to express his feelings nonverbally and in writing.

77. The development of laryngeal cancer is most clearly linked to which of the following factors?

○ 1. High-fat, low-fiber diet.

○ 2. Alcohol and tobacco use.

○ 3. Low socioeconomic status.

○ 4. Overuse of artificial sweeteners.

78. Which of the following measures should the nurse perform in relation to suctioning a tracheostomy tube?

○ 1. Apply suction while inserting the suction catheter into the tube.

○ 2. Change the tracheostomy tube after suctioning the client.

○ 3. Select a suction catheter that approximates the diameter of the tracheostomy tube.

○ 4. Administer high concentrations of oxygen before suctioning the client.

79. To more easily remove thick, tenacious secretions when suctioning a tracheostomy, the nurse would liquefy the secretions before suctioning by instilling the tracheostomy tube with 1 to 2 mL of sterile

○ 1. water.

○ 2. normal saline solution.

○ 3. bacteriostatic water.

○ 4. diluted hydrogen peroxide.

80. While suctioning a client's laryngectomy tube, the nurse should insert the catheter

○ 1. about 1 to 2 inches.

○ 2. until resistance is met.

○ 3. until resistance is met, and then withdraw it 1 to 2 cm.

○ 4. until the client begins coughing.

81. The longest period the nurse should suction a client at one time is

○ 1. 5 to 10 seconds.

○ 2. 11 to 15 seconds.

○ 3. 21 to 25 seconds.

○ 4. 26 to 30 seconds.

82. After suctioning a client's tracheostomy tube, the nurse waits a few minutes before suctioning again. The nurse would use intermittent suction primarily to help prevent

○ 1. stimulating the client's cough reflex.

○ 2. depriving the client of sufficient oxygen supply.

○ 3. dislocating the tracheostomy tube.

○ 4. obstructing the suctioning catheter with secretions.

83. When suctioning a tracheostomy or laryngectomy tube, it is recommended that the nurse use a

○ 1. sterile catheter with each suctioning, and then discard it.

○ 2. sterile catheter for all suctioning during an 8-hour period.

○ 3. sterile catheter for all suctioning during a 24-hour period.

○ 4. clean catheter with each suctioning, and disinfect it between uses.

84. Outcome criteria for evaluating the effectiveness of airway suctioning would include which of the following?

○ 1. Respirations unlabored.

○ 2. Hollow sound on chest percussion.

○ 3. Decreased mucus production.

○ 4. Breath sounds clear on auscultation.

85. Which of the following should the nurse include in a postoperative teaching plan for a client with a laryngectomy?

○ 1. Instructing the client to avoid coughing until the sutures are removed.

○ 2. Telling the client to speak by covering the stoma with a sterile gauze pad.

○ 3. Reassuring the client that normal eating will be possible after healing has occurred.

○ 4. Instructing the client to control oral secretions by swabbing them with tissues or by expectorating into an emesis basin.

86. A client with a new laryngectomy decides to learn about esophageal speech. The speech therapist would explain that this communication technique involves

○ 1. holding an electronic instrument against the esophagus.

○ 2. providing an access route from the trachea to the esophagus.

○ 3. filling the esophagus with air.

○ 4. replacing the larynx with scar tissue.

87. Which of the following health-promoting activities should the nurse teach the client with a new laryngectomy?

○ 1. Cleanse the mouth three times a day.

○ 2. Avoid taking tub baths.

○ 3. Develop an aggressive program of exercise to increase airway functioning.

○ 4. Dehumidify the air for comfort.

88. The client says to the nurse "I don't want my family seeing me this way. This opening in my throat is disgusting." Based on the client's statements, which of the following nursing diagnoses would be most appropriate?

○ 1. Knowledge Deficit about the care of a stoma.

○ 2. Personal Identity Disturbance related to change in appearance.

○ 3. Body Image Disturbance related to neck surgery.

○ 4. Hopelessness related to irreversible changes in body functioning.

89. Which of the following home care activities would be appropriate for a client with a laryngectomy?
○ 1. Keep the stoma opening covered at all times.
○ 2. Participate in activities such as walking and golfing.
○ 3. Stay inside in an air-conditioned environment in the summer.
○ 4. Avoid showering, and take tub baths instead.

The Client With Burns

A client is admitted to the hospital after sustaining burns to the chest, abdomen, right arm, and right leg.

90. Which of the following would provide the best emergency care for a burn victim at the accident site?
○ 1. Pouring cool water over the burned area.
○ 2. Applying clean, dry dressings to the area.
○ 3. Rinsing the area with a warm, mild soap solution.
○ 4. Applying a mild antiseptic ointment to the area.

91. The shaded areas in the diagram below indicate the burned areas on the client's body. Using the "rule of nines," the nurse would determine that about what percentage of the client's body surface has been burned?
○ 1. 18%
○ 2. 27%
○ 3. 45%
○ 4. 64%

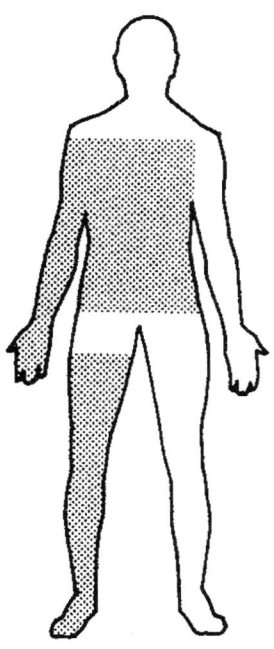

92. The nurse assesses the client for fluid shifting. Fluid shifts that occur during the emergent phase of a burn injury are due to fluid moving from the
○ 1. vascular to interstitial space.
○ 2. extracellular to intracellular space.
○ 3. intracellular to extracellular space.
○ 4. interstitial to vascular space.

93. The nurse should recognize that the fluid shift results from an increase in the
○ 1. permeability of capillary walls.
○ 2. total volume of intravascular plasma.
○ 3. total volume of circulating whole blood.
○ 4. permeability of the kidney tubules.

94. When bandaging the client's hand, the nurse should make certain that
○ 1. the bandage is free of elastic.
○ 2. the hand and finger surfaces do not touch.
○ 3. the hand and fingers are not elevated above the level of the heart.
○ 4. the bandage material is moistened with sterile normal saline solution.

95. A priority nursing diagnosis category for this client during the emergent period would be
○ 1. Fluid Volume Excess.
○ 2. Altered Nutrition: Less Than Body Requirements
○ 3. High Risk for Injury (Falls).
○ 4. High Risk for Infection.

96. Which of the following fluid and electrolyte imbalances would the nurse anticipate that the client would be particularly susceptible to in the emergent phase of burn care?
○ 1. Hemodilution.
○ 2. Metabolic alkalosis.
○ 3. Hypernatremia.
○ 4. Hyperkalemia.

97. During the first 48 to 72 hours of fluid resuscitation therapy after a major burn injury, the intravenous infusion rate will be adjusted by evaluating the client's
○ 1. daily body weight.
○ 2. hourly body temperature.
○ 3. hourly urine output.
○ 4. hourly urine specific gravity.

98. When the open method is used for treating burns, which of the following actions should the nurse take to help prevent discomfort caused by air currents over the client's burned skin surfaces?
○ 1. Keep the client well sedated.
○ 2. Add humidity to the room air.
○ 3. Support the bed linens on a cradle.
○ 4. Keep the door and windows closed in the room.

99. The nurse assesses the client's burned right arm and notes increasing edema, absence of a radial pulse,

and decreased sensation in the fingers. Based on these data, the nurse's priority response should be to
- ○ 1. Document findings and recheck in 1 hour.
- ○ 2. Elevate extremity on one pillow.
- ○ 3. Notify the physician immediately.
- ○ 4. Implement passive range-of-motion exercises.

100. Which of the following activities should the nurse include on the client's care plan to be carried out about one-half hour before his daily whirlpool bath and dressing change?
- ○ 1. Soak the dressing.
- ○ 2. Remove the dressing.
- ○ 3. Administer an analgesic.
- ○ 4. Slit the dressing with blunt scissors.

101. The client with a major burn injury receives total parenteral nutrition (TPN). The primary reason for this therapy for this client is to help
- ○ 1. correct water and electrolyte imbalances.
- ○ 2. allow the gastrointestinal tract to rest.
- ○ 3. provide supplemental vitamins and minerals.
- ○ 4. ensure adequate caloric and protein intake.

102. The client asks the nurse what the word *eschar* means. Which of the following descriptions by the nurse best defines eschar?
- ○ 1. Scar tissue in a developmental stage.
- ○ 2. Crust formation without a blood supply.
- ○ 3. Burned tissue that has become infected.
- ○ 4. Visible living tissue with a rich blood supply.

103. An advantage of using biologic burn grafts, such as porcine (pigskin) grafts, is that they appear to help
- ○ 1. encourage formation of tough skin.
- ○ 2. promote the growth of epithelial tissue.
- ○ 3. provide for permanent wound closure.
- ○ 4. facilitate development of subcutaneous tissue.

104. Which of the following factors would have the least influence on the survival and effectiveness of a burn victim's porcine grafts?
- ○ 1. Absence of infection in the wounds.
- ○ 2. Adequate vascularization in the grafted area.
- ○ 3. Immobilization of the area being grafted.
- ○ 4. Use of analgesics as necessary for pain relief.

105. While caring for the client with a burn injury, the nurse should observe for signs and symptoms of which complication believed to be due primarily to hypersecretion of gastric acid?
- ○ 1. Paralytic ileus.
- ○ 2. Gastric distention.
- ○ 3. Hiatal hernia.
- ○ 4. Gastrointestinal ulceration.

106. When instructing the client about proper nutrition, the nurse would encourage him to eat which of the following meals?
- ○ 1. Chicken breast, salad, iced tea.
- ○ 2. Roast beef sandwich, milkshake, cottage cheese.
- ○ 3. Hamburger, orange, coffee.
- ○ 4. Pasta salad, carrots, iced tea.

107. An autograft is taken from the client's left leg. The nurse should care for the resulting donor site by
- ○ 1. covering it with an occlusive dry dressing.
- ○ 2. keeping the site clean and dry.
- ○ 3. applying a pressure dressing.
- ○ 4. wrapping the extremity with an elastic bandage.

108. The nurse would plan to begin rehabilitation efforts for the burn client
- ○ 1. immediately after the burn has occurred.
- ○ 2. after stabilization of the client's circulatory status.
- ○ 3. after grafting of the burn wounds has occurred.
- ○ 4. after the client's pain has been eliminated.

CORRECT ANSWERS AND RATIONALE

The letters in parentheses following the rationale identify the step of the nursing process (A, D, P, I, E), cognitive level (K, C, T, N), and client needs (S, G, L, H). See the Answer Grid for the key.

The Client With Cataracts

1. 2. The most common cause of cataracts is aging, followed by eye injury. Other causes include ingestion of injurious substances, such as naphthalene, and systemic diseases, such as diabetes. (P, C, G)

2. 3. The lens focuses light rays onto the retina. The process of bringing light rays into focus from both near and far objects is called *accommodation*. The ciliary bodies secrete aqueous humor. The retina houses the rods and cones. The iris regulates the amount of light entering the eye. (I, C, G)

3. 2. The nurse should give a client who seems fearful of surgery an opportunity to express her feelings. Only after identifying the client's concerns can the nurse intervene appropriately. Premature explanations and clichés do not provide needed assessment data and ignore the client's feelings. (I, T, L)

4. 3. A client with a cataract usually complains of blurred and hazy vision. This vision distortion is due to opacity of the lens, which blocks light rays from reaching the retina. (A, T, G)

5. 1. The accepted abbreviation for the right eye is OD, which stands for oculus dexter. OS (oculus sinister) refers to the left eye. OU (oculus uterque) refers to both eyes. RE is not an accepted abbreviation for the right eye. (I, T, S)

6. 2. Instilled in the eye, phenylephrine hydrochloride acts as a mydriatic, causing the pupil to dilate. It also constricts small blood vessels in the eye. (I, T, G)

7. 4. A prescribed antiemetic should be administered as soon as the client who has undergone cataract extraction complains of nausea. Vomiting can increase intraocular pressure, which should be avoided after eye surgery because it can cause complications. (I, T, S)

8. 3. The client should be instructed to bend at the knees and keep the head up and back straight when picking up objects from the floor. The eye shield is usually worn only at night. The client may watch television and read in moderation. Lifting should be restricted for the first week to less than 15 pounds. (E, N, H)

9. 4. Promoting safety is a priority goal for this client.

Her vision will not be clear, and she may need to wear an eye patch after surgery. Orienting the client to the physical environment, assisting her during ambulation, and following other safety precautions to reduce the risk of injury are required. (P, T, S)

10. 3. Safety of the client is the major concern on the return home. The home environment should be assessed for safety hazards, and steps to decrease potential hazards should be implemented. Arrangements for home care, if necessary, should be made before surgery. Oral pain medication should control the client's discomfort. The client is usually able to return to the activities of daily living rapidly, so diversional activity deficits and self-feeding deficits would not typically be anticipated. (D, N, H)

11. 4. After cataract surgery, a client must relearn to judge distances accurately to walk safely. The client will need glasses or contact lenses to restore vision, and cataract glasses do correct vision by magnifying objects; however, these points are not as important in discharge planning as is relearning to judge distance accurately. (I, T, H)

12. 1. Applying pressure against the nose at the inner canthus of the closed eye after administering eye drops prevents the medication from entering the lacrimal (tear) duct. If the medication enters the tear duct, it can enter the nose and pharynx, where it may be absorbed and cause toxic symptoms. Eye drops should be placed in the eye's lower conjunctival sac. (I, T, S)

13. 2. Coughing is contraindicated after cataract extraction because it increases intraocular pressure. Other activities that are contraindicated because they increase intraocular pressure include turning to the operative side, sneezing, crying, and straining. Lying supine, ambulating, and deep breathing do not affect intraocular pressure. (P, T, G)

14. 4. Bending over the sink to wash hair is contraindicated after cataract surgery because it increases intraocular pressure. The client should be taught to tilt her head backward slightly when washing her hair. Activities such as walking, lying in bed on the nonoperative side, and performing isometric exercises are not contraindicated. (I, T, G)

15. 4. Sudden, sharp pain after eye surgery should suggest to the nurse that the client may be experiencing intraocular hemorrhage. The physician should be notified promptly. (A, T, G)

16. 3. Decreasing intraocular pressure is the primary concern after cataract removal. Vision will remain

unclear temporarily after surgery. Infection, although it may occur, is not anticipated. Parenteral pain medication at home is not required. (E, N, G)

The Client With a Retinal Detachment

17. 2. The spots, or floaters, commonly reported by clients with retinal detachment are blood cells released into the vitreous humor by the detachment. (A, T, G)

18. 3. In retinal detachment, the two layers of the retina separate as a result of a small hole or tear, trauma, or degeneration. Vitreous humor seeps into the tear and separates the retinal layers. Vitreous humor does not leak out of the eye or cause any direct damage to the optic nerve. Increased intraocular pressure is not associated with retinal detachment. (I, T, G)

19. 1. Patching the eyes helps decrease random eye movements that could enlarge and worsen retinal detachment. (I, T, S)

20. 4. Untreated retinal detachment results in increasing detachment and eventual blindness, but 90% to 95% of clients can be successfully treated with surgery. If necessary, the surgical procedure can be repeated about 10 to 14 days after the first procedure. Many more services are available for newly blind people, but ideally this client will not need them. (I, T, L)

21. 2. After eye surgery, the eyes should be assessed for excessive or purulent drainage, which may indicate infection. Pressure dressings are not applied to the eyes after surgery, although general eye patching may temporarily be used. Coughing should be avoided. Activity may vary but usually is limited to bed rest with bathroom privileges. (I, T, S)

22. 1. The scarring of the retinal tear needs time to heal completely. Therefore, resumption of activity should be gradual; the client may resume his usual activities in 5 to 6 weeks. Successful healing should allow the client to return to his previous level of functioning. (P, T, H)

23. 4. A client with retinal detachment frequently reports flashing lights in the affected eye followed by a loss of vision commonly described as a curtain being slowly drawn across the eye. The detachment is painless, does not involve the eye muscles, and does not cause lacrimation. (A, K, G)

24. 1. After surgery to correct a detached retina, the client requires analgesics for pain management. Decreasing intraocular pressure is another priority goal. Low-sodium diets and providing a darkened environment are not priority goals for this client. (P, N, G)

25. 4. The client's position is determined by the location of the retinal tear. The rationale for rest is the hope that the retina will fall back into place as much as possible before surgery, which will facilitate adherence of the retina to the choroid. Increased intraocular pressure is not a problem in retinal detachment. There should be no external drainage from the eye. (I, T, G)

26. 4. A choroidal scar will form a permanent seal to close the hole or tear in the retina. A scleral buckle serves as a splint to hold the retina and choroid together until this scar can form. Loss of a portion of or the whole retina would interfere with sight. Retinal transplants are not performed. The retina is never stitched to the optic nerve. (P, T, S)

27. 2. Although restful, reading involves too much jerky eye movement and should be avoided during recovery. Watching television, walking outdoors, and visiting with friends are all appropriate activities and can be encouraged. (P, N, H)

28. 1. During recovery, the client should be instructed to avoid abrupt or jarring head movements. Such activities as shampooing or brushing the hair may be restricted. No specific eye exercises are prescribed, and depth perception is not specially affected by this surgery. (E, T, G)

The Client With Glaucoma

29. 2. In chronic open-angle glaucoma, there is an obstruction to the outflow of aqueous humor, leading to increased intraocular pressure. The increased intraocular pressure eventually causes destruction of the retina's nerve fibers. This nerve destruction causes painless vision loss. The exact cause of glaucoma is unknown. (I, C, G)

30. 4. Although chronic open-angle glaucoma is usually asymptomatic in the early stages, peripheral vision gradually decreases as the disorder progresses. (A, C, G)

31. 3. Proper technique for instilling eye drops includes maintaining sterile asepsis of the applicator tip, being in a supine position, and instilling the eye drops in the conjunctival sac. There is no need for the client to blow his nose after eye drop administration. (E, T, H)

32. 3. A miotic agent constricts the pupil and contracts ciliary musculature. These effects widen the filtration angle and permit increased outflow of aqueous humor. Miotics also cause vasodilation of the intraocular vessels, where intraocular fluids leave the eye, also increasing aqueous humor outflow. Mydriatics cause cycloplegia, or paralysis of the ciliary muscle. (I, K, G)

33. 1. Pilocarpine hydrochloride is a commonly prescribed miotic that produces negligible systemic effects. Atropine sulfate and scopolamine hydrobromide have mydriatic effects. Acetazolamide, a carbonic anhydrase inhibitor, decreases secretion of aqueous humor in the eye, thus lowering intraocular pressure. (P, C, G)

34. 3. The most effective health-promotion measure associated with glaucoma is annual intraocular pressure measurements after 40 years of age. People who are at risk for developing glaucoma, such as those with diabetes or hypertension, African Americans, and people with a family history of glaucoma should have their intraocular pressure checked after 35 years of age. Glaucoma is insidious and basically asymptomatic, and must be diagnosed before the client becomes aware of any vision changes. (I, T, H)

35. 2. Tonometry, which measures intraocular pressure, is a simple and painless procedure that requires no particular preparation or postprocedure care and carries no side effects. (I, C, S)

36. 3. Timolol maleate is commonly administered to control glaucoma. The drug's action is not completely understood, but it is believed to reduce aqueous humor formation, thereby reducing intraocular pressure. (P, C, G)

37. 2. The cornea is sensitive and can be injured by eye drops falling onto it. Thus, eye drops should be instilled into the lower conjunctival sac of the eye to avoid the risk of corneal damage. (I, T, H)

38. 4. Miotic agents may compromise a client's ability to adjust safely to night vision. For safety, extra lighting should be added to the home. The client does not need to curtail fluid intake. Bright lights are not harmful to the eyes, and exercise is permitted, although excessive exertion should be avoided. (I, N, H)

39. 2. Atropine sulfate causes pupil dilation. This action is contraindicated for the client with glaucoma because it increases intraocular pressure. The drug does not have this effect on intraocular pressure in people who do not have glaucoma. (P, T, G)

40. 4. To control his increased intraocular pressure, the client will need to continue taking his eye medications the rest of his life. Any loss of vision that the client has suffered will be permanent. Vision loss can occur gradually without any symptoms. (I, T, G)

41. 4. Acute narrow-angle glaucoma produces abrupt changes in the angle of the iris. Clinical manifestations include severe eye pain, colored halos around lights, and rapid vision loss. (A, C, G)

42. 3. Acute narrow-angle glaucoma is a medical emergency that rapidly leads to blindness if left untreated. Treatment typically involves miotic drugs and surgery, usually iridectomy or laser therapy. Both procedures create a hole in the periphery of the iris, which allows the aqueous humor to flow into the anterior chamber. (P, T, G)

The Client Undergoing Nasal Surgery

43. 2. Postoperative nursing assessment of the client after nasal surgery focuses on early detection of complications. Two common complications are airway obstruction and hemorrhage. The nasal packing can slip out of position and occlude the client's airway. Therefore, assessing the client for airway obstruction is a priority assessment. (A, N, S)

44. 4. The best way for the nurse to detect posterior nasal bleeding is to use a penlight to observe the back of the pharynx. The nasal drip pad will remain dry with posterior nasal bleeding. Nausea can occur postoperatively for several reasons, with bleeding being just one of them. Checking the client's hemoglobin and hematocrit every 8 hours will not help detect bleeding in its earliest stages. (A, N, S)

45. 3. To assist in breathing, promote comfort, and decrease edema formation after surgery, the client is most appropriately placed in semi-Fowler's position. (P, T, S)

46. 4. The most effective way to decrease discomfort is to decrease local edema. Cold application, such as an ice compress or ice bag, is effective. Heat dilates local vessels and increases local congestion. Semi-Fowler's position helps decrease edema and prevent aspiration. Nose blowing should be avoided for at least 48 hours after the nasal packing is removed because it can disrupt the surgical site and lead to bleeding. (I, N, H)

47. 2. Because of the dense packing, it is relatively unusual for bleeding to be apparent through the nasal drip pad. Instead, the blood runs down the throat, causing the client to swallow frequently. The back of the throat can be assessed with a flashlight. An accumulation of blood in the stomach may cause nausea and vomiting. Increased respiratory rate occurs in shock but is not an early sign of bleeding in the client after nasal surgery. (A, N, H)

48. 2. The packing helps maintain hemostasis and prevent bleeding. Removing the packing is uncomfortable and must be done carefully. The packing is generally removed the day after surgery. The client must be watched closely for bleeding after removing the packing. (I, C, G)

49. 1. Mouth-breathing dries the oral mucous membranes. Frequent mouth care is necessary for comfort and to combat the anorexia associated with the taste of blood and loss of the sense of smell. Monitoring the temperature every 4 hours and checking the nares for ulcerations are not necessary. Nose drops are not instilled with packing in place. (I, T, H)

50. 1. Although foods as tolerated are encouraged, the nurse should encourage the client with nasal packing to increase fluid intake because fluids are best tolerated at this time. Nasal packing makes eating difficult and uncomfortable. The packing blocks the passage of air through the nose, creating a partial vacuum during swallowing. A sucking action may occur when the client attempts to drink with a straw. Antiemetics are needed only if the client experiences nausea or vomiting. (I, T, G)

51. 3. A water-soluble lubricant offsets dryness and enhances comfort while healing occurs. The lubricant also prevents secretions from drying and crusting in the nose. The client should be cautioned not to disturb clots either with her fingers or applicators because bleeding may occur. (I, N, H)

52. 1. Nasal bleeding gives stools a tarry appearance for several days; the client should be informed of this effect. Epistaxis and nausea are not expected outcomes, and some discomfort can be expected to persist after 24 hours. (I, T, H)

53. 1. The client should be instructed to avoid any activities that cause Valsalva's maneuver (eg, constipation, vigorous coughing, exercise) to reduce bleeding and stress on suture lines. The client should not take aspirin because of its antiplatelet properties, which may cause bleeding. Oral hygiene is important to rid the mouth of old dried blood and to enhance the client's appetite. Cool compresses, not heat, should be applied to decrease swelling and control discoloration of the area. (I, N, H)

54. 2. Constipation can cause straining during defecation, which can induce bleeding. The client should avoid blowing her nose for 48 hours after the packing is removed. Thereafter, she should blow her nose gently using the open-mouth technique to minimize bleeding in the surgical area. She should also take measures to prevent coughing. Showering is not contraindicated. (E, T, H)

55. 4. For the initial management of nosebleed, the client should sit up and lean forward with the head tipped downward. The soft tissues of the nose should be compressed against the septum with the fingers. The traditional head-back position allows blood to flow down the throat and can trigger vomiting. (I, T, H)

The Client With a Hearing Disorder

56. 3. Standing close to and directly in front of the client will greatly facilitate communication. Yelling at the client distorts the voice and further hinders understanding. The nurse should make sure that the client can see the nurse's mouth at all times to facilitate lip-reading, speak slowly and clearly, and mini-

mize distractions in the environment. The nurse should have the client validate his understanding of the conversation by repeating what was said. (I, T, S)

57. 2. Numerous drugs may cause ototoxicity; furosemide is one of these. Other ototoxic drugs include aminoglycoside antibiotics, antineoplastic drugs, and some thiazide diuretics. When teaching the client about ototoxic drugs, the nurse should emphasize the importance of promptly reporting any hearing loss, dizziness, or tinnitus, to help prevent permanent ear damage. (I, N, H)

58. 1. Ear irrigation is considered to be a clean procedure unless the integrity of the tympanic membrane has been damaged. The solution should be at body temperature and, when instilled, should be allowed to run down the side of the ear canal. It should not be allowed to drop directly on the tympanic membrane because this may cause discomfort or damage. Cotton pledgets should be placed loosely in the ear canal so as not to exert pressure on the tympanic membrane. (I, T, S)

59. 3. Hearing aids have limited use for clients with sensorineural hearing loss because these clients experience problems with sound discrimination as well as volume. A hearing aid can make sound louder but not necessarily clearer. (A, C, G)

60. 1. Sensorineural hearing loss involves the inner ear and is a common degenerative problem for elderly people. The ability to hear high-pitched sounds is decreased, as is the ability to discriminate and understand sounds, especially in a noisy environment. Misinterpretation of voice levels causes these clients to speak more loudly than is normal. (A, C, G)

The Client With Meniere's Disease

61. 2. Meniere's disease involves the inner ear and is characterized by episodes of acute vertigo and tinnitus. It can result in progressive and irreversible hearing loss. The severe vertigo can lead to nausea and vomiting. Double vision and headache are not characteristic features of Meniere's disease. (A, C, G)

62. 1. Vertigo is a form of hallucination in which the person perceives the environment to be moving around him, or perceives himself to be moving within the environment. Clients with Meniere's disease are not light-headed and do not faint or black out. (A, C, G)

63. 4. Many clients are able to identify an incipient attack of Meniere's disease by a feeling of fullness in the ear that reflects the evolving congestion. Meniere's disease does not affect vision. Nausea may result once the classic symptoms occur. (A, C, G)

64. 1. A low-sodium diet is frequently an effective mechanism for reducing the frequency and severity of the disease episodes. About three quarters of clients with Meniere's disease respond to treatment with a low-salt diet. A diuretic may also be ordered. (P, C, H)

65. 2. There is no cure for Meniere's disease, but the wide range of medical and surgical treatments allows for adequate control in many clients. The disease often worsens, but it does not spread to the eyes. The hearing loss is usually unilateral. (E, C, G)

66. 4. The client needs to assume a safe and comfortable position during an attack, which may last several hours. The client's location when the attack occurs may dictate the most reasonable position. Ideally, he should lie down immediately in a reclining or flat position to control the vertigo. The danger of a serious fall is real. (I, T, S)

67. 1. A client with Meniere's disease may curtail social activities out of fear of embarrassment from having a dizzy spell in public. This seems likely in this situation, based on the wife's information, but would need to be validated by the client. However, the wife may be a more reliable source of information about social isolation than the client. The other three diagnoses are appropriate in Meniere's disease but are less directly related to social activity. (D, N, L)

68. 4. A wide variety of medications may be used in an attempt to control Meniere's disease, including antihistamines, antiemetics, tranquilizers (especially diazepam), and diuretics. Glucocorticoids play no significant role in disease treatment. (P, T, G)

69. 2. The chronic tinnitus associated with Meniere's disease can be extremely intrusive and frustrating for clients. Quiet environments appear to worsen the client's perception of the problem. Attempting to mask tinnitus with a low-level competing sound, such as music, is often recommended. (I, T, G)

70. 1. Uncontrolled Meniere's disease can lead to irreversible hearing loss. Preventing this is the primary goal of medical treatment. The other options are important goals for both physicians and nurses during the client's care. (E, C, G)

The Client With Cancer of the Larynx

71. 2. Hoarseness occurs early in the course of most intrinsic laryngeal cancers because the tumor prevents accurate approximation of the vocal cords during phonation. Foul breath and expectoration of blood are late symptoms. Large extrinsic tumors eventually produce difficulty and pain in swallowing. A nagging cough has no direct relationship to laryngeal cancer. (A, K, G)

72. 2. The client may have a temporary laryngectomy tube, which remains in place until the wound is healed and a permanent stoma has formed, usually in 2 or 3 weeks. Speech therapy is delayed until healing occurs. Surgery permanently alters the airway and necessitates breathing through the permanent tracheal opening. An endotracheal tube is not used. (I, T, S)

73. 2. After the client's laryngectomy, the nurse needs to establish an alternate communication pattern because the client can no longer speak. The client needs to be able to make his needs known and express himself with dignity. The nurse should encourage him to communicate by writing or using a communication board with letters, words, or pictures, as desired. (D, N, L)

74. 1. Maintaining a patent airway is *the* priority nursing goal in the immediate postoperative period. The client's ability to cough and deep breathe is impaired because the glottis has been removed. Promoting comfort, reducing strain on suture lines, preventing hemorrhage, and providing nutrition are important nursing goals, but maintaining a patent airway is the priority. (P, N, G)

75. 4. A nasogastric tube is usually inserted during surgery to instill food and fluids postoperatively. The tube allows the suture line to heal adequately, minimizes contamination of the pharyngeal and esophageal suture lines, and prevents fluid from leaking through the wound into the trachea before healing occurs. Normal oral feedings are resumed as soon as the nasogastric tube is removed, usually within 10 days after surgery. A tracheoesophageal fistula is a rare potential complication of total laryngectomy and may occur if radiation therapy has compromised wound healing. (P, T, G)

76. 4. The client has undergone body changes and permanent loss of verbal communication. He may feel isolated and insecure. The nurse can encourage him to express his feelings and use this information to develop an appropriate care plan. Discussing the client's behavior with his wife may not reveal his feelings. Exploring future plans is not appropriate at this time because more information about the client's behavior is needed before proceeding to this level. The nurse can respect the client's need for privacy while also encouraging him to express his feelings. (I, T, L)

77. 2. Predisposing factors for laryngeal cancer include chronic irritants such as alcohol, tobacco, and exposure to noxious fumes. About 75% of people develop laryngeal cancer are smokers. The combination of smoking and heavy alcohol intake is even more strongly implicated as a causative agent in the laryngeal cancer. Epidemiologic studies indicate that a high-fat diet may be a major factor in the development of cancer of the breast, prostate, and colon. Low socioeconomic status is a predisposing factor in cervical cancer but not for laryngeal cancer. Artificial sweeteners have been related to the incidence of bladder cancer. (A, K, G)

78. 4. Clients are hyperoxygenated before suctioning to prevent hypoxia. Suction is never applied while inserting the catheter into the airway. The suction catheter should be about half the diameter of the tube; a larger-diameter suction catheter would interfere with air flow during the procedure. Laryngectomy tubes are not changed after suctioning. (I, T, S)

79. 2. Sterile normal saline is the solution of choice for instillation into a tracheostomy tube cannula to help liquefy sticky secretions. Normal saline solution is less irritating to mucous membranes than plain water, dilute hydrogen peroxide, and bacteriostatic water. The nurse may cleanse the area around a laryngectomy stoma with an applicator moistened with diluted hydrogen peroxide but should be careful that none enters the stoma because of its irritating effects on respiratory mucosa. Furthermore, it is important to prevent aspiration. (I, T, S)

80. 3. The proper suctioning technique is to insert the suction catheter until resistance is met, withdraw the catheter 1 to 2 cm, and then begin applying intermittent suction while withdrawing the catheter. The suction catheter is inserted more than 1 to 2 inches. Coughing by a client does not necessarily indicate when to begin or stop suctioning. (I, T, S)

81. 1. A client should be suctioned for no longer than 10 seconds at a time. Suctioning for longer than 10 seconds may reduce the client's oxygen level so much that he may become hypoxic. (I, T, S)

82. 2. After suctioning, the client should rest at least 3 minutes or until respirations return to normal before suctioning is repeated, unless secretions interfere with breathing. Intermittent suctioning prevents oxygen deprivation. Hypoxia can lead to cardiac dysrhythmias and cardiac arrest. The client should receive 100% oxygen between suctionings. (I, T, S)

83. 1. The recommended technique is to use a sterile catheter for each suctioning in a client with a laryngectomy or tracheostomy tube. There is a danger of introducing organisms into the respiratory tract when strict aseptic technique, including a catheter change for each suctioning, is not used. (I, T, S)

84. 4. Auscultating for clear breath sounds is the most accurate way to evaluate the effectiveness of tracheobronchial suctioning. Auscultation should also be done to determine whether the client needs suctioning. Assessing for labored respirations, observing for cough productive of mucus, and percussing

the chest for a hollow sound are not as accurate in evaluating the effectiveness of tracheobronchial suctioning. (E, T, G)

85. 3. Normal eating is possible once the suture line has healed. Coughing is essential to keep the airway patent. Because the larynx has been removed, the ability to speak is lost. Swallowing is usually not affected, nor is the ability to control oral secretions. (I, T, G)

86. 3. Esophageal speech requires filling the esophagus with air and allowing it to vibrate out. An artificial larynx (electrolarynx) is a hand-held speech aid placed against the neck. An access route from the trachea to the esophagus is required for tracheoesophageal shunting. This provides pulmonary power to the pharyngeal sphincter, which provides vibrations for a pseudovoice. Replacing the larynx with scar tissue would not facilitate speech. (P, T, G)

87. 1. Oral hygiene is an important aspect of self-care for the laryngectomy client, who is less able to detect mouth odor. Additionally, the mouth harbors bacteria, and good mouth care reduces the risk of infection. The client is able to take tub baths with careful instruction on ways to avoid slipping, the need to make sure the water is no more than 6 inches deep, and other safety measures. Air should be humidified to enhance comfort. Moderate exercise may be beneficial, but an aggressive exercise program is not usually part of the plan of care. (I, T, H)

88. 3. Body Image Disturbance is the most appropriate nursing diagnosis based on the client's statements at this time. Most clients are concerned about how their family members will respond to the physical changes that have occurred as a result of radical neck surgery. The nurse should allow the client to verbalize any negative feelings or concerns that exist because of the surgery. Referral to a support group for laryngectomy clients may be helpful to the client and family members in coping with the changes in their lives. (D, N, L)

89. 2. The client should be encouraged to participate in activities such as walking, golfing, and other moderate recreational sports. It is not necessary to keep the stoma covered at all times, although a gauze bib can be used to protect the clothes from mucus and to keep irritants from entering the stoma. New laryngectomy clients may find air-conditioning too cool and dry at first and thus should avoid such environments. It is not necessary to remain in air-conditioning in the summer. Clients may shower as long as they cover the stoma to prevent water from entering the airway. (I, T, H)

The Client With Burns

90. 1. The recommended emergency treatment for a heat burn is immersion in cool water or application of clean, cool wet packs. This treatment helps relieve pain and diminishes tissue damage by cooling the tissue. Ice is not recommended because it may cause the victim to become hypothermic and may further damage burn lesions. Clothing should not be removed, nor should ointments be applied. Antiseptics or ointments are contraindicated because they can lead to further tissue damage. (I, T, G)

91. 3. According to the "rule of nines," this client has sustained burns on about 45% of his body surface. His right arm is calculated as being 9%, his right leg is 18%, and his anterior trunk is 18%, for a total of 45%. (A, T, G)

92. 1. In a burn injury, the injured capillaries dilate, and there is increased capillary permeability at the site of the burn. Plasma seeps out into the burned tissue, moving from the vascular space into the interstitial space. (A, C, G)

93. 1. When a burn occurs, the capillaries and small vessels dilate, and cell damage causes a release of a histamine-like substance. This substance causes the capillary walls to become more permeable, and significant quantities of fluid are lost. The initial fluid derangement after a burn is a plasma–to–interstitial fluid shift. (A, T, G)

94. 2. When bandaging the client's fingers and hands, the nurse must ensure that skin surfaces do not touch. Allowing skin surfaces to touch interferes with normal healing and is likely to be irritating. Bandages for burns may be elasticized and often are used to form an occlusive pressure dressing. The bandages may be impregnated with antimicrobial agents but are not ordinarily kept moist with water or normal saline solution. A bandaged hand is ordinarily elevated to prevent edema. (I, T, G)

95. 4. Infection is a priority problem for the burned victim. Fluid volume excess and altered nutrition are not priorities during the emergent period. A high risk for falling is not a priority for this client because the client would be on bed rest and most likely in a critical care unit. (D, N, G)

96. 4. Due to the massive cellular destruction that occurs in burns, potassium is released into the extracellular fluid, leading to hyperkalemia. Hyponatremia is another anticipated electrolyte imbalance because sodium is trapped in edematous fluid. Metabolic acidosis commonly develops due to loss of bicarbonate ions. Hemoconcentration is caused by circulatory dehydration as plasma shifts into the extracellular space. (P, T, G)

97. 3. During the first 48 to 72 hours of fluid resuscitation therapy, hourly urine output is the most accessible and generally reliable indicator of adequate fluid replacement. Fluid volume is also assessed by monitoring mental status, vital signs, peripheral perfu-

sion, and body weight. Pulmonary artery end-diastolic pressure (PAEDP) and even central venous pressure (CVP) are preferred guides to fluid administration, but urine output is best when PAEDP or CVP are not used. After the first 48 to 72 hours, urine output is a less-reliable guide to fluid needs. The victim enters the diuretic phase as edema reabsorption occurs, and urine output increases dramatically. (E, T, G)

98. 3. Bed linens should be kept off a burn wound when the open method of wound care is used. To prevent drafts over the burned areas, it is best to place a cradle on the bed and drape bed linens over the cradle. Adding humidity to inspired air, keeping the client well sedated, and keeping doors and windows closed do not help prevent discomfort due to air currents passing over burned areas. (I, T, G)

99. 3. The absence of a pulse, decreased sensation in the extremity, and increasing edema are all indicative of compromised neurovascular status due to compartment syndrome. Although elevating the extremity may help to decrease edema, any loss of pulse or sensation must be reported immediately to the physician. An escharotomy or fasciotomy may need to be performed to release pressure in the extremity. Other assessments to note include the temperature, capillary refill time, and movement or increasing pain of the affected extremity. (D, N, S)

100. 3. Removing dressings from severe burns will expose sensitive nerve endings to the air, which is painful. The client should be given a prescribed analgesic about one-half hour before the dressing change to promote comfort. (P, T, G)

101. 4. Nutritional support with sufficient calories and protein is extremely important in the client with severe burns because of the loss of plasma protein through injured capillaries and an increased metabolic rate. Gastric dilation and paralytic ileus commonly occur in severe burns, making oral fluids and foods contraindicated. TPN is also administered if the client is unable to take sufficient nourishment orally or by gastric gavage. It then becomes an effective method for supplying the body with nutrients—especially protein, which the burn victim needs in larger-than-average amounts. (I, T, G)

102. 2. Eschar is dead tissue, heavily contaminated with bacteria and without a blood supply. It is tissue that sloughs. Eschar has also been defined as devitalized skin. When eschar sloughs, an open wound that is almost always infected results. (I, T, G)

103. 2. Biologic dressings, such as porcine grafts, serve many purposes for a client with severe burns. They enhance the growth of epithelial tissues and minimize the overgrowth of granulation tissue, prevent loss of water and protein, decrease pain, increase mobility, and help prevent infection. (P, T, G)

104. 4. Analgesic administration to keep a burn victim comfortable is important but is unlikely to influence graft survival and effectiveness. Such factors as the absence of infection, adequate vascularization, and immobilization of the grafted area promote an effective graft. (E, T, G)

105. 4. Gastrointestinal ulceration, also known as Curling's ulcer, occurs in about half of clients suffering from severe burns. The incidence of ulceration appears proportional to the extent of the burns and is believed to be due to hypersecretion of gastric acid and compromised gastrointestinal perfusion. Such complications as infection, gastric dilation, and nitrogen imbalance may occur in clients with burns, but they are not attributed to stress. (A, T, G)

106. 2. A roast beef sandwich, milkshake, and cottage cheese would provide the burn victim with the extra protein and calories needed for healing. The other meals provide less calories or protein and would not be as good choices for the client with severe burns. (I, T, G)

107. 2. It is important to keep donor sites clean, dry, and free of pressure. Single-layer gauze dressings impregnated with petroleum or scarlet red, or biosynthetic dressings may be used to cover the donor site as it heals. Occlusive dressings are not used, nor are elastic bandages. The site usually heals in 1 to 2 weeks if cared for properly. (I, T, S)

108. 1. Rehabilitation efforts are implemented as soon as the client is admitted to the hospital for treatment. These efforts are interdisciplinary in nature and include the client and family members. Early emphasis on rehabilitation is important to decrease complications and to help ensure that the client will be able to make the adjustments necessary to return to an optimal state of health and independence. (P, T, L)

NURSING CARE OF ADULTS WITH MEDICAL AND SURGICAL HEALTH PROBLEMS

TEST 11: The Client With Sensory Health Problems

Directions: Use this answer grid to determine areas of strength or need for further study.

NURSING PROCESS

A = Assessment
D = Analysis, nursing diagnosis
P = Planning
I = Implementation
E = Evaluation

COGNITIVE LEVEL

K = Knowledge
C = Comprehension
T = Application
N = Analysis

CLIENT NEEDS

S = Safe, effective care environment
G = Physiologic integrity
L = Psychosocial integrity
H = Health promotion and maintenance

Question #	Answer #	A	D	P	I	E	K	C	T	N	S	G	L	H
1	2			P				C				G		
2	3				I			C				G		
3	2				I				T				L	
4	3	A							T			G		
5	1				I				T		S			
6	2				I				T			G		
7	4				I				T		S			
8	3					E				N				H
9	4			P					T		S			
10	3		D							N				H
11	4				I				T					H
12	1				I				T		S			
13	2			P					T			G		
14	4				I				T			G		
15	4	A							T			G		
16	3					E				N		G		
17	2	A							T			G		
18	3				I				T			G		
19	1				I				T		S			
20	4				I				T				L	
21	2				I				T		S			
22	1			P					T					H
23	4	A					K					G		
24	1			P						N		G		
25	4				I				T			G		

ANSWER GRID: 1

613

NURSING PROCESS

A = Assessment
D = Analysis, nursing diagnosis
P = Planning
I = Implementation
E = Evaluation

COGNITIVE LEVEL

K = Knowledge
C = Comprehension
T = Application
N = Analysis

CLIENT NEEDS

S = Safe, effective care environment
G = Physiologic integrity
L = Psychosocial integrity
H = Health promotion and maintenance

Question #	Answer #	A	D	P	I	E	K	C	T	N	S	G	L	H
26	4			P					T		S			
27	2			P						N				H
28	1					E			T			G		
29	2				I			C				G		
30	4	A						C				G		
31	3					E			T					H
32	3				I		K					G		
33	1			P				C				G		
34	3				I				T					H
35	2				I			C			S			
36	3			P				C				G		
37	2				I				T					H
38	4				I					N				H
39	2			P					T			G		
40	4				I				T			G		
41	4	A						C				G		
42	3			P					T			G		
43	2	A								N	S			
44	4	A								N	S			
45	3			P					T		S			
46	4				I					N				H
47	2	A								N				H
48	2				I			C				G		
49	1				I				T					H
50	1				I				T			G		
51	3				I					N				H
52	1				I				T					H
53	1				I					N				H
54	2					E			T					H
55	4				I				T					H

NURSING PROCESS

A = Assessment
D = Analysis, nursing diagnosis
P = Planning
I = Implementation
E = Evaluation

COGNITIVE LEVEL

K = Knowledge
C = Comprehension
T = Application
N = Analysis

CLIENT NEEDS

S = Safe, effective care environment
G = Physiologic integrity
L = Psychosocial integrity
H = Health promotion and maintenance

Question #	Answer #	Nursing Process					Cognitive Level				Client Needs			
		A	D	P	I	E	K	C	T	N	S	G	L	H
56	3				I				T		S			
57	2				I					N				H
58	1				I				T		S			
59	3	A						C				G		
60	1	A						C				G		
61	2	A						C				G		
62	1	A						C				G		
63	4	A						C				G		
64	1			P				C						H
65	2					E		C				G		
66	4				I				T		S			
67	1		D							N			L	
68	4			P					T			G		
69	2				I				T			G		
70	1					E		C				G		
71	2	A					K					G		
72	2				I				T		S			
73	2		D							N			L	
74	1			P						N		G		
75	4			P					T			G		
76	4				I				T				L	
77	2	A					K					G		
78	4				I				T		S			
79	2				I				T		S			
80	3				I				T		S			
81	1				I				T		S			
82	2				I				T		S			
83	1				I				T		S			
84	4					E			T			G		
85	3				I				T			G		

ANSWER GRID: 3

NURSING PROCESS

A = Assessment
D = Analysis, nursing diagnosis
P = Planning
I = Implementation
E = Evaluation

COGNITIVE LEVEL

K = Knowledge
C = Comprehension
T = Application
N = Analysis

CLIENT NEEDS

S = Safe, effective care environment
G = Physiologic integrity
L = Psychosocial integrity
H = Health promotion and maintenance

Question #	Answer #	Nursing Process					Cognitive Level				Client Needs			
		A	D	P	I	E	K	C	T	N	S	G	L	H
86	3			P					T			G		
87	1				I				T					H
88	3		D							N			L	
89	2				I				T					H
90	1				I				T			G		
91	3	A							T			G		
92	1	A						C				G		
93	1	A							T			G		
94	2				I				T			G		
95	4		D							N		G		
96	4			P					T			G		
97	3					E			T			G		
98	3				I				T			G		
99	3		D							N	S			
100	3			P					T			G		
101	4				I				T			G		
102	2				I				T			G		
103	2			P					T			G		
104	4					E			T			G		
105	4	A							T			G		
106	2				I				T			G		
107	2				I				T		S			
108	1			P					T				L	

ANSWER GRID: 4

NURSING PROCESS

A = Assessment
D = Analysis, nursing diagnosis
P = Planning
I = Implementation
E = Evaluation

COGNITIVE LEVEL

K = Knowledge
C = Comprehension
T = Application
N = Analysis

CLIENT NEEDS

S = Safe, effective care environment
G = Physiologic integrity
L = Psychosocial integrity
H = Health promotion and maintenance

Question #	Answer #	Nursing Process					Cognitive Level				Client Needs			
		A	D	P	I	E	K	C	T	N	S	G	L	H
Number Correct														
Number Possible	108	20	6	21	51	10	4	18	67	19	23	57	7	21
Percentage Correct														

Score Calculation: To determine your **Percentage Correct,** divide the **Number Correct** by the **Number Possible.**

ANSWER GRID: 5

BIBLIOGRAPHY

Bates, B. (1995). *A guide to physical examination and history taking* (6th ed.). Philadelphia: JB Lippincott.

Beare, C., and Myers, J. (1994). *Principles and practice of adult health nursing.* (2nd ed.). St. Louis: CV Mosby.

Beckingham, A.C. (1993). *Promoting health aging: A nursing and community perspective.* St. Louis: Mosby-Year Book.

Birchenall, J.M., and Streight, M.E. (1993). *Care of the older adult* (3rd ed.). Philadelphia: JB Lippincott.

Black, J.M., and Matassarin-Jacobs, E. (1997). *Medical-surgical nursing: Clinical management for continuity of care* (5th ed.). Philadelphia: WB Saunders.

Bowers, A.C., and Thompson, J.M. (1992). *Clinical manual of health assessment* (4th ed.). St. Louis: Mosby-Year Book.

Bullock, B. (1996). *Pathophysiology: Adaptations and alterations in function* (4th ed.). Philadelphia: Lippincott-Raven.

Carpenito, L.J. (1997). *Handbook of nursing diagnosis* (7th ed.). Philadelphia: Lippincott-Raven.

Carpenito, L.J. (1997). *Nursing diagnosis: Application to clinical practice* (7th ed.). Philadelphia: Lippincott-Raven.

Chernecky, C.C., Berger, B.J., and Krech, R.L. (1993). *Laboratory tests and diagnostic procedures.* Philadelphia: WB Saunders.

Clark, J.B., Queener, S.F., and Karb, V.B. (1992). *Pharmacologic basis of nursing practice.* (4th ed.). St. Louis: Mosby-Year Book.

Clochesy, J.M., Breu, C., Cardin, S., Rudy, E.B., and Whittaker, A. (1996). *Critical care nursing.* (2nd ed.). Philadelphia: WB Saunders.

Craven, R.F., and Hirnle, C.J. (1996). *Fundamentals of nursing: Human health and function.* (2nd ed.) Philadelphia: Lippincott-Raven.

Davis, J., and Sherer, K. (1993). *Applied nutrition and diet therapy for nurses* (2nd ed.). Philadelphia: WB Saunders.

Dossey, B.M., Guzzetta, C.E., and Kenner, C.V. (1992). *Critical care nursing: Body-mind-spirit* (3rd ed.). Philadelphia: JB Lippincott.

Earnest, V.V. (1993). *Clinical skills in nursing practice* (2nd ed.). Philadelphia: JB Lippincott.

Edelman, C.L., and Mandle, C.L. (1994). *Health promotion throughout the lifespan* (3rd ed.). St. Louis: Mosby-Year Book.

Eliopoulos, C. (1996). *Gerontological nursing* (4th ed.). Philadelphia: Lippincott-Raven.

Ferri, R.S. (1992). *Care planning for the older adult: Nursing diagnosis in long-term care.* Philadelphia: WB Saunders.

Fischbach, F. (1996). *A manual of laboratory and diagnostic tests* (5th ed.). Philadelphia: Lippincott-Raven.

Giger, J., and Davidhizar, R. (1995). *Transcultural nursing: Assessment and intervention.* (2nd ed.) St. Louis: Mosby-Year Book.

Grimes, J., and Burns, E. (1992). *Health assessment in nursing practice* (3rd ed.). Boston: Jones and Bartlett.

Groenwald, S.L., Frogge, M.H., Goodman, M., and Yarbro, C.H. (1993). *Cancer nursing principles and practice* (3rd ed.). Boston: Jones and Bartlett.

Gruendemann, B.J., and Fernsebner, B. (1993). *Textbook of perioperative nursing.* Boston: Jones and Bartlett.

Hartshorn, J.C., Lamborn, M., and Noll, M.L. (1993). *Introduction to critical care nursing.* Philadelphia: WB Saunders.

Horne, M., Heitz, U.E., and Swearingen, P.L. (1991). *Fluid, electrolyte, and acid-base balance: A case study approach.* St. Louis: Mosby-Year Book.

Huang, S.H., Kessler, A., McCulloch, C.D., and Dasher, L.A. (1989). *Coronary care nursing* (2nd ed.). Philadelphia: WB Saunders.

Hudak, C.M., Gallo, B.M., and Benz, J.J. (1994). *Critical care nursing: A holistic approach* (6th ed.). Philadelphia: JB Lippincott.

Ignatavicius, D.D., and Bayne, M.V. (1995). *Medical-surgical nursing: A nursing process approach.* (2nd ed.). Philadelphia: WB Saunders.

Jarvis, C. (1992). *Physical examination and health assessment.* Philadelphia: WB Saunders.

Kart, C.S., Metress, E.K., and Metress, S.P. (1992). *Human aging and chronic disease.* Boston: Jones and Bartlett.

Kozier, B., and Erb, G. (1991). *Fundamentals of nursing: Concepts and procedures* (4th ed.). Menlo Park, CA: Addison-Wesley.

Lewis, S., and Collier, I. (1996). *Medical-surgical nursing: Assessment and management of clinical problems* (4th ed.). St. Louis: Mosby-Year Book.

Lippincott's Nursing Drug Guide, 1997. (1996). Philadelphia: Lippincott-Raven.

Lubkin, I.M. (1995). *Chronic illness: Impact and interventions* (3rd ed.). Boston: Jones and Bartlett.

Meltzer, M., and Palau, S.M. (1993). *Reading and study strategies for nursing students.* Philadelphia: WB Saunders.

Metheny, N.M. (1996). *Fluid and electrolyte balance: Nursing considerations* (3rd ed.). Philadelphia: Lippincott-Raven.

Pagana, K.D., and Pagana, T.J. (1995). *Mosby's diagnostic and laboratory test reference* (2nd ed.). St. Louis: Mosby-Year Book.

Pojman, L.P. (1992). *Life and death: Grappling with the moral dilemmas of our time.* Boston: Jones and Bartlett.

Porth, C.M. (1994). *Pathophysiology: Concepts of altered health states* (4th ed.). Philadelphia: JB Lippincott.

Potter, P., and Perry, A. (1995). *Basic nursing theory and practice* (3rd ed.). St. Louis: CV Mosby.

Potter, P., and Perry, A.G. (1997). *Fundamentals of nursing: Concepts, process, and practice* (4th ed.). St. Louis: Mosby-Year Book.

Smeltzer, S.C., and Bare, B.G. (1996). *Brunner and Suddarth's textbook of medical-surgical nursing* (8th ed.). Philadelphia: Lippincott-Raven.

Swearingen, P.L., and Keen, J.H. (1991). *Manual of critical care: Applying nursing diagnoses to adult critical illness* (2nd ed.). St. Louis: Mosby-Year Book.

Taylor, C., Lillis, C.A., and LeMone, P. (1996). *Fundamentals of nursing: The art and science of nursing care* (3rd ed.). Philadelphia: Lippincott-Raven.

Thelan, L.A., Davie, J.K., and Urden, L.D. (1994). *Textbook of critical care nursing: Diagnosis and management* (2nd ed.). St. Louis: Mosby-Year Book.

Tilkian, A.G., and Conover, M.B. (1993). *Understanding heart sounds and murmurs: With an introduction to lung sounds* (3rd ed.). Philadelphia: WB Saunders.

Section TWO

Postreview Tests

Part V

Postreview Comprehensive Tests

These four tests resemble the National Council Examination for Registered Nurses (NCLEX-RN). Just as the examination is comprehensive, so are these tests. After you have completed the four comprehensive tests, refer to the sections entitled "Correct Answers and Rationale" to reinforce or increase your knowledge and to evaluate your success. Study the rationale for each item carefully. Reading the rationale for items that you answered correctly reinforces your knowledge, whereas reading the rationale for items that you answered incorrectly clarifies misconceptions and expands your knowledge.

To evaluate your success on a comprehensive test, make a check mark next to the items you answered incorrectly and then determine the percentage of items you answered correctly. To do so, divide the number of your correct responses by the total number of questions in the test and multiply by 100. For example, if you answered 80 of 90 questions correctly, divide 80 by 90 and multiply by 100. The result is 89%. If you answered more than 75% of the items correctly, you are most likely prepared to take the NCLEX-RN. If, however, you answered less than 75% of the items correctly, carefully examine the items that you answered incorrectly. Did you answer incorrectly because of lack of content knowledge or because you did not read carefully? Errors attributable to not reading the question carefully indicate the need to revise your test-taking strategies (see the introduction to this book). Lack of knowledge indicates the need for further review in that content area. If you identify areas in which you need more concentrated review, you can complete the questions in the section of this book devoted to that clinical area. More information about NCLEX-RN and the format and use of this review is presented in the introduction to this book.

Comprehensive Test 1

Select the one best answer, and indicate your choice by filling in the circle in front of the option.

1. A client who comes to the emergency department complaining of back and left flank pain is tentatively diagnosed with renal calculi. Initially, the pain was dull and constant, but now the client is experiencing periods of complete comfort alternating with periods of excruciating pain. The priority nursing diagnosis for this client would be
   - ○ 1. Activity Intolerance.
   - ○ 2. Pain.
   - ○ 3. Fluid Volume Deficit.
   - ○ 4. Impaired Skin Integrity.

2. A 2-year-old child is brought to the emergency room with a broken arm. Which of the following findings would lead the nurse to suspect child abuse?
   - ○ 1. The child has bruises on the forearms.
   - ○ 2. The child's clothes are dirty and torn and obviously "hand-me-downs."
   - ○ 3. The child's father alters the story of the injury each time he tells it.
   - ○ 4. The child's mother did not come to the hospital with the child.

3. While making a home visit to a multigravida 2 weeks after delivery of viable twins at 38 weeks' gestation, the nurse observes that the client looks pale, has dark circles around her eyes, and is breast-feeding one of the twins. The client's apartment is clean, and nothing appears out of place. The client tells the nurse that she completed three loads of laundry this morning. A priority nursing diagnosis for this client is
   - ○ 1. Anxiety related to inability to cope with twins who are breast-feeding.
   - ○ 2. Potential for Altered Nutrition: Less Than Body Requirements related to twin delivery.
   - ○ 3. Potential for Anemia related to large volume of blood loss and twin delivery.
   - ○ 4. High Risk for Fatigue related to home maintenance and caring for twins.

4. A client has been taking prescribed aspirin in large doses. She complains of stomach irritation, sometimes with vomiting. Of the following foods and beverages, the one most likely contributing to her gastrointestinal irritation would be
   - ○ 1. dry toast several times a day.
   - ○ 2. a hard-boiled egg at least once a day.
   - ○ 3. sweetened tea with each meal.
   - ○ 4. several ounces of wine before her evening meal.

5. A 9-month-old well-nourished boy who lives with his extensive extended family tests positive for tuberculosis. Which of the following is a risk factor for tuberculosis in this client?
   - ○ 1. The infant is a boy.
   - ○ 2. The infant is in the 95% for height and weight.
   - ○ 3. His mother did not receive prenatal care until the second trimester of her pregnancy.
   - ○ 4. The client is an infant.

6. A multipara asks the nurse during a home visit about breast-feeding. She tells the nurse that with her last newborn, her nipples became cracked and sore. The nurse should instruct the client that
   - ○ 1. the newborn's mouth should cover the areola during the feeding.
   - ○ 2. breast-feeding every 4 to 5 hours should decrease nipple soreness.
   - ○ 3. nipples should be washed with a mild soap and rinsed thoroughly.
   - ○ 4. using latex nipple shields that fit over the client's own nipples should alleviate the problem.

7. The client with dual diagnoses of major depression and alcohol abuse states, "I only drink when I can't sleep." An expected outcome for this client is that the client will
   - ○ 1. describe adaptive methods of coping to induce sleep.
   - ○ 2. verbalize negative effects of alcohol on the body.
   - ○ 3. describe dangerous effects when combining alcohol and antidepressant medication.
   - ○ 4. verbalize the desire to stop drinking alcohol.

8. A preschool-aged child who is hospitalized with gastroenteritis has been NPO. The physician has written an order to advance the diet as tolerated. The first feeding the nurse should offer the child is
   - ○ 1. cooked cereal.
   - ○ 2. ice cream shake.
   - ○ 3. clear lemon carbonated beverage.
   - ○ 4. toast.

9. While caring for a multigravida in active labor with no anesthesia, the nurse midwife determines that the client's cervix is completely dilated. The nurse midwife should instruct the client to deliver the fetal head by pushing
   - ○ 1. as soon as a contraction begins.
   - ○ 2. when she has an urge to push.

○ 3. near the end of a contraction.

○ 4. between contractions.

10. Classic signs of rheumatoid arthritis include

○ 1. pain on weight-bearing, rash, and low-grade fever.

○ 2. joint swelling, joint stiffness in the morning, and bilateral joint involvement.

○ 3. crepitus, development of Heberden's nodes, and anemia.

○ 4. fatigue, leukopenia, and joint pain.

11. The nurse will conduct a psychoeducational group for family members on depression. Which of the following topics would be of little help to the family members?

○ 1. Managing the depressed client at home.

○ 2. Drug classifications.

○ 3. Support and self-help groups.

○ 4. Skills for self-preservation.

12. Which of the following statements indicates the client needs further teaching about taking medication to control his cancer pain?

○ 1. "I should take my medication around-the-clock to control my pain."

⊗ 2. "I should skip doses periodically so I don't get hooked on my drugs."

○ 3. "It is okay to take my pain medication even if I am not having any pain."

○ 4. "I should contact the oncology nurse if my pain is not effectively controlled."

13. The nurse is caring for a primipara after a cesarean section delivery 12 hours ago. The nurse observes that the client's fundus is at the umbilicus and firm. The nurse should

○ 1. ask the client if she feels the urge to void.

○ 2. document this as a normal finding.

○ 3. contact the physician for an order for an oxytocic.

○ 4. encourage the client to remain on bed rest.

14. An infant admitted to the hospital with acute rotovirus is having frequent diarrheal stools; on assessment, the nurse notes 40 to 60 bowel sounds per minute. The child has poor skin turgor, and the mucous membranes are dry. The nurse would make a nursing diagnosis of Fluid Volume Deficit related to

○ 1. decreased gastric emptying.

○ 2. insufficient antidiuretic hormone.

○ 3. inability to metabolize nutrients.

⊗ 4. increased gastrointestinal motility.

15. The nurse is conducting an initial nursing history of a client who is experiencing pain related to bone cancer. The most important information to gather in this initial assessment is the

○ 1. nurse's physical assessment of the client.

○ 2. amount of pain medication the client is taking.

⊗ 3. client's self-reporting of her pain experience.

○ 4. family's response to the client's illness.

16. A client has had a cast applied to his arm as an outpatient in the emergency room. Which of the following home care instructions would be appropriate for cast care? The client should

○ 1. use powder on the skin around the cast.

○ 2. smell the cast for foul odors.

○ 3. use a ruler to reach inside and scratch under the cast.

○ 4. apply a heating pad to the arm for 24 hours after the injury.

17. In teaching a client about Alcoholics Anonymous (AA), the nurse states that AA has helped in the rehabilitation of many alcoholics, probably because many people find it easier to change their behavior when they

○ 1. have the support of rehabilitated alcoholics.

○ 2. know that rehabilitated alcoholics will sympathize with them.

○ 3. can depend on rehabilitated alcoholics to help them identify personal problems related to alcoholism.

○ 4. realize that rehabilitated alcoholics will help them develop mechanisms to cope with their alcoholism.

18. The client walks into the mental health clinic and states to the nurse, "I guess I can't make it without my wife. I can't even sleep without her." Which of the following responses by the nurse would be most therapeutic?

○ 1. "Things always look worse before they get better."

○ 2. "I'd say that you're not giving yourself a fair chance."

○ 3. "You can make it, given a little more time. Don't hurry yourself."

○ 4. "I'm interested in knowing more about what you mean when you say that you can't make it without your wife."

19. The nurse preparing to give a child an intramuscular injection chooses to give the injection into the gluteal muscle. The site is acceptable because the child

○ 1. has been walking for 1 year.

○ 2. has small deltoid muscles.

○ 3. is older than 2 years.

○ 4. weighs more than 25 pounds.

20. The primary purpose of administering aminophylline to a client with emphysema is to

○ 1. relieve diaphragm spasms.

○ 2. relax smooth muscles in the bronchioles.

○ 3. promote efficient pulmonary circulation.

○ 4. stimulate chemoreceptors in the medullary respiratory center.

21. An infant who has undergone surgery for bilateral clubfoot returns from the operating room with bilateral casts. After noting that the infant's toes are slightly cool and edematous, the nurse should first

○ 1. cut the casts.

○ 2. elevate the legs on pillows.

○ 3. notify the surgeon.

○ 4. place warm packs on the child's feet.

22. During the conversation with the nurse, a victim of physical abuse says, "Let me try to explain why I stay with my husband." Which of the following reasons would the client be least likely to mention?

○ 1. "I'm responsible for keeping my family together."

○ 2. "When it's not too bad, the abuse adds spice to our relationship."

○ 3. "I have only a sixth-grade education."

○ 4. "I'm not sure I could get a job that pays even minimum wage."

23. The nurse is caring for a primigravida in active labor when the client's membranes rupture spontaneously. The nurse should assess the client for

○ 1. increased intensity of contractions.

○ 2. fetal head engagement.

○ 3. prolapsed cord.

○ 4. a need for an analgesic medication.

24. During a home visit, the client tells the nurse she's not taking prescribed doses of haloperidol (Haldol) because she's tired of bothering with it and doesn't need it. The nurse's best action is to

○ 1. explain the negative effects of skipping the medication.

○ 2. consult with the physician about changing the medication to haloperidol decanoate (Haldol Decanoate) injections.

○ 3. have the client's family begin commitment procedures so that her medication regimen can be supervised more closely.

○ 4. refer the client to a partial hospitalization program so that she can participate regularly in group therapy sessions.

25. A primipara on the postpartum unit 2 hours after a vaginal delivery tells the nurse that she was in labor for 16 hours and pushed for 2 hours before delivery of a viable female neonate. She tells the nurse that she is "thirsty and very happy it is over." A priority nursing diagnosis for this client is

○ 1. Fluid Volume Deficit related to decreased fluid intake during labor.

○ 2. Potential for Altered Parenting related to lack of experience as a mother.

○ 3. Potential for Urinary Retention related to lengthy labor process.

○ 4. Anxiety related to inexperience in the new role of parenting.

26. A priority nursing diagnosis for the client after a total laryngectomy for cancer of the larynx is

○ 1. Altered Gastrointestinal Function.

○ 2. Fluid Volume Overload.

○ 3. Potential for Emboli.

○ 4. Inability to Communicate.

27. A nurse observes a family in the waiting room of a well child clinic. Which of the following behaviors would be considered to be an example of social affective play?

○ 1. The 8-year-old is taking turns playing a hand-held video game with another child he met in the waiting room.

○ 2. The 4-year-old is listening to the mother's chest with a stethoscope.

○ 3. The infant makes happy noises in response to her father speaking to her.

○ 4. The 2-year-old is sitting in her mother's lap hugging a teddy bear.

28. Diuretic therapy with torsemide is started for a client with heart failure. When calling the client 2 days after the drug therapy is started, the nurse evaluates the torsemide as effective when the client says she

○ 1. has an improved appetite and is eating better.

○ 2. weighs 6 pounds less than she did 2 days ago.

○ 3. is less thirsty than she was.

○ 4. has clearer urine after starting the torsemide.

29. A client is 6 hours postoperative an abdominal hysterectomy. Since the surgery, the client has voided three times, about 25 mL each time. Based on these data, the nurse determines that the client

○ 1. is probably dehydrated and needs additional intravenous fluids.

○ 2. is experiencing urinary retention and needs to be catheterized.

○ 3. has a normal postoperative urinary pattern and needs no intervention.

○ 4. has probably developed a urinary tract infection and needs antibiotics.

30. The client has been taking the monoamine oxidase inhibitor (MAOI) phenelzine (Nardil), 10 mg bid. The physician orders a selective serotonin reuptake inhibitor (SSRI), paroxetine (Paxil), 20 mg given every morning. The nurse

○ 1. gives the medication as ordered.

○ 2. questions the physician about the order.

○ 3. questions the dosage ordered.

○ 4. asks the physician to order benztropine (Cogentin) for the side effects.

31. A young woman with a malignant growth on the larynx is admitted to the hospital for a laryngectomy. The client would most likely state that the earliest symptom of her health problem was

○ 1. a sore throat.

○ 2. chronic hoarseness.

○ 3. pain radiating to the ear.

○ 4. difficulty swallowing.

32. The nurse is caring for a client who has experienced severe multiple trauma. The client's arterial blood gases reveal low arterial oxygen levels that are not responsive to high concentrations of oxygen. The nurse is aware that this finding is a major indicator of the development of

○ 1. hypostatic pneumonia.

○ 2. hypovolemic shock.

○ 3. adult respiratory distress syndrome.

○ 4. asthma.

33. After undergoing gastrectomy surgery, the nurse should position the client in bed in which position?

○ 1. Prone.

○ 2. Supine.

○ 3. Low-Fowler's.

○ 4. Right or left Sims'.

34. The clinic nurse is instructing a group of parents about emergency treatment for accidental poisoning. The nurse would need to do further teaching if one of the mother states, "I should

○ 1. flush my child's eye with room temperature tap water for 15 to 20 minutes if a caustic material gets into it."

○ 2. save the emesis if my child vomits."

○ 3. call the poison control center if there are any symptoms."

○ 4. give 2 to 5 teaspoons of clear fluids after administering ipecac."

35. A voluntary client has been taking haloperidol (Haldol) as prescribed. One morning, she refuses to take the Haldol. Which of the following actions should the nurse take?

○ 1. Summon another nurse to help ensure that the client takes her medicine.

○ 2. Tell the client that she can take the medication either orally or by injection.

○ 3. Withhold the medication until it is determined why the client is refusing to take it.

○ 4. Tell the client that she needs to take her "vitamin" to stay healthy.

36. To help promote independence in the area of feeding for a school-aged child in skeletal traction, the nurse would help the child choose which of the following meals?

○ 1. Carrot sticks, celery with cream cheese, roast beef and gravy, peas, gelatin, and milk in a cup.

○ 2. Chicken noodle soup with crackers, grilled cheese sandwich, cole slaw, and chocolate milk in a carton.

○ 3. Chicken nuggets with sauce, carrot sticks, French-fried potatoes, ice cream sandwich, and milk in a carton.

○ 4. Spaghetti and meat sauce, cherry cobbler, and apple juice in a can.

37. A 1-day postpartum client asks the nurse about resuming sexual activity after delivery of a viable male infant. After giving instructions, the nurse determines that the client understands the instructions when she says,

○ 1. "I should refrain from intercourse until I no longer have any vaginal discharge."

○ 2. "Kegel exercises shouldn't be started until 4 weeks postpartum."

○ 3. "Sexual intercourse may be resumed about 3 to 4 weeks postpartum."

○ 4. "Sitz baths once a week can help to heal the episiotomy."

38. The nurse is caring for a primipara who delivered a viable neonate 12 hours ago. While caring for the client, the client says, "Look at all of the beautiful things my family brought for the new baby." The nurse should become concerned if the client has

○ 1. four neonatal receiving blankets.

○ 2. breast-pumping equipment.

○ 3. a soft pillow for the neonate's crib.

○ 4. a clean, but used, infant car seat.

39. A 4-year-old is admitted to the emergency room with sudden onset of a temperature of 103°F, sore throat, and refusal to drink .The child will not lie down and prefers to lean forward while sitting up. Which of the following plans are not appropriate?

○ 1. Give 240 mg acetaminophen (Tylenol) per rectum.

○ 2. Start an intravenous infusion of 5% dextrose in 0.45% saline.

○ 3. Have an appropriate-sized tracheostomy tube and tracheostomy tray available.

○ 4. Obtain a throat culture.

40. A client who has a fractured leg has been instructed to ambulate without weight-bearing on the affected leg. The nurse evaluates that the client is ambulating correctly if he uses which of the following crutch-walking gaits?

○ 1. Two-point gait.

○ 2. Four-point gait.

○ 3. Three-point gait.

○ 4. Swing-to gait.

41. A client with diabetes is explaining to the nurse how he cares for his feet at home. Which statement indicates the client needs *further* instruction on how to care for his feet properly?

○ 1. "I inspect my feet once a week for cuts and redness."

○ 2. "I am not allowed to use a heating pad on my feet."

○ 3. "It is important to dry my feet carefully after my bath."

○ 4. "I should not go barefoot, even in my home."

42. The client is taking fluoxetine (Prozac), 20 mg, at

bedtime. He states that Prozac is not helping him to sleep. The nurse judges

- ○ 1. that the client should take Prozac in the morning.
- ○ 2. that dose is too high.
- ○ 3. that the client's symptoms of depression seem to be getting worse.
- ○ 4. that the client is on the wrong medication.

43. A client, who is a computer operator, has developed carpal tunnel syndrome. The nurse explains to the client that carpal tunnel syndrome is caused by

- ○ 1. decreased circulation to the brachial nerve.
- ○ 2. muscle atrophy resulting from disuse.
- ○ 3. median nerve compression.
- ○ 4. progressive contraction of the wrist.

44. To help prevent hip flexion deformities associated with rheumatoid arthritis, the nurse should help the client assume which of the following positions in bed several times a day?

- ○ 1. Prone.
- ○ 2. Very low Fowler's.
- ○ 3. Modified Trendelenburg's.
- ○ 4. Side-lying.

45. A client with bipolar disorder, manic phase, has a nursing diagnosis of Altered Nutrition: Less Than Body Requirements. To help the client meet recommended daily allowances of nutrients, which of the following nursing interventions would be best?

- ○ 1. Give the client half of a meat and cheese sandwich between meals.
- ○ 2. Inform the client that snacks are available only if he eats properly at mealtime.
- ○ 3. Tell the client to sit alone at mealtime so that he won't be distracted by others.
- ○ 4. Teach the client about proper nutrition.

46. On the second postpartum day, a primipara, who is breast-feeding her neonate, asks the nurse, "How many wet diapers should I plan to change every day?" The nurse should instruct the client that after the first 24 to 48 hours of life, the neonate should have at least

- ○ 1. 2 to 3 wet diapers a day.
- ○ 2. 4 to 5 wet diapers a day.
- ○ 3. 6 to 8 wet diapers a day.
- ○ 4. 9 to 12 wet diapers a day.

47. A 30-year-old female client visits the family planning clinic and desires oral contraceptives. While obtaining the nursing history, the client tells the nurse that she was hospitalized 3 years ago for thrombophlebitis. After giving instructions about contraindications to combined forms of oral contraceptives, the nurse determines that the client understands the instructions when she says,

- ○ 1. "Because I have had thrombophlebitis, I should use another type of contraception."
- ○ 2. "I should start out with the mini-pill, and see if that is effective."
- ○ 3. "I should immediately report any signs of calf tenderness while I am taking the pills."
- ○ 4. "Because of my age, I should probably choose a different method of contraception."

48. When conducting a screening session for hypertension at the retirement center, the nurse encounters a client who has a long history of uncontrolled hypertension. Teaching for this client should include information about how chronic hypertension can lead to eye problems resulting from damage to the eye's

- ○ 1. iris.
- ○ 2. cornea.
- ○ 3. retina.
- ○ 4. sclera.

49. The nurse plans to administer an injection of heparin to a client. Which of the following techniques for heparin administration is appropriate? The nurse

- ○ 1. selects a 1.5-inch, 21-gauge needle for the injection.
- ○ 2. makes the injection into the deltoid muscle.
- ○ 3. applies gentle pressure to the site for 5 to 10 seconds after the injection.
- ○ 4. aspirates with the plunger to check for entry into the blood vessel before injecting the heparin.

50. The nurse observes a neonate at 2 hours after birth and determines that the neonate has acrocyanosis. The nurse should explain to the neonate's parents that this symptom is due to

- ○ 1. cardiac anomalies.
- ○ 2. sluggish peripheral circulation.
- ○ 3. vasomotor instability.
- ○ 4. decreased red blood cell production.

51. An adolescent has just been admitted to the hospital with the probable diagnosis of leukemia. He complains of feeling tired all the time, low-grade fever, and bruises on his arms and legs. The nurse is planning care for him and would include which of the following as a priority nursing diagnosis?

- ○ 1. Impaired Skin Integrity.
- ○ 2. Powerlessness.
- ○ 3. Fatigue.
- ○ 4. Anxiety.

52. A client visits the clinic, and it is determined that she is about 10 weeks' gestation with her first pregnancy. After the nurse has explained exercise during pregnancy, the nurse determines that the client understands the instructions when she says,

- ○ 1. "I should avoid any contact sports."
- ○ 2. "Even if I am pregnant, I can learn how to downhill ski next month."
- ○ 3. "I can go scuba diving with my husband while we are in Florida next week."

4. "I should avoid my usual swimming routine."

53. After teaching the parents of a toddler about appropriate snack foods for toddlers, the nurse would judge that the instructions about not giving the child raisins for snacks are effective when the father states, "Raisins
    1. are low in nutritive value."
    2. can increase tooth decay."
    3. are easily aspirated."
    4. cannot be entirely digested."

54. The nurse has assisted a multigravida with a precipitous delivery of a viable neonate in a local grocery store. While waiting for the ambulance to arrive, the nurse should
    1. wrap the placenta in aluminum foil.
    2. massage the client's fundus continuously.
    3. remain with the client and newborn.
    4. contact the client's family.

55. The nurse is caring for a primigravida who delivered a viable neonate 2 hours ago under epidural anesthesia and a midline episiotomy. Which of the following findings by the nurse would warrant further assessment?
    1. Distended vaginal tissue.
    2. Slight edema around the episiotomy site.
    3. Two perineal pads soaked within 30 minutes.
    4. Yellowish fluid leaking from the breasts.

56. A client admits to using cocaine and says, "When I stop using, I feel bad." Which of the following effects is the client most likely to describe as occurring after he stops using cocaine?
    1. Depression.
    2. Palpitations.
    3. Flashbacks.
    4. Double vision.

57. When inserting a rectal suppository for an adult client, the nurse should
    1. insert the suppository while the client bears down.
    2. place the client in a supine position.
    3. position the suppository along the rectal wall.
    4. insert the suppository 2 inches into the rectum.

58. A primipara 28 hours postpartum is to be given medroxyprogesterone acetate (Depo-Provera) intramuscularly before discharge from the birthing center. Before administering the medication, the nurse should instruct the client that for clients who received this medication
    1. breast-feeding is contraindicated.
    2. amenorrhea is common for the first 6 months.
    3. heavy menstrual bleeding may occur.
    4. blurred vision and seeing spots may occur.

59. The nurse has discussed sexuality issues during the prenatal period with a primigravida at 32 weeks' gestation with one episode of preterm labor before discharge from the birthing center. The nurse determines that the client understands the instructions when she says,
    1. "I can resume sexual intercourse when the bleeding stops."
    2. "I should not get sexually aroused or have any nipple stimulation."
    3. "I can resume sexual intercourse in 1 to 2 weeks."
    4. "I should not have sexual intercourse until I see the doctor at my next prenatal visit."

60. After teaching a client about myasthenia gravis, the nurse would judge that the client has formed a realistic concept of her condition when she says that by taking her medication and pacing her activities,
    1. she will live longer, but ultimately the disease will cause her death.
    2. her symptoms will be controlled, and eventually the disease will be cured.
    3. she should be able to control the disease and enjoy a healthy lifestyle.
    4. her fatigue will be relieved, but she should expect occasional periods of muscle weakness.

61. The nurse planning interventions for the victim of physical abuse would base the plan on knowledge that
    1. a woman in crisis is unlikely to be receptive to professional help.
    2. the client generally can control the batterer.
    3. assessing the client's level of danger is a prerequisite to intervention.
    4. success is least likely with a multidisciplinary approach.

62. The nurse is planning care for a client with Alzheimer's disease. Which of the following activities would be of least benefit to the client?
    1. Reminiscence group.
    2. Walking.
    3. Pet therapy.
    4. Stress management.

63. Health-promotion activities to reduce the incidence of osteoporosis include
    1. teaching women to maintain adequate calcium intake.
    2. teaching women how to administer pain medication safely.
    3. teaching women to increase caffeine intake as a preventive measure.
    4. avoiding estrogen replacement therapy when postmenopausal.

64. The nurse is assessing the neurovascular status of a client's right arm that is newly casted with a short arm cast. Which of the following assessment findings should be reported to the physician?
    1. Nail bed capillary refill time of 10 seconds.
    2. Localized pain in the right arm
    3. Slight swelling of the fingers.

○ 4. No pain on passive movement of fingers.

65. The client is taking clozapine (Clozaril). His pulse is 144 beats/minute. The nurse's best action is
○ 1. give the clozapine, and tell the client to lie down.
○ 2. withhold the clozapine, and tell the client to go to exercise group.
○ 3. give the clozapine, and notify the physician.
○ 4. withhold the clozapine, and notify the physician.

66. A 20-year-old single parent brings her 3-year-old son into the emergency department because "he fell." The child has bruises on his face, arms, and legs; his mother says that she did not witness the fall. The nurse suspects child abuse. While examining the child, the mother says, "sometimes I guess I'm pretty rough with him. I'm alone, and I just don't know how to manage him." Referral to what type of program would be most appropriate for the mother at this time?
○ 1. A program for single parents.
○ 2. A parenting education program.
○ 3. A women's support group.
○ 4. A support group for abusive parents.

67. The nurse in the coronary care unit obtains a pulse rate of 116 before administering digoxin to the client with heart failure. The appropriate action by the nurse is to
○ 1. administer the digoxin.
○ 2. withhold the digoxin, and take the pulse again in 15 minutes.
○ 3. obtain the client's respiratory rate.
○ 4. evaluate the client's cardiac rhythm.

68. A nurse is performing a Denver Developmental Screening Test on a 4-year-old. The nurse determines that the test has resulted in an abnormal score when there are
○ 1. a large number of refusals.
○ 2. more failures than passes along the age line.
○ 3. one sector with two or more failures.
○ 4. two or more sectors with two or more delays.

69. A pregnant client at 12 weeks' gestation visits the clinic for a routine visit. The nurse plans to discuss neonatal nutrition with the client. The nurse should plan to instruct the client that
○ 1. formula feeding provides greater calories to the neonate than breast-feeding.
○ 2. breast-feeding can be successful even if the mother does not want to breast-feed.
○ 3. breast milk is sufficient to provide nutrition for the first 4 months of the neonate's life.
○ 4. no additional daily calories are needed for the breast-feeding mother.

70. A primigravida at 36 weeks' gestation complains of discomfort during a pelvic examination. To help the client relax during the examination, the nurse should instruct the client to

○ 1. breathe in and out with slow deep breaths.
○ 2. hold on tightly to the nurse with both hands.
○ 3. visualize the examination being completed.
○ 4. hold her breath until the speculum is inserted.

71. How can the emergency room nurse quickly estimate the extent of an adult client's burns?
○ 1. By correlating the percentage of the burned area with the client's admission weight.
○ 2. By dividing the body into areas equal to multiples of nine, with the calculation based on areas affected.
○ 3. By calculating the circumference of the body, then measuring and subtracting unburned areas from the total.
○ 4. By measuring the burned area in square inches, then multiplying that total by a factor of 0.862.

72. After completing teaching about sickle cell disease to a mother, the nurse would be concerned when the mother stated,
○ 1. "I need to stop at the health food store to pick up medicines that my child will need."
○ 2. "When my child runs a high fever, I will need to call the physician."
○ 3. "I will be sure to give her a lot of fluids when she gets sick."
○ 4. "I know she does not have as much pain as she acts like she has."

73. The nurse is caring for a multigravida in active labor when the nurse observes a variable fetal heart rate deceleration pattern. The nurse should first
○ 1. administer oxygen by mask at 4 liters.
○ 2. contact the client's physician.
○ 3. change the client's position.
○ 4. document the tracing in the client's record.

74. The nurse plans to teach a client who is receiving radiation therapy how to care for his skin at home. The nurse's instructions should include:
○ 1. "Apply a heating pad to the area to relieve pain."
○ 2. "You may use deodorant soap if you wish to cleanse the area."
○ 3. "Put baby oil on the area after each treatment to keep it from getting dry."
○ 4. "Keep the area covered when you go outdoors."

75. Typically, parents who abuse children
○ 1. were also abused as children.
○ 2. married at a very early age.
○ 3. did not want any children.
○ 4. are disappointed in the sex of the child.

76. Which of the following assessments would be important for the nurse to make to determine whether a client is recovering as expected from spinal anesthesia?
○ 1. Level of consciousness.
○ 2. Rate and depth of respirations.
○ 3. Rate of capillary refill in the toes.

4. Degree of response to pinpricks in the legs and toes.

77. A 64-year-old man is admitted to the emergency room with palpitations, a choking sensation, and tightness in the chest. He is hyperventilating. The nurse analyzes the results of arterial blood gas (ABG) studies. In this situation, the ABG studies would likely reveal excessive loss of
   ○ 1. sodium.
   ○ 2. oxygen.
   ○ 3. potassium.
   ○ 4. carbon dioxide.

78. Which of the following behaviors displayed by a 13-year-old boy dying of leukemia would most clearly indicate his need for emotional support?
   ○ 1. Teasing his sister about her new boyfriend.
   ○ 2. Wanting to have someone with him at all times.
   ○ 3. Having the nurse wait with his bath while he makes a telephone call.
   ○ 4. Complaining about the limited number of choices on the dietary list.

79. During hospitalization, a client with bulimia stops vomiting but becomes fearful that she will gain weight. She tells the nurse, "I can't gain weight. I'm fat enough as it is. I'll be really disgusting if I get fatter." When responding to this client, it would be most therapeutic for the nurse to
   ○ 1. explain that the calories in her prescribed diet are not enough to cause weight gain.
   ○ 2. tell her that she is not fat, and encourage her to negotiate a calorie change with the nutritionist.
   ○ 3. validate her feelings, and help her identify positive aspects of herself other than appearance.
   ○ 4. reassure her that the staff will take complete control of her eating and will prevent her from gaining weight in the hospital.

80. The nurse is caring for a primipara during the first hour after a vaginal delivery of a viable neonate under lumbar epidural anesthesia and intravenous fluids. While assessing the client, the nurse observes that the client has a pulse rate of 65 beats/minute, temperature of 99.9°F, fundus firm at one finger breath above the midline, and a slow trickle of dark red vaginal bleeding on the perineal pad. The client's legs are still somewhat numb. The nurse should
   ○ 1. notify the anesthesiologist who performed the lumbar epidural anesthesia.
   ○ 2. continue to monitor the client's temperature on an hourly basis.
   ○ 3. massage the fundus and contact the client's physician immediately.
   ○ 4. discontinue the client's intravenous fluids if the client is drinking fluids.

81. After talking with the nurse, the client admits to being physically abused by her husband. She says that she has never called the police because her husband has threatened to kill her if she does. She says, "I don't want to get him into trouble because he's the father of my children. I don't know what to do!" Which of the following nursing interventions would be most therapeutic at this time?
   ○ 1. Express concern for the client's safety.
   ○ 2. Help the client identify the behaviors that provoke the abuse.
   ○ 3. Teach the client ways to reduce stress within her family.
   ○ 4. Tell the client that she should leave her husband.

82. An 8-year-old child with severe cerebral palsy is underweight and undersized for his age. He is being fed a diet of pureed foods and liquids through a syringe. An appropriate nursing diagnosis for this child would be Altered Nutrition: Less Than Body Requirements related to
   ○ 1. impaired oral motor control.
   ○ 2. increased metabolism.
   ○ 3. inability to metabolize fats.
   ○ 4. increased intracranial pressure.

83. A school-aged child has her broken arm in a cast. The parents are ready to take her home from the emergency room. Discharge teaching should consist of telling the parents that which of the following would indicate she needed to be brought back to the emergency room?
   ○ 1. The plaster cast does not dry in 4 hours.
   ○ 2. The cast feels too heavy, and it's hard for her to move her arm.
   ○ 3. Her fingers become pale, and she complains of numbness.
   ○ 4. Her pain is not better 30 minutes after taking acetaminophen.

84. A male client with an obsessive-compulsive disorder frequently washes his feet, which often makes him late for meals, group activities, therapy sessions, and other occasions. It probably would be best for the nurse to help the client overcome this habitual tardiness by planning to
   ○ 1. explain how his tardiness for scheduled activities interferes with his getting well.
   ○ 2. help him stop his ritualistic behavior when it is time for him to leave for scheduled activities.
   ○ 3. allow him to decide whether he wishes to attend scheduled activities or do his ritualistic behavior.
   ○ 4. remind him early enough that he can carry out his ritualistic behavior in time to arrive for scheduled activities.

85. A community health nurse has taught a parent in clinic about the ages that children receive immunizations and the reason why certain immunizations are given at different times. The nurse would evalu-

ate the teaching as successful when she overhears this parent tell another parent,

○ 1. "My 6-month-old will have to wait for the MMR (measles, mumps, and rubella) because complete immunity is not achieved until the child is 12 months of age."

○ 2. "Children cannot receive two injections at the same time because it is too traumatic for them."

○ 3. "Children must wait 4 months between MMR and oral polio vaccines."

○ 4. "Your 15-month-old is fortunate that he never has to have another immunization again."

86. The mother of a toddler asks the nurse what she should do with her toddler when she has a temper tantrum. The nurse would advise

○ 1. moving the toddler to her time-out chair.

○ 2. trying to talk her out of the tantrum.

○ 3. leaving her alone during the tantrum as long as she is safe.

○ 4. punishing her for having a temper tantrum.

87. A client with an obsessive-compulsive disorder washes his feet frequently. Which of the following nursing diagnoses is specifically related to this behavior?

○ 1. Self-Care Deficit.

○ 2. High Risk for Impaired Skin Integrity.

○ 3. Ineffective Individual Coping.

○ 4. Anxiety (panic).

88. Which of the following signs would be indicative of peritonitis in a client with diverticulitis?

○ 1. Hyperactive bowel sounds.

○ 2. Rigid abdominal wall.

○ 3. Explosive diarrhea.

○ 4. Excessive flatulence.

89. A client with obsessive-compulsive disorder washes his feet endlessly because they "are so dirty that I can't put on my socks and shoes." The nurse recognizes the client is using ritualistic behavior primarily to relieve discomfort associated with feelings of

○ 1. depression.

○ 2. ambivalence.

○ 3. irrational fear.

○ 4. intolerable anxiety.

90. An 8-year-old child is sent home by the school nurse with pediculosis. The child's mother speaks with the nurse and is obviously upset and embarrassed. Which of the following statements by the mother would indicate to the nurse that she understands how her child got pediculosis?

○ 1. "I brush her hair twice a day."

○ 2. "I am very careful to shampoo her hair daily."

○ 3. "Could this result from sharing batting helmets at T-ball practice?"

○ 4. "We always use a dandruff-control shampoo."

CORRECT ANSWERS AND RATIONALE

The letters in parentheses following the rationale identify the step of the nursing process (A, D, P, I, E), cognitive level (K, C, T, N), client needs (S, G, L, H), and nursing care area (O, X, Y, M). See the Answer Grid for the key.

1. 2. Pain is a priority problem for the client with renal calculi. The pain is typically described as excruciating and intermittent, occurring as the stone moves. Analgesics are a major part of therapy. (D, N, G, M)

2. 3. The nurse should suspect child abuse when the child's caregiver changes the story of the injury each time it is told. A child who is still learning to walk and run often will have bruises on the forearms and shins; bruises on the upper arms and thighs are suspicious. Children often become dirty and tear clothes when they play. A parent may not be able to come to the hospital with the child for many reasons, such as care of other children, illness, or lack of transportation. (D, N, G, Y)

3. 4. Most postpartum clients complain of excessive fatigue after delivery. This multigravida is demonstrating dark circles around the eyes and is pale, which can indicate anemia or excessive sleep deprivation. The client maintains a spotless environment, has completed three loads of laundry, and is trying to breast-feed twins. There is no evidence of anxiety or altered nutrition. Anemia is not a nursing diagnosis. (D, N, H, O)

4. 4. Gastrointestinal irritation is a common side effect of aspirin, especially when taken in large doses. Such signs and symptoms as anorexia, nausea, vomiting, diarrhea, and constipation are also common. The combination of aspirin and alcohol is especially likely to cause gastrointestinal irritation, sometimes to the point of doing direct damage to gastric mucosa. (A, T, G, M)

5. 4. Infants are more susceptible to tuberculosis because of a diminished resistance to infection due to an immature immune system. In later childhood and adolescence, morbidity and mortality are higher in females than males. A higher than average weight and height would indicate that the child has had good nutrition. Poor nutrition is a risk factor for tuberculosis. Prenatal care is unrelated to tuberculosis. (A, C, G, Y)

6. 1. Cracked and sore nipples usually result from the newborn failing to take in the areola or from the nipple being improperly removed from the newborn's mouth. Most clients breast-feed on demand, and increasing the length of time between feedings does not affect nipple soreness or cracking. When one nipple is more sore than the other, the mother should be instructed to begin each feeding with the least sore side first. Nipples should be cleansed only with water because soap makes the nipples drier and more susceptible to cracking. Applying colostrum or breast milk to the nipples after the feeding aids healing. A mild analgesic can be taken before the feeding to ease nipple soreness. (I, T, H, O)

7. 1. The outcome specific to the client's needs is that the client will describe adaptive methods to use instead of drinking alcohol to induce sleep. Relaxation exercises, use of imagery, warm baths, and listening to relaxing music are adaptive methods the client can use. Verbalizing the negative effects of alcohol on the body, describing the dangerous effects of using alcohol with antidepressant medication, and verbalizing the desire to stop drinking alcohol are therapeutic behaviors but not specific to helping the client sleep. (E, N, L, X)

8. 1. A child with gastroenteritis should start to receive soft foods first after resting of the bowel and rehydration. Cooked cereals, vegetables, and meats are recommended. Milk-based foods are not recommended because a child with gastroenteritis may become lactose-intolerant for a period after the acute illness. (I, N, G, Y)

9. 2. During the second stage of labor (the stage of expulsion), uterine contractions often increase in intensity, frequency, and duration for a short period. The woman may immediately feel an urge to push, or it may take time for fetal descent to stimulate stretch receptors. Delivery of the fetal head should be accomplished slowly, about midway between contractions. Ritgen's technique may also be used. With this technique, when the fetal head causes distention of the perineum as it delivers, downward pressure is placed on the occiput, and forward pressure is placed on the neonate's chin. This technique allows for control of the head and facilitates extension of the head to prevent perineal lacerations. Intraabdominal pressure is combined with uterine contractions to expel the fetus. Therefore, pushing at the end of a contraction or between contractions is not as effective. Urging the mother to push before she feels the urge will needlessly tire the woman and prevent expulsion efforts from being as effective as possible. (I, T, G, O)

10. 2. Classic symptoms of rheumatoid arthritis include joint pain, swelling, and warmth. Symptoms are typically bilaterally symmetric. Joint stiffness in the morning lasting longer than 30 minutes is another classic symptom. Rheumatoid arthritis is a systemic disease. Other symptoms can include fatigue, low-grade fever, anemia, and weight loss. Heberden's nodes are present in osteoarthritis (degenerative joint disease). (A, K, G, M)

11. 2. Topics such as managing the depressed client at home, developing skills for self-preservation, and receiving support from self-help groups are helpful to family members. Focusing on antidepressant medications would be helpful, but the topic of drug classifications is too general. (P, T, L, X)

12. 2. The client should not skip dosages of his pain medication to prevent addiction. Clients with cancer pain do not become psychologically dependent on the medication and should not fear becoming addicted. The nurse should allow the client and family members to verbalize their concerns about drug addiction. The other statements indicate an appropriate understanding of pain therapy. (E, N, L, M)

13. 2. Clients who deliver by cesarean section are often given oxytocic medications to prevent uterine atony. The client's fundus located at the umbilicus 12 hours after delivery is a normal sign. There is no evidence of a full bladder, which would cause displacement of the fundus. The client does not need an oxytocic agent if the fundus is firm. Early ambulation is preferred to prolonged bed rest, and clients frequently have an order to be up in a chair soon after cesarean section delivery. (I, T, G, O)

14. 4. Rotovirus is a type of viral infection that affects the gastrointestinal tract. It causes diarrhea, which results in fluid loss. This type of infection can be very serious in infants, who cannot adjust to fluid loss as readily as adults because of their immature kidneys. Treatment is supportive. (D, N, G, Y)

15. 3. Although all the information listed is important to planning the care of the client, the most important component of pain assessment is the client's self-report of the pain. The nurse should have the client describe the quality, location, and intensity of the pain, the client's response to the pain, and alleviating or aggravating factors affecting the pain. (A, T, L, M)

16. 2. The client should be instructed to smell the cast to note foul odors, a sign of potential infection. Powder should not be used around the cast, and nothing should be inserted into the cast. A heating pad is not applied to a fracture; rather, the application of cold may be used to decrease edema and help decrease pain. (I, T, H, M)

17. 1. Membership in Alcoholics Anonymous (AA) is voluntary. Its rehabilitated members are available to support alcoholics, and the understanding and influence of these rehabilitated members often help alcoholics change their own behavior. The role of rehabilitated members does not include helping others abusing alcohol to identify personal problems, sympathizing with them, or helping them develop defense mechanisms to cope with alcoholism. (I, T, L, X)

18. 4. The nurse helps the client explore his feelings by expressing interest in knowing more about his problem in order to make an accurate assessment. Clichés and statements that make unwarranted judgments about the client are not helpful. (I, T, L, X)

19. 1. Muscle mass determines whether or not a muscle can be safely used as an injection site. The gluteal muscle enlarges in response to use in walking. After the child has been walking for a year, it should be safe to use the gluteus maximus for injections. Weight or age have only a minor influence on muscle mass. (I, T, S, Y)

20. 2. Aminophylline, a bronchodilator that relaxes smooth muscles in the bronchioles, is used in treatment of emphysema to improve ventilation by dilating the bronchioles. (I, T, G, M)

21. 2. The nurse's first action here is to elevate the part that is edematous. Decreasing the edema by promoting venous return may help improve circulation and warm the toes. The nurse should follow-up after a short time to evaluate whether the intervention is effective. The toes may also be cool because plaster casts are wet and cool. There is no reason to notify the surgeon at this time, nor should the casts be cut. A warm pack would be contraindicated at this point because it would serve to increase circulation and therefore the potential for edema and further decreasing venous return. (I, N, G, Y)

22. 2. Violence is never acceptable to a victim; this myth condones the use of violence. Often, an episode of battering is followed by a period of pleasant relations between the partners, during which the victim may hope that the violence will never happen again. The victim may stay in the relationship for that reason. Women are conditioned to be responsible for the family's well-being, and this is often a motivation for a battered woman to stay in an abusive relationship. A woman's lack of job skills and financial resources also may cause her to stay. Many women are injured or killed when they try to leave a violent relationship. (E, N, L, X)

23. 3. Whenever the membranes rupture, it is important for the nurse to assess for a prolapsed cord. Prolapse of the umbilical cord is a serious intrapartum complication, occurring in about 1 of 200 pregnancies. The spontaneous rupture of the membranes produces a gush of fluid, and the force can cause the cord to enter the vagina. This is an emergency situation because the compression of the fetal presenting part on the cord can occlude the perfusion of blood to the fetus. After spontaneous rupture of the membranes, the contractions may become more frequent and may increase in intensity, but this is not a priority at this time. There is no evidence that rupture of the membranes shortens labor. Checking whether the fetal head is engaged is not indicated. Once the membranes have ruptured, the client is at risk for chorioamnionitis; therefore, vaginal examinations should be kept to a minimum. (A, T, G, O)

24. 2. For the client who is noncompliant with oral medication, depot medication is advantageous because the client will only need to keep one appointment every 2 to 4 weeks instead of taking medication daily. Education may or may not affect the client's compliance with medication. Long-term commitment is unnecessary at this time. Participation in a partial hospitalization program may be a desirable referral but would affect the client's compliance with medication only indirectly. (I, T, L, X)

25. 1. The most appropriate priority diagnosis for this client is Fluid Volume Deficit. The average length of the second stage of labor is about 1 hour. Analgesia and anesthesia can result in a prolonged second stage of labor. Thirst is a common phenomenon after delivery because clients may be kept NPO during the labor process and may be dehydrated. There is no evidence that the client's inexperience as a mother will affect the bonding process. Although the nurse should monitor the client's intake and output after delivery, there is no evidence of a full bladder due to a lengthy labor process, so urinary retention is not a priority diagnosis at this time. The client has not expressed any evidence of anxiety at this point. (D, N, G, O)

26. 4. Inability to Communicate is a priority nursing diagnosis for the client after a total laryngectomy because the client will have a tracheostomy. These clients frequently require training on ways to communicate after surgery. Altered Gastrointestinal Function, Fluid Volume Overload, and Potential for Emboli are not priorities associated with laryngectomy surgery. (D, T, G, M)

27. 3. Social affective play occurs when infants take pleasure in relationships with people. The 4-year-old is participating in symbolic or pretend play. The 8-year-old is participating in interactive play. The 2-year-old is exhibiting unoccupied behavior. (A, T, H, Y)

28. 2. The primary purpose of a diuretic in a client with heart failure is to promote sodium and water excretion through the kidneys. As a result, the excessive body water that tends to accumulate in a client with heart failure is eliminated, which will cause the client to lose weight. Monitoring the client's weight daily helps evaluate the effectiveness of diuretic therapy. (E, T, G, M)

29. 2. Urinary control may not return for 6 to 8 hours after surgery owing to the effects of anesthesia and bladder manipulation during surgery. Urinary retention is common; voiding small amount of urine after surgery may be indicative of urinary retention. The nurse should further assess for bladder distention by palpating and percussing the bladder and should intervene with catheterization as appropriate. Clients should not be allowed to go longer than 6 to 8 hours without voiding or catheterization after surgery. (D, N, S, M)

30. 2. The nurse questions the physician about the order because the client who has been taking an MAOI such as phenelzine must wait 14 days after stopping the MAOI before starting an SSRI such as paroxetine. Serotonin syndrome, a potentially lethal consequence, can occur when combining an MAOI and an SSRI. The dosage is accurate. Benztropine is not given with an SSRI; it is an antiparkinsonian agent usually ordered for the side effects of antipsychotic medication. (I, T, G, X)

31. 2. Hoarseness that fails to subside with conservative care is an early sign of cancer of the larynx. Difficulty swallowing is a later symptom and occurs as the tumor enlarges to the point that it obstructs swallowing. Sore throat is not an early symptom of laryngeal cancer. Pain radiating to the ear may indicate that the tumor is metastasizing. (A, T, G, M)

32. 3. Adult respiratory distress syndrome (ARDS) frequently develops after a major insult to the body. The major diagnostic indicator is low arterial oxygen levels that are nonresponsive to the administration of high concentrations of oxygen. Early recognition of ARDS is important to increasing the client's chances of recovery, and the nurse should closely assess all clients who are at high risk for developing ARDS. (D, N, G, M)

33. 3. A client who has had abdominal surgery is best placed in low-Fowler's position postoperatively. This positioning relaxes abdominal muscles and provides for maximum respiratory and cardiovascular function. (I, T, G, M)

34. 3. Many poisons do not cause immediate symptoms but require immediate attention. Eyes should be flushed for 15 to 20 minutes with saline or room-temperature tap water. Ipecac should be followed by 10 to 20 mL of clear liquids. Emesis should be saved for analysis, especially if the type or amount of poison ingested is not clear. (E, N, S, Y)

35. 3. The client has a legal right to refuse treatment. When a client refuses medication, the nurse must explore the reason for the refusal; the desire to avoid unwanted side effects is a common reason. Legally, a client cannot be forcibly medicated unless he is a danger to himself or others or there is a court order to treat. Lying to a client about a medication is neither appropriate nor ethical. (I, T, L, X)

36. 3. To promote self-feeding, the nurse should provide the child with foods that can be eaten with the fingers or that do not spill easily. Soups, cottage cheese or puddings, gravies, and small round vegetables can easily spill from a spoon or fork when the child is eating in an unfamiliar position. Fluids should be provided in containers with straws to prevent spillage. (I, T, S, Y)

37. 3. Sexual intercourse may be resumed at about 3 to 4 weeks postpartum. The general rule is that intercourse may be resumed when the episiotomy (if present) is healed and all bleeding has stopped. Usually these two conditions are met by 3 weeks postpartum. The client can be taught how to check the perineal area by using a hand-held mirror or inserting two or three fingers into the vagina. This helps the client to identify if intercourse can be tolerated without a great deal of discomfort. Kegel exercises can begin immediately after birth to tighten the muscles. If the client has decreased vaginal lubrication, the client should be instructed to use K-Y jelly for additional lubrication. Sitz baths should be used three times daily to help heal the episiotomy. (E, T, L, O)

38. 3. Newborn infants should not sleep with a pillow in the crib because this could lead to suffocation. The client should be instructed to avoid the use of a pillow in the infant's crib. Receiving blankets, breast-pumping equipment, and a clean, but used car seat are appropriate items for a neonate to have available. (D, N, G, O)

39. 4. The symptoms point to a diagnosis of epiglottitis. Administering acetaminophen rectally to decrease the temperature, administering intravenous fluids, and having access to tracheostomy equipment are appropriate. When any type of croup is suspected, however, especially epiglottitis, it is inappropriate to put any object in the back of the mouth or throat. This includes tongue blades and cotton tip applicators used to obtain a throat culture. The stimulation of the back of the throat may result in laryngospasm or occlusion of the airway by a swollen epiglottis. (P, N, S, Y)

40. 3. The three-point gait, in which the client advances the crutches and the affected leg at the same time while weight is supported on the unaffected extremity, is the appropriate gait of choice. This allows for non-weight-bearing on the affected extremity. The

remaining gaits all require some weight-bearing on both legs. (E, T, S, M)

41. 1. Clients with diabetes should be taught to inspect their feet visually on a daily basis. The remaining options reflect an accurate understanding of diabetic foot care. (E, T, H, M)

42. 1. Fluoxetine should be taken as early in the day as possible so as not to interfere with nighttime sleep because it may cause nervousness in some clients. The dose is therapeutic and not too high. There is no evidence in this situation to justify the conclusions that the client's depression is worsening or that the client is on the wrong medication. (E, N, G, X)

43. 3. Carpal tunnel syndrome is a condition on which the median nerve becomes compressed in the wrist. Carpal tunnel syndrome may be the result of a systemic disease such as rheumatoid arthritis or diabetes mellitus, or it may be an occupational hazard for people whose jobs require repetitive hand movements. (I, C, G, M)

44. 1. To help prevent flexion deformities, a client with rheumatoid arthritis should lie in a prone position in bed for about one-half hour several times a day. This positioning helps keep the hips and knees in an extended position and prevents joint flexion. (I, T, H, M)

45. 1. Here, the best nursing intervention is giving the client finger-foods high in protein and calories that he can eat while he paces or walks. Informing the client that snacks are available if he eats properly at mealtime is inappropriate because the client is too busy and distracted to sit and eat an entire meal. Telling the client to sit alone at mealtime to decrease distractions will not help him. Teaching the client about proper nutrition ignores his need for adequate intake. The client would be unable to focus on the nurse's teaching. (I, T, L, X)

46. 3. Both breast-fed and formula-fed neonates should produce at least 6 to 8 wet diapers each day after the first 24 to 48 hours of life. This indicates that the neonate is adequately hydrated. The neonate should regain any weight loss by 7 to 14 days of life. (I, T, G, O)

47. 1. Thrombophlebitis, cardiovascular disease, cancer, and liver disease are contraindications to use of any type of oral contraceptives. The client's age does not preclude the use of oral contraceptives. (E, N, G, O)

48. 3. The retina is especially susceptible to damage in a client with chronic hypertension. The arterioles supplying the retina are damaged. Such damage can lead to vision loss. (P, T, H, M)

49. 3. Heparin is administered subcutaneously, never intramuscularly. A 25- or 26-gauge, $\frac{1}{2}$- to $\frac{5}{8}$-inch needle is most appropriate for heparin administration. The fatty layer of the abdomen is the preferred injection site. The nurse should select a site 1 to 2 inches away from the umbilicus, scar tissue, or any bruises. To decrease the risk of hematoma formation and tissue damage, aspiration of the plunger should be avoided. Gentle pressure should be applied after the injection, but the area must not be massaged. (E, T, S, M)

50. 2. Acrocyanosis, or localized cyanosis of the hands and feet, is common in the neonate and is due to sluggish peripheral circulation. Persistent circumoral cyanosis that persists with feeding or crying may be indicative of cardiac anomalies. Mottling is a result of vasomotor instability. (I, N, G, O)

51. 4. The priority diagnosis at this time is Anxiety. The adolescent and family both will have a great deal of anxiety about diagnostic procedures and the diagnosis itself. Impaired Skin Integrity, Powerlessness, and Fatigue are also appropriate nursing diagnoses at this time but are not the priority. (D, N, S, Y)

52. 1. The client understands the nurse's instructions about exercise when she says she should avoid contact sports because injury may result. Now is not the time for the client to learn how to ski downhill because of potential injury. The client should avoid scuba diving because of the depth pressures. Swimming and walking at normal speeds are excellent exercises during pregnancy. Prolonged exercise in hot, humid environments should be avoided. (E, T, G, O)

53. 2. Raisins are sticky and have high sugar content. The raisin can stick to the teeth and act like high sugar candies in promoting tooth decay. Although anything can be aspirated, round, hard, smooth foods are more easily aspirated. (E, N, H, Y)

54. 3. The nurse should remain with the client and neonate until the ambulance arrives. If a blanket is available, the client and newborn should be kept warm. If the client desires to breast-feed the neonate, the nurse should put the neonate to the client's breast. Neonatal sucking will induce the release of natural oxytocin, which will help to contract the uterus and control uterine bleeding. One complication of a precipitous delivery is decreased uterine tone, particularly with a multigravida. The umbilical cord should not be cut. The client and fetus should be transferred to a health care facility for assessment. The placenta does not need to be wrapped in aluminum foil. Although the client's family should be notified, this is not a priority at this time. Massage of the fundus should be done gently and frequently but not continuously. Massaging the fundus continuously can lead to decreased uterine tone and postpartum hemorrhage. (I, T, G, O)

55. 3. Two perineal pads soaked within 30 minutes may be indicative of early postpartum hemorrhage and warrants further investigation. The most frequent cause of early postpartum hemorrhage is uterine atony or a "boggy fundus." The nurse should gently massage the fundus and call for assistance if the lochia continues. Distended vaginal tissue, slight edema around the episiotomy, and yellowish fluid leaking from the breasts (colostrum) are normal findings. (I, N, G, O)

56. 1. Depression typically occurs after a person stops using cocaine. Some people experience "cocaine bugs" and describe bugs crawling under the skin. Flashbacks, double vision, and palpitations are not associated with cocaine withdrawal. (A, C, L, X)

57. 3. The client should be placed in a side-lying position and encouraged to take a deep breath during the insertion of the suppository. The nurse should insert the suppository 3 to 4 inches into the rectum of an adult client, positioning the suppository along the rectal wall. Avoid placing the suppository into a fecal mass. (I, T, S, M)

58. 3. As with other contraceptives that are progestin-based, heavy menstrual bleeding during the menstrual periods has been associated with Depo-Provera injections. Breast-feeding is not contraindicated. Amenorrhea has been reported after 1 year of use (four injections, 3 months apart). Blurred vision is associated with pregnancy-induced hypertension, not Depo-Provera. (I, T, H, O)

59. 2. This client has already had one episode of preterm labor at 32 weeks' gestation. Sexual intercourse, arousal, and nipple stimulation may result in the release of oxytocin, which can contribute to continued preterm labor and early delivery. The client should be advised to refrain from these activities until closer to term, which is 6 to 8 weeks later. There is no indication of when the client's next prenatal visit is scheduled, so choice 4 is inappropriate. Telling the client that intercourse is acceptable after the bleeding stops is incorrect and may lead to early delivery of a preterm neonate. (E, T, G, O)

60. 3. With a well-managed regimen, a client with myasthenia gravis should be able to control symptoms, maintain a normal lifestyle, and achieve a normal life expectancy. Myasthenia gravis can be controlled, not cured. Episodes of increased muscle weakness should not occur if treatment is well managed. (E, T, H, M)

61. 3. Assessing the client's level of danger is a prerequisite to intervention, which usually requires a multidisciplinary approach. A woman is more open to change and more receptive to professional intervention during a crisis. At other times, it is easier for her to deny the problems and maintain usual patterns of interaction. The client cannot control the batterer, only her responses to the batterer and to her situation. (P, C, L, X)

62. 4. Stress management would not be beneficial to the client with Alzheimer's disease because of cognitive impairment, confusion, and short-term memory loss. (P, T, L, X)

63. 1. Many factors may contribute to the development of osteoporosis. A regular program of exercise is one activity thought to reduce disease incidence. Weight-bearing exercises may be recommended as a preventive or treatment measure. Proper diet instruction would be another health-promotion activity. Pain management by medication is not a health-promotion activity. Bed rest and caffeine intake are considered contributing factors to osteoporosis. (I, T, H, M)

64. 1. Normal capillary refill is 3 to 5 seconds. A capillary refill time of 10 seconds is prolonged and should be reported. Localized pain immediately after a fracture is to be expected. Slight swelling of the fingers is also expected and can be relieved by elevating the extremity. The absence of pain on passive movement of the client's fingers is a normal, desirable finding. (D, N, S, M)

65. 4. Clozapine may cause tachycardia. The nurse should hold the medication if the pulse rate is greater than 140 per minute and notify the physician. (I, T, G, X)

66. 2. Referral to a parenting education program is the most appropriate measure at this time because this client is expressing problems with parenting. (I, T, L, X)

67. 4. The appropriate action by the nurse is to evaluate the cardiac rhythm of the client. Digoxin has negative chronotropic and dromotropic effects and acts to slow the heart rate and conduction. For this reason, it may be administered to the client with sinus tachycardia or atrial fibrillation. A sign of digitalis toxicity is atrial fibrillation, sometimes with a heart rate of more than 100 beats/minute. Before administering the medication, the nurse needs to collect further data to determine the reason that digoxin is being administered to the client and to evaluate the possibility of digitalis toxicity. Other signs and symptoms of digitalis toxicity include bradycardia, anorexia, nausea, vomiting, headache, and general malaise. Urine output should also be carefully monitored in a client taking digitalis preparations who has poor renal function and electrolyte depletion. (E, T, G, M)

68. 4. An abnormal score is given when there are two or more sectors with two or more delays. Failed items need to be considered in relation to where the age line crosses the item box. Large numbers of refusals result in an untestable score. (D, T, H, Y)

69. 3. Breast milk is sufficient to provide the neonate's nutrition for the first 4 months of life. Specific nutrient supplements include vitamin K, vitamin D, fluoride, and iron. Breast milk also may provide protection against infections and against allergies, and may enhance the maternal−infant bonding process. Formula feeding does not provide higher calories than breast-feeding. Breast-feeding will not be successful if the mother does not want to breast-feed. Breast-feeding mothers require an additional 500 calories per day. (P ,T, H, O)

70. 1. The nurse should assist the client to relax by instructing her to breathe in and out slowly. This relaxes the muscles and allows for easier insertion of the moistened speculum. Telling the client to hold the nurse tightly with both hands increases muscular tension. Holding her breath until the speculum is inserted is not appropriate. Visualization requires training and usually involves visualizing a pleasant scene. (I, T, L, O)

71. 2. The rule of nines is used to determine the extent of burns quickly. A chart with the body areas divided into areas equal to multiples of nine is used. Affected areas are shaded, and the total shaded areas are calculated. Other, more detailed charts can be used later for more specific calculation. It is impractical to measure the body when critical care is indicated. Weight is not a reliable parameter to use when measuring the extent of burns. (A, C, G, M)

72. 4. Hemodilution is an important aspect of sickle cell crisis prevention. Calling the physician when the child has a high fever would be appropriate in this situation. Homeopathic treatment can be appropriate as long as the child is not placed in any danger and accepted medical therapy is also followed. (I, T, H, Y)

73. 3. A variable deceleration pattern of the fetal heart rate is usually due to cord compression. This may be a result of the cord around the presenting part, a short cord, or maternal position. Treatment involves changing the maternal position. If this does not resolve the variable heart rate pattern, the physician or nurse midwife should be notified. Oxygen may be needed at a rate of 8 to 12 liters. Amnioinfusion may be ordered to decrease cord compression. After treatment, the condition and results of treatment should be documented in the client's record. (I, T, G, O)

74. 4. The irradiated area should be protected from temperature extremes. No lotion, perfumes, or oils should be applied to the area without the consent of the radiologist. Such preparations can increase the skin irritation that results from the radiation treatments. Heat should not be applied, and only mild soaps should be used. (P, T, S, M)

75. 1. Child abuse can be a vicious cycle because abused children often become abusive parents. Marrying at an early age, being disappointed at the child's sex, and having unwanted children are not necessarily associated with child abuse. (A, C, L, X)

76. 4. Sensations in the toes and legs mark recovery from spinal anesthesia. The anesthesia should not alter skin color. Because the client receiving spinal anesthesia is conscious, he will not ordinarily be disoriented, nor will his respiratory rate be affected unless a complication is present. (A, C, S, M)

77. 4. Hyperventilation causes the excessive loss of carbon dioxide through respirations. This results in a decreased carbonic acid content of the blood. The kidneys will try to compensate by eliminating bicarbonate to maintain a normal carbonic acid–to–bicarbonate ratio, but this takes several days. If compensatory efforts are insufficient, the client will develop respiratory alkalosis. (E, N, G, M)

78. 2. A client who wants to have someone with him at all times is displaying dependency. For the client described in this item, who is 13 years old, the behavior illustrates regression. It would be considered normal for a 13-year-old boy to tease a sister, make the nurse wait while he uses the telephone, and complain about his dietary choices. (A, T, L, X)

79. 3. Bulimia involves low self-esteem and a belief that one's appearance is the only attractive aspect of oneself. Thus, this client needs to change her self-concept and challenge her negative self-perceptions. Reassurance about weight gain misses the point and probably will be rejected. Changing calories perpetuates the need to focus on eating and weight. Emphasizing the staff's control detracts from the client's sense of responsibility and capability to heal herself. (I, T, L, X)

80. 3. A slow, dark-red trickle of blood after a delivery is a symptom of postpartum hemorrhage and should be reported and treated immediately. If the cause is due to uterine atony, the nurse should gently massage the fundus, call for assistance, and prepare to administer oxytocic drugs. If the cause is due to massive blood clots in the uterus, the client may need to have the clots manually extracted. The client's temperature is normal for this stage of the postpartum period. It is not unusual for the client's legs to still be numb. If the client has an intravenous line, this should not be discontinued until the bleeding is under control because the client may need intravenous fluids or blood replacement therapy to prevent shock. Hemorrhage is one of the three leading causes of maternal mortality. The other two causes are infection and pregnancy-induced hypertension. (I, N, G, O)

81. 1. The nurse's expression of concern for the client's safety may help the client validate her fears and choose to take action. Telling her to leave her husband is inappropriate advice. The idea of leaving the marriage may be so overwhelming that it may push the client away from the nurse as a support person. Talking to the client about changing her behavior or reducing family stress are forms of victim blaming. They reinforce the message that the client is responsible for the abuse. She is likely getting the same message from the abuser and others. (I, T, L, X)

82. 1. A child with severe cerebral palsy often has a lack of oral motor control that interferes with tongue control, chewing, and swallowing. This is the reason that this child is being fed pureed foods and fluids. Lack of tongue control often causes the child to push the food back out of the mouth while trying to chew and swallow. This child should be able to absorb and metabolize ingested nutrients. A child with cerebral palsy has a nonprogressive central nervous system insult. Ongoing, increased intracranial pressure is not related to cerebral palsy, nor is the client's metabolism altered. (D, N, G, Y)

83. 3. The plaster cast will take longer to dry than 4 hours, and it will feel heavy. Acetaminophen may not be a strong enough medication to relieve the pain, or it may take 45 minutes before she has any pain relief, particularly if she has just eaten. New complaints of tingling and noticing pale fingers would indicate a more serious problem that needs immediate attention. (I, T, G, Y)

84. 4. Coping with compulsive behavior can be frustrating. Interfering with the client's behavior is not helpful and may cause him to become negative and more firmly committed to the behavior. Nor does it help to explain how his behavior may interfere with getting well. Allowing the client to decide whether he will carry out his behavior or attend meals, group activities, therapy sessions, and the like usually means that he will favor his compulsive behavior over activities that he requires for healthful living. Therefore, in this situation, it would be best for the nurse to remind the client in sufficient time so that he can carry out his ritualistic behavior and arrive on time for scheduled activities. (P, T, L, X)

85. 1. Research studies have shown that complete immunity for the MMR vaccine is not achieved until the child is 12 months of age. Therefore, the normal, healthy child should not receive it before then. Children can receive two injections at the same time. There is no 4-month waiting period between MMR and oral polio vaccines. (E, T, H, Y)

86. 3. Toddlers have temper tantrums in their attempt to develop autonomy. Toddlers should be left alone as long as they are safe during a tantrum. Talking to the toddler, punishing, or moving the child reinforces the behavior. (I, T, H, Y)

87. 2. The nursing diagnosis High Risk for Impaired Skin Integrity related to frequent foot washing is indicated. The skin of the feet can become red and raw, providing an entry for infection. The ritualistic behavior provides relief for the client's anxiety and keeps it in check. Panic could result if the client is not allowed to perform his ritualistic behavior. (D, T, L, X)

88. 2. Diverticular rupture causes peritonitis from the release of intestinal contents (chemicals and bacteria) into the peritoneal cavity. The inflammatory response of the peritoneal tissue produces severe abdominal rigidity and pain, diminished intestinal motility, and retention of intestinal contents (air, fluid, and stool). (A, C, G, M)

89. 4. The client with an obsessive-compulsive disorder has an uncontrollable and persistent need to perform behavior that helps relieve intolerable anxiety. An irrational fear is called a *phobia. Ambivalence* refers to two simultaneous opposing feelings. In *depression,* the client feels extreme sadness. (D, C, L, X)

90. 3. Pediculosis, or head lice, is commonly spread by the sharing of headwear, combs, and brushes. The adult lice can also travel from one person to another if contact is close. The adult lice lay eggs, or nits. These nits are "glued" to the hair and cannot be removed unless treated with special shampoo that is formulated for just this purpose. The hair is then combed with a fine-toothed comb to remove the nits. Cleanliness does not prevent the acquisition of pediculosis. Because head lice spread so easily, a child is usually kept out of school until he or she is treated and found to be free of nits. (E, N, H, Y)

NURSING CARE COMPREHENSIVE TEST

TEST 1

Directions: Use this answer grid to determine areas of strength or need for further study.

NURSING PROCESS

A = Assessment
D = Analysis, nursing diagnosis
P = Planning
I = Implementation
E = Evaluation

COGNITIVE LEVEL

K = Knowledge
C = Comprehension
T = Application
N = Analysis

CLIENT NEEDS

S = Safe, effective care environment
G = Physiologic integrity
L = Psychosocial integrity
H = Health promotion and maintenance

NURSING CARE AREA

O = Maternity and newborn care
X = Psychosocial health problems
Y = Nursing care of children
M = Medical and surgical health problems

Question #	Answer #	Nursing Process					Cognitive Level				Client Needs				Care Area			
		A	D	P	I	E	K	C	T	N	S	G	L	H	O	X	Y	M
1	2		D							N		G						M
2	3		D							N		G					Y	
3	4		D							N				H	O			
4	4	A							T			G						M
5	4	A						C				G					Y	
6	1				I				T					H	O			
7	1					E				N			L			X		
8	1				I					N		G					Y	
9	2				I				T			G			O			
10	2	A					K					G						M
11	2			P					T				L			X		
12	2					E				N			L					M
13	2				I				T			G			O			
14	4		D							N		G					Y	
15	3	A							T				L					M
16	2				I				T					H				M
17	1				I				T				L			X		
18	4				I				T				L			X		
19	1				I				T		S						Y	

NURSING PROCESS

A = Assessment
D = Analysis, nursing diagnosis
P = Planning
I = Implementation
E = Evaluation

COGNITIVE LEVEL

K = Knowledge
C = Comprehension
T = Application
N = Analysis

CLIENT NEEDS

S = Safe, effective care environment
G = Physiologic integrity
L = Psychosocial integrity
H = Health promotion and maintenance

NURSING CARE AREA

O = Maternity and newborn care
X = Psychosocial health problems
Y = Nursing care of children
M = Medical and surgical health problems

Question #	Answer #	| Nursing Process					| Cognitive Level				| Client Needs				| Care Area			
		A	D	P	I	E	K	C	T	N	S	G	L	H	O	X	Y	M
20	2				I				T			G						M
21	2				I					N		G					Y	
22	2					E				N			L			X		
23	3	A							T			G			O			
24	2				I				T				L			X		
25	1		D							N		G			O			
26	4		D						T			G						M
27	3	A							T					H			Y	
28	2					E			T			G						M
29	2		D							N	S							M
30	2				I				T			G				X		
31	2	A							T			G						M
32	3		D							N		G						M
33	3				I				T			G						M
34	3					E				N	S						Y	
35	3				I				T				L			X		
36	3				I				T		S						Y	
37	3					E			T				L		O			
38	3		D							N		G			O			
39	4			P						N	S						Y	
40	3					E			T		S							M
41	1					E			T					H				M
42	1					E				N		G				X		
43	3				I			C				G						M
44	1				I				T					H				M

NURSING PROCESS

A = Assessment
D = Analysis, nursing diagnosis
P = Planning
I = Implementation
E = Evaluation

COGNITIVE LEVEL

K = Knowledge
C = Comprehension
T = Application
N = Analysis

CLIENT NEEDS

S = Safe, effective care environment
G = Physiologic integrity
L = Psychosocial integrity
H = Health promotion and maintenance

NURSING CARE AREA

O = Maternity and newborn care
X = Psychosocial health problems
Y = Nursing care of children
M = Medical and surgical health problems

Question #	Answer #	Nursing Process					Cognitive Level				Client Needs				Care Area			
		A	D	P	I	E	K	C	T	N	S	G	L	H	O	X	Y	M
45	1				I				T				L			X		
46	3				I				T			G			O			
47	1					E				N		G			O			
48	3			P					T					H				M
49	3					E			T		S							M
50	2				I					N		G			O			
51	4		D							N	S						Y	
52	1					E			T			G			O			
53	2					E				N				H			Y	
54	3				I				T			G			O			
55	3				I					N		G			O			
56	1	A						C					L			X		
57	3				I				T		S							M
58	3				I				T					H	O			
59	2					E			T			G			O			
60	3					E			T					H				M
61	3			P				C					L			X		
62	4			P					T				L			X		
63	1				I				T					H				M
64	1		D							N	S							M
65	4				I				T			G				X		
66	2				I				T				L			X		
67	4					E			T			G						M
68	4		D						T					H			Y	
69	3			P					T					H	O			

ANSWER GRID: 3

Nursing Process

A = Assessment
D = Analysis, nursing diagnosis
P = Planning
I = Implementation
E = Evaluation

Client Needs

S = Safe, effective care environment
G = Physiologic integrity
L = Psychosocial integrity
H = Health promotion and maintenance

Cognitive Level

K = Knowledge
C = Comprehension
T = Application
N = Analysis

Nursing Care Area

O = Maternity and newborn care
X = Psychosocial health problems
Y = Nursing care of children
M = Medical and surgical health problems

Question #	Answer #	Nursing Process					Cognitive Level				Client Needs				Care Area			
		A	D	P	I	E	K	C	T	N	S	G	L	H	O	X	Y	M
70	1				I				T				L		O			
71	2	A						C				G						M
72	4				I				T					H			Y	
73	3				I				T			G			O			
74	4			P					T		S							M
75	1	A						C					L			X		
76	4	A						C			S							M
77	4					E				N		G						M
78	2	A							T				L			X		
79	3				I				T				L			X		
80	3				I					N		G			O			
81	1				I				T				L			X		
82	1		D							N		G					Y	
83	3				I				T			G					Y	
84	4			P					T				L			X		
85	1					E			T					H			Y	
86	3				I				T					H			Y	
87	2		D						T				L			X		
88	2	A						C				G						M
89	4		D					C					L			X		
90	3					E				N				H			Y	

NURSING PROCESS

A = Assessment
D = Analysis, nursing diagnosis
P = Planning
I = Implementation
E = Evaluation

COGNITIVE LEVEL

K = Knowledge
C = Comprehension
T = Application
N = Analysis

CLIENT NEEDS

S = Safe, effective care environment
G = Physiologic integrity
L = Psychosocial integrity
H = Health promotion and maintenance

NURSING CARE AREA

O = Maternity and newborn care
X = Psychosocial health problems
Y = Nursing care of children
M = Medical and surgical health problems

Question #	Answer #	Nursing Process					Cognitive Level				Client Needs				Care Area			
		A	D	P	I	E	K	C	T	N	S	G	L	H	O	X	Y	M
Number Correct																		
Number Possible	90	13	15	8	35	19	1	9	54	26	12	38	23	17	20	22	19	29
Percentage Correct																		

Score Calculation: To determine your **Percentage Correct,** divide the **Number Correct** by the **Number Possible.**

ANSWER GRID: 5

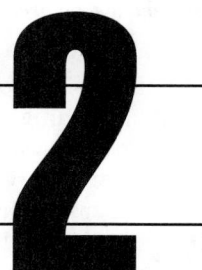
Select the one best answer, and indicate your choice by filling in the circle in front of the option.

1. A 30-year-old multigravida with prolonged rupture of membranes is diagnosed with endometritis 36 hours after delivery of a viable neonate. While assessing the client after intravenous antibiotic therapy is initiated, the nurse notes that the client's temperature is 100°F, pulse rate is 124 beats/minute, and respirations are 24 breaths/minute. The nurse should
○ 1. administer an analgesic as ordered.
○ 2. provide the client with clear liquids.
○ 3. monitor the vital signs every 4 hours.
○ 4. contact the physician immediately.

2. A 4-year-old child with hemophilia is brought to the pediatrician's office with spontaneous soft tissue bleeding of the right knee. Immediately on the child's arrival, the nurse would plan to
○ 1. administer aspirin for discomfort.
○ 2. elevate the right knee.
○ 3. immobilize the knee in a dependent position.
○ 4. do a type and cross-match for platelets.

3. The nurse is caring for a primigravida at 28 weeks' gestation who is admitted with a diagnosis of preterm labor. The client's contractions are occurring every 15 to 20 minutes, lasting 25 seconds. The membranes are intact. The nurse should plan to
○ 1. place the client on bed rest on her left side.
○ 2. obtain equipment for an amniotomy.
○ 3. prepare terbutaline in an intravenous solution.
○ 4. request assistance from the neonatal resuscitation team.

4. Which of the following nursing actions would be least helpful for a battered client?
○ 1. Helping the client displace her feelings.
○ 2. Giving her information about a safe home and a crisis help line telephone number.
○ 3. Teaching the client about the cycle of violence.
○ 4. Discussing the client's legal and personal rights.

5. The client with a cognitive disorder tells the nurse, "Everyone is after me. They want to kill me." The nurse's best response is
○ 1. "Why do you think someone wants to kill you?"
○ 2. "No one wants to kill you. We like you."
○ 3. "You're frightened. This is a hospital and these people are staff members. You're safe here."
○ 4. "Don't worry, we'll protect you. No one can come here to harm you."

6. A primigravida at 26 weeks' gestation visits the clinic and tells the nurse that her lower back aches when she arrives home from work. The nurse should suggest that the client perform
○ 1. leg lifting.
○ 2. tailor sitting.
○ 3. shoulder circling.
○ 4. squatting.

7. The nurse caring for a child with leukemia should place priority on
○ 1. preventing injury.
○ 2. monitoring the child's temperature.
○ 3. monitoring the child's platelet count.
○ 4. encouraging increased fluid intake.

8. The nurse is caring for a primipara who delivered a viable neonate vaginally 12 hours ago. The client is diagnosed with class II heart disease. The nurse should instruct the client to
○ 1. remain on bed rest continuously.
○ 2. allow the nursing staff to assist her in baby care.
○ 3. avoid breast-feeding because this may cause exertion on the heart.
○ 4. keep fluid intake to a minimum to avoid fluid overload.

9. A 6-month-old comes to the clinic with a high fever and cold symptoms, and she is pulling at her left ear. She is scheduled to receive her 6-month immunizations, which are diphtheria-pertussis-tetanus (DPT) with *Haemophilus influenzae* (H-flu) and hepatitis vaccines. The mother asks the nurse if she will receive them. The nurse's best response would be
○ 1. "She will receive just her hepatitis immunizations."
○ 2. "She can wait until she comes back in 3 weeks to have her ear rechecked."
○ 3. "She will receive her DPT with H-flu and hepatitis today."
○ 4. "She will receive her hepatitis and H-flu immunization only today."

10. Radiation therapy is instituted for a client with Hodgkin's disease; after 1 week, the radiation site becomes red and irritated. Which of the following statements would indicate that the client treated the area appropriately at home? "I applied
○ 1. aloe vera lotion to the area."

647

○ 2. moist cool soaks to the area."
○ 3. nothing to the area; I just kept it dry."
○ 4. a hot-water bottle to the area."

11. At an emergency shelter, an earthquake victim tells the nurse that he is going to spend the night in his own bed at home. Which defense mechanism is the client exhibiting?
○ 1. Intellectualization.
○ 2. Denial.
○ 3. Rationalization.
○ 4. Undoing.

12. The nurse is caring for a multigravida in active labor with continuous electronic fetal heart rate monitoring. As the client begins to push, the nurse observes that the fetal heart rate shows a deceleration pattern that mirrors the contractions. The nurse should
○ 1. continue to monitor the client and fetus.
○ 2. turn the client to her left side.
○ 3. ask the client to push in the squatting position.
○ 4. administer oxygen by mask at 8 liters.

13. The primary nursing goals for a client with myasthenia gravis are to conserve the client's energy and to
○ 1. ensure a safe environment.
○ 2. maintain respiratory function.
○ 3. provide psychological support and reassurance.
○ 4. promote comfort and relieve pain.

14. For a child receiving steroids in therapeutic doses over a long period, the nurse should
○ 1. decrease the child's ingestion of potassium-rich foods.
○ 2. give the drug on an empty stomach.
○ 3. monitor the child's serum glucose level.
○ 4. monitor the child's temperature to assess for infection.

15. While assessing a primipara during the immediate postpartum period, the nurse plans to use both hands to assess the client's fundus to
○ 1. promote uterine involution.
○ 2. hasten the puerperium period.
○ 3. prevent uterine inversion.
○ 4. determine the size of the fundus.

16. Which of the following signs and symptoms would indicate that a client with human immunodeficiency virus (HIV) infection has developed acquired immunodeficiency syndrome (AIDS)?
○ 1. Severe fatigue at night.
○ 2. Pain on standing and walking.
○ 3. Weight loss of 10 pounds over 3 months.
○ 4. Herpes simplex ulcer persisting for 2 months.

17. A parent calls the clinic saying her 3-year-old has chickenpox. The parent asks how to care for the lesions. The nurse would advise that the child
○ 1. soak in a hot tub for 30 minutes three times a day.

○ 2. take an antihistamine and use calamine lotion on lesions.
○ 3. can return to preschool in 3 days.
○ 4. will not appear very ill.

18. While caring for a neonate 2 days after birth, the nurse observes a swelling on the neonate's head that appears to have blood between the bone and the periosteum and does not cross the cranial suture line. The nurse should explain to the parents that this will
○ 1. require several surgeries to repair.
○ 2. remain swollen for at least 6 months before receding.
○ 3. be a normal symptom of a skull fracture that occurred during the delivery.
○ 4. resolves without treatment by 6 weeks of age.

19. A 5-year old will have an appendectomy shortly. The nurse would tell the child and parents
○ 1. that this is a painful surgery.
○ 2. that when the child returns from surgery, there will be a tube in the nose.
○ 3. that the child will get a shot before going to surgery.
○ 4. where the incision will be with the use of a doll.

20. Two adolescents come to the school nurse's office to talk about their friend. They are concerned because he seems to be using several different drugs. One of the adolescents asks how he would be able to tell if his friend was using cocaine. The nurse replies that his
○ 1. eyes would be red and bloodshot.
○ 2. pupils would be constricted to pinpoints.
○ 3. pupils would be large.
○ 4. eyes would look tired.

21. A nurse working in a community center counsels a husband and wife referred to the center because of suspected abuse of their 3-year-old daughter. The couple also have three older daughters at home. During counseling, the nurse should recognize that the parents give a typical description of an abused child when they say that their daughter
○ 1. tends to lie and cheat frequently.
○ 2. always keeps running away from home.
○ 3. does not show respect for authority.
○ 4. has always been different from her sisters.

22. A client with class II cardiac disease in active labor is planning on epidural anesthesia for labor and delivery. After the anesthesiologist has explained the procedure and potential complications, the nurse determines that the client needs *further* instructions when she says,
○ 1. "I may need to lie flat for 6 hours and drink plenty of fluids after I deliver."
○ 2. "Sometimes, the labor process is slower after the epidural anesthesia is administered."

○ 3. "If my bladder gets full, I may need to be catheterized."

○ 4. "The second stage of labor may be prolonged as a result of the anesthesia."

23. The nurse is planning an educational program about the prevention of osteoporosis for a group of women at the local community center. Which of the following preventive measures would be appropriate for the nurse to include in the teaching plan?

○ 1. Encouraging weight-bearing exercise on a regular basis.

○ 2. Increasing daily intake of protein.

○ 3. Ingesting 2000 mg of calcium supplements daily.

○ 4. Sunbathing for 1 hour a day during the summer months.

24. The nurse should plan to include which of the following interventions in the plan of care for a child admitted to the hospital with a medical diagnosis of febrile seizure?

○ 1. Keep the child supine.

○ 2. Keep the room temperature low and bedclothes to a minimum.

○ 3. Place the child in respiratory isolation and restrict visitors.

○ 4. Place a padded tongue blade at the bedside.

25. Outcome criteria for the client with osteoarthritis should include

○ 1. Joint degeneration arrested.

○ 2. Joint range of motion improved.

○ 3. Able to self-administer gold compound safely.

○ 4. Feels better than on hospital admission.

26. The nurse planning care for a child in vasoocclusive crisis because of sickle cell disease would include increasing fluid intake in the list of interventions because

○ 1. decreased blood viscosity prevents the sickling process.

○ 2. children with sickle cell disease lose more water than is normal through diaphoresis.

○ 3. hemodilution increases normal red blood cell life span.

○ 4. increasing fluid intake increases hemolysis.

27. A multigravida is admitted to the labor area for induction with intravenous oxytocin because she is 42 weeks' pregnant. The nurse should instruct the client that during the process of labor,

○ 1. continuous fetal heart rate monitoring will be implemented.

○ 2. frequent ultrasound examinations will be performed.

○ 3. at least 5 to 10 fetal scalp pH tests will be performed.

○ 4. oligohydramnios will be carefully evaluated.

28. A client describes anxiety attacks that usually occur shortly after work when he is preparing his evening meal. Which of the following questions would be most appropriate for the nurse to ask the client first in an effort to learn how he can be helped?

○ 1. "When during the day do you most often think of your wife?"

○ 2. "Where do you feel most uncomfortable when you're anxious?"

○ 3. "Why do you think you feel anxious when returning from work?"

○ 4. "What do you do when you're anxious to help yourself feel better?"

29. A toddler with croup is given a Vaponefrin updraft because of increasing respiratory distress. The nurse evaluates the treatment as being effective when the child's

○ 1. color is normal.

○ 2. heart rate is 100 beats/minute.

○ 3. pulse oximeter reads 90.

○ 4. retractions are less severe.

30. The client's nursing diagnosis is Chronic Low Self-Esteem Secondary to Self-Doubt as evidenced by self-deprecatory statements. Which of the following expected outcomes specifically relates to this diagnosis? The client will

○ 1. demonstrate reality-based thinking.

○ 2. use relaxation exercises.

○ 3. continually ask for approval from others.

○ 4. accept encouragement from others.

31. The nurse is caring for a primigravida at about 9 weeks' gestation. After explaining self-care measures for common discomforts of pregnancy, the nurse determines that the client understands the instructions when she says,

○ 1. "If I start to leak colostrum, I should cleanse my nipples with soap and water."

○ 2. "If I have a vaginal discharge, I should wear nylon underwear."

○ 3. "Leg cramps can be alleviated if I put an ice pack on the area."

○ 4. "Nausea and vomiting can be decreased if I eat a few crackers before arising."

32. The nurse is preparing to administer promethazine (Phenergan) intramuscularly to a client in active labor. The nurse should explain to the client that one of the effects of this medication is

○ 1. increased fetal heart rate.

○ 2. decreased nausea and vomiting.

○ 3. increased neonatal sucking reflex.

○ 4. increased blood pressure in the client.

33. Which of the following is an early symptom of glaucoma?

○ 1. Hazy vision.

○ 2. Loss of central vision.

○ 3. Impaired peripheral vision.

○ 4. Blurred or "sooty" vision.

34. A school-aged child is admitted to the hospital with newly diagnosed insulin-dependent diabetes mellitus. On admission at 10:00 AM, his blood sugar is 180 mg/dL. His urine tests negative for ketones. He receives 10 units of regular Humulin insulin subcutaneously at 10:30 AM. The nurse should plan to

- ○ 1. assess the child beginning at 12:30 PM for shakiness, feelings of anxiety, or decreased level of consciousness.
- ○ 2. carefully regulate an intravenous solution of normal saline and Lente insulin at 12:30 PM.
- ○ 3. encourage the child to drink at least 500 mL of a sugar-free clear liquid by 11:30 AM.
- ○ 4. begin intravenous administration of 5% dextrose in water at 11:00 AM.

35. A primigravida visits the clinic at 12 weeks' gestation and tells the nurse that she has a cold and her nose is stuffy. The nurse should instruct the client to treat the nasal stuffiness by using

- ○ 1. oral antihistamines.
- ○ 2. oral decongestants.
- ○ 3. ice packs to the nasal area.
- ○ 4. saline nose drops.

36. The nurse teaches the client who is wheelchair-bound due to a spinal cord injury to reduce the risk of pressure ulcer formation by

- ○ 1. bathing daily.
- ○ 2. eating a high carbohydrate diet.
- ○ 3. shifting his or her sacral pressure every 15 minutes.
- ○ 4. moving from the bed to the wheelchair every 2 hours.

37. For a client with a sucking stab wound in the chest wall, the nurse should first

- ○ 1. start administering oxygen.
- ○ 2. prepare to do a tracheostomy.
- ○ 3. prepare for endotracheal intubation.
- ○ 4. cover the wound with a petroleum-impregnated dressing.

38. The nurse attempts to interact with the client who barely responds with yes or no. The client states, "Don't bother me. I want to die." The nurse's best action is to

- ○ 1. sit with the client for 10 minutes.
- ○ 2. leave the client alone.
- ○ 3. send another staff member to interact with the client.
- ○ 4. turn the television on for the client.

39. The nurse is performing chest percussion on a child. The nurse should

- ○ 1. firmly but gently strike the chest wall to make a popping sound.
- ○ 2. gently strike the chest wall to make a slapping sound.
- ○ 3. percuss over an area from the umbilicus to clavicle.

- ○ 4. place a folded baby blanket between the nurse's hand and the child's chest.

40. A mother asks the nurse if the lesions around her child's mouth could be impetigo. To verify the mother's suspicions, the nurse would look for

- ○ 1. erythema and formation of pus around hair follicles.
- ○ 2. honey-colored crusts, vesicles, and reddish maculae on the skin.
- ○ 3. increased warmth, intense redness, swelling, and firmness of the skin.
- ○ 4. macular erythema with a sandpaper-like texture of the skin.

41. A client who is receiving chemotherapy expresses concern at the thought of losing her hair. The nurse's best response would be:

- ○ 1. "Don't worry about your hair loss. A good wig can disguise that."
- ○ 2. "No one knows how long it will take your hair to grow back. You will have to learn to cope with its loss."
- ○ 3. "Your hair loss will be temporary. Would you like to tell me about your concerns?"
- ○ 4. "A little hair loss shouldn't concern you. You have more serious things to worry about."

42. The client is taking risperidone (Risperdal) to treat the positive and negative symptoms of schizophrenia. Which of the following negative symptoms will improve?

- ○ 1. Abnormal thought form.
- ○ 2. Hallucinations and delusions.
- ○ 3. Bizarre behavior.
- ○ 4. Asocial behavior and anergia.

43. The nurse teaches a client scheduled for an intravenous pyelogram (IVP) what to expect when the dye is injected. The nurse would know that the client has correctly understood the teaching when he states that when the dye is injected, he may experience

- ○ 1. a metallic taste.
- ○ 2. flushing of the face.
- ○ 3. cold chills.
- ○ 4. chest pain.

44. The occupational health nurse is screening employees for symptoms of carpal tunnel syndrome. Symptoms indicative of carpal tunnel syndrome most commonly include

- ○ 1. difficulty flexing fingers.
- ○ 2. paresthesia in the thumb and first and second fingers.
- ○ 3. decreased capillary refilling.
- ○ 4. numbness in the forearm.

45. During a precipitous delivery, the nurse assists a multigravida to deliver the fetal head. The nurse should tell the client that it is necessary to determine if the fetal umbilical cord is around the neck to prevent

○ 1. rupture of the cord.

○ 2. spontaneous separation of the placenta.

○ 3. decreased oxygenation to the fetus.

○ 4. slow delivery of the fetal shoulder.

46. A client has a total serum cholesterol level of 326 mg/dL. The nurse explains to the client that this level

○ 1. is normal and requires no further treatment.

○ 2. is low and requires no further treatment.

○ 3. is borderline normal and may require dietary modification.

⌀ 4. is high and will require dietary modification.

47. A client calls the physician's office 2 days after a herniorrhaphy to report that his scrotum is swollen and painful. To promote comfort, the nurse should instruct the client to

○ 1. apply a snug binder on his abdomen.

○ 2. have him wear a truss to support the scrotum.

○ 3. elevate the scrotum and place ice bags on the area intermittently.

○ 4. have him lie on his side and place a pillow between his legs.

48. The client, with an Axis I diagnosis of Schizophrenia: disorganized type, walks into group naked. The nurse's best action is

○ 1. instruct the client to go to his room and to put on some clothes.

○ 2. wrap a blanket around him and tell him to be seated for the remainder of group.

○ 3. ask a male client to take off his sweater and wrap it around the client's waist.

○ 4. lead the client to his room, and help him dress if he needs assistance.

49. A client with emphysema is receiving continuous oxygen therapy. Depressed ventilation is likely to occur unless the nurse ensures that the oxygen is administered

○ 1. warmed.

○ 2. humidified.

○ 3. at a low flow rate.

○ 4. through a nasal cannula.

50. The nurse makes a home visit to a primigravida on the fourth postpartum day after delivery of a viable neonate. When the nurse enters the house, the nurse finds the client sitting in a chair, crying inconsolably, while the neonate is crying in another room. The client tells the nurse that she hasn't been sleeping well, and she has been hearing voices. The nurse determines that the client is most likely experiencing

○ 1. normal reactions to being a new mother.

○ 2. the "baby blues."

○ 3. postpartum depression.

○ 4. postpartum psychosis.

51. The nurse admits a multigravida in active labor to the birthing center. The client has had no prenatal care with this pregnancy. The nurse determines that the client's cervix is 9 cm dilated and completely effaced. The fetus is at 0 station with a face presentation. After explaining to the client about face presentations, the nurse determines that the client needs *further* instructions when she says,

○ 1. "Face presentation is associated with a small maternal pelvis."

○ 2. "Anencephalic fetuses commonly present by face presentation."

○ 3. "If the baby's face is looking toward my umbilicus, I can have a vaginal delivery."

○ 4. "If the baby's chin faces my back, a vaginal delivery is likely."

52. A child is receiving long-term steroid therapy. The nurse should instruct the parents to expect the child to

○ 1. exhibit his usual behavior and temperament.

○ 2. lose weight.

○ 3. develop truncal obesity.

○ 4. experience a growth spurt.

53. A client receiving digoxin for congestive heart failure undergoes cardiac catheterization to evaluate his condition further. The procedure reveals a cardiac output of 2.2 liters per minute. The nurse would evaluate this cardiac output as

○ 1. high, due to the effects of digoxin.

○ 2. within normal limits; the digoxin is effective.

○ 3. within normal limits, but not adequate to support strenuous activity.

○ 4. low, requiring further medical intervention.

54. A client has been admitted to the hospital with acute osteomyelitis in the left leg. He complains of acute pain in the left leg that intensifies when he moves it. The nurse notes a temperature of 101°F and a reddened, warm area in the mid-calf region over the shaft of the tibia. Based on this information, which of the following nursing diagnoses would be most appropriate for this client?

○ 1. Anticipatory Grieving related to possible left lower leg amputation.

⌀ 2. Activity Intolerance related to severe left leg pain.

○ 3. Body Image Disturbance related to left leg swelling and inflammation.

○ 4. Fluid Volume Deficit related to elevated temperature of 101°F.

55. The nurse admits a primigravida in active labor to the birthing center. To assess the frequency of the client's contractions, the nurse should assess the interval between the

1. acme of one contraction to the beginning of the next contraction.
2. beginning of one contraction to the end of the contraction.
3. end of one contraction to the end of the next contraction.
4. beginning of one contraction to the beginning of the next contraction.

56. During a health history, a 59-year-old male client with non–insulin-dependent diabetes mellitus says he is "not feeling right." Which of the following client statements is most probably unrelated to diabetes mellitus?
1. "I have this cut on my hand that doesn't want to heal."
2. "No matter how much I drink, I'm still thirsty all the time."
3. "I seem to be unable to get an erection. I've never been impotent before."
4. "In the past couple of weeks, I've been having a lot of trouble urinating."

57. A 4-year-old is brought to the clinic for a checkup. It is determined that the family does not have fluoridated water. The nurse would advise which of the following when using fluoride supplements?
1. Give with meals.
2. Do not eat or drink for 30 minutes after the supplement.
3. Be sure to take the supplement with milk.
4. Have the child swallow the tablet immediately after putting it in the mouth.

58. The nurse is suctioning the tracheostomy of a 3-year-old client in a pediatric intensive care. The nurse should
1. insert the catheter slightly beyond the end of the tracheostomy tube.
2. insert the catheter with the suction port of the catheter closed.
3. keep the catheter straight as it is removed from the tracheostomy tube.
4. use clean technique while suctioning.

59. The nurse should plan care for the client with cancer based on the fact that an important principle of using medication to manage cancer pain is to
1. individualize the medication therapy to the client.
2. avoid giving the client addictive medications.
3. provide the medications as soon as the client requests them.
4. discontinue the medications periodically to discourage the development of drug tolerance.

60. The nurse is caring for a multigravida in active labor with a fetus in a frank breech presentation. The

nurse should notify the physician if the nurse observes
1. intense uterine contractions during the transition phase of labor.
2. fetal bradycardia at any time during the labor process.
3. maternal tachycardia during a contraction.
4. meconium-stained amniotic fluid during the second stage of labor.

61. A 14-year-old girl with Type I diabetes is monitoring her blood glucose level at home. Which of the following indicates that she understands appropriate care management strategies for a blood glucose level of 250 mg/dL? She will
1. take insulin and drink water.
2. skip the next dose of insulin and drink fruit juice.
3. eat a high-carbohydrate meal and exercise.
4. inject glucagon and rest.

62. A child newly diagnosed with rheumatic fever is to receive penicillin therapy. Which of the following statements by the parents would lead the nurse to judge that the parents understand the teaching about penicillin as part of the treatment plan for rheumatic fever?
1. "How long will it take for the penicillin to help relieve the joint discomfort?"
2. "Our child should take the medication until the physician discontinues it."
3. "We need to also give these pills to our other children to prevent them from getting rheumatic fever."
4. "We should give our child the medication on a full stomach."

63. The nurse assessing a multigravida at 36 weeks' gestation plans to assess the client for symptoms of pregnancy-induced hypertension. The nurse should plan to first assess the client's
1. face.
2. reflexes.
3. pulse.
4. ankles.

64. A parent group is discussing different types of punishment. The parents ask the nurse to discuss corporeal punishment. The nurse tells the group that corporeal punishment
1. does not physically harm the child.
2. reinforces the idea that violence is not acceptable.
3. can result in children becoming accustomed to spanking and require more severe punishment for the same results.
4. can be beneficial in teaching children what they should do.

65. If a nursing goal is to increase a child's protein intake, the nurse would encourage the child to eat which of the following foods that the child likes?
- ○ 1. A bacon, lettuce, and tomato sandwich.
- ⊗ 2. Fruit-flavored yogurt.
- ○ 3. Nacho chips and salsa.
- ○ 4. Crackers with butter and jelly.

66. Two days after a client's wife and child were found dead in a flood, the client returns to the crisis center and says he thinks it would be better to "end it all right now and join my wife and kid, wherever they are." The nurse has already determined that the client has no history of psychiatric problems. In terms of the seriousness of the client's suicide threat, his risk should be considered as
- ○ 1. very low; as long as the client speaks of suicide, he is unlikely to carry out the act.
- ○ 2. low; a person who has not had psychiatric problems in the past rarely carries out a first suicide threat.
- ○ 3. moderate; the client appears to be making an effort to gain attention and extra support.
- ○ 4. high; the client's suicide threat can be considered a call for help and should be taken seriously.

67. Which one of the following would the nurse evaluate as an expected outcome for a client who has undergone surgical repair of an inguinal hernia?
- ○ 1. The client will verbalize understanding of instructions to avoid lifting for 2 to 6 weeks after surgery.
- ○ 2. The client's voiding patterns will return to normal within 6 months after surgery.
- ○ 3. The client will use a cane for assistance with ambulation for 2 to 6 weeks after surgery.
- ○ 4. The client will remain on a soft diet until the wound is healed.

68. A 10-month-old child with bronchitis is taken out of the 30% oxygen tent for breakfast because he refuses to eat unless in a high chair. During the feeding, the nurse notes that the child's respiratory rate has increased, he is becoming more irritable, and he is using accessory muscles to breathe. The first action of the nurse should be to
- ○ 1. assess the pulse rate and respirations and notify the physician.
- ○ 2. discontinue the feeding and place the child back in the tent.
- ○ 3. perform postural drainage and then complete the feeding.
- ○ 4. suction the child's nose with a bulb syringe.

69. A public health nurse has realized that there is an increase in the number of children involved in automobile accidents who were not wearing seat belts. What would be the nurse's best strategy to reduce the number of accidents?
- ○ 1. Contact the local state representative to discuss new legislation.
- ○ 2. Attend a school board meeting and advocate for classes to teach seat belt safety to the children.
- ○ 3. Call the town mayor's office with this information so the mayor can discuss it with the media.
- ○ 4. Start a letter-writing campaign addressed to the school superintendent about the importance of wearing seat belts.

70. After a period of depression and preoccupation with his son's impending death, a father has started to adjust to the idea of life without his son. This phenomenon of emotionally reacting to a person's death before it actually occurs is known as
- ○ 1. dysthymia.
- ○ 2. acute grief reaction.
- ○ 3. pathologic mourning.
- ○ 4. anticipatory mourning.

71. A mother brings her 2-year-old adopted Korean child to the clinic for an initial checkup. The child has been living with the adopted family for several weeks. The nurse notes an irregular area of deep blue pigment on the child's buttocks extending into the sacral area. The nurse should
- ○ 1. ask the mother in private how the bruise occurred.
- ○ 2. do nothing concerning this finding.
- ○ 3. notify social services of a case of possible child abuse.
- ○ 4. question the mother about the family's discipline style.

72. According to Erikson's theory of development, a 13-year-old client dying of cancer normally would be expected to be resolving which of the following psychosocial issues?
- ○ 1. Lifetime vocation.
- ○ 2. Social conscience.
- ⊗ 3. Personal identity.
- ○ 4. Sense of industry.

73. Which of the following nursing diagnoses would receive the greatest priority in the care of an unconscious client with a head injury?
- ⊗ 1. Ineffective Airway Clearance related to inability to remove respiratory secretions.
- ○ 2. Impaired Gas Exchange related to shallow, irregular breathing.
- ○ 3. High Risk for Injury related to disorientation and decreased level of consciousness.
- ○ 4. Sensory-Perceptual Alterations related to decreased level of consciousness.

74. The nurse is taking a nursing history on a preoperative client. Which of the following pieces of information would most likely have a significant impact on the client's recovery postoperatively? The client

- ○ 1. had a cold 6 weeks ago.
- Ⓧ 2. has smoked 1 pack of cigarettes a day for 12 years.
- ○ 3. drinks about two beers a week on a regular basis.
- ○ 4. is 10 pounds overweight.

75. A child admitted to the hospital with a serum sodium level of 160 mmol/L is receiving 5% dextrose with 0.45 normal saline solution. The mother asks the child's nurse why the child is receiving sodium. The nurse's best reply would be, "Your child's sodium is

- ○ 1. high; I'll stop the infusion and check with the physician."
- ○ 2. high; but if serum sodium level is decreased too rapidly, it may cause seizures."
- ○ 3. low; we need to give some more sodium intravenously."
- ○ 4. normal; the solution will maintain the level."

76. A priority nursing goal for the client presenting with pelvic inflammatory disease is

- ○ 1. Alteration in Nutrition.
- ○ 2. Self-Care Deficit.
- ○ 3. Alteration in Comfort.
- ○ 4. Alteration in Skin Integrity.

77. A client is admitted to the inpatient psychiatric unit. He is unshaven, has body odor, and has spots on his shirt and pants. He moves slowly, gazes at the floor, and has a flat affect. The nurse's highest priority in assessing the client on admission would be to ask him

- ○ 1. how he sleeps at night.
- ○ 2. if he is thinking about hurting himself.
- ○ 3. about recent stresses.
- ○ 4. how he feels about himself.

78. A 37-year-old Hispanic client visits the clinic for the first time. She is about 12 weeks' pregnant, and this is her first pregnancy. The nurse instructs the client that one of the tests that will most likely be ordered for the client is a

- ○ 1. chorionic villi sampling.
- ○ 2. glucose tolerance test.
- ○ 3. urine culture and sensitivity.
- ○ 4. hepatitis D test.

79. A mother and her infant are being seen by the clinic nurse. Which of the following will negatively influence the mother's transition to a parenting role with this child?

- ○ 1. The child is characterized by the mother as being "easier" than her first child.
- ○ 2. The child is a healthy baby.
- ○ 3. The father was supportive of the mother during pregnancy.

- ○ 4. The mother complains that her husband allows his mother to make all the child care decisions.

80. The nurse judges the client to no longer need constant one-to-one observation for self-directed violence when the client

- ○ 1. stops putting his head in the toilet to drown himself.
- ○ 2. begins to interact with the nurse.
- ○ 3. displays a sudden elevation in mood.
- ○ 4. eats his meals in the dining room.

81. A 10-year-old is sent home for pediculosis after being at camp for 1 week. The mother thinks others at camp have it. The mother asks the camp nurse how her son could have gotten pediculosis. The nurse would reply,

- ○ 1. "I don't think he got it here, there are no other cases."
- ○ 2. "He probably got it in boxing class."
- ○ 3. "Usually the kids get it at camp by sharing towels in the shower."
- ○ 4. "Children who go on an overnight and sleep close to someone who has it get it more easily."

82. The nurse is conducting a mental status examination on a client with a cognitive disorder. Which of the following statements does the nurse judge to be an impairment in abstract thinking? The client's

- ○ 1. ability to remember her wedding day.
- ○ 2. memories regarding her vacation 5 years ago.
- ○ 3. inability to find a similarity between a bird and a butterfly.
- ○ 4. inability to state her home address.

83. A client is admitted to the emergency room with a cut finger that is bleeding profusely. She displays signs of alcohol intoxication, and a blood test confirms this. After the client's wound is sutured but before she leaves the emergency room, it would be best for the nurse to ensure that the client

- ○ 1. takes a nap.
- ○ 2. does some exercising.
- ○ 3. restricts fluid intake.
- ○ 4. drinks generous amounts of black coffee.

84. The nurse is caring for a 38-year-old primigravida in the third trimester of pregnancy. The nurse plans to assess the client for symptoms of

- ○ 1. pregnancy-induced hypertension.
- ○ 2. pelvic inflammatory disease.
- ○ 3. ruptured membranes.
- ○ 4. cardiac overload.

85. A hyperactive client uses the telephone as often as several times an hour. In a nursing team conference, the team decides the best course of action would be to

- ○ 1. take the client back to his room each time he goes to the telephone.
- ○ 2. explain to the client that because he abused his

telephone privileges, he can no longer use the telephone.

○ 3. work out a plan with the client about the number of telephone calls he can make each day.

○ 4. allow the client to use the telephone when he likes until he begins to show improvement from therapy.

86. To decrease anxiety in a young child admitted overnight for observation, the nurse should do which of the following when caring for him?

○ 1. Move quickly around the child.

○ 2. Keep the child away from the center of activity.

○ 3. Avoid using a night light.

○ 4. Avoid making loud noises.

87. A client with insulin-dependent diabetes mellitus is being considered for the tight-control program. In determining whether the client is a candidate for this program, the nurse and health care team evaluate the

○ 1. client's daily dietary requirements.

○ 2. client's previous compliance history.

○ 3. client's family support system.

○ 4. length of time the client has had diabetes mellitus.

88. A client is admitted to the emergency room hyperventilating. A physical examination is essentially

negative. The client's medical diagnosis is acute anxiety attack. While planning nursing care for this client, the nurse's behavior should reflect

○ 1. calmness.

○ 2. sympathy.

○ 3. cheerfulness.

○ 4. friendliness.

89. Which of the following statements that the nurse could make to a client suspected of being abused would most likely encourage her to admit and describe her abuse?

○ 1. "How did you hurt yourself?"

○ 2. "When were you in an accident?"

○ 3. "Who is doing this to you?"

○ 4. "How long have you had these bruises?"

90. Two boys in their early teens come to the crisis center. One says, "Can you help? Our friend is sick in the car. We don't know what's wrong but he uses lots of stuff to feel better." After bringing the client into the center, the nurse judges that the client has most probably been using marijuana because his eyes

○ 1. are bloodshot.

○ 2. have dilated pupils.

○ 3. have pinpoint pupils.

○ 4. show rapid movement.

CORRECT ANSWERS AND RATIONALE

The letters in parentheses following the rationale identify the step of the nursing process (A, D, P, I, E), cognitive level (K, C, T, N), client needs (S, G, L, H), and nursing care area (O, X, Y, M). See the Answer Grid for the key.

1. 4. The nurse should contact the physician immediately because the client is demonstrating danger signals of septic shock. Tachycardia, or a pulse rate greater than 120 beats/minute; tachypnea, or respirations of 24 breaths/minute or higher; hypotension; changes in the level of consciousness; and decreased urine output are all danger signs of septic shock. Antipyretics and analgesics can assist the client's comfort but are not critical at this time. The vital signs should be monitored more frequently if the client is developing septic shock or the spread of infection. (I, N, G, O)

2. 2. The goal is to decrease the bleeding. This can be aided by decreasing circulation to the area. Elevating the part and applying cold decreases circulation to the area. The child will also receive cryoprecipitate. Lack of platelets is not the problem in children with hemophilia. Aspirin is contraindicated for clients who have bleeding disorders because it increases capillary fragility. (P, N, G, Y)

3. 1. This client is experiencing early signs of preterm labor. The nurse should plan to place the client on bed rest on her left side, which promotes uterine placental perfusion. The client should be encouraged to keep well hydrated either by drinking fluids or by intravenous therapy. The client should be encouraged to keep her bladder empty through frequent voiding. If progressive dilation occurs, or if the contractions become stronger and more frequent, other forms of more aggressive therapy may be initiated, such as ritodrine or magnesium sulfate. Amniotomy, or rupture of the membranes, will not be performed unless delivery is necessary due to an infection or fetal compromise. The neonatal resuscitation team should be alerted to the client's admission and potential delivery, but their assistance is not needed at this time. (P, N, G, O)

4. 1. When working with a battered woman, the nurse should help her share and discuss her anger, frustration, guilt, shame, and other feelings. Displacing or placing feelings onto another person or object is not helpful to the client and is not a healthy way for her to handle her feelings. Informing the client of safe homes and crisis lines, teaching her about the cycle of violence, and informing her about legal and personal rights are some of the issues the nurse should address with the battered client. (I, T, L, X)

5. 3. The nurse does not argue with the client having delusions. The nurse addresses the client's underlying feeling and presents reality to promote the client's trust, comfort, and sense of reality. "Why do you think someone wants to kill you" challenges the client and further distances the client from reality. "No one wants to kill you, we like you" defends the staff and does not address the client's feeling. "Don't worry, we'll protect you, and no one can come here to harm you" validates the client's delusion, does not address the client's feeling, and may further confuse the client. (I, T, L, X)

6. 2. Tailor sitting is an excellent exercise that helps to strengthen the client's back muscles and also prepares the client for the process of labor. The client should be encouraged to rest periodically during the day and avoid standing or sitting in one position for a long time. Leg lifts are helpful for leg aches, and shoulder circling exercises are helpful for neck and upper backaches. Squatting is not helpful for alleviating lower backaches. (I, T, H, O)

7. 2. The most common cause of death in children with leukemia is infection. The child should be monitored for any signs of infection, including temperature. Bleeding, although a common problem, is not the most common cause of death. (A, N, G, Y)

8. 2. The client diagnosed with class II heart disease may become easily fatigued with exertion. The client should be encouraged to rest frequently and ask for assistance with care of the neonate. The client does not need to remain on bed rest continuously, nor is breast-feeding contraindicated. The client should be encouraged to remain well hydrated by drinking plenty of fluids. (I, T, G, O)

9. 2. The normal immunizations given to a 6-month-old are diphtheria-pertussis-tetanus with *Haemophilus influenzae* vaccine and hepatitis. The third oral polio vaccine can be given at 6 months to 18 months. Generally, immunizations are not given to a child with a severe febrile illness. (I, N, H, Y)

10. 3. Lotions, creams, and powders may increase skin irritation and should be avoided. The area should be kept dry and open to the air. Radiated skin is temperature-sensitive, and a hot-water bottle could cause a burn. (E, N, G, M)

11. 2. *Denial* is an unconscious refusal to admit an unacceptable idea or behavior. It protects the client in this crisis situation by blocking out the earthquake from conscious awareness. *Intellectualization* is the use of logical explanations without feelings. *Rationalization* is the attempt to prove that one's feelings are justifiable. *Undoing* is doing something to make up for a wrongdoing. (D, T, L, X)

12. 1. Early decelerations are decelerations that mirror the contraction pattern. They are caused by pressure on the fetal skull and are not considered an ominous sign. The nurse should continue to monitor the client and fetus. Turning the client to the left side and administering oxygen are not warranted. Pushing in the squatting position should not alter the early deceleration pattern. Early decelerations are common during the second stage of labor. (I, N, G, O)

13. 2. In myasthenia gravis, major respiratory complications can result from weakness in the muscles of breathing and swallowing. The client is at risk for aspiration, respiratory infection, and respiratory failure. Providing a safe environment and emotional support are secondary goals. Pain is not a problem with myasthenia gravis. (P, T, G, M)

14. 3. Steroid use tends to elevate glucose levels, and the child should be monitored for increases. Potassium intake should be increased. The drug should be taken with food or milk to reduce gastrointestinal upset. Because steroids suppress the inflammatory response, temperature measurement is not an effective assessment tool for identifying infections. (I, N, S, Y)

15. 3. Using both hands to assess the fundus is useful for the prevention of uterine inversion. Using both hands does not hasten or promote uterine involution, which lasts about 6 weeks from the time of delivery. Determining the size of the fundus may be important if the client is experiencing excessive lochia because an enlarged fundus may be an indicator of retained blood clots or fragments of the placenta, but the nurse does not need to use both hands to determine this. (P, T, G, O)

16. 4. Herpes simplex with skin ulcerations persisting longer than 1 month is categorized as an AIDS-defining illness. The Centers for Disease Control and Prevention (CDC) list opportunistic diseases that, when found in people with laboratory evidence of HIV infection, are diagnostic of AIDS. (A, C, G, M)

17. 2. Use of an antihistamine and calamine lotion are recommended to help decrease the itching. The child can have a bath in cool water, but soaking will dry out the skin. Use of oatmeal baths also helps decrease itching. Children are contagious from 1 day before the lesions break out until they are all scabbed over. (I, T, H, Y)

18. 4. The neonate has a cephalohematoma, which usu-

ally resolves without treatment by 6 weeks of age. It is usually not present at birth and begins about 24 hours after delivery. It is caused by pressure on the fetal skull during the birth process. Because of the breakdown of red blood cells within the hematoma, the neonate is at greater risk for hyperbilirubinemia. About 10% to 25% of neonates may have a skull fracture, but the skull fracture is not the cause of the hematoma. The neonate does not need repeated surgeries. (I, N, G, O)

19. 4. The nurse should inform the child and parents of events that will definitely happen. The surgeon may not order an injection or nasogastric tube. If the nurse learns these measures are ordered, then the child and parents can be informed. The nurse should be honest about pain. The use of a doll gives the child concrete information about where the surgery will occur. (I, N, G, Y)

20. 3. Cocaine use causes pupils to dilate. Marijuana causes eyes to be red and appear bloodshot. Heroin causes pupils to be pinpoints. Having tired-looking eyes would not necessarily be caused by drug use. (I, T, H, Y)

21. 4. A typical finding when interviewing the parents of abused children is their description of the abused child as being different from other children, including siblings. They frequently say that the child whines a lot, cries, and is sullen. The nurse often will find other crisis or near-crisis situations in the home of an abused child, such as unemployment, financial strains, alcoholism, and the like. If one child in a family is being abused, siblings are also at risk for abuse. (A, N, L, X)

22. 1. Headache is not a common side effect of epidural anesthesia because the dura mater is not entered. Epidural anesthesia is associated with a decreased urge to void, therefore catheterization of a full bladder may be necessary. Anesthesia and analgesia can slow the process of labor. Because the client is anesthetized, bearing down efforts during the second stage of labor may be less effective, thus the second stage may be prolonged. (E, N, G, O)

23. 1. Exercise, especially weight-bearing exercise such as walking or jogging, is recommended on a regular basis to maintain high-density bone mass. Diet should be high in calcium and vitamin D, but increasing the daily intake of protein is not appropriate. It is recommended that premenopausal women consume about 1000 to 1200 mg of calcium daily. Sunbathing is not recommended. (P, T, H, M)

24. 2. One nursing goal for clients with febrile seizures is to maintain temperature at a low enough level to prevent recurrence of seizures. Decreasing the environmental temperature and removing excess clothing and blankets will help decrease the client's temperature. Respiratory isolation is not necessary unless the child has a condition that warrants such an isolation. There is no reason to keep the child supine; a side-lying position would be acceptable. This action will help decrease intracranial pressure, but a febrile seizure results from abnormal electrical activity in the brain due to elevated body temperature. The child with a fever should have an increased fluid and caloric intake. Strict intake and output monitoring is not necessary at this time. Using tongue blades to separate the teeth in the upper jaw from the lower in an attempt to prevent the child from biting the tongue has proved to be ineffective and may result in broken teeth. (P, N, G, Y)

25. 2. One outcome criterion for the client with osteoarthritis is improved joint mobility. It is probably not possible to arrest the disease. Gold compound is administered to clients with rheumatoid arthritis, not osteoarthritis. Outcome criteria should be specific; feeling better is too general to be useful. (E, T, G, M)

26. 1. Treatment of a child in vasoocclusive crisis from sickle cell disease includes measures to prevent further sickling. Sickling occurs in the presence of decreased oxygen tension and alterations in pH. The hard sickle-shaped cells catch on each other and can eventually occlude vessels, which decreases oxygenation of the area and increases the sickling process. Increasing fluids will increase hemodilution and prevent the clumps of sickle cells from occluding vessels. The life span of a normal red blood cell is 120 days; there is no way to increase this life span. *Hemolysis* refers to the breakdown of red blood cells, something to be avoided in a child with sickle cell disease. (P, N, G, Y)

27. 1. Uteroplacental insufficiency is associated with a postterm fetus; therefore, it is recommended that the fetal heart rate and contraction pattern be monitored throughout the labor and delivery process. In addition, intravenous oxytocin, which is frequently used for induction of labor, may result in hyperstimulation of the uterus; therefore, monitoring the client is critical. These clients generally do not have a decreased amount of amniotic fluid (oligohydramnios). A scalp pH may be performed if there is evidence of fetal bradycardia, particularly late decelerations, but 5 to 10 scalp pH measurements would be highly unusual. One ultrasound may be performed to assess position and confirm gestational age. (I, N, G, O)

28. 4. The nurse should first assess the client who is subject to anxiety attacks by determining what behavior usually relieves his anxiety. Nursing care of an anxious client, however, must ultimately take into account all aspects of the client's anxiety, including what leads to attacks and what happens during an attack. Only then can the nurse help the client understand his anxiety, what personal needs may be unmet, and how to cope with his problem with behavior that is more satisfactory than having an anxiety attack. (I, T, L, X)

29. 4. Vaponefrin is epinephrine in an inhalable form. It is given to decrease inflammation in the upper airway through vasoconstriction. It also has bronchodilator effects. In the case of croup, epinephrine is used to increase the opening of the narrowed airway. A decrease in the severity of retractions is the only answer that indicates a change that reflects an increase in the opening of the airway. Color, heart rate, and oximeter readings could have remained the same before and after the treatment. In addition, epinephrine normally increases heart rate. (E, N, G, Y)

30. 4. The expected outcome that the client will accept encouragement from others specifically relates to the nursing diagnosis of Chronic Low Self-Esteem Secondary to Self-Doubt as evidenced by self-deprecatory comments. Using relaxation exercises relates more to decreasing anxiety. Demonstrating reality-based thinking relates to altered thought processes. Continually asking for approval from others relates to the client with low self-esteem but is more specific to the client with dependency problems. (D, N, L, X)

31. 4. Eating dry crackers before arising can assist in decreasing the common discomfort of nausea and vomiting. Avoiding strong food odors and eating a high-protein snack before bedtime can also help. Nipples should not be cleansed with soap. Cotton underwear, not nylon, should be worn. Leg cramps should be treated with heat not ice. Adequate dairy products can also decrease the incidence of leg cramps. (E, T, H, O)

32. 2. Promethazine is a tranquilizer that also serves as an antinauseant. It is a muscle relaxant that potentiates narcotics and barbiturates. The fetal heart rate and beat-to-beat variability usually decrease after analgesia is administered. Tranquilizers used in labor may have a central nervous system depressant effect on the neonate, and reduced sucking may occur. Tranquilizers used in labor can decrease the client's blood pressure. (I, T, G, O)

33. 3. In glaucoma, peripheral vision is impaired long before central vision is impaired. Hazy, blurred, or distorted vision is consistent with a diagnosis of cataracts. Loss of central vision is consistent with senile macular degeneration but occurs late in glaucoma. Blurred or "sooty" vision is consistent with a diagnosis of detached retina. (A, K, G, M)

34. 1. The onset of the action of insulin is one-half to one hour. The peak action occurs in 2 to 4 hours. The child needs to be checked for a hypoglycemic reaction (shaking, feelings of anxiety, and decreased level of consciousness) 2 hours after the insulin is given. Lente insulin is not given in an intravenous solution. Only Regular insulin is given through the intravenous route. It is not necessary to force fluids on this child. Because there is no information that indicates the child is unable to take fluids and foods by mouth, it is not necessary to give a dextrose solution at this time. (E, N, G, Y)

35. 4. Clients who are pregnant should not take any medications without consulting the health care provider; therefore, oral decongestants and antihistamines should be avoided whenever possible. Ice packs are not helpful in alleviating congestion. Warm moist towels might be helpful. Saline nose drops are a natural remedy and can alleviate the discomfort. The client should also be instructed to drink plenty of fluids. (I, T, G, O)

36. 3. The client who is wheelchair-bound with a spinal cord injury should be taught to make small pressure changes every 15 minutes to decrease the risk of pressure ulcer formation. (I, T, H, M)

37. 4. The first course of action for a client with a sucking chest wound is to stop air from entering the chest cavity, which will cause the lung to collapse. This is best done in an emergency situation by applying an air-occlusive dressing over the wound. Such measures as starting oxygen therapy, preparing for a tracheostomy, and preparing for endotracheal intubation may be necessary later but do not have the same priority on admission as closing the wound. (I, N, S, M)

38. 1. The nurse sits in silence with the client who is severely depressed. The nurse's presence conveys concern for and acceptance of the client and security, increases self-worth, and provides some structure to the client's day. Leaving the client alone, sending another staff member to interact with the client, and turning the television on for the client ignore the client's needs and do nothing to foster trust in the nurse. (I, T, L, X)

39. 1. The nurse should strike firmly with the hand cupped to make a hollow popping sound. This type of sound is produced when percussion is administered correctly. The child should wear a thin piece of clothing over the chest area like a tee shirt, to provide protection of the skin, without diminishing the effect of the percussion. Percussion is delivered over the rib cage to vibrate underlying lung passages to loosen mucus. (I, T, S, Y)

40. 2. Impetigo presents as reddish macules, which turn to vesicles and then erupt and form honey-colored crusts. The lesions can be in any stage. Red-

ness and formation of pus around a follicle describes folliculitis. Cellulitis is described as being warm, intensely red, edematous, and firm. Macular eruption with a sandpaper-like texture describes staphylococcal scalded skin syndrome. (A, T, G, Y)

41. 3. Alopecia, which can occur with the administration of some chemotherapeutic agents, is psychologically disturbing for many clients even though the loss is temporary. Clients should be reassured that their hair will grow back. Their concerns should not be trivialized. The nurse should encourage the client to discuss any concerns and should explore the various options available to the client (eg, wigs, scarfs, turbans). (I, N, L, M)

42. 4. Asocial behavior, anergia, alogia, and affective flattening are some of the negative symptoms of schizophrenia that may improve with risperidone therapy. Hallucinations, delusions, bizarre behavior, and abnormal thought form are positive symptoms of schizophrenia. (E, N, G, X)

43. 2. As the dye is injected, the client may experience a feeling of warmth, flushing of the face, and a salty taste in the mouth. The client should not experience chest pain. (E, T, S, M)

44. 2. Symptoms of carpal tunnel syndrome include pain, numbness, paresthesia, and weakness in the thumb and first and second fingers of the affected extremity (along the median nerve). Symptoms may be more severe at night owing to pressure or flexion of the wrist. Frequently, the dominant hand is affected, although carpal tunnel syndrome can occur bilaterally. (A, C, G, M)

45. 3. Compression of the umbilical cord around the fetal neck or head can result in decreased oxygenation to the fetus. Rupture of the cord, spontaneous separation of the placenta, and slow delivery of the fetal shoulder are not associated with the cord around the fetal neck. (I, T, G, O)

46. 4. A total serum cholesterol level of 326 is high. Normal serum cholesterol is from 140 to 200 mg/dL. A client with a cholesterol level of 326 will require dietary modifications and may be placed on lipid-lowering medication. (E, N, G, M)

47. 3. A swollen, painful scrotum after herniorrhaphy is relatively common. Elevating the scrotum, as on a rolled towel, and placing ice bags on the area intermittently are helpful. Applying a binder or a truss and having the client lie on his side with a pillow between his legs are unlikely to promote comfort when the scrotum is swollen. (I, N, S, M)

48. 4. The best nursing action is to lead the client to his room and assist him with putting on his clothes. The client with disorganized behavior needs the nurse's assistance to protect his self-esteem and dignity and to avoid embarrassment. Instructing the client to go to his room to put his clothes on may not be effective because the client may be too disorganized to follow directions. Wrapping a blanket around the client is helpful but instructing him then to be seated for the remainder of group is inappropriate and demeaning to the client. Asking another client to remove his sweater and wrap it around the other client's waist is inappropriate. (I, T, L, X)

49. 3. The client with emphysema has chronic retention of excessive carbon dioxide; as a result, the normal stimulus for respirations in the medulla becomes ineffective. Instead, peripheral pressoreceptors in the aortic arch and carotid arteries, which are sensitive to oxygen blood levels, stimulate respirations in response to low oxygen levels that have developed over time. If the client then receives high concentrations of oxygen, the blood level of oxygen will rise excessively, the stimulus for respiration will decrease, and respiratory failure may result. (I, N, G, M)

50. 4. The client's symptoms of insomnia, crying inconsolably, and hearing voices (hallucinations) are all symptoms of postpartum psychosis. The client needs immediate treatment to prevent injury to herself and the neonate. Postpartum psychosis occurs in about 1 in 1000 pregnancies; thus, it is relatively rare but serious. Hospitalization, chemotherapy, social support, and psychotherapy are used to treat postpartum psychosis. Prognosis for recovery is good, but the condition may recur with subsequent pregnancies. (D, N, L, O)

51. 4. If the fetal chin is posterior or facing the client's back, a cesarean section is usually warranted. Anencephaly and small maternal pelvis are associated with face presentation. If the face presented is anterior, a vaginal delivery may be accomplished. (E, N, G, O)

52. 3. One of the side effects of steroid therapy is fat deposition on the trunk and face, producing classic Cushing's-like signs. Steroids also can cause altered moods, weight gain, and may inhibit growth hormone action. (I, N, S, Y)

53. 4. Normal cardiac output is 4 to 8 liters per minute. The value does vary with body size, but 2.2 liters per minute is very low and can be life-threatening. For the client with a cardiac output of 2.2 liters per minute, the nurse should anticipate that the physician will adjust the medication regimen. The client may experience symptoms of dyspnea and fatigue, requiring nursing intervention. (E, T, G, M)

54. 2. Based on the data given, the most appropriate nursing diagnosis is Activity Intolerance related to severe left leg pain. The other diagnoses are not supported by the data presented. (D, N, G, M)

55. 4. To assess the frequency of the contractions, the nurse should assess the interval from the beginning of one contraction to the beginning of the next contraction. The duration of a contraction is the interval between the beginning and end of the contraction. The intensity can be assessed by using the fingertips of one hand. The intensity is estimated and classified as mild when uterine muscles are somewhat tense, moderate when the uterine muscles become moderately strong, and strong when the uterine muscles are so firm that the uterus cannot be indented. (A, T, G, O)

56. 4. It is unlikely that trouble urinating is related to diabetes mellitus. Common signs and symptoms of diabetes mellitus include poor wound healing, impotence, thirst, hunger, and frequent voiding. Additional signs and symptoms may include fatigue, itching, blurred vision, irritability, and muscle cramps, especially in the legs. (A, T, G, M)

57. 2. Fluoride supplements should be administered on an empty stomach, with no food or fluids ingested for 30 minutes after taking. They should not be given with calcium-rich foods. A 4-year-old would probably not be able to take a tablet, but if the child were able to, the table should be chewed and swished for 30 seconds before swallowing. (I, T, H, Y)

58. 1. The catheter should only be inserted just slightly beyond the end of the tracheostomy tube to prevent damage to the carina. The catheter should be inserted with the suction port open and removed while turning the catheter with the suction port closed. Tracheostomy suctioning in children is an aseptic procedure in acute care settings. In some circumstances, it can be a clean procedure in the home. (I, T, S, Y)

59. 1. The most important principle related to the management of cancer pain is to individualize the therapy to the client. Fear of client addiction to pain medication is unfounded. Medications should not be discontinued or given on a p.r.n. basis, but instead should be given on a regular, around-the-clock schedule, with increasing dosages as drug tolerance increases. (P, T, G, M)

60. 2. The client with a breech presentation needs to be carefully monitored for fetal distress or fetal bradycardia, which is often associated with umbilical cord compression. It is not unusual to see an increased intensity and frequency of contractions during the transition stage of labor. Meconium-stained amniotic fluid is not unusual with a breech presentation. (I, T, G, O)

61. 1. A blood glucose level of 250 mg/dL is indicative of diabetic ketoacidosis. The client should contact her health care provider, take insulin to lower glucose levels, and drink water to prevent dehydration. Hypoglycemic episodes are managed by ingesting foods or beverages with high sugar content; glucagon is used when the client is unconscious. (E, T, H, Y)

62. 2. Penicillin is given to children with rheumatic fever to eradicate the hemolytic streptococci that triggered the autoimmune response that causes the disease. It does not decrease joint pain. Penicillin should be given on an empty stomach. Prophylactic use of penicillin with siblings is not indicated. (E, N, G, Y)

63. 1. The most consistent signs of pregnancy-induced hypertension are sudden, excessive weight gain and facial and finger edema. Checking the client's pulse, calf muscles, or ankles will not provide the nurse with data related to pregnancy-induced hypertension. Ankle and leg edema are common in pregnant women due to the fluid volume shifts associated with pregnancy. Proteinuria is a sign of progression of hypertension. (A, N, G, O)

64. 3. Corporeal punishment is an aversion technique that teaches children what not to do. Children can often become accustomed to physical punishment, and the punishment must be more severe to get the same results. Corporeal punishment, such as spanking, can reinforce the idea that violence is acceptable in certain circumstances. Often, parents use physical punishment when they are in a rage, and injury to the child can result. (I, C, H, Y)

65. 2. Yogurt is high in protein because it is made from milk. The other choices are much higher in carbohydrates than protein except for bacon, which is higher in fat. (I, T, G, Y)

66. 4. The client who threatens suicide should be considered at high risk, and his threat should be taken seriously as a call for help. It is untrue that a suicide threat is only a bid for attention, that people who talk about suicide will not do it, and that a person without a history of psychiatric problems will be unlikely to carry out a first threat. (D, N, L, X)

67. 1. The client should be instructed to avoid straining and lifting for 2 to 6 weeks after surgery. The client should be able to void without difficulty after the immediate postoperative phase. The client typically can ambulate without assistance and should not require assistive devices, unless such devices were used before surgery. The client returns to a regular diet as tolerated after surgery. Increased dietary fiber intake is suggested to avoid constipation, but the client does not need to remain on a soft diet until the wound heals. (E, T, G, M)

68. 2. The child who has increasing respiratory difficulty after being removed from an increased oxygen environment should be placed back in the environment. The child's pulse rate will most likely be increased. The nurse does not need to notify the physician of the child's status unless no improvement occurs after the child is back in the oxygen tent. It is best to wait until a later time to feed the child because the act of eating takes up energy and oxygen that the child does not have in sufficient supply at the moment. Unless the child has blocked nasal passages, there is no reason to suction the nares. (D, N, G, Y)

69. 2. The public health nurse has identified several helpful strategies. The one strategy that would impact most would be to attend the school board meeting and advocate for educational programming. The programming could be simple and done quickly. (P, N, H, Y)

70. 4. A person who starts to adjust to life without a family member before the member actually dies is experiencing anticipatory grief or mourning. This represents an early "giving up" of the loved one and accomplishes some of the grieving for the loved one before he dies. (D, T, L, X)

71. 2. This lesion is a mongolian spot, which is common in children of Asian or African American heritage. The key word in the description is *pigment*. A bruise results from bleeding into subcutaneous or muscle tissue; it is not a pigment change in the skin. (D, T, G, Y)

72. 3. According to Erikson, a child of 13 years is normally seeking to meet his needs for developing personal identity. (D, C, L, X)

73. 1. A major goal of nursing care in the care of the unconscious client with a head injury is to establish and maintain an open airway. An obstructed airway can lead to hypoxia and carbon dioxide retention, which will further increase intracranial pressure. The other nursing diagnoses are appropriate for this client but are not the highest priority. (D, N, G, M)

74. 2. A client who smokes is at increased risk for atelectasis postoperatively; thus, smoking is the most significant risk factor listed in this item. If the client has completely recovered from the cold he had 6 weeks ago, it would be irrelevant to his postoperative recovery. Although an obese client faces increased surgical risks, an excess of 10 pounds is not significant enough to pose a greater risk than the smoking. (A, N, G, M)

75. 2. The normal serum sodium level for a child is 138 to 146 mmol/L. The value given is high. A rapid decrease in serum sodium level, however, can cause fluid shifts that will result in a rapid increase in intracranial pressure, increasing the risk of seizures. Therefore, the child's sodium level is monitored carefully and decreased slowly. A solution of 0.2%

normal saline in 5% dextrose is most commonly used as a maintenance fluid. (I, K, G, Y)

76. 3. Alteration in Comfort is a priority nursing diagnosis for the client with pelvic inflammatory disease because the disease is associated with severe pain. Alterations in nutrition and skin integrity and self-care deficits are not priorities associated with the disorder. (D, T, G, M)

77. 2. The nurse's highest priority is to ask the client if he is thinking about hurting himself or to assess for suicide. Questioning the client about his sleep pattern, recent stresses, and feelings about himself are important areas of assessment for the depressed client but not as immediate a priority as assessing the risk for suicide. (I, T, L, X)

78. 2. There is a greater incidence of both gestational diabetes and preexisting diabetes among women older than 35 years. In addition, clients of Native American and Hispanic descent have a greater incidence of gestational diabetes than the general population. The client does not present symptoms that would warrant testing of chorionic villi, urine culture and sensitivity, or hepatitis D. (I, T, G, O)

79. 4. Transition to parenthood is negatively affected by stress, especially marital tension or strife. The best single predictor of postpartum marital adjustment is the level of marital adjustment during pregnancy. Special characteristics of the infant, like a difficult temperament or disability, can add to stress and decrease a smooth adjustment to parenthood. (A, T, H, Y)

80. 1. The nurse judges the client to no longer require constant one-to-one observation when the client stops putting his head in the toilet to drown. Interacting with the nurse and eating meals in the dining room are behaviors that indicate nothing about the client's potential for self-directed violence. A sudden elevation in mood may indicate relief about ambivalent feelings and thoughts about killing himself and may be a signal to the nurse that a suicide attempt is imminent. (E, N, G, X)

81. 4. Children at slumber parties are at higher risk for developing pediculosis because of the close contact with others. Pediculosis is spread person to person or on other objects that are shared, such as hats and combs. There may be someone else at camp with pediculosis and the nurse does not know it yet. (I, T,H,Y)

82. 3. Impairment in abstract thinking is demonstrated by the client's inability to find a similarity between a bird and a butterfly. The client's ability to remember her wedding day and vacation 5 years ago demonstrate intact long-term memory. The client's inability to state her home address demonstrates impairment in short-term memory. (E, N, L, X)

83. 1. It is best to overcome the effects of excessive alcohol intake by sleeping. Alcohol is not used directly by muscle cells; therefore, physical activity does not affect the rate at which alcohol is removed from the bloodstream. Restricting fluids or drinking black coffee does not hasten removal of alcohol from the body. (I, T, L, X)

84. 1. There is a strong association between advanced maternal age and pregnancy-induced hypertension as well as chronic hypertension. The incidence of pregnancy-induced hypertension is greatest among primigravidas. Although the older client is also at risk for preterm labor and birth, this client does not present any symptoms of preterm labor. (P, N, H, O)

85. 3. A hyperactive client needs help in setting limits on behavior. The best course of action when this client abuses telephone privileges is to work out a plan with him about the number of calls he can make each day. The agreed-on plan should then be followed. (P, T, L, X)

86. 4. Caregiver behaviors that decrease a child's fears and anxieties include moving slowly around the child, keeping the child near the center of activity, using night lights, and avoiding loud noises. (I, T, L, X)

87. 2. The tight-control program for clients with diabetes mellitus involves frequent testing of serum glucose and insulin administration (every 2 to 4 hours in some cases). The tight-control program has been found to be effective in reducing vascular complications associated with diabetes mellitus. For a client to be able to be placed on this program, it would be essential to evaluate the client's previous ability to be compliant with the diabetic regimen. (E, T, G, M)

88. 1. A nurse caring for an anxious client should be calm and sufficiently authoritative to help the client understand that she or he can provide controls for the client when he cannot do so on his own. If possible, the client should be kept in a quiet, relatively small room because he is already overwhelmed by external stimuli. (P, T, L, X)

89. 3. A question from the nurse that helps the client describe her health problem is most helpful when abuse is suspected. Statements that help the client avoid the issue are least helpful. Even if the client does not want to discuss the cause of her bruises, helping her to express her thoughts in a supportive atmosphere often helps open channels of communication. (I, T, L, X)

90. 1. Marijuana causes dilation of arterioles, and this causes a marked redness of the eyes. Heroin characteristically causes pinpoint pupils, cocaine causes dilation of the pupils, and phencyclidine (PCP) causes rapid eye movements. (A, C, L, X)

NURSING CARE COMPREHENSIVE TEST

TEST 2

Directions: Use this answer grid to determine areas of strength or need for further study.

NURSING PROCESS

A = Assessment
D = Analysis, nursing diagnosis
P = Planning
I = Implementation
E = Evaluation

CLIENT NEEDS

S = Safe, effective care environment
G = Physiologic integrity
L = Psychosocial integrity
H = Health promotion and maintenance

COGNITIVE LEVEL

K = Knowledge
C = Comprehension
T = Application
N = Analysis

NURSING CARE AREA

O = Maternity and newborn care
X = Psychosocial health problems
Y = Nursing care of children
M = Medical and surgical health problems

Question #	Answer #	Nursing Process					Cognitive Level				Client Needs				Care Area			
		A	**D**	**P**	**I**	**E**	**K**	**C**	**T**	**N**	**S**	**G**	**L**	**H**	**O**	**X**	**Y**	**M**
1	4				I					N		G			O			
2	2			P						N		G					Y	
3	1			P						N		G			O			
4	1				I				T				L			X		
5	3				I				T				L			X		
6	2				I				T					H	O			
7	2	A								N		G					Y	
8	2				I				T			G			O			
9	2				I					N				H			Y	
10	3					E				N		G						M
11	2		D						T				L			X		
12	1				I					N		G			O			
13	2			P					T			G						M
14	3				I					N	S						Y	
15	3			P					T			G			O			
16	4	A						C				G						M
17	2				I				T					H			Y	
18	4				I					N		G			O			
19	4				I					N		G					Y	

ANSWER GRID: 1

NURSING PROCESS

A = Assessment
D = Analysis, nursing diagnosis
P = Planning
I = Implementation
E = Evaluation

CLIENT NEEDS

S = Safe, effective care environment
G = Physiologic integrity
L = Psychosocial integrity
H = Health promotion and maintenance

COGNITIVE LEVEL

K = Knowledge
C = Comprehension
T = Application
N = Analysis

NURSING CARE AREA

O = Maternity and newborn care
X = Psychosocial health problems
Y = Nursing care of children
M = Medical and surgical health problems

Question #	Answer #	A	D	P	I	E	K	C	T	N	S	G	L	H	O	X	Y	M
20	3				I				T					H			Y	
21	4	A								N			L			X		
22	1					E				N		G			O			
23	1			P					T					H				M
24	2			P						N		G					Y	
25	2					E			T			G						M
26	1			P						N		G					Y	
27	1				I					N		G			O			
28	4				I				T				L			X		
29	4					E				N		G					Y	
30	4		D							N			L			X		
31	4					E			T					H	O			
32	2				I				T			G			O			
33	3	A					K					G						M
34	1					E				N		G					Y	
35	4				I				T			G			O			
36	3				I				T					H				M
37	4				I					N	S							M
38	1				I				T				L			X		
39	1				I				T		S						Y	
40	2	A							T			G					Y	
41	3				I					N			L					M
42	4					E				N		G				X		
43	2					E			T		S							M
44	2	A						C				G						M

ANSWER GRID: 2

NURSING PROCESS

A = Assessment
D = Analysis, nursing diagnosis
P = Planning
I = Implementation
E = Evaluation

COGNITIVE LEVEL

K = Knowledge
C = Comprehension
T = Application
N = Analysis

CLIENT NEEDS

S = Safe, effective care environment
G = Physiologic integrity
L = Psychosocial integrity
H = Health promotion and maintenance

NURSING CARE AREA

O = Maternity and newborn care
X = Psychosocial health problems
Y = Nursing care of children
M = Medical and surgical health problems

Question #	Answer #	\ Nursing Process A	D	P	I	E	\ Cognitive Level K	C	T	N	\ Client Needs S	G	L	H	\ Care Area O	X	Y	M
45	3				I				T			G			O			
46	4					E				N		G						M
47	3				I					N	S							M
48	4				I				T				L			X		
49	3				I					N		G						M
50	4		D							N			L		O			
51	4					E				N		G			O			
52	3				I					N	S						Y	
53	4					E			T			G						M
54	2		D							N		G						M
55	4	A							T			G			O			
56	4	A							T			G						M
57	2				I				T					H			Y	
58	1				I				T		S						Y	
59	1			P					T			G						M
60	2				I				T			G			O			
61	1					E			T					H			Y	
62	2					E				N		G					Y	
63	1	A								N		G			O			
64	3				I			C						H			Y	
65	2				I				T			G					Y	
66	4		D							N			L			X		
67	1					E			T			G						M
68	2		D							N		G					Y	
69	2			P						N				H			Y	

ANSWER GRID: 3

NURSING PROCESS

A = Assessment
D = Analysis, nursing diagnosis
P = Planning
I = Implementation
E = Evaluation

COGNITIVE LEVEL

K = Knowledge
C = Comprehension
T = Application
N = Analysis

CLIENT NEEDS

S = Safe, effective care environment
G = Physiologic integrity
L = Psychosocial integrity
H = Health promotion and maintenance

NURSING CARE AREA

O = Maternity and newborn care
X = Psychosocial health problems
Y = Nursing care of children
M = Medical and surgical health problems

Question #	Answer #	Nursing Process					Cognitive Level				Client Needs				Care Area			
		A	D	P	I	E	K	C	T	N	S	G	L	H	O	X	Y	M
70	4		D						T				L			X		
71	2		D						T			G					Y	
72	3		D					C					L			X		
73	1		D							N		G						M
74	2	A								N		G						M
75	2				I		K					G					Y	
76	3		D						T			G						M
77	2				I				T				L			X		
78	2				I				T			G			O			
79	4	A							T					H			Y	
80	1					E				N		G				X		
81	4				I				T					H			Y	
82	3					E				N			L			X		
83	1				I				T				L			X		
84	1			P						N				H	O			
85	3			P					T				L			X		
86	4				I				T				L			X		
87	2					E			T			G						M
88	1			P					T				L			X		
89	3				I				T				L			X		
90	1	A						C					L			X		

ANSWER GRID: 4

NURSING PROCESS

A = Assessment
D = Analysis, nursing diagnosis
P = Planning
I = Implementation
E = Evaluation

CLIENT NEEDS

S = Safe, effective care environment
G = Physiologic integrity
L = Psychosocial integrity
H = Health promotion and maintenance

COGNITIVE LEVEL

K = Knowledge
C = Comprehension
T = Application
N = Analysis

NURSING CARE AREA

O = Maternity and newborn care
X = Psychosocial health problems
Y = Nursing care of children
M = Medical and surgical health problems

Question #	Answer #	Nursing Process					Cognitive Level				Client Needs				Care Area			
		A	D	P	I	E	K	C	T	N	S	G	L	H	O	X	Y	M
Number Correct																		
Number Possible	90	12	11	12	38	17	2	5	45	38	7	48	21	14	20	21	26	23
Percentage Correct																		

Score Calculation: To determine your **Percentage Correct,** divide the **Number Correct** by the **Number Possible.**

ANSWER GRID: 5

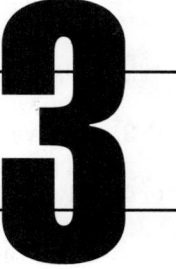
Select the one best answer, and indicate your choice by filling in the circle in front of the option.

1. The client with major depression and borderline personality disorder is hospitalized for self-mutilation and threats of suicide. Which of the following expected outcomes would the nurse judge as therapeutic and realistic for the client? The client will
○ 1. stay in her room when overwhelmed by feelings.
○ 2. leave group to pace when feeling anxious.
○ 3. appropriately verbalize feelings of anger and sadness to the nurse.
○ 4. ask the nurse for a p.r.n. medication when feeling out of control.

2. An 8-year-old child has a fluid restriction of 1000 mL/day. The mother is staying with the child in the room. The nurse should plan to
○ 1. discuss the fluid restriction with the mother and child and allow them to decide how to allocate the fluids over the 24 hours.
○ 2. explain to the mother that only the hospital personnel will be able to provide fluids.
○ 3. let the child drink until the limit is reached and then allow no more fluids.
○ 4. tell the mother exactly how much fluid the child can have each hour.

3. A client agrees to undergo disulfiram (Antabuse) therapy. The nurse would suspect that the client most probably has drunk alcohol while taking disulfiram when the client experiences
○ 1. vertigo.
○ 2. hallucinations.
○ 3. diarrhea and fever.
○ 4. nausea and vomiting.

4. Which of the following nursing actions would be most helpful for the verbally aggressive client to help manage anger appropriately?
○ 1. Role-playing assertive statements with the nurse.
○ 2. Watching a videotape about assertiveness.
○ 3. Describing feelings that occur after aggressive outbursts.
○ 4. Discussing situations that appear to be threatening.

5. A female client comes to the emergency room complaining of a fever and a sore throat. While examining the client, the nurse notes that she has many bruises in various stages of healing. The nurse suspects that she may be an abuse victim. When the client notes that the nurse observes her bruises, she says that her fever caused her to become confused and clumsy and that she fell several times and bruised herself. If the client is being abused and denying it, this behavior is most probably due to
○ 1. gaining pleasure from being abused.
○ 2. fearing that she will be blamed for her plight.
○ 3. believing that because she is ill, the abuse will now end.
○ 4. thinking that she can handle the problem as soon as she is well.

6. While visiting a client with multiple sclerosis, the community health nurse observes that the client looks unkempt and sad. The client suddenly says, "I can't even find the strength to comb my hair," and bursts into tears. Which of the following responses by the nurse would be best?
○ 1. "It must be frustrating not to be able to care for yourself."
○ 2. "How many days have you been unable to comb your hair?"
○ 3. "Why hasn't your husband been helping you?"
○ 4. "Tell me more about how you're feeling."

7. A primigravida at 24 weeks' gestation has received permission from the physician to make a 6-hour automobile trip to visit her parents. After teaching the client about precautions she should take during the trip, the nurse determines that the client needs *further* instructions when she says she should
○ 1. drink plenty of fluids to avoid dehydration.
○ 2. sleep for 1 hour at the halfway point of the trip.
○ 3. take frequent rest breaks every 2 hours.
○ 4. wear the automobile seat belt while traveling.

8. The nurse would judge that a client may be developing Wernicke-Korsakoff syndrome when the client exhibits
○ 1. fear and paranoia.
○ 2. aggression and hostility.
○ 3. short-term memory loss and disorientation.
○ 4. depression and suicidal tendencies.

9. The nurse has provided health teaching to a postpartum client who is bottle-feeding her neonate about physiologic changes that the client can expect during the postpartum period. The nurse determines that the client understands the instructions when the client says,
○ 1. "I can expect to have heart palpitations for several weeks."

○ 2. "It's normal for me to have reddish lochia until my 6-week checkup."

○ 3. "Any varicosities I had during pregnancy will disappear within 2 weeks."

○ 4. "My menstrual flow should resume in 6 to 10 weeks."

10. A 32-year-old female client visits the family planning clinic and requests an intrauterine device for contraception. The nurse should assess the client for history of

○ 1. thrombophlebitis.

○ 2. pelvic inflammatory disease.

○ 3. previous liver disease.

○ 4. coronary artery disease.

11. The nurse is evaluating the effectiveness of teaching about sickle cell disease with a child's mother. The nurse evaluates a need for further teaching when the mother

○ 1. states that she has started to give her child extra fluids with and between meals.

○ 2. is concerned about how the hospital staff will manage her child's pain.

○ 3. tells the nurse that she has placed her child on a soccer team.

○ 4. explains to the child's father that both he and she are carriers of the disease.

12. A female client is experiencing bladder control problems. She and the nurse identify several interventions to promote urinary continence, such as keeping the bedpan within easy reach and developing a drinking and voiding schedule. Which of the following client outcomes would indicate the success of these interventions? The client

○ 1. is continent 24 hours a day.

○ 2. states that her bladder control is improved.

○ 3. monitors herself for urine retention.

○ 4. complies with the drinking and voiding schedule.

13. A pregnant client at about 29 weeks' gestation asks the nurse "What can I do about this dark brown line running down my stomach?" The nurse should instruct the client that this dark-brown line is

○ 1. called *linea nigra* and will fade after the baby is born.

○ 2. indicative of a melanoma and should be evaluated.

○ 3. called the *pigmentation of pregnancy* and will remain dark after delivery.

○ 4. called *stretch marks* and will turn silvery after delivery.

14. A 4-week-old infant is admitted to the hospital with a diagnosis of pyloric stenosis. The nurse would identify which of the following as a priority nursing diagnosis?

○ 1. Constipation.

○ 2. Fluid and Electrolyte Imbalance.

○ 3. Altered Nutrition.

○ 4. Impaired Swallowing.

15. The client just finished talking on the telephone with his wife. He is tense, irritable, and perspiring. Which nursing action is best?

○ 1. Encourage ventilation.

○ 2. Direct the client to a quiet room for time out.

○ 3. Give the client an oral tranquilizer.

○ 4. Prepare for a show of determination.

16. A primipara on the postpartum unit delivered a viable male neonate vaginally under epidural anesthesia. The client asks the nurse, "Why are my baby's breasts so swollen?" The nurse should instruct the client that slight breast engorgement in term neonates is due to

○ 1. maternal hormonal influences.

○ 2. epidural anesthesia.

○ 3. maternal hyperthyroidism.

○ 4. genetic influences from both parents.

17. A child with rheumatic fever has polyarthritis and chorea. An echocardiogram shows fragmentation and swelling of the cardiac tissue. The nurse should

○ 1. explain to the child and family that the chorea will disappear over time.

○ 2. keep the child in a warm environment.

○ 3. perform neurologic checks every 4 hours until the chorea subsides.

○ 4. promote ambulation by giving aspirin every 4 hours.

18. The nurse is talking to a group of parents about drug abuse among adolescents. One parent says that he has heard that you can tell which drug a person is using by how their eyes look. The parent asks how you could tell a person was taking heroin. The nurse replies that the person's

○ 1. eyes would be red and bloodshot.

○ 2. pupils would be constricted to pinpoints.

○ 3. pupils would be large.

○ 4. eyelids would droop.

19. A primigravida in active labor has been diagnosed with chorioamnionitis. The nurse has explained the condition to the client. The nurse determines that the client understands the instructions when the client says

○ 1. "My baby's heart rate is slow because of my infection."

○ 2. "My infection is the cause of my hypertonic labor pattern."

○ 3. "Women who are overweight are more likely to get an infection during labor."

○ 4. "If left untreated, my baby might be born with pneumonia."

20. The nurse is assisting the physician in cardioversion of a client admitted with ventricular tachycardia. Cardioversion differs from defibrillation in that during cardioversion, the shock is

○ 1. unsynchronized with the R wave.

○ 2. synchronized with the R wave.

○ 3. delivered at a higher wattage.

○ 4. delivered with a different machine.

21. The nurse assesses a client with multiple sclerosis for euphoria, looking for which of the following characteristic clinical manifestations?

○ 1. Inappropriate laughter and giddiness.

○ 2. Mood elevation with an exaggerated sense of well-being.

○ 3. Slurring of words when excited.

○ 4. Visual hallucinations and giddiness.

22. A mother of an ill child is concerned because the child "isn't eating well." Of the following strategies devised by the mother to help increase the child's intake, the nurse should advise against

○ 1. allowing the child to choose his meals from an acceptable list of foods she would like him to eat.

○ 2. allowing the child to substitute items on his tray for other nutritious foods.

○ 3. asking the child why he is not eating.

○ 4. telling the child he must eat or he will not get better.

23. The nurse is caring for a client with acute osteomyelitis in the right tibia. Which of the following measures is most appropriate for the nurse to implement when repositioning the client's leg?

○ 1. Hold the leg by the ankle when repositioning to avoid touching the tibia.

○ 2. Have the client move the leg by himself to decrease pain.

○ 3. Support the leg above and below the affected area when positioning.

○ 4. Apply warm moist heat to leg before repositioning.

24. The nurse assesses a primipara who delivered a viable neonate 12 hours ago. The nurse observes that the client's fundus is firm at midline, her breasts are soft, she has scant lochia, and is negative for Homans' sign. The client tells the nurse that she has pain in her lower back. The nurse should

○ 1. contact the physician for an order for a urinalysis.

○ 2. ask the client how long she was in labor.

○ 3. administer an ordered mild analgesic.

○ 4. instruct the client to perform abdominal exercises.

25. A nurse is planning a seminar on injury prevention to be presented to a group of parents of children from 2 to 18 years. The first priority should be placed on discussing the use of

○ 1. child restraints in automobiles.

○ 2. helmets for biking and skating.

○ 3. special locks for cabinets.

○ 4. sunscreen and topical bug repellent in summer.

26. A client with bulimia binges twice a day. These binges would most likely involve

○ 1. feelings of euphoria and gratification.

○ 2. feeling out of control and disgusted with self.

○ 3. leaving traces of food around to attract attention.

○ 4. eating increasing amounts of food, resulting in substantial weight gain.

27. The mother of an infant with a cyanotic heart defect tells the nurse that her child has not been gaining weight even with an increased calorie formula. The mother states that the infant starts out with a good suck but tires and quits after 2 ounces. The infant is receiving oxygen through a nasal cannula as necessary, and is on digoxin therapy. The nurse should suggest that the mother

○ 1. cut a large hole in the nipple.

○ 2. feed the infant every 2 hours.

○ 3. have the infant tested for digoxin toxicity.

○ 4. increase the oxygen for feedings.

28. After a mastectomy for breast cancer, the nurse teaches the client how to avoid the development of lymphedema. The client should be taught to

○ 1. apply an elastic bandage to the affected extremity.

○ 2. limit range-of-motion exercises in the shoulder and elbow.

○ 3. elevate the affected arm on a pillow.

○ 4. take diuretics as necessary to decrease swelling.

29. While using an otoscope to examine the tympanic membrane of a 2-year-old child, the nurse should pull the pinna

● 1. down and back.

○ 2. down and slightly forward.

○ 3. up and back.

○ 4. up and forward.

30. When caring for a client with a fracture of a long bone, the nurse should assess the client for the earliest symptom of fat embolism, which is

○ 1. respiratory distress.

○ 2. confusion.

○ 3. petechiae.

○ 4. fever.

31. A primigravida in active labor received lumbar epidural anesthesia 3 hours ago. The client's cervix is now completely dilated, and she is ready to begin pushing. Before the client begins to push, the nurse should assess her

○ 1. contraction pattern.

○ 2. bladder.

○ 3. temperature.

○ 4. blood pressure.

32. A young child who has undergone a tonsillectomy refuses to let the nurse look at the tonsilar beds to check for bleeding. To assess whether the child is bleeding from the tonsilar beds, the nurse should

○ 1. assess capillary refill.

○ 2. get help to force open the mouth with a tongue blade.

○ 3. monitor for decreased blood pressure.

○ 4. observe for frequent swallowing.

33. A client is admitted to an inpatient psychiatric unit accompanied by his wife, who reports that he has been "on a spending spree; he sent roses to everyone we know. He plays a seductive game with women he meets, telling them that he's next in line for the throne in some country in Europe." The client becomes very active, moves about, and then puts his arm around the nurse in a show of affection and says to her, "I sure like you a lot, honey. I can do a lot for you in the real world out there." In this situation, what would be the nurse's best response?

○ 1. "Let's get some popcorn and a soda."

○ 2. "I'll have to tell my supervisor if you don't stop this minute."

○ 3. "You know you shouldn't do this. It's against the rules of the hospital."

○ 4. "Please stop. I'm very uncomfortable with your display of affection."

34. The nurse instructs the client how to instill nose drops correctly. The nurse evaluates that the client's technique is correct if the client

○ 1. uses sterile technique when handling the dropper.

○ 2. blows the nose gently after instillation of the medicine.

○ 3. lies supine for several minutes after instillation of the drops.

○ 4. uses a new dropper for each instillation of the medication.

35. When assessing a dark-skinned client for cyanosis, the nurse should examine the client's

○ 1. retinas.

○ 2. nail beds.

○ 3. oral mucous membranes.

○ 4. skin on the inner aspects of the wrists.

36. When performing a physical assessment on an 18-month-old child, the nurse should

○ 1. have the mother hold the toddler on her lap.

○ 2. assess the respiratory and cardiac systems first.

○ 3. carry out the assessment from head to toe.

○ 4. assess motor function by having the child run and walk.

37. The mother and nurse are planning a diet to increase protein in a 4-year-old's diet. Which of the following foods are least likely to increase protein intake?

○ 1. Bacon.

○ 2. Cooked dry beans.

○ 3. Peanut butter.

○ 4. Yogurt.

38. A client has been told to take ibuprofen (Motrin, Advil) to relieve the pain of her rheumatoid arthritis. Which of the following statements indicates the client understands how to take this drug safely and effectively?

○ 1. "I should not take aspirin or acetaminophen with ibuprofen unless my doctor tells me to."

○ 2. "I should not take this drug with antacids."

○ 3. "I do not need to worry about this medicine irritating my stomach."

○ 4. "I should notice the effects of this medicine within the first few days of therapy."

39. The priority need for a client experiencing a flashback is

○ 1. physical activity.

○ 2. large amounts of fluid.

○ 3. reassurance in a calm environment.

○ 4. close contact with his friends.

40. While assisting a multipara to the bathroom for the first time 1 hour after a vaginal delivery of a viable neonate, the nurse notes that the client's urine has two small blood clots in the measuring container. The nurse should

○ 1. massage the client's fundus vigorously.

○ 2. ask the client if she passed clots with her previous deliveries.

○ 3. review the client's records to determine the length of the third stage of labor.

○ 4. document this as a normal finding.

41. The nurse is caring for a primigravida in active labor when the client's membranes rupture spontaneously. The nurse should first

○ 1. turn the client to her left side.

○ 2. increase the rate of intravenous fluids.

○ 3. assess the client for a prolapsed cord.

○ 4. instruct the client how to push during contractions.

42. The nurse assesses a primipara on the seventh postpartum day during a home visit. The client tells the nurse that her lochia has been profuse and foul-smelling and she has had chills. During palpation of the uterus, the client indicates that she is very sore. The nurse determines that the client is most likely experiencing

○ 1. normal uterine involution.

○ 2. retained placental fragments.

○ 3. puerperal infection.

○ 4. uterine atony.

43. The nurse teaches a client how to self-administer NPH insulin injections. Which of the following techniques for self-administering insulin is incorrect?

○ 1. Shaking the insulin vial before withdrawing the insulin.

○ 2. Introducing the needle into subcutaneous tissue with a dart-like action.

3. Pulling back on the syringe plunger as soon as the needle is in place in subcutaneous tissue.

4. Holding an antiseptic sponge against the needle when removing it from subcutaneous tissue.

44. Which of the following positions would permit the best assessment of a client's inguinal hernia?

- 1. Standing.
- 2. Sitting.
- 3. Left side-lying.
- 4. Right side-lying.

45. After noting that an 8-month-old child's posterior fontanel is slightly open, the nurse should

- 1. check the child's head circumference.
- 2. consider this a normal finding.
- 3. question the mother about her delivery of this child.
- 4. schedule a radiologic examination of the child's head.

46. While caring for a multigravida in early labor in a birthing center, which of the following foods would be best if the client requests a snack?

- 1. yogurt.
- 2. cereal with milk.
- 3. vegetable soup.
- 4. peanut butter cookies.

47. A 10-year-old child is diagnosed with pediculosis. The mother is concerned about the spread of the lice to children who have been in contact with her child. The nurse asks about the type of contact the child has had with his friends. The nurse would tell the mother to be most concerned about

- 1. contact occurring in a summar craft class.
- 2. contact occurring in a swimming class.
- 3. sharing of batting helmets.
- 4. showering after football practice.

48. An adolescent is admitted to the emergency room with dyspnea related to bronchospasms. The nurse should place the client in which of the following positions?

- 1. High Fowler's.
- 2. Side-lying.
- 3. Prone.
- 4. Supine.

49. Which of the following nursing diagnoses would be most appropriate for a client newly diagnosed with non–insulin-dependent diabetes mellitus?

- 1. High Risk for Infection related to diabetes.
- 2. Altered Nutrition: More Than Body Requirements related to overproduction of insulin in the pancreas.
- 3. Pain related to elevated blood glucose levels.
- 4. Altered Health Maintenance related to lack of knowledge of proper foot care.

50. The nurse should assess for pediculosis capitis (head lice) in a child who

- 1. has spotty baldness.
- 2. has wheals with blistering on the scalp.
- 3. scratches the scalp frequently.
- 4. has dry, scaly patches on the skin.

51. The nurse and parents of a child with juvenile rheumatoid arthritis are planning interventions to reduce joint pain in the morning just after arising. The plan should include

- 1. having the child sleep in a sleeping bag.
- 2. increasing pain medication at bedtime.
- 3. having the child sleep with the joints flexed.
- 4. awakening the child for range-of-motion exercises once during the night.

52. A client in an inpatient psychiatric unit tells the nurse, "I'm going to divorce my no-good husband. I hope he rots in hell. But I miss him so bad. I love him. When's he going to come get me out of here?" The client is displaying

- 1. ambivalence.
- 2. autistic thinking.
- 3. associative looseness.
- 4. auditory hallucinations.

53. The nurse is assessing a 6-month-old child with a large ventral septal defect. The child has gained 5 pounds in 1 month. The mother reports that the child has not been wetting many diapers in the last week, although the child is taking the prescribed amounts of formula. The mother states she thinks it is because the child seems to sweat so much. Auscultation of the lung fields reveals fine crackles in the bases. The child's digoxin level is 1 ng/mL. The nurse makes a nursing diagnosis of

- 1. Alteration in Nutrition: More Than Body Requirements.
- 2. Fluid Volume Excess.
- 3. High Risk for Injury: Arrhythmias.
- 4. Urinary Retention.

54. After 2 weeks of radiotherapy, a client with Hodgkin's disease becomes discouraged. He tells the nurse that he is so tired that he can barely keep up with his studies. What information related to the nursing diagnosis of Fatigue should the nurse use in planning a response?

- 1. Fatigue is one of the most common problems associated with radiotherapy and will persist throughout therapy.
- 2. Fatigue is a transient problem that will resolve as radiotherapy continues.
- 3. Fatigue is unrelated to the radiotherapy, and another possible cause should be sought.
- 4. Fatigue indicates that the disease is eradicated and that radiotherapy is not needed.

55. An 18-month-old with acquired immunodeficiency

syndrome (AIDS) is seen in the clinic for health maintenance. Which of the following immunizations would the nurse plan to administer to this toddler?

- ○ 1. Diphtheria-tetanus-pertussis.
- ○ 2. Oral polio vaccine.
- ○ 3. Measles, mumps, and rubella.
- ○ 4. Purified protein derivative of tuberculin.

56. After abdominal surgery, a client is reluctant to turn in bed. An appropriate intervention by the nurse would be to

- ○ 1. allow the client to turn when she wants.
- ⊘ 2. explain to the client why turning is important.
- ○ 3. remind her that she must follow her doctor's orders.
- ○ 4. tell her family to encourage her to turn.

57. Parents ask for advice in how to handle the negativism in their 2-year-old son. The nurse would recommend that the parents

- ○ 1. ignore this behavior because it is a stage he is going through.
- ○ 2. set realistic limits and stick to them.
- ○ 3. encourage grandmother to visit frequently to relieve them.
- ○ 4. set strict limits and punish him when he misbehaves.

58. The nurse is caring for a laboring primigravida who is being induced with intravenous oxytocin because she is at 41 weeks' gestation. The nurse observes the fetal heart rate drop to 60 beats/minute at the end of the last two contractions, and then the fetal heart rate rises to 120 beats/minute. The nurse should first

- ○ 1. discontinue the oxytocin infusion.
- ○ 2. position the client on her right side.
- ○ 3. administer oxygen at 3 liters.
- ○ 4. notify the client's physician.

59. Which of the following statements best reflects a 50-year-old client's developmental concerns at this time in his life?

- ⊘ 1. It is time to reevaluate life's goals.
- ○ 2. The selection of a career is important.
- ○ 3. Leisure-time activities are a center of focus.
- ○ 4. Stress associated with illness precipitates a need to "settle down."

60. A nurse develops a care plan that includes interventions aimed at preventing complications of a low platelet count in a child with leukemia. Which of the following is appropriate?

- ○ 1. Consult with a physician about the use of a stool softener.
- ○ 2. Place the child in protective isolation.
- ○ 3. Use heparin instead of saline to flush an intermittent intravenous access device.

- ○ 4. Eliminate raw vegetables and fruits from the child's diet.

61. The nurse is caring for a 15-year-old primipara after vaginal delivery of a viable neonate. The client tells the nurse, "My mother started feeding me rice cereal when I was only 2 weeks old." The nurse should instruct the client that neonates

- ○ 1. can have a small amount of rice cereal once in a while.
- ○ 2. can have rice cereal if it is well mixed into formula.
- ○ 3. should not have rice cereal until they are at least 4 months of age.
- ○ 4. should not have iron-fortified rice cereal until at least 1 year of age.

62. A client with Hodgkin's disease explains to the nurse the monitoring he will be doing at home between radiation treatments. Which of the following statements would indicate that he knows how to detect a major complication?

- ○ 1. "I'll measure my neck circumference every day."
- ○ 2. "I'll take my temperature every day."
- ○ 3. "I'll monitor the loss of body hair every week."
- ○ 4. "I'll check the circulation in my arms every day."

63. A client with chronic schizophrenia is admitted for the third time to a state mental institution under a 72-hour involuntary commitment for evaluation. On admission, the client tells the nurse, "I didn't do anything wrong. I was just carrying out the orders God gave me to paint an X on the door of all sinners." Several hours after being admitted, the client wants to leave the hospital. Besides explaining that the staff is concerned about her health and safety, the nurse would also tell the client that

- ○ 1. it will take about 3 days to complete the evaluation.
- ○ 2. she must stay at least 2 days but then may be able to leave.
- ○ 3. the court has mandated a 72-hour evaluation.
- ○ 4. the court has mandated that she stay until she is well.

64. A client is admitted to the emergency room with complaints of palpitations, a choking sensation, and chest tightness. The nurse notes that he is hyperventilating. During the initial interview he states, "My wife left me with all the chores and I don't know what to do. She died 6 months ago and I didn't realize how much I needed her." The client's medical diagnosis is acute anxiety attack. Of the following nursing diagnoses, which would most accurately reflect the client's behavior?

- ○ 1. Anxiety (panic) related to hopelessness.
- ○ 2. Anxiety (panic) related to loss of wife.
- ○ 3. Sleep Pattern Disturbance related to anxiety.
- ○ 4. Powerlessness related to wife's death.

65. After feedings are resumed in an infant who has undergone a pyloroplasty, the nurse should
- ○ 1. keep the head of the bed flat and the infant supine.
- ○ 2. offer several ounces of an oral electrolyte solution as an initial feeding.
- ○ 3. place the infant prone after feedings.
- ○ 4. start with small feedings (5 to 10 mL) and slowly increase the amounts as tolerated.

66. A pregnant client is diagnosed with a chlamydial infection at 28 weeks' gestation. The nurse should instruct the client that chlamydial infection during pregnancy
- ○ 1. may result in central nervous systems disorders in the fetus.
- ○ 2. is usually treated with a 10-day course of erythromycin.
- ○ 3. usually means that the client will have a cesarean section delivery.
- ○ 4. can result in fetal death before delivery.

67. When teaching a class on health promotion to a group of women, the nurse should instruct them that strategies to reduce the risk of development of osteoarthritis include
- ○ 1. following a high-protein diet.
- ○ 2. exercising at least three times per week.
- ○ 3. preventing obesity.
- ○ 4. taking a multivitamin supplement daily.

68. A client who had an appendectomy for a perforated appendix returns from surgery with a drain inserted in his incisional site. The nurse understands that the purpose of the drain is to
- ○ 1. provide access for wound irrigation.
- ○ 2. promote drainage of wound exudate.
- ○ 3. minimize development of scar tissue.
- ○ 4. decrease postoperative discomfort.

69. Because a mother recently lost a friend, the mother can be expected to react to the impending loss of her child even more intensely than is usually expected. Which of the following concepts best explains this expected grief experience? Losses
- ○ 1. are cumulative in effect.
- ○ 2. take time to resolve.
- ○ 3. affect one's emotional reserves.
- ○ 4. involve objects or people that are significant to oneself.

70. On the second postpartum day, a primigravida who delivered a viable neonate under epidural anesthesia and low forceps tells the nurse that she noticed some blood in her urine. The nurse should
- ○ 1. massage the client's fundus.
- ○ 2. measure the next voiding.
- ○ 3. insert an indwelling catheter.
- ○ 4. contact the client's physician.

71. Which of the following techniques would be least

appropriate for the nurse to implement in crisis intervention?
- ○ 1. Encouraging the client to ventilate feelings.
- ○ 2. Including the client in an effort to find solutions to the problem.
- ○ 3. Using active and flexible approaches.
- ○ 4. Attacking the client's maladaptive defenses.

72. Before being helped to ambulate, a client is first prepared for dangling her feet over the side of the bed. Which of the following measures should the nurse plan to carry out before helping the client dangle?
- ○ 1. Administer a prescribed analgesic.
- ○ 2. Encourage the client to take a short nap.
- ○ 3. Have the client carry out leg exercises for a few minutes.
- ○ 4. Help the client assume high-Fowler's position for a few minutes.

73. A 4-year-old who has been ill for 4 hours is admitted to the hospital. The child is having difficulty swallowing and complains of a sore throat. The apical pulse is 140 beats/minute. The white blood cell count is 16. The temperature is 104°F. The child has severe substernal retractions. The nurse makes a priority nursing diagnosis of
- ○ 1. Anxiety and Fear related to need for immediate hospitalization.
- ○ 2. High Risk for Injury: Airway Obstruction related to edema and inflammation of the epiglottis.
- ○ 3. Impaired Gas Exchange related to excessive respiratory effort.
- ○ 4. Ineffective Airway Clearance related to aspiration.

74. A client with a chronic mental illness who does not always take her medications is separated from her husband and receives Supplemental Security Income. She lives with her mother and older sister and manages her own medication. The client's mother is in poor health and receives Social Security benefits. The client's sister works outside the home, and the client's father is dead. Which of the following issues should the nurse address *first* in this client's care?
- ○ 1. Family.
- ○ 2. Marital.
- ○ 3. Financial.
- ○ 4. Medication.

75. A client's husband is notified of her admission to the emergency room for acute alcohol intoxication. Which of the following statements by the husband would be least typical of his wife?
- ○ 1. "She uses alcohol and tranquilizers to steady her nerves."
- ○ 2. "Whenever she has a problem, she seems to hit the bottle."
- ○ 3. "Her drinking certainly hasn't interfered with her eating."

○ 4. "She has stopped drinking several times; sometimes for as long as 4 months."

76. While preparing a client for surgery, the nurse assesses for psychosocial problems that may cause preoperative anxiety. It is believed that the most devastating fear a preoperative client is likely to experience is a fear of
○ 1. the unknown.
○ 2. changes in body image.
○ 3. the effects of anesthesia.
○ 4. being separated from family members.

77. The nurse answers a call on a telephone hot line from a man who was at the crisis center once in the past when he made a suicide threat. The client says, "Don't try to help me anymore. This is it. I've had enough, and I have a gun in front of me now." He then hangs up the telephone. The nurse's first action in this situation would be to call
○ 1. the client back to try to calm him.
○ 2. the police to request their intervention.
○ 3. his wife at work to suggest that she hurry home.
○ 4. a neighbor to ask him to go to the client's home immediately.

78. Which of the following nursing measures would most help to prevent pressure ulcer formation in an at-risk client?
○ 1. Reposition every hour.
○ 2. Provide a low-protein diet.
○ 3. Ensure generous fluid intake.
○ 4. Massage any reddened areas on the sacral area.

79. A client visits the clinic 2 months after having a Pap smear and beginning oral contraceptives. She tells the nurse that her menstrual flow has decreased since taking the oral contraceptives. The nurse should instruct the client that she most likely needs
○ 1. to have another Pap smear.
○ 2. a thorough endocrine workup.
○ 3. to continue taking the oral contraceptives.
○ 4. a lower dosage of oral contraceptives.

80. The nurse assists the nurse midwife with a vaginal delivery of a term neonate. Immediately after the birth, the nurse plans to
○ 1. place a cord clamp on the umbilical cord.
○ 2. instill an antibiotic ointment into the neonate's eyes.
○ 3. perform a complete neonatal assessment.
○ 4. dry the neonate thoroughly with sterile towels.

81. A parent confides in the nurse that she thinks her infant is anxious or nervous. What advice should the nurse give the mother about how she could lessen the anxiety in her infant?
○ 1. Only hold the infant for feedings.
○ 2. Talk quietly to the infant while he is awake.
○ 3. Play music in his room for most of the day and night.

○ 4. Have a close friend keep the infant for a few days.

82. When assessing a 2-month-old infant, the nurse feels a "click" when abducting the infant's left hip. The nurse should then
○ 1. chart the finding; it is normal for a 2-month-old.
○ 2. check the lengths of the femurs to see if they are equal.
○ 3. instruct the mother to keep the leg in an adducted position.
○ 4. reschedule the child for a follow-up assessment of the hip problem in 3 weeks.

83. A client's belief in her "mission from God" can be referred to as a religious delusion of grandeur. A primary purpose of such a delusion is to provide
○ 1. a sexual outlet.
○ 2. comfort.
○ 3. safety.
○ 4. self-esteem.

84. A 39-year-old multigravida visits the clinic at 14 weeks' gestation and tells the nurse that she has had severe nausea and vomiting since becoming pregnant. The client's fundal measurement is 20 cm. The nurse should assess the client for symptoms of
○ 1. pregnancy-induced hypertension.
○ 2. multifetal pregnancy.
○ 3. increased fetal activity.
○ 4. history of polycythemia.

85. The nurse in a crisis center is helping clients who have suffered from the effects of a severe flood. The nurse interviews a client whose pregnant wife is missing and whose home has been destroyed. The client keeps talking rapidly about his experience and says, "I can't see how I can ever rebuild my life." Which of the following responses by the nurse would be best?
○ 1. "If you start organizing your life now, I'm sure all will be fine."
○ 2. "This has been a bad experience. Tell me more about how you feel."
○ 3. "Let me note a few of the things you said before you continue with your story."
○ 4. "Think some more of what happened tonight, so that we can continue with this tomorrow. For now, let's discuss how you might rebuild your life."

86. A client is admitted to the inpatient psychiatric unit. The nurse observes that he is unshaven, has body odor, has spots on his shirt and pants, moves slowly, gazes at the floor, and has a flat affect. Which observation would point to psychomotor retardation?
○ 1. Slow movements.
○ 2. Flat affect.
○ 3. Unkempt appearance.
○ 4. Avoidance of eye contact.

87. A mother of a child with strabismus brings the child

to the clinic. The physician has prescribed patching. Which of the following actions or statements by the mother would lead the nurse to judge that further teaching concerning this treatment is necessary?

○ 1. The abnormal eye is patched.

○ 2. The mother keeps the patch on even when the child fusses.

○ 3. The mother says she has to watch him when he walks because he is clumsy.

○ 4. The mother tells the nurse that she removes the patch at night.

88. A 70-year-old woman who was recently admitted to a nursing home has developed urinary incontinence. The client's family is concerned and asks the nurse what can be done to help their mother. The nurse's most appropriate response would be

○ 1. "We need to further assess your mother and her environment to determine an appropriate plan of care for her incontinence."

○ 2. "Usually these episodes are self-limiting. After she adjusts to her environment, she should have no further problems with incontinence."

○ 3. "This happens frequently and is not a cause for concern. We can provide her with absorbent pads to keep her dry."

○ 4. "It is difficult to treat urinary incontinence, especially in the elderly. If it continues, a catheter can be used to make her more comfortable."

89. A 16-year-old primigravida at 36 weeks' gestation has had no prenatal care. She has experienced a seizure at work and is being transported to the hospital by ambulance. After the nurse is notified that the client will soon be arriving, the nurse plans to

○ 1. position the client in a supine position.

○ 2. auscultate breath sounds every 4 hours.

○ 3. monitor the vital signs every 4 hours.

○ 4. admit the client to a quiet, darkened room.

90. Which of the following nursing measures would be appropriate when caring for a client in skeletal traction for a fractured femur?

○ 1. Maintain the client in a supine position.

○ 2. Temporarily remove the weights when repositioning the client.

○ 3. Inspect the pin site at least every 8 hours.

○ 4. Maintain the foot in a position of plantar flexion.

CORRECT ANSWERS AND RATIONALE

The letters in parentheses following the rationale identify the step of the nursing process (A, D, P, I, E), cognitive level (K, C, T, N), client needs (S, G, L, H), and nursing care area (O, X, Y, M). See the Answer Grid for the key.

1. 3. The client needs to ventilate and discuss feelings of anger and sadness with the nurse to decrease behaviors of self-harm. Other alternatives like punching the pillow may be helpful to the client in expressing anger and rage. Staying in her room when feeling overwhelmed, leaving group to pace when anxious, and asking for p.r.n. medications when feeling out of control will not help the client to understand herself or her feelings and will not foster growth in autonomy and responsibility for self. (E, N, L, X)

2. 1. The nurse should plan the child's fluid restriction with the mother and child for two reasons. First, the mother and child would best know the child's usual pattern of fluid intake. Second, the mother also needs to feel in control of her child's situation, and this is an area in which the nurse can allow the mother and child some control. It is not advisable to allow a client on fluid restriction to drink all the allotted fluid at once; this may result in many thirsty hours for the client. Also, the nurse should remind the mother to count fluids used when the child takes any medications. (P, N, G, Y)

3. 4. When a client drinks alcohol while taking disulfiram (Antabuse), adverse effects that result include flushing of the face, neck, and upper trunk; hyperventilation; and rapid pulse rate. Nausea and severe vomiting then typically follow. These symptoms are often accompanied by pallor, hypotension, headaches, palpitations, dyspnea, and faintness. (A, N, L, X)

4. 1. The nurse and the client role-play assertive statements to help the client learn how to use assertiveness and to practice behaviors in a safe environment. Watching a videotape on assertiveness, discussing situations that appear threatening, and describing feelings that occur after an angry outburst are less helpful than actually practicing assertiveness. (I, T, L, X)

5. 2. Battered women commonly deny being abused because they are afraid that they will be blamed for their plight. It is a myth that battered women are masochistic and gain pleasure from abuse. Most abused women realize that the abuse is unlikely to stop, and they suffer from fear, shame, hopelessness, and helplessness. (D, N, L, X)

6. 4. By asking the client to tell her more about how she is feeling, the nurse is not making any assumptions about what is troubling the client. The nurse should acknowledge the client's feelings and encourage her to discuss them. (I, N, L, M)

7. 2. The client does not need to take a 1 hour nap at the halfway point of the trip. Travel by automobile is permissible as long as the client has not experienced any complications of pregnancy, such as preterm labor or rupture of the membranes. The client should be encouraged to take frequent rest breaks and stretch her muscles by walking. Drinking plenty of fluids will promote adequate hydration, and wearing the seat belt is recommended for all pregnant women. (E, T, H, O)

8. 3. Short-term memory loss, disorientation, and confabulation are typical signs of Wernicke-Korsakoff syndrome. The syndrome is believed to be due to a vitamin B deficiency and usually occurs in clients with long-standing alcoholism who have poor diets. (D, N, L, X)

9. 4. For clients who are bottle-feeding, menstrual flow usually returns in 6 to 10 weeks. Heart palpitations and reddish lochia for 6 weeks are not normal and warrant further evaluation. Varicosities may fade, but they rarely disappear altogether after delivery. (E, N, H, O)

10. 2. The nurse should assess the client for a history of pelvic inflammatory disease. Intrauterine devices have been associated with an increased risk of pelvic inflammatory disease and perforation of the uterus. Thrombophlebitis, previous liver disease, and cardiovascular disease are contraindications in clients desiring oral contraceptives, not intrauterine devices. (A, T, G, O)

11. 3. Physical and emotional stress can precipitate a sickle cell crisis. Physical exercise like the running involved in soccer would increase the child's risk for a crisis. Children with sickle cell disease need to be kept well hydrated. In addition, these children often have nephrosis related to sickle cell disease. These children have difficulty conserving fluids and therefore need up to 150% of normal fluid intake. Pain control is an issue in sickle cell crisis, and the mother is showing concern for her child by asking how pain will be managed. Sickle cell disease is an autosomal recessive disease. (E, T, G, Y)

12. 1. The goal is to promote urinary continence; an indication that this goal has been met is that the client is continent 24 hours a day. A client's report that her bladder control is improved may indicate that the goal has been attained, but 24-hour-a-day continence is a more definite indication that the goal has been met. Monitoring for urine retention and complying with the drinking and voiding schedule are important but do not reflect achievement of the stated goal. (E, N, G, M)

13. 1. This dark brown line is a darkened pigmentation termed *linea nigra*. The pigmentation will fade after delivery. It is not related to melanoma; it is not called stretch marks, which are reddish or purplish in color; nor is it called the pigmentation of pregnancy. (I, T, H, O)

14. 2. Infants with pyloric stenosis generally have a history of spitting up, which progresses to projectile vomiting, weight loss, decrease in number of stools, and some degree of dehydration. Infants with dehydration need fluid and electrolyte replacement before surgery. There is no difficulty swallowing. (D, N, G, Y)

15. 1. The client is in the triggering phase of the assault cycle. He needs to ventilate or talk about what just occurred on the telephone with his wife and his feelings related to the conversation. The nurse conveys empathetic support, uses clear, simple statements, and instructs the client to maintain control. If the client refuses to talk about the situation and does not calm down, he should then be escorted to the quiet room because he has proceeded to the escalation phase of the assault cycle. An oral tranquilizer may be helpful, and a show of determination is prepared. (I, T, L, X)

16. 1. Slight breast engorgement in term neonates is related to the maternal hormone elevations during pregnancy. Epidural anesthesia and genetic influences have no effect on breast tissue engorgement in the neonate. Hyperthyroidism is frequently associated with preterm labor and low-birth weight infants. It is unlikely that a preterm infant would have breast engorgement. (I, T, H, O)

17. 1. It is important for the child and family to understand that chorea associated with rheumatic fever is not permanent. The clumsiness and uncontrolled actions can be upsetting to both the child and family. It is not necessary to assess the child's neurologic status or to keep the child warm. Because the child has cardiac involvement, ambulation is contraindicated. Aspirin is used primarily as an antiinflammatory drug and secondarily for pain relief. (P, N, G, Y)

18. 2. Heroin causes pupils to be pinpoints. Cocaine use causes pupils to dilate. Marijuana causes eyes to appear bloodshot. Having drooping eyelids would not necessarily be caused by drug use. (P, N, G, Y)

19. 4. Chorioamnionitis is a serious intrapartum infection that may result in fetal tachycardia and a hypotonic labor pattern. If left untreated, infected amniotic fluid in the fetal lungs may result in pneumonia

during the neonatal period. Vaginal birth is preferred to cesarean section delivery. The client is usually treated with intravenous antibiotic therapy. There is no relationship between being overweight and chorioamnionitis. (E, T, G, O)

20. 2. In cardioversion, the shock is synchronous, which means that it is not delivered during the R wave. Cardioversion is used in ventricular tachycardia to prevent the shock from occurring during the R wave and thereby causing ventricular fibrillation. Typically, cardioversion is done at a lower wattage than defibrillation. The same machine is used for cardioversion and defibrillation; the caregiver sets the mode to synchronous or asynchronous. When set on synchronous mode, the machine then automatically synchronizes the shock with the R wave of the client's rhythm. (I, T, G, M)

21. 2. A client with multiple sclerosis may have a sense of optimism and euphoria, particularly during remissions. Euphoria is characterized by mood elevation with an exaggerated sense of well-being. Inappropriate laughter and giddiness, slurring of words when excited, and visual hallucinations and giddiness are uncharacteristic of euphoria. (A, C, L, M)

22. 4. Although nutrition plays a large part in the healing process, it is not advisable to tell a child that he will not get better if he does or does not do a particular activity. Not only is this dishonest, but it also makes the child believe that his own actions are causing the illness. Allowing children choices often helps them feel in control. They also will be more likely to eat foods they have chosen. It is also important to find out the reason the child is not eating. Clients refuse to eat for multiple reasons, and interventions should be devised taking into consideration the reason for the child's refusal. (P, N, L, Y)

23. 3. The most appropriate action when moving an extremity with acute osteomyelitis is to ensure that the extremity is carefully supported above and below the affected area. Acute osteomyelitis can be very painful; therefore, the extremity must be handled carefully when being moved. It is important that the nurse move the extremity slowly and closely monitor the client's response to the activity. The affected extremity may be immobilized with a splint to decrease discomfort. (I, T, S, M)

24. 3. After delivery, it is not unusual for postpartum clients to complain of backache, which results from stretching of the muscles during the labor and delivery process. The nurse can provide the client with a mild analgesic to help alleviate the backache. On the day of delivery, it is too soon for the client to begin abdominal exercises. The client is not demonstrating any evidence of a urinary tract infection at this time. Asking the client how long she was in labor may encourage her to discuss her labor and delivery experience, but that is not alleviating the client's backache. (I, T, G, O)

25. 1. Motor vehicle injuries are the leading cause of death in children older than 1 year of age. Most fatalities are related to nonuse of child restraints and seat belts. Biking and skating safety, prevention of poisoning, and prevention of sunburn and Lyme disease are also important, but motor vehicle safety takes priority in injury prevention. (P, T, S, Y)

26. 2. For the client with bulimia, binges involve loss of control that results in thoughts of self-deprecation. Binges are done secretively, and the person has no desire to attract attention. Because of the purging, substantial weight gain usually does not occur, although weight may fluctuate. (D, C, L, X)

27. 4. All children use energy to ingest and digest nutrients. The body needs oxygen to use the calories taken in to provide energy. Usually, the caloric intake outweighs the energy needed to obtain them. A child with a heart defect that circulates unoxygenated blood to the tissues may need extra oxygen support during times of high energy consumption, such as feeding. Without this extra support, the child may become tired. If the child's suck is good, then enlarging the hole in the nipple will give the child too much volume with each suck and may cause the child to choke. Tiring during feedings is not a symptom of digitoxin toxicity, although lack of appetite may be. (I, N, G, Y)

28. 3. The client should be taught to elevate the affected arm on a pillow. Constriction of the extremity should be avoided. Range-of-motion exercising is not limited; instead, it is encouraged. Diuretics are not used to control lymphedema. (I, T, H, M)

29. 1. When examining the tympanic membrane of a child younger than 3 years, the nurse should pull the pinna down and back. For a child older than 3 years, the nurse should pull the pinna up and back to view the tympanic membrane. (A,T,G,Y)

30. 2. Although all the symptoms listed can manifest in fat embolism syndrome, confusion is the earliest symptom noted. The confusion is due to a low arterial oxygen level. (A, C, G, M)

31. 2. An important nursing measure for a client with lumbar anesthesia is to check the client's bladder. A full bladder can impede the progress of labor, and pushing with a full bladder may result in an injury to the client. Generally, clients with lumbar anesthesia are given intravenous therapy; therefore, the bladder should be checked frequently throughout the labor process. It is important to monitor the contraction pattern and the maternal vital signs throughout labor, but these do not have an effect on the client's ability to push. If the client is completely numb, the nursing responsibility would be to alert the client

that a contraction is occurring and to push with the contraction. (A, T, G, O)

32. 4. By observing for frequent swallowing, the nurse can evaluate whether the child is bleeding. Getting help to force open the mouth can result in broken teeth, tissue damage, and psychological damage. Although a drop in blood pressure is a sign of blood loss, it is a late sign in children. Decreased peripheral perfusion may also be a sign of blood loss; however, it is also a late sign. (A, N, G, Y)

33. 4. The manic client needs limits set on behavior, especially when his behavior is demanding or seductive. The nurse tells the client to stop his behavior and explains her intolerance for it. Telling a seductive client that it is against the rules for clients and nurses to display affection toward each other does not tell the client that his behavior is unacceptable; nor will it help to threaten him by saying the supervisor will be notified. It may become appropriate to divert the client's attention (eg, by suggesting something to eat and drink), but first the nurse should set limits and explain them to the client. (I, T, L, X)

34. 3. The client should be instructed to lie supine with head tilted back for several minutes after instillation of the nose drops. Sterile technique is not necessary. The dropper should be cleaned after each use; a new dropper is not necessary for each instillation. The client should not blow the nose after instilling the nose drops; the nose should be blown before instillation. (E, T, H, M)

35. 3. In dark-skinned clients, cyanosis can best be detected by examining the conjunctiva, lips, and oral mucous membranes. (A, N, G, M)

36. 1. The best strategy for assessing a toddler is to have the parent hold the toddler. Assessment should begin with noninvasive assessments first. Having a toddler run and be active may make it difficult to settle him down after the physical exertion. Starting with the head and working down is more appropriate for an older child. (I, N, G, Y)

37. 1. Yogurt, dry beans, and peanut butter all contain protein in amounts that make them good sources of protein for the child. Bacon contains some protein but consists mostly of fat. (P, T, H, Y)

38. 1. Ibuprofen can be irritating to the stomach and should not be taken with other drugs that are known gastric irritants. Antacids may be taken at the same time as the ibuprofen; they do not affect the drug's absorption. It may take several days to weeks for the drug to be effective in relieving the client's symptoms. (E, T, H, M)

39. 3. A client experiencing a flashback needs reassurance, acceptance, and a calm, quiet environment. Various stimuli, physical activities, and fluids are less likely to provide the kind of environment the client needs at this time. (P, T, L, X)

40. 4. The passage of two small blood clots from a multipara is not an unusual occurrence. The nurse should continue to monitor the client and document this as a normal finding. The nurse should never massage a postpartum client's fundus vigorously. The length of the third stage of labor and whether the client passed any clots with previous deliveries are not relevant. (I, N, G, O)

41. 3. As fluid gushes from the amniotic sac, it may carry the umbilical cord out of the birth canal. Sudden deceleration of the fetal heart rate often signifies prolapsed cord. Prolapse of the umbilical cord is a medical emergency and requires immediate intervention to prevent fetal demise. (I, T, G, O)

42. 3. Symptoms of puerperal infection include profuse, foul-smelling lochia, chills, fever, and a uterus that is larger than expected for the postdelivery day. Infection may spread through the lymphatic system, and antibiotic therapy is necessary. During normal uterine involution, the lochia becomes less profuse and should not be foul-smelling. Uterine atony is relaxation of the uterus and may be a result of retained placental fragments. (D, N, G, O)

43. 1. The client should be instructed to mix the sediment that accumulates in a vial of NPH insulin by rolling the vial gently between the palms or by turning the vial upside down several times. Shaking the vial is not recommended because it produces bubbles, which make it difficult to withdraw accurate doses of insulin. Proper techniques for self-administering insulin include introducing the needle with a dart-like action, pulling back on the plunger as soon as the needle is in place to determine whether the needle is in a blood vessel, and holding an antiseptic sponge against the needle when removing it from tissue to prevent the discomfort of the needle pulling on the skin. (I, T, H, M)

44. 1. For the best assessment of an inguinal hernia, the client should be in a standing position. The sitting and side-lying positions do not help the examiner palpate for the inguinal ring. The client may be asked to lie down after being examined in the standing position to determine whether the hernia can be reduced and its sac contents returned to the abdominal cavity. (A, T, G, M)

45. 1. The posterior fontanel usually closes by age 2 to 3 months. The nurse would measure the head circumference to identify if the child's head is larger than the established norms because hydrocephalus can cause separation of the sutures of the cranium. Another factor that can cause lack of fontanel closure is slow bone growth, which may be related to hypothyroidism. Because the child is 8 months old, the delivery history probably would not be a significant factor. A radiologic examination is not necessary until other data are collected. (D, N, G, Y)

46. 1. In some birth settings, intravenous therapy is not used with low-risk clients. Clients in early labor are encouraged to eat healthy snacks and drink fluids to avoid dehydration. Yogurt provides an excellent source of calcium and riboflavin, is soft, and is easily digested. During pregnancy, gastric emptying time is delayed, and in most hospital settings, clients are allowed only ice chips or clear liquids. Cereal with milk and vegetable soup may be nutritious but can result in potential aspiration if nausea and vomiting occur. Peanut butter cookies are not as nutritious as yogurt for the laboring client. (I, T, H, O)

47. 3. Pediculosis capitis or head lice can be spread by close contact or sharing head gear or combs and brushes with other children. Craft classes, swimming, or showering do not usually involve close contact. (I, T, G, Y)

48. 1. The goal of the intervention is to decrease the child's work of breathing by decreasing pressure on the diaphragm and increasing chest expansion by increasing the pull of gravity on the diaphragm. Side-lying positions make it more difficult to expand the side of the lung closest to the bed. Prone and supine positions do not decrease the work of breathing unless the head of the bed is raised. (I, T, G, Y)

49. 4. Knowledge of foot care is essential for the client with diabetes mellitus; improper care may lead to serious debilitating complications. Pain is not typically a problem. Overproduction of insulin would cause hypoglycemia; moreover, it would be treated by a physician. Using a medical diagnosis, such as diabetes, as a cause in a nursing diagnosis is not appropriate because a medical diagnosis requires treatment by the physician. (D, N, G, M)

50. 3. A typical sign of pediculosis capitis (head lice) is frequent scratching of the scalp because the condition causes severe itching. Scratch marks are usually easily visible. Because head lice are easily transmitted to others, the child's family members and peers also should be examined for infestation. Spotty baldness is common in various allergic reactions. Scaly lesions are also often allergic in nature. (A, T, G, Y)

51. 1. Sleeping in a sleeping bag keeps the joints warm and therefore more flexible. Increasing bedtime pain medications may help the child sleep but will not decrease early morning stiffness. The child's joints should be kept in an extended position during sleep to maintain function. Lack of sleep is a stressor that can lead to exacerbation of juvenile rheumatoid arthritis. (P, N, G, Y)

52. 1. *Ambivalence* refers to strong, conflicting attitudes or feelings toward an object, person, goal, or situation. *Autistic thinking* involves attributing personal and private meanings to words and situations.

Associative looseness is characterized by simultaneous expression of unrelated, or only slightly related, ideas or thoughts. *Auditory hallucinations* involves hearing sounds, words, or voices not heard by others. (A, T, L, X)

53. 2. The child exhibits characteristics of fluid volume excess that are related to congestive heart failure. (decreased output, diaphoresis, weight gain, rales). The congestive heart failure is related to left to right shunting that occurs when the child has a large ventral septal defect. Altered nutrition is not indicated by the symptoms. The mother has reported that the child is taking in prescribed amounts of formula and is not having good output. The weight gain is related to fluid overload systemically and not urinary retention. The digoxin level is within normal limits. (D, N, G, Y)

54. 1. Fatigue is one of the most common problems associated with radiotherapy. It persists during therapy and for varying periods after therapy ends. Extra rest and a reduction in normal activity are often necessary to maintain a reasonable energy level. Informing the client about the fatigue before treatment enables him to schedule his activities accordingly. (P, N, G, M)

55. 1. Live virus vaccines are not routinely administered to anyone with an altered immune system because multiplication of the virus may be enhanced, causing a severe, vaccine-induced illness. Oral polio and measles, mumps, and rubella are live virus vaccines. Protein-purified derivative of tuberculin is not an immunization but a skin test. Diphtheria, pertussis, and tetanus are killed vaccines. (P, T, H, Y).

56. 2. The most appropriate intervention for the nurse is to reinforce for the client is that turning in bed will decrease the likelihood of postoperative complications developing. It would not be appropriate to allow her to turn when she wants. If the client understands the reason for turning, she may be more inclined to participate in the activity despite the discomfort. (I, T, S, M)

57. 2. A characteristic of a 2-year-old is negativism, which is a response to their developing autonomy. Setting realistic limits is important so that the toddler learns what is and is not acceptable behavior. Having grandmother visit will give the parents a break, but setting limits is more important. (P, T, H, Y)

58. 1. Induction of labor with oxytocin is not without risk. Hyperstimulation of the uterus can lead to fetal distress. The nurse monitors the client's uterine activity and fetal heart rate activity every 15 to 30 minutes. A drop in the fetal heart rate to 60 beats/minute at the end of a contraction may be indicative of late decelerations due to placental insufficiency.

Stopping the oxytocin infusion will reduce uterine activity and improve uteroplacental perfusion. (I, N, G, O)

59. 1. During middle adulthood (age 45 to 55 years), most people go through a process of taking stock of their lives and become very aware of the time left to live. This appears to be especially true of men. Death now becomes more of a reality instead of something that happens only to others. Selecting career goals and leisure-time activities and settling down are more typical concerns of younger adults. (E, N, L, M)

60. 1. A stool softener would assist in preventing damage to the rectal mucosa due to hard stool and thereby decreases the chances of rectal bleeding. The child would not need to be in protective isolation nor avoid raw vegetables or fruits. These interventions would be related to a low neutrophil count. The use of heparin is contraindicated in situations in which there is a possibility of increased bleeding due to low platelets. (P, T, G, Y)

61. 3. Breast milk or formula should provide adequate nourishment for a neonate until 4 to 6 months of age. The client who is breast-feeding may need to provide a supplement of iron, vitamin D, and fluoride, but cereal before the age of 4 months is not easily digested by the neonate and may lead to food allergies and possibly aspiration. (I, T, G, O)

62. 2. Clients with Hodgkin's disease are extremely vulnerable to infection because of the defective immune responses caused by the tumor as well as the bone-marrow depression and low white blood cell count caused by the radiation therapy. Fever is the most sensitive indicator of infection and should be reported immediately so that treatment can be initiated. Loss of hair is unusual in radiation therapy to the neck. Neck circumference and upper extremity circulation are not related to major complications. (E, N, G, M)

63. 3. Clients admitted involuntarily must remain hospitalized for the time allotted for the evaluation. If the treatment team completes the evaluation in less than the allotted time, they may decide to discharge the client or may institute further commitment procedures. Clients cannot sign themselves out of the hospital during this period, nor can family members release them. (I, T, L, X)

64. 2. The appropriate nursing diagnosis is Anxiety (panic) related to loss of wife. The symptoms of hyperventilation, palpitations, choking sensation, and chest tightness relate to a panic level of anxiety or a panic attack. The client stated that his wife died 6 months ago and that he realizes that he needs her. (D, N, L, X)

65. 4. The child who has undergone pyloroplasty often vomits after the first feeding because peristalsis that has been right to left before repair has not reverted to the normal left to right. Peristalsis reverses owing to the tightening of the pyloric sphincter that does not allow stomach contents to enter the small intestine. Therefore, small feedings of 5 to 10 mL are given and slowly increased as tolerated. If there is a chance of vomiting, it is not advisable to place an infant supine with the head of the bed flat. If the infant does vomit, aspiration of stomach contents may occur, and pneumonia may result. The child will have an abdominal incision, so a prone position would be uncomfortable. (I, C, G, Y)

66. 2. Chlamydial infection is usually treated with a 10-day course of erythromycin, tetracycline, or doxycycline. Diagnosis is made by cervical culture. Chlamydial infection during pregnancy has been associated with preterm labor, resulting in a low-birth weight infant, and with preterm rupture of the membranes. The neonate can be infected during passage through the birth canal. Neonatal complications include conjunctivitis, pneumonitis, chronic otitis media, and asthma. There is no evidence to suggest that the client will require a cesarean section delivery, fetal demise is rare, and lack of treatment is not associated with central nervous system disorders. (I, T, G, O)

67. 3. Obesity is a risk factor for development of osteoarthritis because it places increased stress on the joints. A high-protein diet, regular exercise, and vitamin supplements *are not risk factors* for development of osteoarthritis. (P, T, H, M)

68. 2. Drains are inserted postoperatively in appendectomies when an abscess is present or the appendix perforated. The purpose is to promote removal of drainage from the wound. (P, T, S, M)

69. 1. Losses tend to be cumulative. Old losses are re-lived or reexperienced with each new loss and add to the intensity of the present grief experience. (D, T, L, X)

70. 4. Hematuria after the first 24 hours is most commonly associated with urinary tract infection. A history of bacteriuria in pregnancy, an operative delivery, and epidural anesthesia can contribute to urinary tract infections. The nurse should contact the physician or nurse midwife because a urinalysis will most likely be ordered. Hematuria during the first 24 hours after delivery is most likely due to bladder trauma. (I, N, G, O)

71. 4. The nurse should carefully encourage adaptive defenses. Attacking the client's defenses decreases his ability to maintain his self-esteem and ego integrity. Encouraging the client to ventilate feelings increases his awareness of his feelings and reduces tension. Including the client in finding solutions to problems helps the client regain his self-worth and

communicates confidence and respect. Using active and flexible approaches helps the nurse use interventions specific to each crisis situation for a healthy resolution of the crisis. (I, T, L, X)

72. 4. Many clients feel faint and weak when helped to ambulate for the first time postoperatively. The nurse can help prevent these feelings by giving the circulatory system time to adjust before helping the client assume a standing position. This is best done by helping the client into high-Fowler's position in bed for a few minutes. After becoming accustomed to a sitting position, the client can then be helped to dangle the legs at the edge of the bed before ambulating. Such preparations for ambulating help give the client's circulatory system time to adjust to the upright position. (I, N, S, M)

73. 2. The priority diagnosis at this time would be High Risk for Injury. The airway may become completely occluded by the epiglottis at any time. The child will probably be experiencing fear and anxiety, but this is not a priority diagnosis. There is no evidence that any aspiration has occurred, nor does exertion of respiratory muscles cause impaired gas exchange. (D, N, G, Y)

74. 4. Medication noncompliance is a primary cause of exacerbation in chronic mental illnesses. Of the issues listed in this item, noncompliance should be addressed first. Other issues can be addressed as client stabilization is maintained. (P, N, L, X)

75. 3. Alcoholics typically are malnourished. Alcoholics would rather drink than eat, and their caloric intake is made up of empty calories. Poor digestion and absorption of food constituents due to the damaging effect of alcohol on the stomach and small intestine, and subsequently on the liver and pancreas, also seriously compromise nutritional status in the alcoholic. (E, N, L, X)

76. 1. Anxiety in a preoperative client may be caused by many different fears, such as fear of the effects of anesthesia, the effects of surgery on body image, separation from family and friends, job loss, disability, pain, and death. Fear of the unknown, however, most likely looms as the greatest fear because the client feels helpless. Therefore, an important part of preoperative nursing care is to assess the client for anxieties and explore possible causes. Interventions can then be used to offer the client emotional support so that he is in the best possible psychological condition for surgery. (A, T, L, M)

77. 2. The nurse's first responsibility when a client threatens suicide is to do whatever can be done most quickly to protect the client from himself. When the nurse is in a crisis center and the client is at home, it is best to call the police to intervene. They will be able to reach the client quickly and are experienced in handling such situations. Outsiders, such as a neighbor or even the client's wife, may be hurt, especially when the client has a weapon. It is appropriate to err on the side of safety rather than to assume that the client is not serious about a suicide threat. (I, T, L, X)

78. 1. Because pressure ulcers (decubitus ulcers) are caused by pressure to the tissues, the most important measure to prevent them is relieving pressure by repositioning the client every 1 to 2 hours. Adequate caloric and protein intake is also essential. High fluid intake will not prevent ulcer formation. Massaging reddened areas and bony prominences, once thought to reduce risk of pressure ulcer formation, is now known to increase the risk of pressure ulcer formation. The Agency for Health Care Policy Research (AHCPR) has recently published guidelines for pressure ulcer prevention, which all nurses should incorporate into their practice. (I, T, G, M)

79. 3. A common side effect of oral contraceptives is decreased menstrual flow. Other side effects include breast tenderness, irritability, nausea, headaches, cyclic weight gain, and increased vaginal yeast infections. More serious side effects include hypertension, myocardial infarction, and cervical dysplasia. The nurse should instruct the client that decreased menstrual flow is normal. The client does not need another Pap smear because these are usually performed annually. The client does not need an endocrine workup or a lower dosage of oral contraceptives. (I, T, G, O)

80. 4. Immediately after birth, the nurse is responsible for ensuring that the neonate is dried thoroughly, including the head, to prevent heat loss from evaporation. The infant may be placed temporarily in a slight Trendelenburg position to facilitate drainage. Once a clear airway and normal respirations have been established, other procedures may be performed, such as instilling antibiotic ointment into the eyes and performing a thorough assessment. After respirations have been established, the neonate can be positioned in a side-lying position to facilitate drainage of mucus. (P, T, G, O)

81. 2. Infants are sensitive to stress in their caretakers. The best way to handle an anxious infant is to talk quietly to him. Only holding him during feedings will not meet his needs, and having a friend take him for several days will not necessarily take care of the problem either. Playing music most of the day and night will make it difficult for the infant to keep his days and nights straight. (I, T, H, Y)

82. 2. The "click" the nurse feels when abducting the femur is the head of the femur slipping into the acetabulum. This is Ortolani's sign and indicates a dislocated hip. Usual medical treatment involves keeping the hip joint in an abducted position through triple diapering, Pavlik harness, or casting. The goal of treatment is to keep the head of the femur centered in the acetabulum. Other signs of hip dislocation are unequal leg lengths and asymmetry of the gluteal and thigh folds. (A, T, G, Y)

83. 4. Delusions of grandeur provide the client with an exaggerated sense of self-esteem that is unrelated to the client's actual achievements. Other, less grandiose, religious delusions may provide comfort or meaning for the client. Delusions of persecution are frequently related to safety issues. Delusions may also be related to sexual issues. (D, C, L, X)

84. 1. Severe nausea and vomiting that continues throughout the first trimester of pregnancy and on into the second trimester may be indicative of a hydatidiform mole. Early symptoms of pregnancy-induced hypertension and an enlarged fundus are associated with a molar pregnancy, which occurs more often in multigravidas. An enlarged fundus may be associated with multifetal pregnancies but not with the client's symptoms of severe nausea and vomiting. A molar pregnancy is not associated with increased fetal activity because there is no fetus, nor is it associated with polycythemia. (A, N, G, O)

85. 2. At the time of a major crisis, such as the flood described in this item, the client suffering a great loss is best helped by being encouraged to talk about his experience and describe his feelings. Telling the client to think more about what happened for further discussion the next day and suggesting that he start to rebuild his life are nurse-centered rather than client-centered activities and are unlikely to help the client. Asking the client to stop talking so that the nurse can write notes places more emphasis on the nurse's needs than on the client's needs. Clichés such as "everything will be fine" are not helpful. (I, T, L, X)

86. 1. Psychomotor retardation refers to a general slowdown of motor activity commonly seen in a depressed client. Movements appear lethargic, energy is absent or lacking, and performance of activity is slow and difficult. (A, T, L, X)

87. 1. When an eye patch is used to correct strabismus, the normal eye is patched. This forces the child to use the abnormal, or "lazy," eye and increases muscle strength in that eye. The patch can be removed at night while the child sleeps. Patching one eye interferes with depth perception and can cause the child to be clumsy at first. (E, N, G, Y)

88. 1. Urinary incontinence should not be accepted as a normal occurrence in the elderly or in the nursing home. Clients who develop incontinence need to be thoroughly evaluated for an underlying physical cause. The client's physical environment and emotional and social factors also need to be evaluated because these elements can contribute to the development of urinary incontinence. Behavioral interventions can be effective in the treatment of incontinence. Indwelling catheters are not considered the first line of treatment and are to be avoided. (I, N, H, M)

89. 4. Eclampsia is a condition in which convulsions occur in the absence of any underlying cause. Although the actual cause of pregnancy-induced hypertension is unknown, adolescents and women older than 35 years are at higher risk. The client's

environment should be kept as quiet as possible. Clients experiencing eclampsia should be kept on the left side to promote placental perfusion. Vital signs should be monitored at least hourly. Accurate intake and output should be performed. Breath sounds should be monitored every 2 hours to determine the presence of pulmonary edema. (I, N, G, O)

90. 3. The pin site should be inspected for redness, swelling, drainage, pain, and movement at least once a shift. The client may be placed in a semi-Fowler's position and does not have to be kept supine. Skeletal traction is never interrupted. Plantar flexion is to be avoided. (I, T, S, M)

NURSING CARE COMPREHENSIVE TEST

TEST 3

Directions: Use this answer grid to determine areas of strength or need for further study.

NURSING PROCESS

A = Assessment
D = Analysis, nursing diagnosis
P = Planning
I = Implementation
E = Evaluation

CLIENT NEEDS

S = Safe, effective care environment
G = Physiologic integrity
L = Psychosocial integrity
H = Health promotion and maintenance

COGNITIVE LEVEL

K = Knowledge
C = Comprehension
T = Application
N = Analysis

NURSING CARE AREA

O = Maternity and newborn care
X = Psychosocial health problems
Y = Nursing care of children
M = Medical and surgical health problems

Question #	Answer #	Nursing Process					Cognitive Level				Client Needs				Care Area			
		A	D	P	I	E	K	C	T	N	S	G	L	H	O	X	Y	M
1	3					E				N			L			X		
2	1			P						N		G					Y	
3	4	A								N			L			X		
4	1				I				T				L			X		
5	2		D							N			L			X		
6	4				I					N			L					M
7	2					E			T					H	O			
8	3		D							N			L			X		
9	4					E				N				H	O			
10	2	A							T			G			O			
11	3					E			T			G					Y	
12	1					E				N		G						M
13	1				I				T					H	O			
14	2		D							N		G					Y	
15	1				I				T				L			X		
16	1				I				T					H	O			
17	1			P						N		G					Y	
18	2			P						N		G					Y	
19	4					E			T			G			O			

ANSWER GRID: 1

NURSING PROCESS

A = Assessment
D = Analysis, nursing diagnosis
P = Planning
I = Implementation
E = Evaluation

CLIENT NEEDS

S = Safe, effective care environment
G = Physiologic integrity
L = Psychosocial integrity
H = Health promotion and maintenance

COGNITIVE LEVEL

K = Knowledge
C = Comprehension
T = Application
N = Analysis

NURSING CARE AREA

O = Maternity and newborn care
X = Psychosocial health problems
Y = Nursing care of children
M = Medical and surgical health problems

Question #	Answer #	A	D	P	I	E	K	C	T	N	S	G	L	H	O	X	Y	M
20	2				I				T			G						M
21	2	A						C					L					M
22	4			P						N			L				Y	
23	3				I				T		S							M
24	3				I				T			G			O			
25	1			P					T		S						Y	
26	2		D					C					L			X		
27	4				I					N		G					Y	
28	3				I				T					H				M
29	1	A							T			G					Y	
30	2	A						C				G						M
31	2	A							T			G			O			
32	4	A								N		G					Y	
33	4				I				T				L			X		
34	3					E			T					H				M
35	3	A								N		G						M
36	1				I					N		G					Y	
37	1			P					T					H			Y	
38	1					E			T					H				M
39	3			P					T				L			X		
40	4				I					N		G			O			
41	3				I				T			G			O			
42	3		D							N		G			O			
43	1				I				T					H				M
44	1	A							T			G						M

NURSING PROCESS

A = Assessment
D = Analysis, nursing diagnosis
P = Planning
I = Implementation
E = Evaluation

COGNITIVE LEVEL

K = Knowledge
C = Comprehension
T = Application
N = Analysis

CLIENT NEEDS

S = Safe, effective care environment
G = Physiologic integrity
L = Psychosocial integrity
H = Health promotion and maintenance

NURSING CARE AREA

O = Maternity and newborn care
X = Psychosocial health problems
Y = Nursing care of children
M = Medical and surgical health problems

Question #	Answer #	Nursing Process					Cognitive Level				Client Needs				Care Area			
		A	D	P	I	E	K	C	T	N	S	G	L	H	O	X	Y	M
45	1		D							N		G					Y	
46	1				I				T					H	O			
47	3				I				T			G					Y	
48	1				I				T			G					Y	
49	4		D							N		G						M
50	3	A							T			G					Y	
51	1			P						N		G					Y	
52	1	A							T				L			X		
53	2		D							N		G					Y	
54	1			P						N		G						M
55	1			P					T					H			Y	
56	2				I				T		S							M
57	2			P					T					H			Y	
58	1				I					N		G			O			
59	1					E				N			L					M
60	1			P					T			G					Y	
61	3				I				T			G			O			
62	2					E				N		G						M
63	3				I				T				L			X		
64	2		D							N			L			X		
65	4				I			C				G					Y	
66	2				I				T			G			O			
67	3			P					T					H				M
68	2			P					T		S							M
69	1		D						T				L			X		

NURSING PROCESS

A = Assessment
D = Analysis, nursing diagnosis
P = Planning
I = Implementation
E = Evaluation

CLIENT NEEDS

S = Safe, effective care environment
G = Physiologic integrity
L = Psychosocial integrity
H = Health promotion and maintenance

COGNITIVE LEVEL

K = Knowledge
C = Comprehension
T = Application
N = Analysis

NURSING CARE AREA

O = Maternity and newborn care
X = Psychosocial health problems
Y = Nursing care of children
M = Medical and surgical health problems

Question #	Answer #	A	D	P	I	E	K	C	T	N	S	G	L	H	O	X	Y	M
70	4				I					N		G			O			
71	4				I				T				L			X		
72	4				I					N	S							M
73	2		D							N		G					Y	
74	4			P						N			L			X		
75	3					E				N			L			X		
76	1	A							T				L					M
77	2				I				T				L			X		
78	1				I				T			G						M
79	3				I				T			G			O			
80	4			P					T			G			O			
81	2				I				T					H			Y	
82	2	A							T			G					Y	
83	4		D					C					L			X		
84	1	A								N		G			O			
85	2				I				T				L			X		
86	1	A							T				L			X		
87	1					E				N		G					Y	
88	1				I					N				H				M
89	4				I					N		G			O			
90	3				I				T		S							M

NURSING PROCESS

A = Assessment
D = Analysis, nursing diagnosis
P = Planning
I = Implementation
E = Evaluation

COGNITIVE LEVEL

K = Knowledge
C = Comprehension
T = Application
N = Analysis

CLIENT NEEDS

S = Safe, effective care environment
G = Physiologic integrity
L = Psychosocial integrity
H = Health promotion and maintenance

NURSING CARE AREA

O = Maternity and newborn care
X = Psychosocial health problems
Y = Nursing care of children
M = Medical and surgical health problems

Question #	Answer #	Nursing Process					Cognitive Level				Client Needs				Care Area			
		A	D	P	I	E	K	C	T	N	S	G	L	H	O	X	Y	M
Number Correct																		
Number Possible	90	15	12	16	35	12	0	5	49	36	6	44	25	15	20	20	26	24
Percentage Correct																		

Score Calculation: To determine your **Percentage Correct,** divide the **Number Correct** by the **Number Possible.**

ANSWER GRID: 5

Comprehensive Test 4

1. The nurse plans to assess a postpartum client 12 hours after delivery of a viable neonate. This client is breast-feeding the neonate. While assessing the client's breasts during a physical assessment, the nurse would expect to find that the breasts are
   ○ 1. soft, not tender.
   ○ 2. filling, slightly firm.
   ○ 3. firm with beginning milk production.
   ○ 4. firm, tender to touch.

2. The nurse is caring for a 27-year-old primigravida at 20 weeks' gestation. The client asks the nurse if she should plan to attend childbirth preparation classes. The nurse should explain to the client that women who have attended childbirth preparation classes have expressed that they had
   ○ 1. a decreased length of labor.
   ○ 2. a need for less pain medication in labor.
   ○ 3. greater control over their birth plans.
   ○ 4. increased support from their significant other.

3. A nurse working in a community health center is interviewing a family. The nurse suspects that the 20-month-old is being abused. Which of the following behaviors would make the nurse think of abuse? The toddler
   ○ 1. does not cry while being examined.
   ○ 2. clings to the parent during the examination.
   ○ 3. plays with the toys on the floor in the examination room.
   ○ 4. talks easily to the nurse.

4. A nurse prepares to present a community program about women who are victims of physical abuse. Which of the following facts could the nurse stress about the incidence of battering? Battering
   ○ 1. rarely results in death.
   ○ 2. is a major cause of injury to women.
   ○ 3. occurs primarily in lower socioeconomic groups.
   ○ 4. rarely occurs in pregnant women.

5. A client has had an upper gastrointestinal radiograph series. Which of the following statements indicates the client understands what to expect after the test?
   ○ 1. "I can expect to have stomach pains for about 2 days after the test."
   ○ 2. "I should limit my diet to soft foods until my first bowel movement after the test."
   ○ 3. "I will experience white stools about 24 hours after the test."

   ○ 4. "I should limit my activity for 24 hours after the test."

6. A neonate is delivered vaginally to a multigravida. While assessing the neonate, the nurse observes that the neonate has one artery and one vein in the umbilical cord. The nurse plans to assess the neonate further for
   ○ 1. cardiovascular anomalies.
   ○ 2. respiratory anomalies.
   ○ 3. facial anomalies.
   ○ 4. limb anomalies.

7. The nurse is caring for a primigravida who is in active labor. Her cervix is dilated to 5 cm and is completely effaced. The client is using the Lamaze method of prepared childbirth during labor. The client has been using slow paced breathing and tells the nurse that this does not appear to be helping her during a contraction. The nurse should suggest to the client that she use
   ○ 1. deep abdominal breathing.
   ○ 2. pant-and-blow breathing.
   ○ 3. open-glottis breathing.
   ○ 4. modified-pace breathing.

8. A client suspected of being an abuse victim returns to the emergency room and, sobbing, tells the nurse, "I guess you really know that my husband beats me and that's why I have bruises all over my body. I don't know what to do. I'm afraid he'll kill me one of these times." Which of the following responses would best show that the nurse recognizes the client's needs at this time?
   ○ 1. "The fear that your husband will kill you is unfounded."
   ○ 2. "We can begin by discussing various options open to you."
   ○ 3. "You can legally leave your husband because he has no right to hurt you."
   ○ 4. "We can begin by listing ways to avoid making your husband angry with you."

9. Mechanical ventilation is associated with which of the following complications?
   ○ 1. Gastrointestinal hemorrhage.
   ○ 2. Immunosuppression.
   ○ 3. Increased cardiac output.
   ○ 4. Pulmonary emboli.

10. When caring for a client receiving haloperidol (Haldol), the nurse should plan to assess for

691

○ 1. hypertensive episodes.

○ 2. extrapyramidal symptoms.

○ 3. hypersalivation.

○ 4. oversedation.

11. Risk factors for development of pressure ulcers include which of the following?

○ 1. Ambulating less than twice a day.

○ 2. Anchored urinary catheter.

○ 3. Decreased serum albumin.

○ 4. Elevated white blood cell count.

12. A client with a 4-year history of severe bulimia is admitted to a psychiatric unit. The nurse would anticipate that the client's signs and symptoms most likely will include

○ 1. amenorrhea, binge-eating episodes, vomiting, and high serum potassium level.

○ 2. normal weight, binge-eating episodes, vomiting, and low serum potassium level.

○ 3. severe weight loss, vomiting, compulsive exercising, and tachycardia.

○ 4. amenorrhea, laxative abuse, diet pill abuse, and vomiting.

13. A multigravida visits the clinic because she suspects that she is pregnant but is unable to tell the nurse when her last menstrual period began. The client has a history of preterm delivery. The nurse instructs the client that the gestational age of the fetus can be estimated by

○ 1. amniocentesis.

○ 2. percutaneous umbilical blood sampling.

○ 3. alpha-fetoprotein level.

○ 4. ultrasonography.

14. At 36 weeks' gestation, a multigravida is diagnosed with polyhydramnios. The nurse has instructed the client about possible complications related to polyhydramnios. The nurse determines that the client needs *further* instructions when the client says,

○ 1. "Because I have polyhydramnios, I can expect to have more edema in my feet."

○ 2. "Polyhydramnios has been associated with gastrointestinal disorders in the fetus."

○ 3. "I need to watch for signs of preterm labor."

○ 4. "Polyhydramnios has been associated with renal anomalies in the fetus."

15. A client tells the nurse, "Everybody smiles at me because they know that I was chosen by God for this mission." This statement reflects

○ 1. an idea of reference.

○ 2. a thought insertion.

○ 3. a visual hallucination.

○ 4. a neologism.

16. A 25-year-old client tells the nurse that she would like to become pregnant, but she has been diagnosed with blocked fallopian tubes due to pelvic inflammatory disease. The nurse should suggest that the client explore an infertility treatment termed

○ 1. gamete intrafallopian transfer.

○ 2. surrogate transfer.

○ 3. menotropins (Pergonal) therapy

○ 4. in vitro fertilization.

17. A 2-month-old child returns from a cardiac catheterization. The child's fontanel is flat, and the diaper is dry. The respiratory rate is 20 breaths/minute, breath sounds are decreased bilaterally, and the child is limp, although the child moves all extremities when stimulated. The dressing over the insertion site is intact, clean, and dry. The pedal pulses are palpable bilaterally and equal to the heart rate. The nurse makes a nursing diagnosis of

○ 1. Altered Tissue Perfusion related to thrombus formation.

○ 2. Fluid Volume Deficit related to inability to take in fluids.

○ 3. High Risk for Injury related to disruption of vessel integrity.

○ 4. Ineffective Breathing Pattern related to sedation.

18. An adolescent client immobilized in a spica cast complains of having trouble breathing after meals. The nurse should

○ 1. encourage the client to drink more between meals.

○ 2. teach the adolescent pursed-lip breathing.

○ 3. give the client a laxative after meals.

○ 4. offer the client small feedings several times a day.

19. The client with a burn injury is assessed using the "rule of nines" to determine the

○ 1. amount of body surface area burned.

○ 2. rehabilitation needs.

○ 3. ventilatory assistance needs.

○ 4. type of intravenous infusion required.

20. A child with rheumatic fever has polyarthritis and chorea. An echocardiogram shows fragmentation and swelling of the cardiac tissue. The nurse would plan which of the following interventions for this child?

○ 1. Explaining to the child and family that the chorea will disappear over time.

○ 2. Performing neurologic checks every 4 hours until the chorea subsides.

○ 3. Promoting ambulation by giving aspirin every 4 hours.

○ 4. Keeping the child in a slightly cool environment.

21. A client admits herself to a rehabilitation program for alcoholics. Plans are made to care for her if she begins to have alcohol-withdrawal delirium. An appropriate intervention for the nurse to take when alcohol-withdrawal delirium occurs is to

○ 1. help the client remain awake.

○ 2. place the client in restraints.

○ 3. keep the client's room well lighted.

○ 4. deny the client's visual misinterpretations.

22. When teaching a sexuality class at a community center, the nurse should instruct class participants that human immunodeficiency virus (HIV) transmission can be greatly reduced by which of the following behaviors?

○ 1. Avoiding inhalant drugs.

○ 2. Avoiding prolonged sex.

○ 3. Using latex condoms during sexual intercourse.

○ 4. Douching after sexual intercourse.

23. During a home visit to a primipara 4 days after delivery, the breast-feeding client tells the nurse that her breasts are hard and tender from engorgement. The nurse should instruct the client to

○ 1. discontinue breast-feeding and use bottle-feeding during the night.

○ 2. apply ice packs to the breasts just before breast-feeding the newborn.

○ 3. take a moderately strong analgesic after breast-feeding on both sides.

○ 4. express a small amount of breast milk by hand or with a pump before breast-feeding.

24. The nurse judges the client to need *further* teaching regarding clozapine (Clozaril) when the client states,

○ 1. "I need to have my blood checked only when I think I have the flu."

○ 2. "I need to sit on the side of the bed for a while when I wake up in the morning."

○ 3. "The sleepiness I feel will decrease as my body adjusts to clozapine.

○ 4. "I need to call my doctor when I start to feel ill."

25. Which of the following nursing interventions is appropriate for preventing the development of pressure ulcers?

○ 1. Cleanse the skin daily using mild soap and hot water.

○ 2. Perform a systematic skin assessment at least once a day.

○ 3. Massage bony prominences gently every shift.

○ 4. Encourage the client to sit in a chair as much as possible.

26. A child is brought to the clinic for a well-infant checkup and the DPT (diphtheria-pertussis-tetanus) and OPV (oral polio vaccine) immunizations. The child is recovering from a cold and is afebrile. The child's sibling has cancer and is receiving chemotherapy. Nursing considerations would include

○ 1. giving only the DPT and withholding the OPV.

○ 2. giving both the DPT and OPV.

○ 3. postponing both the immunizations until the sibling is in remission.

○ 4. withholding both immunizations until the child recovers from the cold.

27. Arterial blood gas (ABG) values of a client with emphysema are monitored closely during hospitalization. Which of the following $PaCO_2$ values would indicate the need for immediate intervention in this client?

○ 1. 35 mm Hg.

○ 2. 45 mm Hg.

○ 3. 60 mm Hg.

○ 4. 80 mm Hg.

28. When asked how she cut her finger, a client with a cognitive disorder says, "While cutting flowers in our garden." The client's husband later tells the nurse that they do not have a flower garden. Filling in gaps of memory, as the client has done, is called

○ 1. displacement.

○ 2. confabulation.

○ 3. disorientation.

○ 4. flight of ideas.

29. To prevent osteomyelitis in a child who has a fracture and is in skeletal traction, the nurse should plan to

○ 1. encourage good nutrition.

○ 2. keep the child positioned in correct alignment.

○ 3. keep the child in protective isolation.

○ 4. protect the child from visitors with colds.

30. A cerclage procedure is performed on a client at 20 weeks' gestation who is diagnosed with cervical incompetence. Before releasing the client from the hospital unit, the nurse plans to instruct the client to monitor herself for

○ 1. Braxton Hicks contractions.

○ 2. nausea and vomiting.

○ 3. symptoms of infection.

○ 4. transient hypotension.

31. When dressing the wounds of a child who has sustained serious burns, the nurse would likely note which characteristic of full-thickness burns?

○ 1. Blanching to the touch.

○ 2. Excessive bleeding.

○ 3. Little pain.

○ 4. Blisters and moist appearance.

32. Which of the following goals should be of highest priority during the first 24 hours postoperatively for the client who had a total laryngectomy owing to cancer of the larynx?

○ 1. Provide adequate nourishment.

○ 2. Prevent skin breakdown.

○ 3. Maintain proper bowel elimination.

○ 4. Maintain a patent airway.

33. A client has been using crutches at home for 1 week. He tells the health clinic nurse that he is having trouble using the crutches because his armpits hurt and his fingers tingle. The nurse's most appropriate response would be,

○ 1. "You need to do more arm exercises. It sounds like your muscles need strengthening."

○ 2. "That's normal. As you adjust to the crutches, the discomfort will diminish."

○ 3. "Be sure to take your pain medication before ambulating. That will help your discomfort."

○ 4. "Let me watch you ambulate. Your technique may need some adjustment."

34. The nurse teaches the parents of a 3-year-old child who has undergone cleft palate repair how to use elbow restraints. The nurse would evaluate the teaching as successful when the parents state,

○ 1. "The restraints should remain in place continuously until the doctor says it's okay to remove them."

○ 2. "The child should wear the restraints at night but can have them off while playing."

○ 3. "The restraints should be taped right to the arms so they will stay in place."

○ 4. "We'll take the restraints off at least three times a day to look for any redness or swelling, and then put them right back on."

35. A multigravida who is at 28 weeks' gestation and has a history of pregnancy-induced hypertension asks the nurse about traveling overseas. The client's father lives in a rural village in India, and the client wishes to visit him before the delivery of the neonate. The nurse should advise the client that

○ 1. traveling overseas is permissible if the client is not having any complications.

○ 2. if traveling is not fatiguing to the client, it is acceptable to visit India.

○ 3. air travel at 28 weeks' gestation can lead to preterm birth.

○ 4. with the client's history of pregnancy-induced hypertension, traveling is not advisable.

36. For a client with a demand pacemaker, the nurse should explain that this pacemaker functions by providing

○ 1. stimuli to the heart muscle only when the heart begins to beat irregularly.

○ 2. continuous stimuli to the heart muscle, resulting in a predetermined heart rate.

○ 3. stimuli to the heart muscle only when the heart rate falls below a specified level.

○ 4. continuous stimuli to the heart muscle whenever ventricular fibrillation occurs.

37. The parent of a 2-week infant brings the infant to the clinic for a checkup. The parent expresses concern about the baby's breathing. The parent reports the infant breathes fast for a while then breathes slowly. The nurse would advise the parent that the breathing

○ 1. is normal in infants this age.

○ 2. is abnormal, and the infant needs to be on an apnea monitor.

○ 3. may be normal, but the mother should watch the infant closely.

○ 4. is not normal, and the infant needs a chest radiograph.

38. In the event of evisceration of an abdominal wound, which of the following actions should the nurse implement first?

○ 1. Call the physician immediately.

○ 2. Reinsert the protruding viscera into the abdominal cavity.

○ 3. Place the client in reverse Trendelenburg's position.

○ 4. Cover the wound with a sterile dressing moistened with sterile normal saline solution.

39. An 18-month-old has just returned to the pediatric unit after having a ventriculoperitoneal shunt placed. The nurse would *first*

○ 1. ask the child to state his name.

○ 2. palpate his anterior fontanel.

○ 3. place him on his side opposite the shunt site.

○ 4. check his pupil size.

40. After abdominal surgery, the nurse should use which of the following measures to determine if a school-aged child is ready to drink oral fluids?

○ 1. Asking if the child wants something to drink.

○ 2. Auscultating the child's abdomen for bowel sounds.

○ 3. Determining that the child has a gag reflex.

○ 4. Palpating the epigastric area for discomfort.

41. The nurse is caring for a primigravida in active labor who is diagnosed with outlet dystocia due to a narrow pubic arch. The term fetus is estimated to be average for gestational age, and the presenting part is at +2 station. In planning for the client's delivery, the nurse should plan for a delivery by

○ 1. mid-forceps.

○ 2. cesarean section.

○ 3. low forceps.

○ 4. high forceps.

42. The nurse is caring for a 1-day-old neonate who was delivered at 27 weeks' gestation. The mother planned on bottle-feeding the infant. The nurse should explain to the parents that gavage feeding of the neonate is necessary because

○ 1. the neonate has difficulty coordinating sucking, swallowing, and breathing.

○ 2. the neonate requires high-fat and -calorie formula that can more easily be provided by gavage feeding.

○ 3. hyperglycemia can be prevented more easily using the gavage method.

○ 4. the neonate may experience cold stress if bottle-feedings are given.

43. A 33-year-old primigravida at 12 weeks' gestation tells the nurse that she has smoked two packs of cigarettes daily for the last year. An appropriate goal for the client is to
○ 1. smoke only cigarettes that have a filter on them.
○ 2. decrease the smoking to one pack a day.
○ 3. quit smoking during the pregnancy.
○ 4. smoke only when she feels stressed.

44. The mother of a 15-month-old telephones the clinic to ask advice for her child she suspects has croup. The nurse would advise her when the child is coughing and having trouble breathing to
○ 1. administer acetaminophen every 4 hours.
○ 2. take the child into the bathroom and run the hot shower.
○ 3. give cough medicine every 6 hours.
○ 4. get the child to take as many fluids as possible.

45. A preadolescent is going to receive 48 hours of chemotherapy. Nausea and vomiting are frequent side effects of the chemotherapy drugs. The nurse would administer an antiemetic
○ 1. 30 minutes after the chemotherapy has started, then every 4 to 6 hours.
○ 2. 30 minutes before the chemotherapy starts, then every 4 to 6 hours.
○ 3. when the preadolescent requests medication for nausea.
○ 4. when the nurse starts the chemotherapy and then routinely.

46. The nurse is caring for a primipara who plans to breast-feed. During the first breast-feeding session, the client asks the nurse, "When will my milk come in?" The nurse should instruct the client that breasts begin to fill with milk within
○ 1. 12 hours after delivery.
○ 2. 24 hours after delivery.
○ 3. 48 to 72 hours after delivery.
○ 4. 1 week after delivery.

47. Clients receiving total parenteral nutrition (TPN) are at risk for the development of which of the following complications?
○ 1. Hypostatic pneumonia.
○ 2. Excessive constipation.
○ 3. Diabetes mellitus.
○ 4. Fluid imbalances.

48. Which of the following abilities that the nurse may possess is best suited to helping provide a therapeutic milieu for clients? The ability to
○ 1. display leadership and persuasiveness.
○ 2. set goals for the clients' final recovery.
○ 3. accept behavior as meaningful and motivated.
○ 4. meet the nurse's own needs while helping clients meet their needs.

49. The nurse tells a rape victim that even if she was protected against pregnancy by a contraceptive and has no intention of taking any legal action against her assailant, she should still be checked by a physician. This postrape physical examination is recommended for early detection of
○ 1. venereal disease.
○ 2. anxiety reaction.
○ 3. periurethral tears.
○ 4. menstrual difficulties.

50. The nurse is collaborating with the physician in the development of a drug regimen for a client with cancer. Which of the following medications should be avoided in the treatment of cancer pain?
○ 1. Meperidine (Demerol).
○ 2. Morphine.
○ 3. Acetaminophen (Tylenol)
○ 4. Hydrocodone.

51. The nurse is caring for a low-risk multigravida in active labor during a home birth who has begun pushing, and the fetal head is beginning to crown. To prevent perineal lacerations during the delivery, the nurse should
○ 1. stretch the perineal tissues with sterile, gloved fingers.
○ 2. hold the fetal head back with a sterile, gloved hand.
○ 3. tell the client to stop pushing during the next two contractions.
○ 4. ask the client to hold her breath while pushing during the entire contraction.

52. As the nurse is administering a tap-water enema, the client begins to complain of abdominal cramping. Which of the following actions should the nurse implement *first?*
○ 1. Stop infusing the enema, and allow the client to evacuate the fluid.
○ 2. Temporarily stop the infusion until the cramping subsides.
○ 3. Tell the client to hold his breath, and continue infusing the enema.
○ 4. Turn the client onto his back, and continue infusing the enema.

53. The client is being discharged on lithium, 300 mg tid. Which of the following client statements does the nurse judge to be accurate?
○ 1. "I need to eliminate salt from my diet."
○ 2. "If I forget to take a dose of medication, I can double the dose the next time I take it."
○ 3. "I need to call my doctor immediately if I have vomiting, extreme hand tremors, dizziness, or muscle weakness or feel sedated."
○ 4. "I need to drink five or six 8-ounce glasses of water each day."

54. During an appointment with the nurse, a client says,

"I could hate God for that flood." The nurse responds, "Oh, don't feel that way. We're making progress in these sessions." The nurse's statement demonstrates a failure to

○ 1. look for meaning in what the client says.

○ 2. explain to the client why he may think as he does.

○ 3. add to the strength of the client's support system.

○ 4. give the client credit for being able to solve his own problems.

55. The nurse is preparing a health education plan for a family that lives in a rural area where the drinking water is not fluoridated. Health teaching for the family should include informing them that a significant amount of fluoride can be obtained in

○ 1. tea.

○ 2. yogurt.

○ 3. citrus juices.

○ 4. natural cheeses.

56. The nurse planning a screening clinic for scoliosis would target

○ 1. preadolescents at the beginning of a growth spurt.

○ 2. toddlers who have diets low in calcium and vitamin D.

○ 3. preschoolers who are entering kindergarten.

○ 4. infants whose mothers have had no prenatal care.

57. After hearing a client with bulimia talk about her bizarre eating binges of raw pancake batter and bowls of whipped cream, the nurse feels disgusted and feels like telling her to "snap out of it." At this point, it would be best for the nurse to

○ 1. share her or his feelings with the client, and point out that her behavior alienates people.

○ 2. ask the client to talk more about her eating habits, and try harder to understand her underlying problem.

○ 3. suggest that another nurse work with the client because this relationship is no longer therapeutic.

○ 4. discuss her or his feelings with another nurse and try to resolve them.

58. A 23-month-old pulled a pan of hot water off of the stove onto her chest and arms. Her mother was right there when it happened. The mother should immediately

○ 1. apply ice to the burned areas.

○ 2. place the child in the bathtub in cool water.

○ 3. apply antibiotic ointment to the burned areas.

○ 4. call the neighbor to come over and help her.

59. Two hours ago, a multigravida laboring without anesthesia was examined. Her cervix was determined to be 5 cm dilated and completely effaced; the presenting part was at 0 station, with membranes intact. The nurse caring for the client now observes

that the client is irritable and has had some nausea with one episode of vomiting. The nurse determines that the client is most likely experiencing

○ 1. a precipitous labor pattern.

○ 2. the transition phase of labor.

○ 3. fear and anxiety related to the labor outcome.

○ 4. spontaneous rupture of the membranes.

60. When assessing a healthy adolescent client, the nurse should

○ 1. obtain a detailed prenatal and early developmental history.

○ 2. discuss sexual preferences and behaviors with the parents present for legal reasons.

○ 3. obtain most of the information from the parents, and gather any other necessary information from an interview with the adolescent.

○ 4. interact primarily with the adolescent, and gather any other necessary information from an interview with the parents.

61. Which of the following goals would be appropriate for a client with aplastic anemia? The client will

○ 1. perform activities of daily living without excessive fatigue or dyspnea.

○ 2. learn how to administer weekly vitamin B_{12} injections.

○ 3. describe correctly how to take prescribed anticoagulant drug therapy.

○ 4. describe self-care behaviors that will prevent spread of the disease to family members.

62. A client with chronic renal failure tells the nurse that his skin feels dry and is constantly itching. Based on these data, an appropriate nursing diagnosis would be

○ 1. Altered Health Maintenance related to poor hygiene.

○ 2. Chronic Pain related to skin irritation.

○ 3. High Risk for Impaired Skin Integrity related to severe pruritus.

○ 4. Ineffective Individual Coping related to manifestations of chronic illness.

63. A preschooler is diagnosed with tinea, and treatment is begun with griseofulvin. The nurse would teach the parents to

○ 1. give the medication before a meal.

○ 2. have the child avoid intense sunlight.

○ 3. give the medication for 10 days.

○ 4. drink lots of liquids with this medicine.

64. The nurse is caring for a primigravida at 30 weeks' gestation. The client has been diagnosed with mild hyperthyroidism before the pregnancy. The nurse should instruct the client to

○ 1. continuing taking methimazole as prescribed until delivery.

○ 2. contact the physician immediately if bradycardia occurs.

○ 3. discontinue taking propylthiouracil until birth of the neonate.

○ 4. notify the physician if regular contractions begin.

65. At 3 AM, the mother of a 3-year-old calls the emergency room nurse and reports the child has a temperature of 101°F, a runny nose, and a barky cough that "gets going and won't stop." The mother states that she just gave the child Tylenol. The nurse should recommend that the mother try

○ 1. sitting with the child in a steamy bathroom.

○ 2. running a steam vaporizer near the child's bedside.

○ 3. giving the child an over-the-counter decongestant.

○ 4. giving the child aspirin in 2 hours.

66. When the nurse documents the initial care of a suspected abuse victim, which of the following statements would be *least* helpful for others caring for the client?

○ 1. "Requests that her bruises not be described to a doctor."

○ 2. "Seems fearful to discuss how bruises on her body had been caused."

○ 3. "Asks that her husband not be called at work because she says she knows he is very busy."

○ 4. "Refuses a follow-up appointment because she states that she has a child at home who needs her care."

67. A clinic's nursing staff is planning to conduct prenatal and parenting classes. Child care will be provided for the children of the parents attending the classes, who range in age from 12 months to 6 years. The clinic has a playroom. The staff should plan which of the following activities for the children?

○ 1. Free play with adult supervision.

○ 2. A group sing-along.

○ 3. Drawing and painting projects.

○ 4. Viewing of cartoon videos.

68. The nurse should teach a client who is taking warfarin sodium (Coumadin) to

○ 1. not have dental work without consulting the physician.

○ 2. avoid the use of toothbrush during oral hygiene.

○ 3. use rectal suppositories to avoid straining for bowel movements.

○ 4. eat green leafy vegetables.

69. The client with paranoid schizophrenia is withdrawn, suspicious of others, and projects blame. The client's behavior reflect problems in which of Erikson's stages of development?

○ 1. Trust versus mistrust.

○ 2. Autonomy versus shame and doubt

○ 3. Initiative versus guilt.

○ 4. Intimacy versus isolation.

70. While examining a 12-month-old child, the nurse notes that the child can stand independently but cannot walk without support. The nurse should

○ 1. ask the mother if the child uses a walker at home.

○ 2. do nothing; this is a normal finding in a child this age.

○ 3. initiate a consultation with a developmental specialist.

○ 4. tell the mother that the child may have a developmental delay.

71. What would be the priority nursing intervention for a client admitted to the emergency room with estimated 27% burns?

○ 1. Inserting a large-caliber intravenous line.

○ 2. Administering an intramuscular morphine injection.

○ 3. Establishing an airway.

○ 4. Administering tetanus toxoid.

72. In which of the following instances would the nurse anticipate that a client who has been sexually assaulted will have future adjustment problems and the need for additional counseling?

○ 1. When she becomes upset when talking about the rape to anyone.

○ 2. When she seeks support from formerly ignored relatives and friends.

○ 3. When her parents show shame and suspicion about her part in the rape.

○ 4. When her life becomes focused on helping other rape victims like herself.

73. A client comes to the emergency department with multiple bruises on her face and arms, a black eye, and a broken nose. She says that these injuries occurred when she "fell down the stairs." The nurse suspects that the client may have been physically assaulted. The nurse's best action is to

○ 1. ask the client specifically about the possibility of physical abuse.

○ 2. tell the client that it is difficult to believe that such injuries resulted from a fall.

○ 3. ask the client what she did to make someone beat her.

○ 4. discuss with the client what she can do to de-escalate the situation next time.

74. When some clients fail to clean the hospital's recreation room after using it, a client government meeting is held to discuss the problem. In this situation, it is best for staff members to assume a role of

○ 1. offering their view but agreeing to the group's decision.

○ 2. coleading the meeting with assistance from any one of the clients.

○ 3. remaining silent while observing the group's process of decision making.

○ 4. allowing a client the leadership role but requiring staff approval of the group's decision.

75. A nurse must be able to distinguish cholinergic crisis (too much medication) from myasthenic crisis (too little medication) in a client receiving anticholinesterase drug therapy. Which of the following symptoms are present in cholinergic crisis?
- ○ 1. improved muscle strength after intravenous edrophonium chloride (Tensilon) administration.
- ○ 2. increased strength of skeletal muscles.
- ○ 3. respiratory embarrassment.
- ○ 4. decreased salivation.

76. A parent calls the poison control center because her 3-year-old has eaten 10 to 12 chewable acetaminophen tablets. The nurse should tell the parent to take the child to the emergency room but first
- ○ 1. give the child 6 to 8 ounces of milk, and keep the child awake.
- ○ 2. give the child 6 to 8 ounces of water and 3 teaspoons of ipecac.
- ○ 3. give the child 1 teaspoon of baking soda in 4 ounces of water.
- ○ 4. withhold fluids and position the child on either side.

77. The physician has determined that a primigravida needs a cesarean section delivery due to prolonged labor and cephalopelvic disproportion. After the cesarean delivery of a male neonate, it is important for the nurse to assess the neonate for
- ○ 1. decreased muscle tone.
- ○ 2. high-pitched cry.
- ○ 3. head circumference.
- ○ 4. nasopharyngeal secretions.

78. The nurse is caring for a 3-day-old neonate who is receiving phototherapy to treat jaundice. The nurse plans to
- ○ 1. turn the neonate every 6 hours.
- ○ 2. encourage the mother to discontinue breast-feeding.
- ○ 3. notify the physician if the skin becomes bronze in color.
- ○ 4. check the vital signs every 2 to 4 hours.

79. About 2 weeks after receiving care in the emergency room, a client admits to her husband that she has a drinking problem and that she has "decided to do something about it." Of critical importance for her successful rehabilitation is
- ○ 1. her emotional support system.
- ○ 2. her motivation to change her behavior.
- ○ 3. the presence of self-help groups in the community.
- ○ 4. the presence of local health centers for alcoholics.

80. The nurse is admitting a 4-month-old with congestive heart failure and congenital heart disease. The priority nursing diagnosis is

- ○ 1. Activity Intolerance.
- ○ 2. Altered Health Maintenance.
- ○ 3. Potential for Infection.
- ○ 4. Impaired Mobility.

81. The nurse would judge correctly that a male client with bipolar disorder, manic phase, is nearing readiness for discharge when
- ○ 1. he sleeps 4 hours per night.
- ○ 2. he is able to differentiate between reality and unrealistic situations.
- ○ 3. he telephones his wife and asks for a divorce.
- ○ 4. his affect is labile.

82. A primigravida has been in labor for 12 hours when it is determined that the client's cervix is now 10 cm dilated and the presenting part is at 0 station. The nurse should inform the client and family members that the
- ○ 1. first phase of labor is over.
- ○ 2. client is now in transition phase.
- ○ 3. delivery will occur in the next few minutes.
- ○ 4. second stage of labor is now beginning.

83. The nurse is teaching the parents of a 5-year-old boy who has leukemia how to talk with their child about death and dying. The parents have age-appropriate expectations about their child's reaction to his impending death when they state that their child
- ○ 1. is too young to understand what is happening to him.
- ○ 2. might think he can cause his death because he has misbehaved.
- ○ 3. will accept his death as caused by his disease.
- ○ 4. will understand how much his siblings will miss him.

84. When preparing a client for a scheduled colonoscopy, the nurse would include
- ○ 1. inserting a nasogastric tube 12 hours before the procedure.
- ○ 2. cleansing the bowel with laxatives or enemas.
- ○ 3. administering an antibiotic to decrease the risk of infection.
- ○ 4. spraying a local anesthetic into the client's throat to calm the gag reflex.

85. A community health nurse is creating a program to decrease the primary cause of disability and death in children. The nurse would
- ○ 1. encourage the state legislator to draft legislation to promote prenatal care.
- ○ 2. encourage the health department to make immunizations available at no cost to all children.
- ○ 3. teach health and safety practices to children and parents.
- ○ 4. use blood tests to screen for cancer in school-aged children.

86. The nurse caring for a client with insulin-dependent diabetes mellitus would use which of the following

assessment tools to determine how well the child's insulin, diet, and exercise are balanced?
- ○ 1. Fasting serum glucose level.
- ○ 2. 1-week diet recall.
- ○ 3. Home log of blood glucose levels.
- ○ 4. Glycosylated hemoglobin level.

87. The nurse is caring for a client who has an acute case of stomatitis. Which of the following nursing interventions is most appropriate?
- ○ 1. Use a soft toothbrush to provide oral hygiene.
- ○ 2. Rinse mouth with commercial mouthwash before and after each meal.
- ○ 3. Cleanse gums and oral mucosa with lemon-glycerin swabs every shift.
- ○ 4. Keep dentures in place to decrease development of edema.

88. Initial nursing interventions for a child admitted to the hospital with a diagnosis of meningitis should include
- ○ 1. keeping the child well hydrated.
- ○ 2. maintaining a quiet, cool environment.
- ○ 3. keeping the child positioned flat in the bed.
- ○ 4. placing the child in enteric isolation.

89. Which one of the following people is at highest risk for developing a urinary tract infection?
- ○ 1. A 45-year-old woman who has had two children.
- ○ 2. A 75-year-old man with an indwelling urinary catheter inserted for incontinence.
- ○ 3. A 50-year-old man with a history of renal calculi.
- ○ 4. A 28-year-old woman with a history of well-controlled diabetes mellitus.

90. The nurse is caring for a client with third-degree burns on 35% of his body. When developing a care plan for pain control, the nurse would anticipate
- ○ 1. using oral analgesics because third-degree burns are painless due to nerve destruction.
- ○ 2. relying on nonpharmacologic measures to avoid respiratory depression.
- ○ 3. sedating the client to an unconscious state to decrease awareness of pain.
- ○ 4. administering intravenous opioid analgesics, such as morphine.

CORRECT ANSWERS AND RATIONALE

The letters in parentheses following the rationale identify the step of the nursing process (A, D, P, I, E), cognitive level (K, C, T, N), client needs (S, G, L, H), and nursing care area (O, X, Y, M). See the Answer Grid for the key.

1. 1. The client is 12 hours postpartum, therefore the breasts should still be soft and nontender. Breast milk production does not begin until the second or third postpartum day, at which time the breasts become larger, firm, and tender to touch. (A, T, H, O)

2. 2. It is believed that childbirth education classes are critically important in the empowerment of women through knowledge of the choices they may have to make during the birth experience. This may serve to enhance their self-esteem and decrease dissatisfaction with the birth experience. The single documented effect of childbirth preparation is the use of less pain medication in labor. Childbirth preparation classes do not affect the length of labor, the support provided by the significant other, or the mother's control over her birth plans. (I, N, H, O)

3. 1. Children who are being abused demonstrate behaviors such as withdrawal, apparent fear of parents, and lack of reaction to frightening events, such as an examination, appropriately with crying and attempting to get away. (A, T, S, Y)

4. 2. Battering is a major cause of injury to women. Although battering occurs in all socioeconomic groups, it may appear to be more common in members of lower socioeconomic groups because they are more likely to use emergency room services. Pregnant women are frequent victims of battering. (P, C, L, X)

5. 3. The client will experience white stools about 24 to 48 hours after the upper gastrointestinal series due to the passage of barium. It is not necessary to eat soft foods or limit activity after this test. Abdominal pain would not be expected and should be reported to the physician. (E, T, H, M)

6. 1. The umbilical cord normally has two umbilical arteries and one vein. When there is an absence of an artery, the nurse should plan to assess the neonate for cardiovascular anomalies. Other common congenital problems associated with congenital absence of an artery include renal anomalies, central nervous system lesions, tracheoesophageal fistulas, and trisomy 13 and 18. (P, N, G, O)

7. 4. With time, habituation may occur, making slow-paced breathing less effective. The nurse should suggest to the client that she switch to modified pace breathing, which is performed as an upper chest breath either through her nose or mouth. A frequently taught method is three breaths, then a soft blow. Open-glottis breathing is useful for the delivery process, and pant-and-blow breathing is useful during the transition stage. Deep breathing is useful in early labor. (I, T, G, O)

8. 2. This client is asking for help when she says that she does not know what to do about being abused by her husband. The nurse's best course of action is to explain the various options available to her. This helps the client make decisions based on appropriate knowledge. (I, T, L, X)

9. 1. Gastrointestinal hemorrhage occurs in about 25% of clients receiving prolonged mechanical ventilation. Other possible complications include incorrect ventilation, oxygen toxicity, fluid imbalance, decreased cardiac output, pneumothorax, infection, and atelectasis. (A, C, G, M)

10. 2. Haloperidol is associated with a high incidence of severe extrapyramidal reactions. Other side effects of haloperidol include blurred vision, dry mouth, urine retention, and skin rash. Haloperidol is associated with a low incidence of sedation and a low incidence of cardiovascular effects at therapeutic dosages. Hypersalivation is a paradoxical effect of clozapine. (P, T, G, X)

11. 3. Risk factors for the development of pressure ulcers include malnourishment indicated by a decreased serum albumin level. According to the Guidelines for Pressure Ulcers published by the Agency for Healthcare Policy Research, other risk factors include immobility, incontinence, and decreased sensation. (A, C, S, M)

12. 2. Manifestations of bulimia always include eating binges, usually include vomiting, and often include low serum potassium level secondary to the vomiting. Amenorrhea, severe weight loss, and compulsive exercise are signs of anorexia. Laxative abuse and diet pill abuse are sometimes seen in clients with bulimia. (A, C, L, X)

13. 4. An ultrasound can provide a fairly accurate estimate of the fetal gestational age through various measurements of fetal landmarks. Amniocentesis is appropriate for determining genetic deviations and fetal lung maturity (lecithin-to-sphygomyelin ratio). Alpha-fetoprotein studies are performed between the 15th and 20th weeks of gestation to determine if neural tube defects are present. Percutaneous umbilical blood sampling is used to detect inherited blood disorders, acidosis, or infection. (A, T, G, O)

14. 4. Polyhydramnios is an abnormally large amount of amniotic fluid. The client needs further instructions if she states that polyhydramnios is associated with renal anomalies in the fetus. Renal anomalies are associated with oligohydramnios or an abnormally small volume of amniotic fluid. Polyhydramnios is a risk factor for preterm labor. This condition is also associated with large-for-gestational-age neonates, maternal diabetes, multifetal pregnancies, Rh isoimmunization, and other congenital anomalies of the gastrointestinal system and central nervous system. There is some evidence that polyhydramnios is associated with neonates born with tracheoesophageal fistulas. (E, T, G, O)

15. 1. An idea of reference is a person's view that other people recognize that he or she has an important characteristic or power. Thought insertion is a person's belief that others, or a specific other, can put thoughts into his or her mind. Visual hallucinations involve seeing objects or persons not based in reality. A neologism is a word or phrase that has meaning only to the person using it. (A, T, L, X)

16. 4. The client should be encouraged to explore in vitro fertilization. With this procedure, the ova are removed surgically from the client, then are fertilized outside the uterus. After fertilization, the fertilized ova are introduced vaginally through a special tube through the cervix to the uterus for implantation, completely bypassing the fallopian tubes. Gamete intrafallopian transfer is not therapeutic for a client with blocked fallopian tubes. Menotropins therapy is appropriate if there is ovarian dysfunction. Surrogate transfer is not a treatment for infertility. The correct term is *surrogate mother,* in which a female client agrees to be artificially inseminated, usually by the client's husband's sperm, and the surrogate mother then carries the fetus to term for the couple. (I, N, H, O)

17. 4. The defining characteristics of ineffective breathing pattern are a decrease in respiratory rate and chest expansion, limpness or unresponsiveness, and changes in mental status. In this situation, sedation used during the catheterization is the probable cause of the ineffective breathing pattern. A thrombus is unlikely if pedal pulses are palpable. A disruption in vessel integrity would lead to bleeding at the site and circulatory or neurologic deficit in the affected leg. (D, N, G, Y)

18. 4. A spica cast extends up over the abdomen. When a child eats large meals, the abdomen distends; because the abdomen is in a fixed space, the distention pushes the abdominal contents against the diaphragm. This results in decreased chest expansion, and the client may experience some respiratory distress. The best way to prevent the distress is to de- crease abdominal distention. Because the client's complaints are associated with meals, it may be assumed that decreasing the amount of food consumed at any one time may help decrease the distress. By offering small, frequent meals, the nurse can provide nutritional support while minimizing distention. (I, N, G, Y)

19. 1. The rule of nines is used to determine the amount of the client's body surface area that was burned. Medical treatment, including fluid volume replacement therapy, is based on the percentage of body surface area burned. (A, T, G, M)

20. 1. It is important for the child and family to understand that chorea associated with rheumatic fever is not permanent. It is not necessary to assess the child's neurologic status or to keep the child in a slightly cool environment. Because the child has cardiac involvement, ambulation is contraindicated. Aspirin is used primarily as an antiinflammatory drug and secondarily for pain relief. (P, N, G, Y)

21. 3. Alcohol-withdrawal delirium often occurs after the client who has been abusing alcohol does not drink alcohol for about 24 to 72 hours. It is a serious, possibly even life-threatening, complication. The client should be kept in a private room, which should be well lighted to reduce shadows and visual hallucinations. A calm, nonstressful environment is recommended, and the client should be given the prescribed sedation. Restraints are used only as a last resort. It is preferable that the nurse calm the client with reassurance and a constant presence. The nurse's attitude of acceptance and support is important. One way to help strengthen the client's link with reality is to explain her visual misinterpretations rather than deny them. (I, T, L, X)

22. 3. Using a latex condom and a spermicide during sexual intercourse greatly reduces the risk of HIV transmission. Because HIV is most concentrated in blood and vaginal and seminal fluids, protective measures during intercourse are necessary to prevent transmission. Sharing unsterile needles for drug injections is another major mode of HIV transmission. (I, T, H, M)

23. 4. The client should be instructed to express milk from the nipples either by hand or with a breast pump. As soon as the areola is soft, the client should begin to breastfeed. Continued breast-feeding is not contraindicated. Frequent feedings with complete emptying of the breasts should alleviate engorgement. Ice packs can be used to relieve edema and pain but should be used between feedings, not immediately before a feeding. Warm compresses may also stimulate milk flow. (I, T, G, O)

24. 1. The client on clozapine therapy needs to have weekly complete blood count tests to monitor for declines in white blood cell counts because agranulocytosis is a serious adverse effect. (E, N, G, X)

25. 2. Daily skin inspection is essential to preventing the development of pressure ulcers. Hot water is irritating to skin and should be avoided. Massaging bony prominences is contraindicated. Prolonged, uninterrupted chair sitting should be avoided; the client's position should be adjusted at least every hour. (I, T, S, M)

26. 1. At this time, the child should be given the DPT only. The fact that the child's sibling is immunosuppressed due to chemotherapy should alert the nurse not to give a live vaccine like the OPV. The virus can be shed in the stool of the vaccinated child and infect the immunosuppressed child. The fact that the child has a cold is not grounds for delaying the immunizations. If the child had a fever, the immunizations would be delayed. (I, N, G, Y)

27. 4. Normal $PaCO_2$ values range from 35 to 45 mm Hg. The client with long-standing emphysema has chronic carbon dioxide retention, leading to elevated $PaCO_2$ levels. The client with emphysema and a $PaCO_2$ level of 60 mm Hg may not be in immediate danger, but the nurse would want to further evaluate the client with a level of 60 mm Hg. A $PaCO_2$ level of 80 mm Hg is life-threatening and always requires immediate intervention, possibly mechanical ventilation, to reduce the $PaCO_2$ level. (E, N, G, M)

28. 2. Making up stories to fill in memory gaps is called *confabulation*. *Displacement* is a defense mechanism that refers ideas and feelings to something or someone not responsible for them. *Disorientation* is a loss of understanding in relation to place, time, or identity. *Flight of ideas* is a rapid shift of thoughts from one subject to another before any idea has been finished. (D, T, L, X)

29. 1. The best strategy for preventing osteomyelitis is to maintain skin integrity and promote good nutrition. Protective isolation is not necessary for this child and could lead to social isolation. Antibiotics are not administered prophylactically when pins are inserted for traction, unless the child already has a bacterial infection. Osteomyelitis is caused by bacteria invading bone tissue. Colds are caused by a virus. (P, N, G, Y)

30. 3. Placement of a cerclage or pursestring suture may be used to maintain cervical closure. The procedure is performed between 12 and 20 weeks' gestation in the presence of a congenital cervical problem, or during the second trimester when the cervix appears to be normal. There is some risk of maternal infection; therefore, the client should be taught to contact the health care provider if she experiences pain, fever, or changes in the vaginal discharge. The

client should be advised to maintain modified bed rest and vaginal rest. Braxton Hicks contractions are normal during pregnancy. Nausea and vomiting are not associated with cerclage, nor is transient hypotension. (P, T, G, O)

31. 3. Full-thickness burns are serious injuries in which all the skin layers are destroyed. Lack of pain is characteristic of full-thickness burns. Because blood supply is destroyed, blanching and bleeding are absent. Blisters and moist appearance characterize partial-thickness burns. (A, T, G, Y)

32. 4. Maintaining a patent airway is a priority goal for the client after a total laryngectomy. After a total laryngectomy, the client will have a tracheostomy with increased secretions and will require suctioning and tracheostomy care to maintain oxygenation. (P, T, G, M)

33. 4. The nurse should reevaluate the client's use of his crutches. Pressure on the axillae from the crutches can lead to "crutch paralysis" due to pressure on the brachial plexus nerves. Axillae pressure can result from inappropriate use of the crutches or crutches that are sized incorrectly for the client. There should be two to three finger widths between the axillae and the top of the crutches when the crutches are placed 6 to 8 inches in front of the feet. When walking, the client's weight should be on the palms of the hands, not on the axillae. (D, N, S, M)

34. 4. Elbow restraints help keep the child from placing fingers or any other object in the mouth that would cause injury to the operative site. The restraints are worn at all times, except when they are removed to check the skin. It is best to advise parents to remove only one restraint at a time and to keep hold of the child's hand on the unrestrained side. Toddlers are quick and usually want to explore the area in the mouth that the surgery has made feel different. Taping the restraints directly to the skin is not advised because of the skin breakdown that can occur when tape is reapplied to the same area over several weeks. The restraints can be fastened to clothing to keep them from slipping. (E, T, S, Y)

35. 4. With the client's previous history of pregnancy-induced hypertension, traveling to India is not advisable. The client may be in jeopardy if complications arise if medical care is not available, and some insurance companies will not cover costs in foreign countries. There is no correlation between air travel and premature births. Any travel that causes fatigue should be avoided. (I, T, G, O)

36. 3. In contrast to a fixed-rate pacemaker, a demand pacemaker functions only when the heart rate falls below a certain level. A fixed-rate pacemaker stimulates heart contractions at a constant rate independent of the client's heart rate. This type is much less common than the demand pacemaker. (I, T, G, M)

37. 1. Periodic breathing is normal in infants this age, who typically alternate short periods of rapid, louder respirations with periods of slower, quieter respirations. (I, T, H, Y)

38. 4. In the event of wound evisceration, the nurse should first cover the wound with a sterile towel or dressing that has been moistened with sterile normal saline solution. The client is placed supine with knees flexed. Vital signs are monitored for possible signs of shock. The nurse should not attempt to reinsert any protruding viscera. The physician should be notified and the client prepared for surgery. (I, N, S, M)

39. 3. As soon as the child returns to his room, he needs to be positioned appropriately, in this case on the side opposite of the shunt placement. He may or may not be able to state his name. Palpating his fontanel and checking pupils are part of the neurologic assessment, which would be done next. (A, T, S, Y)

40. 2. After an uncomplicated abdominal surgery, fluid intake is resumed early in the postoperative period. But before providing fluids, the nurse should auscultate the child's abdomen for bowel sounds; fluids should be withheld until bowel sounds are heard. Asking the child if he is thirsty, making sure he is fully conscious, and palpating the abdomen for pain will not help determine whether he has bowel sounds and is ready to take oral fluids. Having a gag reflex is usually not a concern in a normal child who has had abdominal surgery and who is alert. (A, T, G, Y)

41. 3. If cephalopelvic disproportion is not present and fetal distress is not occurring, the client can anticipate a delivery with low forceps when the fetal presenting part is at +2 station. A cesarean section is not necessary unless there is fetal compromise. Midforceps and high forceps delivery are dangerous, and few deliveries are performed in this manner. (P, T, G, O)

42. 1. Many complications of preterm neonates make it impossible to bottle-feed or breastfeed them. These neonates have difficulty coordinating sucking, swallowing, and breathing, and may aspirate or become fatigued. Increased respiratory distress may also occur when attempting to suck from a bottle. (I, T, G, O)

43. 3. An appropriate goal, while difficult, is to encourage the client to quit smoking during the pregnancy. The client should be informed about the effects of smoking on the fetus, such as low birth weight. Often, if the client is able to quit smoking during the pregnancy, she remains smoke free after delivery.

Smoking has also been associated with sudden infant death syndrome, which affects children up to 3 years of age. (P, T, G, O)

44. 2. With difficulty breathing, the child should be taken into the shower and hot water should be run to make the bathroom steamy. That should relieve some of the respiratory distress. Giving acetaminophen and fluids is important but will not ease difficult breathing. (I, T, G, Y)

45. 2. Administering an antiemetic before beginning chemotherapy and then routinely around the clock helps prevent nausea and vomiting. Waiting until the client requests it may be too late in that nausea is already present. (P, T, G, Y)

46. 3. The clients who is breastfeeding usually has breast milk by 48 to 72 hours after delivery if she breastfeeds early and often from the time of birth. (I, T, G, O)

47. 4. Clients receiving TPN are at risk for a number of complications, including fluid imbalances such as fluid overload and hyperosmolar diuresis. Other common complications include hyperglycemia, sepsis, pneumothorax, and air embolism. (A, C, G, M)

48. 3. The milieu should provide an atmosphere that fosters growth, change, and self-responsibility. The nurse needs to accept behavior as meaningful and motivated. Staff interventions should also be flexible and open, and should encourage clients to achieve their own potential. Displaying leadership and persuasiveness, setting goals for clients, and meeting one's own needs while helping clients meet their needs are not well-suited for a therapeutic milieu. (E, N, L, X)

49. 1. Venereal diseases can be spread through rape. If the victim or the rapist was not using a contraceptive, postcoital contraceptive methods should be discussed. (P, T, L, X)

50. 1. Meperidine is useful for short-term treatment of acute pain and should be avoided in the treatment of cancer pain. Morphine is the most commonly used opioid drug. Hydrocodone is another appropriate drug of choice. Acetaminophen may be used to treat mild to moderate pain. (P, C, G, M)

51. 1. Sterile gloves should always be worn by birth attendants to prevent infection to the laboring client and the fetus. Stretching of the perineal muscles can decrease the incidence of tearing or lacerations. Holding the fetal head back, telling the client not to push for two contractions, and asking her to hold her breath are not appropriate nursing actions. Holding the breath while pushing may result in a Valsalva maneuver, which may compromise the fetus. (I, T, G, O)

52. 2. When the client initially begins complaining of abdominal cramping during an enema, it is usually most appropriate to temporarily stop the infusion until the cramping subsides. If on resuming the flow of enema fluid, the client continues to complain of cramping or inability to retain further fluid, the nurse should then discontinue the enema. (I, T, S, M)

53. 3. The client's statement regarding signs of lithium toxicity reflects accurate knowledge about lithium. Eliminating salt from the diet, doubling the dose at the next scheduled time when a dose is skipped, and drinking only five or six 8-ounce glasses of water per day can lead to lithium toxicity. (E, N, G, X)

54. 1. Such clichés as "don't feel that way" are not helpful because they ignore the client's feelings and his interpretation of the situation in which he finds himself. They fail to focus on the client and what he feels, and are judgmental. (E, N, L, X)

55. 1. Tea contains a significant amount of fluoride. Most foods contain limited amounts. In most communities, water is fluoridated, an effective and safe practice that helps prevent dental caries. Fluoride drops or tablets may also be given to provide fluorine; however, the nurse should observe careful safety measures because children may accidentally take them in sufficient quantities to cause serious toxicity. (I, T, H, M)

56. 1. Preadolescents are at greatest risk for scoliosis. Incidence is higher in girls than in boys and increases during periods of rapid growth. A toddler with a diet low in vitamin D is prone to develop rickets. There is no relation between poor prenatal care and scoliosis. (P, T, G, Y)

57. 4. This is a countertransference reaction that can only be resolved by self-reflection and discussion with other professionals. It is inappropriate for the nurse to tell the client about her feelings; it might perpetuate the client's low self-esteem. Continuing to struggle with the problem without analyzing her or his own reactions is counterproductive for the nurse. Asking another nurse to work with the client may solve the problem momentarily, but the nurse will encounter similar problems and clients, and the client may feel rejected. (I, T, L, X)

58. 2. The emergency treatment of both minor and major burns includes stopping the burning process by immersing the burned area in cool, but not cold, water. Neither ice nor antibiotic ointment should be applied to the burned area at this time. The mother can call the neighbor for help after she has removed her child from the bathtub. (I, T, S, Y)

59. 2. Irritability, nausea, vomiting, and often the urge to push are all signs that the client is beginning the transition phase of labor, which occurs when the client is 7 to 10 cm dilated. A multigravida generally progresses more rapidly than a primigravida; there-

fore, it would not be unusual for a client's cervix to dilate from 5 cm to 7 or cm or more within a 2-hour period. Rupture of the membranes may occur at any time in the labor process. There is no evidence of a precipitous labor or fear and anxiety related to the labor outcome. (D, N, G, O)

60. 4. When assessing an adolescent, it is appropriate to first obtain information from the adolescent and then interview the parents for additional information. No legal reason would prohibit the nurse from discussing sexuality with the adolescent without the parents present. Obtaining prenatal and early developmental history information is usually not important for a healthy adolescent. (A, N, H, Y)

61. 1. An appropriate goal for the client with aplastic anemia would be to strive to perform activities of daily living without excessive fatigue or dyspnea. It is important for the client to learn to schedule rest periods throughout the day to conserve energy and reduce oxygen requirements. The client needs adequate vitamin B_{12} in the diet but typically does not require vitamin B_{12} injections. Anticoagulants are contraindicated in clients with low platelet counts, which often occurs in aplastic anemia. Aplastic anemia is not contagious. (P, T, G, M)

62. 3. Clients with chronic renal failure are susceptible to uremia, an accumulation of nitrogenous waste products in the blood. Clinical manifestations include dry, itchy skin that can be severe in nature. Due to the irritation of the skin and the inclination to scratch, clients are prone to impaired skin integrity. (D, N, G, M)

63. 2. Griseofulvin is better absorbed when administered after a high fat meal. Avoid exposure to intense sunlight. There are no indications that a lot of fluids affect absorption. (I, T, G, Y)

64. 4. Hyperthyroidism has been associated with preterm labor and low-birth-weight infants; therefore, the client should contact the physician if contractions begin. Thyroid storm usually results in tachycardia, not bradycardia. Propylthiouracil is the treatment drug of choice during pregnancy and should not be discontinued. (I, N, G, O)

65. 1. The child has symptoms of laryngotracheal bronchitis. The mother should try to decrease the inflammation in the upper airway by exposing her child to a warm, steamy environment. The safest method is to steam up the bathroom and stay with the child. Steam vaporizers work by boiling water and can cause severe burns if the child comes in close contact with the steam or the vaporizer spills. A decongestant may assist in decreasing the rhinorrhea but will not decrease the inflammation in the upper airway. Laryngotracheal bronchitis is caused by a virus, and aspirin is contraindicated in children with viral infection because this combination is implicated in Reye's syndrome. (I, N, G, Y)

66. 2. Information documented on a client's record should be as objective as possible so that other health personnel can verify findings as necessary. Stating that a client seems fearful to discuss how bruises on her body were caused is a subjective statement that expresses the nurse's opinion. Rather than stating an opinion, the nurse should state exactly what the client said. (E, N, L, X)

67. 1. Planning any single activity that will appeal to children from ages 12 months to 6 years is next to impossible. Toddlers have short attention spans and probably will not cooperate in a group play situation for long. Drawing and painting would be an inappropriate activity for a toddler. It would be best to allow these children to participate in free play with adult supervision. (P, N, H, Y)

68. 1. Clients who are on anticoagulant therapy should consult the physician before undergoing any dental work. The dentist should also be aware that the client is on anticoagulants. A soft toothbrush is desirable for oral hygiene. Green leafy vegetables should not be eaten in excess owing to their vitamin K content, which may alter the effectiveness of the anticoagulant therapy. Rectal suppositories are contraindicated during anticoagulant therapy; stool softeners may be used to prevent straining that may promote bleeding. (P, T, H, M)

69. 1. The client who is withdrawn, suspicious, and projects blame is exhibiting problems in trust versus mistrust. (D, N, L, X)

70. 2. A child aged 12 months is expected to cruise, but not necessarily walk without support. Even if the child's development in walking is slow, this fact is not sufficient data on which to make a diagnosis of developmental delay. A developmental specialist consult is not necessary. Using or not using a walker does not significantly affect independent walking. (D, N, H, Y)

71. 3. Establishing a patent airway is the priority intervention in burn trauma cases. Prophylactic intubation is initiated if heat has been inhaled or if the neck, head, or face is involved. Swelling of the upper airways can progress to obstruction. After the airway has been established, circulatory support is the next priority. Fluid replacement is best accomplished using two large-caliber peripheral catheters. One peripheral line and one central line are preferable, however, if the burn is large or complicated by inhalation injuries. Partial-thickness burns are painful, but morphine sulfate, the analgesic of choice, is not administered until the client is stable; furthermore, the intravenous route is used. Tetanus pro-

phylaxis is begun in the emergency room but is not the priority intervention. (I, N, G, M)

72. 3. The potential for problems in adjusting after a rape will be increased when those around the victim treat her as though she is to blame for the rape, especially when she already may feel some guilt and shame about it. A rape victim is likely showing adjustment to her experience when she is upset about her experience, when she seeks out formerly ignored relatives and friends for support, or when she attempts to help other rape victims. (D, N, L, X)

73. 1. It is important to determine whether abuse is occurring to provide appropriate nursing care and support for the client. Many clients are hesitant to talk about abuse and need help to do so. The nurse should ask directly about abuse when it is suspected with sensitivity, empathy, and compassion. Telling the client that it's difficult to believe her injuries resulted from a fall is not helpful. Asking the client what she did to make someone hit her and discussing what she can do the next time blames and alienates the client. (I, T, L, X)

74. 1. The milieu should foster relationship development and decision-making abilities among clients. Staff members need to encourage client discussion and decision making by offering their view but agreeing to abide by the group's decision concerning unit (but not hospital) policies and issues. Coleading a client government meeting, remaining silent during a meeting, and requiring staff approval of the group's decision are not the most therapeutic roles for staff members in the milieu setting and may hinder effective client government. (I, T, L, X)

75. 3. Extreme muscle weakness is present in both cholinergic and myasthenic crisis. In cholinergic crisis, intravenous edrophonium chloride, a cholinergic agent, does not improve muscle weakness; in myasthenic crisis, it does. The muscarinic effects of pyridostigmine bromide (Mestinon) overdosage cause respiratory embarrassment, abdominal cramps, and excessive salivation in cholinergic crisis. (E, C, G, M)

76. 2. The first treatment for ingestion of nonprescription medication is to empty the stomach. This can be achieved by giving syrup of ipecac and water. If the child does not vomit in 30 minutes, then the dose should be repeated. It is important that the parent attempt to empty the child's stomach before or during transport to the emergency room. (I, N, S, Y)

77. 4. A neonate delivered by cesarean section has not had the benefit of the squeezing action of a vaginal birth, which helps remove nasopharyngeal secretions. Decreased muscle tone is related to analgesia or anesthesia. A high-pitched cry is usually related

to neurologic involvement or drug withdrawal and is not directly related to cesarean section delivery. During assessment of the neonate, both head and chest circumference are routinely measured whether the birth is a cesarean section delivery or vaginal delivery. (A, T, G, O)

78. 4. While caring for an infant under a bilirubin light (eg, Bililite) for treatment of jaundice, it is important to check the vital signs every 2 to 4 hours because hyperthermia can occur. The infant should be turned every 2 to 4 hours to expose all body surfaces to the lights. Breast-feeding does not need to be discontinued, but the infant needs adequate hydration. The skin of the neonate may become bronze as a result of phototherapy, but this is a benign condition with no adverse effects and disappears when therapy is discontinued. (I, T, G, O)

79. 2. The client with an alcohol problem must be motivated to change her behavior before rehabilitation can be successful. Such other factors as a support system in the home, a community health center for alcoholics, and self-help groups can play an important role, but they cannot be expected to help unless the client wants to solve her alcohol abuse problem. (P, N, L, X)

80. 1. An infant with congenital heart disease and congestive heart failure would have as a priority nursing diagnosis activity intolerance. These infants usually tire rapidly and thus need nursing care that allows them frequent rest periods. These infants are not necessarily at risk for more infections that other infants. Impaired mobility and altered health maintenance are not a problem for these heart clients. (D, N, G, Y)

81. 2. The client is approaching discharge when he is able to differentiate between reality and unrealistic situations. Sleeping 4 hours per night and exhibiting a labile affect are indications that the client is still acutely ill. Asking for a divorce could indicate the client's poor judgment and inability to perceive his situation realistically. (E, N, L, X)

82. 4. A primigravida whose cervix is 10 cm dilated has completed the first stage of labor, which lasts from the beginning of cervical dilation to complete dilation (10 cm). Usually, the second stage of labor (pushing) for a primigravida lasts about 1 to 2 hours. If the client is a primigravida, and the presenting part is at 0 station, delivery is not imminent. The transition phase of the first stage of labor occurs when the client is 7 to 10 cm dilated. (I, T, H, O)

83. 2. A 5-year-old child is in the preoperational stage of cognitive development and thinks of death as temporary and, because of thinking about behavior as often magical, may think that behavior can cause death. Generally, children under 3 years of age are unable to differentiate death from temporary separation; logical thinking occurs during Piaget's stage of concrete operations, which occurs between ages 6 and 12 (E, T, L, Y)

84. 2. A colonoscopy is the visual examination of the large bowel. Typically, the client will be placed on a liquid diet 24 hours before the procedure and kept NPO after midnight the night before the procedure. The bowel is cleansed through the use of laxatives and enemas. Introducing a nasogastric tube is not part of the preparation for a colonoscopy. The client does not usually receive antibiotics before the procedure. (I, T, G, M)

85. 3. The primary cause of disability and death in children is injury from accidents. Teaching safety measures is a way to decrease injury and accidents. (P, T, H, Y)

86. 4. A fasting serum glucose level gives a picture of the child's recent glucose level. A glycosylated hemoglobin level gives the nurse data about the average blood glucose level over 2 to 3 months. (A, N, G, Y)

87. 1. A soft toothbrush, Toothette, or gauze pad should be used to provide oral hygiene at least every 2 hours to promote client comfort and prevent superinfection. Commercial mouthwash is contraindicated owing to its high alcohol content, which is irritating to inflamed mucosa. Lemon-glycerine swabs are drying and can also promote bacterial growth. Dentures should be removed if the client is experiencing pain. (I, T, S, M)

88. 2. The child with meningitis should be kept in a quiet, cool environment to decrease intracranial pressure. Any fluid deficit should be corrected, and then the child should be kept on low fluid maintenance to prevent cerebral edema. To decrease intracranial pressure, the child should be positioned with the head of the bed elevated and the head midline to facilitate venous return. A child with meningitis does not need to be in enteric isolation but should be in respiratory isolation until the causative agent is identified and treated. (I, N, G, Y)

89. 2. Indwelling catheters are considered to be a major contributor to nosocomial infections, and any client with an indwelling catheter is at high risk for developing a urinary tract infection. A history of previous childbirths does not necessarily predispose a client to urinary tract infections. Clients with diabetes mellitus are at a higher risk for developing urinary tract infections, but this risk can be decreased by maintaining good control over blood glucose levels. Clients with a history of renal calculi are not necessarily at risk for developing urinary tract infections, unless the renal calculi recur. (D, N, G, M)

90. 4. The pain associated with burns can be excruciating. Pain control most commonly involves the use of intravenous opioid analgesics. The intramuscular or subcutaneous route is not used owing to edematous tissue, which limits absorption of medications. Nonpharmacologic measures may be used in conjunction with analgesia but would not be relied on to provide pain relief. It is not appropriate to sedate the client to the point of unconsciousness because this may promote the development of other complications. (P, T, G, M)

NURSING CARE COMPREHENSIVE TEST

TEST 4

Directions: Use this answer grid to determine areas of strength or need for further study.

NURSING PROCESS

A = Assessment
D = Analysis, nursing diagnosis
P = Planning
I = Implementation
E = Evaluation

COGNITIVE LEVEL

K = Knowledge
C = Comprehension
T = Application
N = Analysis

CLIENT NEEDS

S = Safe, effective care environment
G = Physiologic integrity
L = Psychosocial integrity
H = Health promotion and maintenance

NURSING CARE AREA

O = Maternity and newborn care
X = Psychosocial health problems
Y = Nursing care of children
M = Medical and surgical health problems

Question #	Answer #	___Nursing Process___					__Cognitive Level__				__Client Needs__				__Care Area__			
		A	**D**	**P**	**I**	**E**	**K**	**C**	**T**	**N**	**S**	**G**	**L**	**H**	**O**	**X**	**Y**	**M**
1	1	A							T					H	O			
2	2				I					N				H	O			
3	1	A							T		S						Y	
4	2			P				C					L			X		
5	3					E			T					H				M
6	1			P						N		G			O			
7	4				I				T			G			O			
8	2				I				T				L			X		
9	1	A						C				G						M
10	2			P					T			G				X		
11	3	A						C			S							M
12	2	A						C					L			X		
13	4	A							T			G			O			
14	4					E			T			G			O			
15	1	A							T				L			X		
16	4				I					N				H	O			
17	4		D							N		G					Y	
18	4				I					N		G					Y	
19	1	A							T			G						M

Answer Grid

NURSING PROCESS

A = Assessment
D = Analysis, nursing diagnosis
P = Planning
I = Implementation
E = Evaluation

COGNITIVE LEVEL

K = Knowledge
C = Comprehension
T = Application
N = Analysis

CLIENT NEEDS

S = Safe, effective care environment
G = Physiologic integrity
L = Psychosocial integrity
H = Health promotion and maintenance

NURSING CARE AREA

O = Maternity and newborn care
X = Psychosocial health problems
Y = Nursing care of children
M = Medical and surgical health problems

Question #	Answer #	A	D	P	I	E	K	C	T	N	S	G	L	H	O	X	Y	M
20	1			P						N		G					Y	
21	3				I				T				L			X		
22	3				I				T					H				M
23	4				I				T			G			O			
24	1					E				N		G				X		
25	2				I				T		S							M
26	1				I					N		G					Y	
27	4					E				N		G						M
28	2		D						T				L			X		
29	1			P						N		G					Y	
30	3			P					T			G			O			
31	3	A							T			G					Y	
32	4			P					T			G						M
33	4		D							N	S							M
34	4					E			T		S						Y	
35	4				I				T			G			O			
36	3				I				T			G						M
37	1				I				T					H			Y	
38	4				I					N	S							M
39	3	A							T		S						Y	
40	2	A							T			G					Y	
41	3			P					T			G			O			
42	1				I				T			G			O			
43	3			P					T			G			O			
44	2				I				T			G					Y	

ANSWER GRID: 2

709

NURSING PROCESS

A = Assessment
D = Analysis, nursing diagnosis
P = Planning
I = Implementation
E = Evaluation

COGNITIVE LEVEL

K = Knowledge
C = Comprehension
T = Application
N = Analysis

CLIENT NEEDS

S = Safe, effective care environment
G = Physiologic integrity
L = Psychosocial integrity
H = Health promotion and maintenance

NURSING CARE AREA

O = Maternity and newborn care
X = Psychosocial health problems
Y = Nursing care of children
M = Medical and surgical health problems

Question #	Answer #	Nursing Process					Cognitive Level				Client Needs				Care Area			
		A	D	P	I	E	K	C	T	N	S	G	L	H	O	X	Y	M
45	2			P					T			G					Y	
46	3				I				T			G			O			
47	4	A						C				G						M
48	3					E				N			L			X		
49	1			P					T				L			X		
50	1			P				C				G						M
51	1				I				T			G			O			
52	2				I				T		S							M
53	3					E				N		G				X		
54	1					E				N			L			X		
55	1				I				T					H				M
56	1			P					T			G					Y	
57	4				I				T				L			X		
58	2				I				T		S						Y	
59	2		D							N		G			O			
60	4	A								N				H			Y	
61	1			P					T			G						M
62	3		D							N		G						M
63	2				I				T			G					Y	
64	4				I					N		G			O			
65	1				I					N		G					Y	
66	2					E				N			L			X		
67	1			P						N				H			Y	
68	1			P					T					H				M
69	1		D							N			L			X		

NURSING PROCESS

A = Assessment
D = Analysis, nursing diagnosis
P = Planning
I = Implementation
E = Evaluation

COGNITIVE LEVEL

K = Knowledge
C = Comprehension
T = Application
N = Analysis

CLIENT NEEDS

S = Safe, effective care environment
G = Physiologic integrity
L = Psychosocial integrity
H = Health promotion and maintenance

NURSING CARE AREA

O = Maternity and newborn care
X = Psychosocial health problems
Y = Nursing care of children
M = Medical and surgical health problems

Question #	Answer #	Nursing Process					Cognitive Level				Client Needs				Care Area			
		A	D	P	I	E	K	C	T	N	S	G	L	H	O	X	Y	M
70	2		D							N				H			Y	
71	3				I					N		G						M
72	3		D							N			L			X		
73	1				I				T				L			X		
74	1				I				T				L			X		
75	3					E		C				G						M
76	2				I					N	S						Y	
77	4	A							T			G			O			
78	4				I				T			G			O			
79	2			P						N			L			X		
80	1		D							N		G					Y	
81	2					E				N			L			X		
82	4				I				T					H	O			
83	2					E			T				L				Y	
84	2				I				T			G						M
85	3			P					T					H			Y	
86	4	A								N		G					Y	
87	1				I				T		S							M
88	2				I					N		G					Y	
89	2		D							N		G						M
90	4			P					T			G						M

ANSWER GRID: 4

NURSING PROCESS

A = Assessment
D = Analysis, nursing diagnosis
P = Planning
I = Implementation
E = Evaluation

COGNITIVE LEVEL

K = Knowledge
C = Comprehension
T = Application
N = Analysis

CLIENT NEEDS

S = Safe, effective care environment
G = Physiologic integrity
L = Psychosocial integrity
H = Health promotion and maintenance

NURSING CARE AREA

O = Maternity and newborn care
X = Psychosocial health problems
Y = Nursing care of children
M = Medical and surgical health problems

Question #	Answer #	Nursing Process					Cognitive Level				Client Needs				Care Area			
		A	D	P	I	E	K	C	T	N	S	G	L	H	O	X	Y	M
Number Correct																		
Number Possible	90	15	10	19	34	12	0	7	50	33	11	48	18	13	20	20	26	24
Percentage Correct																		

Score Calculation: To determine your **Percentage Correct,** divide the **Number Correct** by the **Number Possible.**

ANSWER GRID: 5

State Boards of Nursing

For information about the dates, requirements, and specifics of writing the examination in your state, contact the appropriate state board of nursing. The address and telephone number for each state board of nursing are provided below.

ALABAMA
Board of Nursing
RSA Plaza
Suite 250, 770 Washington Avenue
Montgomery, Alabama 36130
(205) 242-4060

ALASKA
Board of Nursing
Dept. of Commerce and Economic
   Development
Div. of Occupational Licensing
3601 C Street, Suite 722
Anchorage, Alaska 99503
(907) 561-2878

**For Examination, License
   Verifications, and Information:**
Alaska Board of Nursing
P.O. Box 110806
Juneau, Alaska 99811-0806
(907) 465-2544

AMERICAN SAMOA
Health Service Regulatory Board
LBJ Tropical Medical Center
Pago Pago, American Samoa 96799
(684) 633-1222 Ext. 206

_____

For further information about NCLEX-RN,
write to the National Council of State Boards
of Nursing, Inc.:

National Council of State Boards of Nursing,
   Inc.
676 North St. Clair Street
Suite 550
Chicago, Illinois 60611
(312) 787-6555

ARIZONA
Board of Nursing
2001 W. Camelback Road
Suite 350
Phoenix, Arizona 85015
(602) 255-5092

ARKANSAS
Arkansas State Board of Nursing
Univ. Tower Bldg.
Suite 800, 1123 South University
Little Rock, Arkansas 72204
(501) 686-2700

CALIFORNIA RN
Board of Registered Nursing
P.O. Box 944210
Sacramento, California 94244-2100
(916) 322-3350

CALIFORNIA VN
Board of Vocational Nurse and
   Psychiatric Technician Examiners
1414 K. Street, Suite 103
Sacramento, California 95814
(916) 445-0793

COLORADO
Board of Nursing
1560 Broadway, Suite 670
Denver, Colorado 80202
(303) 894-2430

CONNECTICUT
Board of Examiners for Nursing
150 Washington Street
Hartford, Connecticut 06106
(203) 566-1041

For Exam Information:
Examinations and Licensure Division
   of Medical Quality Assurance
Dept. of Health Services
150 Washington Street
Hartford, Connecticut 06106
(203) 566-1032

DELAWARE
Board of Nursing
Margaret O'Neill Building
P.O. Box 1401
Dover, Delaware 19903
(302) 739-4522

DISTRICT OF COLUMBIA
Board of Nursing
614 H. Street, N.W.
Washington, District of Columbia
   20001
(202) 727-7468

For Exam Information:
(202) 727-7454

FLORIDA
Board of Nursing
111 Coastline Drive, East, Suite 516
Jacksonville, Florida 32202
(904) 359-6331

For Exam Information:
Dept of Professional Regulation
1940 N. Monroe Street
Tallahassee, Florida 32399-0750
(904) 488-5952

GEORGIA PN
Board of Licensed Practical Nurses
166 Pryor Street, S.W.
Atlanta, Georgia, 30303

(404) 656-3921

For Exam Information:
Exam Development & Testing Unit

(404) 656-3903

GEORGIA RN
Board of Nursing
166 Pryor Street, S.W.
Atlanta, Georgia 30303

(404) 656-3943

GUAM
Board of Nurse Examiners
P.O. Box 2816
Agana, Guam 96910

011-(671) 734-7295(6)
011-(671) 734-7304

HAWAII
Board of Nursing
P.O. Box 3469
Honolulu, Hawaii 96801

(808) 586-2695

IDAHO
Board of Nursing
280 North 8th Street, Suite 210
Boise, Idaho 83720

(208) 334-3110

ILLINOIS
Dept. of Professional Regulation
320 West Washington Street
3rd Floor
Springfield, Illinois 62786

(217) 785-9465
(217) 785-0800

For Exam Information:
Application Requests
Licensure Information
Asst. Nursing/Act Coordinator

(217) 782-0458
(217) 782-8556
(217) 785-9465

INDIANA
Board of Nursing
Health Professions Bureau
402 West Washington Street
Room 041
Indianapolis, Indiana 46204

(317) 232-2960

IOWA
Board of Nursing
State Capitol Complex
1223 East Court Avenue
Des Moines, Iowa 50319

(515) 281-3255

KANSAS
Board of Nursing
Landon State Office Building
900 S.W. Jackson, Suite 551-S
Topeka, Kansas 66612-1256

(913) 296-4929

KENTUCKY
Board of Nursing
312 Wittington Parkway, Suite 300
Louisville, Kentucky 40222-5172

(502) 329-7000

LOUISIANA RN
Board of Nursing
912 Pere Marquette Building
150 Baronne Street
New Orleans, Louisiana 70112

(504) 568-5464

LOUISIANA PN
Board of Practical Nurse Examiners
Tidewater Place
1440 Canal Street, Suite 1722
New Orleans, Louisiana 70112

(504) 568-6480

MAINE
Board of Nursing
State House Station 158
Augusta, Maine 04333-0158

(207) 624-5275

MARYLAND
Board of Nursing
4201 Patterson Avenue
Baltimore, Maryland 21215-2299

(301) 764-4741

MASSACHUSETTS
Board of Registration in Nursing
Leverett Saltonstall Building
100 Cambridge Street, Room 1519
Boston, Massachusetts 02202

(617) 727-9962

MICHIGAN
Bureau of Occupational and
 Professional Regulation
Dept. of Commerce
Ottawa Towers North
611 West Ottawa
Lansing, Michigan 48933

(517) 373-1600

For Exam Information:
Office of Testing Services
Department of Commerce
P.O. Box 30018
Lansing, Michigan 48909

(517) 373-3877

MINNESOTA
Board of Nursing
2700 University Avenue, West #108
St. Paul, Minnesota 55114

(612) 642-0567

MISSISSIPPI
Board of Nursing
239 N. Lamar Street, Suite 401
Jackson, Mississippi 39201-1311

(601) 359-6170

MISSOURI
Board of Nursing
P.O. Box 656
Jefferson City, Missouri 65102

(314) 751-0681

MONTANA
Board of Nursing
Dept. of Commerce
Arcade Building, Lower Level
111 North Jackson
Helena, Montana 59620-0407

(406) 444-4279

NEBRASKA
Bureau of Examining Boards
Dept. of Health
P.O. Box 95007
Lincoln, Nebraska 68509

(402) 471-2115

NEVADA
Board of Nursing
1281 Terminal Way, Suite 116
Reno, Nevada 89502

(702) 786-2778

NEW HAMPSHIRE
Board of Nursing
Health & Welfare Building
6 Hazen Drive
Concord, New Hampshire 03301-6527
(603) 271-2323

NEW JERSEY
Board of Nursing
P.O. Box 45010
Newark, New Jersey 07101
(201) 504-6493

NEW MEXICO
Board of Nursing
4253 Montgomery Blvd., Suite 130
Albuquerque, New Mexico 87109
(505) 841-8340

NEW YORK
Board of Nursing
State Education Department
Cultural Education Center,
Room 3023
Albany, New York 12230
(518) 474-3843/3845

For Exam Information:
Div. of Professional Licensing
    Services
State Education Department
Cultural Education Center
Albany, New York 12230
(518) 474-6591

NORTH CAROLINA
Board of Nursing
P.O. Box 2129
Raleigh, North Carolina 27602
(919) 782-3211

NORTH DAKOTA
Board of Nursing
919 South 7th Street, Suite 504
Bismarck, North Dakota 58504-5881
(701) 224-2974

NORTHERN MARIANA ISLANDS
Commonwealth Board of Nurse
    Examiners
Public Health Center
P.O. Box 1458
Saipan, MP 96950
011-670-234-8950

OHIO
Board of Nursing
77 South High Street, 17th Floor
Columbus, Ohio 43266-0316
(614) 466-3947

OKLAHOMA
Board of Nurse Registration &
    Nursing Education
2915 North Classen Blvd., Suite 524
Oklahoma City, Oklahoma 73106
(405) 525-2076

OREGON
Board of Nursing STE 465
800 NE Oregon St. #25
Portland, Oregon 97232
(503) 731-4745

PENNSYLVANIA
Board of Nursing
P.O. Box 2649
Harrisburg, Pennsylvania 17105
(717) 783-7142

PUERTO RICO
Commonwealth of Puerto Rico
Board of Nurse Examiners
Call Box 10200
Santurce, Puerto Rico 00908
(809) 725-8161

RHODE ISLAND
Board of Nurse Registration &
    Nursing Education
Cannon Health Building
Three Capitol Hill, Room 104
Providence, Rhode Island 02908-5097
(401) 277-2827

SOUTH CAROLINA
Board of Nursing
220 Executive Center Drive, Suite 220
Columbia, South Carolina 29210
(803) 731-1648

SOUTH DAKOTA
Board of Nursing
3307 South Lincoln Avenue
Sioux Falls, South Dakota 57105-5224
(605) 335-4973

TENNESSEE
Board of Nursing
283 Plus Park Blvd.
Nashville, Tennessee 37247-1010
(615) 367-6232

TEXAS RN
Board of Nurse Examiners
P.O. Box 140466
Austin, Texas 78714
(512) 835-4880

TEXAS VN
Board of Vocational Nurse Examiners
9101 Burnet Road, Suite 105
Austin, Texas 78758
(512) 835-2071

UTAH
Board of Nursing
Div. of Occupational & Prof. Licensing
P.O. Box 45805
Salt Lake City, Utah 84145-0805
(801) 530-6628

VERMONT
Board of Nursing
Redstone Building
26 Terrace Street
Montpelier, Vermont 05602-1106
(802) 828-2396

VIRGIN ISLANDS
Board of Nurse Licensure
P.O. Box 4247, Veterans Drive Station
St. Thomas, U.S. Virgin Islands 00803
(809) 776-7397

VIRGINIA
Board of Nursing
1601 Rolling Hills Drive
Richmond, Virginia 23229-5005
(804) 662-9909

WASHINGTON RN
Board of Nursing
Dept. of Health
P.O. Box 47864
Olympia, Washington 98504-7864
(206) 753-2686

WASHINGTON PN

Board of Practical Nursing
1300 S.E. Quince Street
P.O. Box 47865
Olympia, Washington 98504-7865

(206) 753-2807

WEST VIRGINIA RN

Board of Examiners for Registered
Professional Nurses
101 Dee Drive
Charleston, West Virginia 25311-1688

(304) 558-3596

WEST VIRGINIA PN

Board of Examiners for Practical
Nurses
101 Dee Drive
Charleston, West Virginia 25311-1688

(304) 558-3572

WISCONSIN

Bureau of Health Service Professions
1400 East Washington Avenue
P.O. Box 8935
Madison, Wisconsin 53708-8935

(608) 266-0257

WYOMING

Board of Nursing
Barrett Building, 2nd Floor
2301 Central Avenue
Cheyenne, Wyoming 82002

(307) 777-7601

Lippincott's Review for NCLEX-RN, 6th Edition Disk Instructions

System Requirements

A PC-compatible computer with an Intel 386 or better processor.

Windows 3.1 or better.

4 Megabytes of RAM (minimum), but recommend 8 MB RAM on Windows 3.1; 8 Megabytes of RAM (minimum), but recommend 12 MB RAM minimum on Windows '95; 3 Megabytes of available hard disk space.

Installing NCLEX-RN for Windows

1. Start up Windows.

2. Insert the *NCLEX-RN* disk into the floppy disk drive.

3. From the Program Manager's File menu, choose the Run command.

4. When the Run dialog box appears, type a:\setup (or b:\setup if you're using the B drive) in the Command Line box. Click OK or press the Enter button.

5. The installation process will begin. A dialog proposing the directory "NCLEXRN" on the drive containing Windows will appear. If the name and location are correct, click OK. If you want to change this information, type over the existing data, then click OK.

6. When the *NCLEX-RN* setup routine is complete, a new group called "NCLEX-RN Exam Review" will appear on your desktop.

7. Start the *NCLEX-RN* disk program by double clicking on its icon.

Lippincott's Review for NCLEX-RN, 6th Edition Disk Program

The *NCLEX-RN* disk program contains 100 questions that review the content covered in ***Lippincott s Review for NCLEX-RN, 6th Edition.***

This is a not timed test. Take your time; consider the questions and the possible answers carefully.

To begin a test, press the **Start Over** button from the Main Menu screen. To continue a test that you have already begun, press the **Resume** button. To restart the exam and erase all the results from your previous session of that exam, press the **Start Over** button. To review the answers you have given and compare them with the correct answers, press the **Answers** button.

When you press either the **Start Over, Resume,** or **Answers** button, the test and the program's Toolbar will appear.

Lippincott's Review for NCLEX-RN, 6th Edition Toolbar

The Toolbar contains a series of buttons that provide direct access to all test program functions. When you move the cursor over a button, an explanation of its function displays in the Status Bar, which is immediately above the Toolbar.

To get help at any time during the test, choose the Program Help button. Program Help reviews basic functions of the program.

Answer each question by clicking on the oval to the left of an answer selection or by selecting the appropriate letter on the keyboard (eg, A, B, C, D, etc.). When an answer is selected, its oval will darken. If you change your mind about an answer, simply select your choice, by mouse or keyboard, again.

To register your answer selection and proceed to the next question, click on the Right Arrow button or press Return.

After taking the test and receiving your score, you may review your answers by clicking on the Answers button on the Main Menu screen.

If you are unsure about an answer to a particular question, the program allows you to mark it for later review. Flag the question by clicking on the Mark button. To review all marked questions for a test, click on the Table of Contents button, which is immediately to the right of the Mark button.

The Table of Contents window lists every question included on the test and summarizes whether it has been answered, left unanswered, or marked for later review. Click on an item in the Table of Contents window and the program will move to that test question.

Use the Arrow buttons to move to the first, previous, next, or last question.

At any time during the test or when you are finished taking the test, click on the Stop button. If you wish, you may return to the session at a later time without erasing your existing answers by clicking on the Resume button on the Main Menu.

After taking the test, view the correct answer for each test question by using the Answers button on the Main Menu. This will take you back to the test, but you will not be able to modify the answers you have given. Click on the Q/A button (to the right of the Stop button) and a window will pop up, explaining the correct answer to the question. (The Q/A button will only appear when you are in the "Answers" section of the test.) You may also wish to use the Table of Contents button to show you which questions you marked for review.

To exit the *NCLEX-RN* program, click the Quit button on the Main Menu.

Good luck and enjoy practicing on this disk before you take the real examination!